Fractures and Dislocations

CLOSED MANAGEMENT

John F. Connolly, M.D.
Director of Medical Education, Department of Orthopaedic Surgery
Orlando Regional Medical Center, Orlando, Florida
and Clinical Professor, Department of Orthopaedic Surgery and Rehabilitation
University of Miami School of Medicine, Miami, Florida

Fractures and Dislocations

CLOSED MANAGEMENT

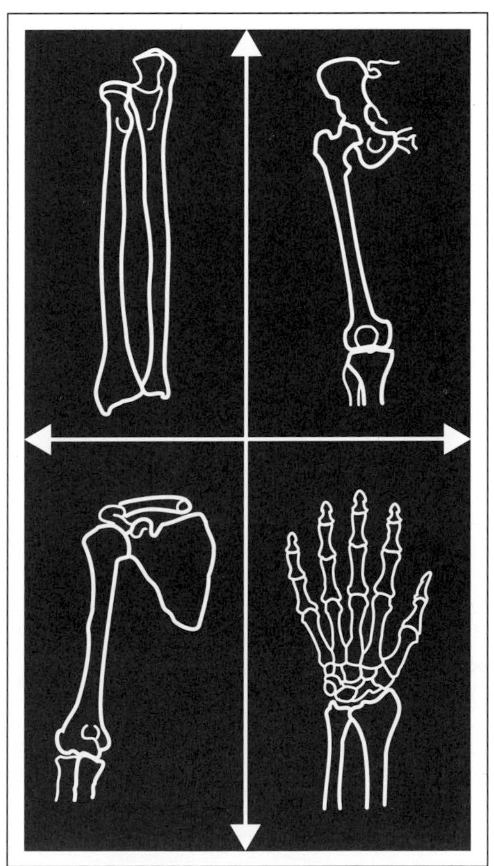

VOLUME 2

W.B. SAUNDERS COMPANY
A Division of Harcourt Brace & Company

W.B. SAUNDERS COMPANY
A Division of
Harcourt Brace & Company

The Curtis Center
Independence Square West
Philadelphia, Pennsylvania 19106

Library of Congress Cataloging-in-Publication Data

Connolly, John F.

Fractures and dislocations—closed management / John F. Connolly.

p. cm.

ISBN 0–7216–2601–7

1. Fracture fixation. 2. Dislocations—Treatment. I. Title. [DNLM: 1. Dislocations—therapy. 2. Fracture Fixation. WE 175 C752f 1995]

RD103.F58C66 1995 617.1′5–dc20

DNLM/DLC 95–11489

Fractures and Dislocations—Closed Management

Volume 1 ISBN 0–7216–6618–3
Volume 2 ISBN 0–7216–6619–1
Two-Volume Set ISBN 0–7216–2601–7

Printed in the United States of America

Last digit is the print number: 9 8 7 6 5 4 3 2 1

Dedication

This text is dedicated to all my teachers but especially to two:

D. Kay Clawson, M.D., who by his example and enthusiasm inspired me to see the exciting challenges in orthopedic surgery.

Augusto Sarmiento, M.D., who more than anyone has advanced the science and the techniques of closed fracture management.

Preface

Skeletal repair processes have proved crucial for survival of vertebrates throughout eons of evolution. Processes of skeletal repair and remodeling have evolved into efficient methods of not only healing but also restoring normal skeletal structure after most injuries. Consequently, the classical view has been that the physician should treat a fracture more as a gardener than as a carpenter; that is, because the fractured bone is much like a tree with roots in surrounding soft tissues, the role of the physician should be to cultivate healing rather than impose it.

Only since the early 1960s has the functional benefit of open surgical treatment of some skeletal injuries been shown to be significant in relation to the risk. Nonetheless, the hazard involved in invading the fracture milieu and disrupting the skeletal vascular support systems remains significant. When operative intervention becomes necessary, it must be carried out with the understanding that the surgeon is significantly assaulting and potentially impeding the normally efficient processes of skeletal repair. Therefore, the functional advantages of open surgical treatment must be significant in relation to its real disadvantages in order to justify its use.

The technology of closed or minimally invasive fracture treatment has also been improved significantly by basic and clinical research since the early 1960s. Closed reduction and fracture fixation with the use of casts, fracture-braces, external fixators, or minimally invasive internal fixation techniques have enabled us to minimize risk and maximize benefits for our patients. When the outcome of fracture treatment can be anticipated to be equal to that of either closed or open methods, the closed methods prove best for most patients and most surgeons.

The science of closed management and the art of caring for patients during the time required for a fracture to heal are difficult to teach in standard textbook format. Consequently, the majority of fracture texts now seem to focus on more readily illustrated surgical intervention techniques. In this text, the author has relied on a pictorial atlas to demonstrate the step-by-step methods of closed functional treatment. This approach enables the illustration of common techniques designed to cultivate rather than conflict with the efficient healing processes. Ultimately, such methods offer our patients the highest benefit-risk advantage for most common fractures.

In this text, the author has avoided radiographic classifications of fracture, which often prove variable from observer to observer and are therefore difficult to apply consistently. His approach to classification is based more on mechanisms of injury, either direct or indirect, that produce the fracture or dislocation. Once mechanisms or causes are understood, as with any disease, these mechanisms can be reversed in order to reduce and treat the fracture.

After the fracture is reduced and satisfactory alignment is achieved, reliable methods of maintaining reduction are illustrated. If internal fixation is needed to stabilize or maintain reduction, the text briefly illustrates available techniques with further references to the many excellent references that detail these methods.

The choice of either closed or open fracture management, whenever possible, is based on clinical as well as basic research. Basic research frequently provides knowledge that may seem to conflict with commonsense observations, much like the discovery that the earth was really round and not the center of the universe. In the past, the commonsense approach to closed fracture management dictated the need for continuous, prolonged rest and the imposition of absolute immobilization to heal the fracture. An important basic "uncommonsense" concept regarding acute fracture management emphasized in this text is that many fractures do not necessitate rigid immobilization in order to heal. In fact, well-vascularized bones, such as the humerus, femur, and tibia, can be stimulated to heal by a controlled amount of functional motion during the early phases of fracture repair. Such basic understanding of fracture healing has led to better clinical methods of treatment.

Closed treatment methods continue to evolve, just as the skeletal system has evolved. This text also continues to reflect an evolution of the author's own thinking and analysis of techniques that work best for him. It is presented in the same way as one would offer reasonably proven concepts and reliable methods to residents, students, and colleagues.

The reader is advised that this presentation is not intended to be an exhaustive survey of all possible methods of treating fractures and dislocations. Rather, it is an atlas of techniques that have been most effective in the author's own experience, as well as in the rich store of scientific literature on the subject.

John F. Connolly

Acknowledgments

This is to acknowledge my sincere appreciation for the many skilled people at the W.B. Saunders Company and at Orlando Regional Medical Center who helped me in the production of this text.

In particular, I want to thank Ed Wicklund, former Medical Editor, and Kim Kist, the current Medical Editor, for their advice and encouragement during this production. Linda R. Garber, Production Manager, and Anne Ostroff, Copy Editor, were constantly supportive in careful editing and production of the entire text. Kate Fisher was invaluable as the Illustration Specialist in coordinating the many illustrations with the manuscript. Ellen Zanolle, Designer, and Patti Maddaloni, the Page Layout Artist, also provided invaluable assistance in the arrangement and organization of the text. Julie Figures compiled the index, which is always an important part of any textbook of this length and nature.

I also thank Patti Durfee, who has contributed almost a thousand new illustrations to this edition. She deserves considerable thanks for being able to work closely with the author and transcribe the techniques into pictures that were worth more than a thousand words. Finally, to Ann Nangle, our transcriptionist and coordinator, I owe a great debt of thanks because of her constant support and accuracy. She was invariably understanding and patient, enduring the numerous manuscript revisions, reviews, and retypings of the text.

John F. Connolly, M.D.

Contents

Volume 1

Volume 2

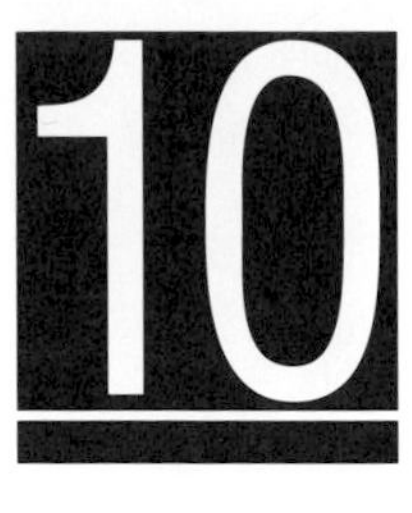

Injuries of the Ankle: Sprains, Dislocations, and Fractures

ANATOMIC FEATURES AND MECHANISMS OF INJURIES

REMARKS

Injuries to the ankle produce the most common joint instability problems, particularly in young active individuals.

Depending on the mechanism, the ankle injury may cause either a sprain or a fracture. Sprains are commonly the result of inversion mechanisms, whereas excessive eversion or external torsion of the ankle produces fractures.

The reason for these differences can best be explained by a review of the functional anatomy of the ankle joint.

Functional Anatomy of the Ankle Joint

Bony Components

Bony Configuration of the Ankle Joint

1. Articular surface of the tibia forms the top of the mortise.
2. Internal and external malleoli form the sides of the mortise.
3. Note the length of the internal malleolus compared with the
4. Length of the external malleolus, which flanks the entire side of the talus.

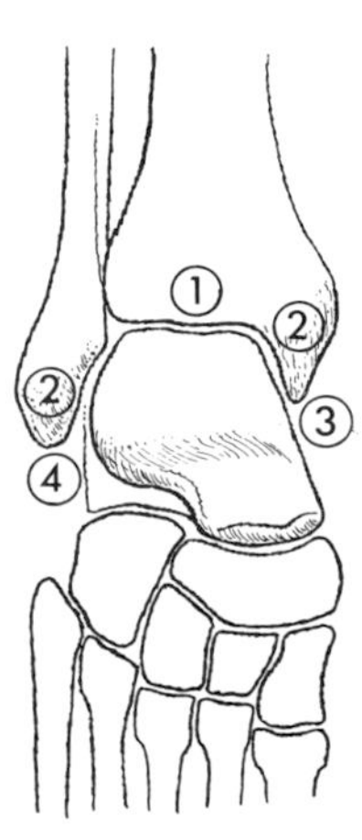

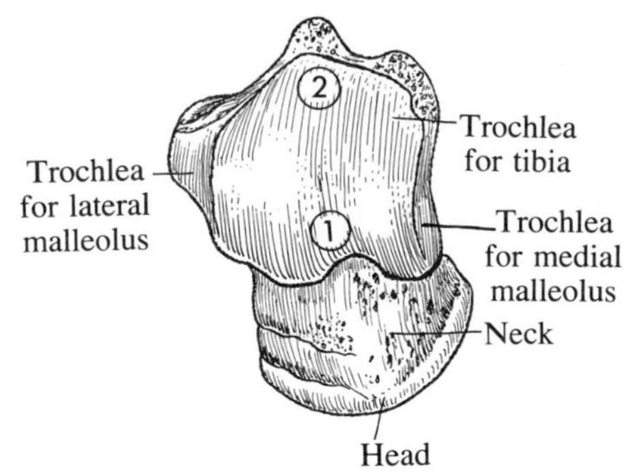

Body of the Talus

1. Anterior portion of the body is wider than the
2. Posterior portion of the body.

Widening of the Mortise With Ankle Flexion and Extension

Despite its wedge shape, the talus does not loosen in the ankle joint mortise during plantar flexion of the foot.

The articular surfaces of the malleoli remain in close contact with the sides of the talus throughout the total arc of motion.

As dorsiflexion takes place, the malleoli separate in regular increments up to 1.5 mm. This is accomplished by a medial rotation of the tibia on the talus and a relatively lateral rotation of the fibula with respect to the tibia.

Widening of the ankle mortise up to 1.5 mm is accomplished during dorsiflexion by

1. Slight internal rotation of the tibia about the talus.
2. Relative lateral rotation of the fibula with respect to the tibia.
3. The elasticity of the tibiofibular ligaments, which allows rotation and widening of the malleoli.

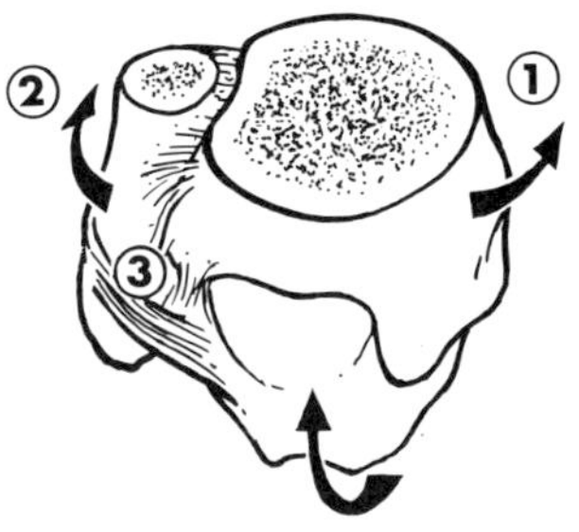

Note: Anatomically, the lateral malleolus is much more susceptible to posterior displacement than to anterior displacement because of the groove in the tibia in which the fibula lies. This groove has a prominent anterior border formed by the distal anterior tibial tubercle but only a shallow posterior boundary (see page 819). The prominent anterolateral tubercle is sometimes called the tubercle of Tillaux-Chaput.

Ligaments on the Posterior Aspect of the Ankle Joint

1. Posterior tibiofibular ligament is a thickened portion of the
2. Interosseous membrane.
3. Posterior talofibular ligament is rarely injured.
4. Calcaneofibular ligament may be injured with severe ankle sprain.
5. Posterior tibiotalar portion of the deltoid ligament supports the talus against lateral displacement.

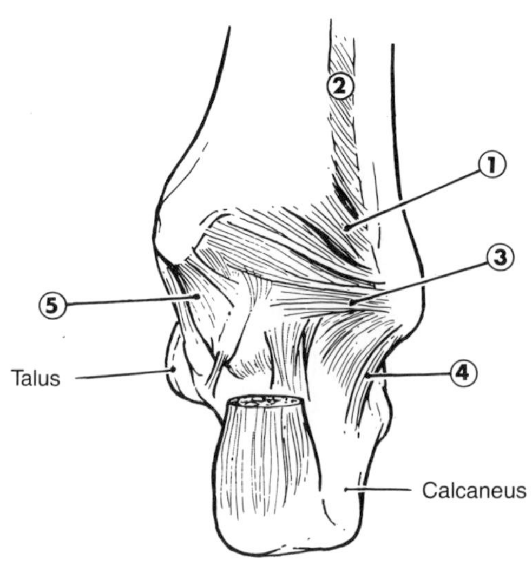

Note: The posterior and anterior ligaments are designed to support against inversion and eversion but allow maximal flexion and extension of the joint.

Ligaments on the Lateral Aspect of the Ankle Joint

1. Anterior tibiofibular ligament permits slight rotation of the tibia and fibula during dorsiflexion. It is most often injured by mechanisms that fracture the ankle rather than produce sprain.
2. Anterior talofibular ligament is relatively weak and injured by forceful inversion.
3. Calcaneofibular ligament is located posterior to the axis of the ankle and is injured with the ankle in dorsiflexion and supination.
4. Talocalcaneal ligament is infrequently torn, except in the more severe sprains.
5. Posterior talofibular ligament is also rarely torn by inversion with the ankle in dorsiflexion.

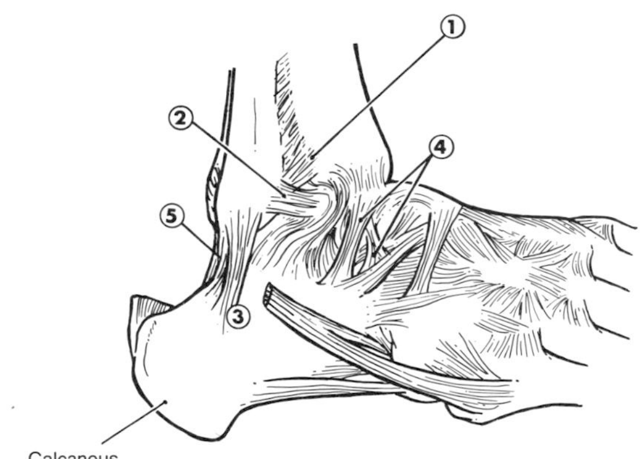

When the foot is dorsiflexed, the
1. Wide anterior portion of the body is gripped firmly by the
2. Internal and external malleoli. The mortise is in its widest position.
3. In plantar flexion, narrow posterior portion of the talus advances into the mortise.
4. Malleoli remain in close contact with the talus to prevent excessive looseness of the joint.

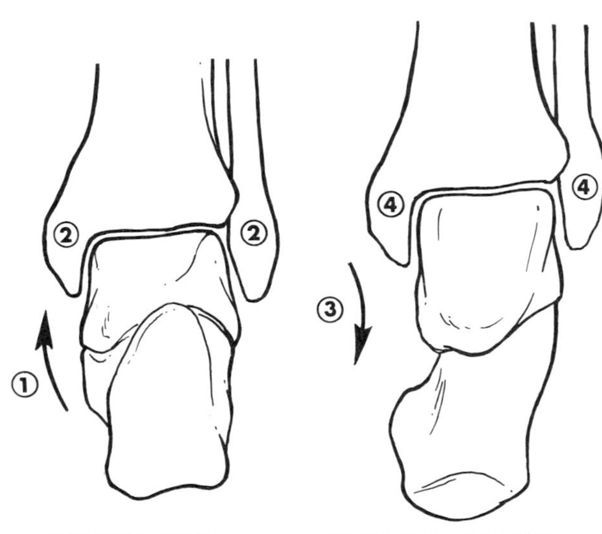

Ligaments

The ligamentous supports are essential for the stability and mobility of the ankle joint.

The anterior and posterior tibiofibular ligaments must be sufficiently elastic to permit tibial and fibular rotation during ankle flexion and extension.

The medial and lateral ligaments support the ankle against inversion and eversion overload. The lateral ligaments, particularly the anterior talofibular ligament, are relatively weak and frequently subject to isolated tears or sprains.

The medial or deltoid ligament is a strong, complex ligament that is rarely injured by itself but usually only after the talofibular or tibiofibular ligament or the fibula fails.

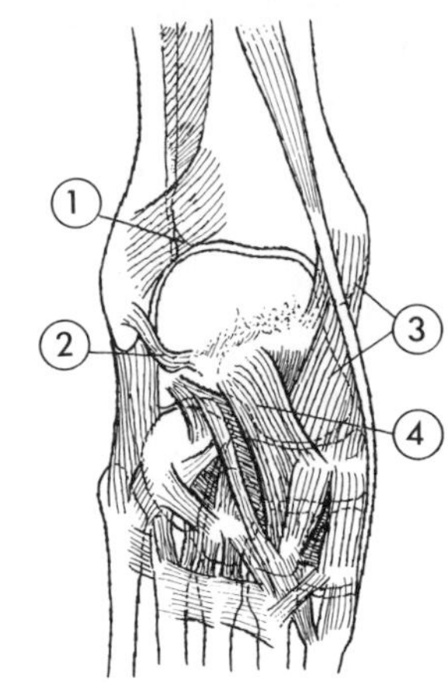

Ligaments on the Anterior Aspect of the Ankle Joint

1. Anterior tibiofibular ligament.
2. Anterior talofibular ligament.
3. Deltoid ligament.
4. Talonavicular ligament.

Ligaments on the Medial Aspect of the Ankle Joint

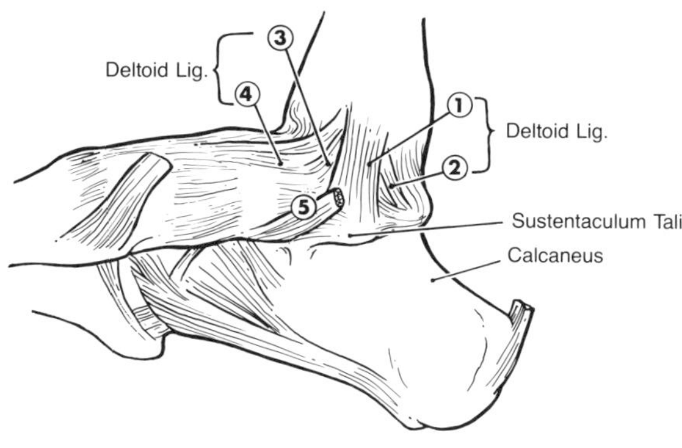

The deltoid ligament is a complex structure that consists of a

1. Tibiocalcaneal portion, a
2. Posterior tibiotalar portion, an
3. Anterior tibiotalar portion, and a
4. Tibionavicular portion.
5. To repair the posterior tibial portion of the deltoid, the tendon of the tibialis posterior must be retracted forward.

ANKLE SPRAINS

Mechanisms

REMARKS

The bony articulations of its mortise make the ankle resistant to failure in the mediolateral direction, i.e., in abduction or adduction.

Most ankle injuries are produced by torsional overloading.

Because of the anatomy with the elongated lateral malleolus, ankle sprains are primarily injuries to the lateral ligaments produced by inversion and internal rotation.

External rotation or eversion injuries most characteristically cause malleolar fractures.

Internal Torsion Mechanism That Produces Grade I, II, or III Injuries

Internal torsional injuries occur

1. After the heel strikes with the ankle plantar flexing.

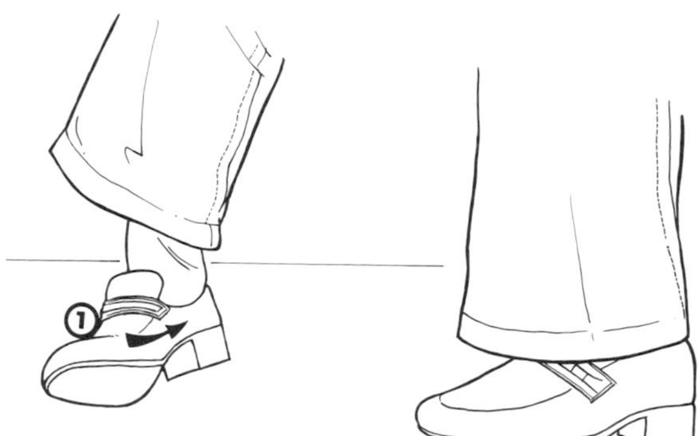

Pathologic Findings in Grade I Injuries

2. Fibula quickly abuts against the distal anterior tibial tubercle of the groove.
3. Resultant strain is absorbed primarily by the weak anterior talofibular ligament.

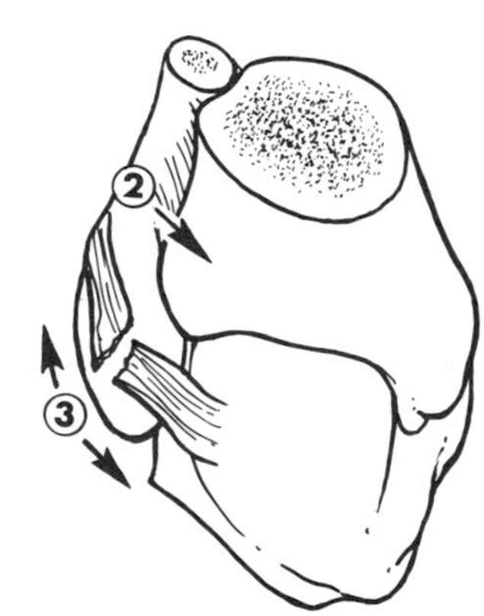

Pathologic Findings in Grade II Injuries

1. Complete tear of the anterior talofibular ligament allows anterior instability.
2. If the injury is produced by forceful plantar flexion, the anterior deltoid ligament may be damaged, and the patient presents with a bimalleolar ankle sprain.
3. Major portion of the calcaneofibular ligament is intact and prevents inversion instability.

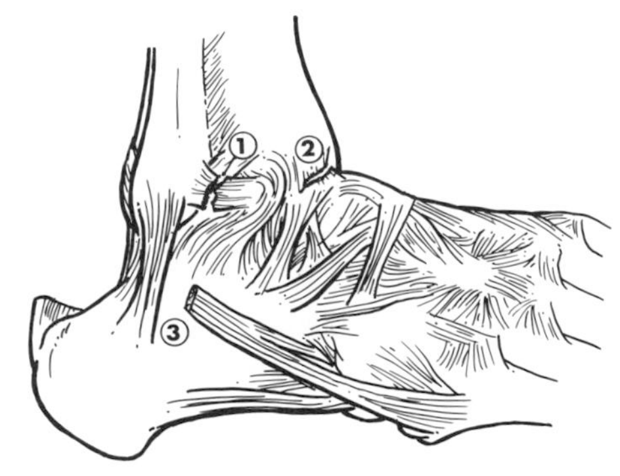

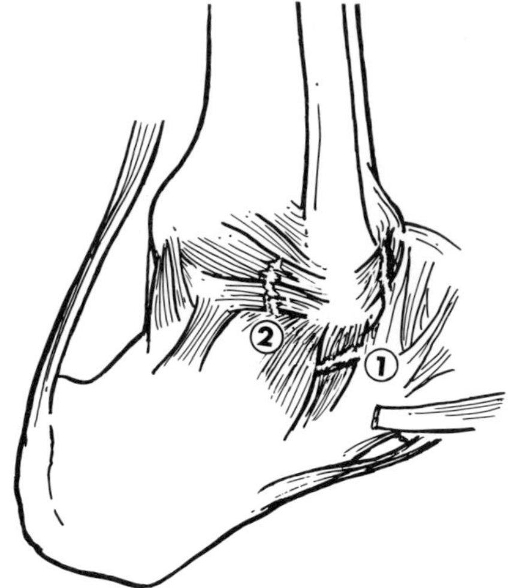

Pathologic Findings in Grade III Injuries

Continued inversion overloading during stance phase leads to
1. Disruption of the calcaneofibular ligament and
2. Disruption of the talocalcaneal ligaments.

Note: Chrisman and Snook showed that both the anterior talofibular and the calcaneofibular ligaments must be torn for gross inversion instability to be evident on stress x-rays.

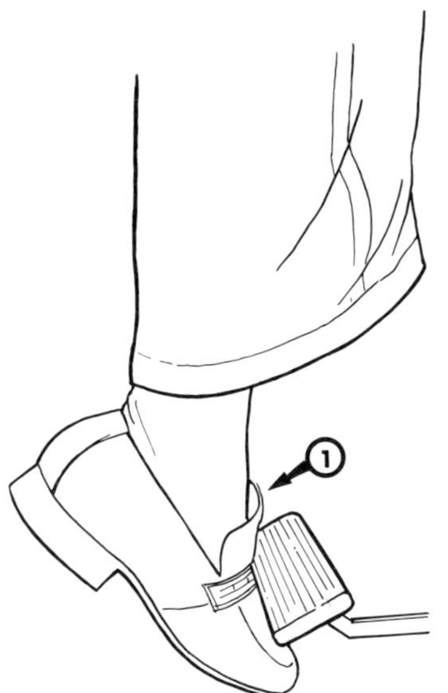

Other Mechanisms

1. Forceful plantar flexion injury to the ankle disrupts the

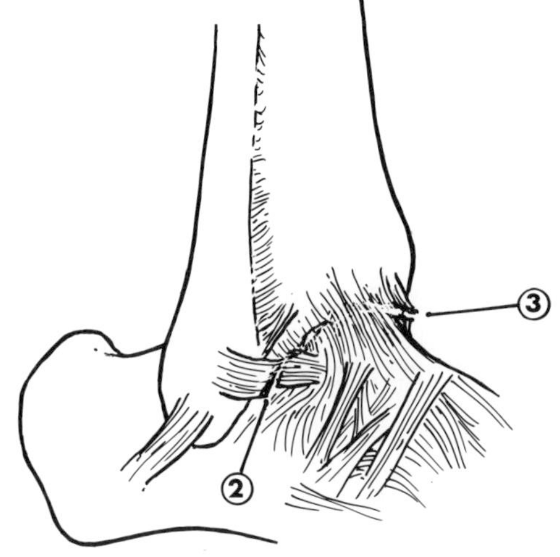

2. Anterolateral or fibulotalar ligament and the
3. Anteromedial portion of the deltoid ligament.

Note: These patients present with bimalleolar symptoms.

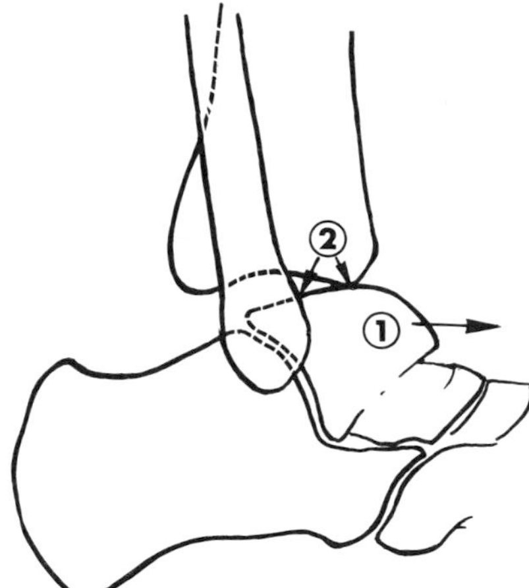

This mechanism results in

1. Abnormal anterior displacement of the talus in the mortise and
2. Caudad displacement of the talus as its dome rides forward under the anterior articular margin of the tibia.

Note: The bimalleolar ankle sprain involves a greater degree of anterior subluxation than does the more common sprain of the lateral ankle ligaments.

■ Evaluation and Management of Acute Ankle Sprains

REMARKS

By far, most ankle sprains involve the anterior talofibular ligament with excellent prognosis for prompt recovery.

The more severe injuries involve the talocalcaneal or fibulocalcaneal ligament and the subtalar joint and anterior talofibular ligament. These produce diffuse pain, swelling, and some instability.

Examination

Physical examination includes assessment of localized areas of tenderness both anterolaterally and anteromedially. The more diffuse the tenderness, the more likely the injury is to be extensive.

Stress test for inversion instability and anterior drawer testing are also sometimes indicated in the physical examination. However, such tests are infrequently useful in the acute injury and are best reserved to evaluate chronic problems of instability.

Anteroposterior and lateral x-rays of the sprained ankle are most important to rule out subtle fractures that can be confused with ligamentous injuries. These include osteochondral fractures of the talus, fractures of the talar processes both laterally and posteriorly (os trigonum), avulsion or fleck fractures of the fibula, and fractures of the calcaneus and base of the fifth metatarsal. All of these can be confused clinically with symptoms of ligamentous sprain.

Clinical Tests

1. Ankle is carefully palpated to locate any areas of tenderness laterally or medially.
2. Dorsiflexion and plantar flexion are tested to determine if the injury is in the anterior capsule.

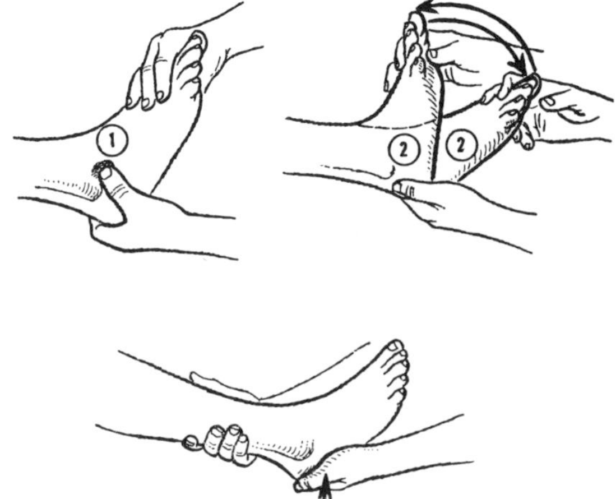

3. Heel is carefully palpated and adducted to determine if the injury involves the calcaneofibular or talocalcaneal ligaments.

Stress Testing

This can usually be done in the acutely injured ankle without anesthesia.

ANTERIOR DRAWER SIGN

1. Injured ankle should be tested at a right angle, not in plantar flexion, which would tighten the injured ligaments.
2. Examiner's hand stabilizes the distal tibia and palpates the anterior ankle joint.
3. Examiner's other hand is placed behind the heel and pushes the talus forward out of the joint.

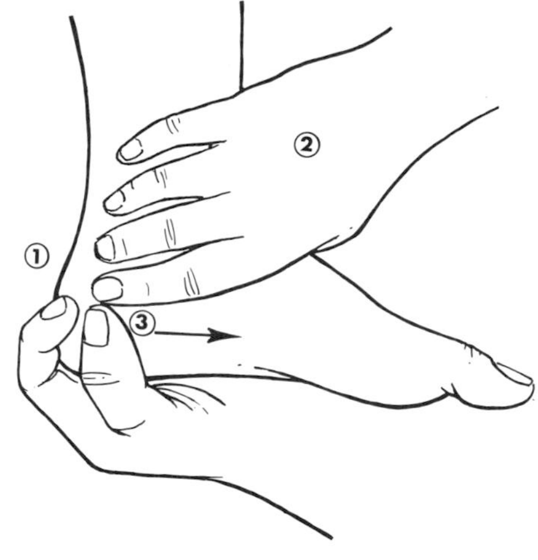

Abnormal drawer test result is indicated by

1. Anterior displacement of the talus from 4–16 mm more than the opposite side, as evidenced by direct palpation or by x-ray.

Note: Bimalleolar ankle sprains should be carefully assessed for this displacement.

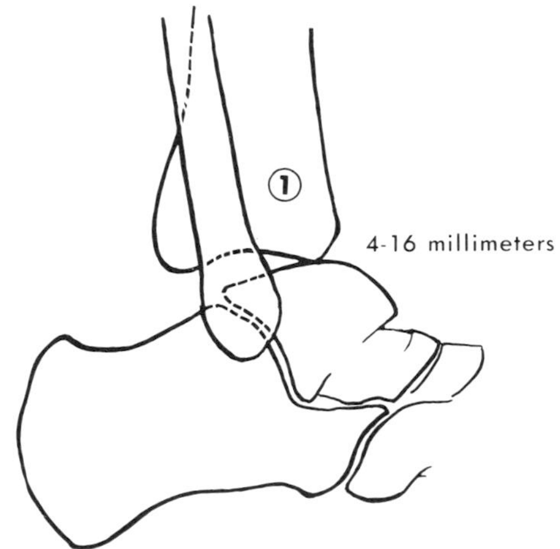

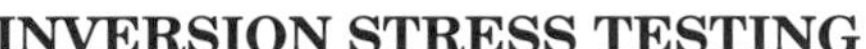

INVERSION STRESS TESTING

1. Ankle is held in neutral.
2. Examiner supports the distal tibia while palpating the anterolateral joint space.
3. Forceful inversion is applied by pushing on the talus and calcaneus.

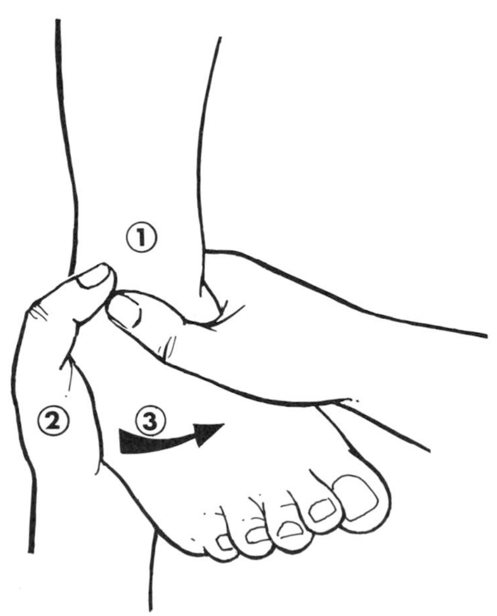

Alternative Method (Gungor Test)

If the patient is unable to relax during the test, try the Gungor maneuver.

1. Patient is asked to lie prone with the ankle extending beyond the edge of the table.
2. With one hand, the surgeon presses the heel forward steadily. If the anterior capsule is ruptured, the talus will move forward further than on the uninjured side.
3. Vacuum effect of negative pressure occurs as a result of the change in the talus position. This draws the skin inward on both sides of the calcaneal tendon on the injured side compared with the uninjured side.

Note: To confirm the test, take a lateral x-ray with the heel in this position and with it pushed forward.

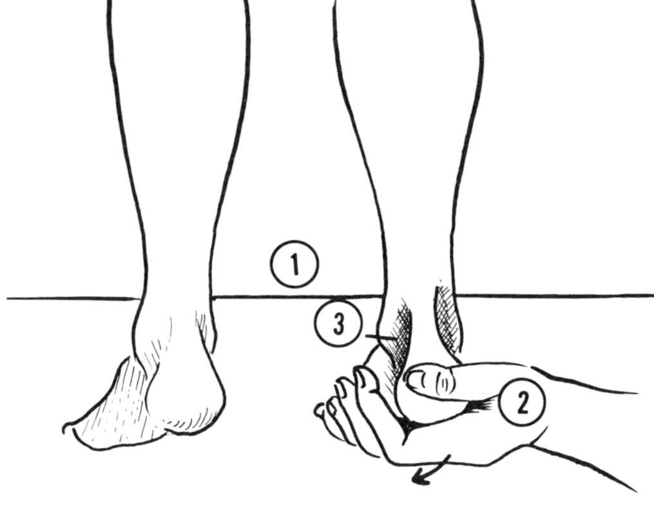

X-Ray Evaluation

The major need for the x-ray is to rule out fractures that can be confused with ankle sprains and may need surgical treatment. These include

1. Osteochondral fractures of the talus, which often may not be recognized on x-ray for the sprained ankle but should always be kept in mind.
2. Fractures of the posterior or lateral process of the talus. These are fairly common in basketball players and are also confused as sprains.
3. Fractures of the os calcis and fifth metatarsal are also sometimes confused clinically with ankle sprains.

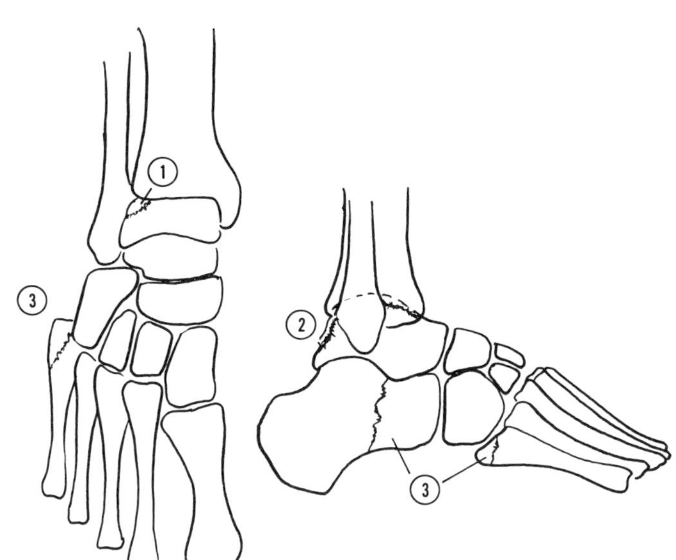

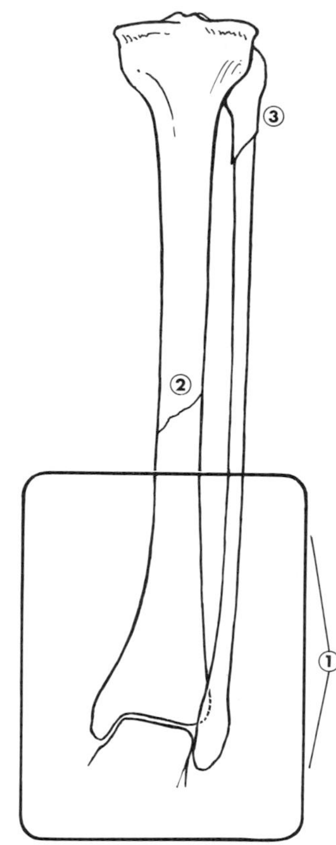

Caution: There may be other fractures associated with "ankle sprains."

1. Occasionally, x-rays are coned diligently to visualize what is assumed to be only an ankle sprain, but
2. Fractures of the proximal tibia or
3. Fractures of the proximal fibula are missed.

Note: Careful physical examination is necessary to rule out missed fractures proximal to the area of x-ray.

Stress X-Rays

Stress x-rays of the sprained ankle are best reserved for the chronically symptomatic problem.

The symptomatic ankle should always be compared with the asymptomatic side because many individuals have lax ankles that allow the talus to tilt in the mortise.

1. Tilting of the talus 10° more than the opposite side is considered an abnormal indicator of chronic laxity.

Note: Patients with chronic symptoms may also suffer from instability of the subtalar joint, which may be difficult to detect on a stress x-ray.

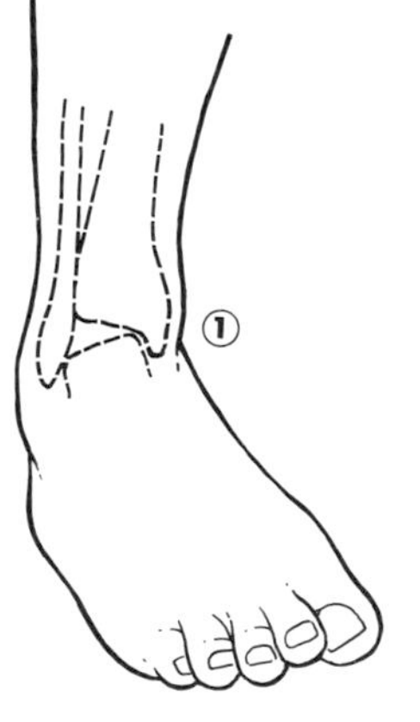

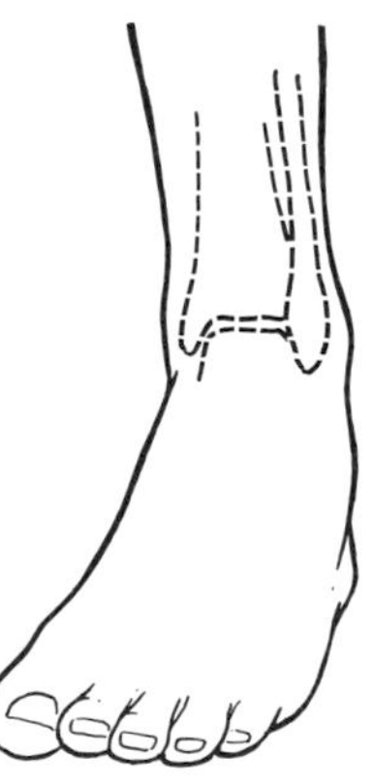

Management

REMARKS

With hardly any exceptions, sprained ankles of most patients can be treated with the RICE technique. This includes rest, ice application, compression dressing, and elevation.

When the acute swelling has subsided, the patient may be then treated with support, such as an Aircast or ankle taping for 1–2 weeks.

For the less frequent more severe injuries with diffuse tenderness throughout the ankle medially, laterally, and posteriorly, cast immobilization may be indicated after the acute swelling subsides.

Operative treatment is not indicated to repair the acute ankle sprain in most individuals, except one who has an acute injury on top of a long-standing chronic problem of instability.

Operative treatment may be indicated for avulsion fractures of the fibula or talar processes and for loose osteochondral fragments within the ankle joint.

RICE Management

1. Basic treatment of almost all ankle sprains for the first 3–5 days is rest, ice application, compression dressing, and elevation. The patient may be up on crutches but should avoid allowing the ankle to hang down, which only increases the swelling.

Caution: Also avoid application of heat to the ankle, which greatly increases the swelling.

The acutely sprained ankle should not be wrapped with a tight cicumferential dressing. This may cause sufficient occlusion of circulation to produce a compartment syndrome.

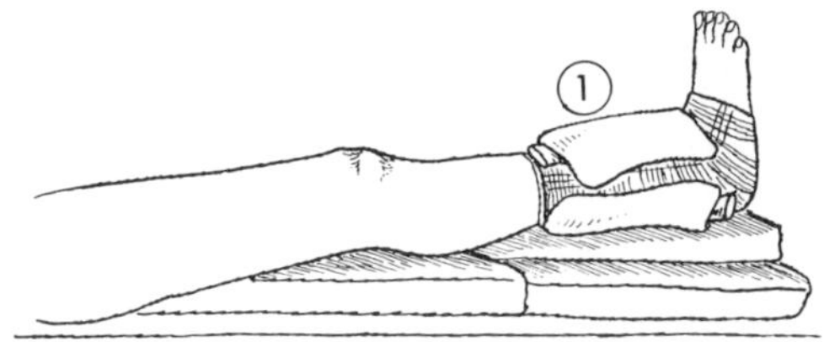

■ Subsequent Management

REMARKS

After the swelling has started to subside, the ideal treatment is to support the ankle with an Aircast device, which allows ankle flexion and extension but resists inversion strain.

If an Aircast is not available, an alternative method is to tape the ankle. This, however, tends to be more uncomfortable for patients, most of whom prefer the Aircast (Summit, NJ) device.

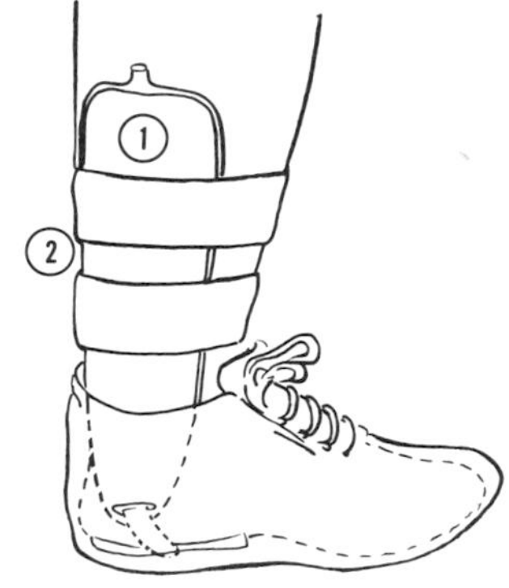

1. Aircast consists of medial and lateral air-filled supports.
2. Supports are wrapped and held with Velcro straps.

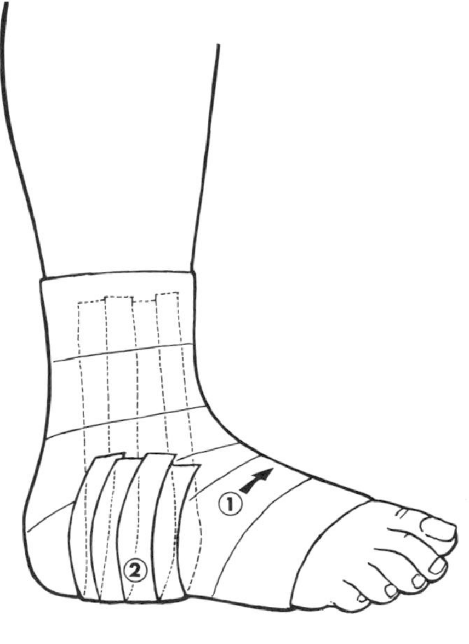

Alternative Method

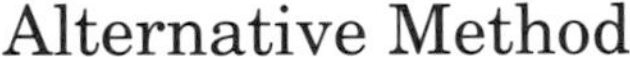

1. Ankle is wrapped with an elastic bandage.
2. Full roll of 1-in (2.5-cm) tape is applied over the bandage with the ankle everted. Tape strips are applied mainly over the lateral and medial aspects of the ankle.

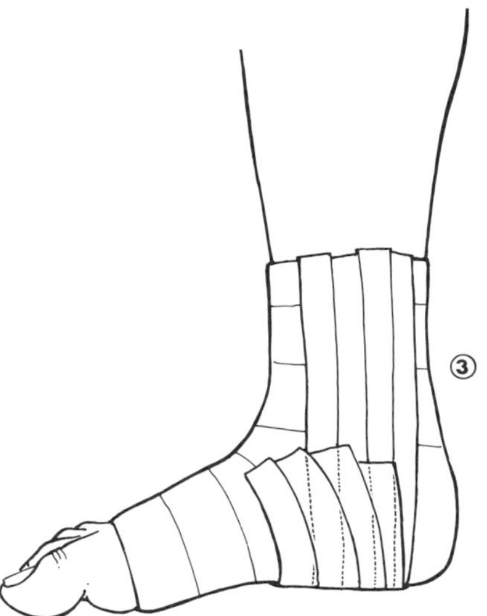

3. Ankle should be free to move in flexion and extension but limited in inversion.

Note: The wrapping is primarily for the patient's comfort. If swelling or irritation of the ankle occurs, the patient should be advised to relieve the taping with scissors. Non–weight-bearing ambulation with crutches tends to produce a symptomatic tight heel cord, which should be avoided. Encourage the patient to bear partial weight with crutches.

Follow-Up Management

REMARKS

Functional instability of the ankle after a sprain may be diminished by early range-of-motion exercises. These exercises are designed to develop coordination of the calf muscles and overcome any proprioceptive defects from the injury.

The patient should be encouraged to bear weight on the injured ankle with crutches and with support at the earliest possible time.

Usually, the support can be removed by 2 weeks, and exercises can be started to regain normal control and balance in the ankle.

Patients with more severe acute injuries to the ankle ligaments medially, laterally, or to the distal tibiofibular ligaments may require a longer recovery time.

It is important to emphasize that weight bearing on the injured side aids rather than impedes recovery and avoids problems of disuse atrophy or even Sudeck's atrophy.

Approximately one in five patients with acute sprains have recurrent problems. These recurrent symptoms may require operative repair to avoid subsequent arthritic breakdown of the joint.

Rehabilitation

REMARKS

When the pain and acute swelling have subsided and the patient is bearing weight with comfort on the ankle, start a rehabilitation program to strengthen the ligaments about the ankle and proprioceptive control of balance.

The exercise program should emphasize inversion and eversion strengthening and heel cord stretching.

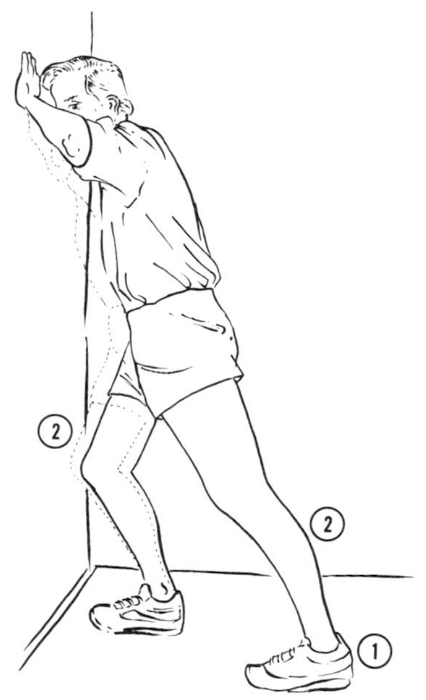

Heel Cord Stretching Exercises

1. Heel cord stretching is an important exercise to prevent recurrent sprain. This is done by maintaining the foot to be stretched posteriorly with the foot flat. The toes are pointed straight ahead.
2. Patient flexes forward on the opposite leg, keeping the knee on the rear leg in extension and the foot flat on the floor, thereby stretching out the tight calf muscles and heel cord.

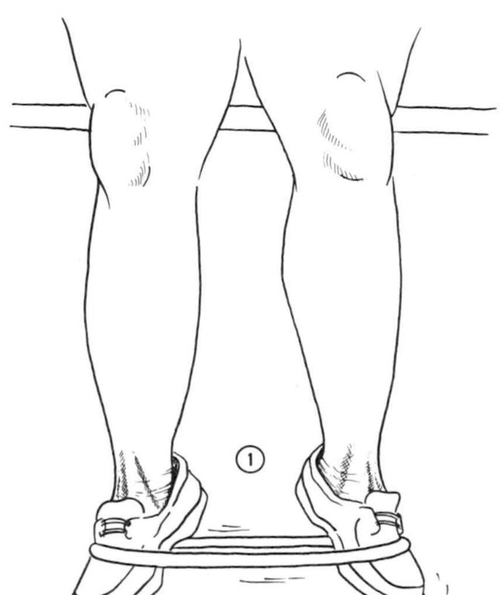

Eversion Muscle Strengthening

1. Peroneal muscles and dorsiflexors can be strengthened by resistive exercises.

■ Management of More Severe Ankle Sprains (Grades II and III)

REMARKS

Frequently, the sprained ankle is classified into three types or grades of injury. However, because most acute ankle sprains are best treated in a similar manner, the advantages of this grading are dubious.

Grade I injury is considered the mild common injury to the anterolateral fibulotalar ligament. Grades II and III are associated with more extensive disruption of the anterolateral and posterolateral support structures on the ankle.

Clinically, grades II and III present with diffuse swelling of the ankle. Anterior instability and lateral tilting of the talus may also be demonstrated.

These more severe injuries are characteristically seen in active young athletes, such as basketball players or individuals with a history of recurrent ankle instability.

With few exceptions, more severe injuries can also be treated by the RICE nonoperative method. The injury requires a longer period of recovery and more intense rehabilitation, but few patients go on to long-term problems.

Rare indications for operative repair of the acute grade II or III ankle injury include the active athlete with recurrent problems or any individual who desires correction of recurrent ankle sprain.

Additional indications for acute operative intervention include avulsion fractures from the fibula or talus, which can lead to peroneal instability or discomfort from the loose bony prominence.

Although effective operative repair techniques are available, it is usually preferable to allow recovery from the acute injury and perform reconstructive procedures only for the more chronic problems. A number of studies have shown that reconstructive repair is satisfactory in the ankle, and the outcome and postoperative stability are predictable.

Mechanism of Grades II and III Sprains

1. Injury occurs most often in an active young adult who twists the ankle while jumping.
2. Complete rupture of the anterior talofibular ligament occurs.

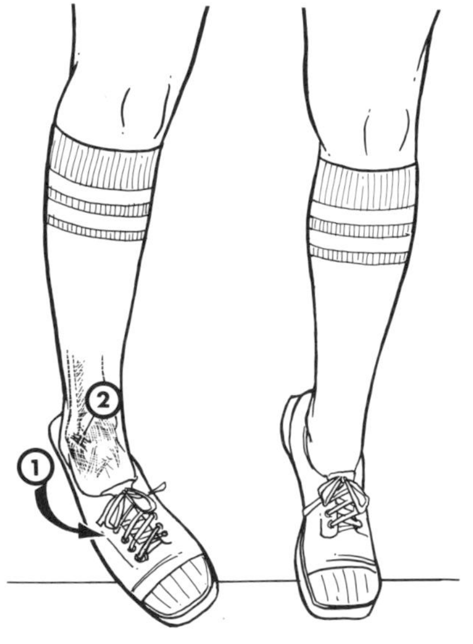

3. Continued inversion of the ankle as it starts to dorsiflex
4. Disrupts the calcaneofibular ligament and, occasionally, the posterior talofibular ligament.

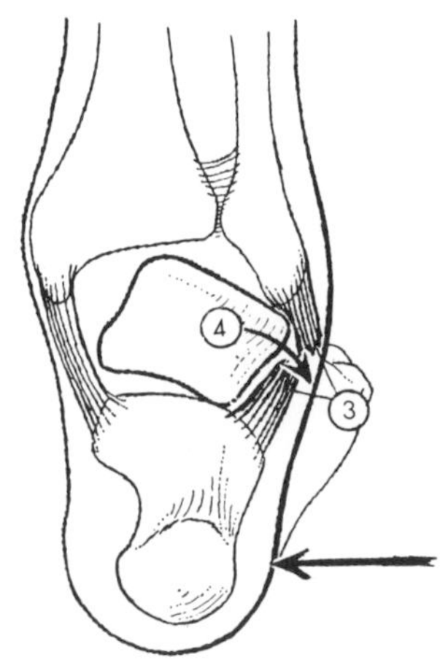

Clinical Tests

1. Tenderness is located both over the talofibular ligament and
2. Over the calcaneofibular ligament.
3. On inversion stress testing, the ankle is relatively painless and excessively mobile in comparison with the opposite side.

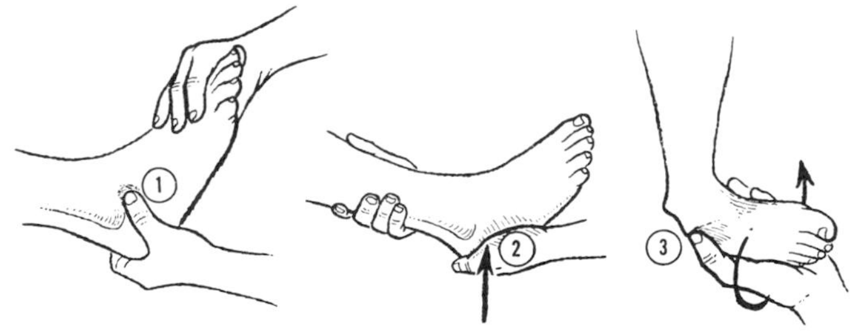

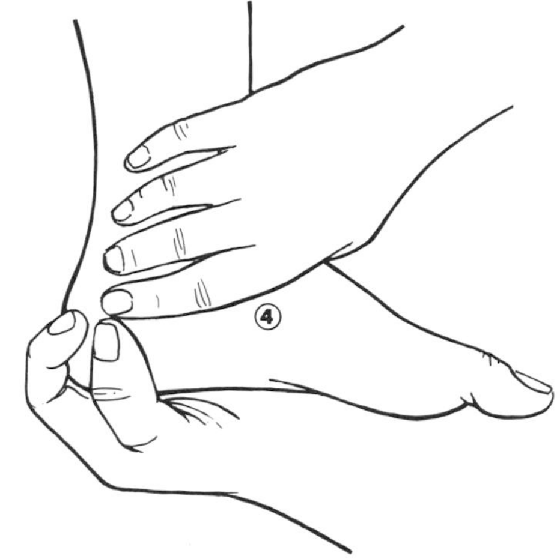

4. Anterior drawer sign is also evident.

Alternative Method (Gungor Test)

If the patient is unable to relax during the drawer test, try the Gungor maneuver.

1. Patient is asked to lie prone with the ankle extending beyond the edge of the table.
2. With one hand, the surgeon presses the heel forward steadily. If the anterior capsule is ruptured, the talus will move further forward than on the uninjured side.
3. Vacuum effect from negative pressure is created by the change in the talus position. This draws the skin inward on both sides of the calcaneal tendon on the injured side compared with the uninjured side.

Note: To confirm the test, take a lateral x-ray with the heel in this position and with it pushed forward.

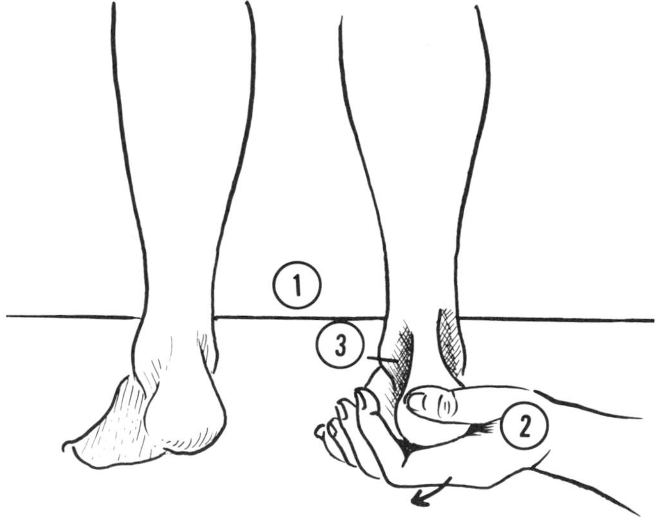

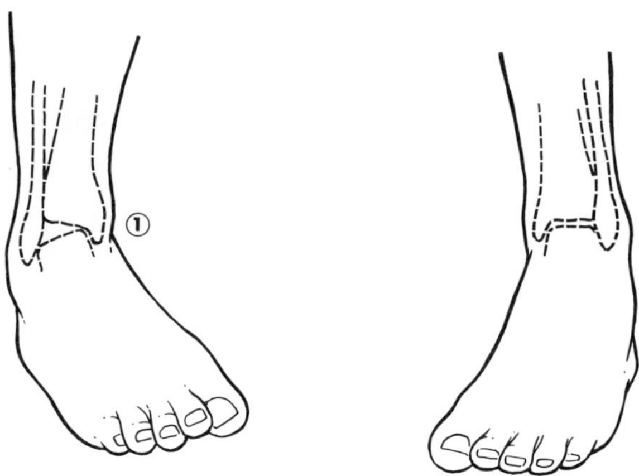

Appearance on X-Ray

1. After the initial injury, stress testing of the ankle demonstrates increased tilting of the talus, at least 10° more than is evident on the opposite, uninjured side.

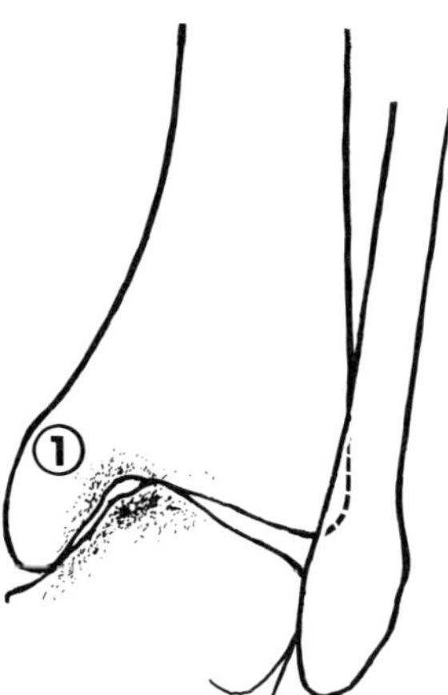

X-RAY OF LONG-STANDING ANKLE INSTABILITY

1. X-rays after many episodes of recurrent instability of 10 or more years' duration show narrowing of the medial joint space and arthritic changes.

Cast Treatment for Severe Injuries

REMARKS

If the patient is active and needs more support than the aircast provides or if an Aircast is not available, a short-leg cast may be applied temporarily.

Avoid applying a cast or any restrictive device to an acutely swollen ankle.

Put the limb at complete rest, and elevate it for 24–48 hours.

Apply a compressive bandage and ice.

After swelling has subsided in 24–48 hours, a short-leg walking cast may be applied.

1. The cast extends from below the knee to the toes.
2. The foot is at a right angle to the leg.
3. The heel is slightly everted.
4. The toes are free.

Note: The patient should also use crutches for 1 week to protect the ankle and elevate the leg when not walking. If the leg is allowed to hang down, the ankle inevitably swells and becomes painful.

Keep the cast on for a minimal period of time because the earlier the ankle can be allowed to move, the faster rehabilitation occurs. In most instances, the cast can be removed by 1–2 weeks, and the ankle rehabilitation program can be begun, as previously described.

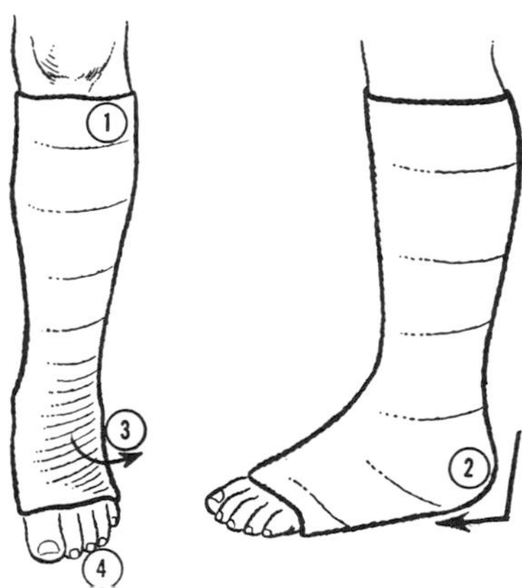

Cast Treatment for Grade III Injuries

The cast is removed after 1–2 weeks, and exercises are begun, as described previously.

If the ankle is still tender after cast removal, it may be wrapped and taped as described previously.

1. Support the ankle to prevent inversion injury.
2. Elevate the heel with a 6.4-mm outer heel wedge to hold the ankle in slight eversion.

Note: The patient should be followed closely and advised that recurrent episodes of ankle instability can be corrected by operative repair. Approximately one in four patients with grade III injuries treated nonoperatively have recurrent ankle instability and may need reconstruction of the lateral supports.

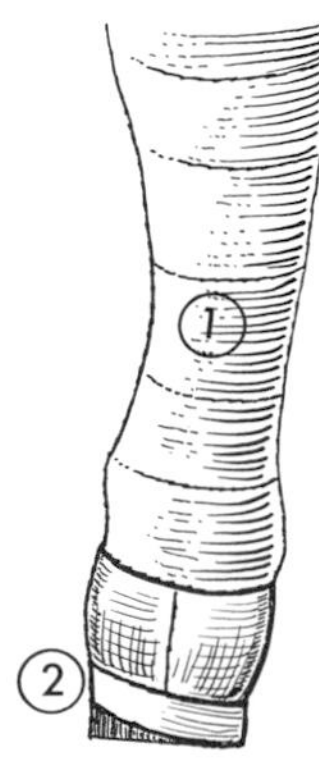

Operative Management

REMARKS

Most ankle sprains, even the more severe grades II and III, can be treated by the RICE method.

Although cast immobilization has been recommended in the past, recent studies show that support with methods such as the Aircast is preferable because these devices allow limited range of motion of the ankle while supporting the injured ligaments.

Operative repair may be indicated for the active individual who has a history of recurrent ankle instability.

Individuals with an ankle sprain and evidence of avulsion fractures of the fibula or talus might also be advised to have an operative repair to avoid persistent symptoms of instability or peroneal dislocations.

In addition, the individual with long-standing ankle instability should undergo a reconstructive procedure to avoid the problems of ankle joint arthritis that Harrington and others found to be associated with chronic ankle instability.

Indications for Operative Repair of the Acute Ankle Sprain

1. The most common indication for acute repair is an individual with a history of repeated instability and evidence of a laxity in anterior lateral capsule. This can be tightened up by a direct surgical approach to the anterolateral aspect of the capsule.
2. Repair of the anterior talofibular ligament is necessary to correct the instability and avoid long-term problems of ankle joint arthritis.

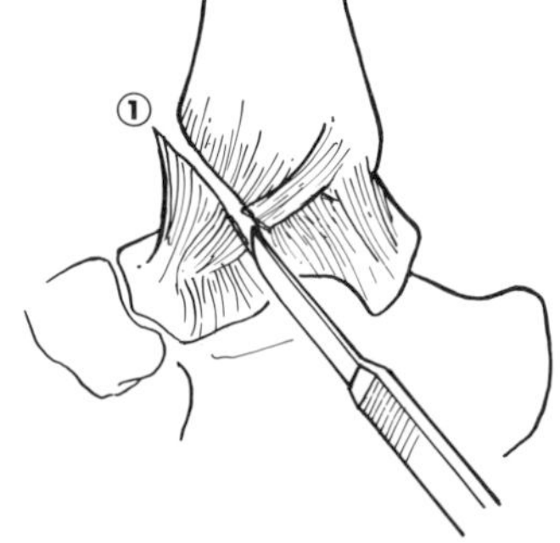

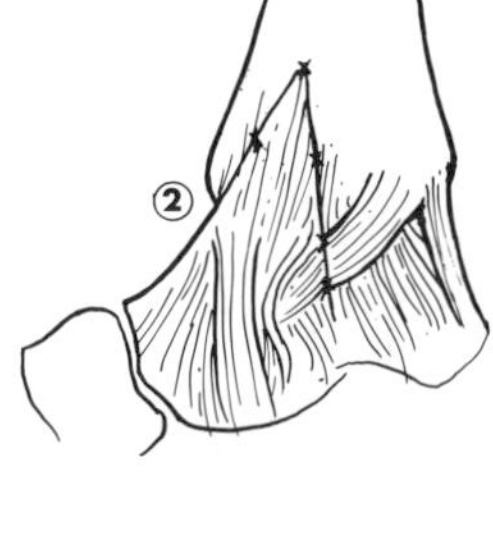

■ Other Indications for Operative Repair

Fractures of the Os Fibulare

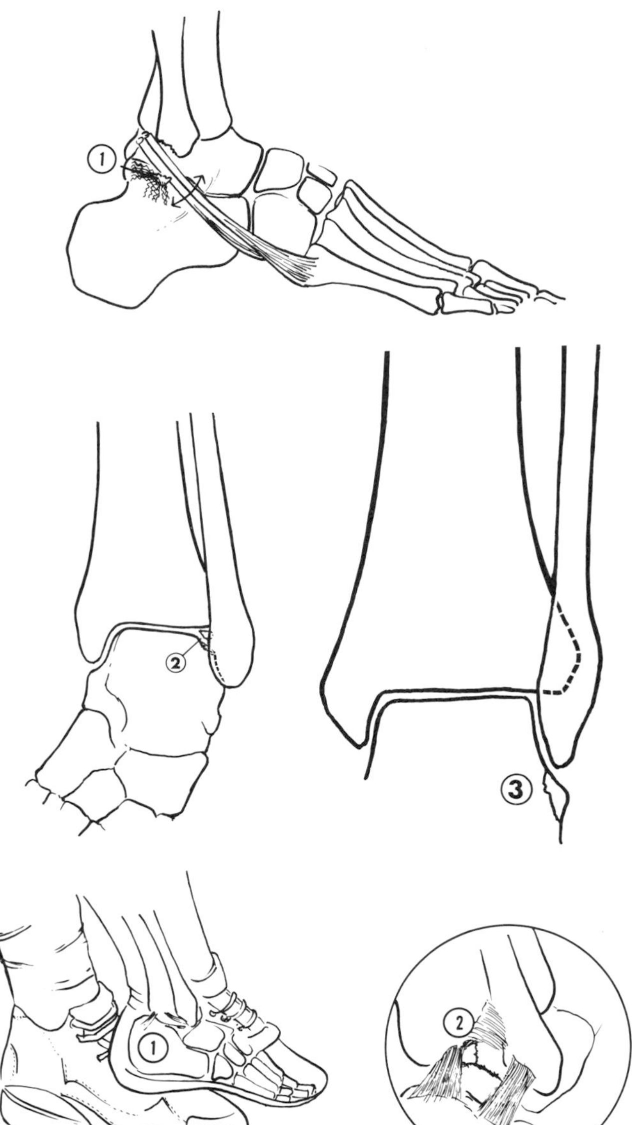

1. Fleck fractures of the fibula, which are sometimes confused with a sesamoid bone (os subfibulare), are associated with disruption of the peroneal retinaculum.

This can go on to chronic symptoms from peroneal tendon instability and is best prevented by early repair.

2. Osteochondral fractures of the lateral talus may be associated with 5 per cent of sprained ankles and should be carefully looked for.
3. Fractures of the posterior facet of the talus may be missed or may be confused with ankle sprains.

1. In addition to the os fibulare or fleck fracture of the fibula, a severe ankle sprain may be associated with a fracture of the posterior process of the talus. This is also called an os trigonum. This results from a forceful plantar flexion of the foot when an athlete lands off balance while jumping.
2. Posterior talus is caught between the calcaneus and the posterior tibia, resulting in a fracture of the posterior process or os trigonum.

Management

The early diagnosis of the os fibulare or fleck fracture of the fibula as a cause of ankle pain is usually the exception rather than the rule.

Frequently, the patient is seen by a wide variety of physicians because the true nature of the condition is usually not recognized initially.

If the fracture of the posterior talar process is recognized acutely, it usually responds to cast immobilization for approximately 4–6 weeks.

If the condition is recognized only after a chronic problem has occurred, it can be treated initially by cast support and nonsteroidal anti-inflammatory medications.

If the symptoms persist for more than 4–6 months, particularly in the active athlete, operative excision is usually necessary. However, if the fragment is unusually large and involves the subtalar joint, internal fixation may be preferable.

Fractures of the Os Peroneum

REMARKS

Peterson and Stinson reported that fracture of the os peroneum results from forceful supination and plantar flexion injuries. They think that these fractures may be more frequent than recognized because the injuries and symptoms are similar to ankle sprains.

The os peroneum is a sesamoid bone in the peroneus longus found fractured in 5–26 per cent of anatomic and radiographic studies.

Patients with these fractures typically complain of pain over the lateral aspect of the foot with running or walking on uneven ground. They may also complain of the ankle giving out, which causes the symptoms to be confused with ankle sprain.

The diagnosis can be made by oblique x-rays of the lateral aspect of the foot. Typically, there are bilateral sesamoids with the affected side more irregular and enlarged compared with the opposite unaffected side.

When in doubt, bone scans are helpful to localize the source of the pain.

In most instances, these injuries are recognized late and are best treated by surgical excision because the fractured sesamoid heals poorly.

1. Os peroneum is typically located in the long peroneal tendon as it curves plantarward onto the cuboid.
2. Care should be taken to distinguish this problem from rupture of the peroneus longus tendon or fracture of the calcaneus. The fractured sesamoid is best managed in the symptomatic patient by surgical excision of the fracture fragments.

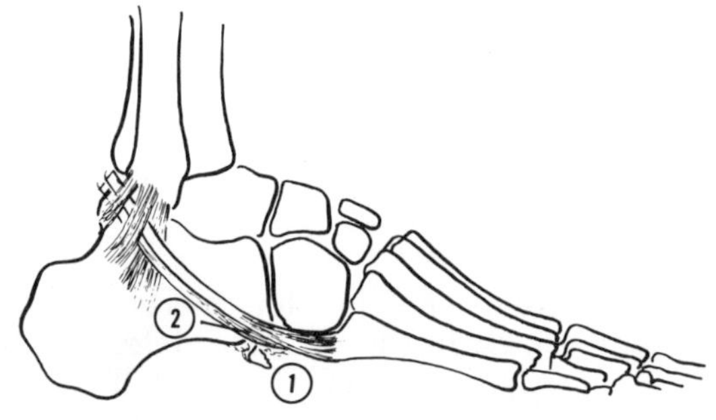

Deltoid Ligament Injuries

REMARKS

Significant isolated injuries to the deltoid do not occur. This is due to the key stabilizing role of the lateral malleolus.

Yablon et al. demonstrated that the talus faithfully follows the lateral malleolus. Injury sufficient to displace the talus laterally occurs only with displaced fractures of the lateral malleolus.

Staples pointed out that, even after complete excision of the deltoid ligament, i.e., after an open fracture, a stable ankle is possible provided that the lateral malleolus remains intact.

The cause of any lateral talar displacement must be carefully sought and corrected because it is a prime factor in unsatisfactory results after ankle injuries.

Occasionally, a plantar flexion injury disrupts the anteromedial deltoid and the anterior talofibular ligament and produces anterior ankle instability. The patients who present with bimalleolar rather than isolated deltoid sprains can usually be treated by cast support.

Lateral talar displacement does not result from an isolated deltoid ligament tear.

1. Avulsion injury of the deltoid ligament is evident on x-ray.
2. Talus is shifted laterally, as indicated by widening of the medial joint space.
3. Subtle angulated fracture of the lateral malleolus is the basic cause of the talar shift and needs to be corrected.

Note: Repair of deltoid ligament tears associated with lateral malleolar fracture is discussed subsequently.

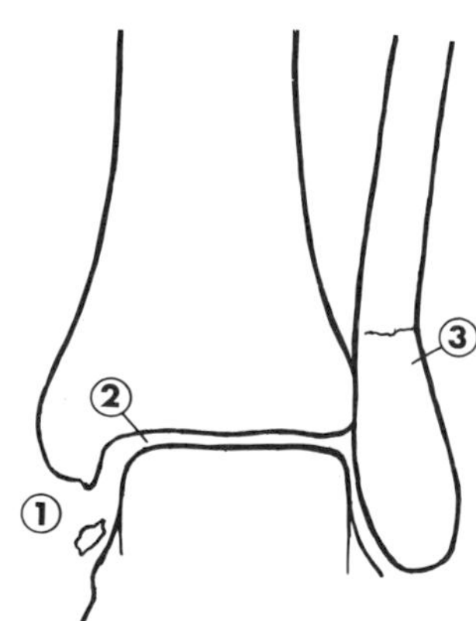

Tear of the Distal Tibiofibular Ligament That Causes Ankle Diastasis Without Fibular Fracture

REMARKS

Although disruption of the syndesmosis rarely occurs without fracture of the fibula, Edwards and DeLee described ankle diastasis without fracture.

These injuries can be divided into two general types: latent and frank.

In latent diastasis, standard x-rays are normal, but the ankle mortise is widened when abduction or external rotation stress is applied.

A frank diastasis presents with a visible diastasis on the initial x-rays.

Latent ankle diastasis requires no reduction and can generally be treated by cast immobilization for 4–6 weeks. This is in contrast to the usual sprained ankle without ankle diastasis, which generally does not require cast immobilization.

Frank diastasis is visible on the x-ray and requires closed reduction and sometimes operative stabilization.

Type I diastasis includes

1. Disruption of the anterior tibiofibular ligament and
2. Tear of the deltoid ligament, sometimes with inversion of the ligament into the ankle joint, which causes
3. Consistent widening of the mortise and diastasis of the distal tibiofibular syndesmosis.

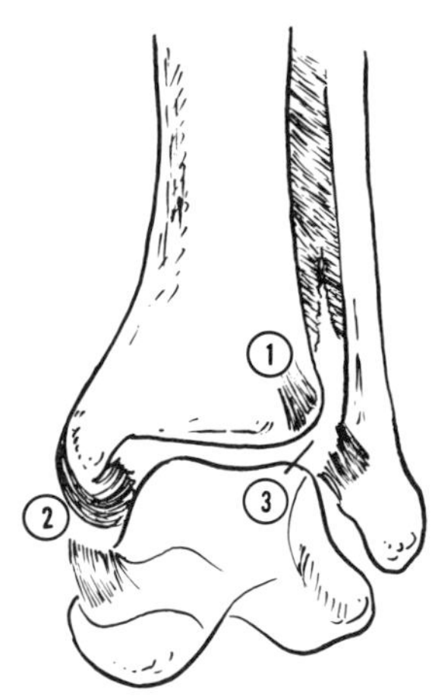

1. The type II latent diastasis is characterized by disruption of the anterior talofibular ligament,
2. Tear of the deltoid ligament, and
3. Plastic deformation of the fibula, which causes diastasis of the syndesmosis, which cannot be corrected by manipulation.

Note: This rare type of injury requires operative treatment to osteotomize the fibula and correct the plastic bending to restore the normal mortise.

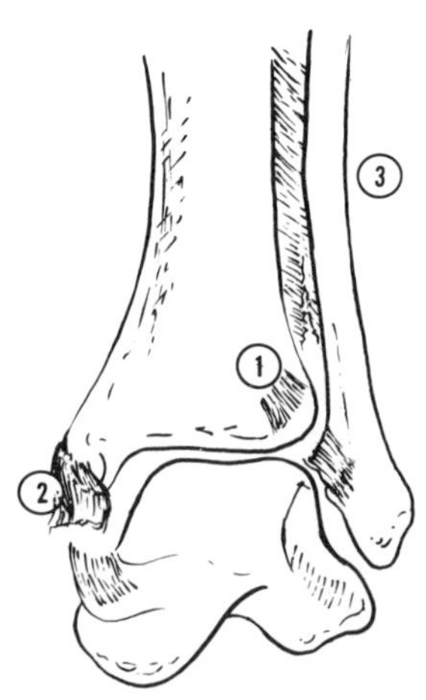

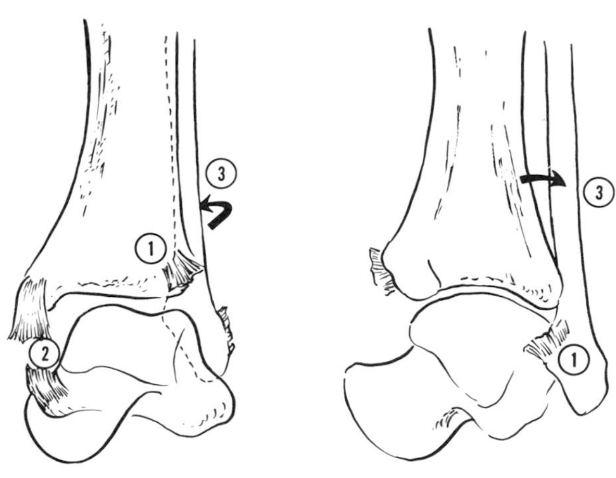

A type III frank ankle diastasis is characterized by
1. Tear of the anterior tibiofibular ligament,
2. Tear of the medial deltoid ligament, and
3. Rotatory subluxation of the fibula seen on a routine unstressed x-ray.

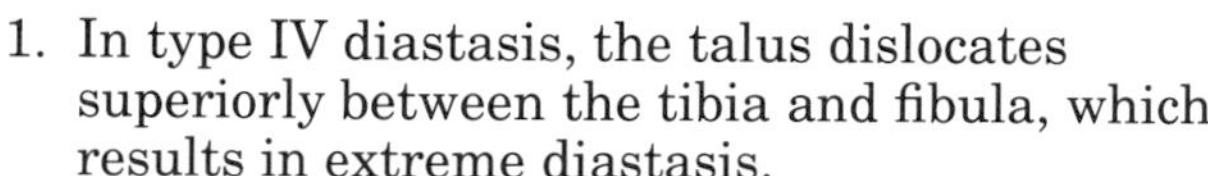

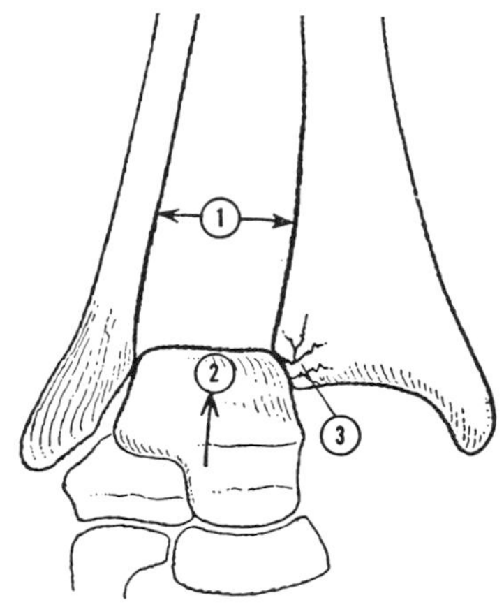

1. In type IV diastasis, the talus dislocates superiorly between the tibia and fibula, which results in extreme diastasis.
2. Talofibular ligaments and interosseous membrane are torn.
3. Deltoid is disrupted but the medial malleolus is usually not fractured. However, there may be a fracture of the lateral portion of the tibial articular surface.

Note: Although this injury may occasionally be treated by closed methods, its severity warrants open reduction and repair of the disrupted structure.

Management

REMARKS

Type I injuries are usually best treated by open reduction, removal of interposed soft tissue, and stabilization of the tibiofibular joint.

Type II injuries also require open reduction; however, an osteotomy of the fibula is usually necessary to correct the bowing.

The rare types III and IV can be treated by closed manipulation and immobilization. If the ankle diastasis persists, however, occasionally tibiofibular screw fixation is necessary.

Postreduction X-Ray

1. Talus fits accurately under the tibia and in the ankle mortise.
2. Fibula is secured to the tibia with a transfixion screw.
3. Fibula fits snugly against the tibia.

Note: Although closed or open reduction may work for the injury without damage to the articular surface, frequently the shearing injury to the joint surface results in traumatic arthritis.

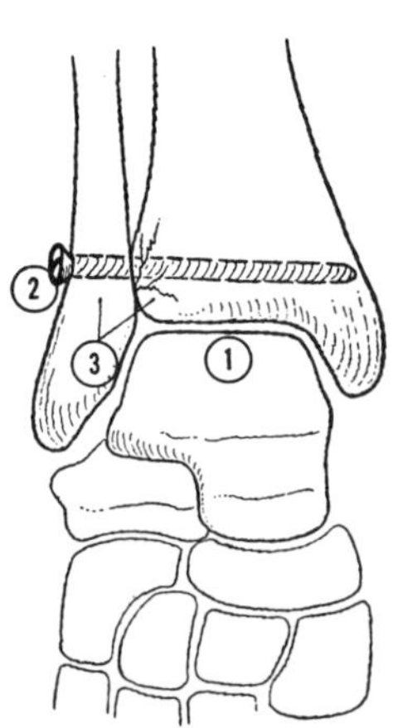

Recurrent Instability of the Lateral Ligaments

REMARKS

Persistent ankle instability is a well-known disability of athletes and active adults.

The evaluation of ankle instability by x-ray is subject to several difficulties, including a definition of what amount of talar tilt evident on stress x-rays of the ankle is normal. In general, more than 10° of tilt in comparison with the opposite ankle can be considered evidence of significant lateral instability.

Stress x-rays do not demonstrate subtalar instability, which can be a significant cause of problems for some patients.

Chrisman and Snook pointed out that the stress x-rays of a clinically unstable ankle are like myelography in the diagnosis of a ruptured intervertebral disc. The results are not always reliable but are a useful adjunct.

More important than radiographic studies in diagnosis of recurrent instability are

- A history of recurrent sprain or "giving way" during mild activity and
- A palpable sulcus in the anterolateral aspect of the ankle joint on inversion.

Arthritic Changes Associated With Long-Standing Lateral Ligament Instability

Harrington showed that long-standing (for 10 years or more) lateral instability results in unbalanced loading and frequently in osteoarthritic changes. Patients with this instability characteristically develop increased ankle pain and radiographic evidence of degenerative arthritis of the medial half of the tibial and talar surfaces.

These changes may be only minimally apparent unless weight-bearing x-rays are made.

Weight-Bearing X-Ray of Advanced Arthritis in a Symptomatically Lax Ankle

1. Medial joint space is narrowed. There is sclerosis of the subchondral bone in the medial half of the joint.

Note: Operative reconstruction of the lateral ligaments can relieve symptoms in the mildly to moderately arthritic ankle and possibly can reverse changes that are already manifest.

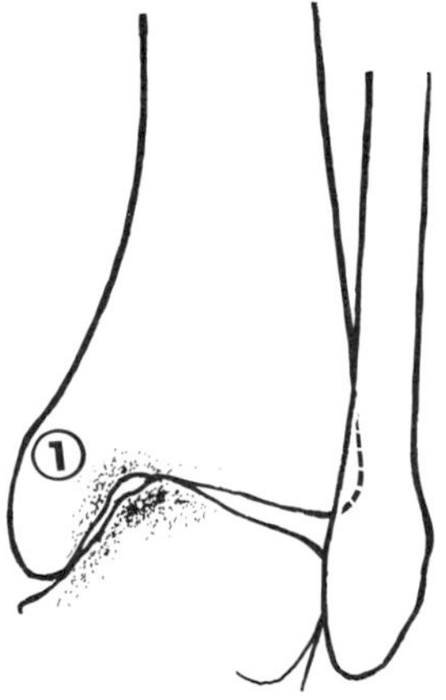

Weight-Bearing X-Rays of Early Degenerative Changes

ANTEROPOSTERIOR VIEW

1. There is early grooving of the medial tibial palfond and
2. Spurring of the medial aspect of the talus and medial malleolus.

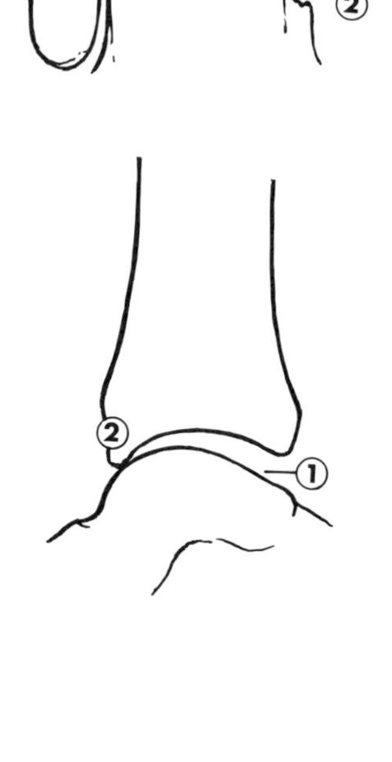

LATERAL VIEW

1. Anteroposterior stress instability secondary to chronic anterior talofibular disruption and
2. Anterior tibial spurring are evident.

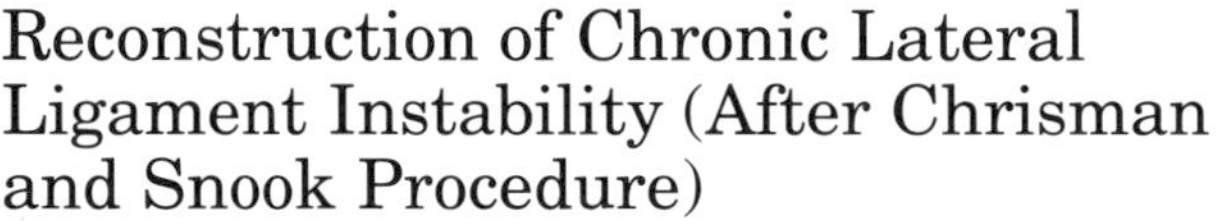

Reconstruction of Chronic Lateral Ligament Instability (After Chrisman and Snook Procedure)

1. Among the reliable procedures to restore stability to the ankle is that developed by Chrisman and Snook, which uses half of the peroneus brevis tendon. This is left attached distally and passed through a drill hole in the distal fibula.
2. Tendon is then fixed to the calcaneus, thereby reinforcing the subtalar joint and the tibiotalar joint.
3. Lax anterolateral structures may also be repaired simultaneously.

Note: This procedure is a reliable way to restore ankle stability and, therefore, can be recommended for patients with symptomatic recurrent instability. Ideally, the reconstruction should be carried out before the symptoms develop into arthritic breakdown of the joint.

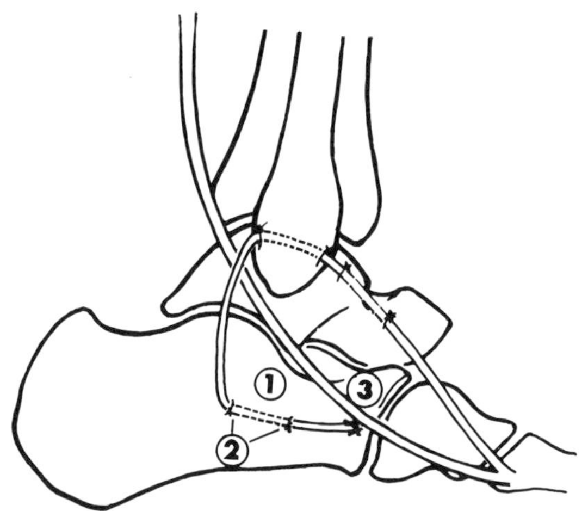

Other Complications

Persistent Pain and Weakness After Ankle Sprains

REMARKS

In addition to recurrent instability, some patients with ankle sprains experience slow resolution of their pain and weakness.

The most common reason for this is failure to bear weight early after ankle sprains so that there is residual heel cord tightening and disuse of the foot and ankle.

Occasional problems result from unrecognized fractures of the talus, the calcaneus, the metatarsals, or other bones of the foot.

A rare cause of persistent weakness after ankle sprain is a stretch injury to the peroneal nerve. Internal torsion of the distal foot and ankle can occasionally stretch the peroneal nerve as it passes around the head and neck of the fibula. The result is a weakness of the ankle and toe dorsiflexors as a result of the traction injury.

Persistent pain and weakness may also occur as a result of a posterior compartment syndrome. This rarely may be seen from severe swelling with an ankle sprain or fracture, particularly if the swollen limb is wrapped in a rigid dressing.

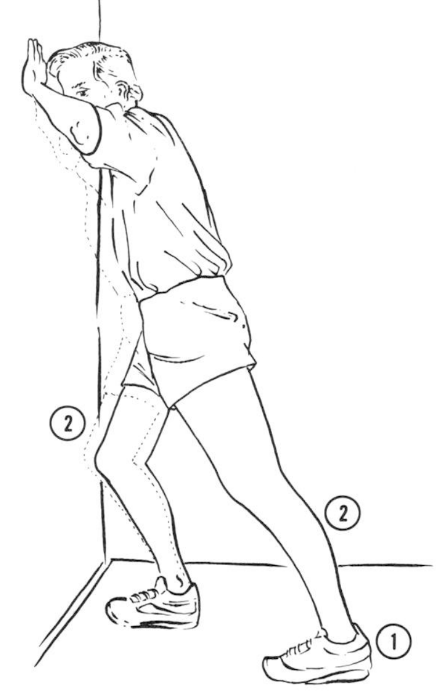

1. A common cause of prolonged disability after ankle sprain is the patient's fear of bearing weight after prolonged use of crutches.
2. This causes the heel cord and other soft tissue structures about the ankle to tighten if the patient maintains a non–weight-bearing status for more than 2–3 weeks. This problem can be combated by heel cord stretching and other exercises.

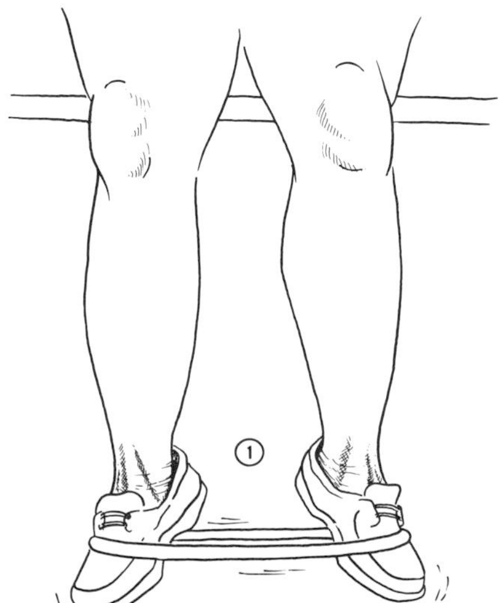

Eversion Muscle Strengthening

1. The peroneal muscles and dorsiflexors can be strengthened by resistive exercises.

Unrecognized Fractures

Other Complications

UNRECOGNIZED FRACTURES THAT CAUSE PROLONGED SYMPTOMS AFTER ANKLE SPRAIN

1. Take care to rule out persistent pain being caused by unrecognized subtle osteochondral fractures of the anterolateral of the dome of the talus or the
2. Posterior aspect of the talus.
3. Stress fractures or other injuries to the calcaneus or the metatarsals may also be a source of persistent pain, which may be confused with an ankle sprain.

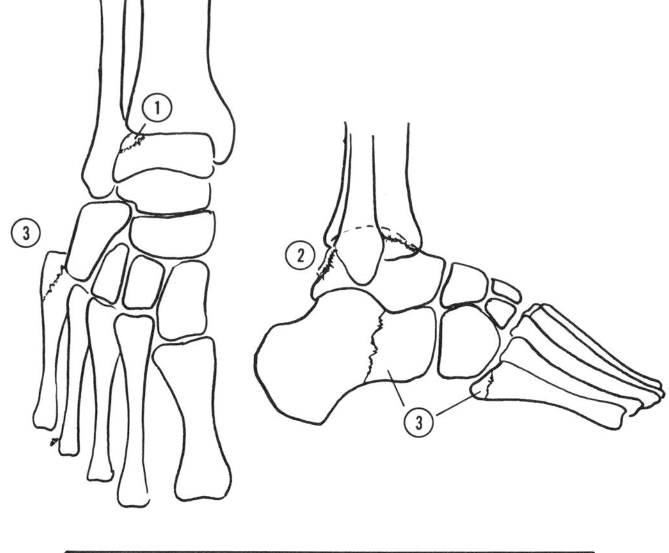

Bone Scan for Unrecognized Fractures

1. For the patient with persistent symptoms after a "sprained ankle," bone scan may detect that the problem is related to a fracture of the posterior talus or fractures in other areas of the talus or calcaneus, which may not be immediately recognized on plain x-ray.

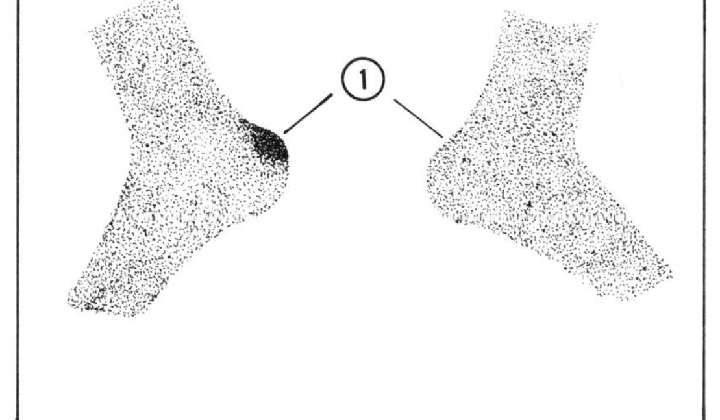

Posterior Compartment Syndrome

POSTERIOR COMPARTMENT SYNDROME WITH SPRAINED ANKLE

1. Rigid dressing applied to a severely swollen ankle may occasionally produce a posterior compartment syndrome. This is characterized by cavus of the entire foot,
2. Adduction of the forefoot, and
3. Claw toes.

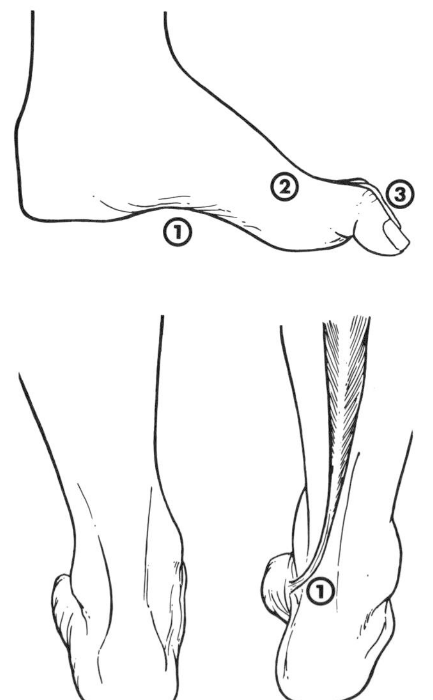

1. Contracture of the posterior tibial muscle particularly contributes to the cavovarus deformity.

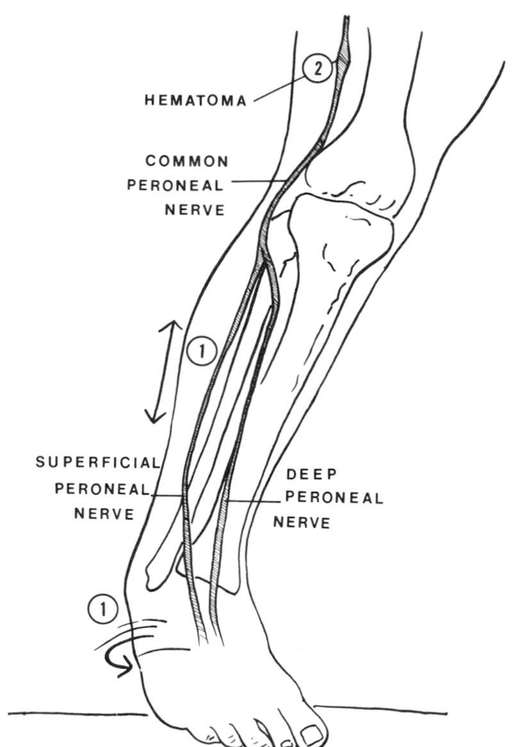

Nerve Injury

NERVE INJURY

1. Severe inversion injury to the ankle or distal tibia can cause an acute palsy by stretching the peroneal nerve around the neck of the fibula.
2. Rarely, the injury may rupture the nutrient vessels and cause delayed palsy as the hematoma expands.

Management of Complications

REMARKS

Persistent pain as a result of refusal to bear weight can be overcome by a well-supervised therapy program to stretch the heel cord and encourage the patient to resume functional activities.

If the cause is an unrecognized fracture of the talus or stress fracture elsewhere in the foot, management should be directed at this specific fracture problem.

For the rare patient with a posterior compartment syndrome associated with an ankle sprain, early fasciotomy of the posterior compartment is indicated. However, if the condition is seen late, the preferable treatment is stretching or lengthening of the contracted muscles.

Traction injuries of the peroneal nerve are usually temporary and recover spontaneously. In most instances, a period of support in an ankle brace is indicated to prevent equinus deformity.

Rarely, pain from peroneal nerve injury may be almost like causalgia from bleeding within the nerve. This may occasionally require exploration of the nerve to decompress any intraneural hematoma.

FRACTURES OF THE ANKLE

REMARKS

Just as sprains result most often from internal torsion or inversion mechanisms, fractures of the ankle are produced by eversion or external torsional injuries. These displace the ankle externally, posteriorly, and laterally.

The anatomy of the distal tibiofibular joint, with the groove preventing anterior fibular displacement with internal rotation but allowing posterior fibular displacement with external torsion, has been discussed previously (see page 816). This anatomic arrangement places the ligaments at risk for internal torsion but the bony supports of the ankle at risk for external torsion.

Less frequently, pure pronation-abduction injuries and supination-adduction injuries fracture the nkle without torsional displacement.

The most complete and applicable system for classifying ankle fractures according to mechanism is that of Lauge-Hansen, as reviewed by Yde. This classification is well worth reviewing to select appropriate treatment and evaluation results. It is based on the ankle mortise's being a ring around which varying injuries occur.

Ankle Mortise Ring

REMARKS

The support structures and ankle mortise, including three bones and uniting ligaments, can be looked at as a continuous ring.

The position of the foot at the time of fracture determines the ligament or bony structure most likely to fail first.

The force of injury then proceeds around the ring, which causes failure of the support structures in proportion to the amount of force applied.

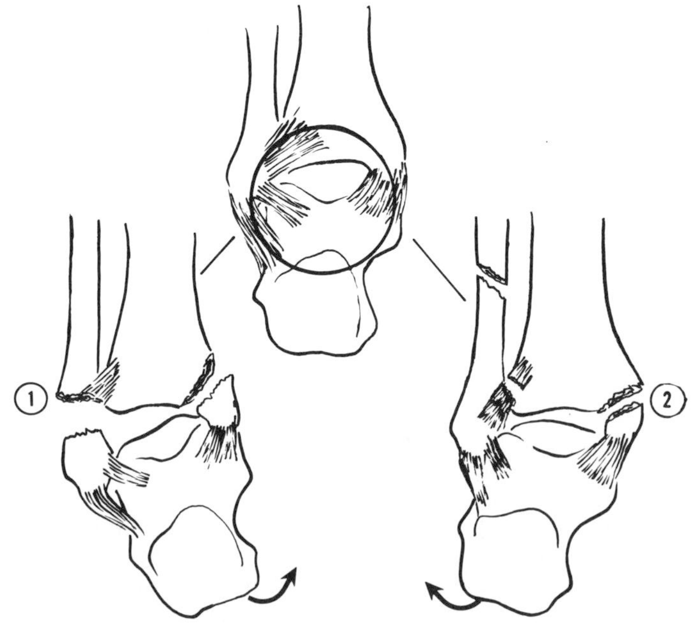

1. With the foot supinated, the lateral support structures fail first and medial structures fail last.
2. With the foot in pronation, the medial support structures are the first to fail.

Classification of the Ankle Fractures

Lauge-Hansen Mechanistic Classification of Ankle Fractures (After Yde)

REMARKS

This classification should be based on adequate x-rays, including mortise views with the foot internally rotated 15° and lateral and oblique studies.

The first word in this classification takes into consideration the position of the foot at the time of the injury, and the second word refers to the direction of the injury force on the talus.

Between 50–60 per cent of ankle fractures occur when the foot is supinated and external rotational force is applied to the talus (S-EX fracture).

Twenty per cent result from pure supination-adduction mechanisms (S-AD fracture).

Pronation and abduction (P-AB) or pronation and external rotation (P-EX fracture) mechanisms cause the remaining 20 per cent.

The distribution of these types varies in many series, but the predominance of the S-EX types is evident in all reports.

The characteristics of the fibular fracture, when present, indicate the nature of the mechanism.

Stages of Ankle Fractures (Lauge-Hansen)

The severity of an ankle fracture depends on the stage to which the injury has advanced and on the mechanism.

This staging may seem unduly complex, but it is logical and important to understand to anticipate what combination of bone and ligamentous injuries is likely.

Stages of S-EX Fractures (Most Common Mechanism)

Forceful external rotation of the ankle with the foot supinated causes the following clockwise sequence of injuries to the structures about the ankle:

Stage I produces an injury to the anterior part of the anterior tibiofibular ligament or an avulsion fracture of its attachment to either the fibula or the tibia.

Stage II results in a typical spiral fracture of the lateral malleolus that runs from the anterior margin in a dorsoproximal direction and includes the stage I injury.

Stage III produces a fracture of the posterior tibial margin and includes stages I and II.

Note: It is not necessary to have a fracture of the posterior margin before the injury advances to a stage IV fracture.

Stage IV produces a fracture of the medial malleolus or rupture of the deltoid ligament and includes stages I and II and sometimes stage III.

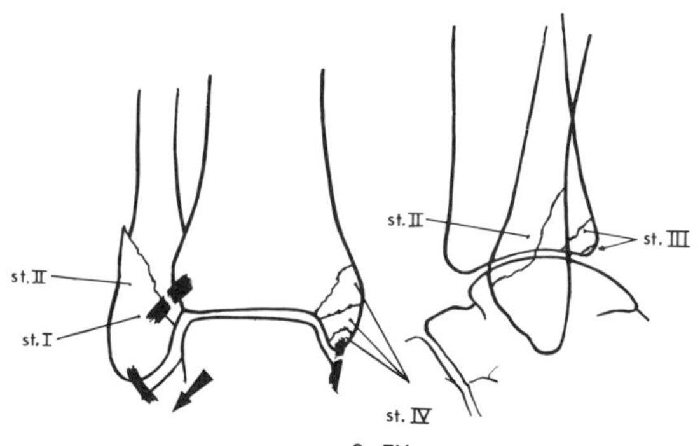

Stages of S-AD Fractures

An adduction injury to the supinated foot produces the following stages of damage to the bone and ligamentous structures of the ankle.

Stage I is a fracture of the lateral malleolus at or distal to the level of the tibiotalar joint or a rupture of the anterior talofibular or calcaneofibular ligament.

Stage II results in a fracture of the medial malleolus and includes stage I. Most of these fractures are oblique or vertical, but some may be transverse. Frequently, the fracture includes the posteromedial tibial surface.

Note: S-AD fracture is the only type associated with medial displacement of the talus. All the other types tend to displace the talus laterally or posterolaterally.

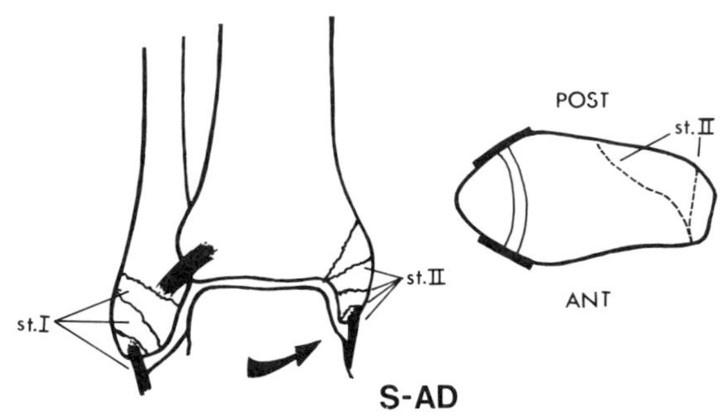

Stages of P-AB and P-EX Fractures

Abduction or external rotation injuries to the pronated foot tend to produce the same initial stages of injury. They differ primarily in the type of fibular fracture that results.

Stage I is a fracture of the medial malleolus or rupture of the deltoid ligament. These are identical for both P-AB and P-EX injuries.

Stage II is a rupture of the distal tibiofibular syndesmosis and includes stage I. Occasionally, avulsion fracture of the posterior tibial tubercle or the anterior tibial tubercle may be found at this stage in both mechanisms.

The difference between P-AB and P-EX fractures is determined by the type of fibular fracture produced at this stage. Characteristically, P-AB mechanism causes a low transverse supramalleolar fracture of the fibula and also includes stages I and II.

A P-EX fracture of stage III is characterized by a high supramalleolar fracture of the fibula and includes stages I and II. The level of the fracture varies, but no fracture is less than 2.5 cm above the tibiotalar joint. Characteristically, the fracture line runs from the anterior fibular margin in a distal direction.

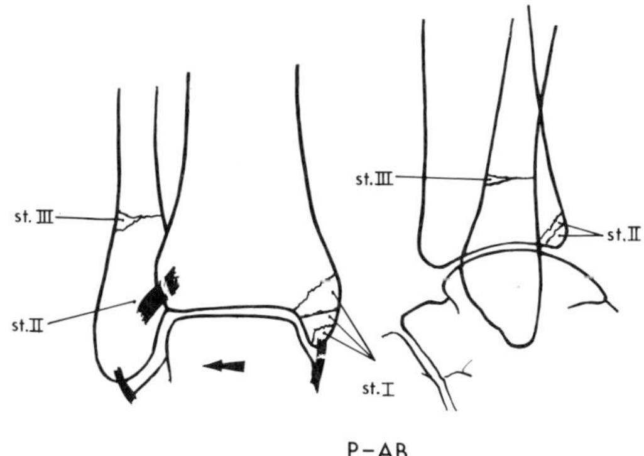

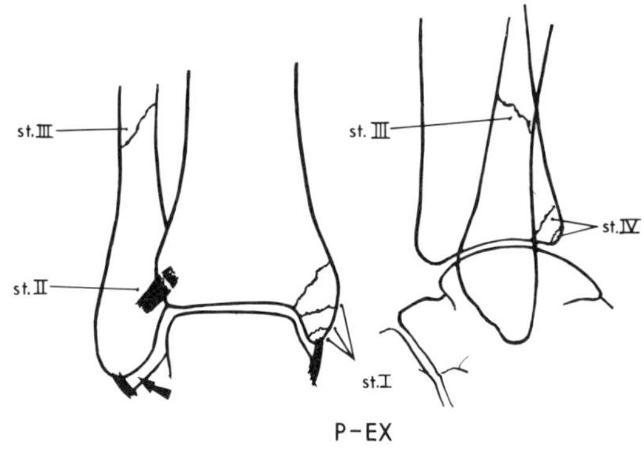

P-EX stage IV is an avulsion fracture of the posterior tibial margin, most often involving more than 25 per cent of the surface.

P-AB mechanisms produce avulsions of the posterior tibiofibular ligament rather than fractures of the tibia.

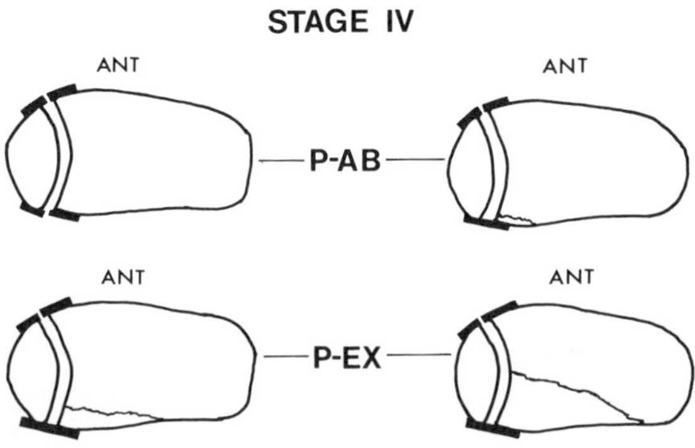

Classification by the Pattern of the Fibular Fracture

REMARKS

A number of groups have classified ankle fractures by the pattern of the fibular fracture.

As a general rule, fibular fractures below the tibiofibular syndesmosis do not require stabilization.

Tibial fractures above the level of the syndesmosis are usually associated with more severe instability of the ankle and require adequate reduction, usually with internal fixation.

The pattern of the fibular fracture can reveal the nature of the original mechanism, according to the Lauge-Hansen method.

Classification by Characteristics of Fibular Fracture

1. S-EX fracture is characterized by a spiral oblique fracture of the fibula that runs from the anterior distal margin up to the posterior superior cortex below the level of the syndesmosis.

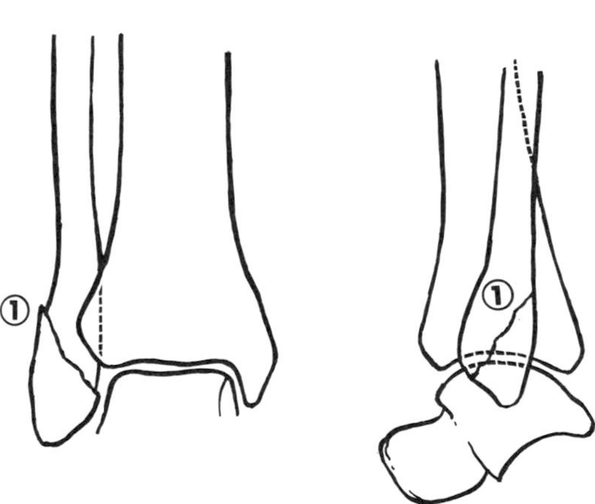

SUPINATION EXTERNAL ROTATION

2. P-EX fracture involves the fibula above the syndesmosis and is associated with diastasis of the tibiofibular joint. The fracture of the fibula runs from the superior anterior cortex down to the posterior inferior cortex. The location of this fracture varies but never is less than 2.5 cm above the tibiotalar joint.

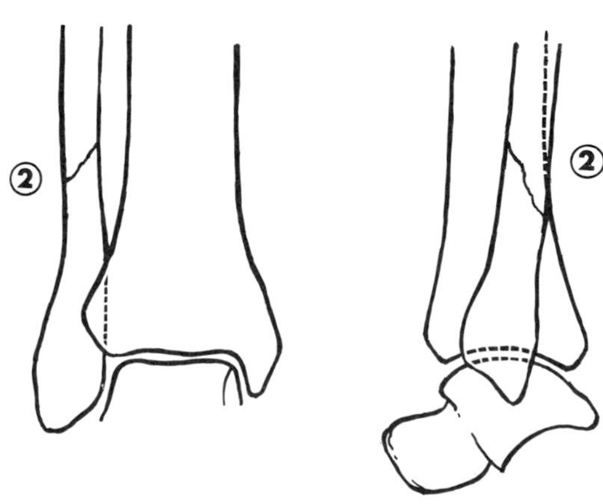

PRONATION EXTERNAL ROTATION

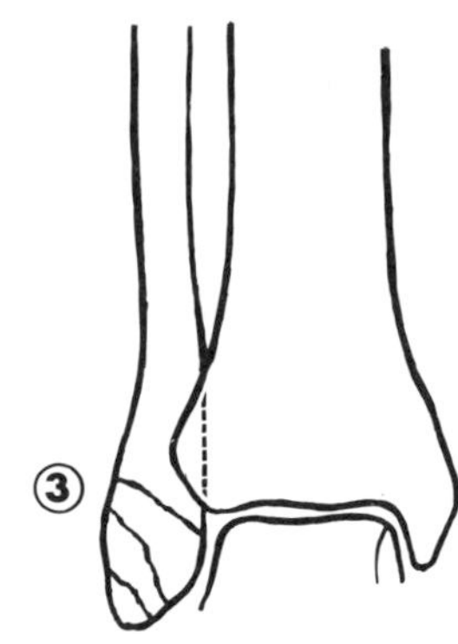

3. S-AD fracture is a characteristic transverse or oblique fibular fracture slightly distal to the mortise or occasionally an avulsion fracture of the tip of the fibula.

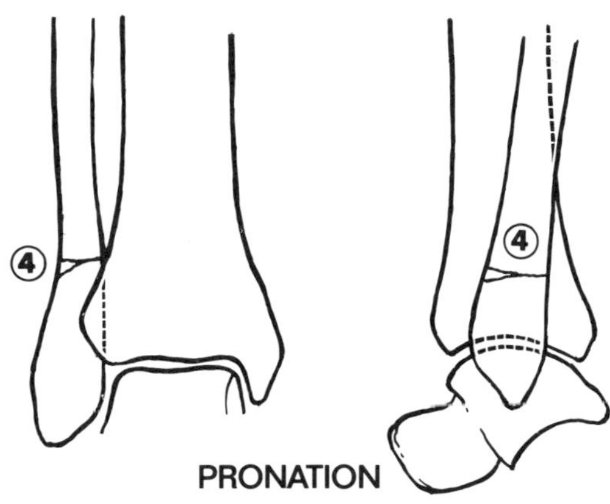

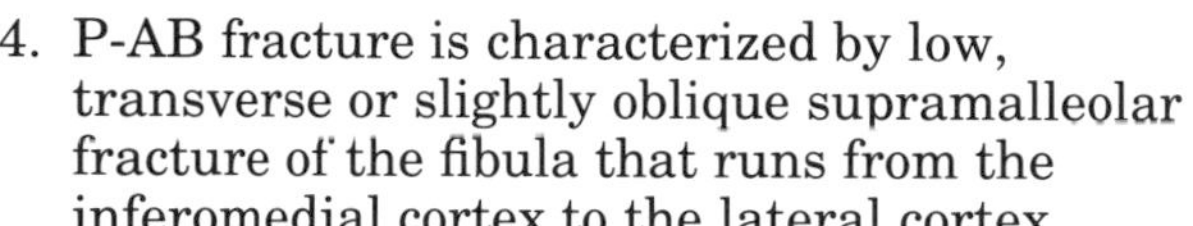

4. P-AB fracture is characterized by low, transverse or slightly oblique supramalleolar fracture of the fibula that runs from the inferomedial cortex to the lateral cortex.

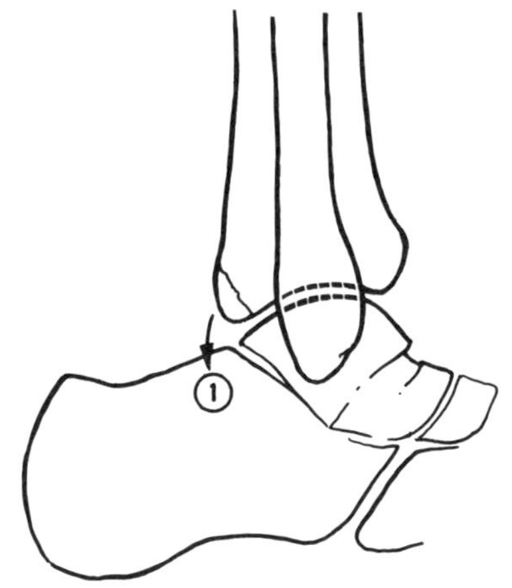

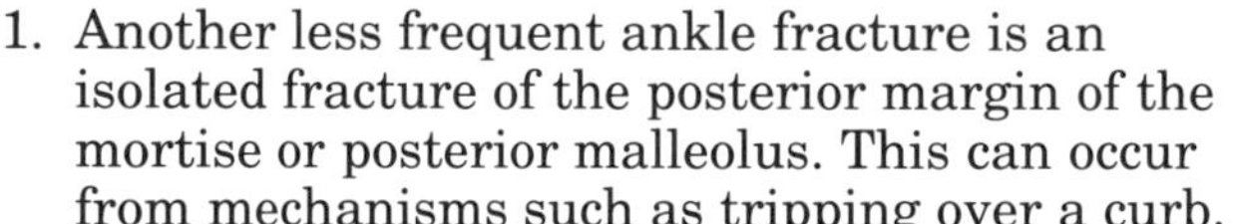

1. Another less frequent ankle fracture is an isolated fracture of the posterior margin of the mortise or posterior malleolus. This can occur from mechanisms such as tripping over a curb.

Other Types of Ankle Fractures

PRONATION-DORSIFLEXION INJURIES (PILON FRACTURE)

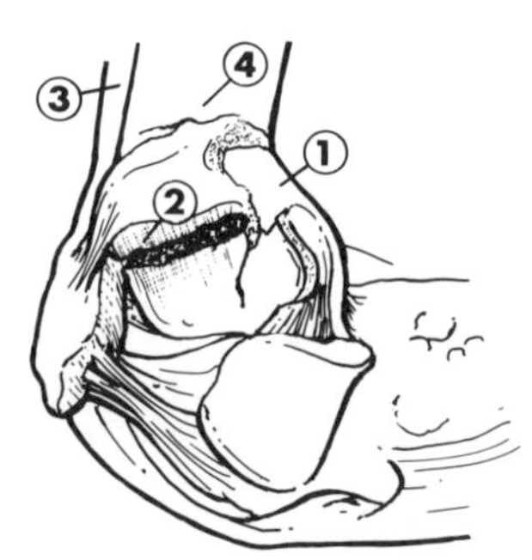

1. Forceful impact loading on the distal tibial articular surface with the talus in pronation produces a pronation-dorsiflexion fracture. This begins with a fracture of the medial malleolus at its base.
2. Anterior metaphyseal region of the tibia fractures at stage II.
3. Supramalleolar fibular fracture then occurs.
4. Transverse fracture of the dorsal tibia completes this unstable injury.

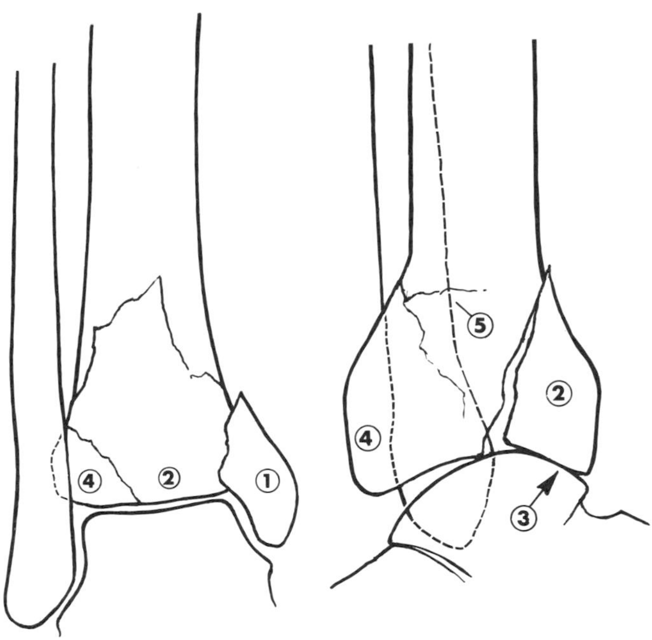

Appearance on X-Ray

1. Fracture of the medial malleolus.
2. Comminuted fracture of the anterior margin of the tibia.
3. Forward displacement of the talus with the marginal fracture.
4. Lateral tibial cortex remains attached to the fibula.
5. Fibula fractures or angulates posteriorly as the talus displaces anteriorly.

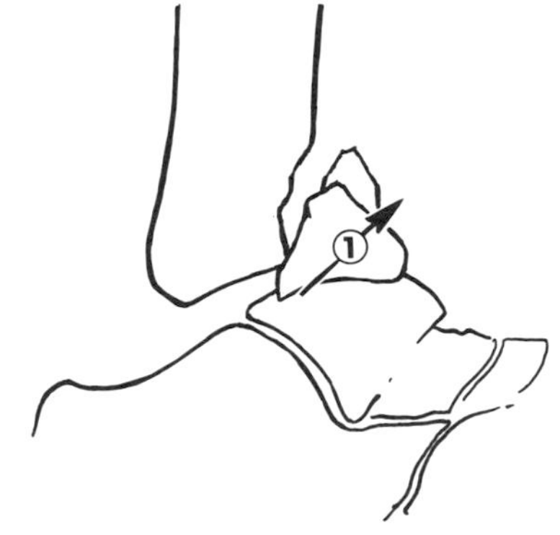

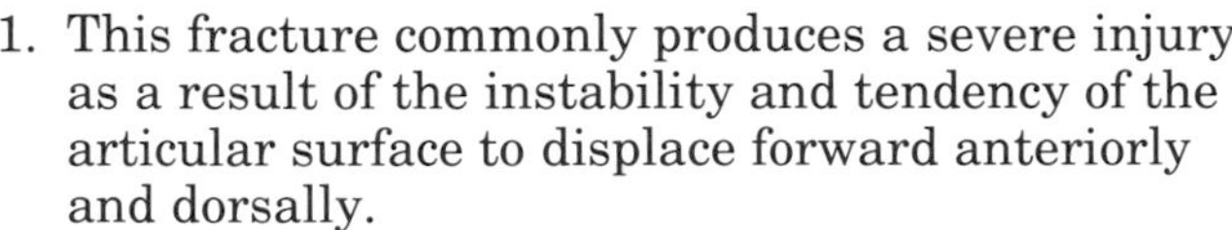

1. This fracture commonly produces a severe injury as a result of the instability and tendency of the articular surface to displace forward anteriorly and dorsally.

Note: The pronation-dorsiflexion fracture is also called a "pilon," the French term for the roof or ceiling of the ankle.

Impaction Fracture of the Lateral Weight-Bearing Surface of the Tibia (Coonrad Fracture)

Coonrad pointed out that unrecognized compression fractures of the lateral plafond occur sometimes in severe trimalleolar fractures with a dislocation.

A shearing injury in which the talus is impacted laterally against the tibial plafond compresses the subchondral bone and impacts or displaces the lateral articular portion superiorly.

Frequently, there is also a posterior malleolar fragment associated with this lateral fracture. Less frequently, an anterior margin fragment may be fractured.

The extent of this injury may be underestimated if the assessment of the posterior fragment is based strictly on a lateral x-ray. For this reason, oblique x-rays are also needed to assess the extent of involvement of the posterior and lateral articular surfaces.

These fractures are associated with a high frequency of unsatisfactory results caused by breakdown of the articular cartilage and early traumatic arthritis of the ankle.

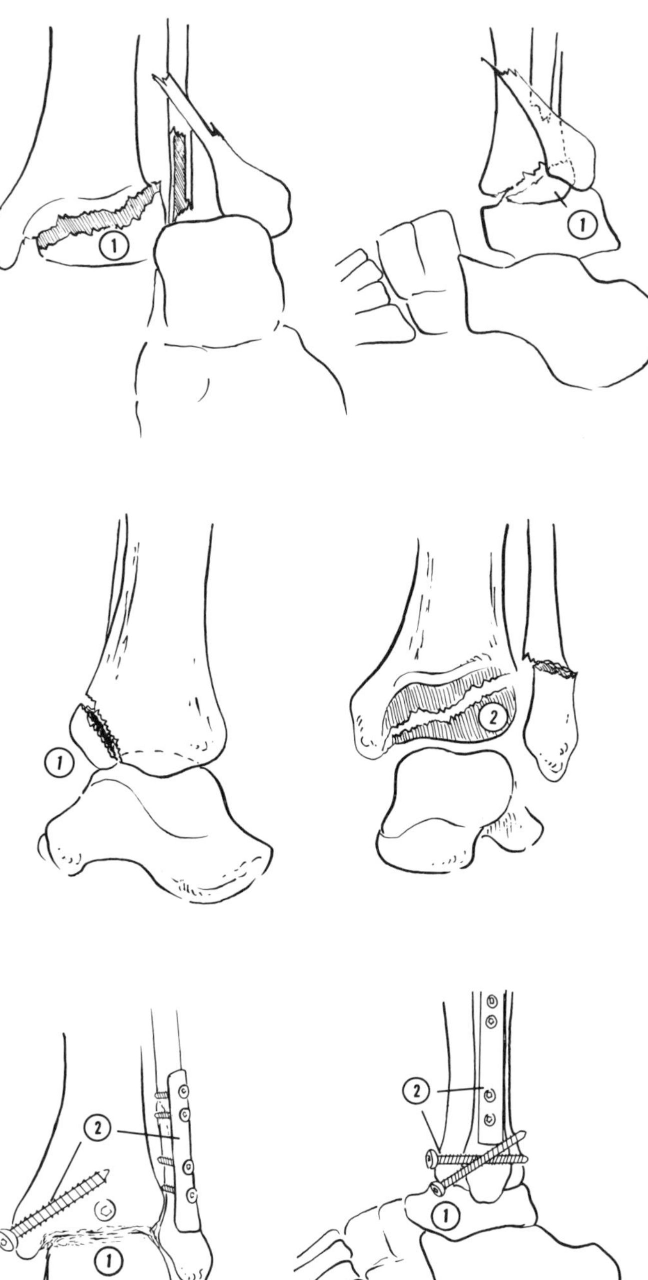

Other investigators have also shown a clear relationship between involvement of the posterior tibial margin and the incidence of post-traumatic osteoarthrosis. The long-term results after anatomic reduction and internal fixation, on the whole, are considerably better than the results after nonoperative treatment of these fractures.

1. Injury that shears off the articular surfaces is frequently a P-EX mechanism that causes direct impact against the posterolateral weight-bearing surface of the tibia. This shearing load on the joint cartilage often produces irreparable damage to the articular cartilage, as does a pilon fracture.

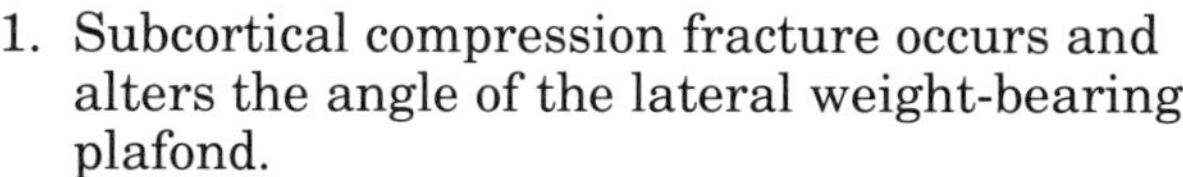

1. Subcortical compression fracture occurs and alters the angle of the lateral weight-bearing plafond.
2. Superficial assessment may focus on the fracture of the lateral malleolus rather than the more significant fracture of the weight-bearing surface of the tibia.

Post-Traumatic Arthritis From Fracture-Dislocations With Shearing Injury

1. Articular surface is frequently destroyed by these injuries, which results in rapid loss of joint space within the first year after treatment.
2. This is seen despite the fact that these fractures may be treated adequately by operative reduction and internal fixation.

Management of Ankle Fractures

Significance of the Lateral Talar Shift

REMARKS

The major concern in regard to the management of ankle fractures is the degree of instability of the talus.

Most frequently, the talus is displaced laterally or posterolaterally by the mechanism of the injury. Only with the S-AD mechanism is medial displacement of the talus likely.

Disruptions of the lateral bony support and of either the medial ligamentous or the medial bony support are necessary to cause the common problem of a lateral shift of the talus.

The degree of talar displacement is best measured on a mortise view taken with the foot internally rotated 15°.

Identifying the mechanism by the characteristics of the fibular fracture helps to separate the stable from the unstable injury.

Management of Ankle Fractures Based on Mechanisms and Stages

REMARKS

Comprehending the mechanisms that produce common ankle fractures is important for proper management. If the surgeon recognizes the mechanisms and stages, the extent of injury may be better appreciated, and the choice of closed or open management may be guided appropriately.

The key to classification of the type of ankle fractures is the pattern of the lateral malleolar fracture (see page 849). Reduction of the lateral malleolus is also key to the restoration of ankle stability. Displacement of the talus faithfully follows the displacement of the lateral malleolus.

Mortise View of the Ankle

1. X-ray is taken with the ankle internally rotated 15°.
2. Medial joint space should be approximately the same as the
3. Superior joint space.

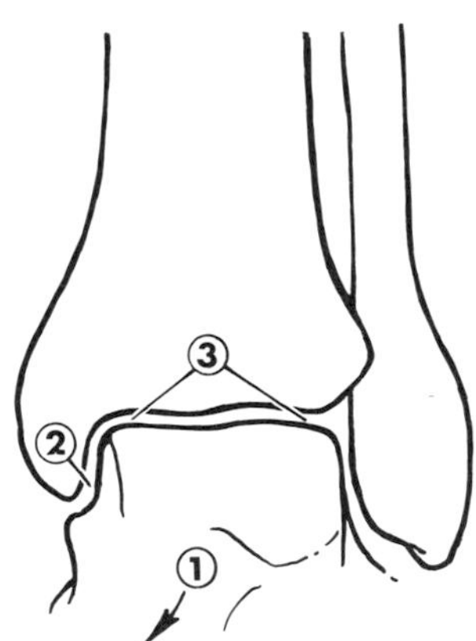

Changes in Tibiotalar Contact Caused by Lateral Shift

1. In the normal articulation, the tibiotalar contact extends across the breadth of the talus and is wide on the lateral side and narrow on the medial side.
2. Once the talus displaces laterally 1 mm, contact occurs only on the medial and lateral prominences of the talus. No contact occurs in the midportion.

Note: The key to the correction of lateral talar shift is to restore the bony support provided by the lateral malleolus.

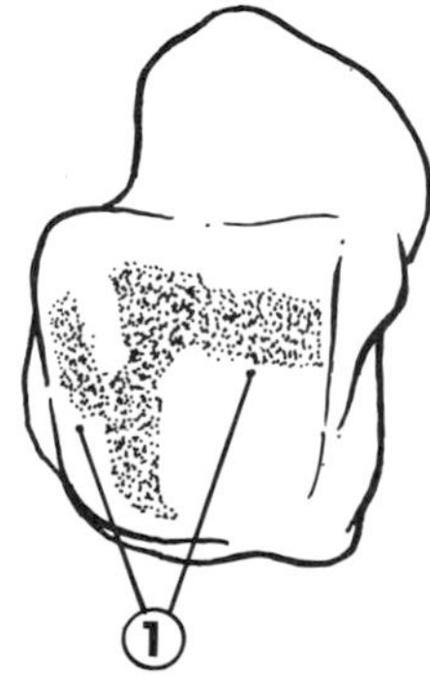

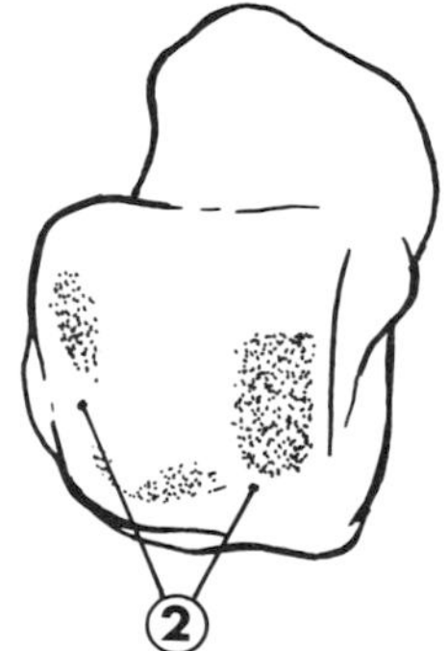

Fracture of the Lateral Malleolus Without Lateral Displacement

REMARKS

If the lateral malleolus is fractured or the anterior talofibular ligament is torn, the talus may not displace, provided that the medial portion of the mortise circle remains intact.

Many of these stage II rotational fractures may be overtreated by internal fixation.

The long-term outcome from this fracture stage is usually better than with severe ankle sprains. These fractures may be treated with minimal immobilization to relieve symptoms followed by early mobilization of the ankle.

Appearance on X-Ray

A. 1. Spiral fracture of the lateral malleolus (displacement is insignificant).
   2. Talus has not shifted.
   3. Tibiofibular joint is not widened.

B. 1. Avulsion of the lateral malleolus (transverse fracture).
   2. No shift of the talus.
   3. No tibiofibular diastasis.

Note: These x-rays may indicate either S-EX or S-AD mechanisms.

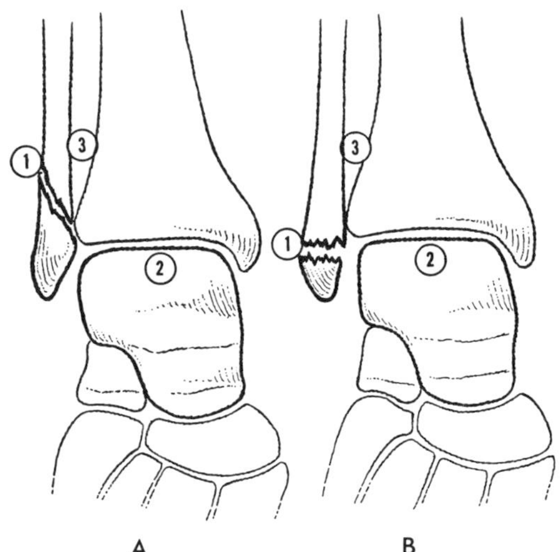

Staging of Undisplaced Lateral Malleolar Fractures

LAUGE-HANSEN (S-EX) STAGE II FRACTURE

The mechanism of S-EX injures the ankle as follows:

Stage I is a tear of the anterior tibiofibular ligament in its substance or from its bony attachment.

Stage II is a spiral oblique fracture of the fibula that is undisplaced and continues to support the talus.

Note: Always examine carefully for injuries to the posterior tibial margin or to the medial deltoid ligament associated with stage II of this mechanism and indicative of greater instability than is evident on initial x-ray (see page 856).

LAUGE-HANSEN (S-AD) STAGE I FRACTURE

S-AD mechanism injures the ankle as follows:

Stage I is an avulsion fracture of the lateral malleolus distal to the level of the tibiotalar joint. This may or may not be associated with a tear of the anterior talofibular ligament.

Note: These are both stable injuries because only the lateral support of the ankle is injured.

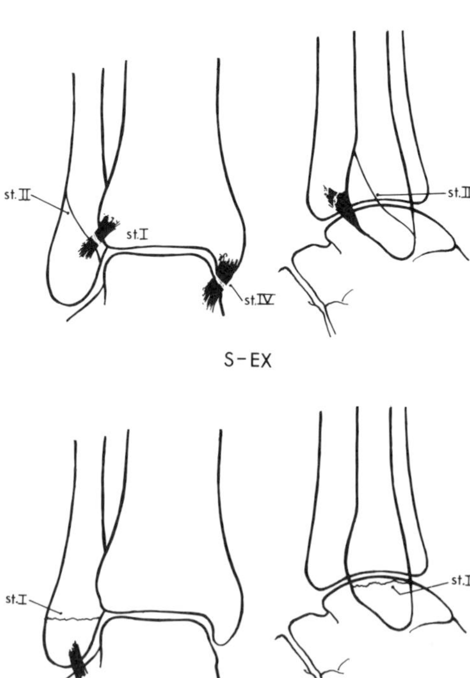

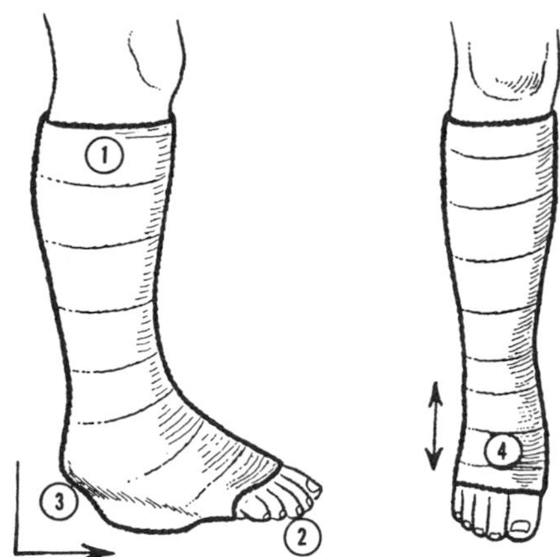

Management of Undisplaced Fractures

1. Apply a below-knee, well-fitting, nonpadded plaster walking cast.
2. Toes are free.
3. Foot is at a right angle to the leg.
4. Foot is in a neutral position.

Subsequent Management

Allow weight bearing as tolerated after the cast hardens.

The cast is primarily used to relieve the symptoms of the acute ankle injury. As soon as these symptoms subside, usually by 2–3 weeks, the cast may be removed.

The ankle may then be supported with an Aircast or similar device to allow range-of-motion exercises, as previously discussed for grade III ankle sprain.

Fracture of the Lateral Malleolus With Lateral Displacement

Prereduction X-Ray

ANTEROPOSTERIOR VIEW

1. Spiral fracture of the lateral malleolus.
2. Widening of the interval between the medial malleolus and the talus.
3. Lateral shift of the talus.

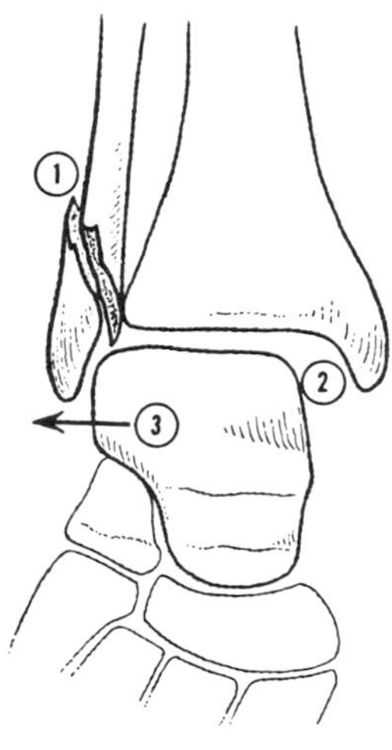

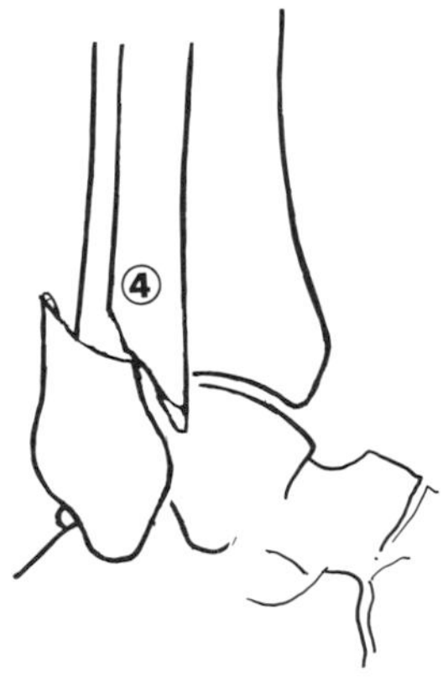

LATERAL VIEW

4. Fibular fracture may be locked in a shortened and externally rotated position, which prevents closed reduction.

Staging of Displaced Fractures: Lauge-Hansen (S-EX) Stage IV Fracture

The mechanism of S-EX injures the ankle as follows.

Stage I is disruption of the anterior talofibular ligament.

Stage II is the spiral oblique fracture of the lateral malleolus.

Stage III is an injury to the posterior tibiofibular ligament or fracture of the posterior articular margin.

Note: It is not necessary to have a fracture of the posterior margin before the injury advances to a stage IV.

Stage IV is a fracture of the medial malleolus or, in this instance, a disruption of the deltoid ligament.

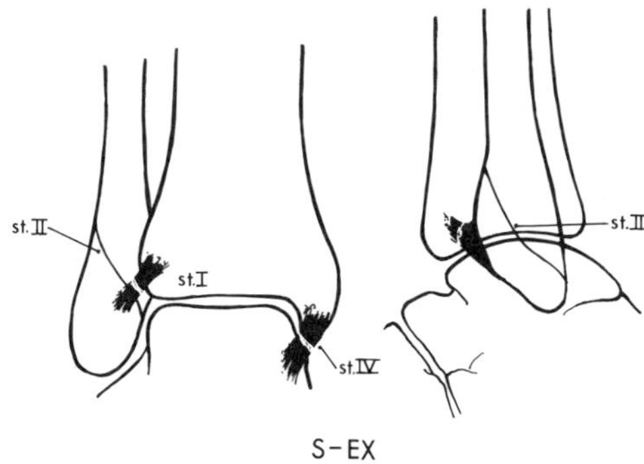

S-EX

Choice of Closed or Open Reduction

Most long-term studies of S-EX ankle fractures indicate that the results are equivalent whether closed or open reduction is used.

Closed reduction is particularly effective in the younger individual with good bony structure to permit stable reduction.

Fractures in older individuals with osteoporotic bone are more difficult to reduce and hold by closed technique. These are frequently best managed by open reduction and stabilization of the lateral and medial support structures.

A particularly difficult and troublesome fracture is the unstable injury in the adult patient with type I long-standing diabetes. In these injuries, internal fixation should be done carefully, and the fractured ankle should be protected until solid union is achieved. Otherwise, neurotrophic breakdown or Charcot joint changes may frequently develop.

Manipulative Reduction of Displaced Fractures

1. Limb hangs over the end of the table.
2. Place one hand over the medial aspect of the leg and the
3. Other hand over the lateral aspect of the foot and the lateral malleolus.
4. Push the foot strongly inward.

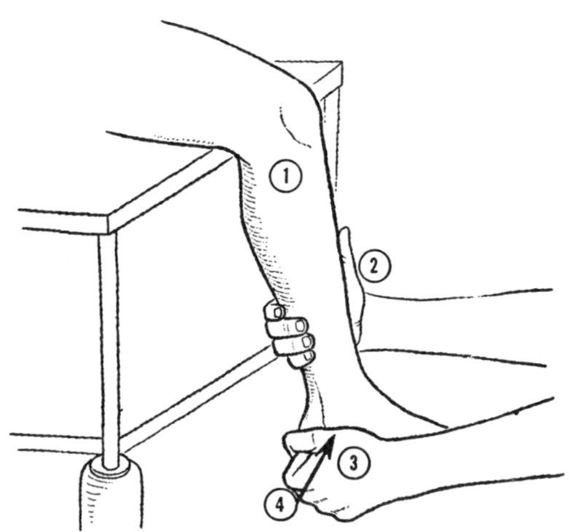

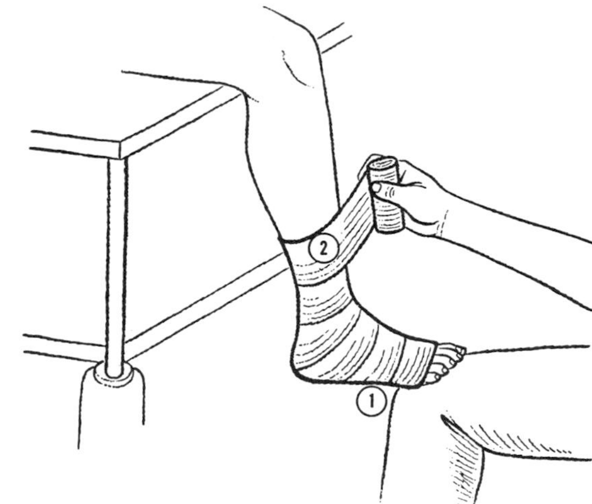

1. While the foot rests on the surgeon's knee,
2. A below-knee plaster cast is applied.

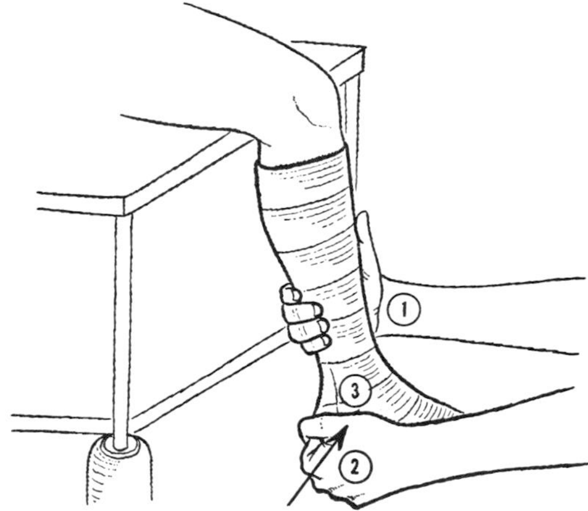

1. While the plaster is setting, the limb is steadied with one hand on the medial aspect of the leg, and the
2. Other hand applies steady, strong pressure inward over the lateral malleolus and foot.
3. Plaster is molded well over and around the malleoli.

Note: Inward pressure should be maintained until the plaster has set.

Evaluation of Reduction and Restoration of the Ankle Mortise: The Talocrural Angle

REMARKS

Sarkisian and Cody showed that the reduction of the ankle mortise can be best evaluated by carefully measuring the talocrural angle on the fractured side in comparison with the uninjured side. A difference greater than 2° indicates failure to restore the ankle mortise to normal and an increased likelihood of a poorly functioning joint.

This talocrural measurement is based on the fact that the fibular side of the joint is the key to reduction. Rotational and longitudinal alignment of the fibular fracture must be exact to maintain the integrity of the mortise.

The talocrural angle is formed by the intersection of two lines, i.e.,

1. One drawn parallel to the tibial articular surface and
2. One drawn between the tips of the two malleoli on the mortise view.
3. The ankle control measurement varies between 8° and 15°.

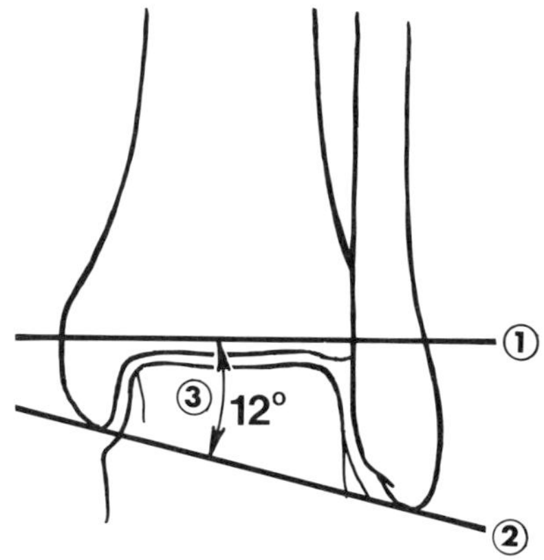

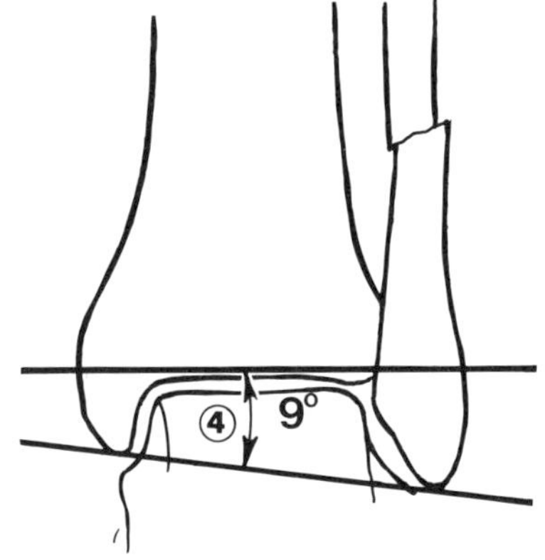

4. Variation of 2° or more between the fractured and the unfractured ankles indicates incomplete restoration of the ankle mortise as a result of shortening or malrotation of the fibula.

Alternative Method to Reduce Displaced Fractures: Quigley Traction

If there is severe swelling of the ankle, this method allows elevation of the limb and also reverses the S-EX mechanism by pronation and internal rotation of the foot and ankle.

1. Long-leg stockinette is rolled over the fracture and then prepared with benzoin.
2. Foot of the fractured ankle is suspended by balanced weights. The knee is supported by a sling to prevent hyperextension.
3. Pull of gravity inverts the position of the ankle to reduce the fracture while allowing swelling to subside.

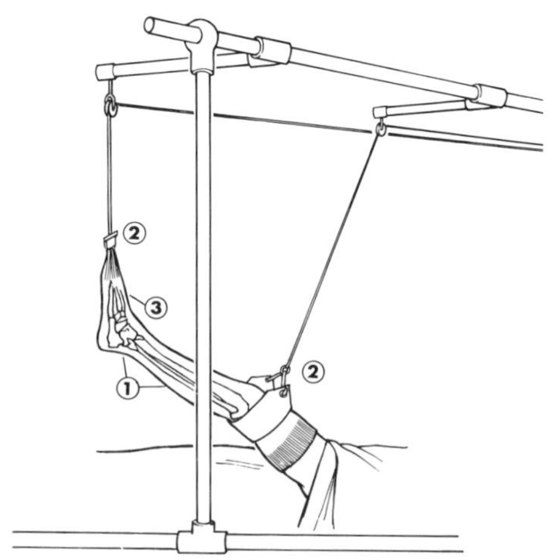

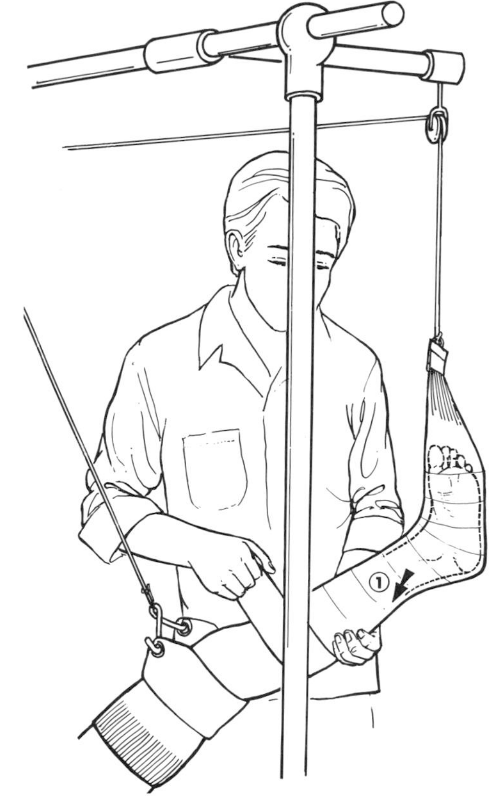

Immobilization

If reduction is satisfactory in Quigley traction,

1. Apply a long cast with the foot held in the inverted position.

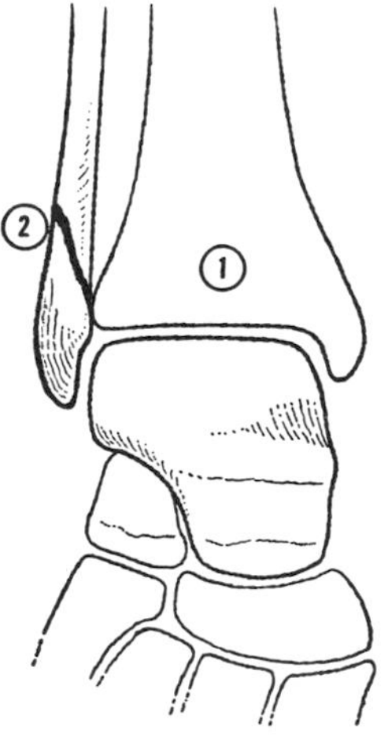

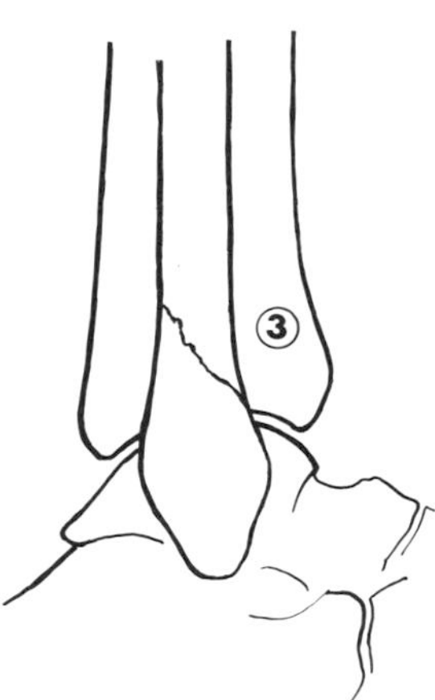

Postreduction X-Ray

1. The talus occupies its normal position in the mortise.
2. The lateral malleolus has been corrected.
3. Always check reduction on the lateral x-ray to ensure that the posterior displacement of the malleolus has been corrected.

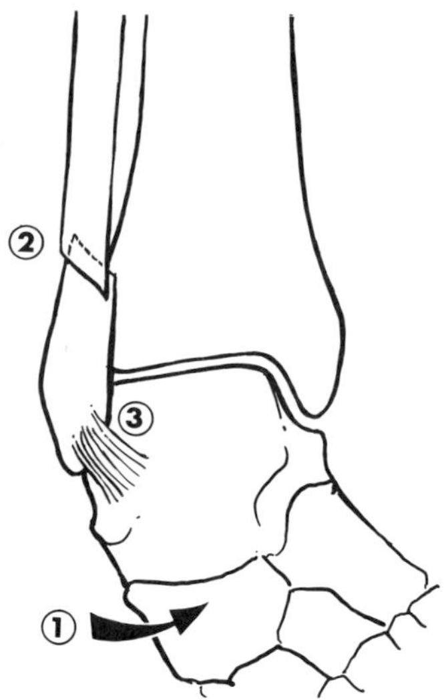

Caution: The key to reduction is to restore the fibula to its proper length and rotational alignment (see page 862).

1. Occasionally, repositioning of the talus can be achieved by the forceful internal rotation of the ankle but without
2. Complete reduction of the fibula.
3. This only stretches the lateral capsule and may lead to redisplacement of the talus.

Careful evaluation of the lateral view is necessary to show that the fibula has been restored to normal length after reduction. The external rotational malalignment should also be corrected.

Management After Closed Reduction

The patient may be allowed to walk on crutches without bearing weight on the fractured leg.

Reevaluate the reduction by x-ray within the first week. If reduction of the ankle mortise is lost at any time, open reduction should be carried out.

Avoid repeated manipulations, which are most likely to result in poor ankle function.

The cast is changed at 4 weeks, and the foot is taken out of the inverted position. Reevaluate by x-rays at this time to be sure that the reduction of the lateral malleolus is maintained.

The cast can be removed 8 weeks after fracture, and the patient can be started on active exercises and physical therapy to restore ankle motion.

Operative Treatment

REMARKS

Operative treatment is the most common method to manage unstable S-EX fractures, particularly as effective and reliable techniques have become availabie.

Operative treatment does not necessarily provide better long-term results than does accurate closed treatment. However, operative treatment does minimize the need for repeated manipulation and cast changes for the unstable injury.

Open reduction and internal fixation are particularly useful in the elderly patient with osteoporotic bone.

Open reduction and accurate internal fixation are also most effective in the patient with multiple injuries.

An additional indication in which operative fixation is generally superior to closed nonoperative treatment is in the ankle fracture in a type I diabetic patient. In this unusual and difficult situation, the risk of neurotrophic (Charcot) joint changes is high, and this risk warrants careful internal stabilization and prolonged non–weight-bearing therapy until the fracture heals.

The outcome after an ankle fracture is determined as much by the degree of initial injury to the soft tissues and particularly to the articular surface as it is to the management (see Coonrad fracture).

The more severely displaced the fracture or the more difficult the underlying problems, including multiple trauma problems and diabetic problems, the more likely it is that the outcome can be improved with careful open reduction and internal fixation.

1. Elderly patient with osteoporotic bone is particularly a candidate for prompt open reduction and internal fixation.
2. Failure of the soft bone prevents adequate reduction of the lateral and medial support structures of the ankle and tends to leave the elderly patient with a less than satisfactory ankle after closed treatment.
3. Patients with multiple fractures are also best managed by early operative stabilization of the ankle fracture and other injuries.

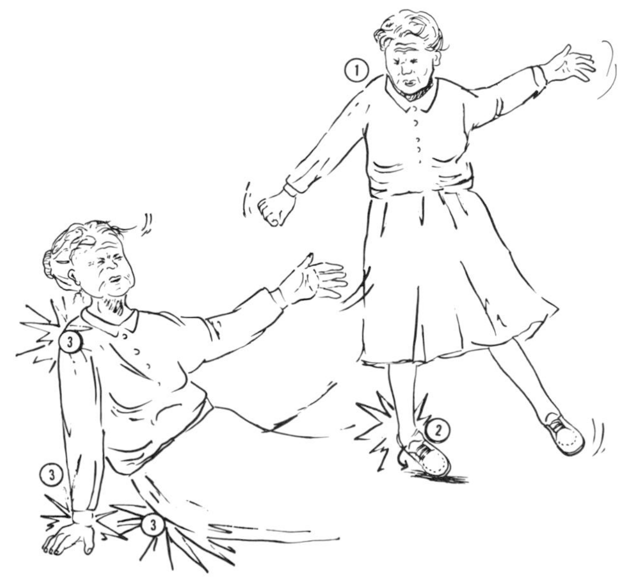

Charcot Joint Changes After Fractures in Diabetic Patients

1. Fracture of the ankle in a diabetic patient can proceed to a serious breakdown of the joint due to neurotrophic (Charcot) joint changes.
2. Rapid destruction of the articular surface and deformity of the joint follows either closed or open treatment of these ankles. However, open treatment is preferred to stabilize these ankles, which can become rapidly unstable, even if they are initially undisplaced.

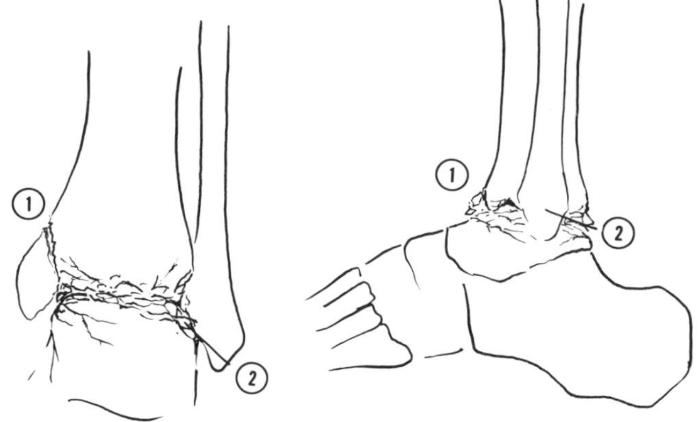

1. Operative fixation of the unstable fracture should be directed primarily to restoration of the length and rotational alignment of the fibula. This is best accomplished with small plate fixation.
2. Syndesmosis or tibiofibular ligaments can usually be repaired directly.
3. Ankle mortise is restored to normal alignment, primarily by stabilization of the lateral structures.
4. Medial malleolar fracture or deltoid ligament or capsular tear should also be repaired and stabilized.
5. Unstable fractures of the posterior malleolus are also reduced and fixed internally.

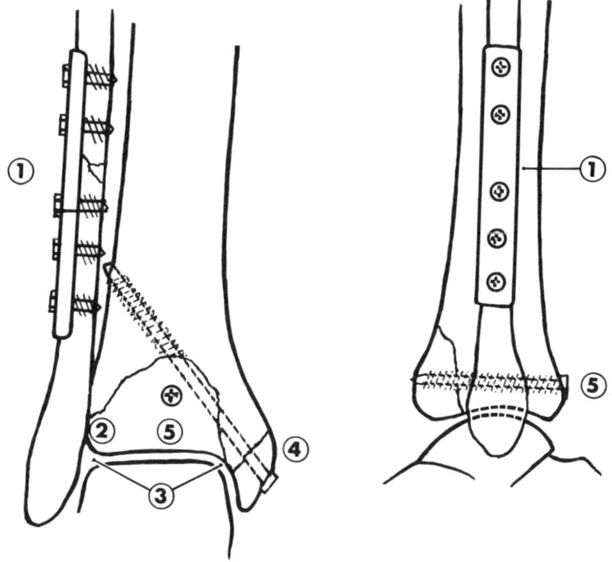

Isolated Fractures of the Medial Malleolus

REMARKS

Isolated fractures of the medial malleolus are characteristically stage I lesions from a P-AB or P-EX mechanism.

The mechanism may advance to stage II and rupture the anterior tibiofibular ligament, but this would not be evident on x-ray.

Because of the intact fibular support, the talus does not displace.

Closed reduction is frequently successful if a reasonable approximation of the malleolar fragments is achieved.

The malleolar fracture heals slowly without periosteal callus; frequently, clinical stability precedes radiographic evidence of union by several months with closed treatment.

Operative fixation may be indicated for widely displaced fragments that are not reduced by closed manipulation.

Appearance on X-Ray

1. Transverse fracture of the medial malleolus.
2. Oblique fracture of the medial malleolus.
3. Talus is in its normal position.
4. There is wide separation of malleolar fragments.

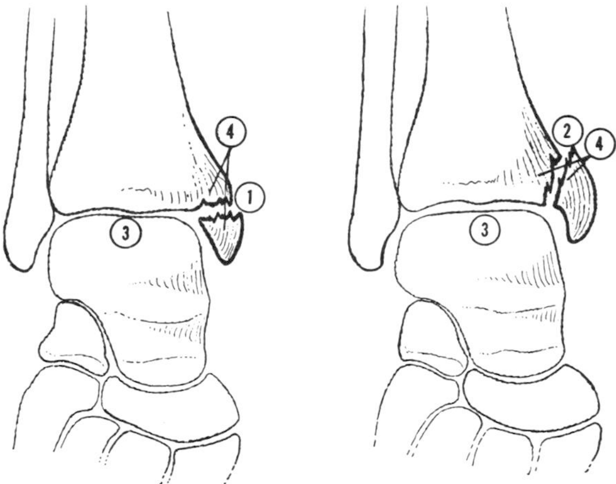

Staging of Medial Malleola Fracture: Lauge-Hansen P-AB or P-EX Fracture, Stage I or II

P-AB and P-EX mechanisms injure the ankle in the following stages.

Stage I avulses the medial malleolus or sometimes the deltoid ligament.

Stage II causes rupture of the distal tibiofibular syndesmosis, which may not be evident on x-ray.

Note: This injury involving only the medial support of the ankle is stable and can usually be treated by a closed method if adequate reduction of the malleolus is achieved.

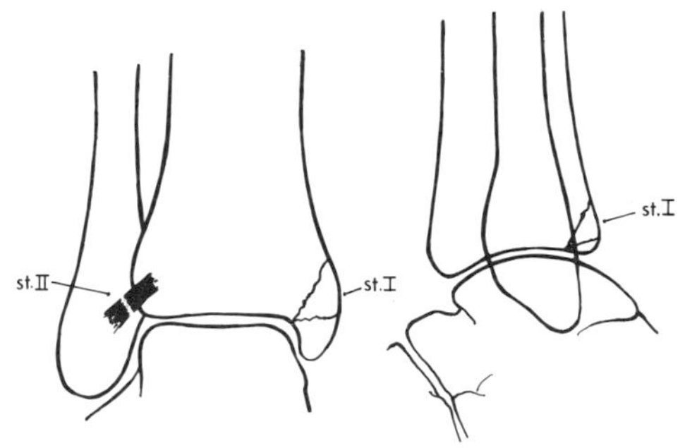

P-AB & P-EX

Technique of Closed Reduction of Medial Malleolar Fracture

1. Limb hangs over the end of the table.
2. With both thumbs, the surgeon manipulates the fragments into normal position.
3. Then, with the heels of the hands, the surgeon compresses both malleoli firmly.

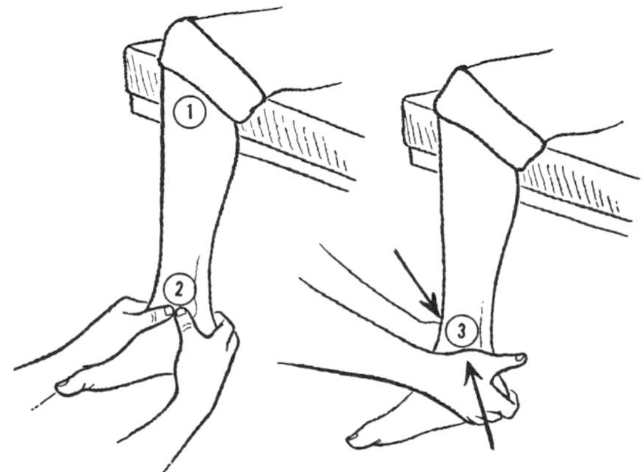

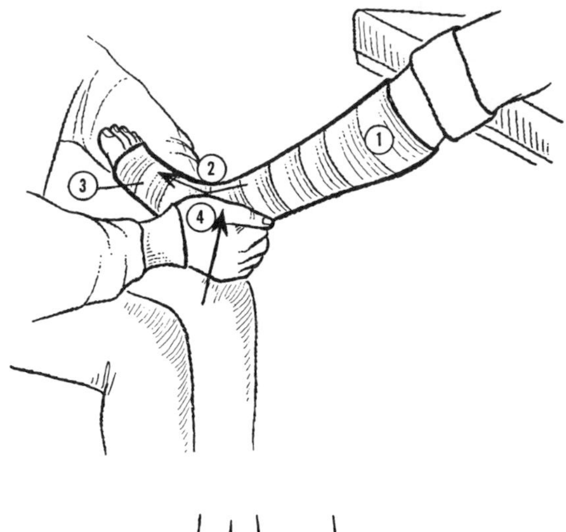

While the foot rests on the surgeon's knee, a

1. Short-leg plaster cast is applied.
2. Foot is at a right angle to the leg.
3. Foot is in a neutral position in regard to inversion and eversion.
4. While the plaster is setting, firm pressure is applied over the medial malleolus, pushing it inward.

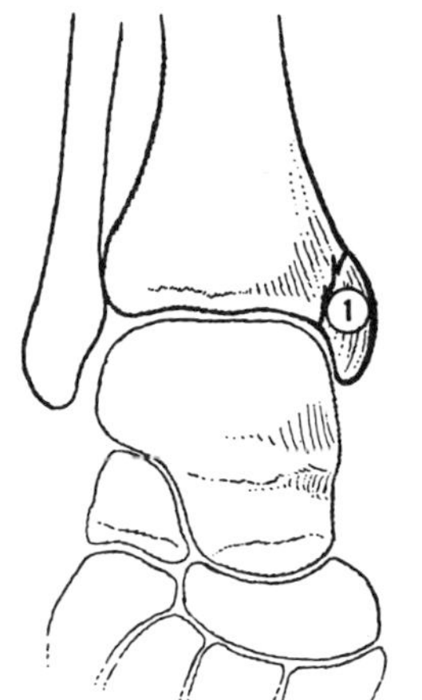

Postreduction X-Ray

1. The malleolus is restored to its normal position.

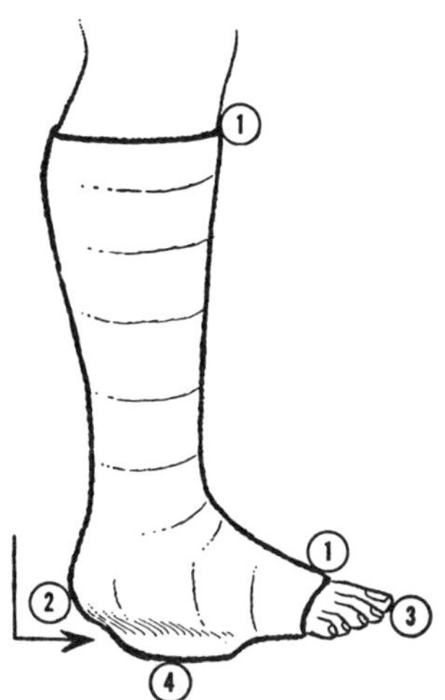

Immobilization

1. Plaster cast extends from below the knee to behind the metatarsal heads.
2. Foot is at a right angle to the leg.
3. Foot is in a neutral position.
4. Heel for walking is incorporated in the cast.

Management

Allow partial weight bearing with crutches.

Insist on active exercises for the toes.

Remove the cast at the end of 6–8 weeks.

Institute active exercises to restore ankle and foot movements.

Surgical Treatment

REMARKS

Failure to restore the malleolar fragment to its anatomic position justifies surgical intervention.

In some instances, a periosteal flap that lies between the fragments precludes manipulative reduction; it must be removed under direct vision.

Always check for avulsion fractures of the posterior tibial surface. This may occur in stage II of a P-EX injury and requires fixation if more than 25 per cent of the joint surface is involved (see page 848).

In most instances, single-screw fixation of the medial malleolar fracture is adequate to reduce and hold these fairly stable injuries.

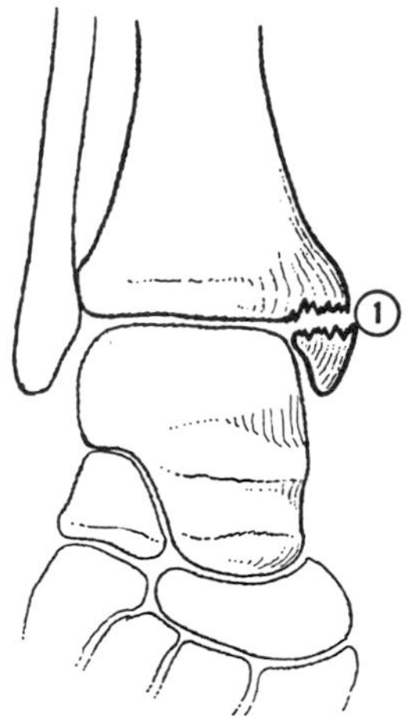

Preoperative X-Ray

1. Wide separation of malleolar fragments (manipulative measures failed in this case).

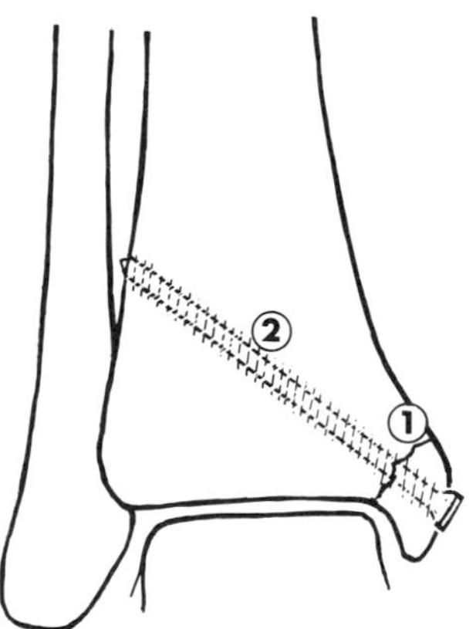

Postoperative X-Ray

1. Malleolar fragment is in perfect anatomic position.
2. There is a transfixion screw across the fracture in the medial malleolus.

Subsequent Management

After a short-leg cast is applied, the patient is allowed out of bed to walk with two crutches.

Subsequently, the cast may be removed, on average, within 5 weeks.

After removal of the plaster cast, the patient generally regains normal range of motion in the ankle promptly.

Removal of the screws is usually unnecessary unless they are causing pain or discomfort.

Fracture of the Medial Malleolus With Rupture of the Lateral Ligament

REMARKS

Fracture of the medial malleolus with rupture of the lateral ligament is the result of an S-AD mechanism. It is the only mechanism that will displace the talus medially, and it can result in an unstable mortise.

Because both the medial and the lateral support structures are lost, operative fixation is desirable to restore mortise stability.

Appearance on X-Ray

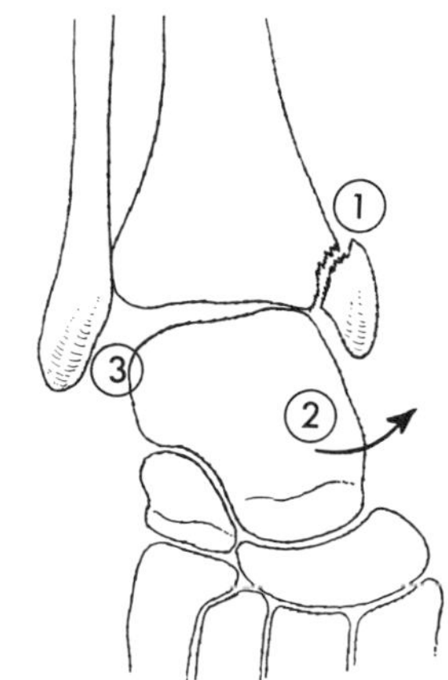

1. There is an oblique fracture of the medial malleolus.
2. Talus is tilted and displaced medially.
3. Joint space is widened laterally and is consistent with a tear of the talofibular ligament.

Note: A fracture of the lateral malleolus may also occur.

Staging of Injury: Lauge-Hansen S-AD Fracture Stage II

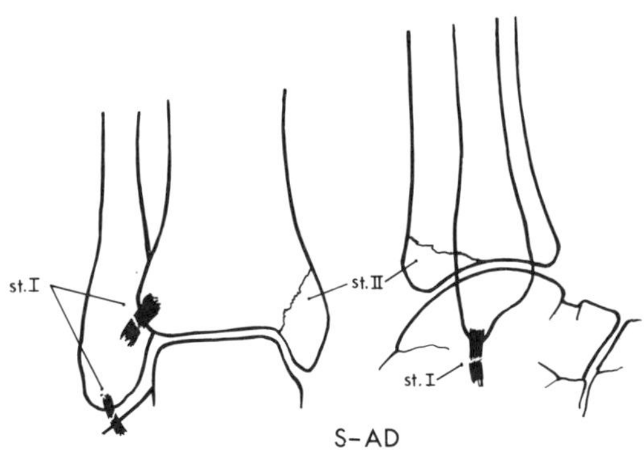

An S-AD injury to the ankle produces the following stages of injury.

Stage I injures the anterior talofibular and calcaneofibular ligaments.

Stage II fractures the medial malleolus, most characteristically with an oblique fracture line. Frequently, the fracture also involves the posteromedial tibial surface.

Closed Reduction Technique

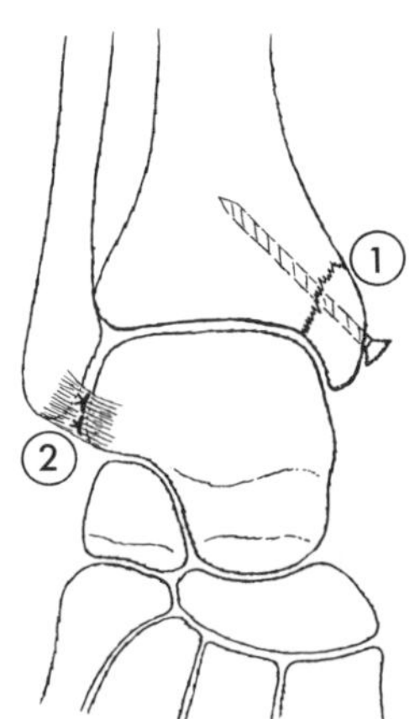

The techniques of reduction and immobilization for this injury are the same as those described for isolated fractures of the medial malleolus. Operative treatment is preferable for the unstable injury.

Operative Management

1. Medial malleolus is fixed with a screw.
2. Lateral ligament is repaired.

Bimalleolar Fractures

REMARKS

Fractures of both malleoli result most commonly from S-EX mechanisms.

P-AB mechanisms also produce fractures of both malleoli at or below the level of the syndesmosis.

Both S-EX and P-AB mechanisms cause lateral displacement of the talus.

S-AD mechanisms also cause bimalleolar fractures but tend to produce medial displacement.

Closed reduction is possible with bimalleolar fractures produced by P-AB or S-AD mechanisms without torsional deformity.

S-EX fractures are frequently associated with rotational shortening and impingement of the lateral malleolus on the proximal fibula that prevents the talus from resuming its normal anatomic position. Consequently, open reduction of the lateral malleolus is indicated to restore fibular alignment and return the talus to its normal articulation.

The fibular fracture can be stabilized by screws, plates, intramedullary pins, or tension-band wiring.

The medial malleolar fracture should also be stabilized to permit early functional ankle exercises.

In all bimalleolar fractures, the posterior articular surface of the tibia should be evaluated by x-ray to determine whether it is fractured or injured enough to cause ankle instability.

Fractures of Both Malleoli With Lateral Displacement of the Talus

Prereduction X-Ray

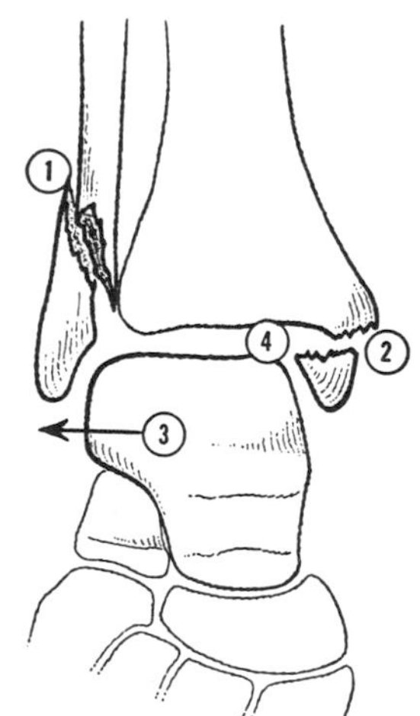

S-EX MECHANISM STAGE IV

1. Oblique spiral fracture of the lateral malleolus runs from the anterior margin in a dorsal proximal direction.
2. Fractures of the medial malleolus and the
3. Talus are displaced laterally.
4. Anteromedial clear space of the joint is widened.

S-EX mechanisms produce injury to the ankle in the following stages.

Stage I is avulsion of the anterior tibiofibular ligament.

Stage II is an oblique spiral fracture of the lateral malleolus that runs from the anterior edge to the posterosuperior cortex.

Stage III is a fracture of the posterior tibial margin.

Note: It is not necessary for this fracture to occur before the injury advances to a stage IV fracture.

Stage IV is a fracture of the medial malleolus.

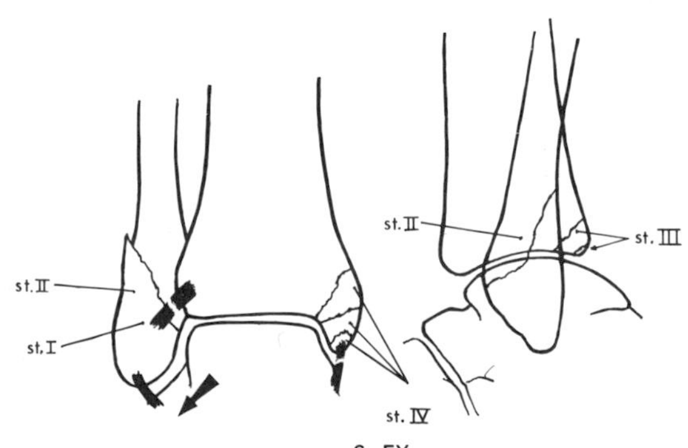

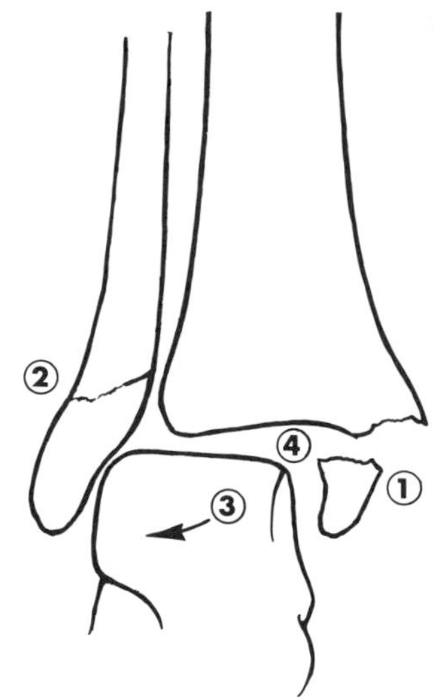

P-AB MECHANISM

1. Fracture of the medial malleolus.
2. Low-transverse supramalleolar fracture of the fibula.
3. Talus is shifted laterally.
4. Anteromedial clear space is widened.

Staging of Injury

P-AB mechanism produces injury to the ankle in the following stages.

Stage I is a fracture of the medial malleolus or a rupture of the deltoid ligament.

Stage II is a rupture of the distal tibiofibular syndesmosis.

Stage III includes the fracture in the supramalleolar region of the fibula. The fracture is characteristically transverse or slightly oblique and extends in an inferomedial direction.

Note: P-AB mechanisms may rupture the posterior tibiofibular ligament but rarely produce significant fractures of the articular surface.

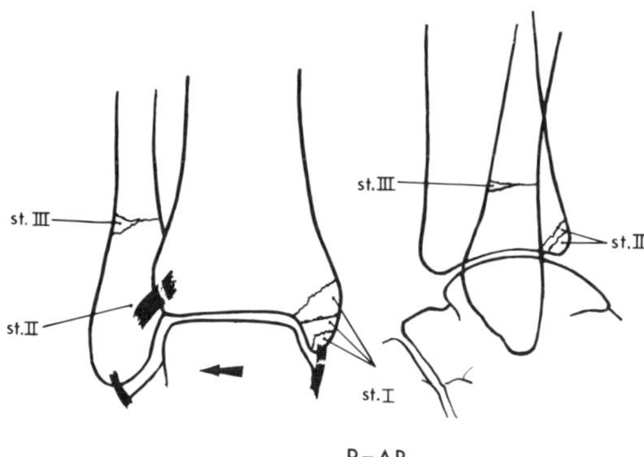

P–AB

Fracture of Both Malleoli With Medial Displacement of the Talus: Supination-Adduction (S-AD) Fracture

REMARKS

The S-AD mechanism is the only type of ankle fracture that produces medial displacement of the talus.

This mechanism may occur in children and cause a type IV epiphyseal fracture.

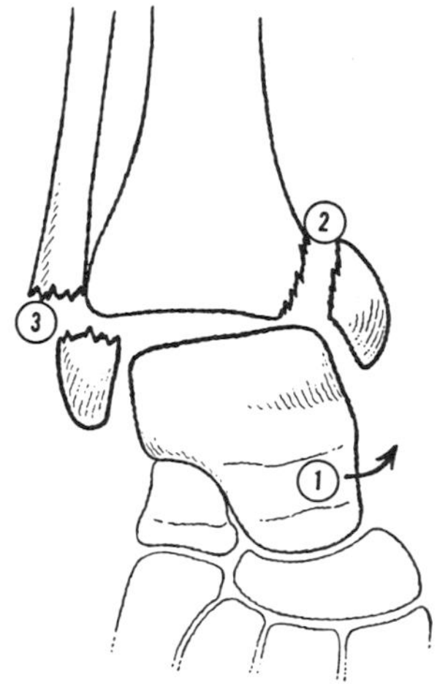

Prereduction X-Rays

1. Talus is displaced medially as a result of the mechanism.
2. Medial malleolus has a characteristic shearing fracture.
3. Lateral malleolus is avulsed.

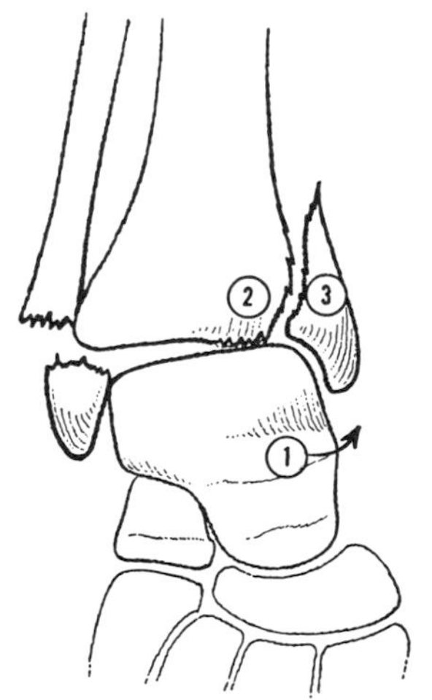

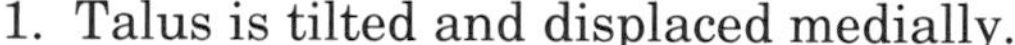

1. Talus is tilted and displaced medially.
2. Fracture line is comminuted and extends around posteriorly.
3. Medial malleolar fragment includes part of the posteromedial articular surface.

S-AD Fracture in a 12-Year-Old Boy

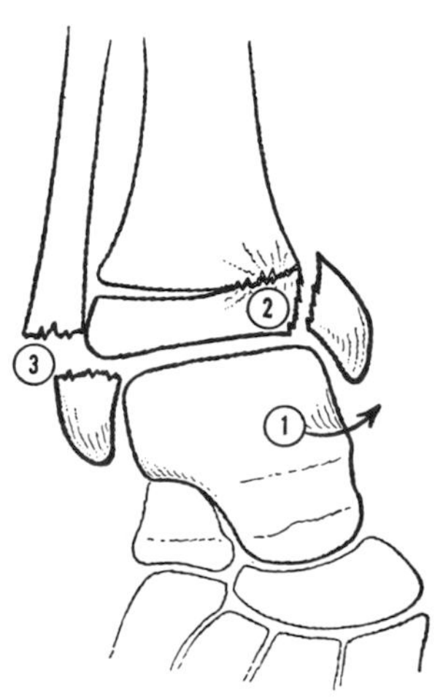

This lesion may cause premature arrest of growth on the medial side of the tibial epiphysis (see Chapter 2).

1. Talus is displaced medially.
2. Medial side of the epiphyseal plate is crushed.
3. Lateral malleolus is avulsed.

The resultant asymmetric growth arrest and varus ankle deformity have been discussed in Chapter 2. Because the tendency is medial displacement, the key determinant of the reduction is the medial malleolus. If this is not satisfactorily returned to its normal position, operative fixation is indicated. This is especially important for the epiphyseal fractures.

Staging of S-AD Fracture

Stage I includes a fracture of the lateral malleolus at or distal to the level of the tibiotalar joint.

Stage II includes a fracture of the medial malleolus. This may extend posteriorly to involve the articular surface.

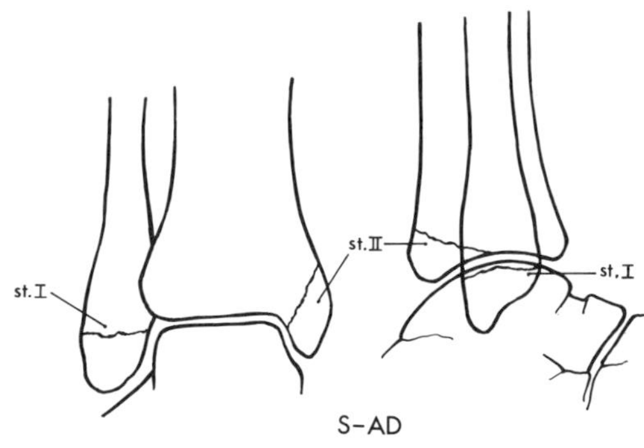

Operative Treatment

Both malleoli should be fixed internally to permit early postoperative range-of-motion exercises.

For a laterally displaced talus, the stability of the fibula is key. For a fracture with medial talar shift, the medial malleolus is a primary concern.

Postreduction X-Ray

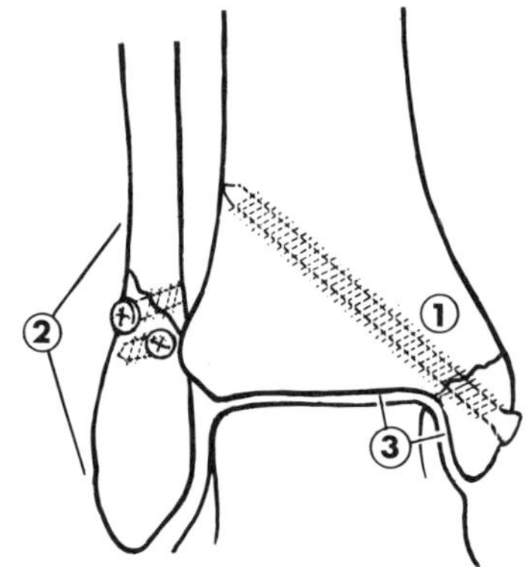

1. Medial malleolus is in its normal position and transfixed with a screw.
2. Lateral malleolus has been restored to its length and anatomic alignment and is held with two screws or a plate.
3. Talus occupies its normal position in the mortise.

Note: Reduction should be accurately evaluated by a comparison of the talocrural angles in the fractured and unfractured ankle.

Any avulsion or injury to the tibiofibular ligaments should also be repaired.

Options for fixation of the lateral malleolar fracture range from screws, as illustrated here, to tension-band wires, plates, and intramedullary pins.

Postoperative Immobilization

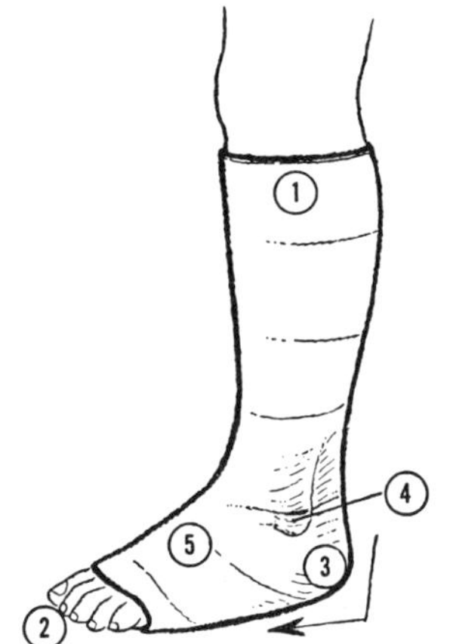

1. Short-leg cast is applied.
2. Toes are free.
3. Ankle is at a right angle.
4. Malleoli are well molded.
5. Ankle is in a neutral position in regard to inversion or eversion.

Subsequent Management

The period of cast immobilization depends on the degree of initial injury and the rigidity of fixation achieved by the surgery.

In most instances, the patient is able to discard the plaster by 6–8 weeks but should continue on crutches for 6 weeks longer.

Most ankle fractures have healed satisfactorily by the end of 12 weeks, and the patient should be regaining full motion.

The internal fixation need not be removed unless it is causing symptoms.

Fracture of the Fibula Proximal to the Tibiofibular Syndesmosis

REMARKS

These injuries, according to the Lauge-Hansen classification, are most often produced by P-EX mechanisms. However, Pankovich showed that, depending on the position of the foot at the time of injury, an S-EX or P-AB mechanism may also fracture the fibula above the syndesmosis.

The specific mechanism may be identified by the characteristics of the fibular fracture.

Identification of the mechanism is helpful in the selection of treatment because the fibular fracture produced by supination may not have associated medial injuries and can be treated closed. Fibular fracture that results from pronation mechanisms always has associated disruption of the medial support structure and generally requires internal stabilization.

When the fibula is fractured above the syndesmosis, the tibiofibular ligaments and the intraosseous membrane are usually disrupted. The key to reduction, however, is to stabilize the fibular fracture because the distal talofibular ligament remains intact and the talus faithfully follows the fibula.

The syndesmosis can be repaired by direct suture. Fibulotibial screw fixation should generally be avoided because it restricts the rotation in the syndesmosis necessary to allow dorsiflexion (see page 817).

S-EX Fracture Stage II

1. Slight widening of the syndesmosis.
2. Characteristically, the fibular fracture line spirals from the anterior edge of the cortex in a posterosuperior direction.
3. Medial joint space is normal.

Note: This injury involves the lateral ankle support structure and is usually stable. It often may be treated closed. The surgeon must carefully evaluate for clinical signs of medial ligament pain, progressive increase in the medial clear space, or shortening of the fibula, any of which is indicative of a more advanced stage that requires operative fixation.

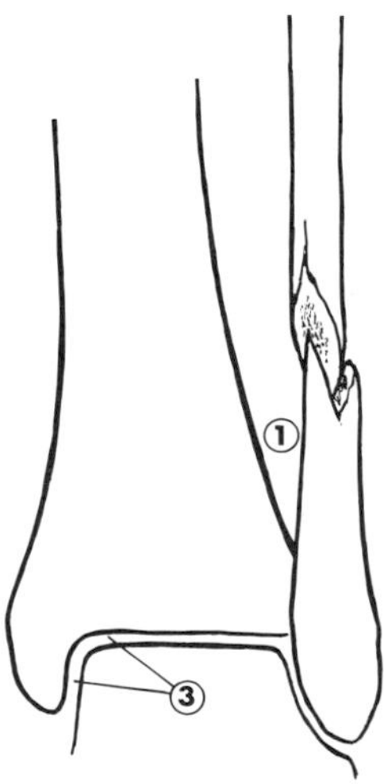

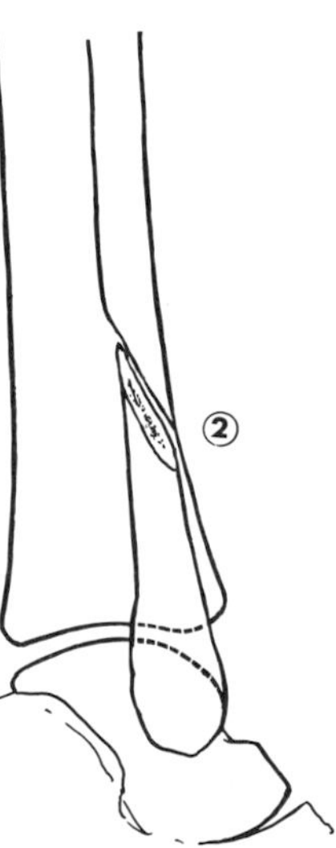

Stages of S-EX Fracture of the Fibula Proximal to the Syndesmosis (After Pankovich)

Because the deltoid ligament is relaxed in supination, a fracture of the fibula occurs before medial disruption.

Stage I is a rupture or avulsion of the anterior tibiofibular ligament associated with rupture of the intraosseous ligament.

Stage II is a fracture of the fibula above the syndesmosis. This is characterized by a typical spiral fracture extending from the anterior edge in a posterosuperior direction.

Stage III is a rupture of the posterior tibiofibular ligament or a fracture of the posterior tubercle of the tibia.

Stage IV is a rupture of the deltoid ligament or a fracture of the medial malleolus.

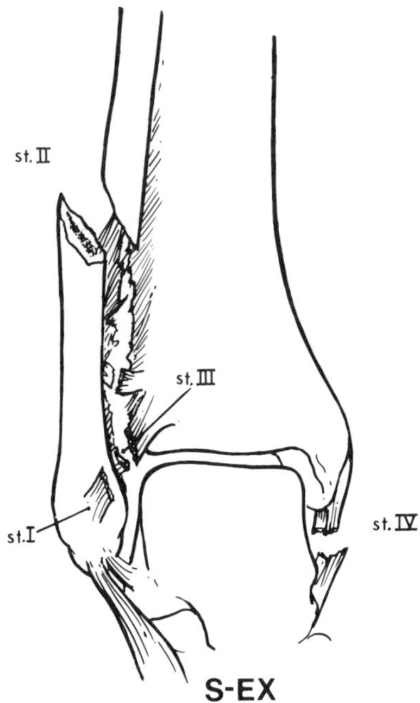

Stages of P-AB Fracture of the Fibula Proximal to the Syndesmosis

With the foot in pronation, the deltoid ligament ruptures first followed by complete diastasis of the syndesmosis and then a fracture of the fibula.

Stage I is a rupture of the deltoid ligament or a fracture of the medial malleolus.

Stage II is a rupture of all ligaments of the syndesmosis or avulsion fractures of their bony insertions.

Stage III is a fracture of the fibula proximal to the syndesmosis.

The fracture is characterized as a transverse or slightly oblique line that runs from the lateral surface in an inferomedial direction.

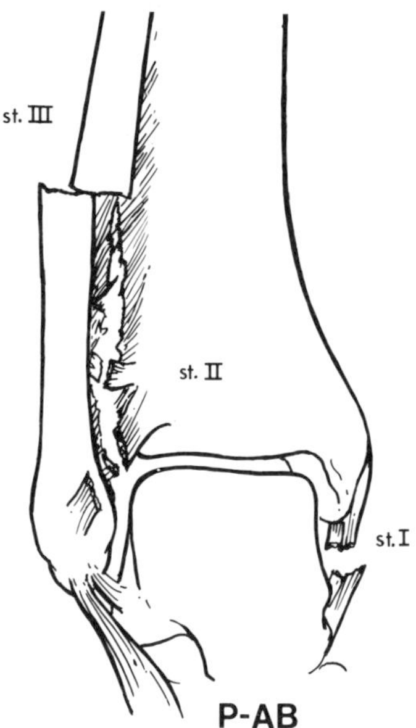

Stages of P-EX Mechanisms That Produce Fractures of the Fibula Proximal to the Syndesmosis

This mechanism applies strong tension to the deltoid ligament or medial malleolus and then continues to disrupt the tibiofibular and intraosseous ligaments, frequently fracturing the posterior tibial attachment of the ligament, and finally fracturing the fibula.

Stage I is a fracture of the medial malleolus or a rupture of the deltoid ligament.

Stage II is a rupture of the anterior tibiofibular ligament or its bony insertion that is associated with rupture of the intraosseous ligament.

Stage III is a fracture of the fibula above the syndesmosis. This is characterized by a fracture line that runs from the anterior edge in a posteroinferior direction.

Stage IV is a fracture of the posterior tubercle of the tibia or a rupture of the posterior tibiofibular ligament. This injury frequently involves a large portion of the posterior articular surface.

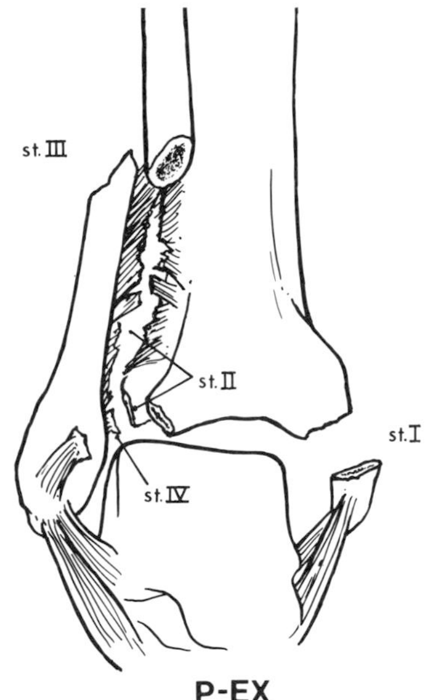

P-EX

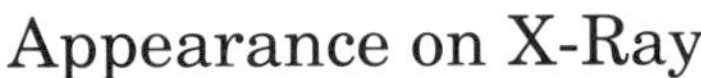

Appearance on X-Ray

P-EX FRACTURE STAGE IV

1. Wide separation of the talus from the medial malleolus indicates disruption of the deltoid.
2. Gross posterolateral displacement of the fibula indicates disruption of the tibiofibular ligament and intraosseous ligament.
3. Fibular fracture line runs from the anterior cortex in a posteroinferior direction, characteristic of the P-EX mechanism.
4. Talus displaces posterolaterally with the fibula.

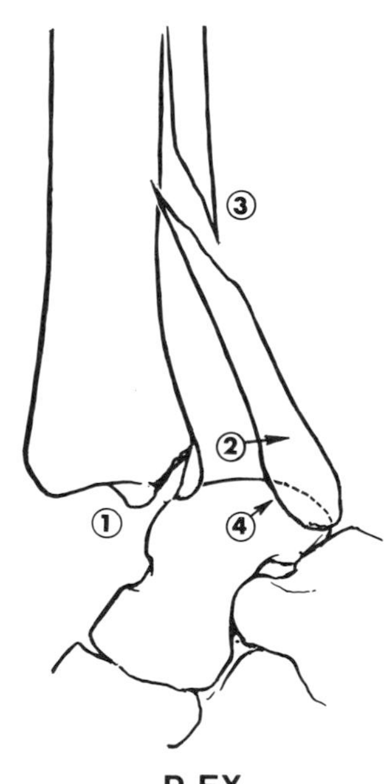

P-EX

P-AB FRACTURE STAGE III

1. Widening of the medial joint space indicates deltoid ligament rupture.
2. Diastasis of the syndesmosis.
3. Fibular fracture line characteristically runs transversely or slightly obliquely from the lateral cortex in an inferomedial direction.

Note: These injuries to the medial and lateral support structures are sufficiently unstable to require operative fixation.

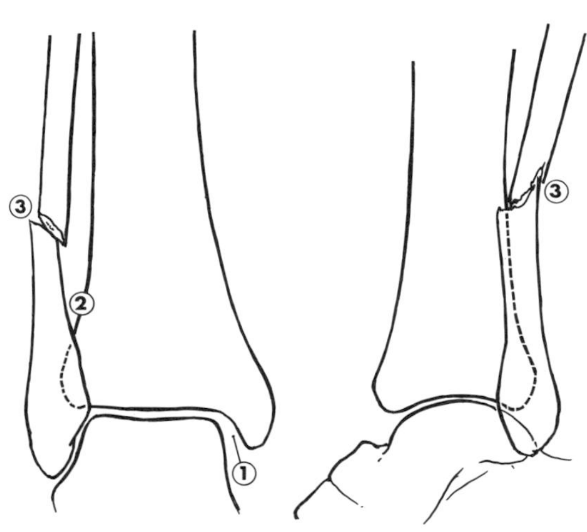

Management of Fibular Fractures Proximal to the Syndesmosis

REMARKS

S-EX stage I, II, or III injuries are stable if the fibula does not shorten and the medial joint space is normal. They may be treated by cast immobilization. Be certain that the fibular fracture is restored to length by closed reduction. Shortening of the fibula results in tilting of the talus and an unsatisfactory result (see page 860).

S-EX stage IV injuries are unstable because the medial and the lateral supports of the ankle are disrupted. These generally require internal fixation of both the medial and lateral structures to ensure satisfactory ankle support.

P-AB and P-EX injuries are unstable because both the medial and lateral support structures are involved. Operative fixation is usually the treatment of choice with these injuries.

The key to stabilization of the ankle mortise is to restore the fibula to normal length and alignment.

The intraosseous ligament can be repaired by direct suture. Transosseous screw fixation across the fibula into the tibia should be avoided because this decreases rotation in the syndesmosis that is necessary for normal ankle dorsiflexion (see page 817).

P-EX mechanisms are particularly likely to produce large posterior tibial articular surface fractures that involve more than 25 per cent of the joint surface. These require internal fixation to stabilize the posterior articular surface.

Keep in mind that fractures of the fibula above the syndesmosis are sometimes associated with shearing injuries to the articular surface (Coonrad fracture). The consequence is that traumatic arthritis may occur despite adequate reduction and internal fixation (see page 851).

Operative Fixation

1. Fibular fracture is reduced and stabilized with a semitubular five-hole plate.
2. Reduction should restore the normal length of the lateral malleolus on the fractured side (compared with the unfractured side.

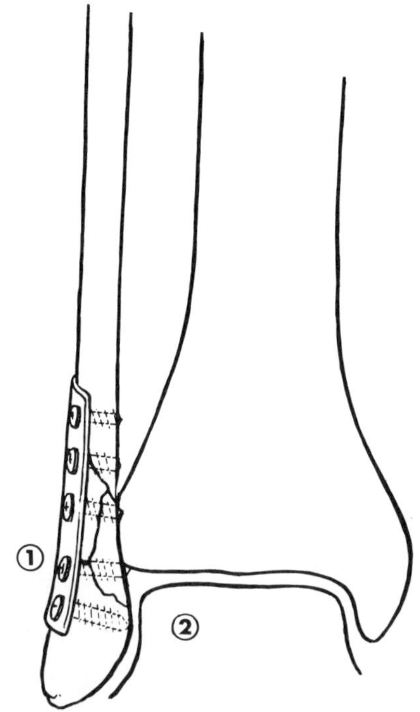

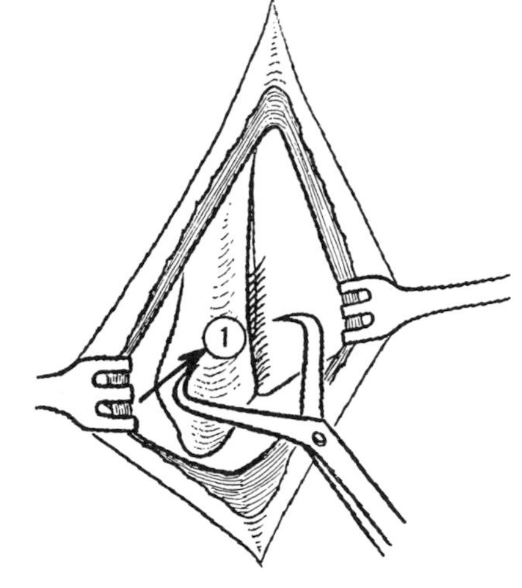

Operative Reduction and Internal Fixation

1. Tibiofibular syndesmosis is also explored, and stability is tested.

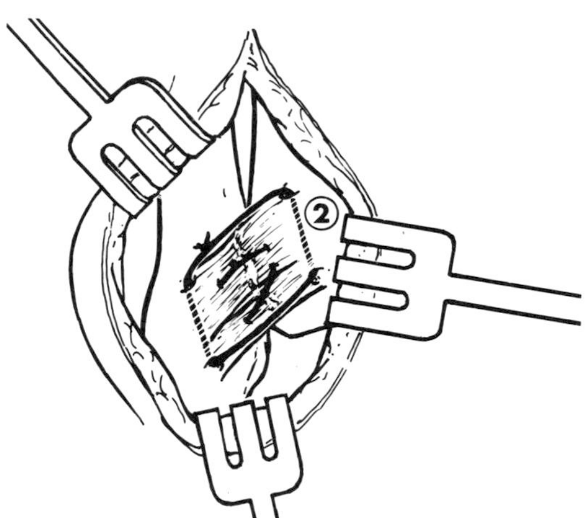

2. If the distal fibula is unstable, the tibiofibular ligament is sutured, or

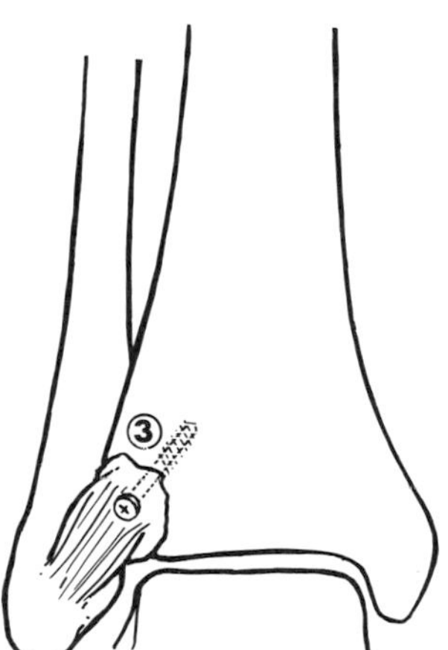

3. There is an avulsion fragment from the bony attachment, it is reattached with a screw.

Fixation of Posterior Tibial Articular Fracture

If the fragment of the posterior tibial articular surface involves more than 25 per cent of the surface, it should be stabilized. This can be done from front to back.

1. Reduction is achieved using Weber's reduction forceps.
2. Two cancellous screws are inserted at slightly different levels using a lag screw effect.

Note: This technique eliminates the need for a posterior approach but may not allow an exact reduction. Fixation is satisfactory to permit early postoperative range-of-motion exercises.

If reduction is not satisfactory by this method, a posterolateral exposure by Henry's approach permits direct visualization of the fracture. The patient must, however, be prone for this exposure.

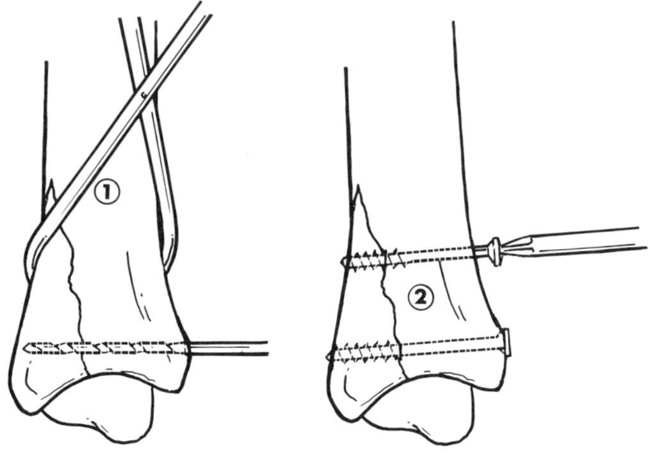

Postreduction X-Ray

P-EX FRACTURE WITH FRACTURE OF THE POSTERIOR ARTICULAR SURFACE

1. Fibula is stabilized by the plate.
2. Distal tibiofibular syndesmosis has been restored by direct suture of the tibiofibular ligament.
3. Restoration of fibula length and alignment has restored the talus to its normal position.
4. Medial malleolus is reduced anatomically and fixed with a screw.
5. Posterior tibial fragment is fixed by a screw inserted from anterior to posterior.

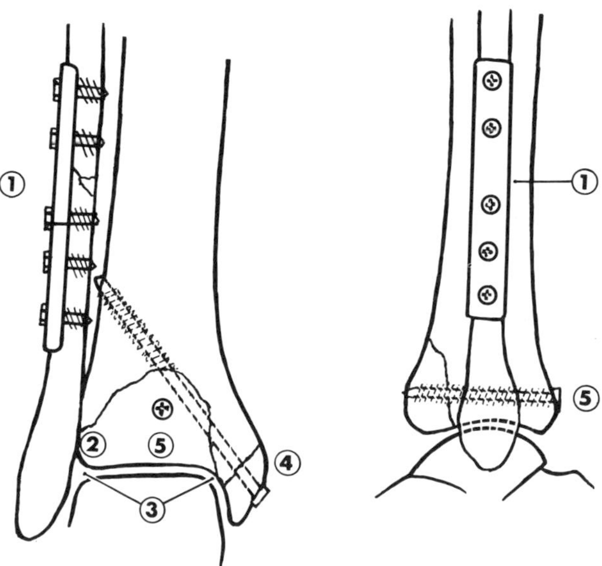

P-AB FRACTURE WITH DISRUPTION OF THE SYNDESMOSIS

1. Fibula has been fixed with a semitubular plate.
2. Avulsion fracture of the tibiofibular ligament is fixed with a screw.
3. Talus has been restored to proper position.
4. Medial malleolar fragment is fixed with a screw.

Note: Reduction can be most accurately evaluated by comparing the talocrural angles in the fractured and unfractured ankles (see page 858).

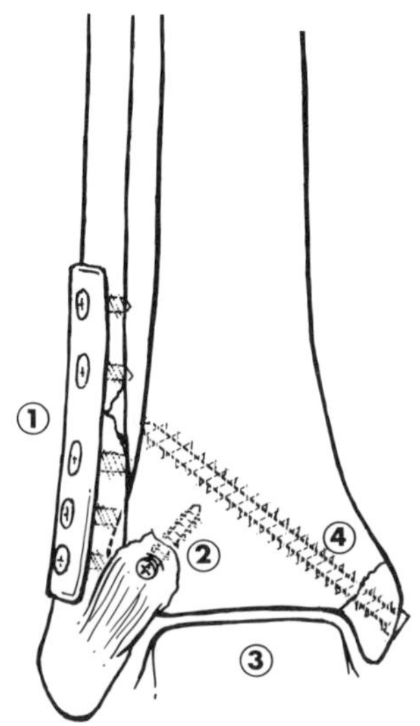

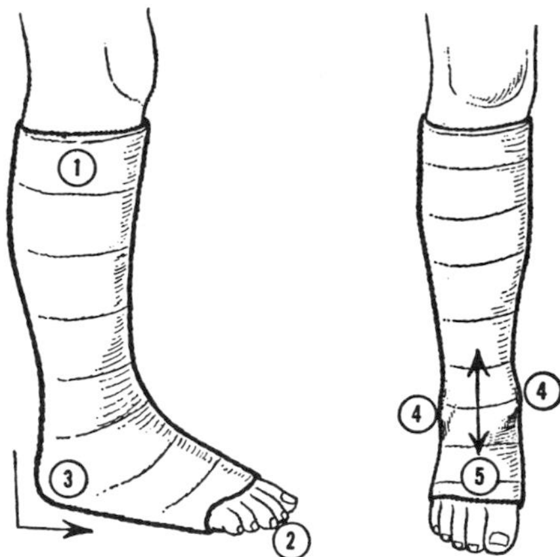

Postoperative Care

1. Short-leg cast is applied.
2. Toes are free.
3. Ankle is at a right angle.
4. Malleoli are well molded.
5. Ankle is in a neutral position in regard to inversion or eversion.

Subsequent Management

The period of cast immobilization depends on the degree of initial injury and the rigidity of fixation achieved by the surgery.

In most instances, the patient is able to discard the plaster by 6–8 weeks but should continue on crutches for 6 weeks longer.

Most ankle fractures have healed satisfactorily by the end of 12 weeks, and the patient should be regaining close to normal motion.

The internal fixation need not be removed unless it is causing symptoms.

Significance of Injuries to Distal Tibiofibular Ligaments

REMARKS

The tibiofibular joint in the leg is analogous to the radioulnar joint in the forearm in its need for rotational mobility. Rotation of the fibula on the tibia is necessary to allow full range of dorsiflexion of the talus in the ankle mortise.

Injury to the distal tibiofibular ligaments may rarely cause diastasis without fracture (see page 838).

In most instances, the distal tibiofibular ligaments are injured by supination or pronation-rotational mechanisms, which also fracture the lateral or medial malleoli.

Any lateral shift or instability thought to be due to disruption of the tibiofibular ligament can usually be corrected by anatomic reduction and stabilization of the fractured fibula along with direct repair of the torn tibiofibular ligament.

In general, it is best to avoid transosseous screw fixation of the fibula to the tibia because this can lead to stiffening of the ankle by blocking full range of motion of the talus in the mortise.

Chronic Diastasis and Malunion Treated With Transosseous Screw Fixation

PREOPERATIVE X-RAY

1. Chronic malunion of an ankle injury has resulted from fibular shortening and
2. Lateral displacement of the talus with the fibula.

Note: To correct the lateral displacement of the talus, the fibula must be repositioned and fixed internally. Fibular and tibial screw fixation can aid in the repositioning of the talus in its normal articulation with the tibia (see page 853).

Postoperative X-Ray

1. In most instances, ankle stability can be restored to anatomic position by adequate reduction and fixation of the lateral malleolus.
2. Additional internal fixation by transosseous screw closes down the tibiofibular ligament and prevents rotation.
3. This leads sometimes to limitation of dorsiflexion of the ankle as a result of the talus being locked in the ankle mortise by narrowing of the tibiofibular space. Therefore, the transosseus screw should be inserted with the ankle held in maximal dorsiflexion.

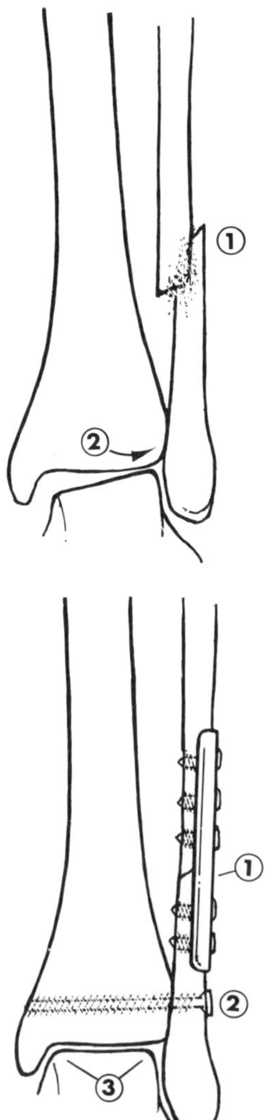

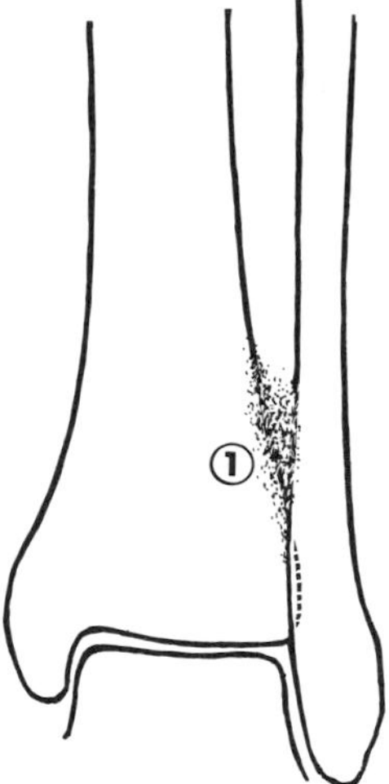

1. Bony ankylosis from an injury to the distal tibiofibular syndesmosis causes ankle stiffness and pain with prolonged walking.

Note: These ankle symptoms can be relieved by excision of the bony ankylosis and interposition of a free fat graft between the distal fibula and tibia to restore ankle mobility.

Maisonneuve Fracture of the Proximal Fibula Without Diastasis of the Ankle

REMARKS

According to Pankovich, this injury is more common than generally appreciated. Forceful external rotation of the foot produces the lesion in five stages.

The interosseous ligament transmits the torsional load from the ankle to the proximal fibula. However, the ligament itself does not rupture.

In most instances, the interosseous ligament only ruptures with grossly displaced fractures of the tibia and fibula.

See also the section on diastasis of the tibiofibular joint without fracture (see page 838).

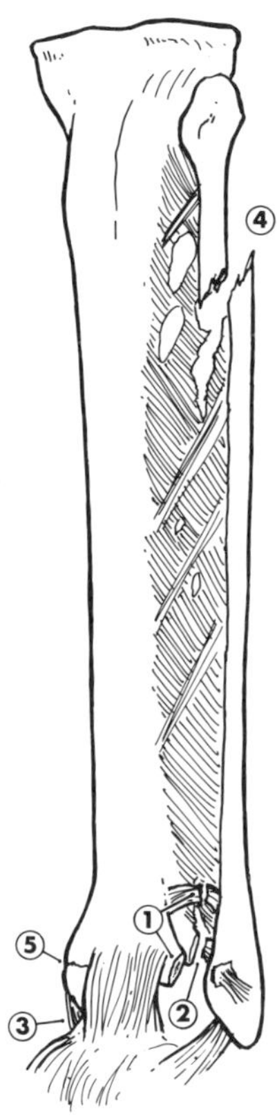

1. Rupture of the anterior tibiofibular ligament or avulsion of its bony insertion is usually not associated with rupture of the interosseous ligament.
2. Fracture of the posterior tibial tuberosity or rupture of the posterior tibiofibular ligament.
3. Rupture of the anteromedial joint capsule or avulsion fracture of its bony insertion.
4. Fracture of the fibula in its proximal third.
5. Rupture of the deltoid ligament or fracture of the medial malleolus.

Clinical Evaluation

The Maisonneuve fracture may be easily overlooked.

The examiner should look carefully for a lesion of the proximal fibula if there is

- An isolated fracture of the posterior tibial tubercle, particularly with associated anteromedial capsular tenderness.
- Deltoid ligament rupture or fracture of the medial malleolus without a fracture of the lateral malleolus.
- Tenderness over the syndesmosis and anteromedial capsule.

Management

Most Maisonneuve fractures of the proximal fibula with or without diastasis of the ankle can be treated by cast immobilization for 3 weeks.

For the more advanced stages of this lesion, particularly if there is wide diastasis and instability of the ankle, operative fixation is indicated.

The lateral support should be restored first by repairing the tibiofibular ligament. The intraosseous ligament may also be sutured, but transosseous screw fixation should be avoided. It is usually unnecessary if adequate ligamentous suturing is accomplished.

After repair of the lateral ligaments, the anteromedial capsule is repaired by a separate incision.

Preoperative X-Ray

1. Maisonneuve fracture of the proximal fibula associated with
2. Wide diastasis of the distal tibiofibular syndesmosis and
3. Avulsion of the deltoid ligament.

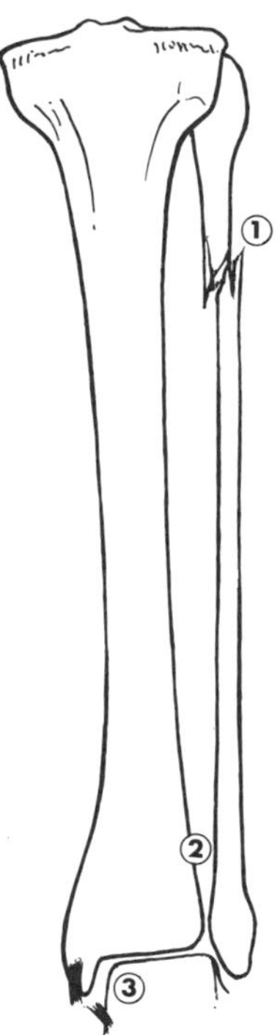

Postoperative X-Ray

1. Widening of the distal tibiofibular joint has been reduced by repair of the anterior ligament and
2. Repair of the deltoid ligament.
3. Anteromedial clear space of the mortise has been restored to normal.
4. Proximal fibula fracture need not be stabilized.

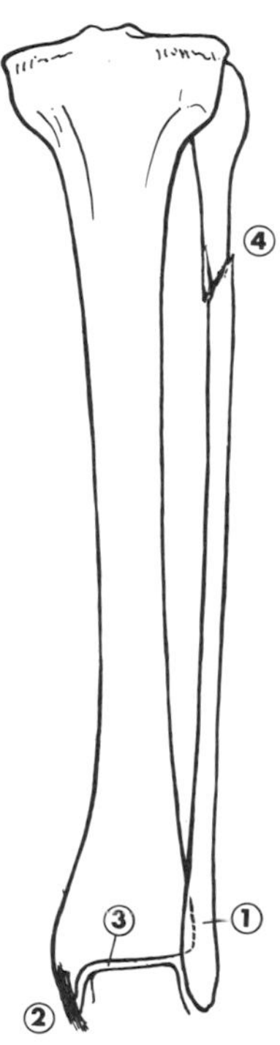

Posterior Dislocation of the Foot With Posterior Marginal Fracture of the Tibia

REMARKS

Posterior marginal or malleolar fractures result frequently from torsional mechanism. Although the fracture fragments are usually small, if they are sufficiently large to cause instability, they warrant internal fixation.

The unreduced posterior marginal or malleolar fracture is a common source of unsatisfactory outcome with ankle fractures. Therefore, when in doubt about the significance or size of a lesion, internal fixation is usually indicated.

The posterolateral shearing fracture (Coonrad fracture) is particularly a source of unsatisfactory results that may or may not be improved by internal fixation (see page 851).

In general, the posterior marginal fractures that result from the S-EX mechanism are usually smaller and cause less instability than do those from pronation mechanisms.

In adolescents, at the time of growth plate closure, the P-EX mechanism can produce a two-fragment epiphyseal fracture. In this instance, a lateral fragment includes part of the epiphysis and posterior tibial metaphysis. These fragments displace posterolaterally. The medial malleolar portion of the epiphysis remains in continuity with the tibial shaft.

Mechanisms

S-EX Mechanism Stage IV

PREREDUCTION X-RAY

1. Spiral oblique fracture of the lateral malleolus is characteristic of the S-EX mechanisms.
2. Medial malleolus has been avulsed.
3. Talus is shifted laterally and posteriorly with the lateral malleolus.
4. Both the posterior marginal fracture and
5. Talus have displaced posteriorly.
6. Articular surfaces of the talus and the tibia are not congruous.

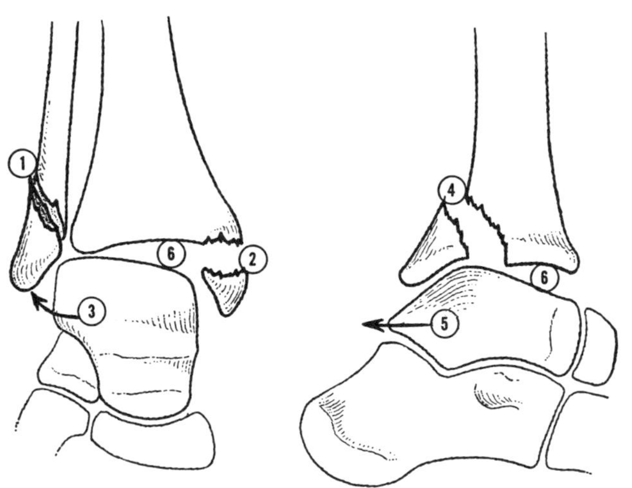

P-EX Mechanism Stage III

PREREDUCTION X-RAY

1. Avulsion of the medial malleolus.
2. Fracture of the shaft of the fibula above the syndesmosis that runs obliquely from the anterior edge in a posteroinferior direction.
3. Lateral displacement of the talus.
4. Fracture of the fibula at the high level indicates rupture of the tibiofibular ligament; diastasis of the tibiofibular joint results.
5. Posterior marginal fracture of the tibia.
6. Posterolateral displacement of the talus, which follows the displaced lateral malleolus.

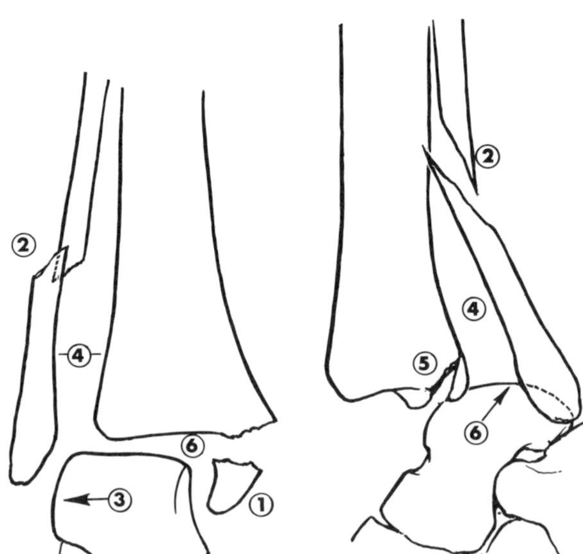

P-EX Epiphyseal Fracture in an Adolescent

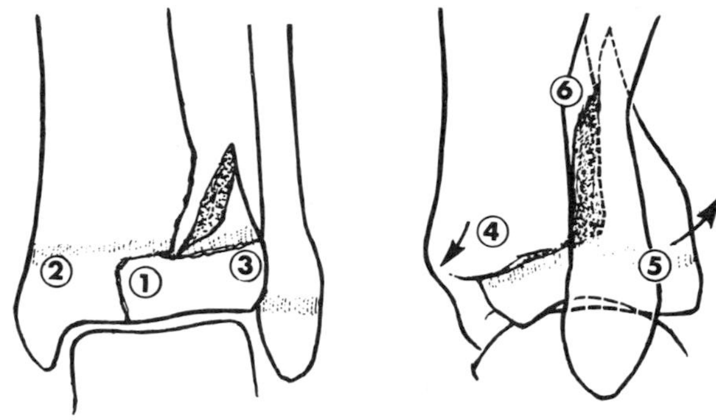

PREREDUCTION X-RAY

1. Anteroposterior tomogram shows a fracture through the epiphysis with displacement.
2. Medial malleolar portion remains in continuity with the tibial shaft.
3. Lateral portion of the epiphysis displaces externally.
4. On lateral x-ray, the medial malleolus displaces anteriorly with the shaft, and the
5. Lateral fragment, including the remainder of the epiphysis and a portion of the posterior metaphysis, is displaced posteriorly.
6. Fibula is usually intact but may be fractured and angulated anteriorly.

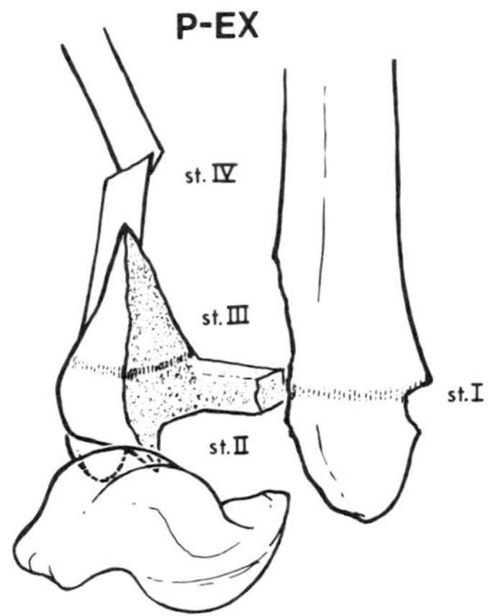

STAGING OF INJURY

P-EX mechanisms in an adolescent lead to a sequence different from that in adults.

Stage I is a rupture of the anterior tibiofibular ligament.

Stage II is a type III epiphyseal fracture.

Stage III is a fracture up through the posterior metaphysis with posterior displacement of the lateral epiphyseal fragment, the metaphyseal fragment, and the fibula.

Stage IV is a greenstick fracture of the fibula with anterior angulation caused by the posterior displacement of the fragment.

S-AD Mechanism Stage II

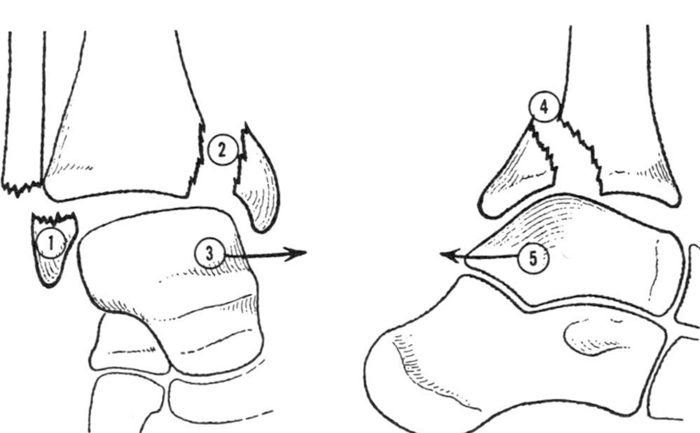

PREREDUCTION X-RAY

1. Avulsion of the lateral malleolus.
2. Shearing of the medial malleolus.
3. Talus is displaced medially.
4. Posteromedial marginal fracture of the tibia.
5. Posterior displacement of the talus.

STAGING OF INJURY

S-AD mechanism injures the ankle in the following stages:

Stage I is a fracture of the lateral malleolus at or distal to the level of the tibiotalar joint, or rupture of the anterior talofibular and calcaneofibular ligaments.

Stage II is a fracture of the medial malleolus, usually of an oblique nature. The S-AD mechanism involves the posteromedial articular surface rather than the posterolateral articular surface.

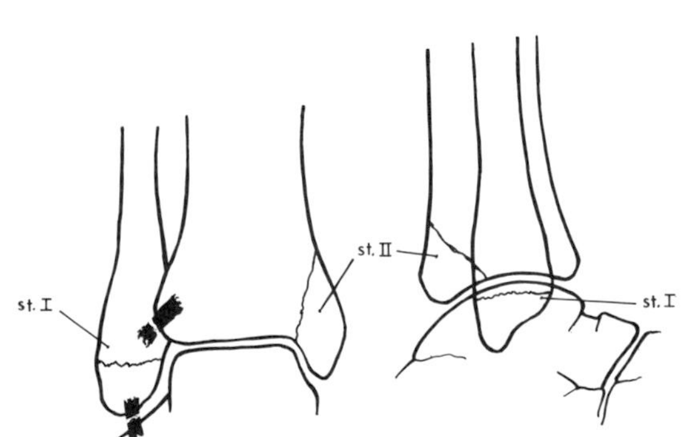

Operative Reduction

INDICATIONS

Most posterior marginal fractures with posterior dislocation of the talus are unstable and require fixation for adequate stability of the ankle.

If there is doubt about the size of the posterior fragment and its contribution to ankle stability, operative fixation is wise because the fragment is frequently larger than is apparent on x-ray.

The distal epiphyseal fracture in adolescent patients may generally be treated by closed reduction, but the reduction should be anatomic. If the epiphyseal fracture is associated with a fibular fracture, operative reduction is usually necessary.

The fractures of the lateral and medial malleoli are fixed first (see page 876.) Stabilization of the fibula frequently adds stability to the posterolateral articular fragment because the posterior tibiofibular ligament remains intact.

An alternative approach is to expose the posterior and lateral malleoli by posterolateral incision, which allows the posterior rim fracture to be reduced under direct vision.

Prereduction X-Ray

P-EX FRACTURE STAGE IV WITH POSTERIOR DISLOCATION

1. Dislocation of the talus from the medial malleolus indicates disruption of the deltoid.
2. Gross posterolateral displacement of the fibula indicates disruption of the tibiofibular ligament and intraosseous ligament.
3. Fibular fracture line runs from the anterior cortex in a posteroinferior direction, characteristic of the P-EX mechanism.
4. Talus displaces posterolaterally with the posterior marginal fracture.

Note: The size of the posterior marginal fracture is underestimated from this x-ray projection.

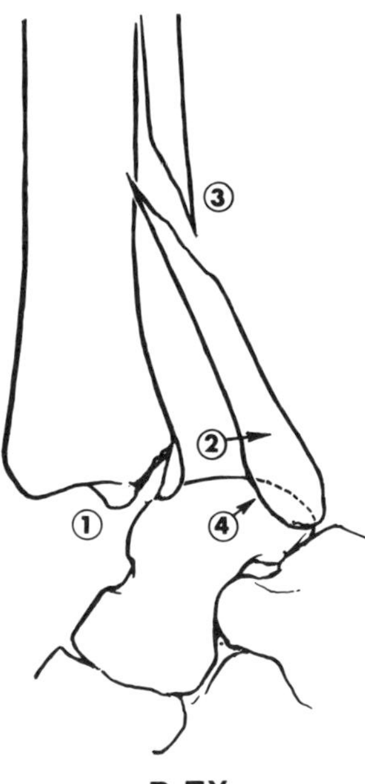

P-EX

Operative Technique: Anterior Approach

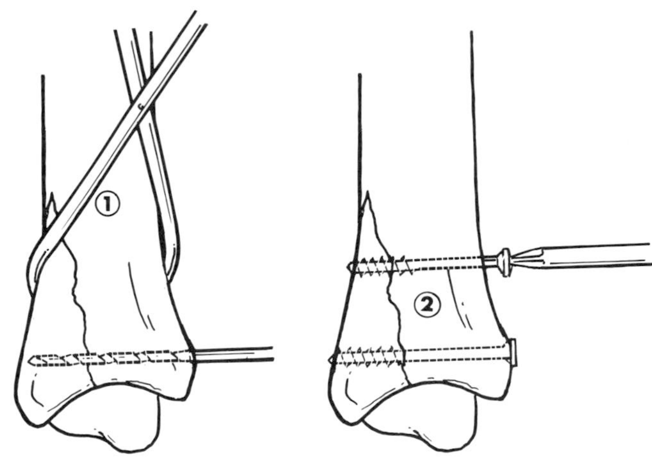

Note: The medial and the lateral malleoli are fixed under direct vision.

1. Reduction of the posterolateral fragment is achieved using Weber reduction forceps.
2. Two cancellous screws are inserted at slightly different levels from the anteromedial cortex by the lag screw method.

Note: If reduction by this method is not satisfactory, the posterolateral exposure by Henry's approach permits direct visualization of the fracture.

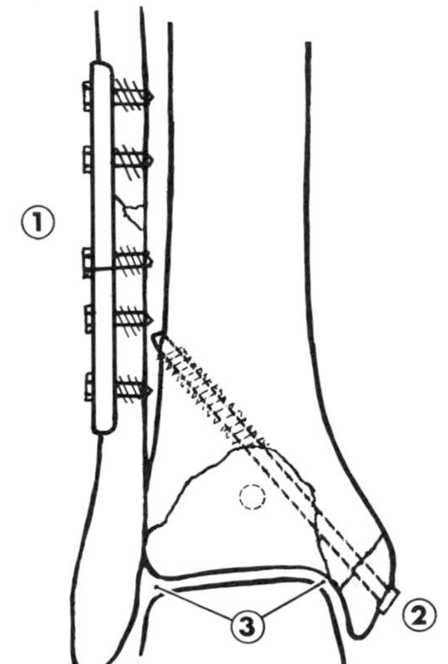

Postreduction X-Ray

1. Fibular fracture has been stabilized with the plate.
2. Medial malleolar fracture is fixed with a screw.
3. Talus is in its normal position in the mortise.

Other Posterior Marginal Fractures (Curbstone Fracture)

REMARKS

Isolated fractures may occur from sudden avulsion injury when the individuals strike their dorsiflexing toes during the swing phase. Most often, this is done by stumbling over a curbstone.

The considerable force generated by the foot, which is accelerating at this point up to 4 G, is sufficient to avulse the posterior articular surface of the tibia.

Typically, this is an undisplaced fracture and requires only symptomatic treatment, usually with cast support for 3 weeks.

Mechanism of Injury

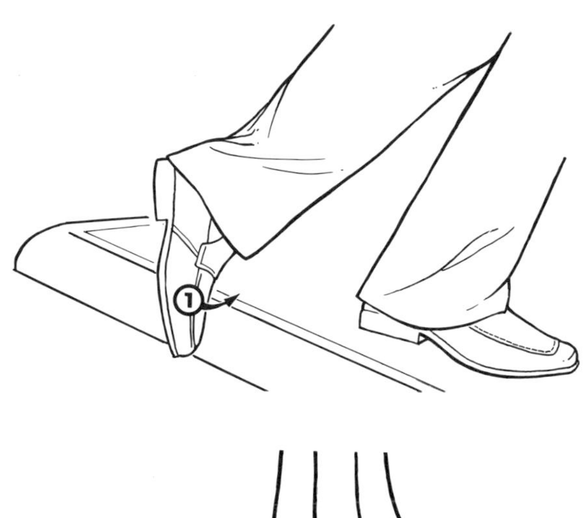

1. Foot strikes the curbstone while accelerating during swing phase.

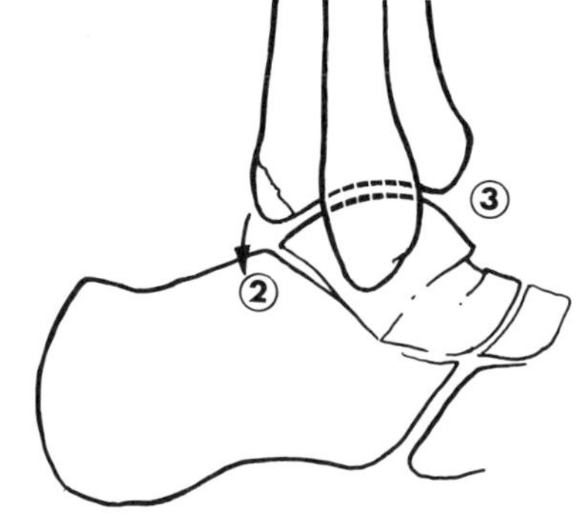

2. Pull of the posterior capsule avulses the posterior articular fragment. This is usually less than 10 per cent of the joint surface.
3. Remaining medial and lateral articular structures are undamaged.

Immobilization

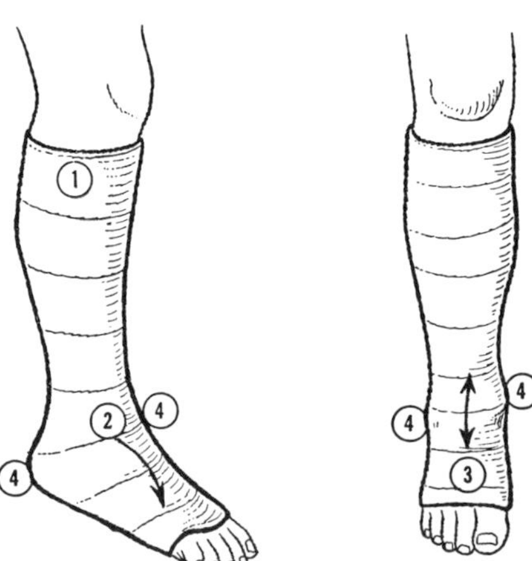

1. Apply a circular plaster cast from the base of the toes to just below the knee.
2. Foot is in 10° of plantar flexion.
3. Foot is in neutral position in regard to inversion and eversion.
4. Plaster is molded well around the heel, in front of the foot, and around the malleoli for the patient's comfort.

Management

Treatment should be symptomatic to relieve the discomfort in the ankle.

Most frequently, the patient is comfortable with a short-leg walking cast maintained for 3 weeks.

Pronation-Dorsiflexion Injuries

Anterior Marginal Fractures With Anterior Subluxation of the Talus (Pilon Fractures)

REMARKS

Pilon fractures are invariably produced by forceful dorsiflexion of the ankle as in a fall from a height or in an automobile collision.

If the foot is pronated at the time of dorsiflexion injury, the talus acts as a wedge against the anterior and medial articular surfaces. Lauge-Hansen described this as an additional mechanism of pronation and dorsiflexion that is characterized by a large fragment torn from the anterior tibial lip with forward subluxation of the talus and a fracture of the base of the medial malleolus.

These injuries, although infrequent, can be among the most difficult ankle fractures to manage. The fracture tends to explode the articular surface, so that traumatic arthritis is the common sequela.

In selecting management, the surgeon should distinguish pronation-dorsiflexion fractures from other types of comminuted distal tibial fractures, particularly those produced by external or internal torsion. These other injuries are entirely different from the pronation-dorsiflexion injury both in mechanism and prognosis.

Fractures of this type are also called pilon (pē'-lon), which is the French term for pestle, as in mortar and pestle. A preferable term is tibial plafond, which means "ceiling" of the ankle joint.

Pathologic Findings

Pronation-dorsiflexion injuries occur in four stages:

1. Stage I is fracture of the medial malleolus.
2. Stage II is avulsion of a large fragment from the anterior lip of the tibia.

Note: Because of this fracture, the lateral tibial plafond remains attached to the fibula and displaces with it. This is in contrast to the usual fibular fracture proximal to the syndesmosis, which is associated with diastasis of the fibulotibial articulation (see pages 848 and 871).

3. Stage III is a supramalleolar fracture of the fibula. Characteristically, the fibula angulates posteriorly as the talus displaces anteriorly.
4. Stage IV is a transverse fracture of the tibia at the level of the proximal margin of the anterior tibial fragment.

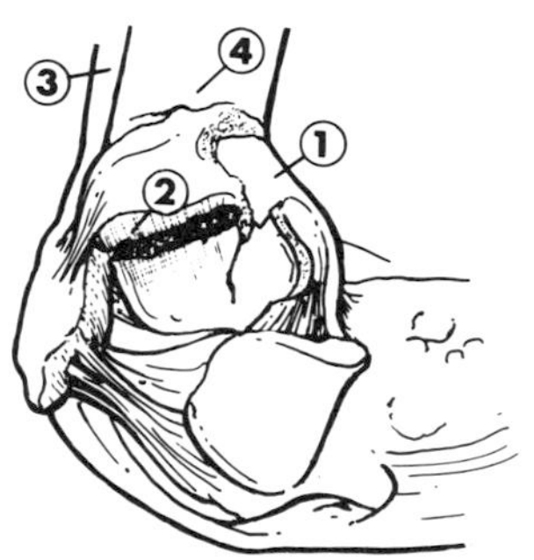

Appearance on X-Ray of Unstable Injury

1. Fracture of the medial portion of the tibia may be comminuted.
2. Anterior margin of the tibia displaces forward.
3. Talus and ankle mortise is extremely unstable, and this is associated with extensive soft tissue damage and, frequently, an open fracture.
4. There is lateral tibial comminution, although a small fragment remains with the fibula.
5. Fibular fracture displaces laterally.

Many of the fractures to this extent are open, particularly on the medial side. Occasionally, stabilization of the fibula may help restore the alignment of the mortise, but frequently these fractures are extremely complication prone.

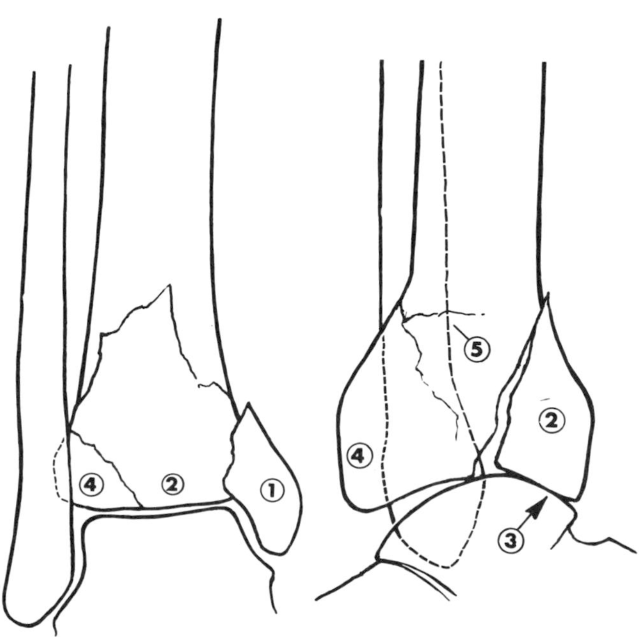

Management

REMARKS

For most of pilon injuries, open reduction and operative stabilization are necessary to restore ankle mortise stability. However, these intraarticular fractures are among the most difficult to treat surgically.

Skin slough is common after open reduction because of significant soft tissue swelling.

The more comminuted type of fracture is frequently associated with open wounds and has a high risk of infection. For these injuries, nonoperative treatment with skeletal traction or external fixation is frequently the most effective compromise method of management.

Closed reduction and cast treatment are generally not indicated, except for the fracture with a single fragment that is relatively undisplaced. For the most part, operative reduction with internal fixation or external fixation with percutaneous screw fixation is the treatment of choice.

Closed Treatment (Single Large, Relatively Stable Fragment)

Prereduction X-Ray

1. Anterior marginal fragment is displaced upward.
2. Talus is displaced forward.
3. Articular surfaces of the talus and the tibia are not congruous.

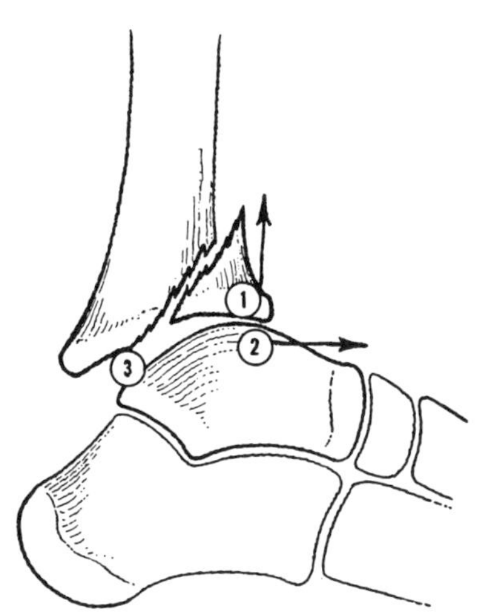

Manipulative Reduction

1. Patient's leg hangs over the edge of the table.
2. Operator grasps the forefoot with one hand and the heel with the other.
3. Operator makes strong traction downward and, at the same time,
4. Forcibly plantar flexes the foot.

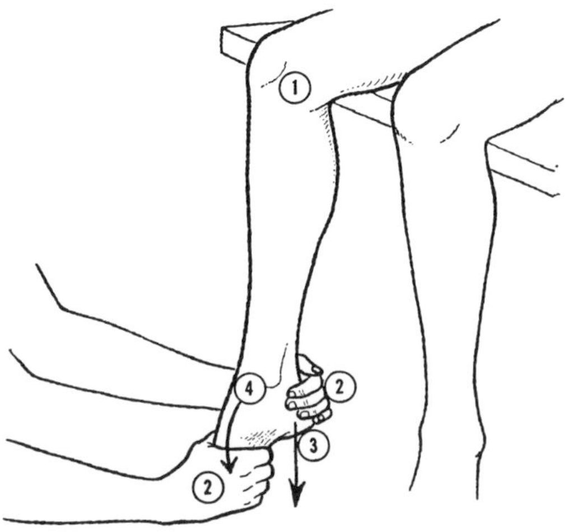

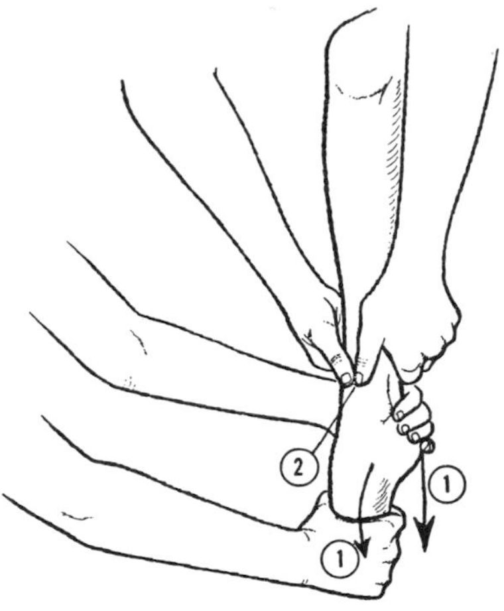

Manipulative Reduction Technique

1. While the operator maintains downward traction and plantar flexion of the foot, the
2. Assistant makes direct pressure on the fragment with both thumbs, molding the fragment into place.

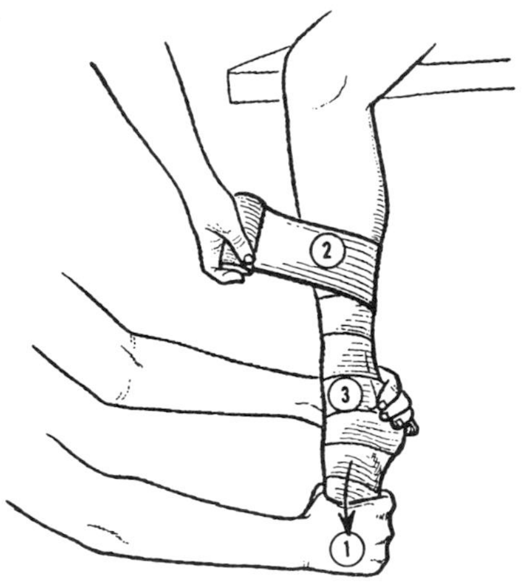

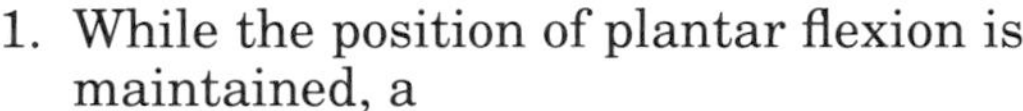

1. While the position of plantar flexion is maintained, a
2. Lightly padded below-knee plaster cast is applied, and the
3. Plaster is molded well over the front of the ankle and around both malleoli.

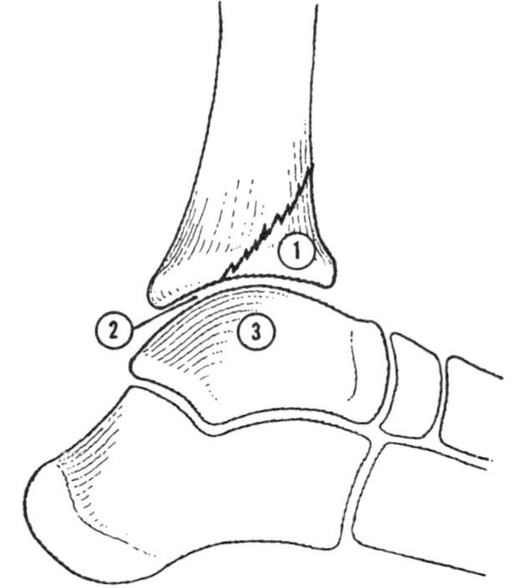

Postreduction X-Ray

1. Anterior marginal fragment is restored to its anatomic position.
2. Articular surfaces of the talus and the tibia are congruous.
3. Forward displacement of the talus is corrected.

Postreduction Management

Check reduction with x-rays immediately after the application of the plaster cast. Follow closely with repeat x-ray because displacement may recur in the cast.

After 3 weeks, apply a new cast, and reduce the amount of plantar flexion.

Six weeks after the reduction, remove the second cast, and bring the foot to a right angle with the leg.

Permit weight bearing in plaster at the end of 10 weeks.

Remove the last cast at the end of 12 weeks.

Now institute active exercises and physical therapy to restore normal movements of the ankle and tarsal joints.

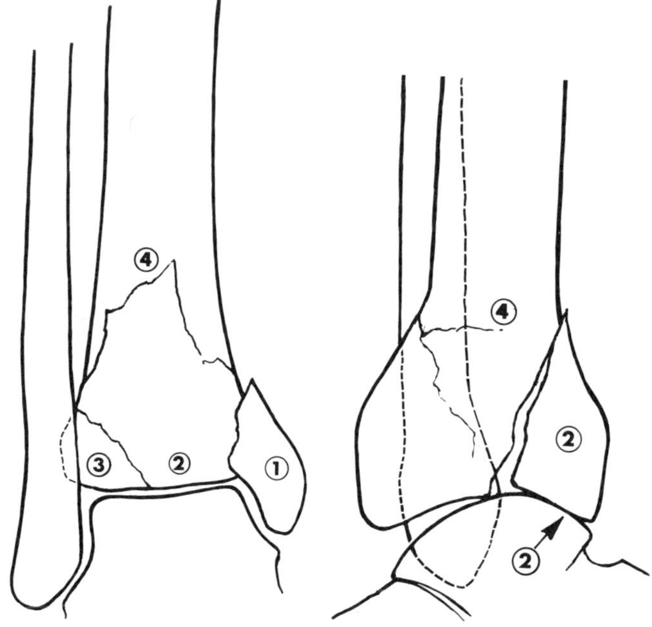

Operative Management

PREOPERATIVE X-RAY

1. Fracture of the medial malleolus.
2. Anterior cortical fragment allows anterior subluxation of the talus.
3. Lateral tibial plafond remains attached to the fibula.
4. Metaphyseal fracture without fracture of the posterior tibial cortex.

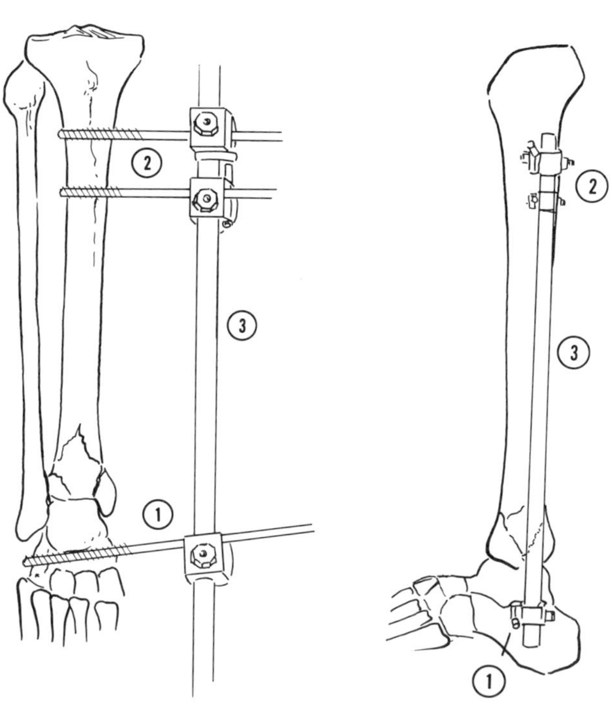

Reduction by External Fixation, Using Ligamentotaxis

Such a pronation-dorsiflexion comminuted fracture is best reduced initially by external fixation with ligamentotaxis to align the multiple fracture fragments.

1. Under operating room technique and x-ray control, a transverse pin is inserted in the calcaneus.
2. One or two pins are inserted in the proximal tibia.
3. External fixation device is used to distract the ankle and align the fracture fragments by the use of ligamentotaxis.

Note: Once the fracture fragments are reduced, they may be fixed internally by screw or plate fixation. Percutaneous fixation may also be possible with cannulated screws.

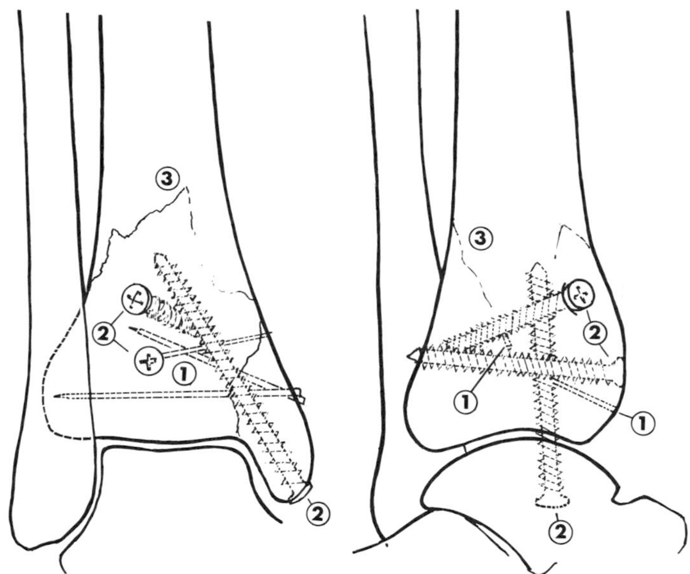

Postoperative X-Ray

1. The small fragments on the anterior cortex are fixed first with Kirschner wires.
2. Major fragments from the anterior cortex and the medial malleolus are fixed with screws.
3. Fixation of the metaphyseal fracture is not necessary once the key fragments have stabilized. Occasionally, cancellous bone grafting may be necessary to fill in defects in the metaphysis. External fixation is continued until the fracture consolidates (usually 6–8 weeks).

Note: Cannulated screws might be used with percutaneous fixation.

Severe Comminution of the Inferior Articular Surface of the Tibia (Explosion Fracture)

REMARKS

With severe compression violence, the entire lower end of the tibia may be disrupted as the talus is driven into the lower subchondral bone.

Restoration of a normal articular surface is usually impossible by either closed or open methods. In addition, attempted open reduction and internal fixation is frequently associated with an unacceptably high complication rate from infection and wound slough.

Because of this, a compromise solution is indicated.

Os calcis traction, which allows the patient to elevate the limb and exercise the ankle, can provide a satisfactory joint with normal function.

The newer alternative technique is external fixation with the Ilizarov method.

Both skeletal traction and external fixation use ligamentotaxis to align the comminuted articular surface.

Both these methods allow the surgeon to gain time and allow the swelling and wound inflammation to subside. If reduction cannot be achieved by ligamentotaxis, operative fixation may still be carried out at a time when soft tissue swelling has diminished and wound slough is less likely.

Prereduction X-Ray

1. Severe comminution of the articular surface of the tibia.
2. Fracture of both malleoli.
3. Talus is displaced upward and
4. Forward.

Note: Attempted operative intervention in this severely comminuted fracture would probably be unsuccessful and might increase the potential for wound necrosis or infection.

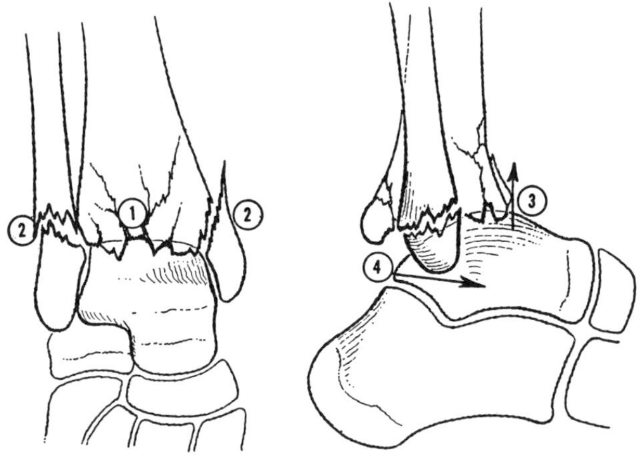

Os Calcis Traction

1. A 2-mm Steinmann pin is inserted through the os calcis.
2. Limb is elevated on a frame or suspended in a sling to diminish edema.
3. Apply 11 lb (5 kg) of traction to the calcaneus.
4. Patient may be allowed to extend and flex the ankle gently while in traction.

Note: An alternative, preferred method is external fixation.

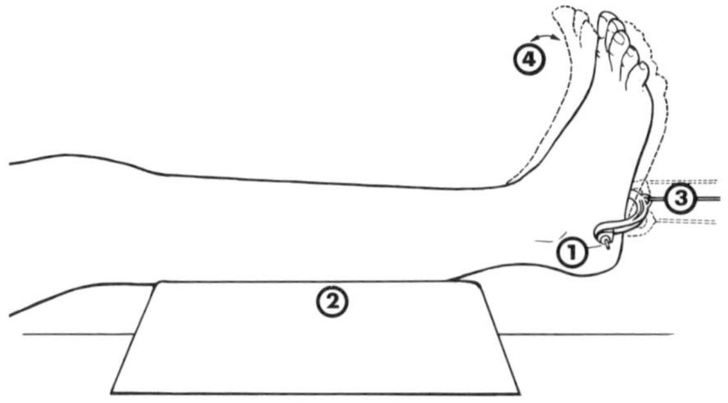

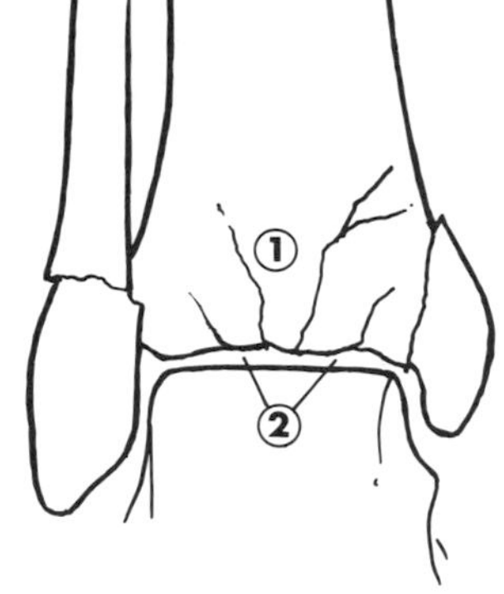

Postreduction X-Ray After 2 Days of Traction

1. Articular fragments are still incompletely reduced, but the position is improved.
2. Joint space is widened owing to the traction.

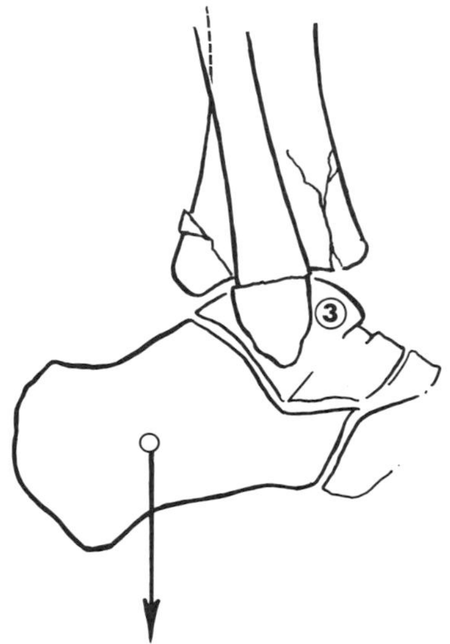

3. Talus is no longer displaced forward and upward.

Alternative Technique: Ilizarov External Fixation

REMARKS

An Ilizarov or similar type of frame is applied with circular rings above and below the ankle mortise.

Percutaneous pins may be inserted with olives to reduce the fracture further (see page 910).

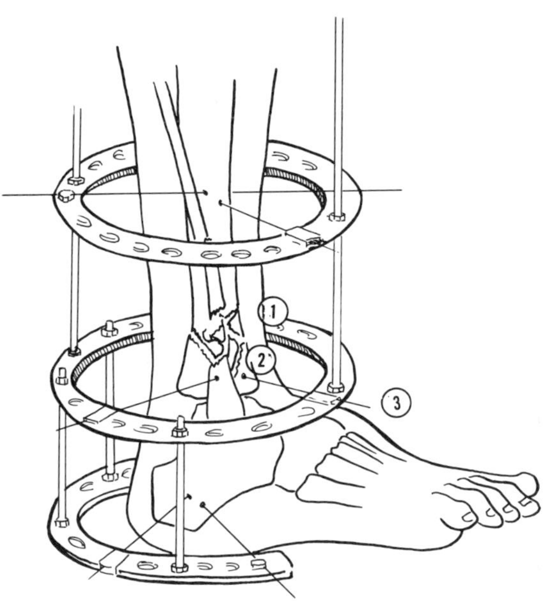

Postreduction X-Ray

1. Mortise should be restored to a reasonable alignment by ligamentotaxis provided through the external fixator.
2. Width of the joint space is restored.
3. Alignment has been improved by the percutaneous pins inserted through the comminuted fracture.

Subsequent Management

The patient is maintained in traction for 4–6 weeks. After this time, the traction is removed, and a cast is applied.

If an external fixator is applied, it should be maintained for approximately 10 weeks.

However, if the fracture alignment remains unacceptable and the ankle mortise remains unstable, operative fixation may be elected after the swelling has subsided.

The prognosis for these injuries is guarded. Nevertheless, there is frequently a minimal correlation between the appearance on x-ray and the symptoms of the patient.

The patient who is free of symptoms for the first year has a good prognosis. If painful arthritis occurs during this time and prevents weight bearing, joint arthrodesis should be recommended.

Arthrodesis of the Ankle for Comminuted Pilon Fractures

REMARKS

Primary arthrodesis should be avoided even with the severely comminuted distal tibial fracture because the degree of radiographic changes of arthritis may not correlate with the degree of clinical symptoms.

After careful observation for 6–12 months after the ankle fracture, if the patient has persistent pain and inability to bear weight satisfactorily, an arthrodesis should be recommended.

Technique of Ankle Arthrodesis After Pilon Fractures

1. Frequently, the anterior comminuted surface requires bone grafting.
2. Internal fixation with screws maintains a satisfactory weight-bearing position of the ankle that is symptomatic from traumatic arthritis.

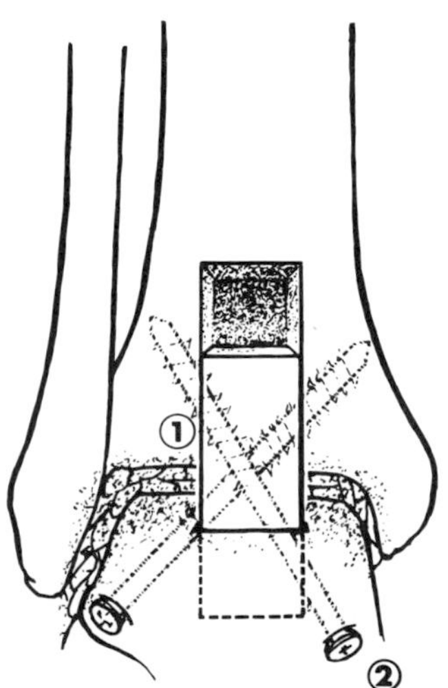

Other Fractures of the Distal Tibial Articular Surface

REMARKS

A pronation-dorsiflexion injury should be distinguished from fractures of the distal tibia produced by external or internal rotational mechanisms.

With these injuries, the talus displaces with the fibula. This is in contrast to pronation-dorsiflexion injuries in which the talus displaces anteriorly with the cortical fracture of the articular surface of the tibia.

P-EX Fracture of the Distal Tibia

PREREDUCTION X-RAY

1. Fracture of the medial malleolus or avulsion of the deltoid ligament.
2. Compression fracture of the lateral palfond of the distal tibia rather than an avulsion of the tibiofibular ligament.

Note: In this fracture, the lateral tibial plafond remains attached to the fibula and displaces with it. Consequently, the talus rotates posterolaterally with the fibula rather than anteriorly with the anterior cortical margin. This displacement also contrasts with the usual fibular fracture proximal to the syndesmosis associated with diastasis of the tibiofibular articulation (see pages 848 and 871).

3. Fracture of the fibula above the syndesmosis is characterized by an oblique pattern that runs from the posteroinferior to the anterosuperior cortex.
4. Fracture of the tibial metaphysis above the level of the articular surface fracture.

Note: The key to reducing this fracture is to restore and stabilize the fibula to length.

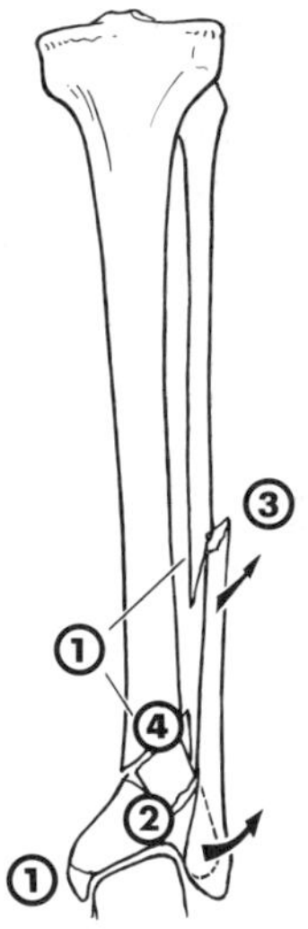

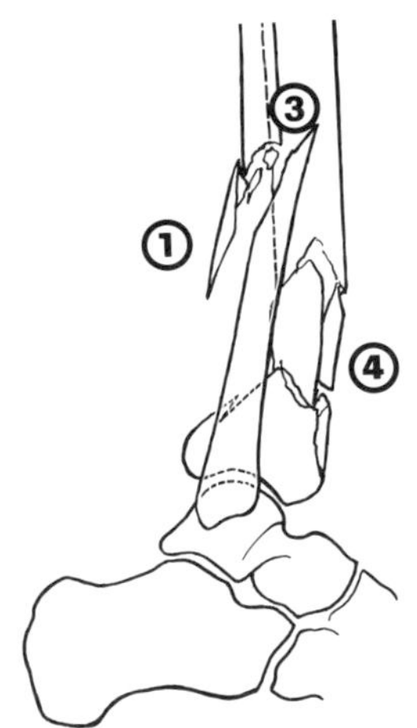

X-Ray After Stabilization

1. Intramedullary pin fixation of the fibula restores length and rotational alignment to the lateral support of the ankle.
2. Lateral plafond fracture, which is still attached to the fibula, is reduced by reduction of the fibula.
3. Talus is restored from its displaced position by reduction of the fibula.
4. Metaphyseal fracture of the tibia can be treated by closed means.

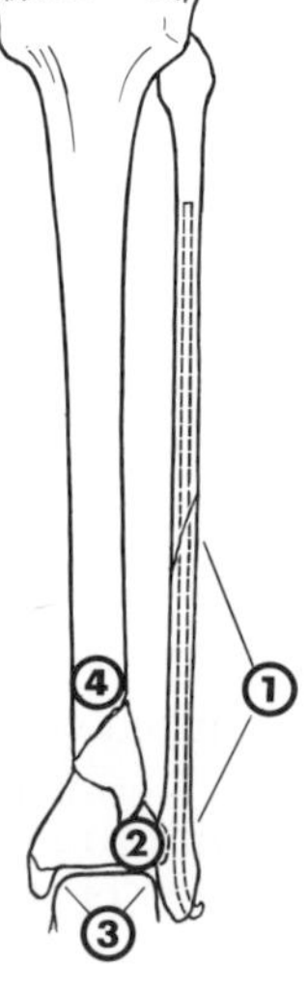

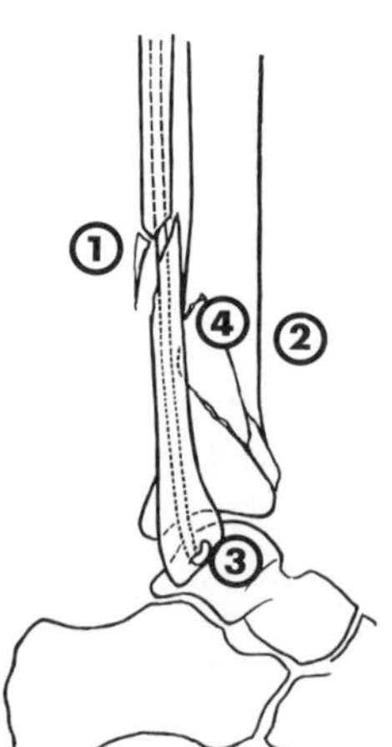

Other Distal Fractures Affecting the Ankle: Internal Rotation Fracture of the Tibia

Other comminuted fractures of the distal tibial shaft that can be confused with pronation-dorsiflexion injuries are those that result from internal torsional mechanisms.

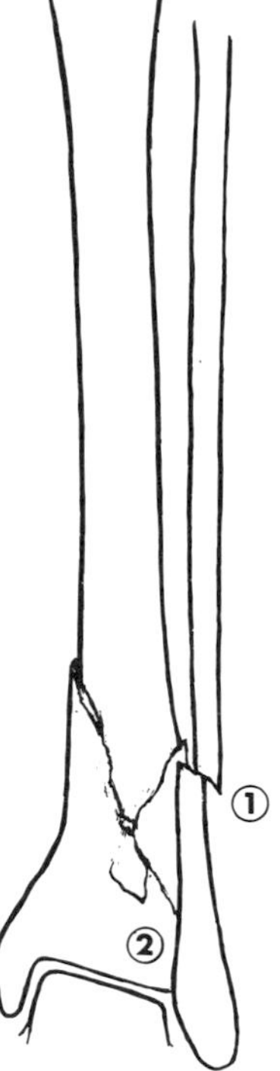

Prereduction X-Ray

1. Fracture of the fibula at or below the level of the tibia or, occasionally, an intact fibula.
2. Comminuted fracture of the tibia that runs from the distal lateral to proximal medial cortex.

Note: These fractures, which are produced by an internal torsional mechanism, are reduced by external rotation of the distal fragment. Stabilization of the fibular fracture will not aid in reduction and may frequently promote "varus drift" of the fracture.

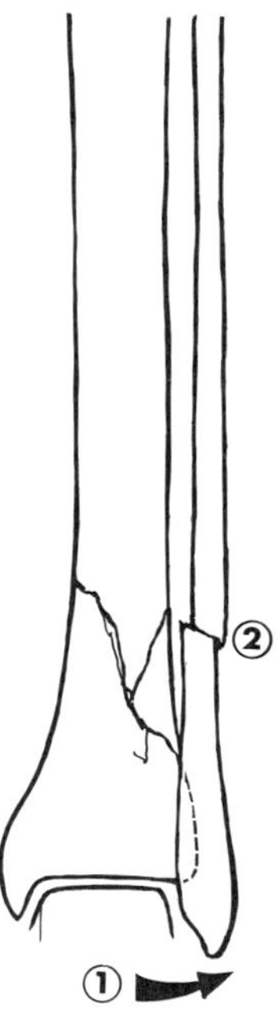

Postreduction X-Ray

Comminuted fracture of the distal tibia produced by internal torsional mechanisms is reduced closed by external rotation of the distal fragment.

1. Reduction and cast immobilization with the foot externally rotated prevents "varus drift" of the fracture.
2. Fibular fracture should be fixed internally if anatomic reduction is not achieved.

DISLOCATIONS OF THE ANKLE JOINT

Posterior Dislocation of the Ankle Joint

REMARKS

Although posterior dislocation is rare, it is the most common of all dislocations of the ankle joint.

The lesion is the result of severe plantar flexion of the foot with a strong forward thrust of the leg.

In most instances, the dislocation is accompanied by a fracture of one or both malleoli or posterior marginal fracture of the tibia.

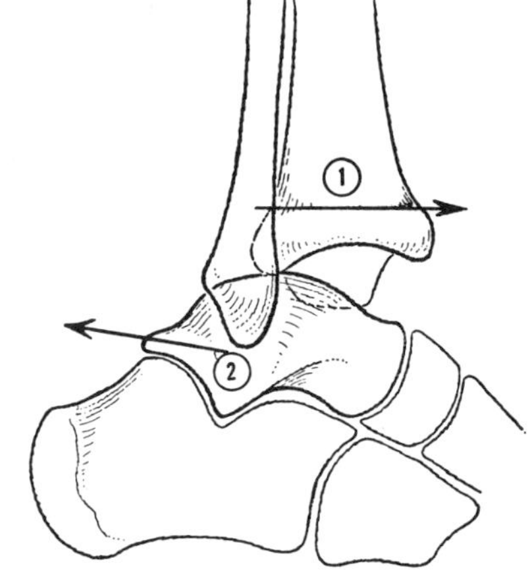

Prereduction X-Ray

1. Tibia and fibula are displaced forward.
2. Talus and foot are displaced backward.

Manipulative Reduction (Under General Ancsthesia)

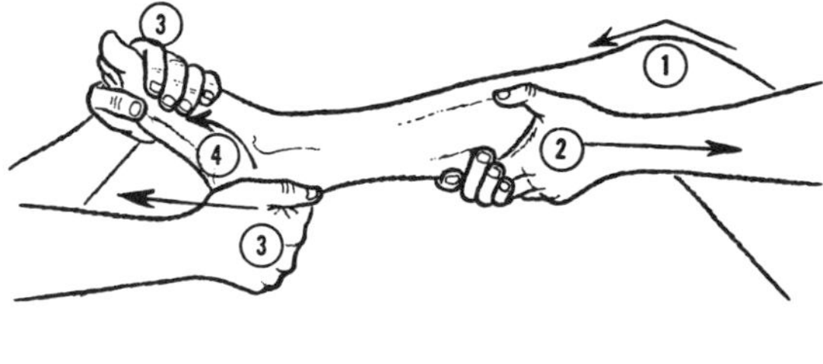

1. Knee is flexed.
2. Assistant applies countertraction on the leg.
3. Grasp the forefoot with one hand and the heel with the other.
4. Foot is slightly plantar flexed.

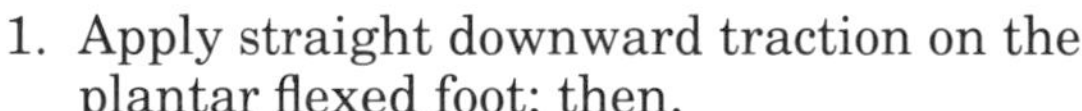
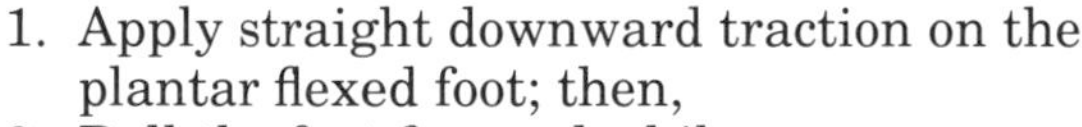

1. Apply straight downward traction on the plantar flexed foot; then,
2. Pull the foot forward while a
3. Second assistant applies counterpressure on the front of the lower leg.

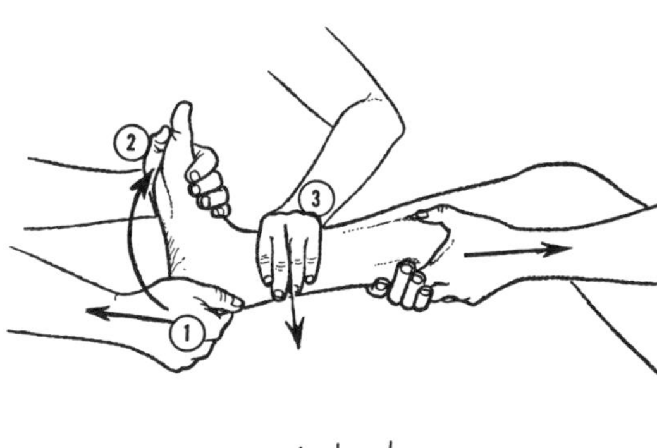

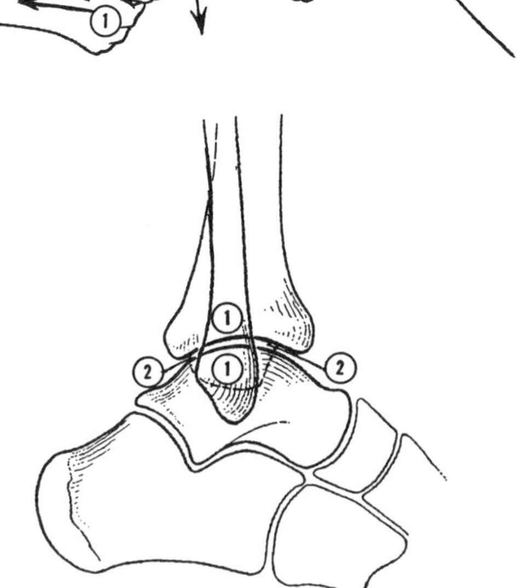

Postreduction X-Ray

1. Talus is in its correct relationship to the tibia.
2. Articular surfaces of the talus and the tibia are congruous.

Immobilization

1. Apply a circular plaster cast from the base of the toe to just below the knees.
2. Foot is dorsiflexed 90°.
3. Foot is in a neutral position in regard to inversion and eversion.
4. Mold the plaster well around the heel and the front of the foot and the malleoli.

Caution: If the ankle is extremely swollen, apply anterior and posterior splints until the swelling subsides, and then apply the cast (see page 901).

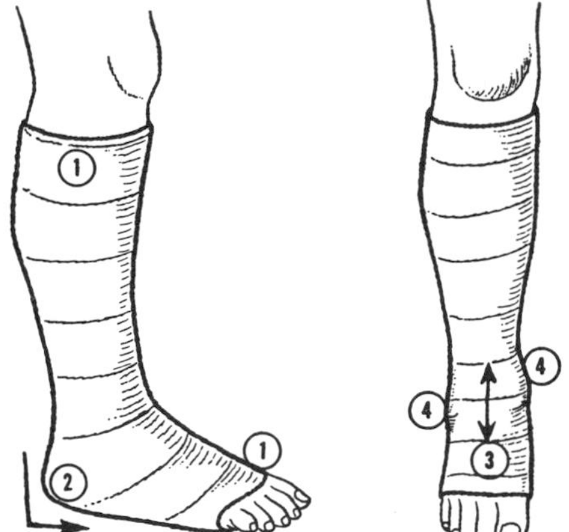

Postreduction Management

REMARKS

The patient should be kept at bed rest and the limb elevated for 3–5 days to diminish swelling, which occurs frequently after these injuries. During this time, the foot should be monitored for changes in circulation or motor or sensory function.

The duration of cast immobilization depends on the stability or instability evident at the time of reduction.

Stable ankles require cast immobilization for 2–3 weeks.

Unstable ankles may require immobilization for 4–6 weeks to achieve satisfactory healing of torn ligaments.

Anterior Dislocation of the Ankle Joint

REMARKS

Anterior dislocation of the ankle joint is indeed rare. When it occurs, it is frequently accompanied by a fracture of the anterior margin of the tibia.

The lesion is produced by forcible dorsiflexion of the foot or a fall on the heel with the foot in dorsiflexion.

Fracture of one or both malleoli may be concomitant lesions.

In this lesion, the anterior capsule may be separated from the neck of the talus.

Prereduction X-Ray

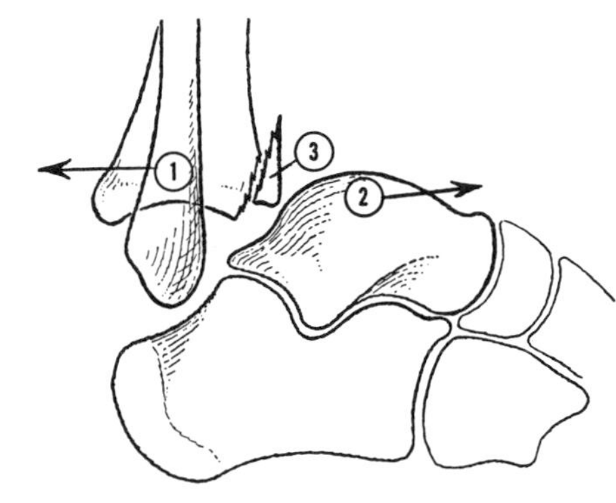

1. Backward displacement of the tibia and the fibula.
2. Forward displacement of the talus.
3. Small marginal fracture of the anterior tip of the tibia.

Manipulative Reduction (Under General Anesthesia)

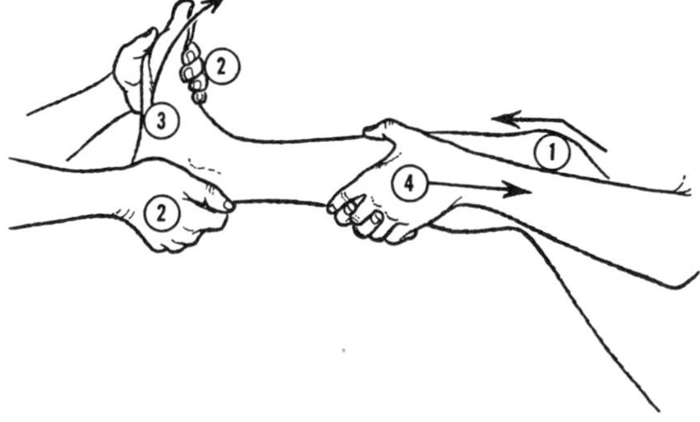

1. Knee is flexed.
2. Operator grasps the forefoot with one hand and the heel with the other.
3. Dorsiflexion of the foot is slightly increased (to disengage the talus).
4. Assistant applies countertraction on the leg.

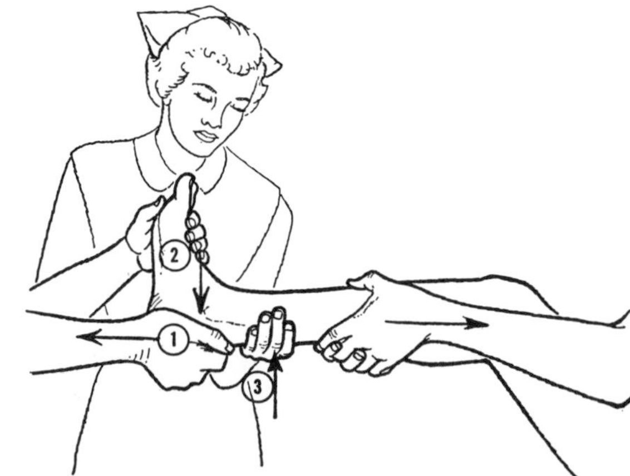

1. Straight downward traction is applied.
2. Then the foot is pushed directly backward while
3. A second assistant applies countertraction on the back of the lower leg.

Postreduction X-Ray

1. Talus is in a normal relation to the tibia.
2. Articular surfaces of the talus and the tibia are congruous.
3. Small anterior marginal fragment is in its anatomic position.

Note: Because of the considerable risk of circulatory damage with this injury, the distal circulation should be monitored carefully before and after reduction.

Occasionally, as a result of the extreme swelling with this injury, compartment syndrome may develop in the foot and require release of the fascia.

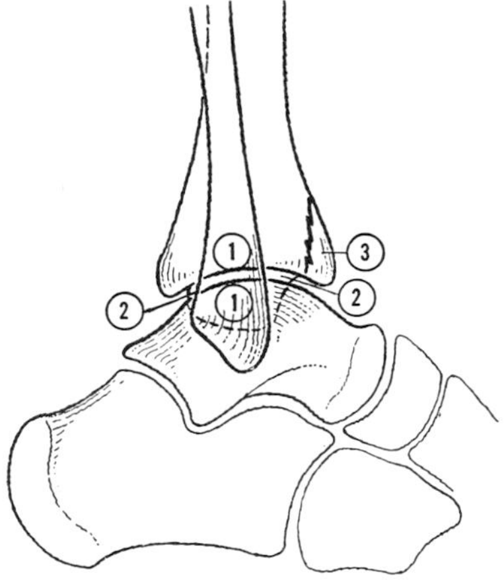

Immobilization

1. Apply a well-padded cast with the foot in slight equinus.
2. Bivalve the cast promptly to accommodate for swelling with these injuries.

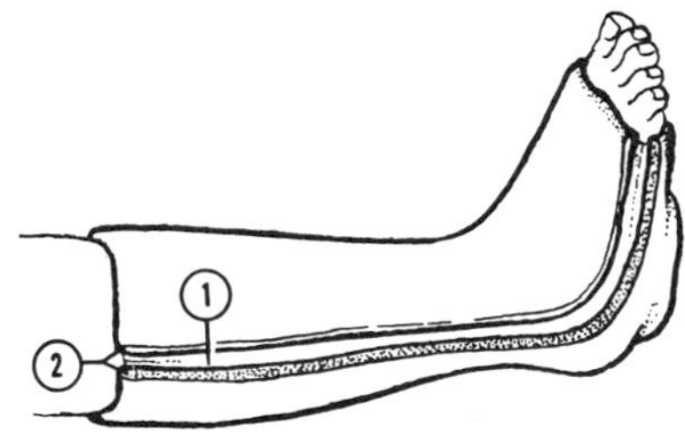

3. Bivalved cast can be wrapped loosely, and the limb should be elevated for 5–7 days. During this time, the foot should be checked periodically for signs of compartment syndrome as a result of extreme swelling. If compartment syndrome develops, fasciotomy of the muscle compartments of the foot may be necessary.

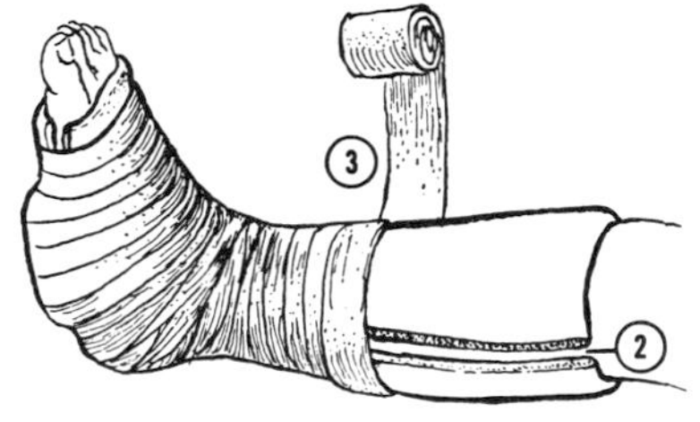

COMPLICATIONS

Compartment Syndrome After Severe Fractures to the Distal Tibia and Ankle

REMARKS

Extreme swelling of severe fractures about the ankle can lead to compartment syndrome of the foot.

This is particularly true if the patient has allowed the foot to hang dependently and has not elevated the limb to diminish swelling.

The diagnosis of compartment syndrome of the foot is made on the basis of severe pain, tight swelling, paralysis, and loss of function similar to that described previously in regard to compartment syndromes (see Chapter 1).

If this condition develops after a severe injury, release of the fascial compartments of the foot may be necessary.

Fasciotomy for Compartment Syndrome of the Foot

1. Multiple dorsal incisions can be used to release the fascia of the tightly swollen compartments of the foot.
2. The area of the fasciotomy can be temporarily covered by fine mesh gauze. This compression dressing is also used to minimize edema. The wound can later be closed with a split-thickness skin graft.

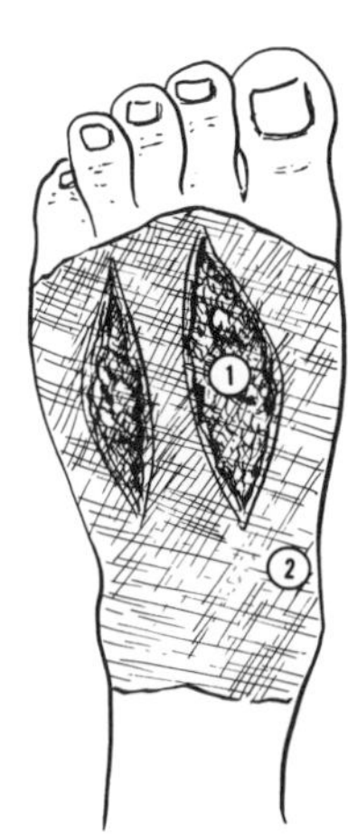

Irreducible Fractures of the Lateral Malleolus

REMARKS

In rare instances, widening of the ankle mortise may not be corrected entirely by reduction of the lateral malleolus.

This may be the result of rupture of the medial ligament or avulsion of the medial malleolus with displacement of the posterior tibial tendon or posterior tibial artery and nerve between the intact portion of the medial malleolus and the talus.

Always suspect such a possibility when, in a fracture of the lateral malleolus with lateral displacement of the talus, the talus cannot be accurately reduced.

Prereduction X-Ray

1. Fracture of the lateral malleolus.
2. Lateral shift of the talus.
3. Avulsion of the tip of the medial malleolus.

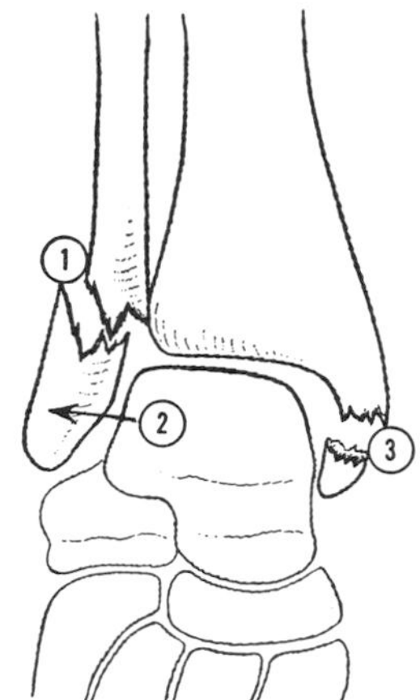

Pathologic Findings

1. Posterior tibial tendon is trapped between the medial malleolus and the talus.
2. Talus is displaced laterally.
3. There is a fracture of the lateral malleolus.
4. There is an avulsion of the tip of the medial malleolus.

Note: This requires operative correction.

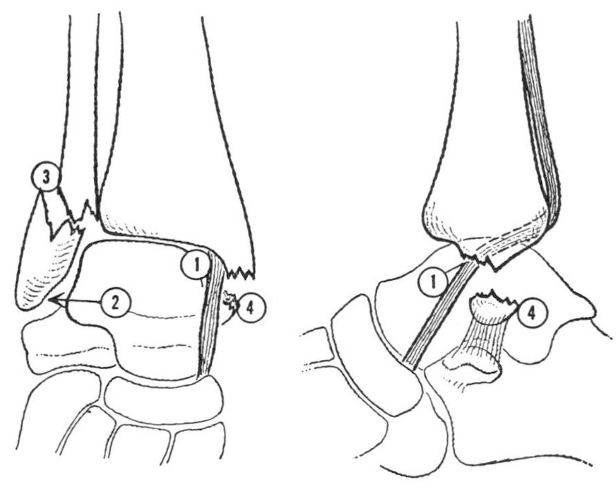

Postreduction X-Ray After Operative Reduction

1. Talus is in its normal position in the mortise.
2. Lateral malleolus is secured by screws.
3. Medial malleolus is secured by a screw.
4. Articular surfaces of the talus and the tibia are congruous.

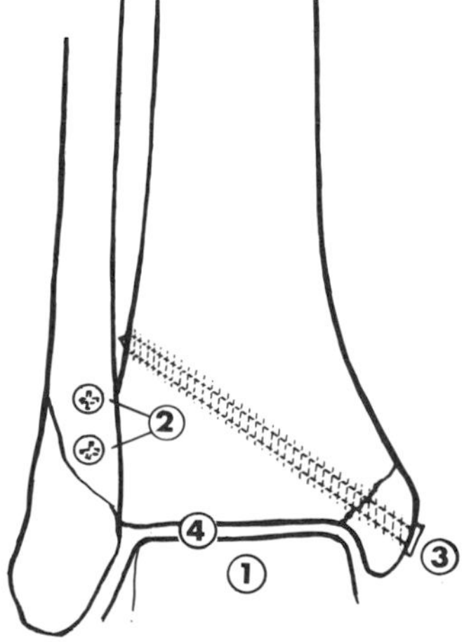

Irreducible Posterior Fracture-Dislocation of the Ankle Joint (Bosworth Fracture)

REMARKS

Occasionally, in posterior fracture-dislocations, the proximal end of the fractured fibula becomes displaced behind the tibia and locked there.

The usual mechanism is a severe external rotational injury, which forces the talus back out of the mortise. The fibula generally sustains a characteristic S-EX fracture with the fracture line running from the distal anterior cortex to the proximal posterior cortex. The fibula may sometimes remain intact and become dislocated behind the tibia.

Most often, the proximal fibular fragment becomes trapped, either in the posterolateral ridge of the tibia with a posterior malleolar fracture, or in the interosseous membrane.

Once the fibula is freed from its entrapment, it will snap back into correct position.

Owing to the extreme rotation of the foot, the x-ray may be misleading. The anteroposterior x-ray may be mistaken for a lateral one or vice versa. The relationship of the tibia to the proximal fibular fragment may be considered normal or caused by improper positioning. Correct orientation, particularly if the knee joint is included on the x-ray, will prevent the physician's being misled by the position of the fibula, malleolus, and talus.

Mayer and Evarts showed that, with a correct diagnosis, closed reduction is possible by traction and medial rotation of the foot while the fibular shaft is pressed on laterally.

If closed reduction fails, a lateral approach to the fractured fibula is sufficient to allow adequate reduction and internal fixation of the injury.

Prereduction X-Ray

LATERAL VIEW

1. Medial malleolus.
2. Lateral malleolus is rotated externally and is not superimposed on the medial malleolus as it should be in a normal lateral.
3. Distal end of the fibular shaft is trapped posteriorly.
4. Typical oblique fracture of the fibula (S-EX mechanism).
5. Position of the patella aids in the proper orientation of the x-ray.

ANTEROPOSTERIOR VIEW

1. Medial malleolus.
2. Lateral malleolus and fibular shaft are displaced posteriorly.
3. Foot is rotated externally.

Note: If true anteroposterior and lateral views are not used, the overlap may not be demonstrated on the anteroposterior view, and the posterior displacement may not be demonstrated on the lateral view.

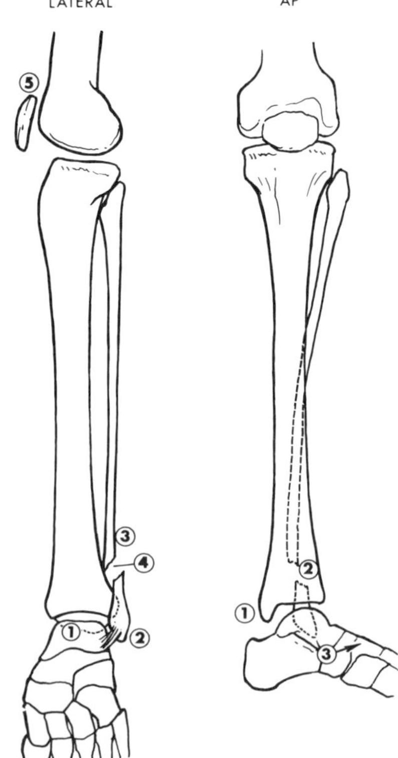

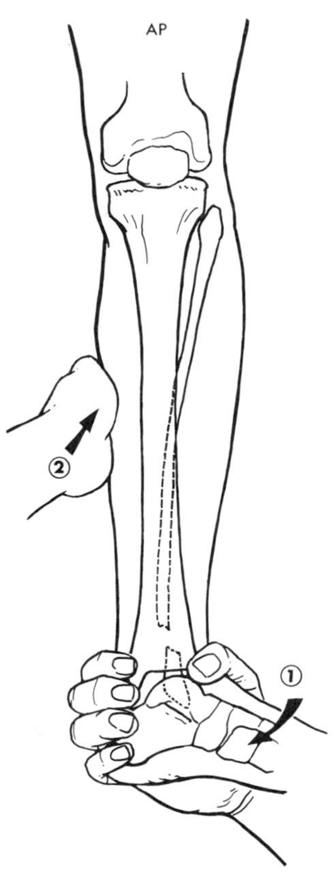

Technique of Closed Reduction (After Mayer and Evarts)

Under adequate anesthesia, the

1. Surgeon's right hand is used to apply axial traction and to rotate the foot internally.
2. Heel of the surgeon's left hand applies an anterolaterally directed force to the fibula.

A snap is heard as the ankle reduces; usually, the joint returns to a stable and acceptable position.

If a fracture of the fibula or medial malleolus remains displaced, internal fixation should then be carried out.

Subsequently, a long-leg cast is applied, and the injury is treated as previously described.

If closed reduction is not possible, open reduction should be performed by a lateral approach.

■ Vascular Impairment That Results From Posterior Fracture-Dislocation of the Ankle

Tipton and D'Ambrosia reported that the dorsalis pedis artery can be trapped by the extensor retinaculum with posterior dislocation of the fibula. This is especially serious if there is also a simultaneous injury to the posterior tibial artery.

Prompt reduction of the fibula releases the entrapped vessel and restores distal arterial flow.

Prereduction Relationship

1. Posterior dislocation of the fibula
2. Tightens the extensor retinaculum and
3. Traps the dorsalis pedis artery. Closed reduction should be done promptly as described in the preceding section.

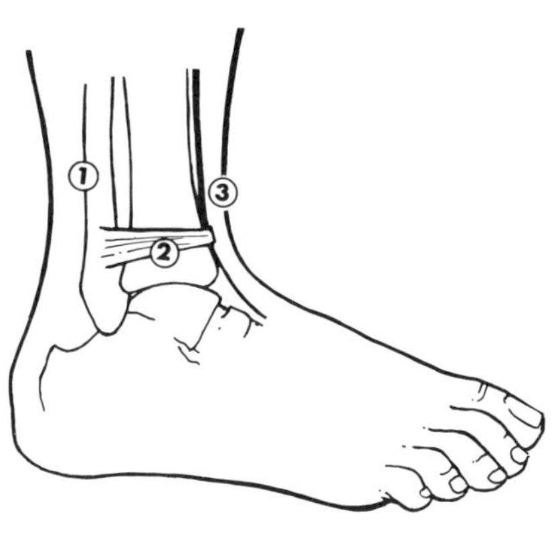

Postreduction Relationship

1. Fibula is restored to normal position.
2. Extensor retinaculum is no longer tight.
3. Release of the dorsalis pedis artery restores distal flow to normal.

Note: If the posterior fibular dislocation cannot be reduced by closed manipulation, perform operative reduction promptly.

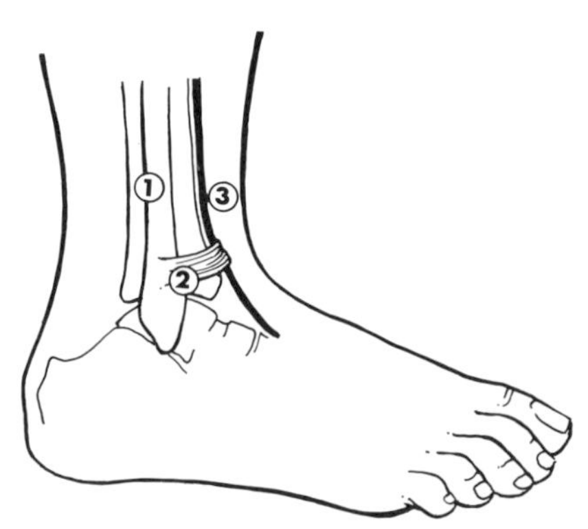

Open Fractures and Fracture-Dislocations of the Ankle Joint

REMARKS

Because of the superficial position of the malleoli, marked displacement of the foot to one side or the other frequently causes rupture of the soft tissues and skin on the side opposite the displacement.

A fall from a height may drive the ends of the tibia and the fibula through the skin.

Circulation to the skin in this area is frequently tenuous, particularly in older patients. Further skin loss or excision should be avoided during wound management.

The principles of management for open ankle fractures are the same as those outlined for open tibial fractures (see Chapter 9). After thorough irrigation and cleansing of the contaminated wound, most should be left open and drained adequately.

Prophylactic broad-spectrum antibiotics are indicated as an adjunctive measure but should not be substituted for thorough wound cleansing. Repetition of debridement and cleaning of the ankle fracture should be planned within 2–3 days postoperatively and secondary closure carried out.

If the ankle itself is unstable, internal fixation may be used on the side opposite from the open wound.

Open ankle fractures carry a poorer prognosis for healing and restoration of ankle function than do similar closed fractures; however, if infection is avoided and adequate ankle stability is achieved, the surgeon may anticipate satisfactory results.

Typical Case

1. Ragged open wound on the outer aspect of the ankle.
2. Foot is markedly inverted.
3. Fractured end of the fibula and the articular surface of the tibia are exposed.

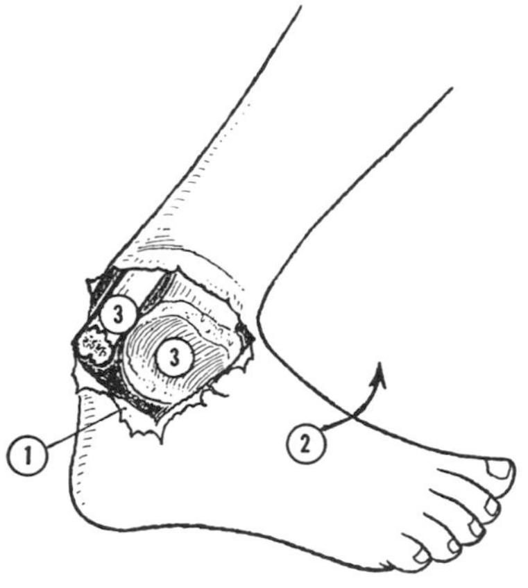

Prereduction X-Ray

1. Talus is displaced upward and inward.
2. Medial and lateral malleoli have followed the talus.
3. Exposed end of the proximal fragment of the fibula.

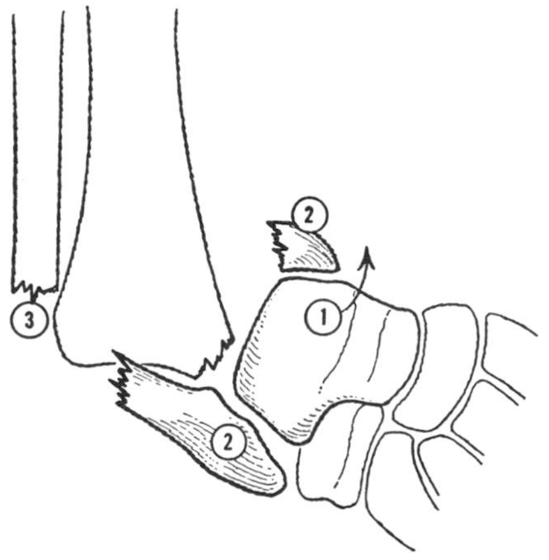

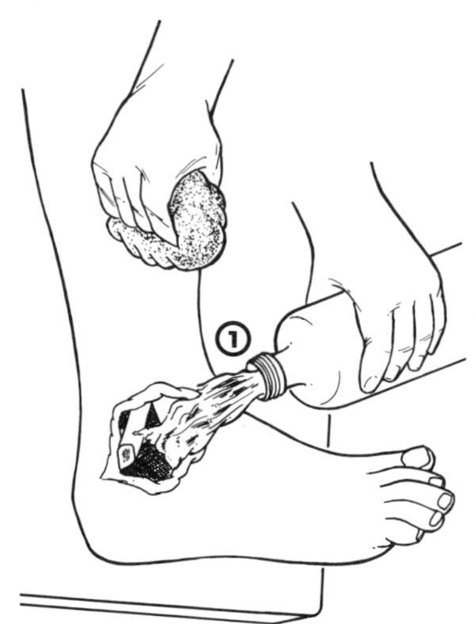

Preparation of the Area (Under Anesthesia)

1. Initial irrigation should be with copious amounts of water to cleanse the leg of all dirt accumulated at the time of injury. This is purely a mechanical washing requiring 10–15 L of fluid.

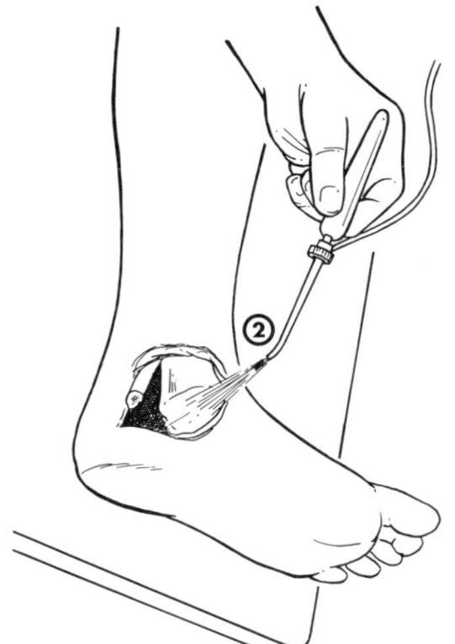

2. Pressure irrigation system is helpful to remove dirt fixed in deep tissue and bone after the injury.

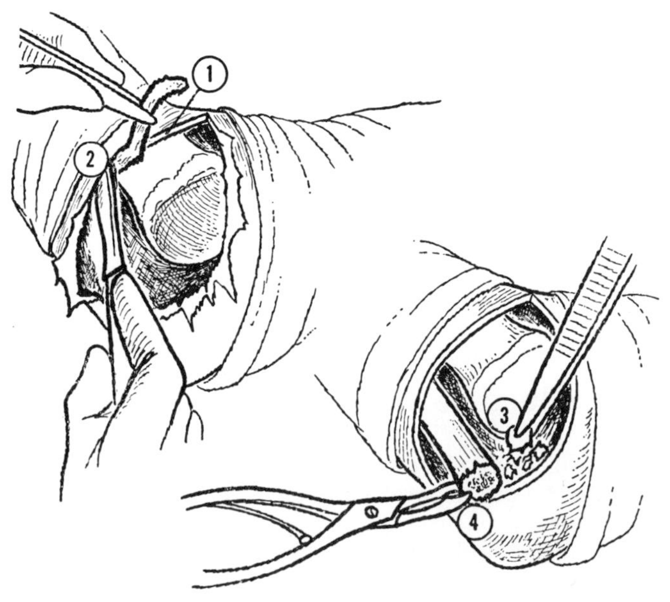

1. Excise the skin edges but spare as much skin as possible.
2. Excise all devitalized soft tissue.
3. Bone excision should be minimal. Remove only loose small bits and pieces. Large loose fragments should be thoroughly cleansed and reinserted into the fracture site to help in stabilization.
4. Remove contaminated dirty ends of bone with a rongeur or a sharp curette.

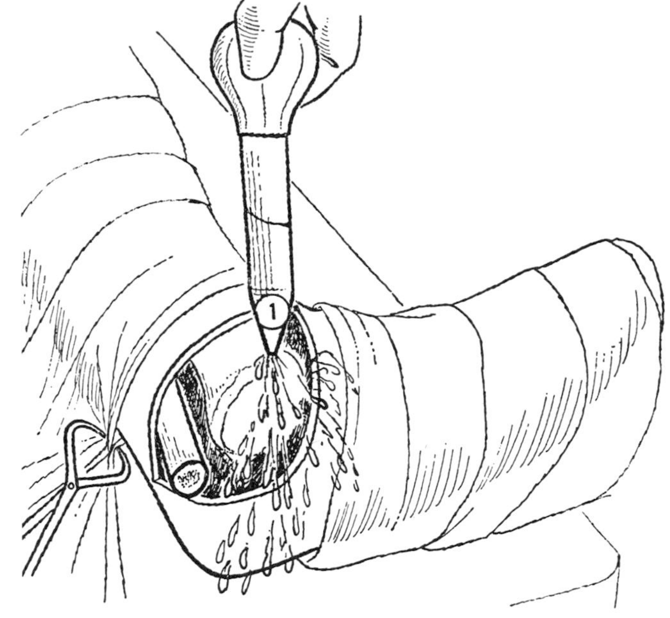

1. Before reducing the fracture, flush the wound again with 8–10 L of saline followed by an antibiotic solution that contains broad-spectrum antibiotics.

Reduction

Depending on the type of dislocation or fracture-dislocation, use the same methods depicted for the closed lesions of the same types.

Give preference to methods that do not use internal fixation if at all possible.

After reduction, the

1. Wound over the ankle is left open but held with 3–0 stainless steel wire suture to prevent retraction of the wound edges.
2. Drain is inserted into the ankle wound to encourage adequate drainage.

Note: Most of these wounds are extremely contaminated and require repeat frequent debridements within 24–48 hours after initial debridement. Secondary closure may be accomplished at that time if the wound is clean. In addition, start broad-spectrum antibiotics to cover the wide number of organisms that can contaminate these wounds and adjust the antibiotic coverage until the wounds are healed satisfactorily.

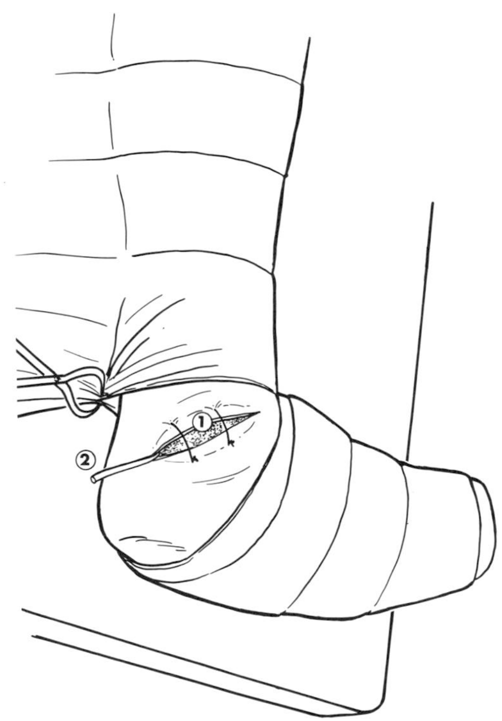

Stabilization of the Unstable Open Ankle Fracture

REMARKS

If the open wound of the medial or lateral malleolus is not contaminated and is grade I, internal fixation may be carried out after primary wound debridement.

For the grossly contaminated grade II or III wounds, the preferred treatment now is a temporary period of external fixation.

If an external fixator is not suitable or available, the pins-in-plaster technique may be used.

When the soft tissue wounds have healed adequately, delayed internal fixation may be carried out to stabilize the unstable injury.

Rarely, with very unstable, open, transarticular injuries, a vertical pin may be the only method suitable for stabilization.

Ilizarov External Fixator for Unstable Ankle Fractures

1. Ilizarov technique for the treatment of unstable fractures is also valuable with the open injury.
2. Apparatus uses three rings.
3. Small malleolar fractures can be reduced by olive wires connected to the appropriate ring.

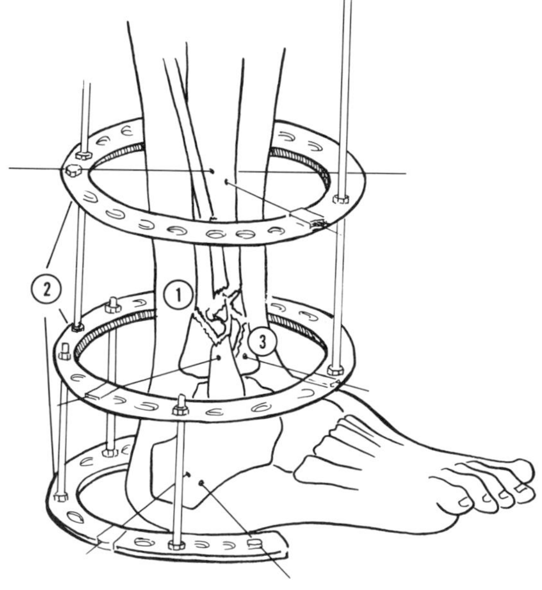

Technique of Steinmann Pin Fixation (Pins-in-Plaster Technique)

The fracture is manipulated, and x-rays are taken in the operating room after wound treatment to show adequate reduction of the fracture.

1. Then, a 3-mm smooth Steinmann pin is inserted into the proximal tibia just distal to the tibial tuberosity.
2. Second pin is inserted 2 cm distal and 2 cm posterior to the tip of the lateral malleolus transversely through the calcaneus.
3. Then, 2-cm^2 felt pads are placed about the exit points of each pin.
4. Cast is applied that incorporates the Steinmann pins while it holds the reduction of the fracture.

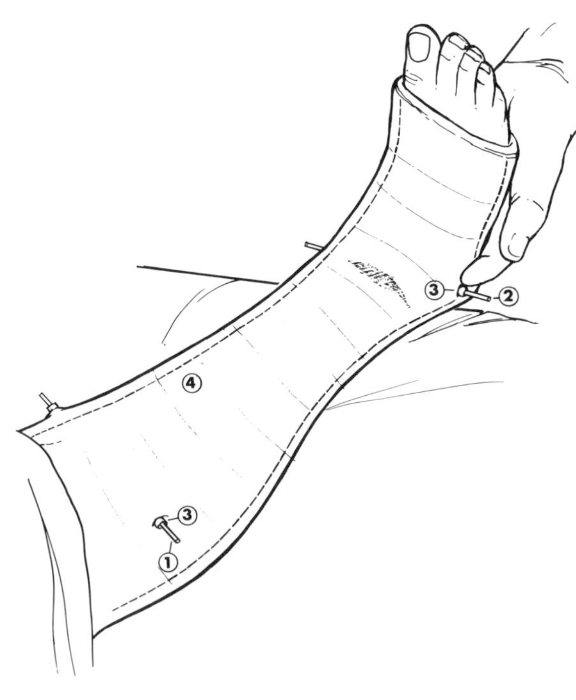

Alternative Method: Vertical Transarticular Pin Fixation (After Childress)

Note: This technique should be restricted to injuries with extensive skin loss.

1. Fracture-dislocation of the ankle is reduced, and the foot is placed in slight equinus. This aids in directing the pin toward the posterior portion of the talus.
2. Kirschner wire is drilled 10 cm upward through the calcaneus into the talus but does not cross the ankle joint. This pin is aimed toward the center of the tibia and should contact the inferior region of the calcaneus about 2.5 cm posterior to the calcaneocuboid joint.

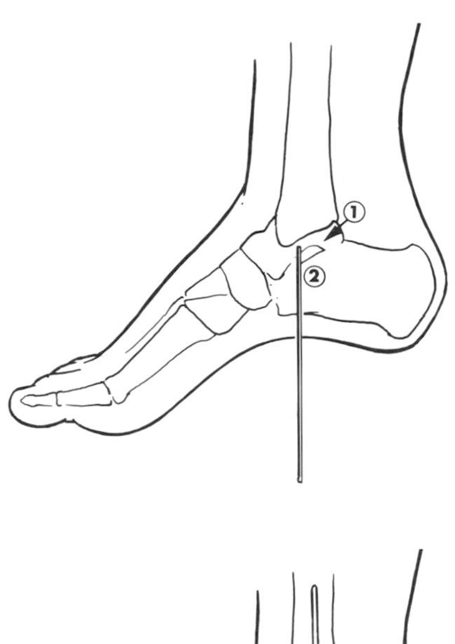

Note: X-rays in two planes are then taken to determine the adequacy of the reduction and the location of the wire. If it is decided to use the vertical pin, the Kirschner wire is used as a guide, and a 3-mm Steinmann pin is inserted with an air-powered drill.

1. Steinmann pin is driven into the distal tibia, and the
2. Pin is allowed to protrude 2.5 cm through the skin; this is bent at a right angle.

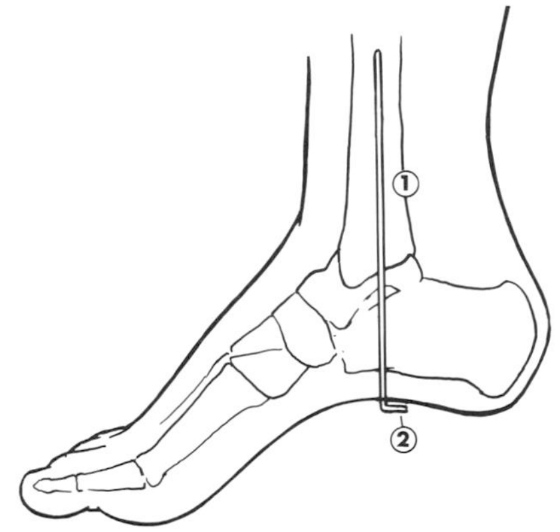

Note: The transarticular pin should not be incorporated in the plaster, and all weight bearing should be prevented until the pin is removed.

Alternative Method: Immediate or Delayed Internal Fixation

If the open ankle fracture is a grade I, which has been adequately debrided, internal fixation may be carried out initially. The open wound should be left open or drained adequately to avoid abscess formation.

It is preferable, if possible, to apply the internal fixation away from the open wound. For example, the usual bimalleolar fracture, which is open on the medial side, can be stabilized by fixing lateral malleolus.

When in doubt about the extent of the soft tissue wound, avoid primary internal fixation. If the wound is healing sufficiently by 7–10 days, delayed internal fixation may be carried out once there is no evidence of infection.

Example of Internal Fixation of Open Fracture

POSTREDUCTION X-RAY

1. Bimalleolar fracture that was open on the lateral side can be stabilized by medial fixation.
2. Talus and ankle mortise have been reduced, and the wound has been left open on the open lateral side. Supplemental cast support is used over the lateral open injury.

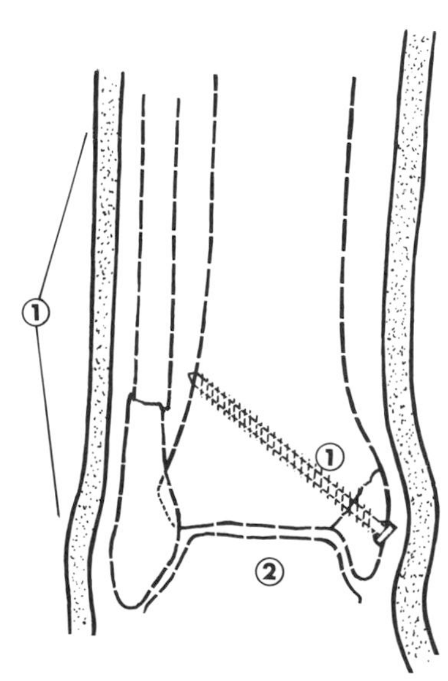

Malunion, Traumatic Arthritis, and Neuropathic (Charcot) Joint

REMARKS

Although most ankle fractures heal satisfactorily, the complications can be diverse and many.

Malunion, when it occurs, is usually the result of shortening and rotational angulation of the lateral malleolus or fibula.

Traumatic arthritis can occur, particularly from a shearing type of injury, which damages the articular surface (see Coonrad fracture).

An increasingly common complication seen with an ankle fracture in diabetic patients is a neuropathic joint problem. This can result even from undisplaced ankle fractures in the patient with juvenile diabetes and loss of autonomic control of the vascular response to the injury. This results in rapid bone destruction rather than bone formation after the injury.

Malunited Fractures of the Ankle

REMARKS

A number of studies have tried to identify factors that lead to unsatisfactory outcomes after ankle fracture. Consistently, the two predominant factors are the amount of initial injury to the ankle joint surface and the reduction achieved by closed or open means.

P-EX mechanisms are associated frequently with greater displacement of the mortise and a slightly higher frequency of subsequent arthritis. S-EX mechanisms tend to produce less disruption and less unsatisfactory outcomes.

Open fractures of the ankle are more likely to develop symptomatic arthritis and an unsatisfactory result than are closed fractures.

Ankle fractures that occur in patients with type I diabetes are notorious in producing complications and unsatisfactory outcomes from either infections or neurotrophic joint changes. They should be managed cautiously and with prolonged non–weight-bearing techniques to avoid, if possible, these unsatisfactory complications.

In most instances, a good anatomic reduction and stabilization of the ankle injury leads to a satisfactory outcome. Unfortunately, this is not always true. Grossly displaced fractures that shear the articular surface can result in early joint breakdown despite perfect anatomic reduction and internal fixation. These patients tend to have a painful ankle early on after the injury, which persists, worsens, and eventually leads to arthrodesis.

The painful ankle from traumatic arthritis should be distinguished from the ankle that is painful as a result of malreduction. These latter problems can be managed with corrective osteotomy to restore the normal ankle mortise and maintain ankle joint function without the necessity of an arthrodesis.

Example of Traumatic Arthritis After Internal Fixation

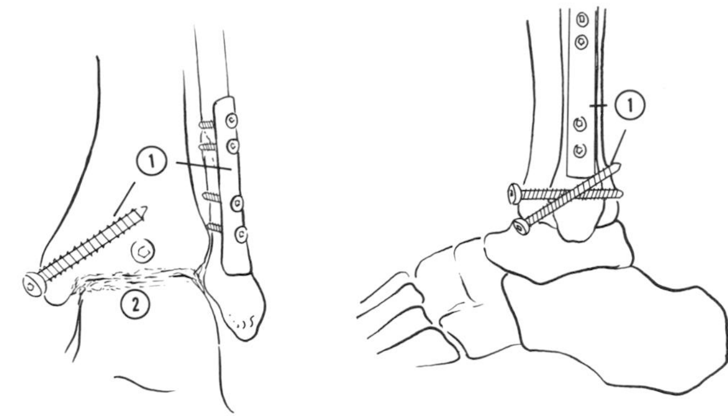

1. P-EX fracture has been stabilized adequately by medial and lateral fixation.
2. Nevertheless, the injury that sheared off the weight-bearing surface has resulted in symptomatic traumatic arthritis, which requires arthrodesis.

Examples of Malunited Fracture-Dislocation Requiring Arthrodesis

Example of Malunion and Persistent Subluxation That Requires Arthrodesis

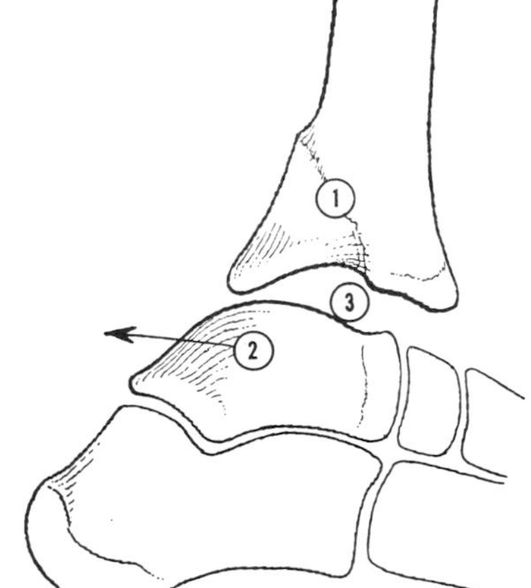

1. Posterior malleolar fracture has healed in the displaced position.
2. Talus has not been reduced and is chronically dislocated posteriorly.
3. Result is constant wear on the articular surface, which causes early breakdown.

Note: The unreduced posterior malleolus is a common contributing factor to early ankle joint breakdown.

Subsequent Breakdown One Year After Injury

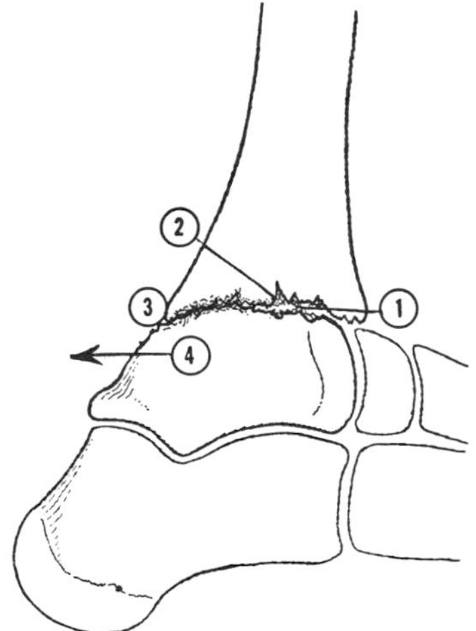

1. Malposition of the ankle has resulted in breakdown of the articular surface.
2. Joint surface is worn out promptly and causes chronic pain.
3. Joint spaces are obliterated.
4. Talus remains in a posterior displaced position.

The preferred treatment to reduce symptoms at this stage is arthrodesis; malunited fracture seen at an earlier stage may be treated by osteotomy.

Examples of Malunited Fractures That Require Corrective Osteotomy

REMARKS

An occasional fracture of the ankle causes persistent aching because of incomplete reduction of the mortise.

Typically, this is due to persistent shortening and external rotation of the fibula. This results in the lateral shifting of the talus and causes the patient pain with weight bearing or prolonged standing.

If this is the case, corrective osteotomy and reconstruction should be considered, no matter what the duration postinjury, if arthritic changes are minimal.

Pain and diminished activity with a malunited fracture is a clear indication for reconstruction.

Such reconstructive procedures, which include correction of the fibular length and rotation and fixation of any nonunions, are well worth considering before an arthrodesis.

The deformity should be carefully evaluated by a measurement of the talocrural (tibiotalar) angle compared with the opposite side to determine the amount of correction needed.

Malreduction Four Months After P-EX Fracture

1. P-EX fracture of the fibula healed with the fibula shortened and externally rotated. This allowed persistent lateral and external displacement of the talus.
2. There is widening of the tibiofibular joint.
3. Patient suffers persistent discomfort with weight bearing because of the rotated malposition of the foot and ankle.
4. There is persistent widening of the medial clear space, but the articular surface has minimal if any signs of arthritis.

Note: This problem requires lengthening of the fibula and correction of the rotational alignment. The medial joint space should also be explored to move any of the deltoid or capsular ligaments that have been trapped in the joint medially.

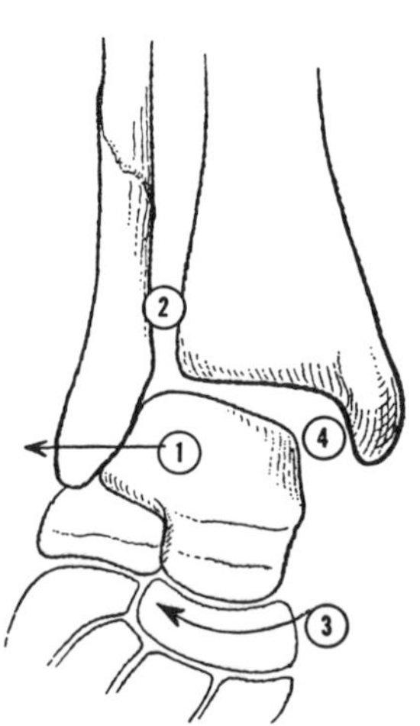

Measurement of Crural Angle

The talocrural angle is formed by the intersection of two lines, i.e.,

1. One drawn parallel to the tibial articular surface and
2. One drawn between the tips of the two malleoli on the mortise view.
3. Ankle control measurement varies between 8°–15°.

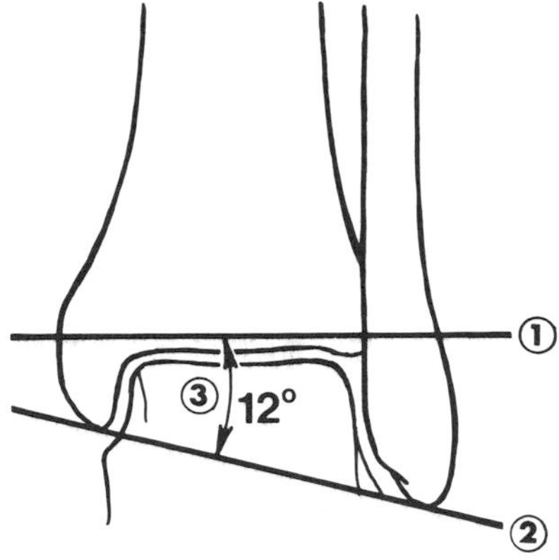

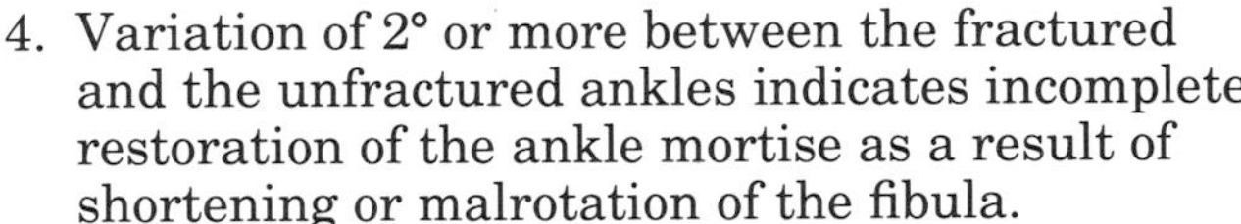

4. Variation of 2° or more between the fractured and the unfractured ankles indicates incomplete restoration of the ankle mortise as a result of shortening or malrotation of the fibula.

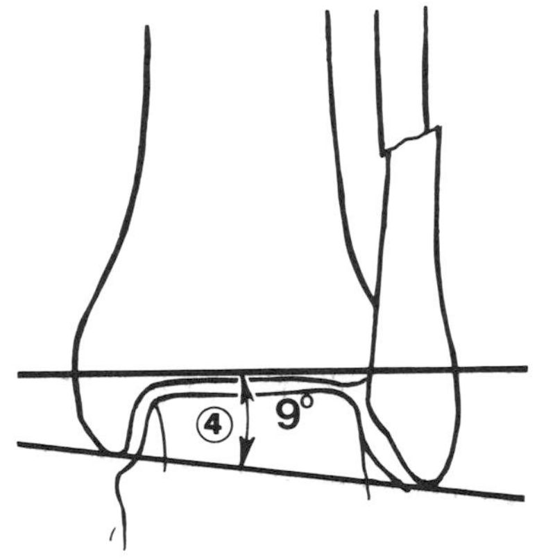

X-Ray After Corrective Osteotomy

1. Fibula has been restored to length by an osteotomy. A bone graft has been used to fill in the space produced by the lengthening osteotomy.
2. Distal tibiofibular syndesmosis has been closed and supported with temporary screw fixation.
3. Clear space in the ankle mortise has been restored to normal by medial debridement of scar tissue in the mortise and repair of the deltoid ligament.

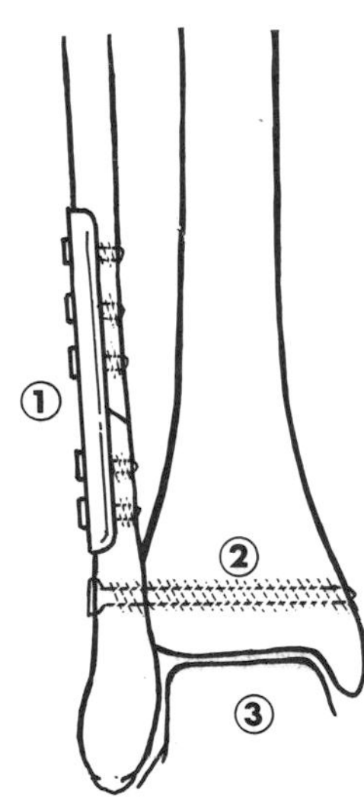

Ankle Fractures Associated With Neuropathic (Charcot) Joints and Other Complications in Diabetic Patients

An Indication for Primary Internal Stabilization

REMARKS

Ankle fractures in adults with juvenile-onset diabetes are notoriously prone to severe complications and deformities.

The tendency has been to treat many of these injuries nonoperatively with a cast because of diabetes and fear of infection. However, when this approach is used, severe swelling, bone resorption, and skeletal deformity that causes pressure sores and subsequent infection often occur.

In a number of these unfortunate patients, the complications have been so severe that below-the-knee amputation has resulted.

Swelling in the diabetic patient has led to gas gangrene in several cases, despite the initial closed nature of the ankle fracture.

An additional complicating factor with these patients is that, in an effort to protect the fractured ankle treated in a cast, the patient bears weight on the opposite uninjured side and rapidly breaks down the opposite ankle.

The susceptibility to these severe complications is typical of the patient with juvenile-onset diabetes but may also occur in those with adult-onset diabetes.

Although commonly the neuropathic changes have been attributed to a loss of protective sensation, a more tenable explanation of the pathologic findings is loss of neurovascular control of blood flow. Hyperemia in these patients who have lost autonomic control of peripheral circulation leads to rapid bone resorption and destruction after minor injuries about the ankle or foot.

Because of this abnormal response to injury and the unsatisfactory outcome of ankle fractures treated nonoperatively, early internal stabilization is recommended for the undisplaced ankle fracture in the adult patient with juvenile-onset diabetes.

Neuropathic Arthropathy in a Diabetic Patient After Undisplaced Bimalleolar Fractures

1. Minimally displaced ankle fracture is treated by closed reduction and cast application in a diabetic patient.
2. Within 5 months, the fracture develops bone resorption and deformity consistent with neuropathic joint changes secondary to extensive bone resorption rather than bone formation.

Note: Ankle fractures in diabetic patients are notorious for developing complications such as this. This is true even with relatively undisplaced injuries. Although operative internal fixation is the treatment of choice for fractures of the ankle in diabetic patients, neurotrophic changes are still possible, even with anatomic reduction.

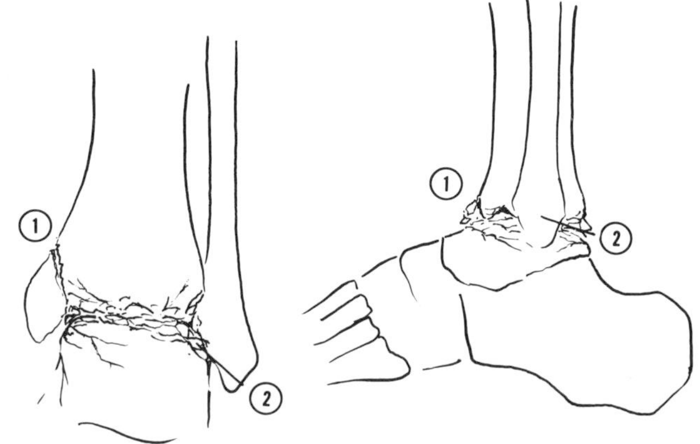

BIBLIOGRAPHY

Ankle Anatomy and Biomechanics of Injury

Close JR: Some applications of the functional anatomy of the ankle joint. J Bone Joint Surg Am 38:761, 1956.

Goergen TG, Danzig LA, Resnick D, et al: Roentgenographic evaluation of the tibiotalar joint. J Bone Joint Surg Am 59:874, 1977.

Lauge-Hansen N: Fractures of the ankle. Arch Surg 60:957, 1950.

Lauge-Hansen N: Fractures of the ankle. Arch Surg 67:813, 1953.

Needleman RL, Skrade DA, Stiehl JB: Effect of the syndesmotic screw on ankle motion. Foot Ankle 10:17, 1989.

Pankovich AM: Fractures of the fibula proximal to the distal tibiofibular syndesmosis. J Bone Joint Surg Am 60:221, 1978.

Ramsey PL, Hamilton W: Changes in tibiotalar area of contact caused by lateral talar shift. J Bone Joint Surg Am 58:356, 1976.

Riegels-Nielsen P, Christensen J, Greiff J: The stability of the tibiofibular syndesmosis following rigid internal fixation for type C malleolar fractures: An experimental and clinical study. Injury 14:357, 1983.

Rolfe B, Nordt W, Sallis JG, et al: Assessing fibular length using bimalleolar angular measurements. Foot Ankle 10:104, 1989.

Staples O: Injuries to the medial ligaments of the ankle. J Bone Joint Surg Am 42:1287, 1960.

Stiehl JB, Skrade DA, Johnson RP: Experimentally produced ankle fractures in autopsy specimens. Clin Orthop 285:244, 1992.

Yablon IG, Heller FG, Shouse L: The key role of the lateral malleolus in displaced fractures of the ankle. J Bone Joint Surg Am 59:169, 1977.

Yde J: The Lauge-Hansen classification of malleolar fracture. Acta Orthop Scand 51:181, 1980.

Ankle Sprains

Amis JA, Gangl PM: When inversion injury is more than a "sprained ankle." J Musculoskeletal Med 68, 1987.

Berg EE: The symptomatic os subfibulare. J Bone Joint Surg Am 73:1251, 1991.

Burkus JK, Sella EJ, Southwick WO: Occult injuries of the talus diagnosed by bone scan and tomography. Foot Ankle 4:316, 1984.

Cass JR, Morrey BF, Katoh Y, et al: Ankle instability: Comparison of primary repair and delayed reconstruction after long-term follow-up study. Clin Orthop 198:110, 1985.

Chrisman OD, Snook GA: Reconstruction of lateral ligament tears of the ankle. J Bone Joint Surg Am 51:904, 1969.

Cox JS: Surgical and nonsurgical treatment of acute ankle sprains. Clin Orthop 198:118, 1985.

Dameron TB: Management of acute ankle sprains. South Med J 70:1166, 1977.

Edwards GS, DeLee JC: Ankle diastasis without fracture. Foot Ankle 4:305, 1984.

Freeman MAR, Dean MRE, Hanham IWF: The etiology and prevention of functional instability of the foot. J Bone Joint Surg Br 47:678, 1965.

Fritschy D, Junet CH, Bonvin JC: Functional treatment of severe ankle sprain. J Traumatol Sport 4:131, 1987.

Harrington KD: Degenerative arthritis of the ankle secondary to long-standing lateral ligament instability. J Bone Joint Surg Am 61:354, 1979.

Hawkins LG: Fracture of the lateral process of the talus. J Bone Joint Surg Am 47:1170, 1965.

Kannus P, Renstrom P: Treatment for acute tears of the lateral ligaments of the ankle. J Bone Joint Surg Am 73:305, 1991.

Keene JS, Lang RH: Diagnostic dilemmas in foot and ankle injuries. JAMA 256:247, 1986.

Konradsen L, Holmer P, Sondergaard L: Early mobilizing treatment for grade III ankle ligament injuries. Foot Ankle 12:69, 1991.

Kym MR, Worsing RA Jr: Compartment syndrome in the foot after an inversion injury to the ankle. A case report. J Bone Joint Surg Am 72:138, 1990.

Landeros O, Frost HM, Higgins CC: Post-traumatic anterior ankle instability. Clin Orthop 56:169, 1968.

Meals RA: Peroneal-nerve palsy complicating ankle sprain. J Bone Joint Surg 966, 1977.

Murr S: Dislocation of the peroneal tendons with marginal fracture of the lateral malleolus. J Bone Joint Surg Br 43:563, 1961.

Nitz AJ, Dobner JJ, Kersey D: Nerve injury and grades II and II ankle sprains. Am J Sports Med 13:177, 1985.

Nobel W: Peroneal palsy due to hematoma in the common peroneal nerve sheath after distal torsional fractures and inversion ankle sprains. J Bone Joint Surg Am 48:1484, 1966.

Paulos LE, Johnson CL, Noyes FR: Posterior compartment fractures of the ankle. A commonly missed athletic injury. Am J Sports Med 11:439, 1983.

Peterson DA, Stinson W: Excision of the fractured os peroneum: A report on five patients and review of the literature. Foot Ankle 13:277, 1992.

Steel J, McKnight D, Greenberg G, et al: Implementation of the Ottawa ankle rules. JAMA 1271:827, 1994.

Stover CN, Bryan DR: Traumatic dislocation of the peroneal tendons. Am J Surg 103:180, 1962.

Ankle Fractures

Ali MS, McLaren CAN, Rouholamin E, et al: Ankle fractures in the elderly: Nonoperative or operative treatment. J Orthop Trauma 1:275, 1987.

Bauer M, Bergstrom B, Hemborg A, et al: Malleolar fractures: Nonoperative versus operative treatment. Clin Orthop 199:17, 1985.

Bauer M, Jonsson K, Nilsson B: Thirty-year follow-up of ankle fractures. Acta Orthop Scand 56:103, 1985.

Beauchamp CG, Clay NR, Thexton PW: Displaced ankle fractures in patients over 50 years of age. J Bone Joint Surg Br 65:329, 1983.

Cedell C: Is closed treatment of ankle fractures advisable? Acta Orthop Scand 56:101, 1985.

Childress HM: Vertical transarticular pin fixation for unstable ankle fractures. Impressions after 16 years of experience. Clin Orthop 120:164, 1976.

Coonrad R: Fracture-dislocations of the ankle joint with impaction injury of the lateral weight-bearing surface of the tibia. J Bone Joint Surg Am 52:1337, 1970.

DeSouza LJ, Gustilo RB, Meyer TJ: Results of operative treatment of displaced external rotation-abduction fractures of the ankle. J Bone Joint Surg Am 67:1066, 1985.

Harper MG, Hardin G: Posterior malleolar fractures of the ankle associated with external rotation-abduction injuries: Results with and without internal fixation. J Bone Joint Surg Am 70:1348, 1988.

Jaskulka RA, Ittner G, Schedl R: Fractures of the posterior tibial margin: Their role in the prognosis of malleolar fractures. J Trauma 29:1565, 1989.

Kristensen KD, Hansen T: Closed treatment of ankle fractures. Acta Orthop Scand 56:107, 1985.

Lantz BA, McAndrew M, Scioli M, et al: The effect of concomitant chondral injuries accompanying operatively reduced malleolar fractures. J Orthop Trauma 5:125, 1991.

Laskin RS: Steinmann-pin fixation in the treatment of unstable fractures of the ankle. J Bone Joint Surg Am 56:549, 1974.

Matti L, Tunturi T: Improvement 2–9 years after ankle fracture. Acta Orthop Scand 61:80, 1990.

Pettrone FA, Gail M, Pee D, et al: Quantitative criteria for prediction of the results after displaced fracture of the ankle. J Bone Joint Surg Am 65:667, 1983.

Phillips WA, Schwartz HS, Keller CS, et al: A prospective, randomized study of the management of severe ankle fractures. J Bone Joint Surg Am 67:67, 1985.

Quigley TB: A simple aid to the reduction of abduction-external rotation fractures of the ankle. Am J Surg 97:488, 1959.

Rowley DI, Norris SH, Duckworth T: A prospective trial comparing operative and manipulative treatment of ankle fractures. J Bone Joint Surg Br 68:610, 1986.

Sarkisian JS, Cody GW: Closed treatment of ankle fractures: A new criterion for evaluation—A review of 250 cases. J Trauma 16:323, 1976.

Stiehl JB, Schwartz HS: Long-term results of pronation-external rotation ankle fracture-dislocations treated with anatomical open reduction, internal fixation. J Orthop Trauma 4:339, 1990.

Tipton WW, D'Ambrosia RD: Vascular impairment as a result of fracture dislocation of the ankle. J Trauma 15:524, 1975.

Yamaguchi K, Martin C, Boden S, et al: Operative treatment of syndesmotic disruptions without use of a syndesmotic screw. Foot Ankle Int 15:407, 1994.

Pilon or Comminuted Pronation-Dorsiflexion Fractures

Bourne RB, Rorabeck CH, Macnab J: Intra-articular fractures of the distal tibia: The pilon fracture. J Trauma 23:591, 1983.

Connolly J, Peterson D: Explosion pronation dorsiflexion fracture dislocation of the ankle—An indication for closed functional traction treatment. Nebr Med J 70:374, 1985.

Dillin L, Slabaugh P: Delayed wound healing, injection, and non-union following open reduction and internal fixation of tibial plafond fractures. J Trauma 26:1116, 1986.

Kellam JF, Waddell JP: Fractures of the distal tibial metaphysis with intra-articular extension—The distal tibial explosion fracture. J Trauma 19:593, 1979.

Moller BN, Krebs B: Intra-articular fractures of the distal tibia. Acta Orthop Scand 53:991, 1982.

Pierce RO Jr, Heinrich JH: Comminuted intra-articular fractures of the distal tibia. J Trauma 19:828, 1979.

Scheck M: Treatment of comminuted distal tibial fractures by combined dual-pin fixation and limited open reduction. J Bone Joint Surg Am 47:1537, 1965.

Complications

Bray TJ, Endicott M, Capra SE: Treatment of open ankle fractures. Immediate internal fixation vs closed immobilization and delayed fixation. Clin Orthop 140:47, 1989.

Brower AC, Allman RM: Pathogenesis of the neurotrophic joint: Neurotraumatic vs. neurovascular. Diagn Radiol 139:349, 1981.

Clohisy DR, Thompson RC: Fractures associated with neuropathic arthropathy in adults who have juvenile-onset diabetes. J Bone Joint Surg Am 70:1192, 1988.

Collins DN, Temple SD: Open joint injuries: Classification and treatment. Clin Orthop 243:48, 1989.

Fogel GR, Sim FH: Reconstruction of ankle malunion—Indications and results. Orthopedics 5:1471, 1982.

Franklin JL, Johnson KD, Hansen ST: Immediate internal fixation of open ankle fractures. J Bone Joint Surg Am 66:1349, 1986.

Hoblitzell RM, Ebraheim NA, Merrit T, et al: Bosworth fracture-dislocation of the ankle. A case report and review of the literature. Clin Orthop 255:257, 1990.

Kelbel M, Jardon OM: Rupture of tibialis posterior tendon in a closed ankle fracture. J Trauma 22:1026, 1982.

Kristiansen B: Ankle and foot fractures in diabetics provoking neuropathic joint changes. Acta Orthop Scand 51:975, 1980.

Marti RK, Raaymakers ELFB, Nolte PA: Malunited ankle fractures—The late results of reconstruction. J Bone Joint Surg Br 72:709, 1990.

Matsen FA, Clawson DK: The deep posterior compartmental syndrome of the leg. J Bone Joint Surg Am 57:34, 1975.

Mayer PJ, Evarts CM: Fracture dislocation of the ankle with posterior entrapment of the fibula behind the tibia. J Bone Joint Surg Am 60:320, 1978.

McMaster JH, Scranton PE: Tibiofibular synostosis. A cause of ankle disability. Clin Orthop 111:172, 1975.

Morrey BF, Wiedman GP: Complications and long-term results of ankle arthrodesis following trauma. J Bone Joint Surg Am 62:777, 1980.

Offierski CM, Graham JD, Hall JH, et al: Late revision of fibular malunion in ankle fractures. Clin Orthop 171:145, 1982.

Ritsema GH: Total talar dislocation. J Trauma 28:692, 1988.

Schatzker J, Johnson RG: Fracture-dislocation of the ankle with anterior dislocation of the fibula. J Trauma 23:420, 1983.

Segal D, Wasilewski S: Total dislocation of the talus. J Bone Joint Surg Am 62:1370, 1980.

Shelton ML, Anderson RL Jr: Complications of fractures and dislocations of the ankle. In Epps CH Jr (ed): *Complications in Orthopaedic Surgery*, 2nd ed. JB Lippincott, Philadelphia, 1986.

Soballe K, Kjaersgaard-Anderson P: Ruptured tibialis posterior tendon in a closed ankle fracture. Clin Orthop 231:140, 1988.

Stein RE: Rupture of the posterior tibial tendon in closed ankle fractures. Possible prognostic value of a medial bone flake: Report of two cases. J Bone Joint Surg Am 67:493, 1987.

Stiehl JB: Concomitant rupture of the peroneus brevis tendon and bimalleolar fracture. A case report. J Bone Joint Surg Am 70:936, 1988.

Tipton WW, D'Ambrosia RD: Vascular impairment as a result of fracture dislocation of the ankle. J Trauma 15:524, 1975.

Toohey JS, Worsing RA Jr: A long-term follow-up study of tibiotalar dislocations without associated fractures. Clin Orthop 239:207, 1989.

Ward AJ, Ackroyd CE, Baker AS: Late lengthening of the fibula for malaligned ankle fractures. J Bone Joint Surg Br 72:714, 1990.

Weber BG, Simpson LA: Corrective lengthening osteotomy of the fibula. Clin Orthop 199:61, 1985.

Wiss DA, Gilbert P, Merritt PO, et al: Immediate internal fixation of open ankle fractures. J Orthop Trauma 2:265, 1988.

Fractures and Fracture-Dislocations of the Bones of the Foot

FRACTURES AND DISLOCATIONS OF THE TALUS

REMARKS

The talus is subject to injury by mechanisms that can be attributed to the extremes of the motion that ordinarily occur between the foot and the leg. These include hyperextension, hyperflexion, inversion, eversion, and compression loading.

Mechanisms

Hyperextension Injuries

Hyperextension mechanisms produce fracture at the junction of the long, exposed talar neck and body.

Peterson and Romanus demonstrated that this fracture results from hyperextension loading on a plantar-flexing foot. Most commonly, this occurs when the victim pushes the foot downward against the floor of a motor vehicle or aircraft in preparing to crash.

The common denominator in all these injuries is the application of force to the plantar surface of the tarsometatarsal area of the foot.

Types of Talar Neck Fracture From Hyperextension Injury

Talar neck fractures from hyperextension injuries may be classified into one of four basic types, depending on the severity of the fracture and the displacement of head and neck fragments.

1. Brake pedal impacts against the arch of the plantar-flexed foot.
2. Extension loading is absorbed entirely by the exposed talar neck, causing it to fracture.
3. Impaction against the articular surface of the tibia is not necessary to produce talar fracture. Usually, the tibia is undamaged.

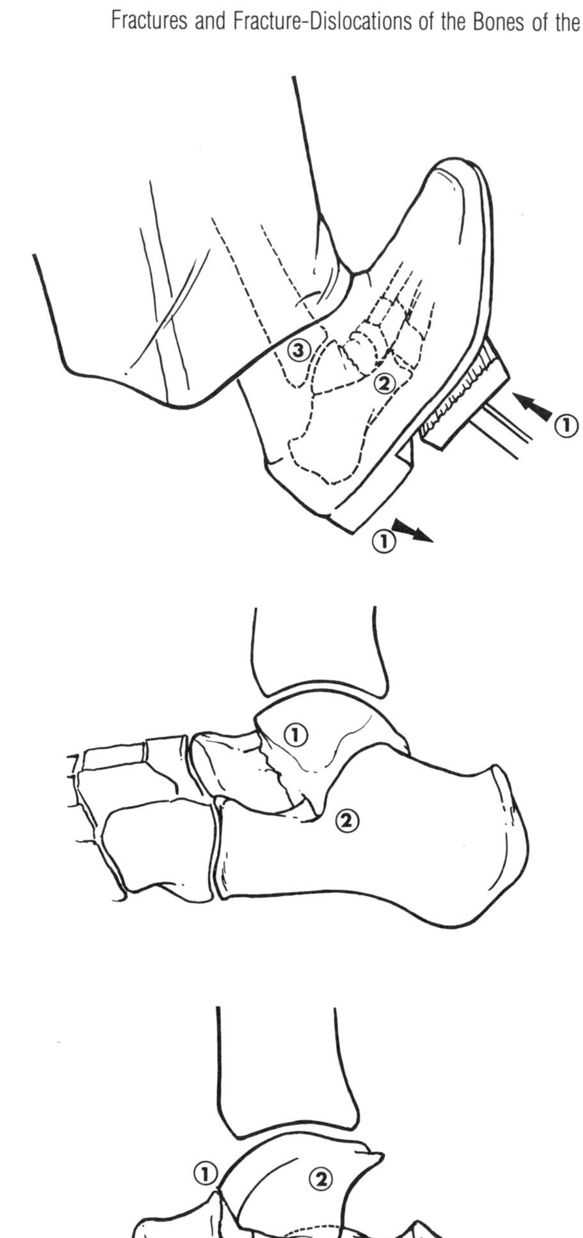

Type I: Undisplaced Fracture

1. Vertical neck fracture of the talus is undisplaced.
2. Subtalar joint is normal.

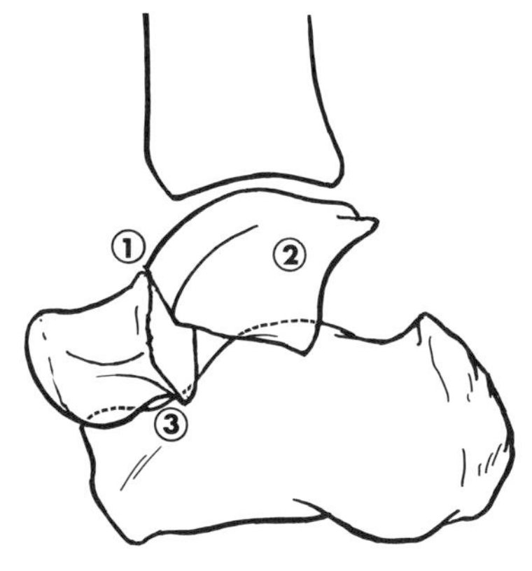

Type II: Displaced Fracture With Subtalar Dislocation or Subluxation

1. Displaced vertical neck fracture.
2. Body displaces, dislocates, or subluxates posteriorly and into equinus.
3. Calcaneus and the remaining portion of the foot subluxate anteriorly with the head fragment.

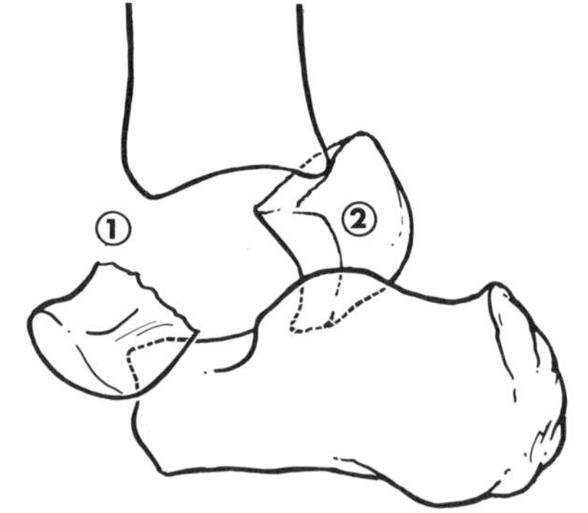

Type III: Displaced Fracture With Complete Dislocation of Body Out of Ankle Mortise

1. Vertical neck fracture is displaced.
2. Body of the talus has dislocated out of the subtalar joint and out of the ankle mortise.

Type IV: Fracture of the Talar Neck With Dislocation of the Body and Dislocation or Subluxation of the Head

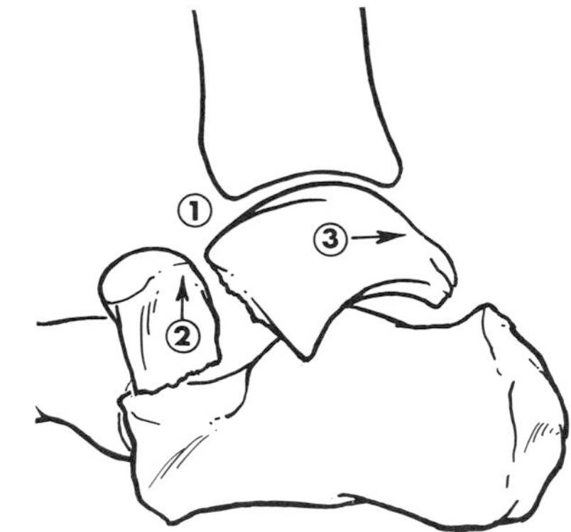

1. Grossly displaced vertical fracture of the neck.
2. Neck fragment is dislocated out of the talonavicular joint.
3. Body fragment subluxates from the subtalar joint or may completely dislocate out of the ankle.

Other Fractures From Hyperextension Injuries: Fractures of the Lateral Process of the Talus

Fractures of the lateral process of the talus are the second most common type of talar fracture, as reported by Hawkins.

The most plausible mechanism is severe hyperextension of an inverted foot. This causes the lateral facet of the calcaneus to shear off the posterior or lateral process of the talus.

This is usually an undisplaced fracture and frequently is not recognized or is confused with an ankle sprain (see Chapter 10.)

1. On the anteroposterior view, a transverse fracture of the lateral process may be obscure.
2. Fracture may be evident only on a lateral view.

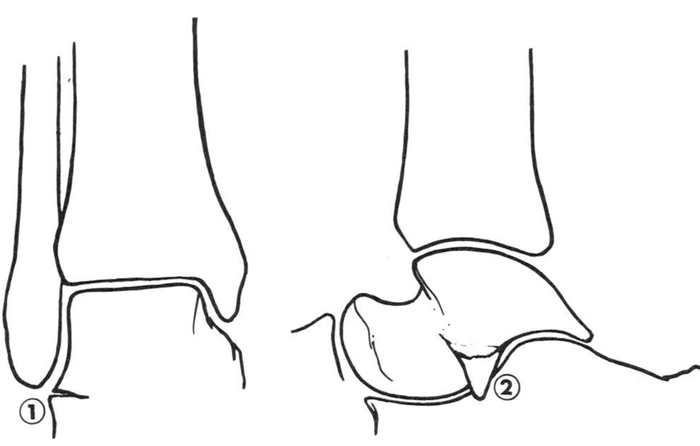

Hyperflexion Injuries

REMARKS

Flexion injuries occur when the force is applied to the heel of the foot behind the posterior tubercle of the talus.

This is a fairly common injury sustained by an athlete while jumping or kicking.

In plantar flexion, a blow to the back of the heel wedges the talus between the posterior calcaneal facet and the posterior tibial margin.

The result is either

1. Fracture of the posterior talar body or

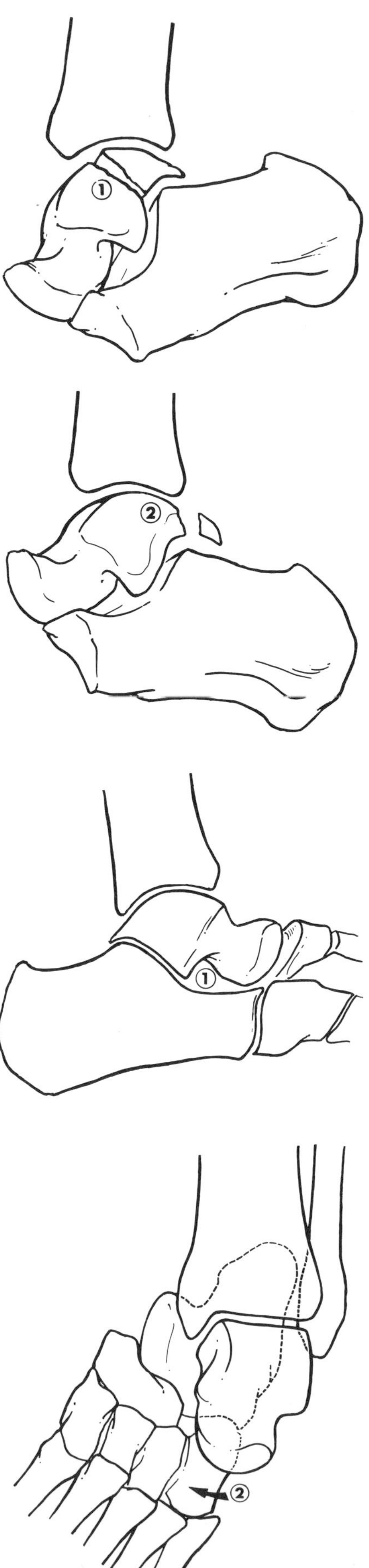

2. Fracture of the posterior talar tubercle.

Note: This undisplaced fracture may be confused with an os trigonum, which can be ruled out by views of the opposite, uninjured ankle.

Inversion Injuries

Forced inversion produces injuries such as

1. Sprain of the calcaneofibular, subtalar, or tibiocalcaneal ligament.

2. Medial dislocation of the subtalar joint.

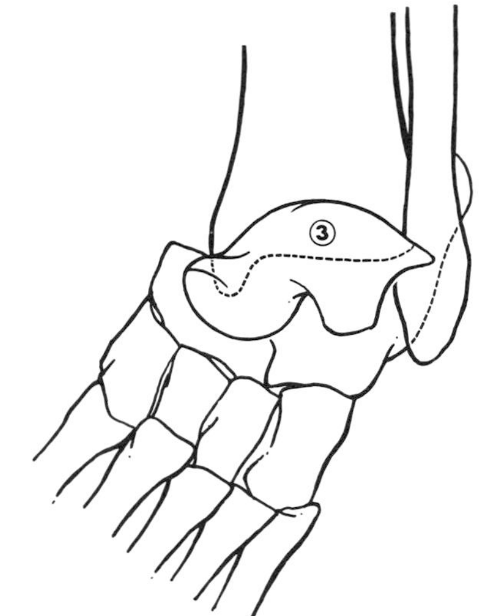

3. Complete anterior dislocation of the talus.

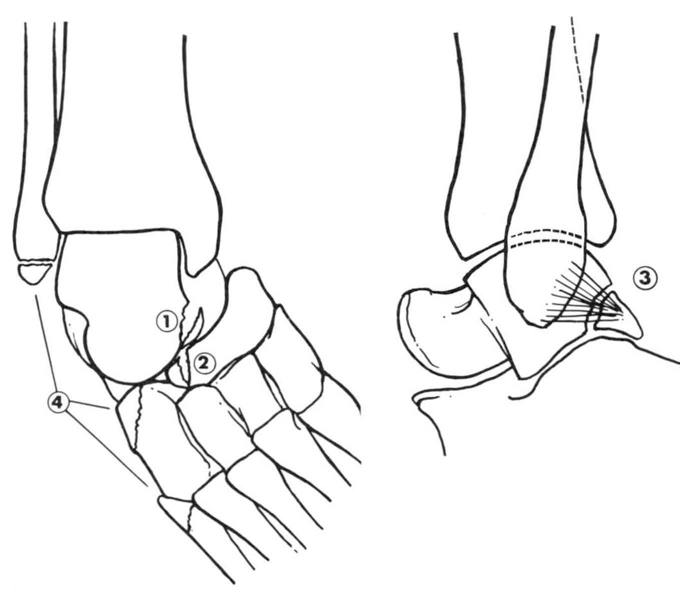

Fractures That Result From Inversion Injury and May Be Associated With Subtalar Dislocation

1. Vertical shear fracture off the talar head or neck.
2. Fracture of the navicular bone.
3. Fracture of the posterolateral talus resulting from avulsion by the posterior talofibular ligament.
4. Fracture of fifth metatarsal, cuboid, or fibula.

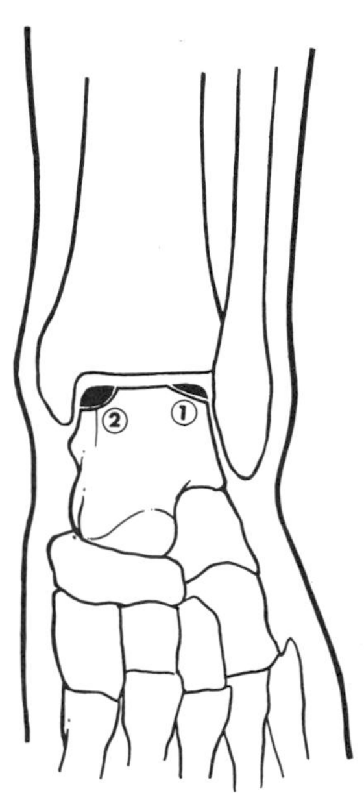

Osteochondral Fractures of the Dome of the Talus That Result From Inversion Mechanisms

Forced inversion, or inversion with hyperextension loading, can produce

1. Fracture of the anterolateral surface of the talus.
2. Fracture of the medial surface of the talus is believed to be produced by inversion and loading in plantar flexion. It may also represent a form of spontaneous osteochondritis dissecans.

Note: Osteochondral fractures of the talus are frequently confused with ankle sprain because the mechanism of the injury and the symptoms are similar (see Chapter 10).

Eversion Mechanisms

REMARKS

Eversion infrequently causes injury to the talus owing to the structural limitations built into the subtalar joint to resist eversion.

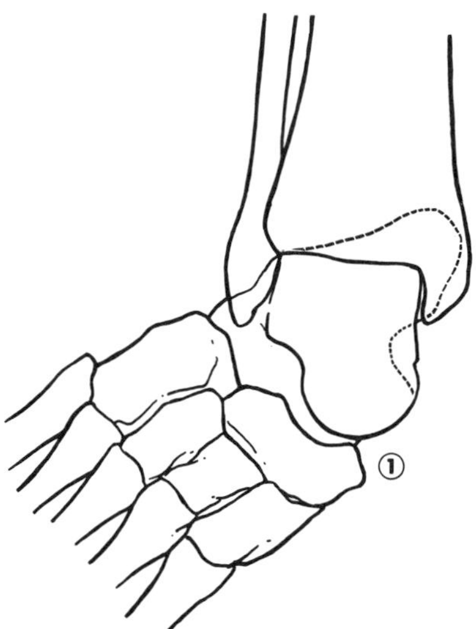

The occasional injuries resulting from eversion mechanisms include

1. Lateral subtalar dislocation.

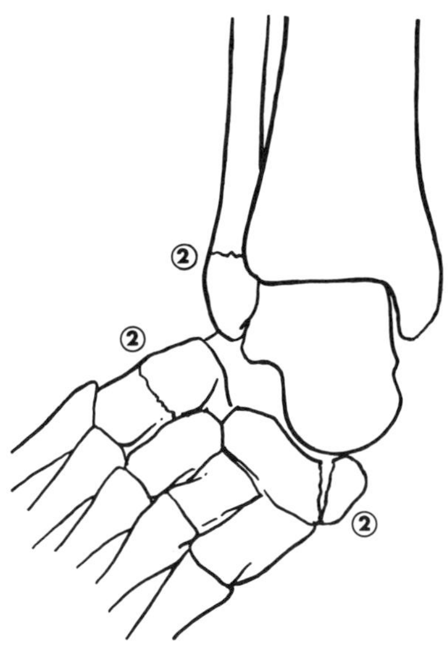

2. Fractures of the lateral malleolus, the navicular bone, or the cuboid associated with lateral subtalar dislocation.

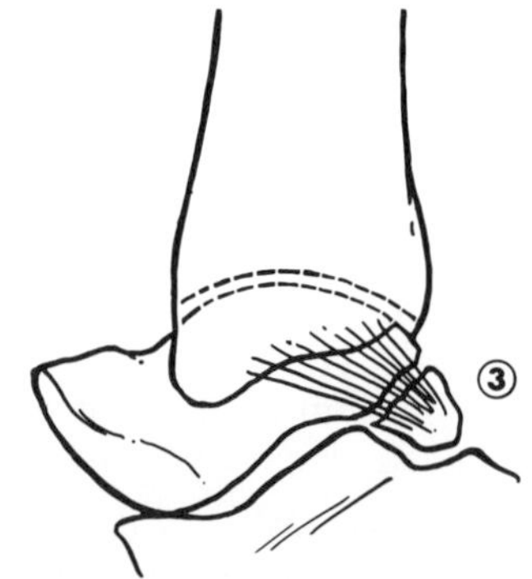

3. Avulsion of the medial side of the posterior talar tubercle produced by the pull of the posterior tibiotalar ligament.

Injuries From Compression or Mixed Mechanisms

REMARKS

Extreme compression loading of the talus causes serious structural damage to both the talus and the surrounding articulations. The result is generally a combination of injuries and mechanisms.

Additional forces may occur in rapid sequence, causing both inversion and eversion injuries.

These might include

1. Comminuted fracture of the talus from hyperextension and compression.
2. Oblique fracture of the medial malleolus from adduction of the ankle.
3. Lateral dislocation of the foot from an eversion mechanism.

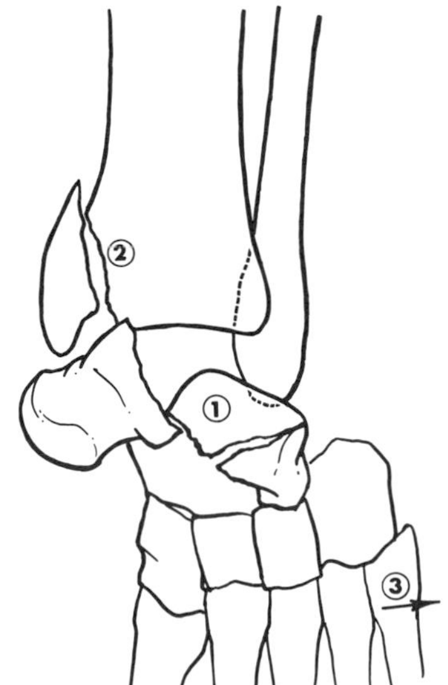

Hyperextension Injuries

Diagnosis of Fractures of the Neck of the Talus

REMARKS

Associated injuries are common in most patients with fractures of the talus. Consequently, the undisplaced fracture of the talus may be overlooked during the management of other injuries that are considered more serious.

Because of the wide diversity of talar fractures, ranging from undisplaced to the completely displaced and open fracture-dislocation, the need for special diagnostic x-rays may vary.

The main use of x-rays is to assess the true amount of displacement in fractures that are initially considered undisplaced. Any degree of displacement of the talar neck fracture is usually associated with subluxation of the subtalar joint, which should be reduced. The outcome of these fractures depends to a great extent on whether a subluxation occurs or persists at the subtalar joint.

Canale and Kelly demonstrated that displacement of the talar neck fracture occurs in two planes.

The head and neck of the talus tend to displace dorsally, leaving a prominence, which can block extension.

A second displacement occurs when the head and neck rotate internally, producing an internal torsion or varus deformity of the foot.

To rule out these displacements, careful x-ray technique is necessary before it is assumed that the fracture is undisplaced.

The outcome of these fractures depends to a great extent on whether any subluxation occurs or persists at the subtalar joint, or the body completely dislocates.

Technique of Anteroposterior X-Ray (After Canale and Kelly)

1. Ankle is placed in maximal equinus position (this is the usual position for reduction of all fractures of the talar neck).
2. Flexion of the hip and knee aids in plantar flexion of the ankle.
3. Foot is pronated 15°.
4. Tube is directed cephalad at a 75° angle from the table top.

Note: This technique allows the physician to detect any step-off or varus deformity of the head and neck of the talus.

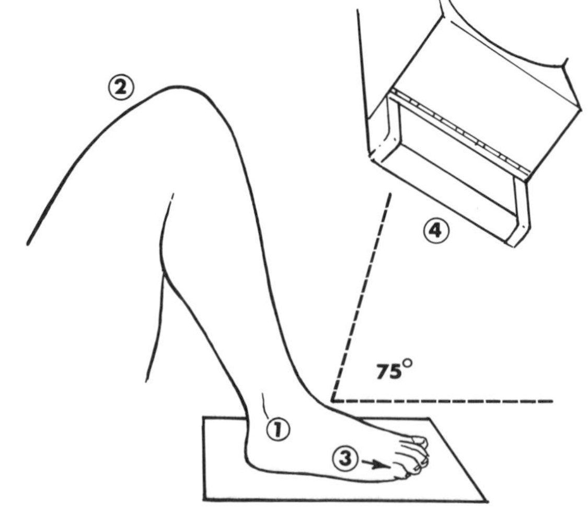

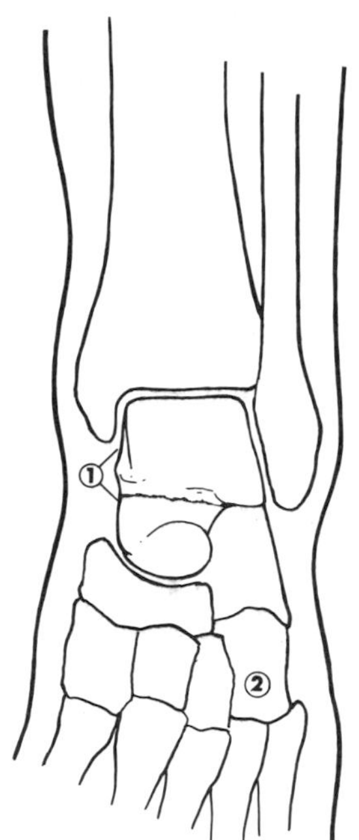

Prereduction X-Rays: Undisplaced Fracture

ANTEROPOSTERIOR VIEW

1. Head-and-neck fragment is aligned with the body fragment without torsional or medial displacement.
2. Forefoot is in a normal relationship with the hindfoot.

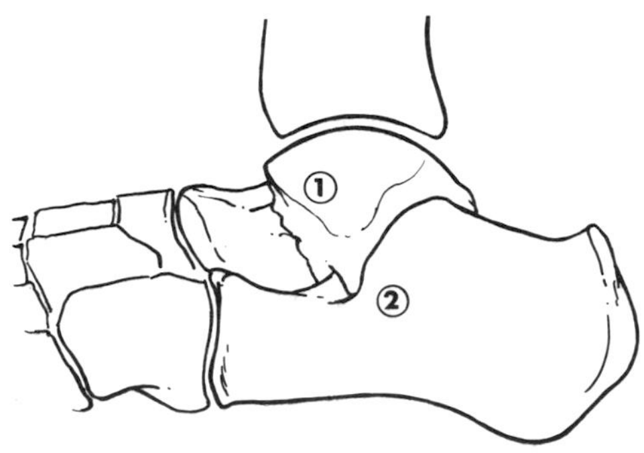

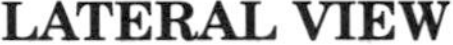

LATERAL VIEW

1. Vertical fracture through the neck of the talus is evident without dorsal displacement of the head-and-neck fragment.
2. Subtalar joint is not subluxated or dislocated.

Type I Injuries: Undisplaced Fractures of the Neck or Body of the Talus

Management

REMARKS

Although the truly undisplaced fracture of the talus can be treated symptomatically by closed methods and early mobilization, most are displaced fractures and are usually treated by open reduction and internal fixation.

If the fracture is thought to be undisplaced, it should be carefully assessed by true lateral and anteroposterior views with the foot in plantar flexion.

A lateral view particularly helps to detect subtalar dislocation or dorsal displacement of the head-and-neck fragment.

Because a main problem with these injuries is subtalar joint stiffening, a reasonable approach is to emphasize early mobilization of the foot and ankle. This requires patient cooperation and protection of the foot from weight-bearing until the fracture heals.

Immobilization

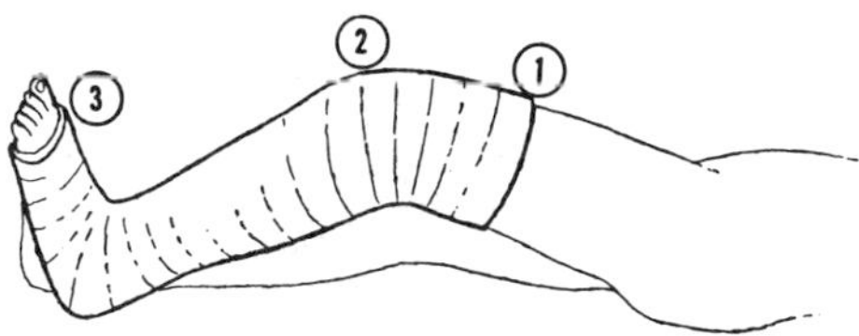

1. Apply a circular plaster cast from behind the metatarsal heads to the midthigh.
2. Knee is flexed 30°.
3. Foot is in slight plantar flexion.

Caution: Follow the fracture carefully, particularly on lateral view, to detect any displacement.

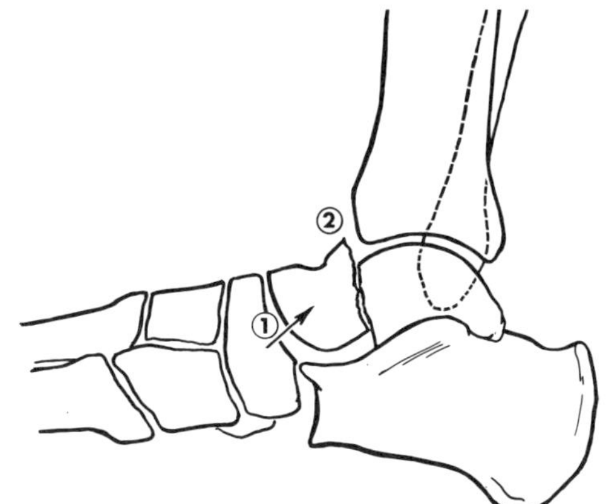

1. When the foot is brought into extension, the distal fragment may displace dorsally if the fracture is not impacted.
2. The result can be a dorsal beak on the talus, which can cause painful limitation of motion. This can and should be corrected by open reduction and internal fixation in the early stages or excision of the dorsal prominence in the healed fracture.

Subsequent Management

Subsequently, the patient is allowed up on crutches but should avoid weight-bearing on the fractured side.

The position of the talar fracture should be monitored carefully to detect dorsal or rotatory displacement.

The cast may be removed by 3–4 weeks and active motion allowed, depending on clinical symptoms. Crutches can be discontinued by 8–10 weeks if the fracture is healed clinically and according to x-ray.

Careful follow-up is necessary because avascular necrosis can occur even in the undisplaced fracture. The patient should be informed of a fairly high likelihood (20–50 per cent) of stiffness of the hindfoot.

Type II Injuries: Fracture of the Neck of the Talus With Subluxation of the Subtalar Joint

REMARKS

Any displacement of the fractured talus or subluxation of the subtalar joint is a general indication for accurate open reduction and internal fixation.

Closed reduction may rarely be successful. It may sometimes be indicated in the patient with multiple injuries that preclude prompt operative fixation of the talus and reduction of the subtalar joint.

The subtalar joint must be carefully assessed on a true lateral x-ray. Fracture alignment in the frontal plane is best evaluated by an anteroposterior x-ray taken with the foot in plantar flexion, as described on page 926.

Prereduction X-Ray

LATERAL VIEW

1. Displaced vertical fracture through the neck of the talus.
2. Body of the talus is displaced into equinus and posteriorly.
3. Os calcis is displaced anteriorly with the neck and body of the talus.

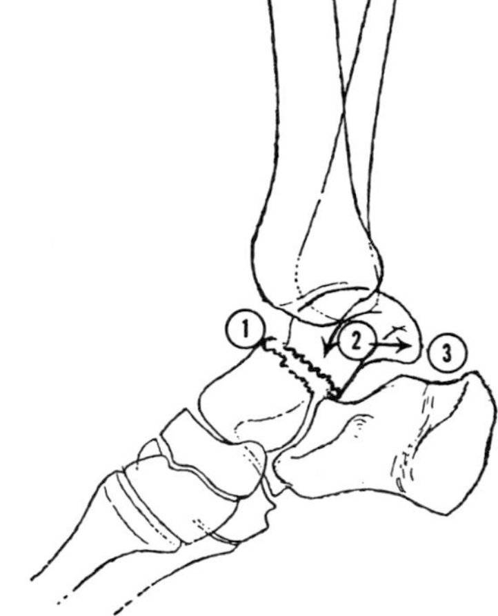

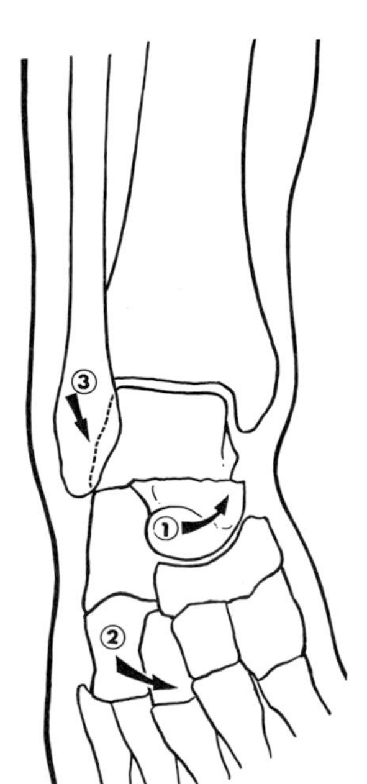

ANTEROPOSTERIOR VIEW IN PLANTAR FLEXION

1. Head-and-neck fragment is rotated internally.
2. Forefoot rotates inward with the head-and-neck fragment.
3. Fibula rotates internally with the talus.

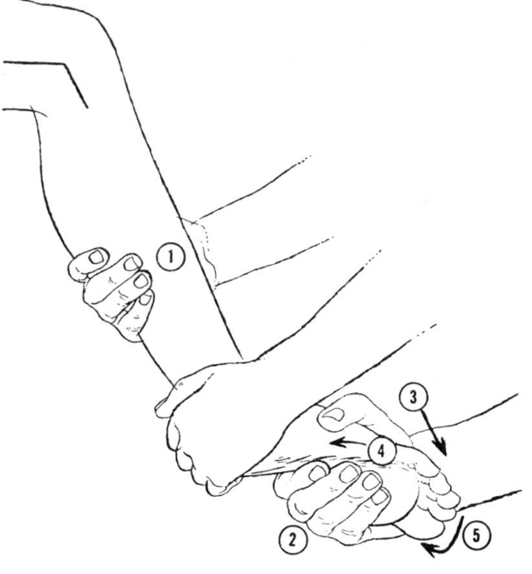

Manipulative Reduction

1. Leg hangs over the end of the table with the knee flexed 45°; an assistant steadies the lower leg.
2. Operator grasps the heel with one hand and the forefoot with the other hand.
3. Operator strongly plantar flexes the foot and at the same time
4. Pushes the foot backward and
5. Everts the foot.

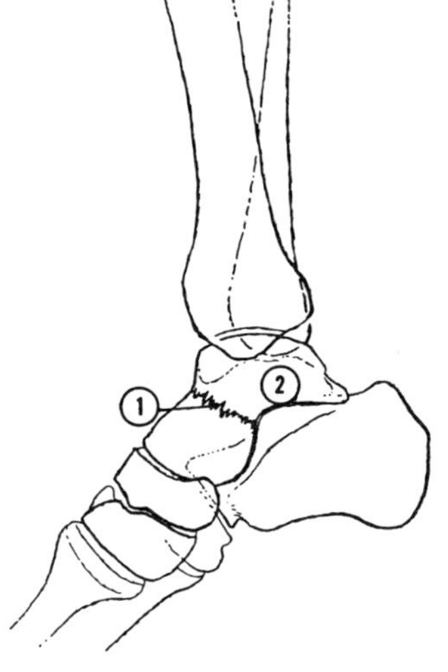

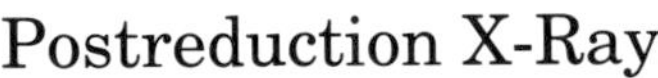

Postreduction X-Ray

LATERAL VIEW

1. Neck and body are in normal position.
2. Articular surfaces of the body and calcaneus are now congruous.

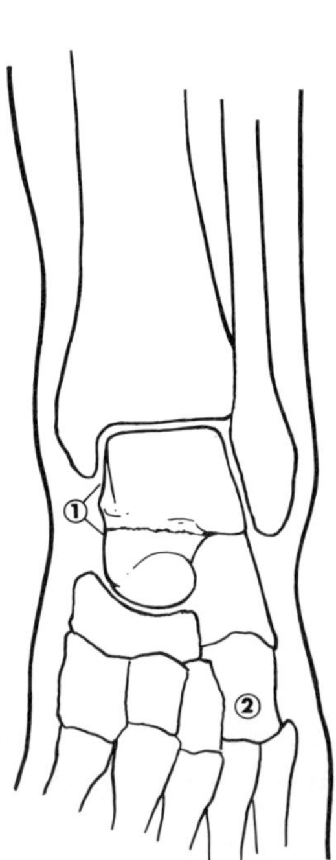

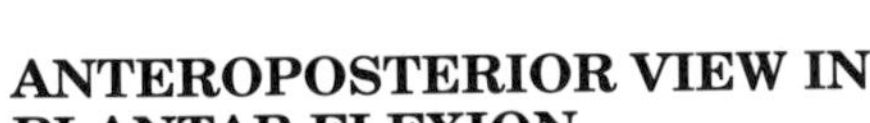

ANTEROPOSTERIOR VIEW IN PLANTAR FLEXION

1. Torsional displacement of the distal head-and-neck fragment has been corrected.
2. Forefoot is in a normal relationship with the hindfoot.

Immobilization

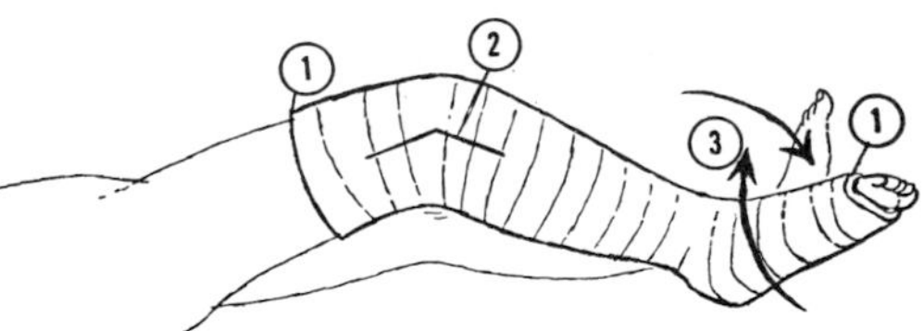

1. Apply a circular cast from behind the metatarsal heads to the midthigh.
2. Knee is flexed 30°.
3. Foot is plantar flexed and everted.

Postreduction Management

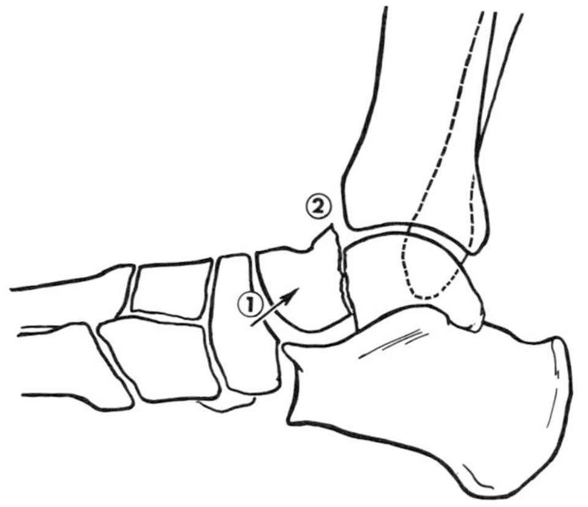

Allow the patient to walk on crutches without bearing weight on the injured limb.

The cast is changed at the end of 4 weeks, and the foot is brought out of the plantar-flexed everted position.

Caution: Avoid dorsal displacement of the neck fragment during the cast change.

1. When the foot is brought out of equinus, the distal fragment may be displaced dorsally.
2. The result can be a dorsal beak on the talus, which causes painful ankle motion and may require excision.

Type III and Type IV Injuries: Displaced Fractures of the Neck With Dislocation of the Head or Body of the Talus

REMARKS

A large percentage of displaced fractures of the neck with dislocation of the head or body of the talus, which are produced by extreme violence, are open and require prompt operative wound treatment and associated internal fixation.

Operative reduction and internal fixation are also indicated for most closed type III or IV injuries.

Early attempts at manipulation may be necessary to relieve skin tension or to improve temporarily the position of the talus while the patient is being treated for life-threatening injuries.

A satisfactory result from closed management is highly unlikely with injuries displaced to this degree. Nonunion or malunion is the rule with closed treatment, and adequate operative reduction and internal fixation is the preferred method.

Prereduction X-Ray

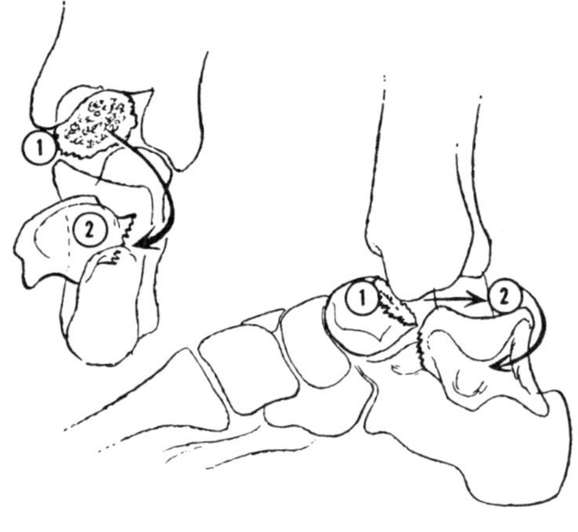

1. Vertical fracture through the neck of the talus with some comminution.
2. Body of the talus is displaced backward and rotated.

Note: Open reduction and internal fixation are necessary for the severely displaced fracture. Attempted closed reduction is usually futile and may add further damage to the skeletal and soft tissue structures.

Preferred Method: Open Reduction and Screw Fixation

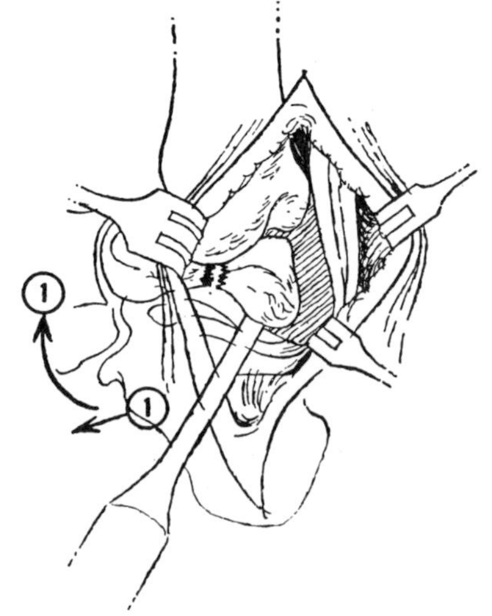

1. A direct approach to the dislocated body is necessary by a medial incision. This allows reduction and visualization of the fracture site.

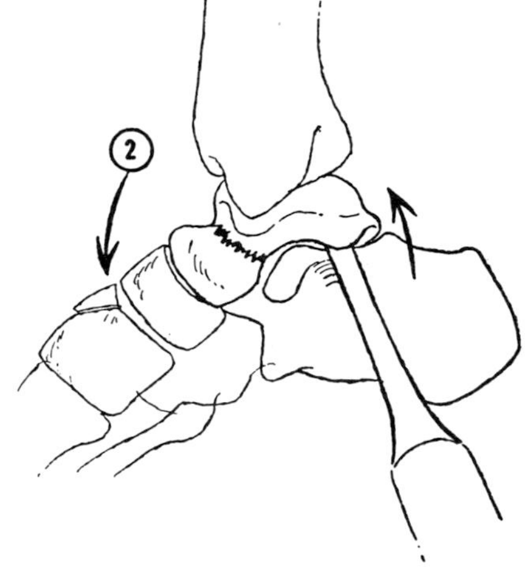

2. Subtalar joint is reduced, and the body is aligned to the head and neck fragment as anatomically as possible.

Fixation is achieved by cannulated screws inserted from the medial and/or lateral sides of the talus.

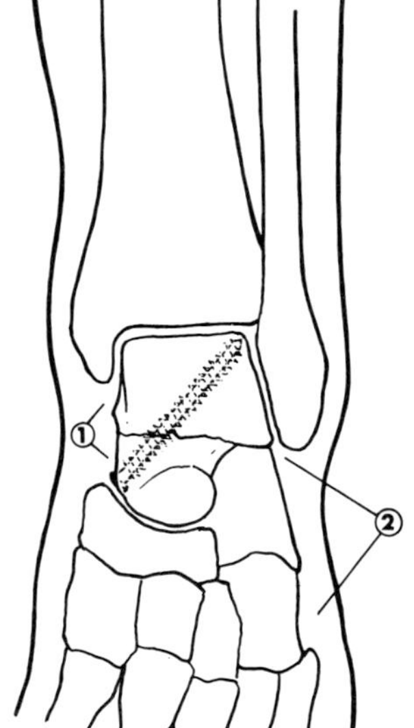

Intraoperative X-Rays

ANTEROPOSTERIOR VIEW IN PLANTAR FLEXION

1. Torsional alignment of the distal fragment has been correctly restored.
2. Forefoot is in a proper relationship with the hindfoot.

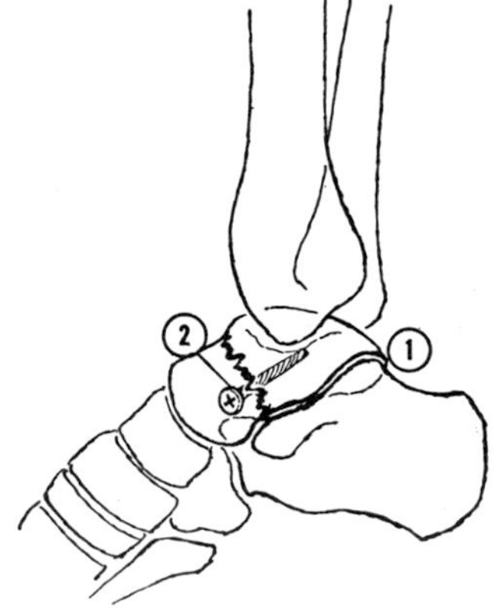

LATERAL VIEW

1. Body of the talus and the calcaneus are in a normal relationship.
2. Screw is transfixing both fragments.

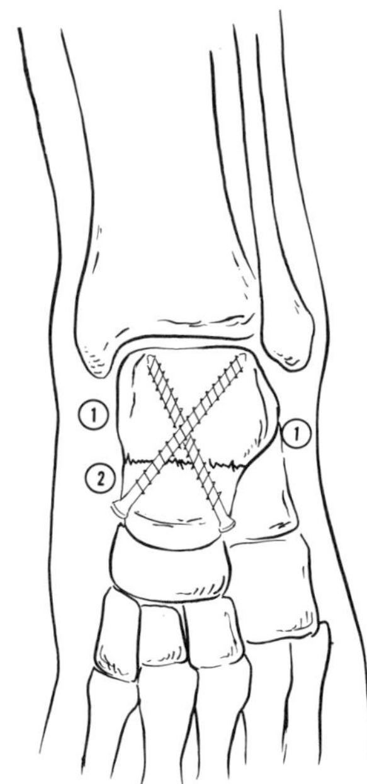

Alternative Method

1. If reduction cannot be anatomically achieved, the fracture site can be opened both from a medial and lateral approach.
2. The fracture can be visualized best and reduced by direct manipulation and visualization from the medial side.

Immobilization

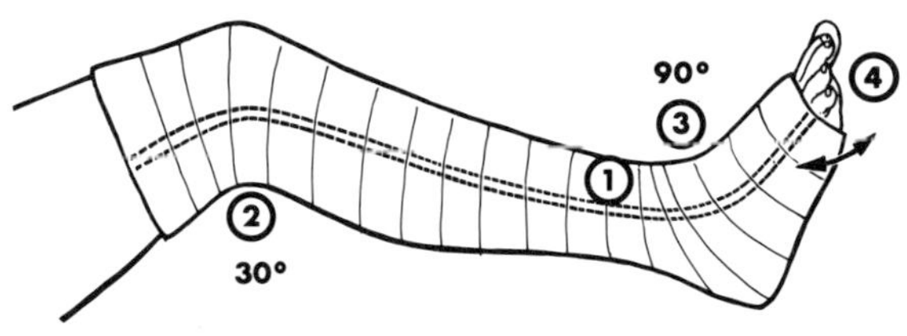

1. Apply anterior and posterior plaster splints to allow for the usual postoperative swelling.
2. Knee is flexed 30°.
3. Ankle is held at 90°.
4. Foot is slightly pronated.

Postoperative Management

The foot is elevated and ice is applied to the foot and ankle.

The circulation should be checked on a regular basis for evidence of any ischemia to the foot.

By 3–5 days, the swelling should be sufficiently diminished, and healing should be occurring adequately to allow careful guarded range-of-motion therapy.

If the swelling has not subsided, range of motion should be delayed until the soft tissue wounds are adequately healed.

The degree of range-of-motion therapy depends on the stability achieved at the fracture site at the time of surgery.

If there is uncertainty as to the stability of the fracture, then cast immobilization should be continued for 4–6 weeks with the foot in a neutral position.

Healing is usually complete and the cast may be discontinued by 8–10 weeks. The patient should be advised to continue on crutches and to bear no weight on the leg but to exercise the ankle and foot actively after cast removal.

Radiographic changes of avascular necrosis should be expected after this significant injury. The patient therefore should be advised to continue to protect the ankle from loading until the circulatory status of the talus is evident on x-ray.

Complications are discussed further later in this chapter.

Fractures of the Lateral Process of the Talus

REMARKS

Hawkins pointed out that, after talar neck fracture, fracture of the lateral process is the second most common fracture of the talus.

The initial diagnosis is frequently missed owing to the sometimes subtle radiographic findings. The patient is then treated for a sprain and has persistent symptoms.

Unexplained and persistent pain about the lateral side of the ankle after a forced dorsiflexion–inversion injury should be carefully evaluated for a fracture of the lateral process of the talus.

Hyperextension Mechanism

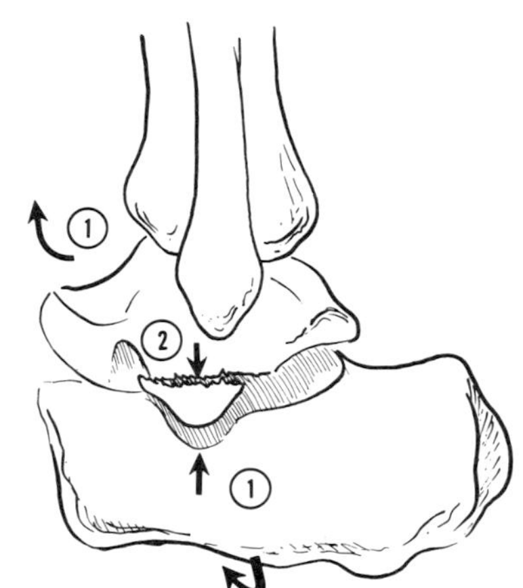

1. With the foot inverted and the ankle dorsiflexed, the
2. Lateral process of the talus can be caught between the fibula and the calcaneus, which produces the fracture.

Note: This frequently can be confused with a sprained ankle and should be considered in anybody with persistent lateral pain after ankle sprain.

Additional helpful x-rays include an anteroposterior view of the ankle mortise with the foot in 45° of internal rotation and 30° of equinus to define the lateral process.

Prereduction X-Ray

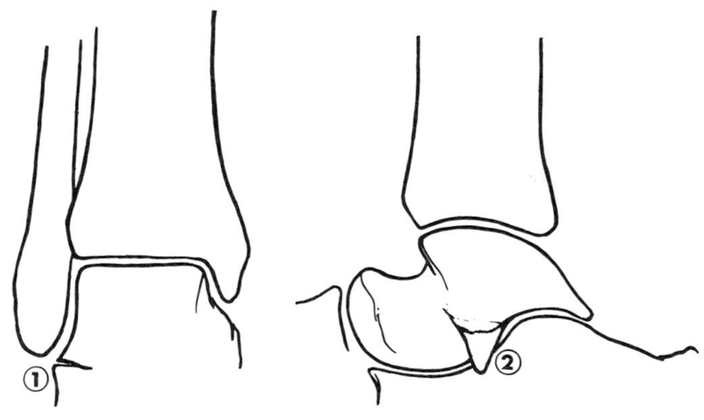

1. On the anteroposterior x-ray, the fracture may be obscure.
2. Lateral x-ray usually shows a chip off the lateral process.

Closed Reduction and Management

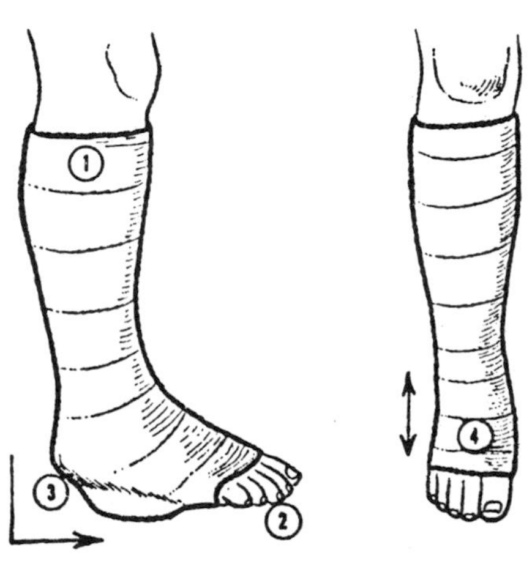

If the fracture is diagnosed promptly, closed reduction should be attempted for all fractures of the lateral process of the talus.

1. Short-leg cast is applied from the toes to the knee.
2. Patient may be allowed to bear weight as tolerated with a walking heel or with a cast boot.
3. Ankle is held at a right angle and a
4. Slightly externally rotated or everted position.

Note: For large fracture fragments that are displaced and do not reduce adequately, open reduction and internal fixation may be necessary. Excision of the fracture fragments may be indicated for fractures in which the diagnosis is delayed. If the diagnosis is delayed 12 weeks or longer, operative excision of the fragment is the treatment of choice.

Subsequent Management

The patient bears weight as tolerated on the walking cast. The cast is continued for 3–4 weeks.

Active exercises should be emphasized to regain subtalar motion because the injury tends to stiffen the subtalar joint if immobilization is prolonged.

Displaced or Unrecognized Fractures

1. For initially displaced or unrecognized fractures or

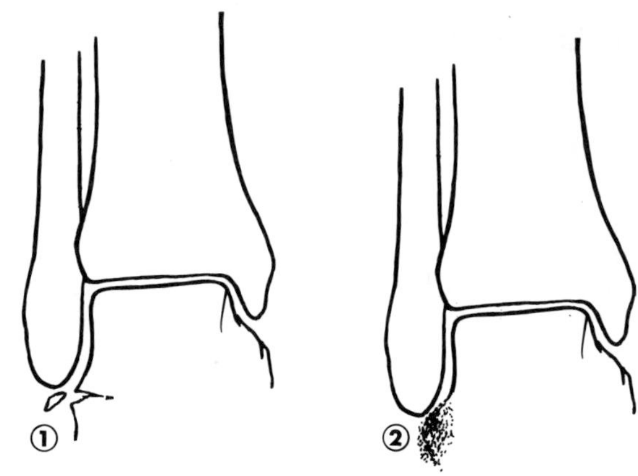

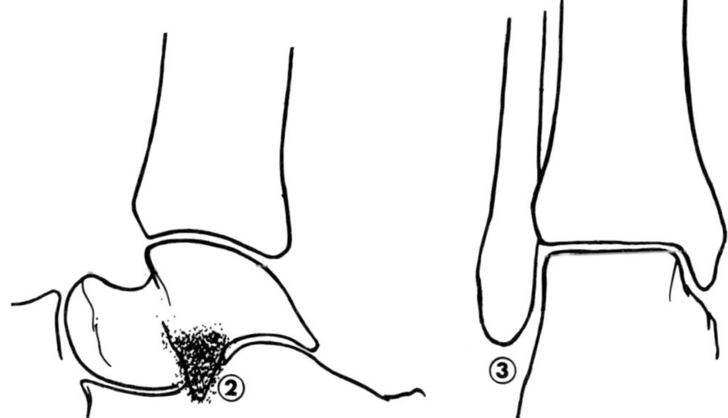

2. Fractures that heal with symptomatic overgrowth,
3. Treatment is by excision of the fragment.

Hyperflexion Injuries

Posterior Compartment Fractures Confused With Ankle Sprains

REMARKS

Hyperflexion injury can occur when a force is applied to the heel behind the posterior tubercle of the talus.

This is a fairly common injury sustained by an athlete while jumping in basketball or kicking in football.

With the ankle plantar-flexed, a blow to the back of the heel wedges the talus between the posterior calcaneal facet and the posterior tibial margin.

The result may be a fracture of the posterior facet of the talus or even the posterior articular surface of the talus.

This injury is commonly confused with an ankle sprain, either because the fracture line is not displaced or the fracture fragment is considered to be an accessory ossicle (os trigonum).

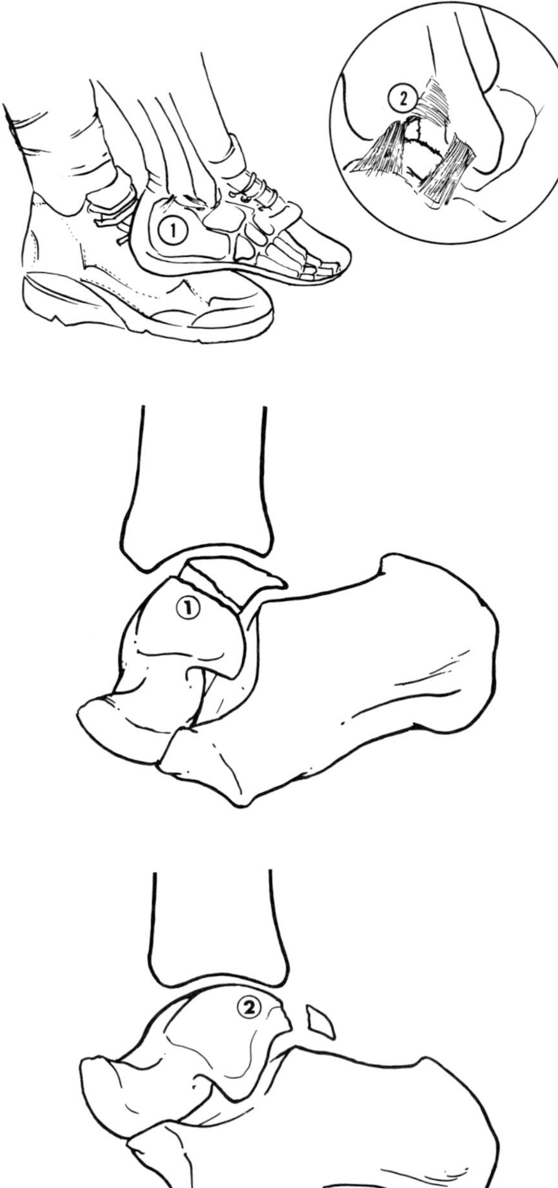

Mechanism of Injury

1. Forceful plantar flexion of the foot occurs when the athlete lands off balance while jumping.
2. Impingement of the posterior talus between the calcaneus and the tibial surface results in a fracture.

Types of Hyperflexion Fractures

1. Fracture of the posterior talar body or

2. Fracture of the posterior talar tubercle.

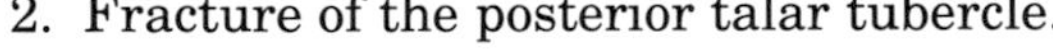

Note: This undisplaced fracture may be confused with an os trigonum, which can be ruled out by views of the opposite, uninjured ankle.

Diagnosis

The diagnosis of a fractured posterior talus is frequently not recognized or is confused with an ankle sprain because of the common mechanism of twisting or "rolling over on the ankle." (See also Chapter 10.)

In active athletes, repeat visits to the physician are common until the diagnosis is considered and recognized with adequate diagnostic studies.

This fracture of the posterior talus may also be confused with a normal sesamoid, the os trigonum.

Clinically, the symptoms are characterized by the following:

1. Significant deep palpable tenderness anterior to the Achilles tendon but posterior to the talus.
2. Posterior pain is reproduced with forceful plantar flexion of the ankle.

Note: These signs should differentiate this condition from the more common causes of recurrent ankle sprain from anterolateral ligament disruption.

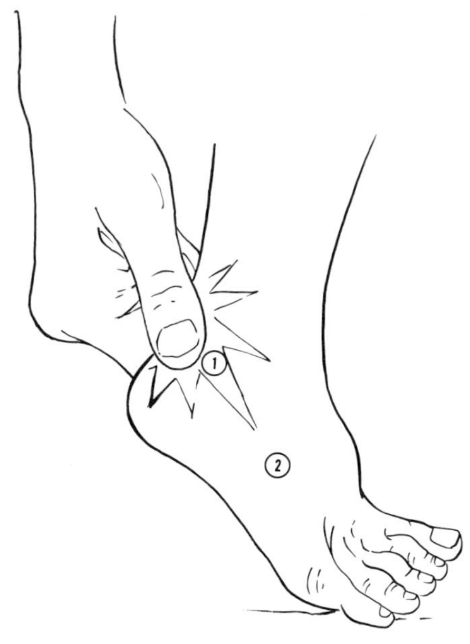

Roentgenographic Diagnosis

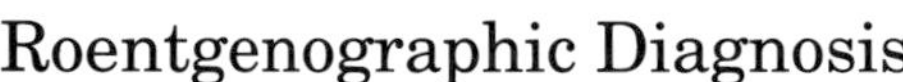

The major differential is between a small posterior process fracture and an os trigonum. The differential, if not made clinically on the basis of well-localized posterior symptoms, can be made on the basis of technetium bone scan.

1. Positive technetium bone scan result helps to distinguish between the normal os trigonum and the fractured posterior process of the talus.

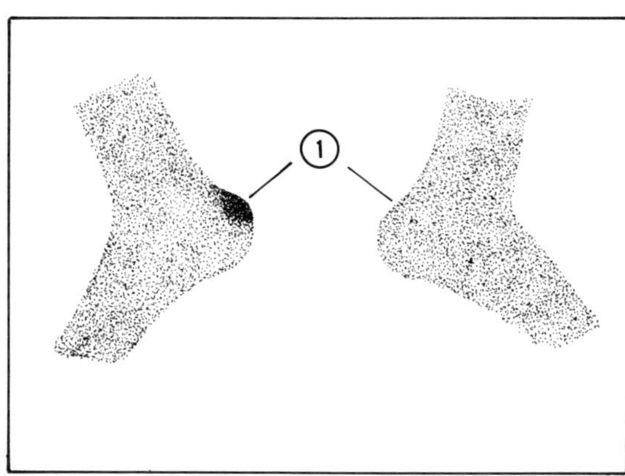

Management

REMARKS

If the injury is diagnosed acutely (the exception rather than the rule), closed reduction and cast immobilization is the treatment of choice for posterior compartment fractures of the talus caused by hyperflexion.

If it is diagnosed late and the patient is willing to try a period of time in a cast, then cast immobilization can be attempted.

In most instances, patients who are seen late require surgical removal of the bone fragment to return to full sports competition.

If the posterior fragment of the talus is sufficiently large or involves the articular surface, internal fixation is indicated.

Closed Reduction Technique

X-RAY OF THE ACUTE INJURY

1. Posterior tuberosity fracture has occurred from a blow to the plantar-flexed heel of a basketball player.

Note: Comparison x-rays of the opposite ankle show that this is a fracture rather than an os trigonum.

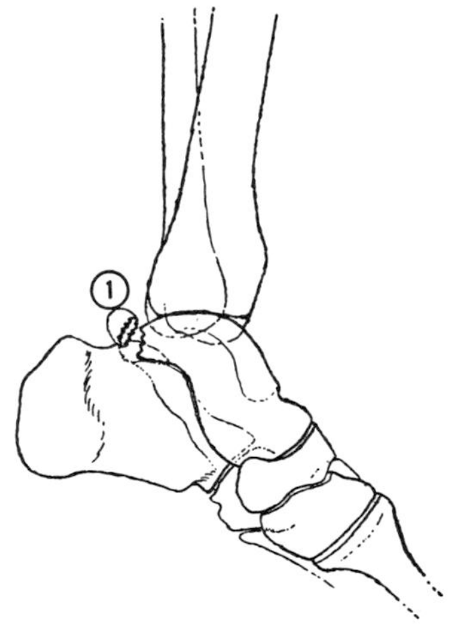

Manipulative Reduction

The patient is in the prone position with the knee flexed 90°.

1. Assistant strongly dorsiflexes the foot while the
2. Operator makes deep downward pressure on either side of the Achilles tendon directly over the displaced fragment.

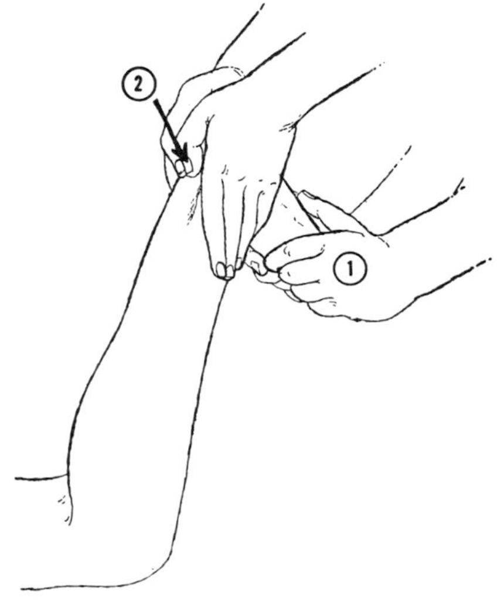

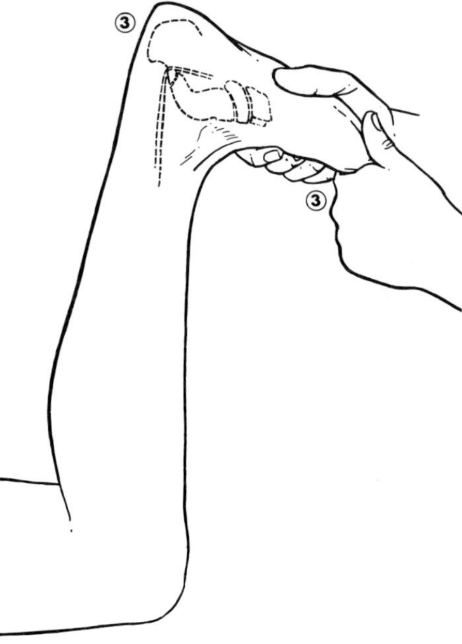

3. Dorsiflexing the big toe aids in the reduction by pulling on the flexor hallucis longus tendon, which runs behind the fragment.

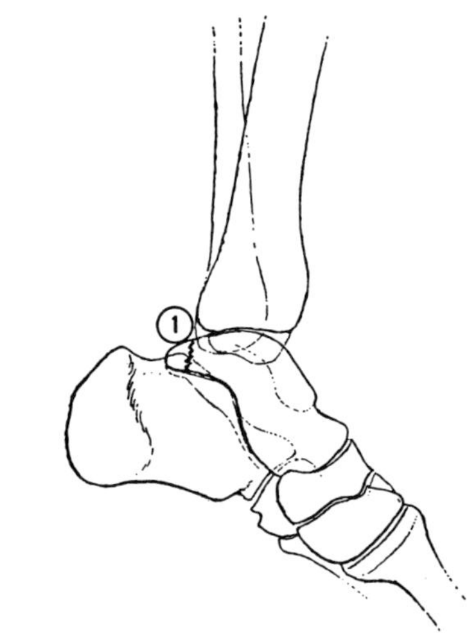

Postreduction X-Ray

1. Posterior process of the talus is in apposition to the body of the talus.

Immobilization

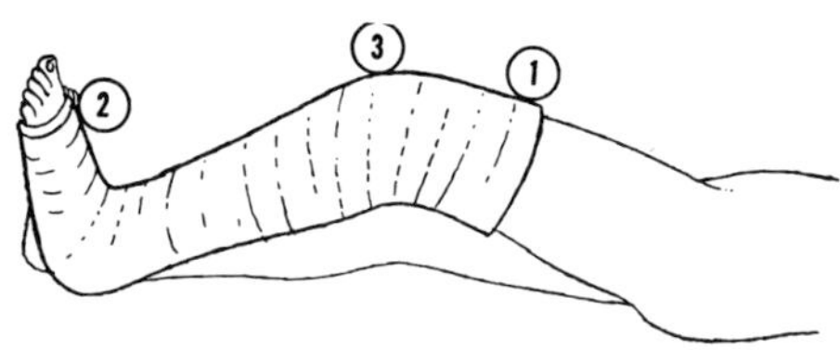

1. Apply a circular plaster cast from behind the toes to midthigh.
2. Foot is slightly dorsiflexed.
3. Knee is flexed 30°.

Postreduction Management

Allow immediate ambulation on crutches with no weight borne on the affected foot.

Remove the cast at the end of 4 weeks and resume weight-bearing.

Persistent symptoms after cast removal may indicate the need for surgical excision.

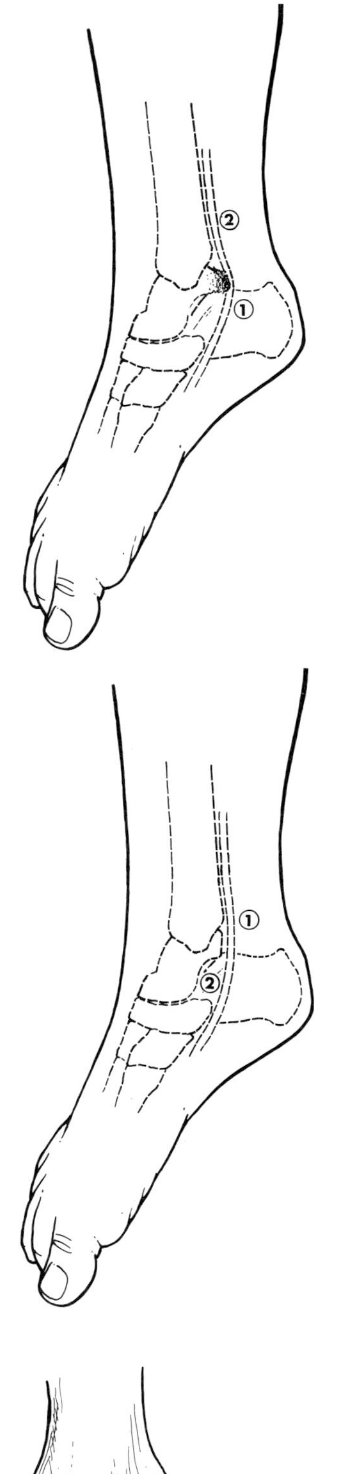

Indications for Surgical Excision of the Fragment

1. Displaced fracture causes sufficient reaction and painful impairment of the flexor hallucis longus in the ankle to prevent active use of the ankle.
2. Frequently, the displaced tuberosity fracture may cause recurrent symptoms and be confused with ankle sprain or tendinitis of the posterior tendons.

X-Ray After Excision of the Fragment

1. Impingement symptoms from the fracture have been relieved.
2. Subtalar joint is unaffected by the excision.

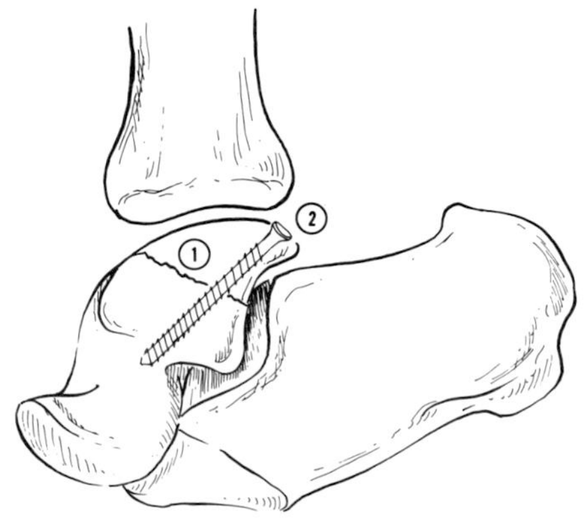

Indications for Internal Fixation

1. Large posterior fracture involving the articular surface is best treated by
2. Internal fixation rather than excision.

Inversion Injuries

REMARKS

Inversion mechanisms produce injuries, including

- Sprain of the subtalar ligaments.
- Medial subtalar dislocation.
- Complete dislocation of the talus.
- Osteochondral lesions of the talus.

Inversion injuries may also produce fractures associated with subtalar dislocation, including

- Shear fracture of the head of the talus.
- Shear fracture of the navicular bone.
- Avulsion fracture of the posterior talus.
- Avulsion of the base of the fifth metatarsal.
- Avulsion of the cuboid.
- Avulsion of the lateral malleolus.

The most common dislocation is a medial subtalar dislocation produced by inversion.

Complete dislocations of the talus out of the ankle mortise are fortunately infrequent but can occur with severe inversion.

Inversion Injuries

1. Forced inversion of the ankle usually tears the anterior fibulotalar ligament.
2. With further loading, however, it can disrupt or sprain any of the subtalar ligaments. With continued inversion force, further injury can occur.

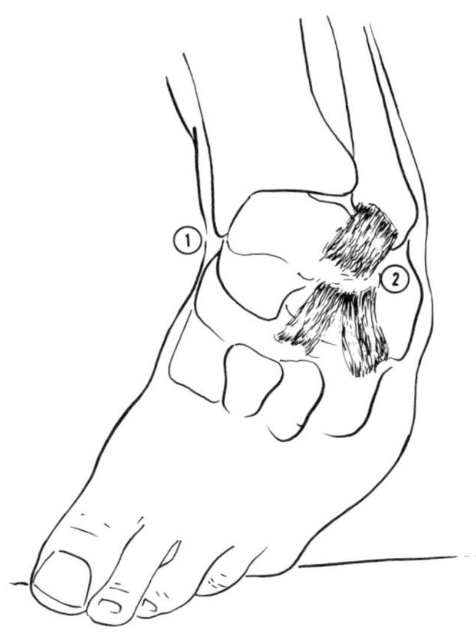

Progressive Injury from Inversion

Forced inversion produces subtalar injuries, such as

1. Sprain of the calcaneofibular, subtalar, or tibiocalcaneal ligament;

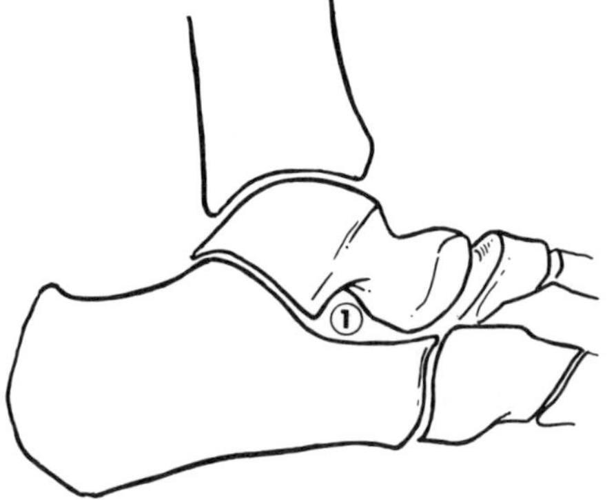

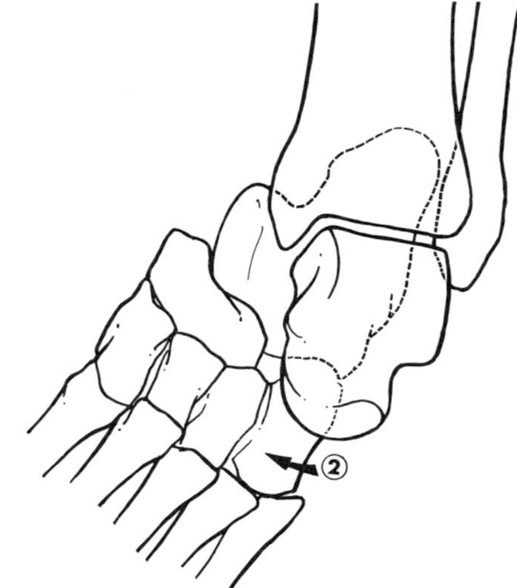

2. Medial dislocation of the subtalar joint; and

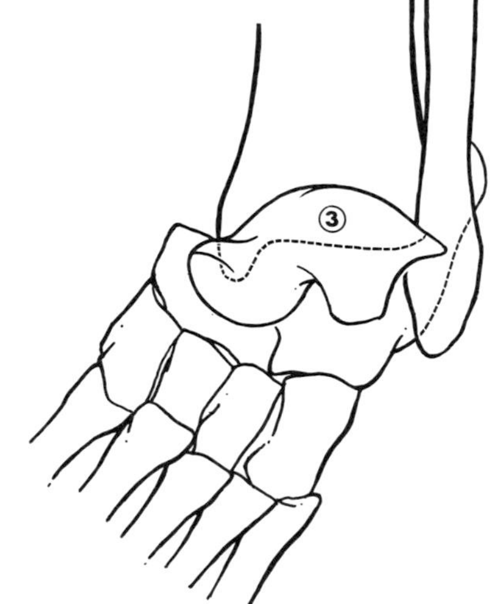

3. Complete anterior dislocation of the talus.

Fractures That Result From Inversion Injury and Are Associated With Subtalar Dislocation

1. Vertical shear fracture off the talar head or neck.
2. Fracture of the navicular bone.
3. Fracture of the posterolateral talus, which results from avulsion by the posterior talofibular ligament.
4. Fracture of fifth metatarsal, cuboid, or fibula.

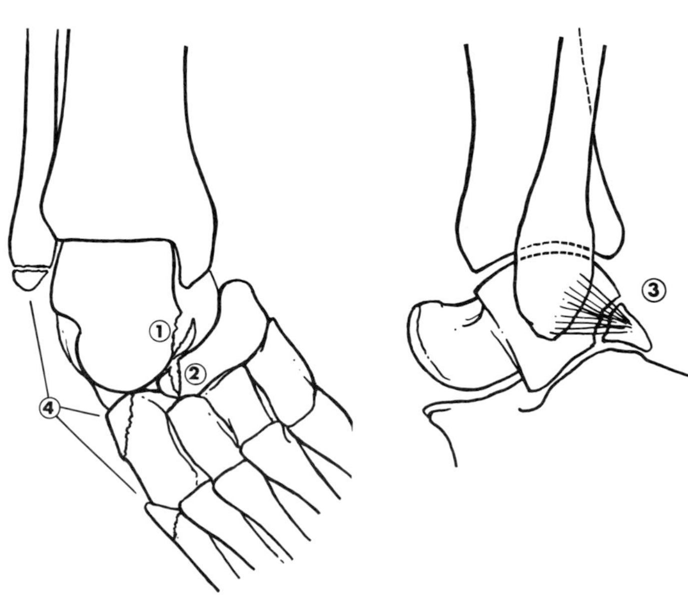

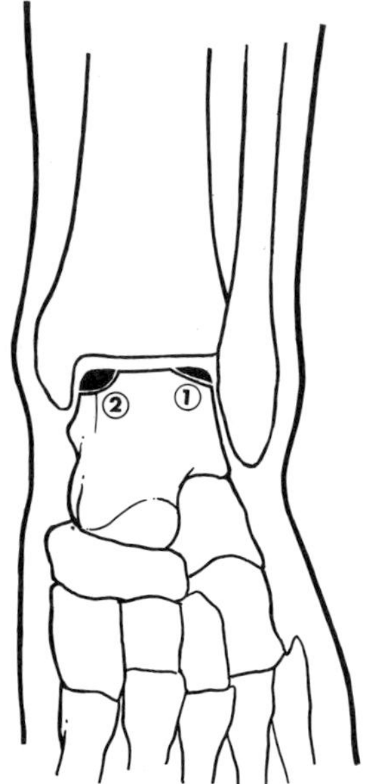

Osteochondral Fractures of the Dome of the Talus That Result From Inversion Mechanisms

Forced inversion, or inversion with hyperextension loading, can produce

1. Fracture of the anterolateral surface of the talus.
2. Fracture of the medial surface of the talus is believed to be produced by inversion and loading in plantar flexion. It may also represent a form of spontaneous osteochondritis dissecans.

Note: Osteochondral fractures of the talus are frequently confused with ankle sprain because the mechanism of the injury and the symptoms are similar (see Chapter 9).

Management of Inversion Injuries That Cause Subtalar Sprains and Dislocations

Treatment of the acute subtalar sprain is similar to that of the tibiotalar sprain. Most of these can be managed with appropriate Aircast support and early immobilization. Operative repair may be necessary for a recurrent problem of instability of the subtalar joint, as described by Chrisman and Snook (see Chapter 10).

Dislocation of the subtalar joint or complete dislocation of the talus requires prompt closed reduction to minimize pressure necrosis of the skin or other complications.

Occasionally, closed reduction may be prevented by the talar head being trapped in the extensor digitorum tendons on the anterolateral aspect of the ankle.

Shear fracture of the talus or of the navicular bone can also lock and prevent reduction of the foot.

Management of Medial Subtalar Dislocation

REMARKS

Medial subtalar dislocation can occur with surprisingly little force in some individuals, such as basketball players. In fact, medial subtalar dislocation has been termed a basketball foot in some reports.

The less forceful type of injury is usually associated with an excellent outcome and minimal long-term signs of subtalar arthritis.

If the injury is sustained as a result of a fall from a height or a high-speed motor vehicle accident, the trauma may be more severe and associated with damage to the articular surfaces and a poor long-term outcome.

It is important in the initial evaluation to look carefully at the x-ray for any associated fractures, which may require operative treatment and adversely affect the outcome.

Occasionally, subtalar dislocation produces an open injury, which also indicates a poorer prognosis. Infection and circulatory compromise are more frequent with the open injury. Therefore, open dislocation requires careful debridement and irrigation before and after reduction.

Prereduction X-Ray

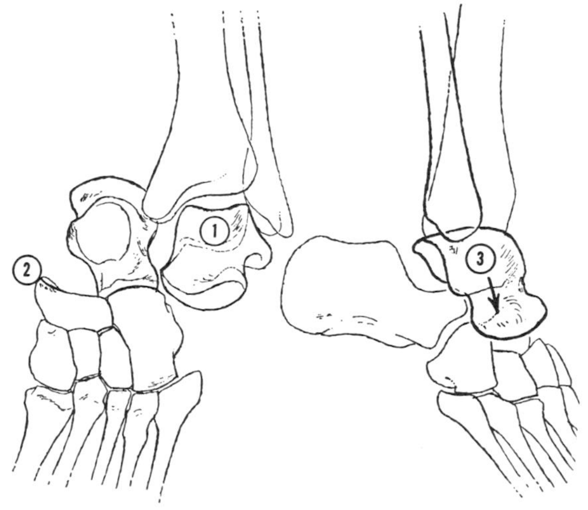

1. Talus is held in the tibiofibular mortise.
2. Foot is displaced medially at the subtalar and talonavicular joints.
3. Talus is in equinus owing to the loss of inferior and anterior support.

Manipulative Reduction

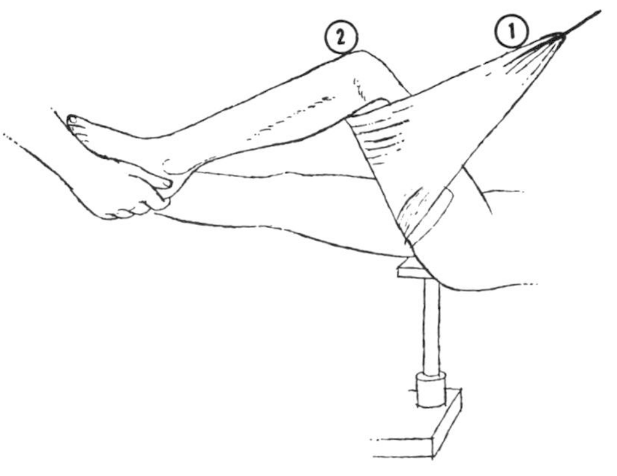

Note: Reduction should be performed promptly. If it is done within a few hours, morphine analgesia is satisfactory. In other cases, general anesthesia may be necessary.

1. Place a well-padded canvas sling under the distal end of the thigh, and suspend it from an overhead crossbar on the fracture table.
2. Knee is flexed 90° to relax the gastrocnemius.

1. Assistant holds and steadies the lower leg.
2. Operator grasps the heel with one hand and the forefoot with the other.
3. Foot is first strongly plantar-flexed; then the
4. Foot is everted and abducted.

Postreduction X-Ray

1. Subtalar and talonavicular dislocations are reduced.
2. Talus is in its normal relation to the navicular bone, calcaneus, and tibia.

Note: Review the postreduction x-rays carefully for any evidence of fractures, which may require surgical removal. These tend to be associated with a poorer long-term prognosis than the usual subtalar dislocation.

If closed reduction is not anatomic or does not occur with reasonable ease, open exploration of the subtalar region is indicated for obstacles to reduction.

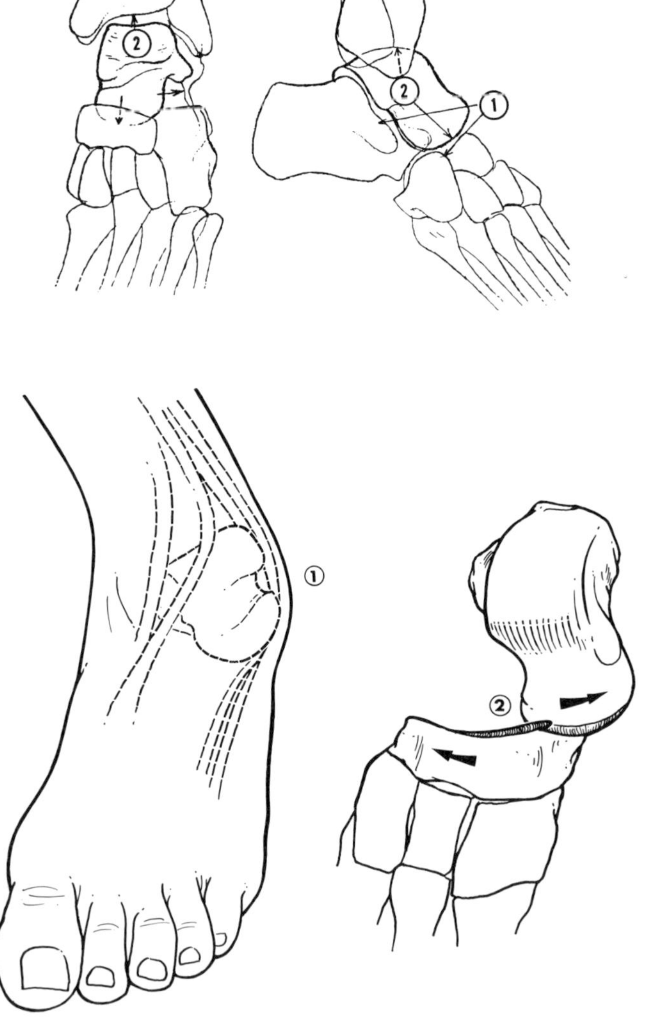

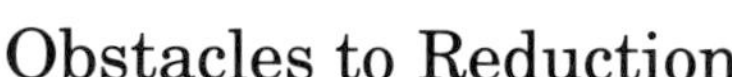

Obstacles to Reduction

Although most subtalar dislocations reduce promptly, approximately 8 per cent of medial subtalar dislocations are irreducible because of
1. Entrapment of the head of the talus in the surrounding soft tissues or
2. Impaction of the fractures of the head of the talus or navicular bone.

Note: Occasionally, the obstacles may be removed by grasping the heel and applying manual traction on the foot while alternating dorsiflexion and plantar flexion manipulation. This should be done carefully, and further fracture of the talus should be avoided. In most instances, operative reduction should be carried out if the subtalar joint is not reduced promptly by careful manipulation.

Immobilization

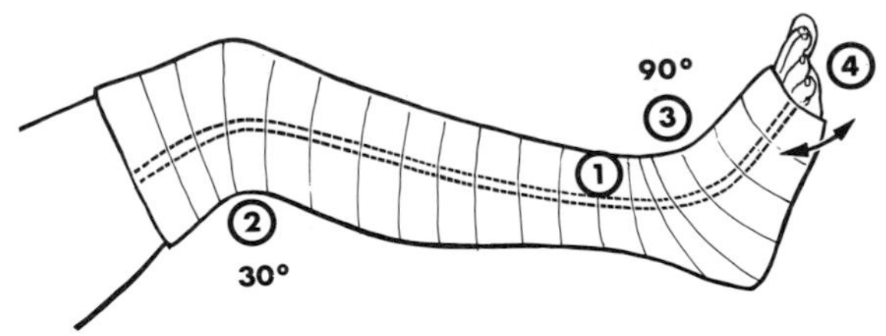

1. Apply anterior and posterior splints to allow for swelling of the foot after reduction.
2. Knee is flexed 30°.
3. Foot is dorsiflexed 90°.
4. Foot is in slight eversion.

Postreduction Management

Elevate the limb on pillows.

Surround the foot with ice bags.

Check the toes frequently for circulatory impairment.

The stability of the foot should be carefully evaluated after reduction to ensure that subluxation does not persist or recur. Most subtalar dislocations are stable and do not require immobilization for more than 2–3 weeks. Early mobilization rather than prolonged immobilization is indicated to prevent fibrosis and stiffness in the subtalar and the other joints of the foot.

The changes of avascular necrosis do not usually complicate this injury. However, if an x-ray shows increased bone density, a period of protective weight-bearing is indicated.

Total Dislocation of the Talus

REMARKS

Total dislocation of the talus represents the ultimate inversion injury to the ankle.

The talus dislocates out of its normal position in the ankle mortise and subtalar joint and displaces anteriorly to the lateral malleolus. Rarely, eversion injuries produce total dislocation with medial displacement of the talus.

These total dislocations are extremely unusual and, in most instances, are open injuries.

All the major blood supply to the talus is disrupted. Therefore, avascular complications are virtually inevitable. Occasionally, ligamentous tissue remains attached to the talus and provides some blood supply.

Because most total dislocations of the talus are open injuries, closed reduction is usually not indicated. However, to achieve an open reduction, a technique of traction and countertraction is usually necessary.

Prereduction X-Ray

1. Body of the talus is in front of the external malleolus.
2. Head of the talus is directed medially.
3. Talus is rotated in its longitudinal axis so that its inferior articular surface faces posteriorly.

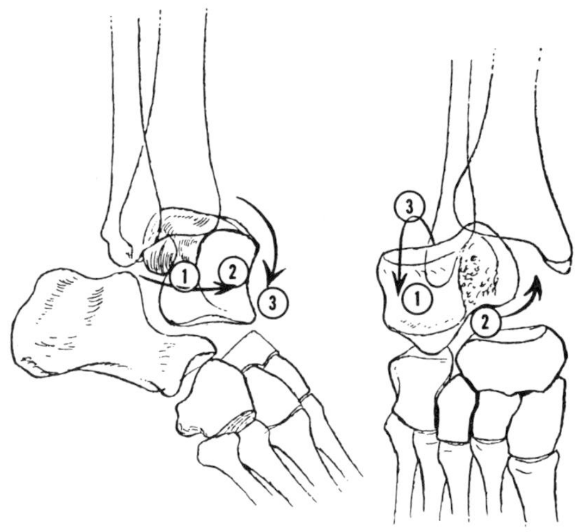

Traction Technique for Reduction of Total Dislocation or Closed Methods

1. External fixator can be applied using pins in the calcaneus and
2. Proximal pins in the tibia for traction and countertraction.
3. These pins are used to distract the ankle joint, thereby allowing
4. Space to permit reduction of the talus.

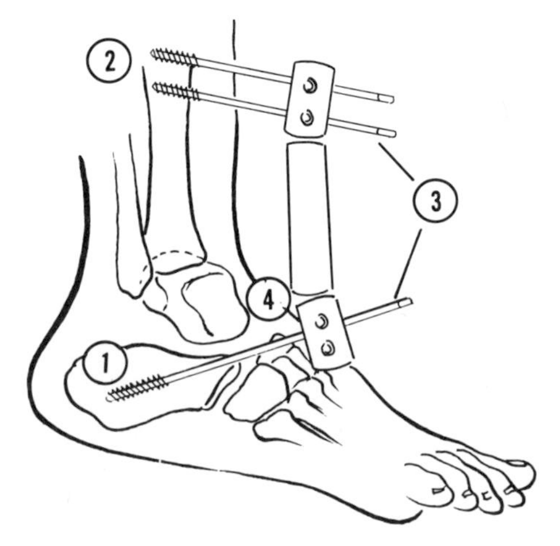

Subsequent Manipulation

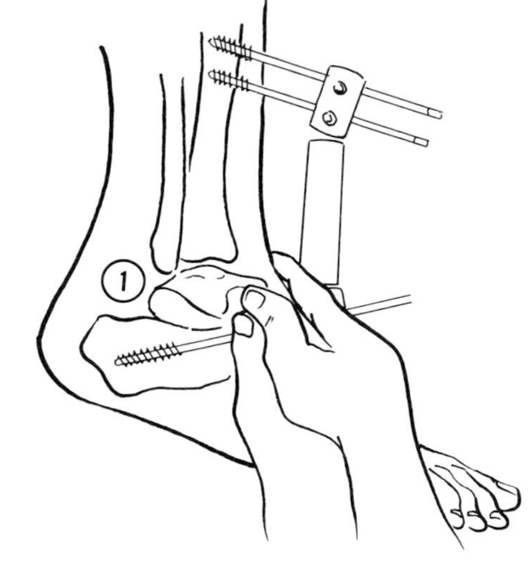

1. The talus is reduced by direct pressure over its head. Once the reduction is obtained, the dislocated talus is usually stable, and the external fixator may be removed.

Caution: Attempted ligamentous repair of the deltoid or other disrupted ligaments after successful closed reduction is not usually indicated acutely because of the risk of producing necrosis of the overlying skin.

If closed reduction of the total dislocation of the talus is unsuccessful, open reduction is mandatory. However, traction with external fixation is often necessary even though an open approach to the talus is carried out.

Immobilization

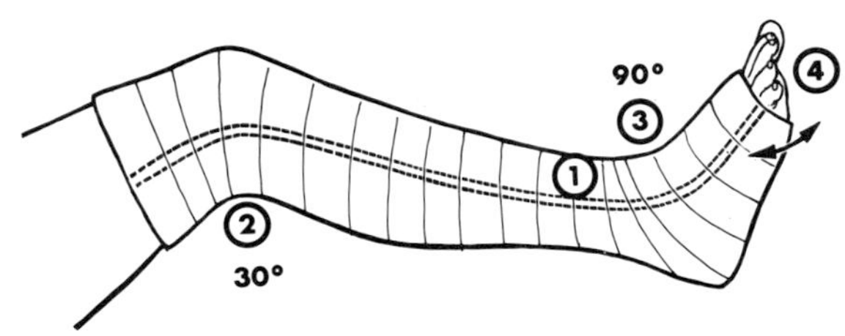

1. Apply anterior and posterior splints to allow for swelling of the foot after reduction.
2. Knee is flexed 30°.
3. Ankle is held at a right angle.
4. Foot is in neutral position in regard to inversion and eversion.

Postreduction X-Ray

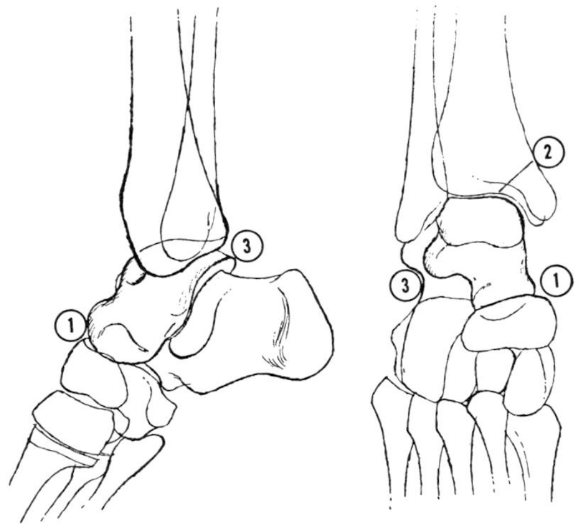

1. Talus is in a normal relationship to the navicular bone.
2. Talus is accurately seated in the tibiofibular mortise.
3. Talus is in a normal relationship to the tibia, calcaneus, and navicular bone.

Subsequent Management

The injury from total talar dislocation is so serious that complications are almost inevitable. Soft tissue infection, osteomyelitis, and arthritis occur with a high degree of frequency after this rare injury, either with closed or open reduction.

Because of its serious nature, a total dislocation of the talus is a surgical emergency. In most instances, open reduction should be done promptly after no more than one or two attempts at closed reduction.

After reduction, maintain the bivalved cast to accommodate the swelling.

If open reduction is necessary or the injury is originally an open injury, repeated wound exploration and redebridement are necessary in the operating room within 2–3 days.

If the soft tissue wounds heal without necrosis or infection, careful follow-up and management of the avascular necrosis is necessary with long-term fracture bracing, as described in the discussion on the complications of fractures of the talus.

Osteochondral Fracture of the Dome of the Talus

REMARKS

Osteochondral fractures of the dome of the talus are small fractures of the articular surface of the medial or lateral domes of the talus that result from inversion mechanisms.

These injuries represent another condition that tends to be confused with a sprained ankle.

The osteochondral lesions are also frequently associated with a fracture of one of the malleoli and may be initially overlooked because of the attention focused on the malleolar fracture.

In most series, the typical patient is a male athlete in the second or third decade.

The osteochondral fracture may initially be minimally symptomatic, particularly if it involves the medial dome of the talus. The symptoms may range from intermittent pain in the joint and limited motion to recurrent swelling, clicking, or merely a weak ankle. Because of these symptoms, often the treatment is for recurrent ankle sprain.

On physical examination, the patient is usually tender anterolaterally or posteromedially in the ankle joint, depending on the location. Inversion and eversion are typically limited by pain or swelling, particularly in the acute injury.

Because of the sometimes difficult differential diagnosis between osteochondral fractures and recurrent sprain, careful roentgenographic evaluation is necessary. This includes a minimum of three views: anteroposterior, lateral, and mortise. If these are nondiagnostic, computed tomography may be necessary when the symptoms and history are typical, particularly in the patient with long-standing symptoms.

Berndt and Harty and Canale and Belding have contributed a great deal to our understanding of the diagnosis and management of these lesions.

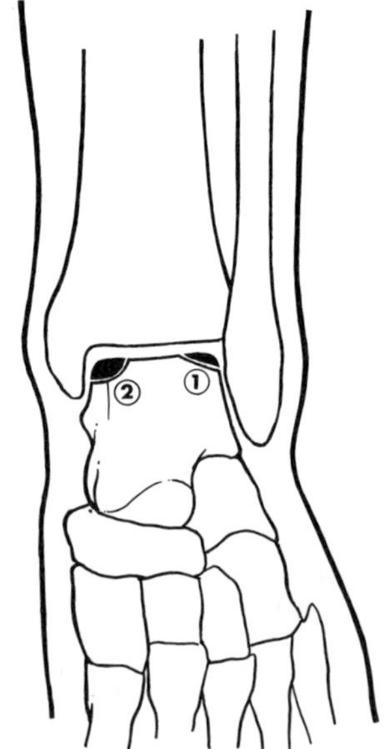

1. Lateral lesions are wafer-shaped and shallow, giving the appearance of being produced by shearing force.
2. Medial lesions are deep and cup-shaped. The depth of the crater is deeper than the width, which suggests that the cause may be other than trauma.

Note: Lateral lesions tend to produce more persistent symptoms and more arthritic changes on x-ray.

Stages of Osteochondral Lesions (After Berndt and Harty)

1. Stage I involves a small area of subchondral compression.
2. Stage II is a partially detached fragment.
3. Stage III is a completely detached fragment remaining in the crater.
4. Stage IV is a fragment that is loose in the joint.

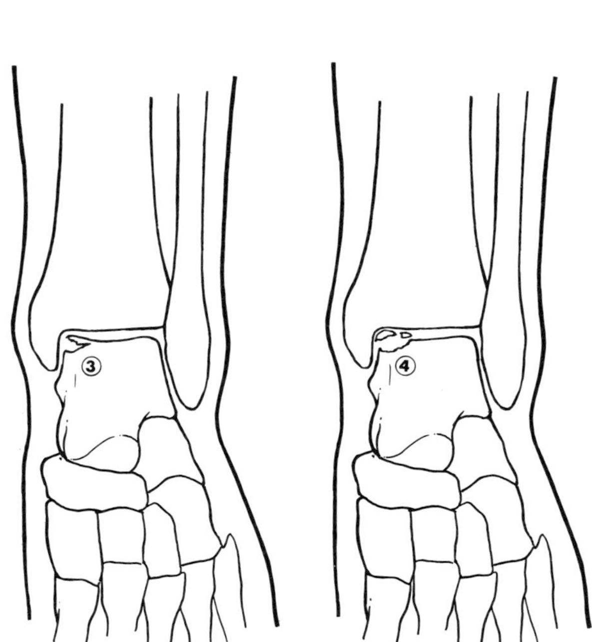

Management According to Stages (After Canale and Belding)

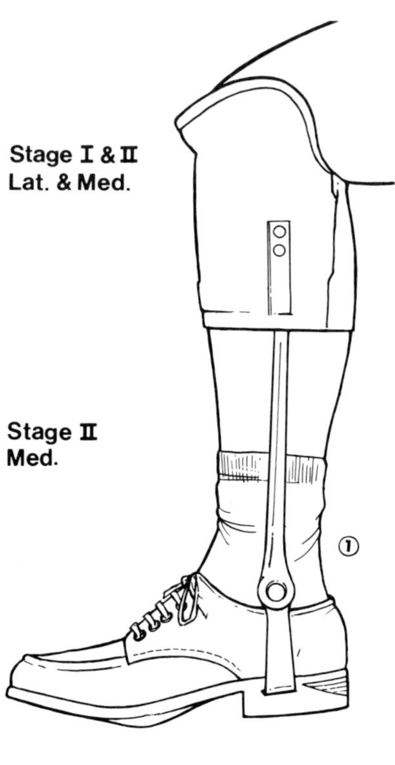

1. Stage I and Stage II lesions regardless of location and Stage III medial lesions can be treated nonoperatively for at least 4 months. A brace, such as a patellar tendon–bearing type, which unloads the ankle but still allows the ankle motion necessary for nourishment of the articular cartilage, is ideal for this purpose, particularly in patients who cannot stay on crutches.

Note: If the ankle causes persistent symptoms for more than 2–3 months, particularly if there is a question about the degree of displacement, operative intervention need not be delayed. In many instances, the lesion can be removed and the defect burred out by the use of arthroscopic techniques. Because of the success of operative versus nonoperative methods, the tendency when there is any question is in favor of operative treatment of these lesions.

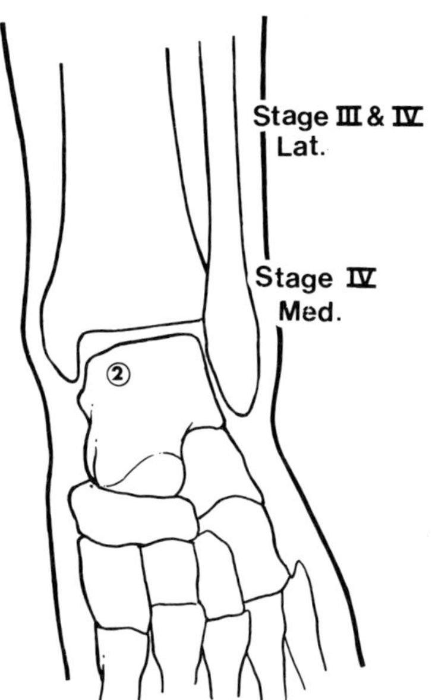

2. Stages III and IV lateral lesions and Stage IV medial lesions should be treated by arthroscopic or open excision and curettage.

Note: Osteotomy of the medial malleolus is frequently necessary to excise medial lesions.

Eversion Injuries

REMARKS

Eversion infrequently causes injury to the talus owing to the structural limitations built into the subtalar joint to resist eversion.

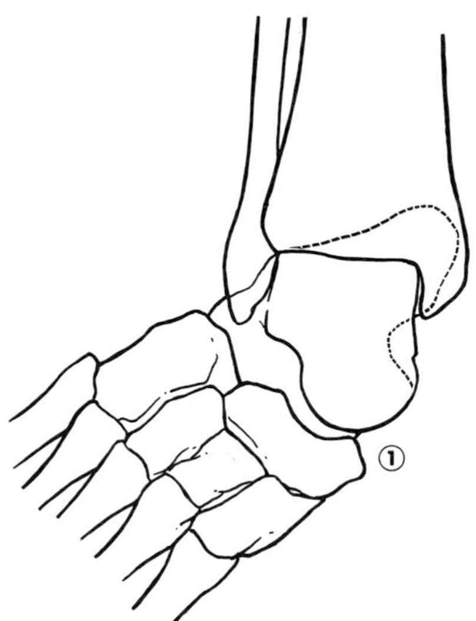

The occasional injuries that results from eversion mechanisms include

1. Lateral subtalar dislocation;

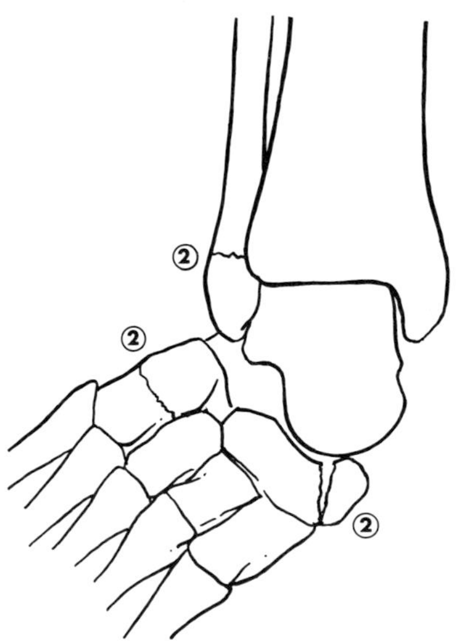

2. Fractures of the lateral malleolus, the navicular bone, or the cuboid associated with lateral subtalar dislocation; and

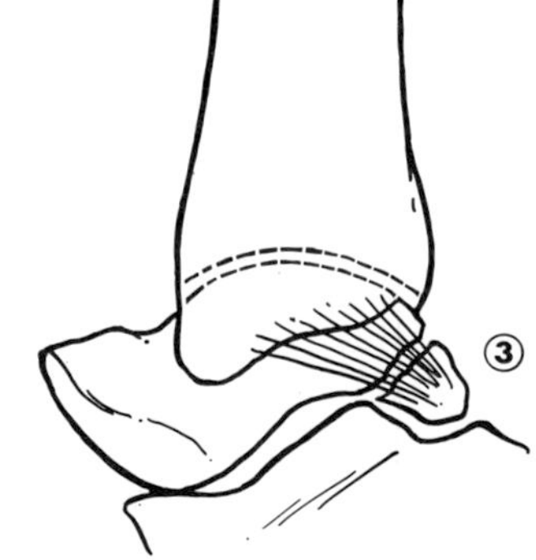

3. Avulsion of the medial side of the posterior talar tubercle produced by the pull of the posterior tibiotalar ligament.

Management

REMARKS

Because of structural limitations to eversion in the subtalar joint, this mechanism infrequently causes a fracture or dislocation of the talus.

Eversion–external rotation injuries are most likely to fracture the ankle (see Chapter 10).

The most common injury to the foot with eversion is a lateral subtalar dislocation.

Occasionally, fractures of the medial side of the posterior talar tubercle are also produced by the pull of the posterior tibiotalar ligament during eversion.

Lateral subtalar dislocation is more likely than medial subtalar dislocation to be associated with obstruction to reduction. This is frequently due to the posterior tibial tendon becoming displaced dorsal and lateral to the neck of the talus.

Leitner described a method of closed manipulation for the locked lateral dislocation. If this technique fails, prompt open reduction is indicated.

Anteroposterior View: Lateral Subtalar Dislocation

1. Subtalar joint is displaced laterally as a result of the eversion injury.
2. Os calcis and foot are also displaced posteriorly.
3. Reduction is obstructed by the posterior tibial tendon wrapping dorsally over the lateral neck of the talus.

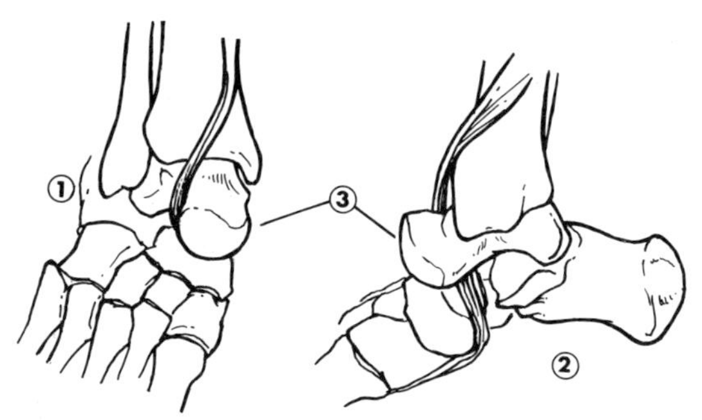

Technique of Closed Reduction (After Leitner)

1. Heel is grasped, and the foot is pulled forward to correct posterior displacement.
2. Foot is then fully dorsiflexed to release the posterior tibial tendon.
3. Foot is pushed medially, and the reduction is completed with the tendon regaining its normal position.

Note: If this maneuver does not reduce the dislocation, open reduction is indicated.

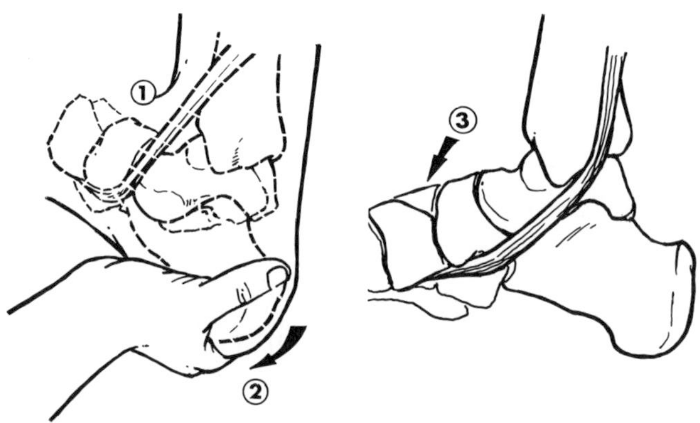

Subsequent Management

The foot is immobilized after reduction in a non–weight-bearing short-leg cast.

Elevate the leg for at least 3–5 days until the swelling has subsided.

The patient may then be up on crutches and should continue with non–weight-bearing crutch walking for 2–3 weeks.

The cast may then be removed, and progressive weight-bearing may be allowed.

Inversion and eversion are consistently limited after this injury, but the result may be satisfactory if avascular necrosis of the talus does not occur.

The patient should be followed by means of periodic x-rays for 6 months to detect signs of avascular necrosis.

■ Compression Injuries

REMARKS

Compression injuries can produce significant comminution and open displacement of the talus and surrounding structures.

If possible, the talus should be reduced and fixed internally, but frequently, this is impossible.

In severely comminuted open fractures of the talus, a primary talectomy and tibiotalar arthrodesis may be indicated.

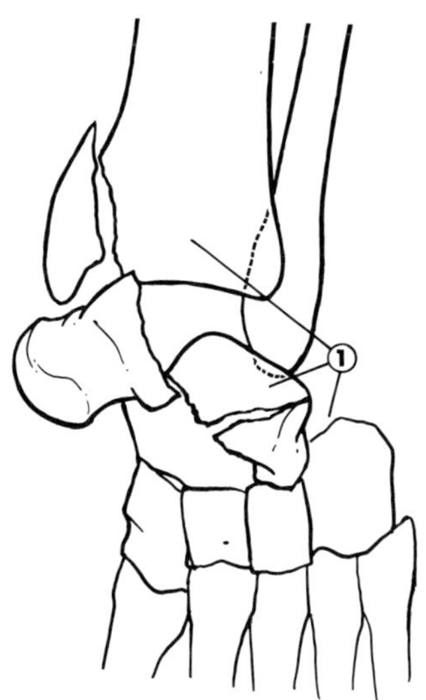

1. Compression injury has comminuted the talus, fractured the medial malleolus, and produced an open subtalar dislocation. The head and neck of the talus were extruded through the open wound.

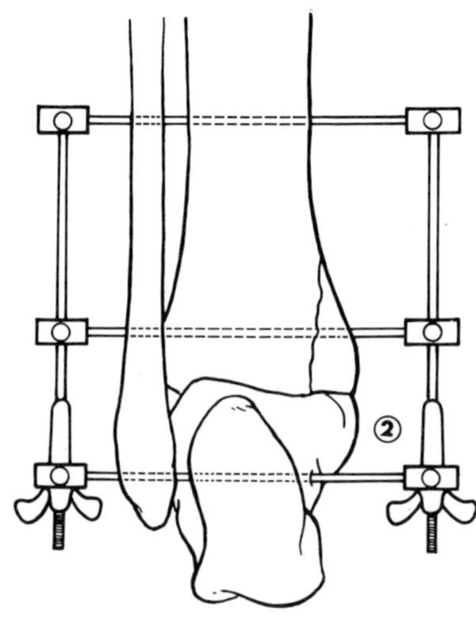

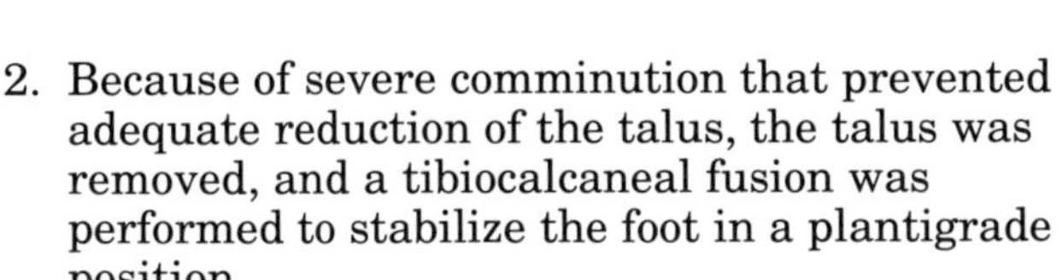

2. Because of severe comminution that prevented adequate reduction of the talus, the talus was removed, and a tibiocalcaneal fusion was performed to stabilize the foot in a plantigrade position.

Complications of Fractures and Fracture-Dislocations of the Talus

REMARKS

Undisplaced fractures of the talus generally heal rapidly without complication.

Displaced fractures or dislocations frequently result in significant problems, which range from infection to malunion, avascular necrosis, and traumatic arthritis, all of which prolong the disability.

Avascular Necrosis

REMARKS

The most common complication after a fracture or dislocation of the talus is avascular necrosis. This is produced by disruption of the blood supply to the talus.

Frequently, this is of more significance radiographically than clinically, particularly if the condition is detected early and the ankle is protected.

The blood supply to the talus is diffuse and arises from three major arteries of the lower leg:
1. Posterior tibial artery,
2. Dorsalis pedis artery, and
3. Peroneal artery.

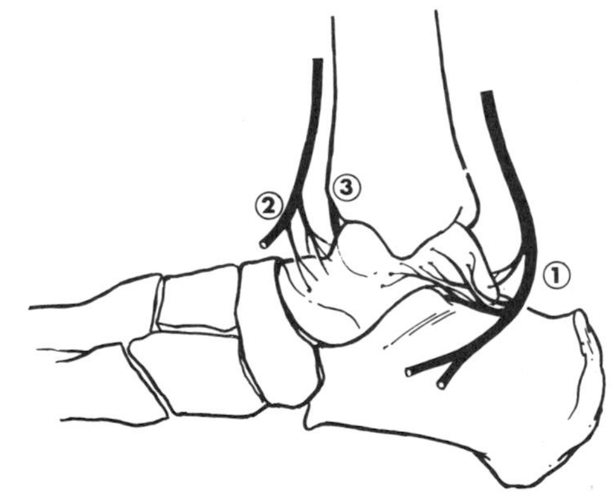

Blood Supply to the Posterior and Medial Talus

There is a rich intraosseous blood supply to the talus, particularly through the tarsal sinus and tarsal canal.
1. Posterior tibial artery gives a branch to the posterior tubercle via its calcaneal branches.
2. These form a plexus over the posterior tubercle along with branches from the peroneal artery.
3. The artery of the tarsal canal arises from the posterior tibial artery 1 cm proximal to the medial and lateral plantar branches. The artery passes between the sheaths of the flexor digitorum longus and flexor hallucis longus into the tarsal canal.
4. A deltoid branch comes off the artery of the tarsal canal to supply the medial surface of the body. This vessel runs between the talotibial and talocalcaneal portions of the deltoid ligament.

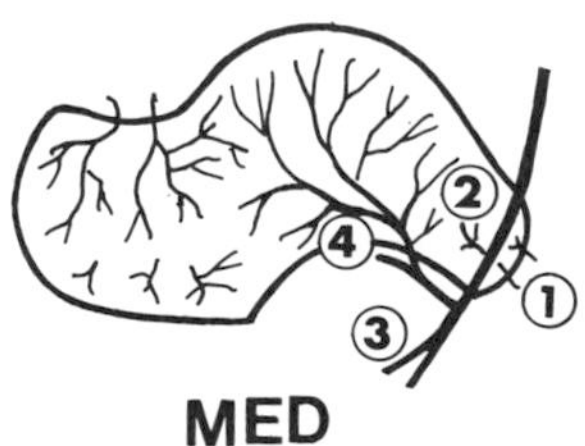

Blood Supply to the Lateral Talus

5. The artery of the tarsal sinus starts from a loop formed between the dorsalis pedis and the lateral tarsal branch of the perforating peroneal artery.
6. The artery of the tarsal sinus gives branches to the head of the talus.
7. It enters the tarsal sinus to give its blood supply to the body and
8. Anastomoses with the artery of the tarsal canal.

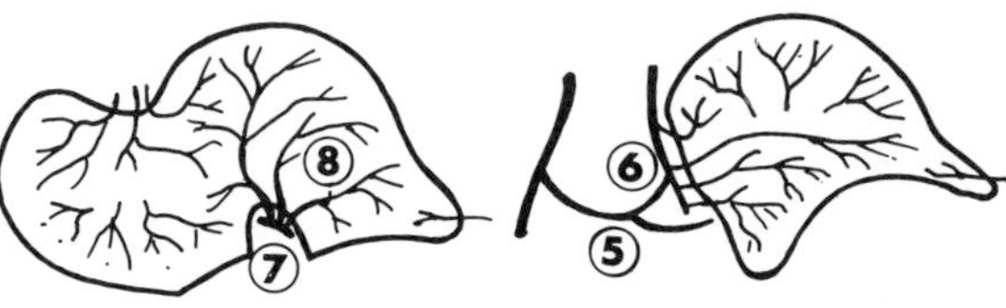

LAT

Effect of Injury on the Blood Supply to the Talus

Most fractures of the neck of the talus do not cause avascular necrosis. The vessels that enter the medial surface of the body and the anterolateral vessels and some of the vessels in the tarsal canal should remain intact.

The incidence of avascular necrosis rises sharply with dislocations and displaced fracture-dislocations of the body associated with extensive soft tissue detachment. Avascular necrosis is virtually inevitable after complete dislocation of the talus.

If the patient bears weight prematurely on a talus subject to avascular necrosis, subchondral collapse and secondary arthritis are likely. However, if weight-bearing is prevented for the period necessary to allow the talus to reconstitute itself, avascular necrosis does not inevitably lead to traumatic arthritis.

Surgical approaches through the tarsal sinus obliterate the major blood supply to the talus from the artery of the tarsal sinus and tarsal canal. Wide medial facet removal also adds to the likelihood of avascular necrosis. This should be kept in mind during operative reduction or any surgical procedure in this area, such as triple arthrodesis.

Diagnosis of Avascular Necrosis of the Talus

Avascular necrosis should be anticipated and suspected with any displaced fracture or dislocation of the talus.

Hawkins pointed out that the time to recognize avascular necrosis is between the sixth and eighth week after the injury. By this time, if the foot has not borne weight, disuse atrophy should be evident on the x-ray of the foot and distal tibia.

Subchondral osteolysis that is evident on the x-ray excludes the possibility of avascular necrosis and indicates the presence of healing revascularization.

Radiographic Signs of Normal Healing (After Hawkins)

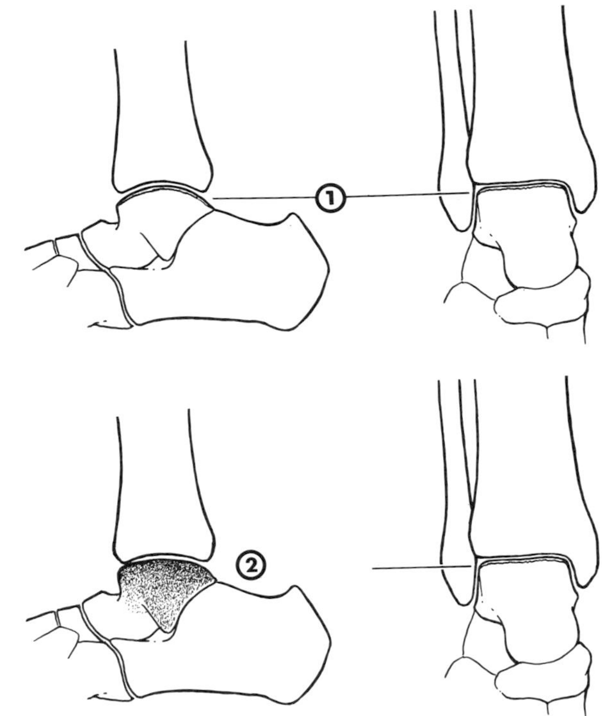

EARLY

1. X-rays of the ankle with the foot out of the cast show subchondral osteolysis of the dome, which indicates the presence of a revascularization response.

Note: Bone scans may also be useful to determine the status of the blood flow to the talus. The significance of bone scans, however, is still under investigation.

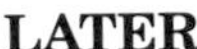

LATER

2. As the contrast between the dead bone of the body of the talus and the surrounding atrophic bone increases, the diagnosis of avascular necrosis can be made readily on a lateral x-ray.

Management of Established Avascular Necrosis

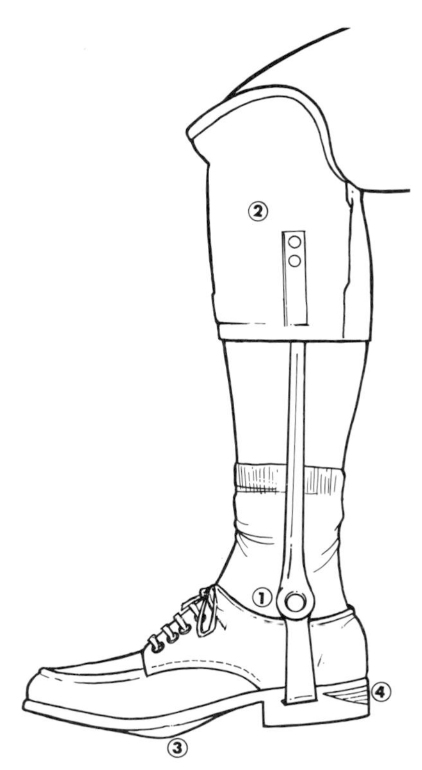

No surgical procedure is effective in the treatment of avascular necrosis once it occurs.

Protected walking with the use of a brace is necessary to allow bony reconstitution and prevent the collapse of the talus and secondary osteoarthritis.

The most effective method of protecting the ankle after the fracture heals is with a patellar tendon–bearing orthosis.

1. Rigid ankle shifts the weight from the talus up to the
2. Proximal tibia by means of the patellar tendon–bearing design.
3. Rocker bottom and
4. Solid ankle cushioned heel allow some heel-toe gait, despite the rigid ankle.

Subsequent Management

The ankle should be protected with crutches or a brace for a minimum of 4–6 months after avascular necrosis is identified.

If there is no evidence of collapse of the talus after the injury, the brace or crutches may generally be discarded after 4–6 months.

The subtalar joint will have some arthritis and definite limitation of motion, but the function of the limb may be satisfactory.

Keep in mind that clinical symptoms do not necessarily or consistently correlate with the changes seen on x-ray.

Nonunion and Malunion

REMARKS

Failure of the fractured talus to heal is infrequent, but delayed union that requires prolonged non–weight-bearing treatment is fairly commonly associated with closed management.

Early operative fixation is necessary for any displaced fracture of the talus, particularly when there is any question about the adequacy of the reduction on either the true lateral or the anteroposterior x-ray of the foot in plantar flexion.

Malunion is a fairly frequent complication that results from fractures of the talus because of the tendency of the head-and-neck fragment to displace dorsally and rotate internally relative to the body fragment.

The dorsal displacement of the fracture limits ankle motion because the fracture impinges on the anterior aspect of the tibia.

The malrotation of the fracture causes the entire foot to rotate internally, which results in a varus position of the entire foot. This makes walking uncomfortable and at times difficult.

Because of these sometimes unrecognized tendencies toward malunion, open reduction and internal fixation of the displaced fracture is usually preferable to closed treatment.

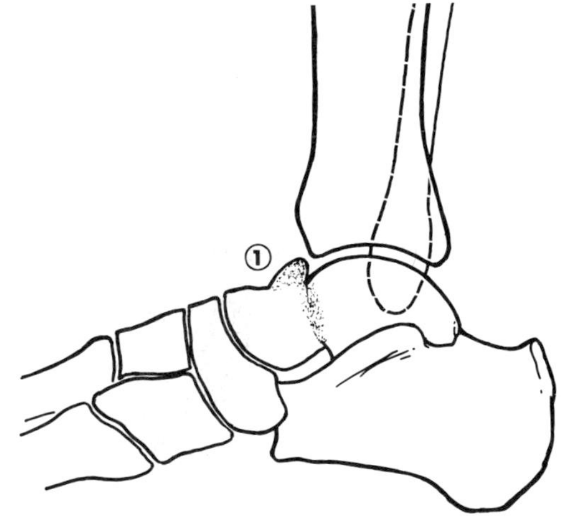

The most common causes of malunion include

1. Dorsal beaking of the talus and

Note: This frequently results when the cast is changed at about 4–6 weeks and the foot is taken out of a plantar-flexed position of reduction.

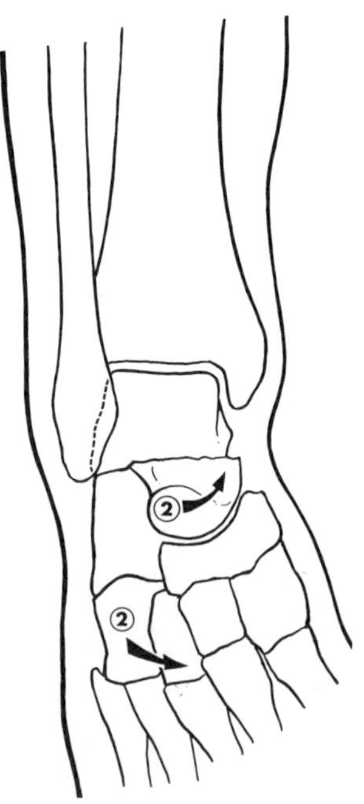

2. Torsional malalignment.

Torsional Malalignment: Effect on Foot Function

1. Healing with the distal fragment internally rotated in relation to the head fragment produces
2. Inversion and a varus position of the foot and causes the patient to walk on the lateral side of the foot.
3. Subtalar arthritis is common with torsional malalignment.

Note: Because the torsional malalignment that occurs with closed cast treatment is frequently not recognized until the patient resumes weight-bearing, open reduction and internal fixation of displaced fractures is preferable. This allows correction of the torsional position of the fracture and maintenance of the correct position to achieve a plantigrade foot.

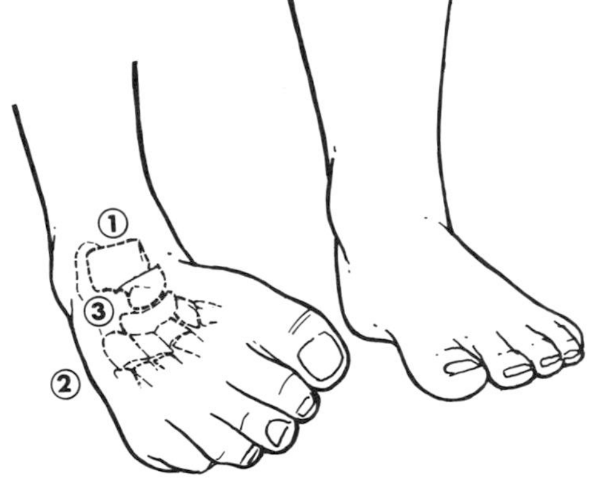

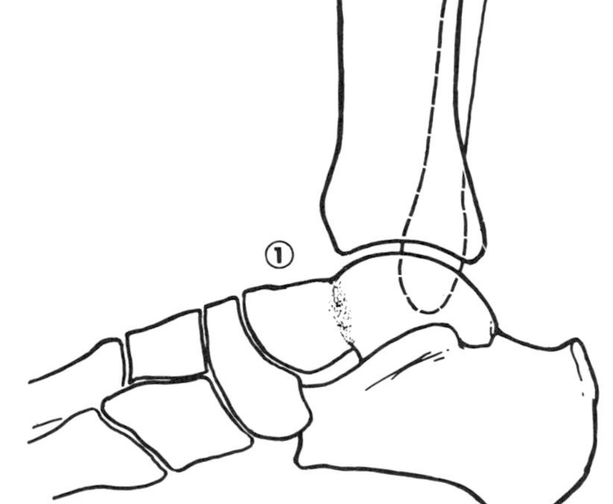

Management

FOR DORSAL BEAKING OF THE TALUS

1. Excision of the dorsal prominence relieves symptoms.

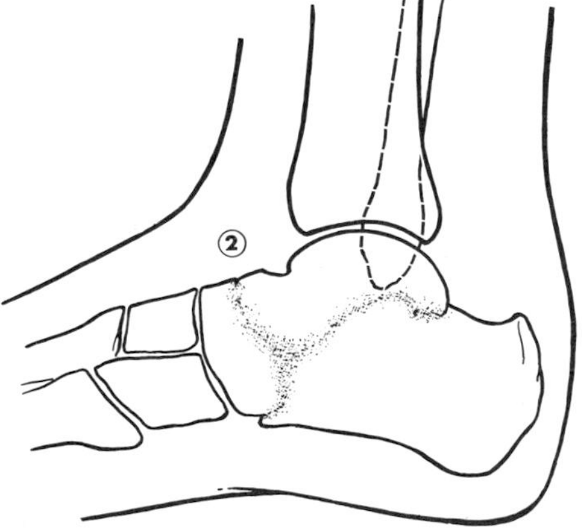

FOR TORSIONAL MALALIGNMENT

2. Triple arthrodesis of the hindfoot is necessary to correct the position of the foot and relieve the symptoms of subtalar arthritis.

Note: Before performing an arthrodesis for painful, traumatic arthritis, the surgeon should determine whether symptoms are also present in the ankle joint. An already arthritic ankle will be overstressed if the subtalar joint is fused.

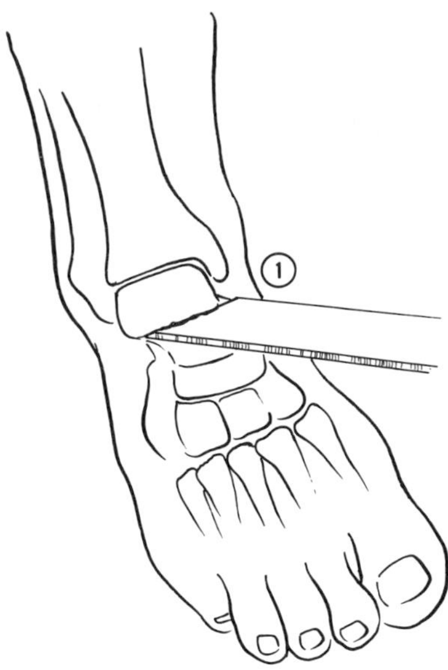

Osteotomy of the Talus for Torsional Malunion

1. If the rotational or torsional deformity is detected early enough after the fracture heals, it may be corrected by an osteotomy through the fracture of the talus.

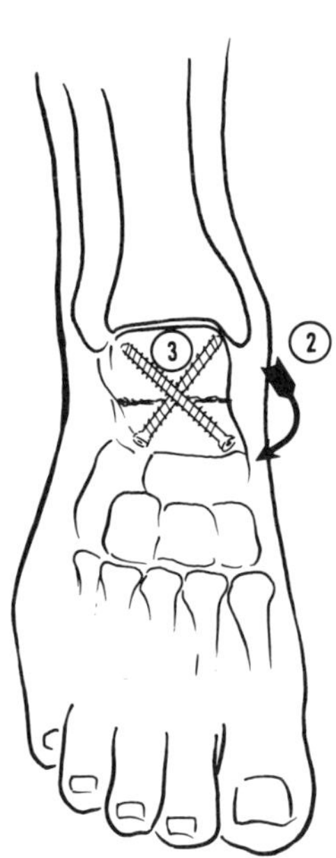

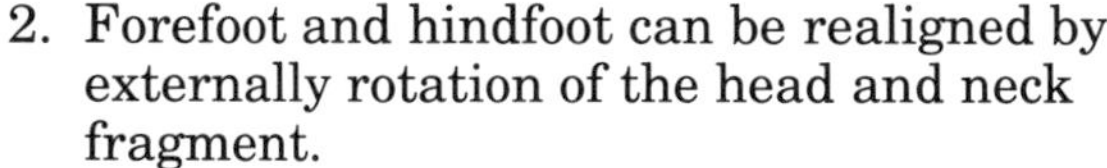

2. Forefoot and hindfoot can be realigned by externally rotation of the head and neck fragment.
3. Alignment can then be maintained with screw fixation.

Note: In most instances, the deformity is not corrected early enough, and arthritis of the subtalar joint requires triple arthrodesis rather than a corrective osteotomy of the talus to relieve the symptoms.

Infection

REMARKS

Because the talus is composed almost entirely of cancellous bone and the injury frequently deprives the talus of its blood supply, infection is disastrous.

Repeated sequestrectomy or attempted excision of draining sinuses is futile for osteomyelitis of the talus.

Talectomy by itself gives unsatisfactory results because of painful instability.

The treatment of choice, once infection occurs after fracture or dislocation of the talus, is talectomy with tibiocalcaneal fusion. This removes the source of infection and still permits functional weight-bearing stability of the foot.

Management of Infection After Fracture-Dislocation of the Talus

1. Compression injury has comminuted the talus, fractured the medial malleolus, and produced an open subtalar dislocation. The head and neck of the talus were extruded through the open wound.

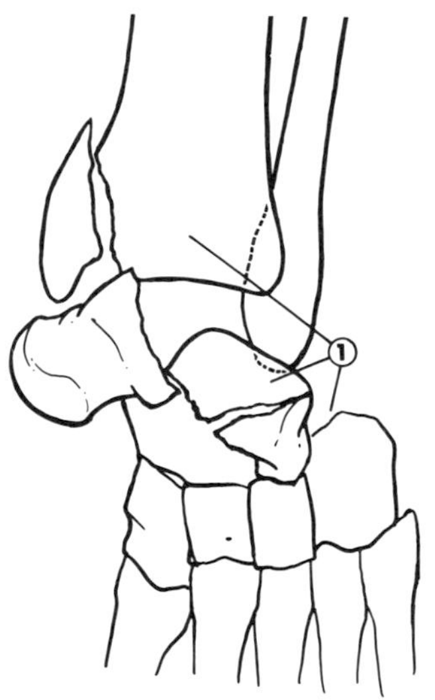

1. Talus is completely excised.
2. Articular cartilages of the calcaneus, the distal tibia, and the malleoli are removed.
3. Calcaneus is held in approximation against the tibia by transverse compression pins using the external fixator technique for immobilization.

Note: Talectomy and tibiocalcaneal fusion are indicated only for infections or severely comminuted talar fractures. Even when complete avascular necrosis develops after a dislocated talus, the functional result is usually better if the talus is left in place and protected long enough for it to heal by creeping substitution. For symptomatic osteoarthritis without infection, a Blair tibiotalar fusion may give better tibiopedal motion and less shortening of the foot than a tibiocalcaneal fusion.

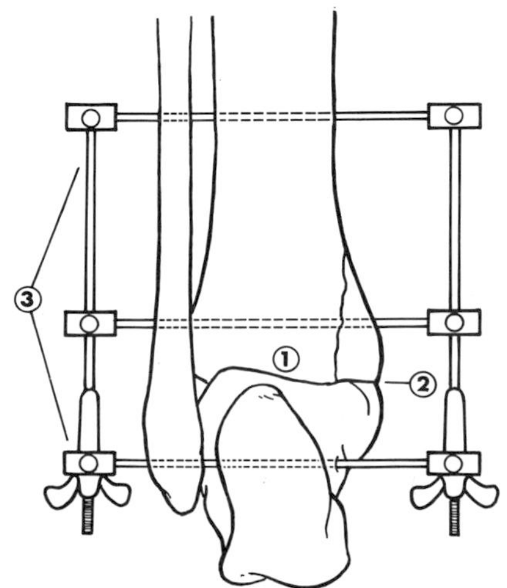

Arthritis of the Subtalar and Tibiotalar Joints

REMARKS

Subtalar arthritis of some degree develops in almost 50 per cent of talar fractures and in 60–70 per cent of fracture-dislocations. The incidence of arthritis appears to be related to the degree of the initial injury, the degree of displacement, and the completeness of reduction. Rotational malalignment particularly leads to arthritis of the hindfoot.

Arthritic involvement of the tibiotalar and the subtalar joint may occur if there has been an injury to the distal tibial articular surface or collapse of the talus secondary to avascular necrosis.

Not all patients with radiographic signs of arthritic changes have significant long-term symptoms. However, malunion, particularly with the foot and subtalar joint internally rotated, causes pain with strenuous activity or walking on uneven ground. These patients then require arthrodesis to correct the foot position and relieve the symptoms.

If the symptoms of arthritis result from collapse of the talus, a Blair tibiotalar arthrodesis can give good or even excellent results.

Blair Tibiotalar Fusion

PREOPERATIVE X-RAY

1. Avascular necrosis and
2. Malunion of the talar fracture has resulted in
3. Tibiotalar arthritis 12 months after the injury.

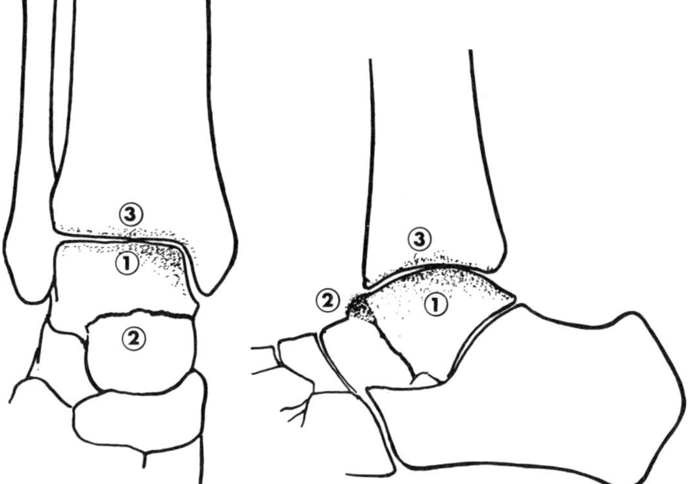

Blair Arthrodesis

1. Blair arthrodesis consists of fusion of the head and neck of the talus to the tibia.
2. The avascular body of the talus and the arthritic ankle joint are excised.
3. Contact between the neck of the talus and the tibia is maintained by screw fixation.

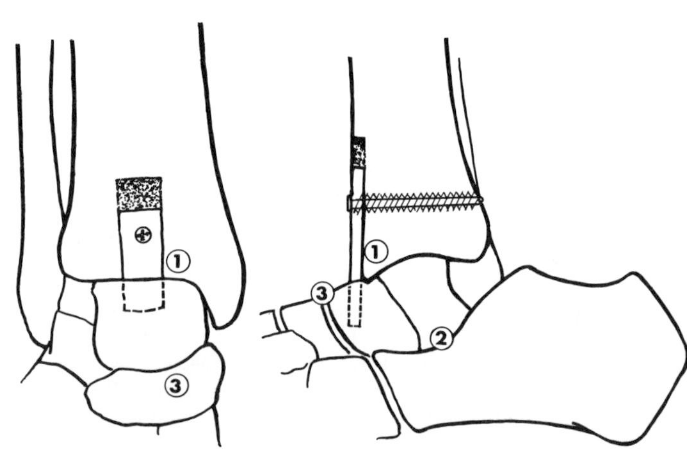

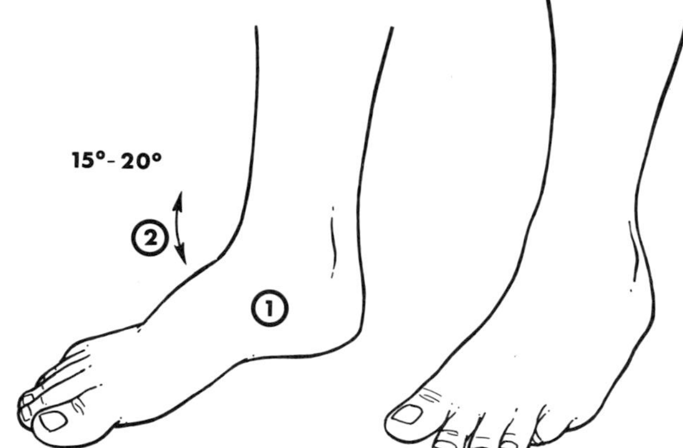

Clinical Result After Blair Arthrodesis

1. The clinical appearance of the foot is good, and
2. Tibiopedal motion of 15°–20° is maintained.

FRACTURES OF THE CALCANEUS

REMARKS

The calcaneus is the largest bone in the foot and the one most frequently fractured. The fracture may be incurred from a minor fall or from major violence.

Os calcis fracture is bilateral in 10–20 per cent of injuries. There are associated fractures of the spine, tibia, or ankle in 20–30 per cent of os calcis fractures. Every patient with an os calcis fracture should therefore be evaluated for fractures elsewhere.

Most of these fractures extend into the subtalar joint and produce varying degrees of joint disruption. Less than 40 per cent involve only the nonarticular portion of the bone.

The treatment of fractures involving the nonarticular portion of the bone is mainly symptomatic. Cast immobilization is useful to relieve pain for a maximum of 2–3 weeks, after which the patient should be encouraged to start active range-of-motion exercises while the injured foot is protected with crutches.

Treatment of the more common fractures, which extend into the articular weight-bearing surface, is more problematic and should be based on detailed assessment of potential complications.

Anatomic Landmarks

1. Böhler's tuberosity joint angle is the angle formed by line A from the highest point on the posterior surface to the most superior part of the calcaneal tuberosity and
2. Line B from the highest point on the anterior process.
3. The intervening angle or Böhler's joint angle is usually between 20° and 40° but is altered considerably with a fracture that involves the posterior articular surface.

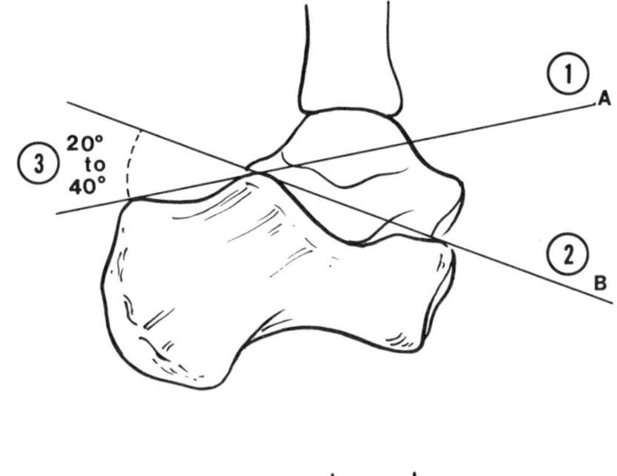

Crucial Angle of Gissane

1. The angle formed by the subchondral density beneath the posterior facet and
2. The subchondral density beneath the anterior and middle facets is called the angle of Gissane.
3. This angle supports the lateral process of the talus and is frequently the site of impact and the primary fracture line when the talus is wedged into the calcaneus in a fall.

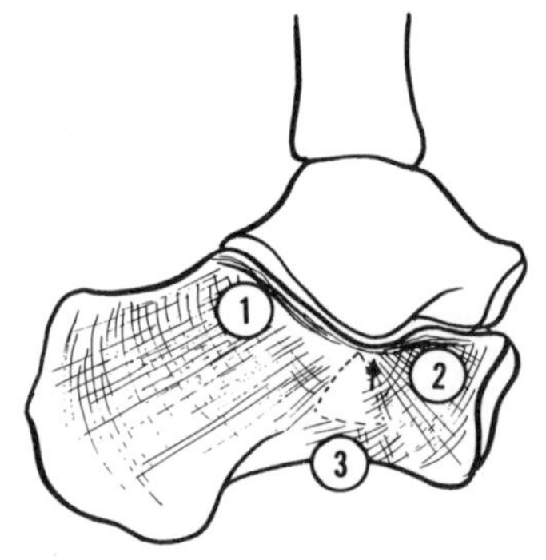

Mechanisms

REMARKS

A typical mechanism is a fall onto the heel from various heights. Frequently (10–20 per cent of the time), both heels are involved.

The type of fracture, either articular or extra-articular, is dependent to some extent on the position of the heel at the time of impact. If the heel is everted, the talus wedges the posterior facet of the calcaneus and produces an intra-articular fracture.

If the foot and heel are inverted at the time of impact, frequently the extra-articular structures, such as the anterior process of the talus or tuberosity or the medial and lateral processes, are fractured without invoving the subtalar joint.

1. If the heel is everted at the time of impact, the talus wedges the posterior facet of the calcaneus.

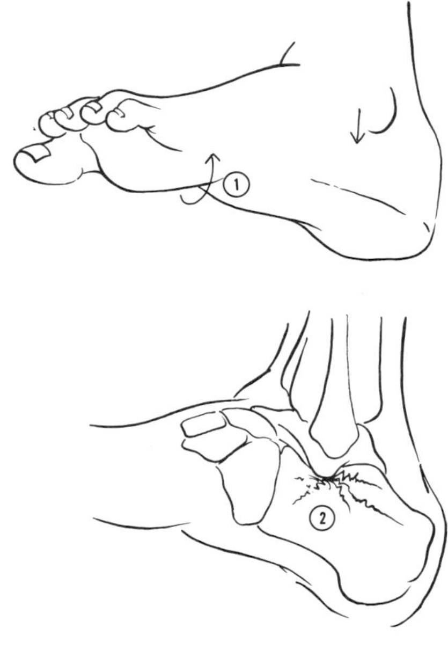

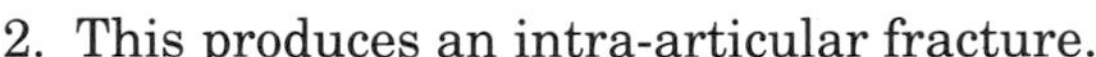

2. This produces an intra-articular fracture.

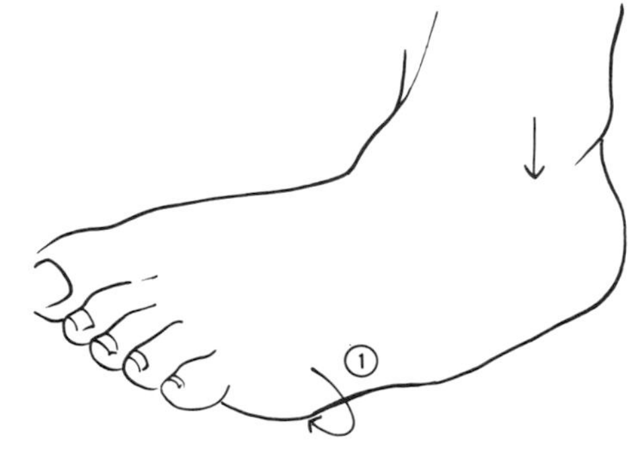

1. If the foot and heel are inverted at the time of impact, the
2. Extra-articular structures, such as the anterior process of the calcaneus or the tuberosity of the calcaneus, are fractured without involving the subtalar joint.

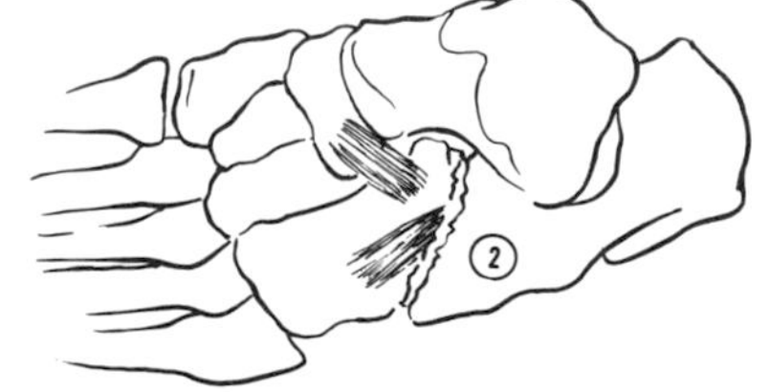

Note: The fracture that does not involve the subtalar joint usually has a considerably better healing time and less long-term symptoms than does the fracture that is intra-articular. This is particularly true if the fracture that involves the posterior facet of the calcaneus is displaced or comminuted.

■ Radiographic Assessment

REMARKS

In addition to standard anteroposterior and lateral views, there are a number of other recommended techniques to visualize the entire callus.

Frequently, coned-down views are necessary to detect isolated extra-articular fractures, such as fractures of the anterior process or tuberosity.

For fractures that involve the subtalar joint, Broden's views are helpful to see the entire posterior facet.

Broden's Projection

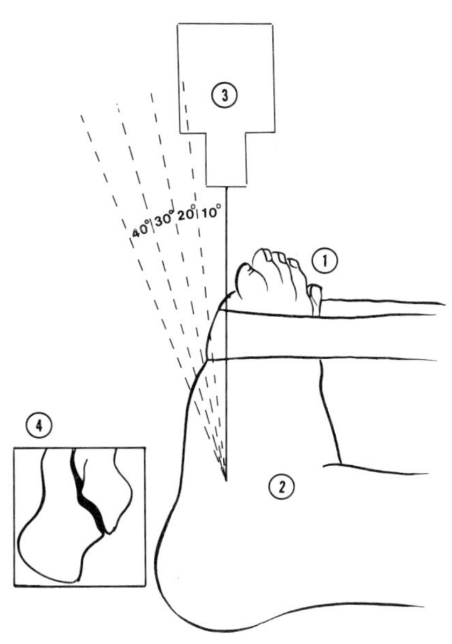

1. Foot is positioned internally rotated 45°.
2. Ankle is dorsiflexed 90°.
3. Four views are taken at 10°, 20°, 30°, and 40°.
4. This allows complete visualization of the posterior lateral facet.

Note: A similar series of Broden's projection can be obtained with the foot externally rotated to see the medial aspect of the joint surface and sinus tarsi.

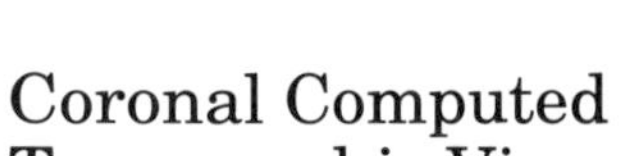

Coronal Computed Tomographic Views

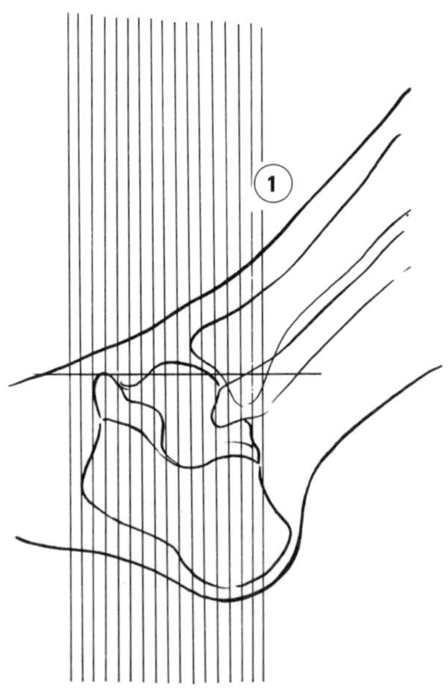

1. Although Broden's view is adequate to visualize most calcaneal fractures, computed tomography is also helpful, particularly if operative intervention may be necessary.

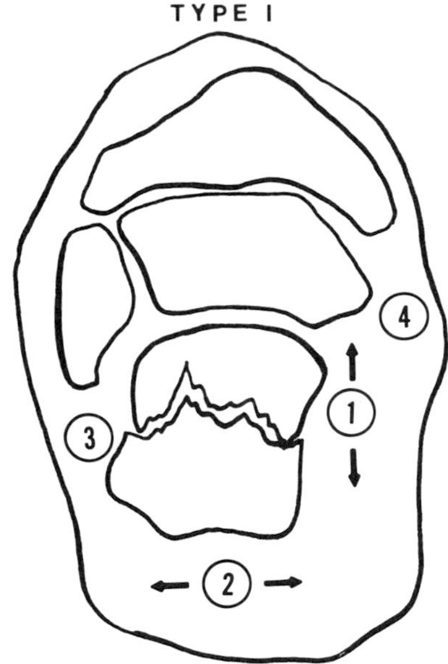

Coronal computed tomography view will show

1. Shortening,
2. Widening,
3. Lateral impingement, and the
4. Extent of posterior facet involved.

Note: Crosby and Fitzgibbons pointed out that extensive involvement of the posterior facet joint indicates a relatively poor prognosis with closed treatment. This finding needs to be studied further but may be a helpful indicator of the possible need for open reduction in some calcaneal fractures.

■ Isolated Fractures of the Calcaneus Without Implication of the Subtalar Joint

REMARKS

Approximately 30 per cent of these calcaneal fractures do not involve the subtalar joint and have minimal to no displacement.

A key problem with these fractures is to distinguish them from sprains of the ankle because the usual mechanism is inversion injury to the ankle.

Persistent or extreme pain after an inversion injury, particularly when it is located in the heel rather than the ankle, should prompt careful evaluation clinically and by x-ray for an undisplaced extra-articular calcaneal fracture.

The most common extra-articular fracture is a minimally displaced fracture of the anterior process.

Other less common fractures include fractures of the tuberosity of the calcaneus or fracture of the sustentaculum tali without displacement.

Common Extra-Articular Calcaneal Fractures

1. Minimally displaced fracture of the anterior process.

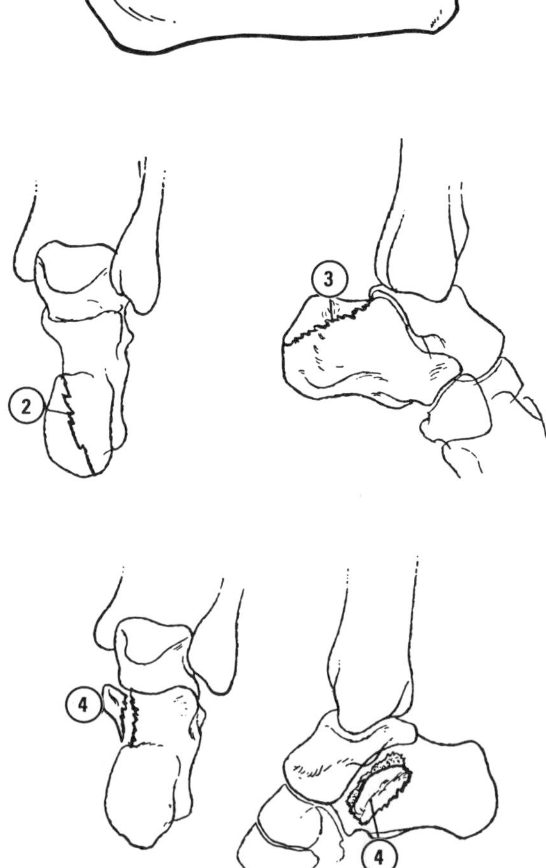

2. Vertical fracture of the tuberosity without displacement.
3. Horizontal fracture of the tuberosity without displacement.
4. Fracture of the sustentaculum tali with minimal displacement.

Management of Extra-Articular Fractures

REMARKS

Most extra-articular fractures can be treated symptomatically.

If the patient is minimally symptomatic, the best treatment is ice, compression dressing, and early mobilization.

Most patients are sufficiently symptomatic to require a brief period of cast immobilization. It should be emphasized that the period of cast immobilization should be brief, usually no longer than 10–14 days followed by early active range of motion.

The fracture heals clinically before it does radiographically. Therefore, treatment should be based on clinical symptoms rather than radiographic signs.

Manipulative reduction is rarely necessary, except for a significantly displaced tuberosity fracture or sustentacular fracture.

Occasionally, horizontal fractures of the tuberosity may rarely require internal fixation.

Immobilization for Symptomatic Undisplaced Extra-Articular Fractures

1. Apply a below-knee plaster cast with a
2. Walking heel.
3. Foot is at a right angle and
4. In neutral in regard to inversion and eversion.

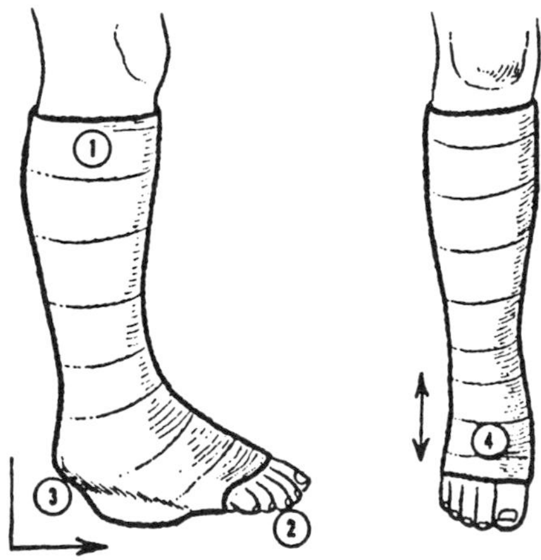

Note: If the patient is minimally symptomatic, a cast may be avoided, and the fracture may be treated simply by compression dressing, ice, early exercises, and crutches.

It is important not to prolong cast immobilization but to use the cast merely as a means to relieve the acute pain symptoms associated with the fracture.

Subsequent Management

Permit weight-bearing as tolerated.

Most of these fractures heal promptly, and disability, if any, is from some residual stiffness. Consequently, cast immobilization should be kept at a minimum, and the cast can generally be removed at the end of 2–3 weeks.

Subsequently, the patient is allowed to continue weight-bearing with crutches, and the crutches are discarded within 2–3 weeks after cast removal.

Apply an elastic ankle support to diminish edema for the first 3–5 weeks after the cast is removed.

Extra-Articular Fractures of the Calcaneus That Require Reduction

REMARKS

Occasionally, a fracture of the sustentaculum or a horizontal or vertical fracture of the tuberosity of the calcaneus may displace sufficiently to warrant an attempt at manipulative reduction.

These all can be treated by minimal manipulation and minimal cast immobilization because the major concern is to avoid stiffening of the foot, particularly the hindfoot and subtalar joint.

The only extra-articular calcaneal fracture that occasionally requires operative reduction is the displaced horizontal fracture of the tuberosity that cannot be reduced by closed methods.

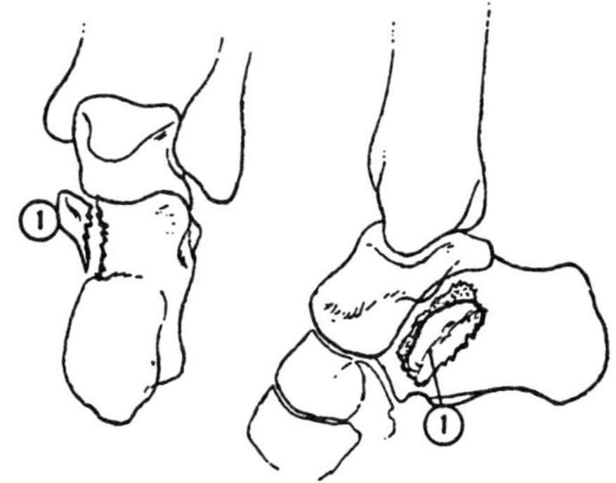

1. Prereduction x-ray of a displaced fracture of the sustentaculum that may require manipulation.

Manipulative Reduction for Displaced Fractures of the Sustentaculum or the Tuberosity of the Calcaneus

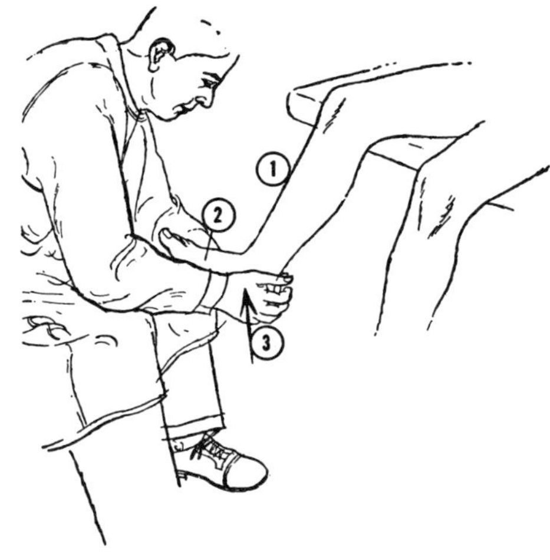

1. Patient's leg is allowed to hang over the edge of the table.
2. Forefoot rests on the operator's knee.
3. Operator inverts the heel and molds the displaced fragment back.

Note: If reduction of the sustentaculum fragment is incomplete, it may still be accepted. There is really no indication for open reduction of these fragments that are extra-articular.

If a symptomatic nonunion develops after a displaced extra-articular fracture, excision of the fragment may occasionally be necessary to relieve the symptoms.

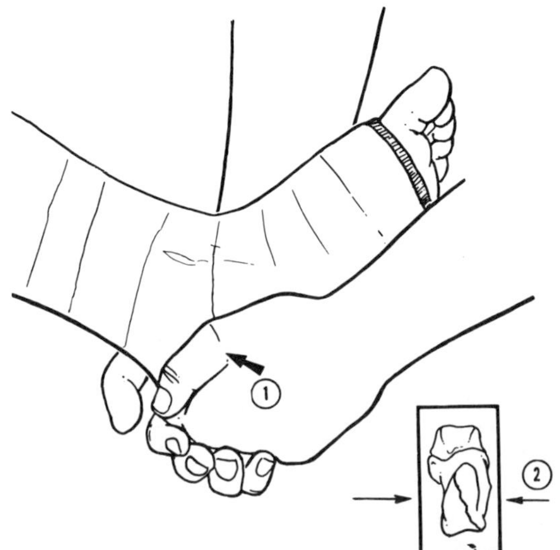

1. Operator compresses the heel with both hands while the plaster sets.
2. Molding of the plaster on the soft tissues and os calcis is sufficient to reduce the fracture.

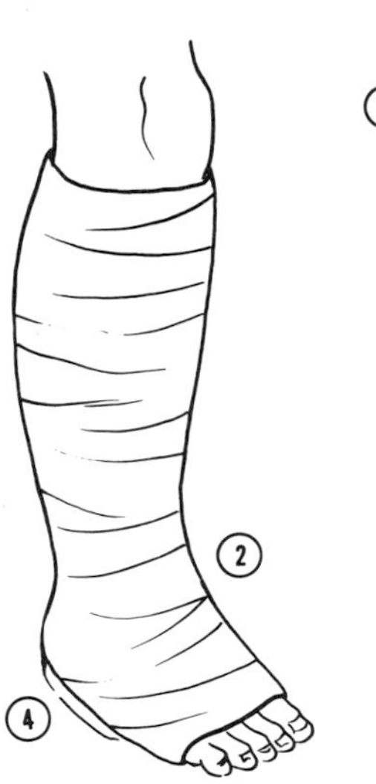

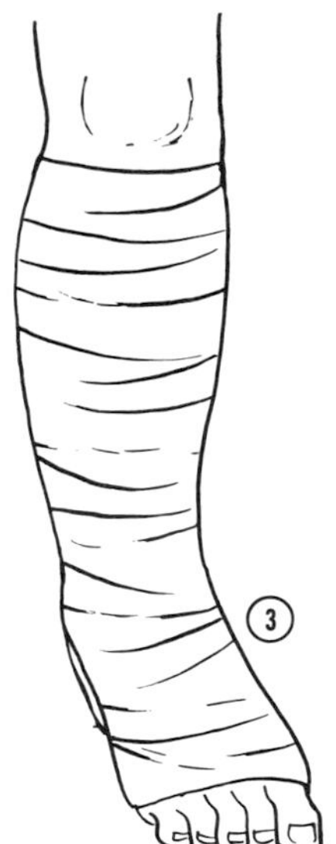

Immobilization

1. Below-knee plaster cast is applied with a
2. Slight equinus position.
3. Heel is slightly inverted.
4. Walking heel is applied.

Subsequent Management

REMARKS

The patient may be allowed to bear weight as tolerated on the cast.

Remove the cast at approximately 3 weeks or as soon as the patient's symptoms subside.

Apply a compression dressing to diminish the persistent swelling of the foot and ankle for several more weeks.

Begin active exercises to restore normal motion to the ankle, subtalar joint, and forefoot.

Note: The fracture should be treated on the basis of clinical symptoms rather than radiographic findings because it heals clinically considerably earlier than it does by x-ray.

Nondisplaced Fracture of the Calcaneus in Diabetic Patients

Caution: If a patient has juvenile-onset diabetes, undisplaced fractures of the calcaneus can occur as a result of neurotrophic changes.

These are notoriously difficult to treat despite their initially benign appearance.

They must be protected against weight-bearing to avoid further severe collapse.

Even with this treatment, progressive resorption and collapse is common.

1. Undisplaced fracture of the tuberosity is evident in a 25-year-old patient with juvenile-onset diabetes.

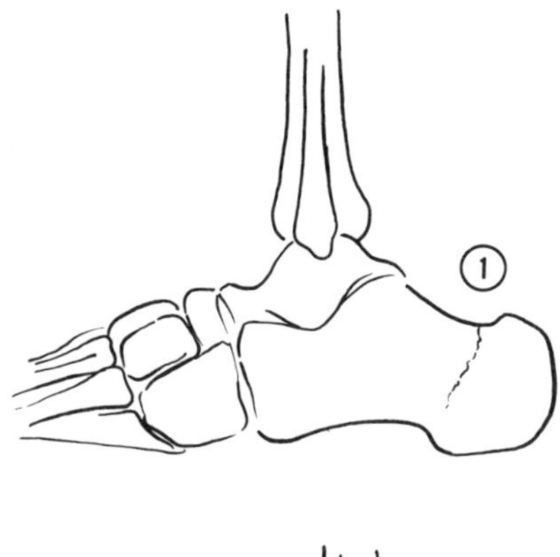

2. Eight months after treatment, despite non–weight-bearing, the foot showed severe progressive neurotrophic destruction and deformity.

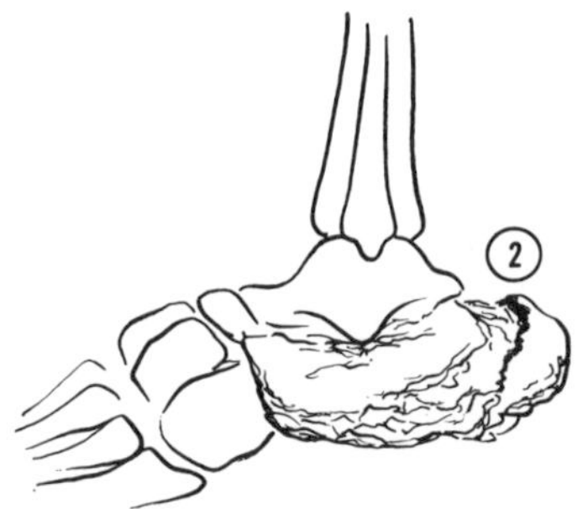

Management

The problem of calcaneal fracture in a diabetic patient almost defies adequate management.

Even with prolonged non–weight-bearing, deformity occurs as a result of the underlying condition, which is abnormal autonomic control of blood flow to the heel. The consequence is bone resorption rather than bone formation after the fracture.

In addition, if the patient is advised not to load the fractured heel, the opposite foot frequently fractures and deforms. This then becomes a secondary problem or complication.

Adequate protection with a patellar tendon–bearing orthosis can diminish the deformity but not eliminate it entirely.

1. A patellar tendon–bearing or similar orthosis is necessary to protect a diabetic patient's foot that manifests neurotrophic fracturing of the heel or other areas.

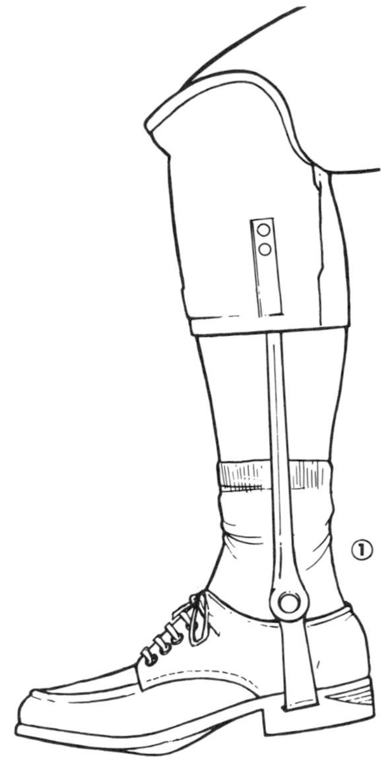

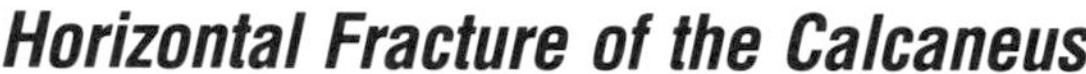

Horizontal Fracture of the Calcaneus

Prereduction X-Ray

1. Horizontal fracture of the tuberosity with upward displacement of the fragment.

Note: This fragment may not include the attachment of the Achilles tendon and, therefore, can be treated by closed manipulation.

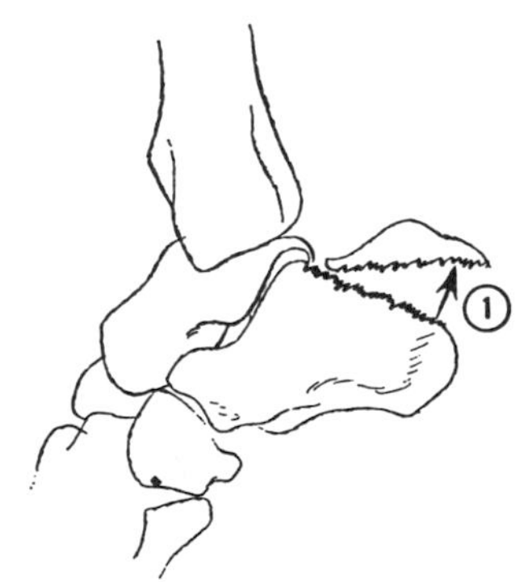

If the patient demonstrates weakness of ankle plantar flexion and loss of passive plantar flexion on squeezing the calf, operative reduction and fixation of the fragment and attached Achilles tendon is usually necessary. If these tests are inconclusive, it is generally safer to explore and fix the fracture fragment rather than rely on closed treatment.

Calf-Squeeze Test to Determine Achilles Tendon Rupture or Avulsion

1. Patient is asked to kneel with the knee on the injured side supported by the examining table.
2. Examiner squeezes the calf on the injured side.
3. Squeezing the calf causes a contraction of the calf muscle and plantar flexion of the ankle and foot if the Achilles tendon is intact.
4. If there is no plantar-flexion response to the calf-squeeze test, this indicates that the Achilles tendon has been avulsed and generally requires surgical repair.

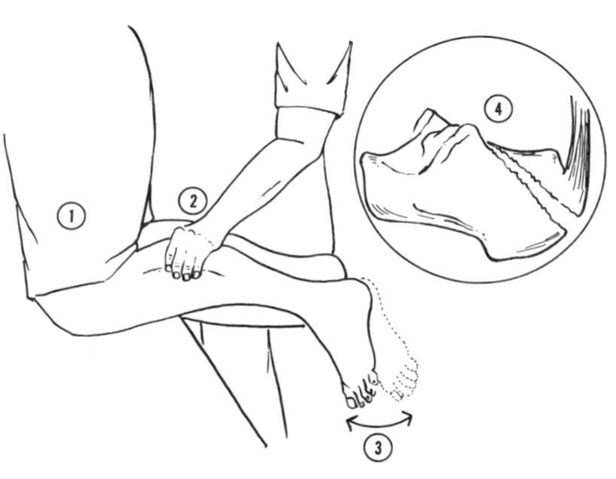

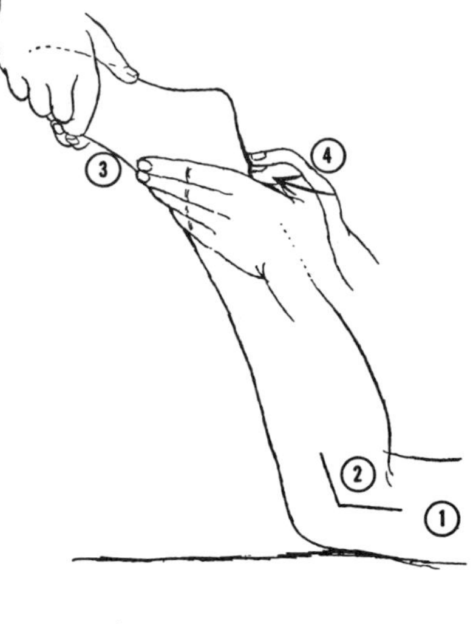

Manipulative Reduction

1. Patient is in the prone position.
2. Knee is flexed 70°.
3. Foot is plantar-flexed.
4. Operator places a thumb on each side of the Achilles tendon and makes firm downward pressure on the displaced fragment.

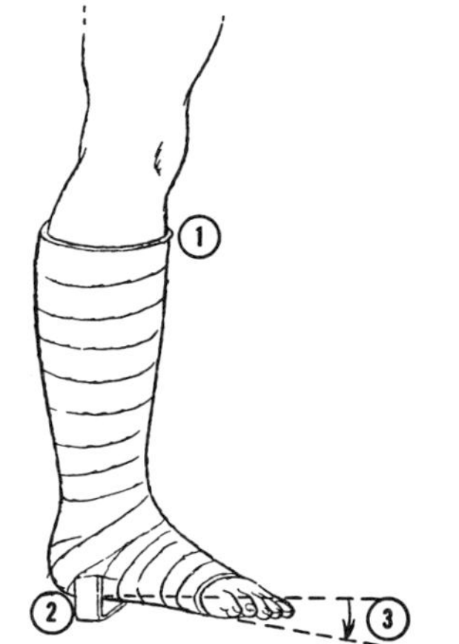

Immobilization

1. Apply a below-knee plaster cast with a
2. Walking heel.
3. Foot is in slight plantar flexion.

Alternative Method: Open Reduction Internal Fixation

Open reduction is usually necessary if the posterior tuberosity fragment is large and displaced.

Most often, this occurs when the fragment includes the attachment of the Achilles tendon.

In these circumstances, it is necessary to restore the tuberosity to its normal position to allow adequate reattachment of the tendon.

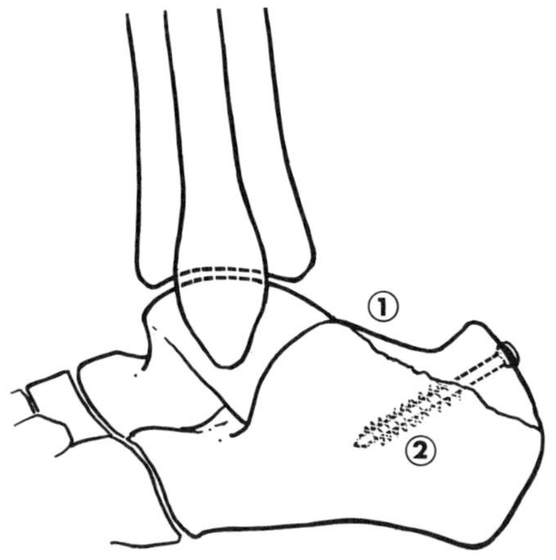

Postreduction X-Ray

1. Fragment is in normal apposition to the rest of the calcaneus.
2. Cancellous lag screw transfixes both fragments.

Fractures of the Calcaneus That Involve the Subtalar Joint

REMARKS

Most os calcis fractures (up to 70 per cent) cause varying degrees of damage to the articular surface of the subtalar joint.

There is a definite pattern to the fragments that is produced by the consistent pathomechanics of the injury and by the architectural relationships of the talus and the os calcis.

Essex-Lopresti showed that the fracture occurs when the talus impacts on the crucial angle of the calcaneus.

This produces a primary fracture line that runs from the crucial angle in the lateral cortex to the plantar calcaneal surface. This may be undisplaced.

If the force continues, a secondary fracture line that extends from the crucial angle of Gissane produces either a joint depression fracture or a tongue-type fracture.

Normal Architecture of the Calcaneus

1. Tuberosity is offset laterally.
2. Sustentaculum is offset medially.

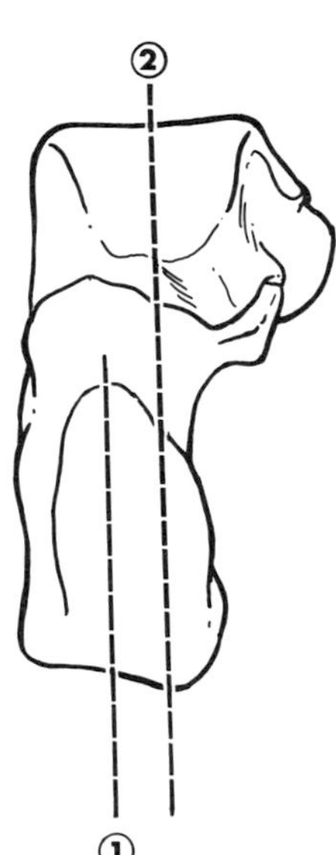

Pathomechanics of an Intra-Articular Fracture

1. Vertical loading of the calcaneus by the talus is concentrated at the crucial angle of Gissane.
2. Posterior subtalar joint is forced into eversion as the lateral process of the talus is driven into the crucial angle.
3. Primary fracture is a line that extends from the crucial angle to the plantar calcaneal surface.

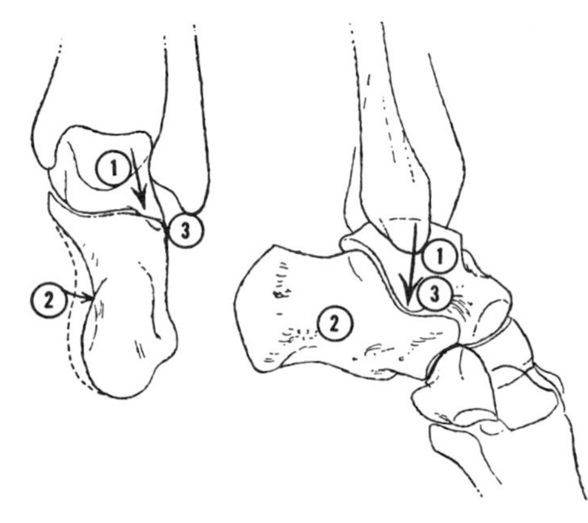

1. If the force is eliminated after the initial fracture occurs, the result is a nondisplaced intra-articular fracture.
2. If the force continues, a secondary fracture line is produced from the angle of Gissane posteriorly. A tongue-type fracture occurs when a secondary fracture line runs straight back from the crucial angle to the posterior border of the tuberosity.
3. If the secondary fracture line runs across the calcaneal body to immediately behind the posterior facet of the subtalar joint, a joint depression fracture occurs.

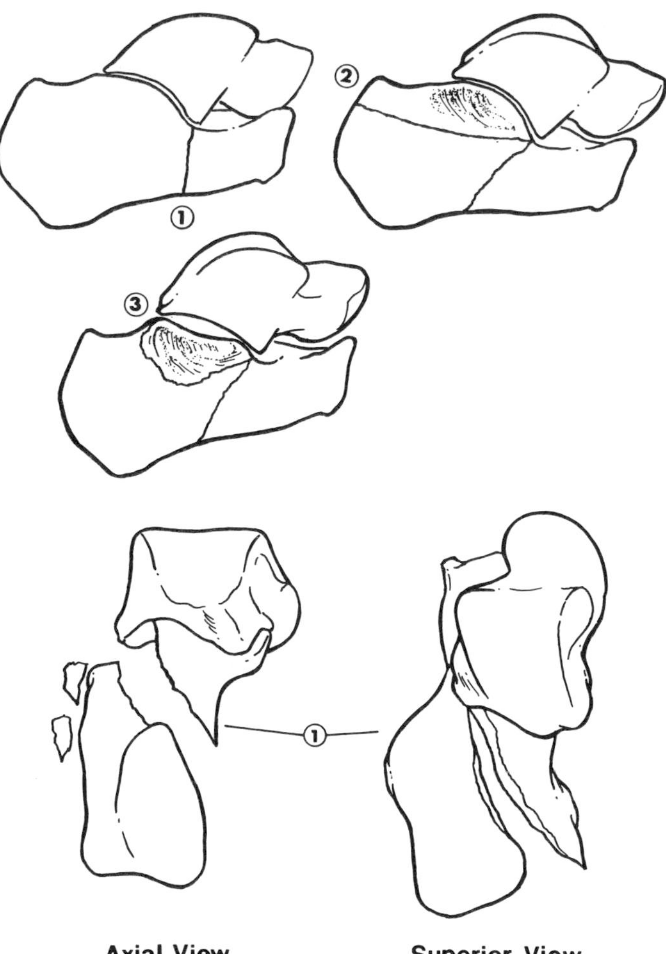

Patterns of Fracture

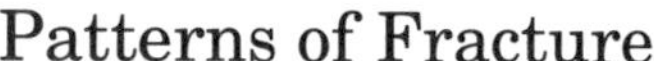

Burdeaux, in biomechanical studies that produced os calcis fractures in cadaver specimens, showed that consistently the

1. Fracture line displaces between the sustentaculum tali and the tuberosity. It produces two major fragments that are seen on the axial view.

The main difference between the tongue or joint depression types is the size of the superolateral fragment.

1. In the tongue type, there is a long fragment that extends to the rear of the tuberosity.

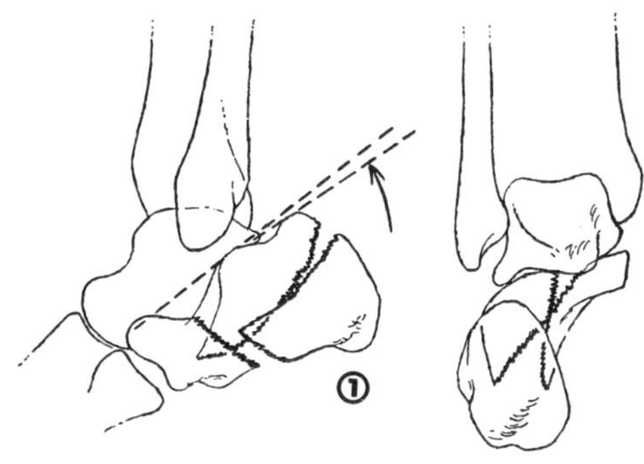

2. In the joint depression type, the fragment is short and extends back only to the end of the posterior facet.

Note: In both types, the fracture line separates the sustentaculum fragment from the tuberosity fragment.

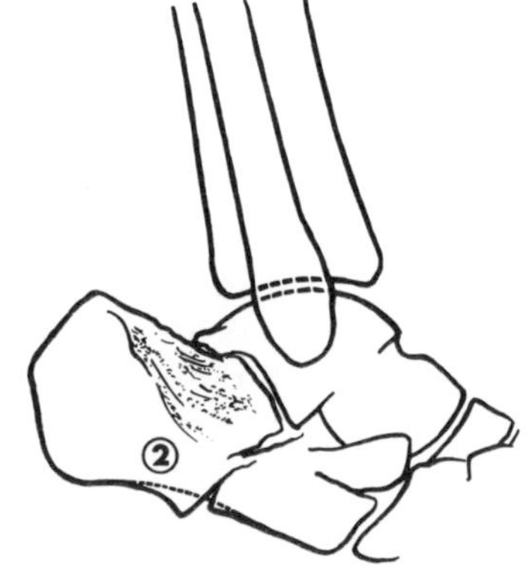

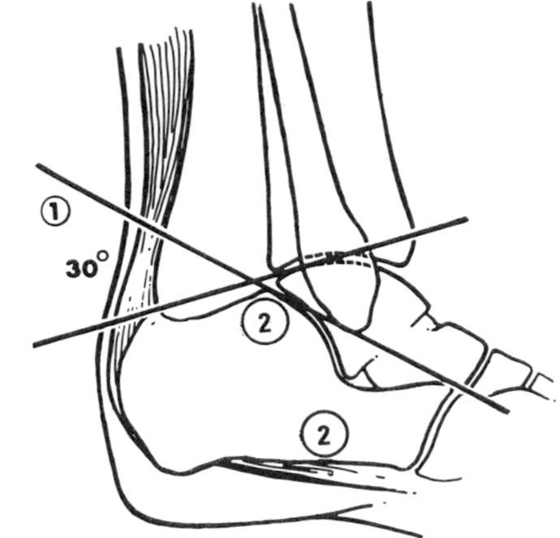

Basic Deformity in Both Tongue Type and Joint Depression Type

1. In a normal foot, the angle formed by the line between the anterior and posterior facets and the line from the superior cortex of the body is normally 30°–40° (Böhler's angle).
2. Vertical compression of the calcaneus decreases this angle by driving the tuberosity upward and

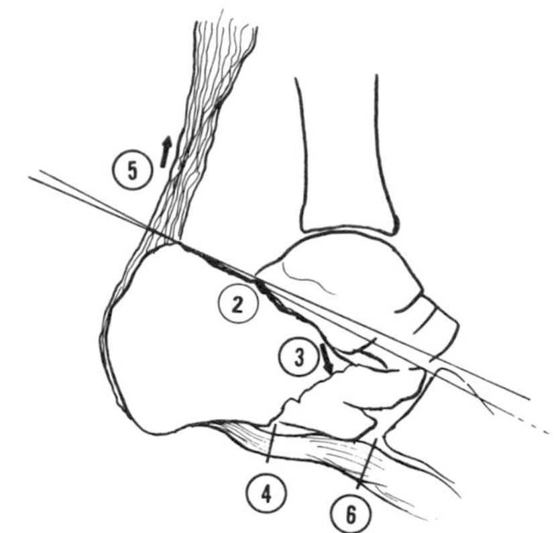

3. Driving the middle articular facet downward.
4. Plantar surface may become prominent.
5. Achilles tendon is functionally lengthened and weakened.
6. Calcaneocuboid joint may also be involved.

Displacement on Axial View

1. In the normal foot, the calcaneus should be in neither a varus nor a valgus position in relation to the ankle.
2. Peroneal tendon sheath is not compressed.
3. After fracture, the vertical fracture line consistently runs between the sustentaculum and the tuberosity fragment.
4. Tuberosity fragment is displaced laterally and usually into varus but sometimes into valgus.
5. Tuberosity is driven upward and laterally to impinge on the lateral malleolus and peroneal tendons.

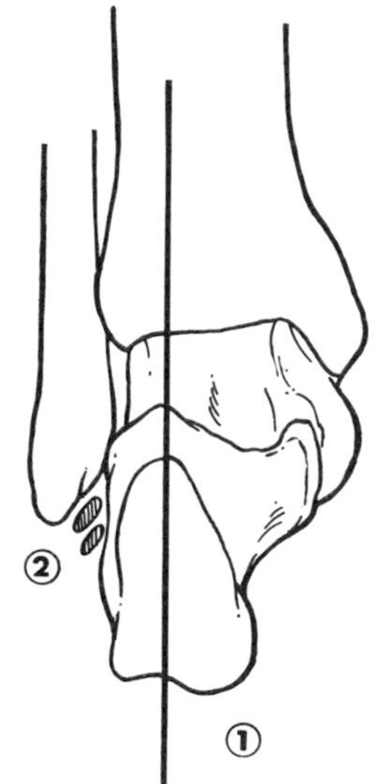

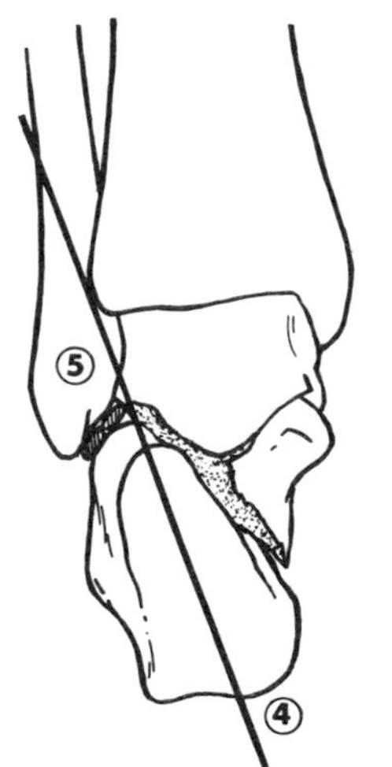

Displacement on Superior View

1. Sustentaculum fragment and talus are driven medially and downward. A characteristic spike of bone protrudes from the sustentaculum fragment medially.
2. Tuberosity fragment moves forward and laterally.
3. This produces shortening and widening of the heel, which is evident particularly when compared with the
4. Normal relationship of the calcaneus to the talus.

Note: The displacement must be considered in three dimensions. The superolateral joint depression or tongue type of fracture involves the subtalar joint. The separation of the sustentaculum and tuberosity fragments causes the heel to be shortened and widened.

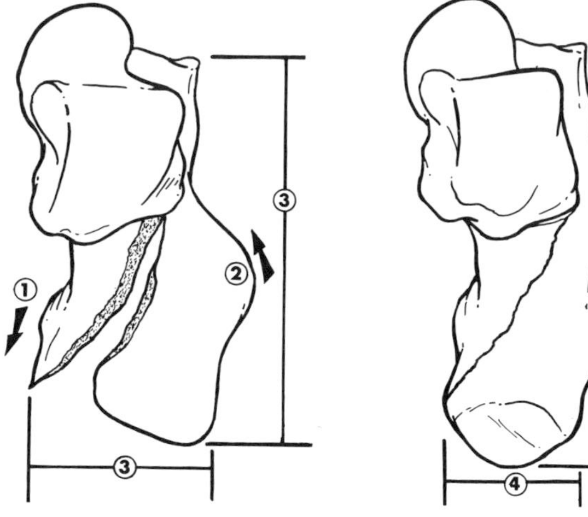

Painful and Tender Hindfoot

1. This is most often located in the lateral peroneal region and results from impingement of the laterally displaced tuberosity fragment on the malleolus and soft tissue structures.
2. Tender heel results from distortion of the plantar surface of the calcaneus, causing either localized pain or
3. Diffuse plantar fasciitis.

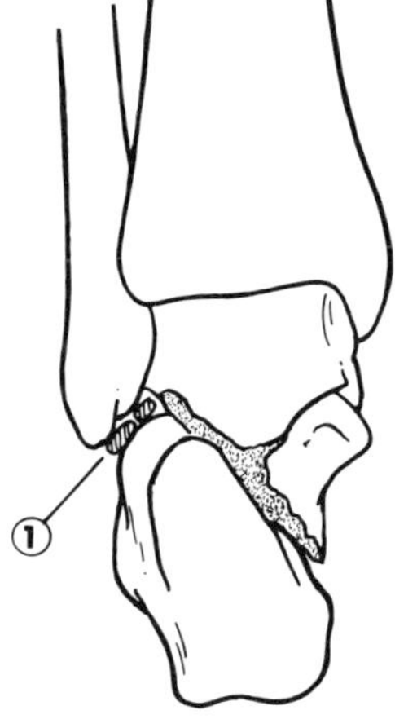

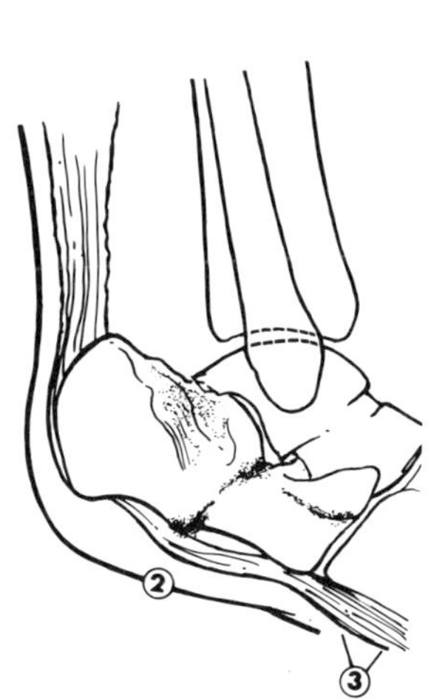

Management of Calcaneal Fractures, Based on Assessment of All Potential Complications

REMARKS

The disability after os calcis fractures may range from minimal to severe.

The degree of subtalar joint disruption does not always correlate with the degree of residual symptoms. Paradoxically, the greater the degree of talocalcaneal involvement, the more likely is spontaneous ankylosis to occur and to eliminate pain from this region.

The subtalar joint is only one of numerous sources of pain likely to occur after a calcaneal fracture.

Consistently, the following problems can be anticipated in patients and should be kept in mind while selecting treatment.

Stiffness of the Foot

1. Stiffness of the foot results from the edema of injury and from prolonged immobilization during treatment. The midtarsal joint, which can accommodate for loss of subtalar motion, is impaired by prolonged immobilization in non-weight-bearing treatment.

Note: Joint stiffness can be minimized by treatment that incorporates early mobilization of the foot.

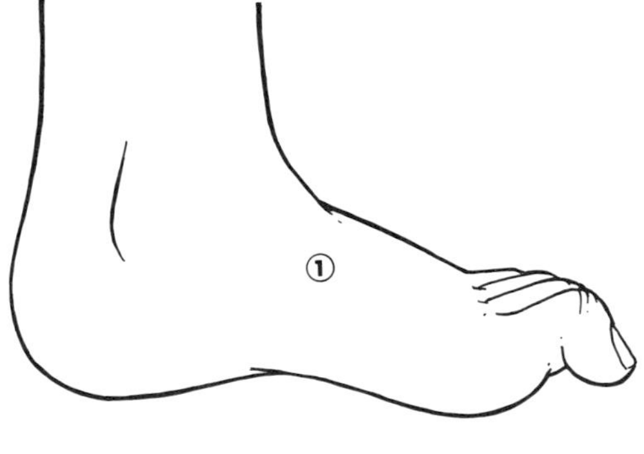

Peroneal Spastic Flat Foot

1. Chronic stenosing tenosynovitis of the peroneal tendon below and lateral to the fibula is likely to follow shortening and widening of the heel after fracture.
2. As a result of the tuberosity fragment, the peroneals contract and pull the forefoot into valgus. This results in lateral foot pain all along the region of the peroneal tendons.

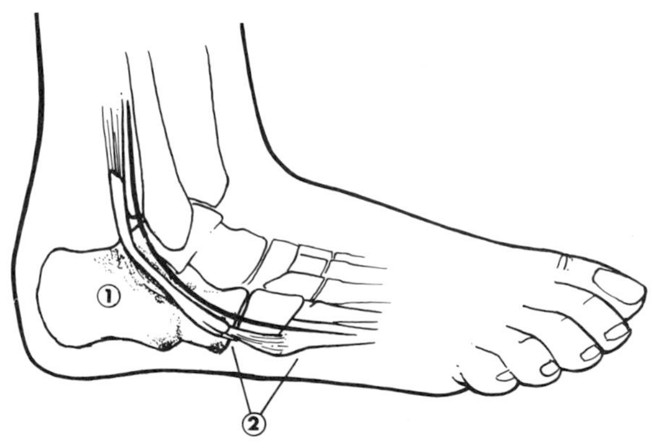

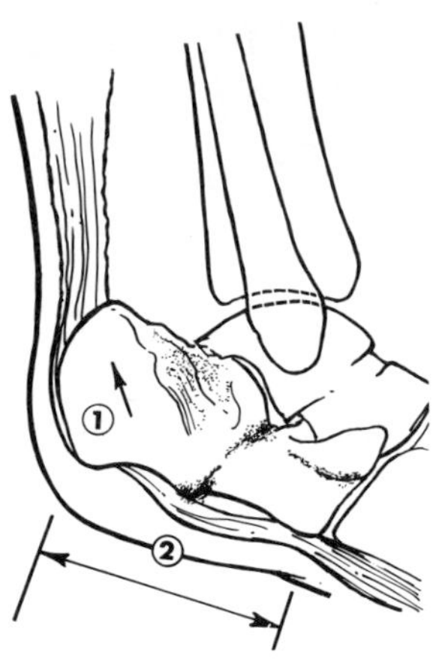

Abnormalities of Gait

A flatfooted (calcaneus) shuffling limp with inability to toe walk is common. This results from

1. Upward displacement of the tuberosity and
2. Shortening of the heel, which impair

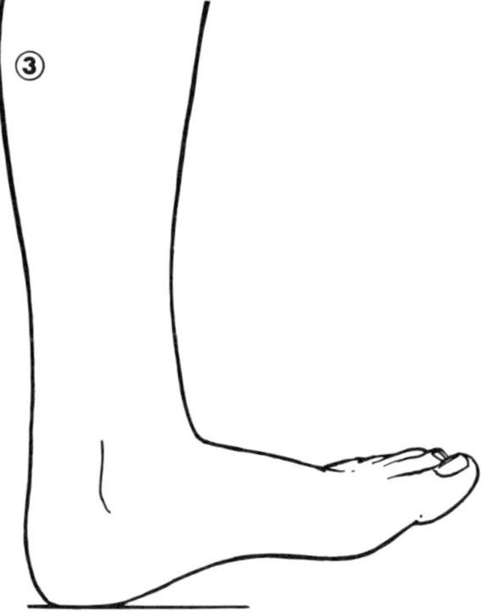

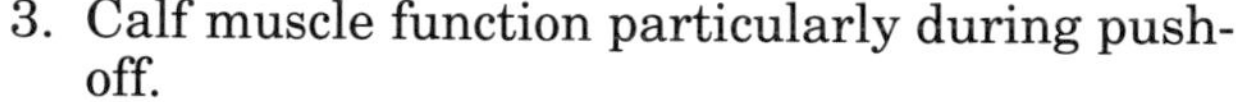

3. Calf muscle function particularly during push-off.

Note: Treatment designed to restore length and reduce the tuberosity fragment is the only effective method of preventing the calcaneus gait. Once muscle impairment is established, there is little that can be done to correct this complication.

Early Mobilization Without Reduction

REMARKS

The therapy advocated for calcaneal fractures has ranged from confirmed conservatism to intrepid intervention.

Most, but not all, can be treated nonoperatively by early mobilization methods. Even when reduction of the fracture is planned, mobilization techniques help to diminish edema and prevent stiffness of the joint.

The concept of early mobilization treatment is based on the fact that a fracture through a large cancellous bone, such as the calcaneus, achieves stability immediately by impaction of the fragments at the time of initial injury. To achieve fracture immobilization, the surgeon need only eliminate the weight-bearing stresses. It is not necessary to immobilize the foot by rigid external or internal fixation.

By emphasizing early mobilization, the surgeon can diminish fracture edema and minimize subsequent joint fibrosis and adhesion formation.

In many instances, no attempt at reduction is necessary because the initial deformity is compatible with good function. However, clinical deformity, particularly heel valgus or lateral bony prominences that might impinge on the peroneal tendons, should be corrected.

Subtalar motion is dependent on continuity between the posterior articular facets of the talus and the os calcis. Extreme displacement of Böhler's tuberosity angle is not likely to yield a satisfactory result if it is treated by early mobilization without fracture reduction.

Weight-bearing too early (sooner than 8 weeks) after early mobilization is also likely to lead to severe displacement and a poor result.

Lance et al. found that the following criteria should be met to select candidates for early mobilization without fracture reduction:

- Normal clinical appearance of the heel without peroneal tendon impingement.
- X-rays that show involvement of the nonarticular portion of the talus or maintenance of reasonable congruity between the posterior articulating facets of the talus and calcaneus.
- Age and general health status also influence the selection. For patients who are older than 60 years or who have been chronically ill, early active motion offers the swiftest and safest return to function.

Technique of Early Mobilization Management

X-rays of the foot to select patients for early mobilization should include lateral, oblique, and axial views to assess the degree of displacement, the shortening of the os calcis, and any incongruity of the posterior articular facets.

Patients should also be thoroughly assessed for other injuries and fractures, particularly of the spine and lower limb.

Early mobilization in treatment is important, even when reduction of the fracture is necessary.

Example of Fracture Treated by Early Mobilization

1. Tongue-type fracture with Böhler's tuberosity angle depressed to 20°.
2. Some displacement is evident, but joint congruity is maintained.
3. Heel has not widened significantly, and there is no significant bony protrusion on the lateral or plantar surface.

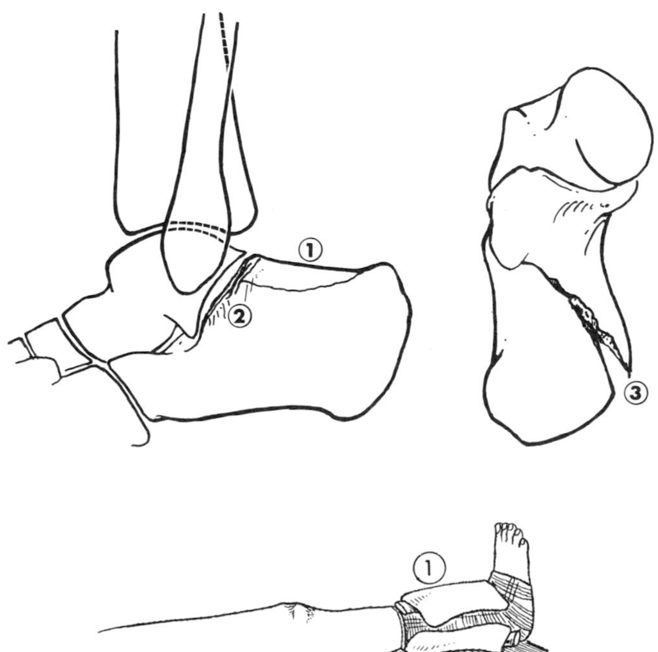

1. Foot and ankle are padded generously with sheet wadding and wrapped with elastic bandage.

The fractured foot is elevated and ice is applied for 5–7 days until the swelling has subsided.

Note: The bandage should be rewrapped several times daily to maintain compression.

Subsequent Management

By day 2 or 3, the patient is encouraged to exercise the toes, tarsal joints, and ankle systematically on an hourly basis within the limits of pain.

By days 3–5, the patient may be up on crutches to go to the bathroom but should be cautioned against weight-bearing or too much dependency of the foot.

At the end of 1 week, the foot should be reexamined for any clinical deformity or area of bony protrusion on the lateral or plantar surface. X-rays should be taken to determine the maintenance of the fracture position. If heel widening or joint asymmetry is evident, reduction of the fracture should be carried out.

Weight-bearing is deferred for 6–8 weeks with linear fractures and 10–12 weeks for fractures with comminution.

The presence or absence of pain is not an adequate criterion to determine the time for weight-bearing because painless displacement of the fracture can occur with premature weight-bearing. Because of other fractures, if the patient needs to put some weight on the side of the fractured os calcis, a weight-bearing plaster cast molded well about the heel may be applied by 7–10 days when the fracture swelling has completely subsided.

Cast Application for Patients With Multiple Injuries in Addition to the Calcaneal Fracture

Note: The cast should be kept on for a minimal time, preferably 4–6 weeks and then followed by early progressive active exercises to the foot and ankle.

1. Cast is molded firmly about the fractured heel.
2. Heel is in a neutral position.

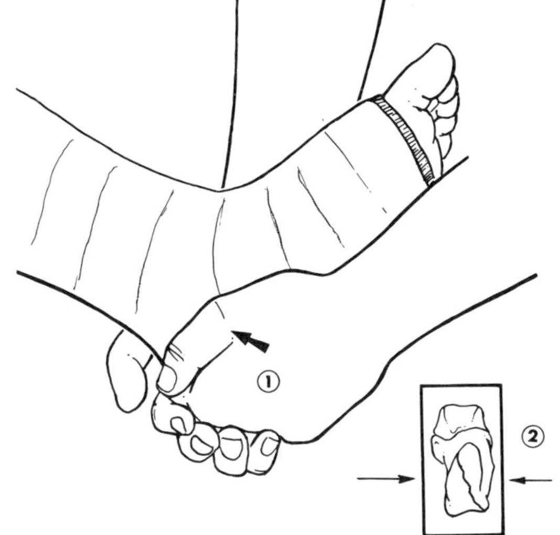

X-Rays After 10 Weeks of Treatment

1. There is good alignment of the articular surface, which correlates with the clinical appearance.
2. There is slight cortical prominence laterally but no impingement on the peroneal tendons.

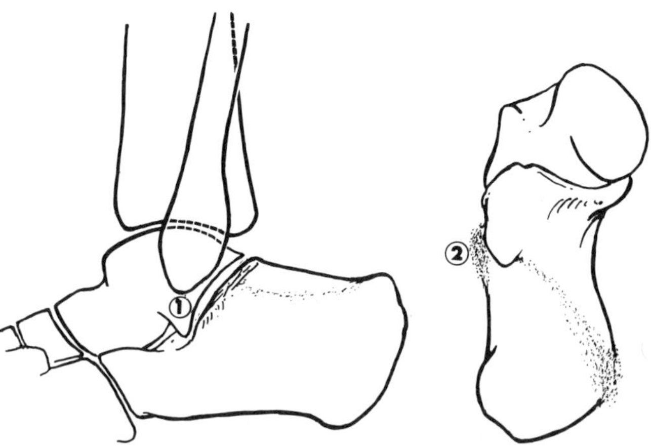

Fracture Reduction Techniques

REMARKS

Overvigorous attempts to reduce calcaneal fractures by clamps or other methods that require forceful heel compression can produce the complications of soft tissue necrosis and should be avoided.

Prolonged cast immobilization also aggravates the tendency of the tarsal joints to stiffen and should be avoided.

Omoto et al. demonstrated an effective method of reduction that can improve the anatomy of the heel without adding to soft tissue impingement problems or joint stiffness.

The method depends on intact medial and lateral calcaneofibular or tibiocalcaneal ligaments.

The objective of this reduction is to improve the joint surface of the posterior articular facet and correct any varus or valgus heel position.

In addition, peroneal tendinitis or nerve impingement can be diminished by reducing the lateral spreading of the heel.

The reduction depends on applying traction or using ligamentotaxis. Therefore, if lateral ligaments were disrupted, the method would be ineffective.

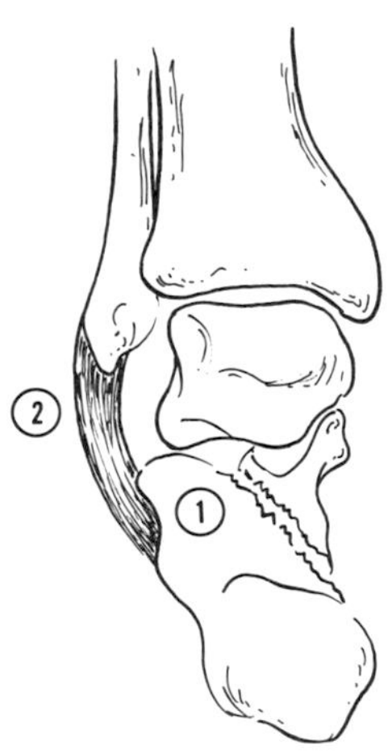

1. As the tuberosity fragment fractures, it displaces upward and laterally.
2. Lateral displacement is usually limited by the lateral fibulocalcaneal ligament.

Note: These ligaments can be used for reduction of the fracture using ligamentotaxis.

Disruption of the Fibulocalcaneal Ligament, Which Leads to Fracture Dislocation

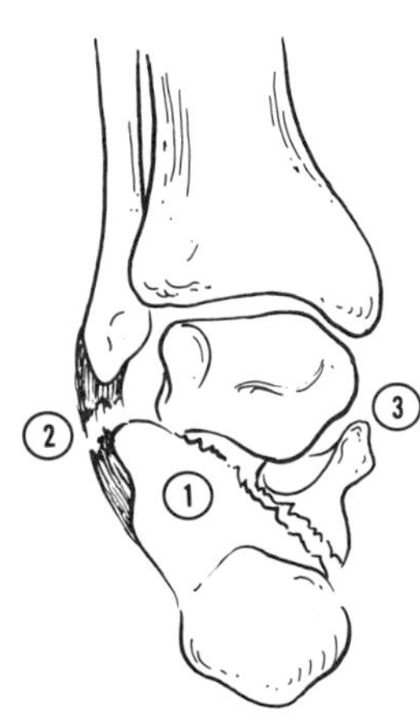

1. Continued force on the heel if it is severe can displace the tuberosity fragment further laterally.
2. This can lead at times to rupture of the lateral fibulocalcaneal ligament.
3. Talus and sustentaculum fragment continue to displace downward.

This is essentially a fracture-dislocation of the calcaneus and is more likely to require internal stabilization than if the fibulocalcaneal ligament is intact.

Technique of Reduction by Ligamentotaxis (After Omoto et al.)

1. Under spinal anesthesia, the patient is placed prone with the knee and injured leg flexed to relax the triceps.
2. An assistant holds the leg while the surgeon cups his or her hands over the lateral and medial calcaneus.
3. The surgeon crosses the fingers of both hands around the heel, compressing the tuberosity fragment and squeezing upward toward the sole, while applying traction.

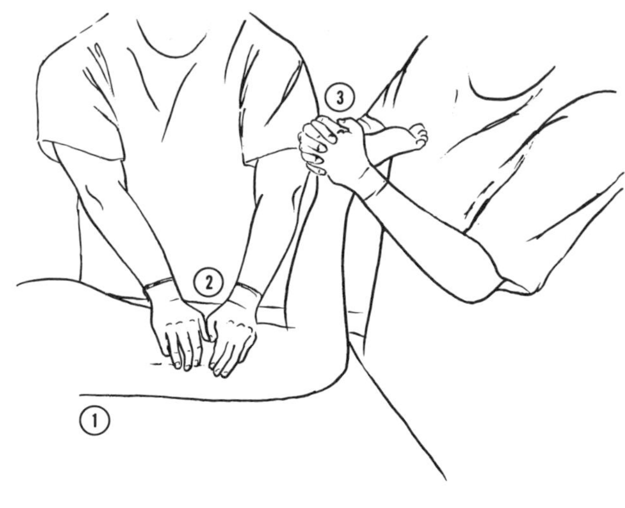

1. Strong traction is continued while the surgeon bends the heel into an inverted and
2. Everted position several times.
3. Crepitations are felt as the fracture is disimpacted in inversion. However, if the ligaments are intact, the joint fragments will not open excessively.

The overall contour of the heel can be molded and restored in this manner.

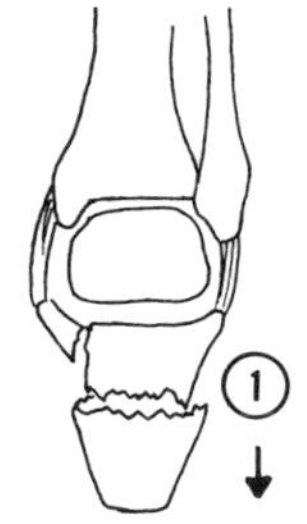

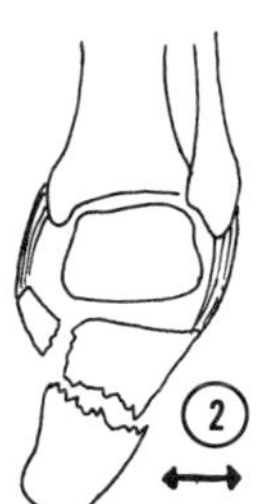

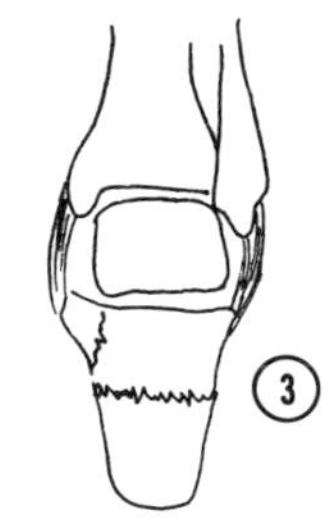

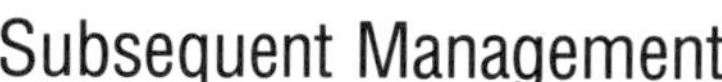

Subsequent Management

Immobilization in plaster should be avoided, if possible.

Wrap the foot and ankle in a compression dressing, apply ice, and elevate the limb to diminish swelling.

By the second or third day, encourage the patient to exercise the toes, tarsal joints, and ankles systematically every hour.

The patient may be up on crutches but should be cautioned against weight-bearing or hanging the foot dependently.

After 1 week, examine the fracture clinically and by x-ray to determine whether there has been any further widening of the heel or displacement of the fracture.

The patient should not bear weight for 6–8 weeks while continuing the exercise program.

On this regimen, 80 per cent of patients usually achieve good results with minor symptoms. Continued improvement can be expected for up to 2 years after the fracture.

Closed Reduction With Skeletal Traction

REMARKS

If shortening and widening of the heel cannot be reduced by Omoto et al.'s technique, skeletal traction may be used.

A skeletal pin is inserted transversely across the tuberosity fragment. The tuberosity is then pulled down to restore heel length and correct the lateral displacement.

A cast is then applied temporarily to maintain reduction until the fragments become stable.

Prereduction X-Ray

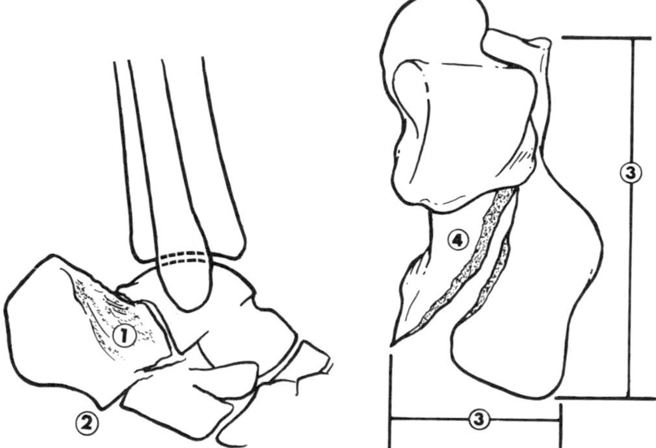

1. Central depression fracture of the calcaneus has depressed the tuberosity angle.
2. Plantar surface has developed a bony prominence.
3. Heel has shortened and widened as a result of upward and lateral displacement of the tuberosity and
4. Downward and backward displacement of the sustentaculum talus.

Technique of Reduction by Longitudinal Traction

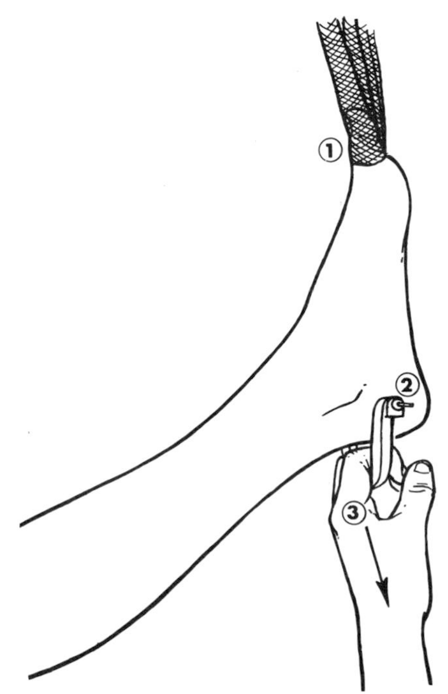

1. Foot is suspended by the toes by means of finger-trap traction.
2. Under fluoroscopic guidance a 3-mm smooth Steinmann pin is inserted from the medial to the lateral side of the tuberosity fragment, with care taken to avoid the plantar neurovascular structures.
3. With a traction bow, the tuberosity is pulled downward and outward to correct its shortening and varus displacement.

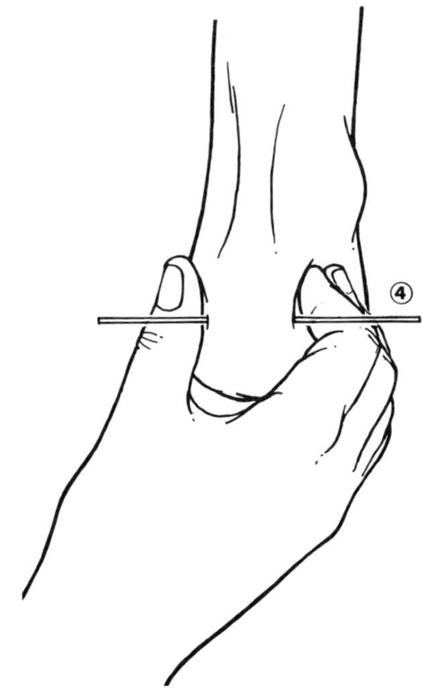

4. All the lateral and plantar bony prominences should no longer be palpable.

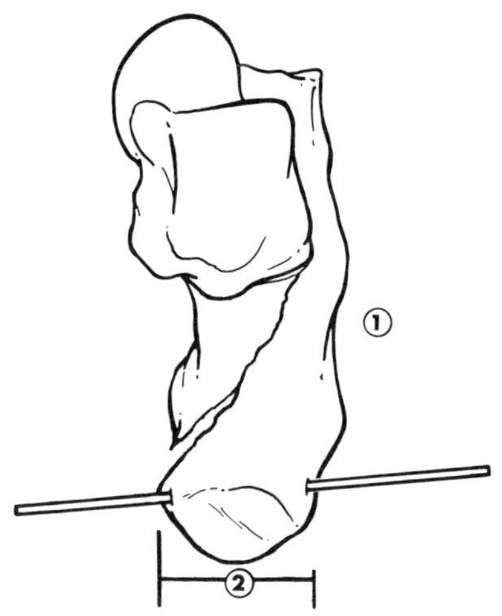

Postreduction X-Rays

1. Calcaneus has been restored to length and
2. Normal width.

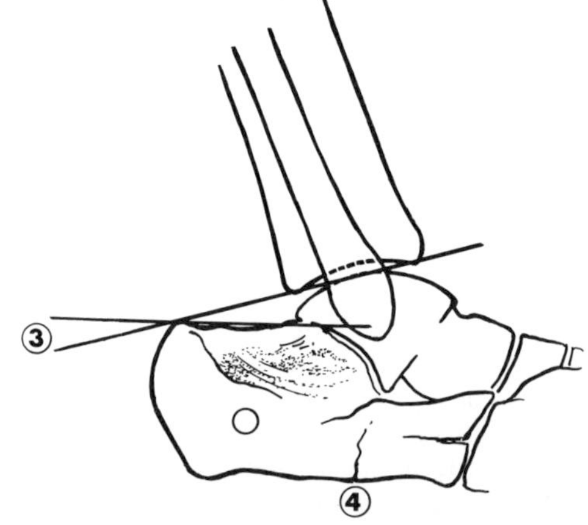

3. Tuberosity angle is corrected, although it has not returned to normal.
4. Plantar and lateral bony prominences have been dispersed.

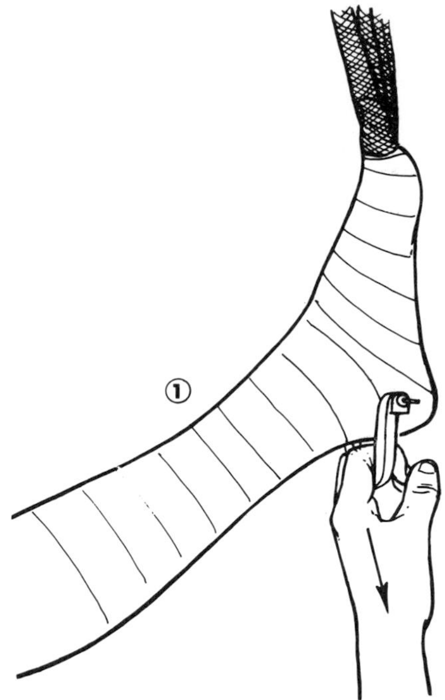

Immobilization

1. Short-leg cast is applied while an assistant maintains traction.

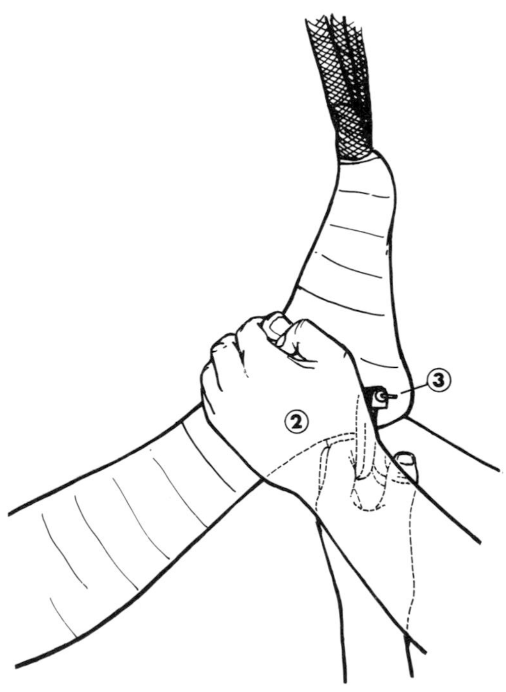

2. Heel is molded to maintain apposition of the tuberosity and the medial spike of the sustentaculum talus.
3. Pin is incorporated in the plaster.

Subsequent Management

The foot is elevated for 2–4 days. Ice is applied to diminish the swelling.

The pin is removed from the cast when the cast is hardened at the end of 2 days. Leaving the pin in longer than this is unnecessary to maintain reduction and may contribute to stiffening of the foot.

It is important to use a smooth pin to allow easy removal through the plaster.

The patient may be up on crutches but should not bear weight on the fractured heel.

Cast immobilization should be minimized and generally can be removed by 2–3 weeks as the swelling subsides. This then allows an active exercise program to regain motion in the hindfoot and forefoot. However, weight-bearing should be avoided for at least 8–10 weeks until adequate consolidation of the fractured heel is evident.

This technique may not completely restore the normal Böhler's angle, but it does achieve the desired goal of restoring the heel to a normal contour.

Alternative Reduction Technique for Tongue-Type Fractures

Essex-Lopresti showed an alternative reduction method to be effective for displaced tongue-type fractures of the calcaneus.

The technique can be used if the joint surfaces and posterior facet remain incongruous after the previously described closed reduction methods.

Prereduction X-Ray

1. Primary fracture between the sustentaculum and tuberosity fragment.
2. Tongue-shaped fragment is depressed anteriorly and elevated posteriorly.
3. Secondary fracture line through the body of the calcaneus.
4. Loss of tuber angle. (The normal angle is 35°–40°.)

Manipulative Reduction and Pin Fixation

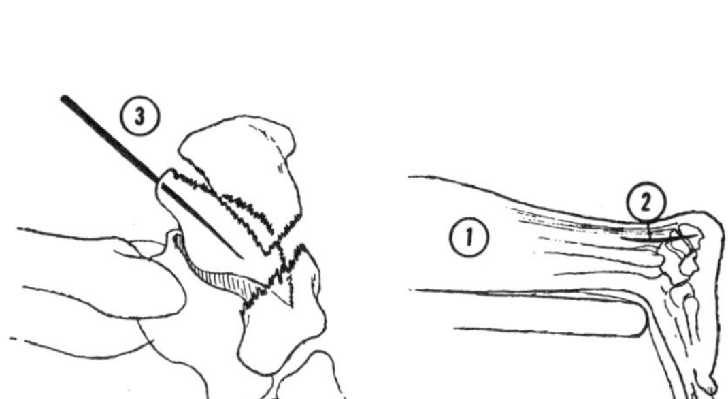

1. Patient is in a prone position.
2. Make a small incision over the calcaneus lateral to the Achilles tendon.
3. Insert a heavy Steinmann pin into the tongue fragment; the pin is directed in a longitudinal direction slightly to the lateral side.

Note: At this point, check the position of the pin by x-ray.

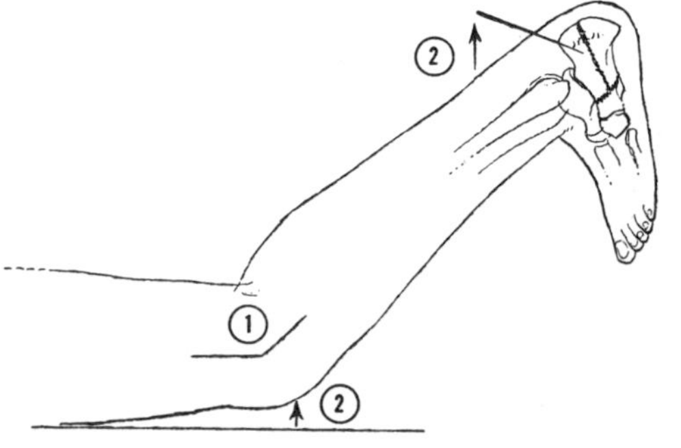

1. Flex the knee 45°.
2. Lift upward on the pin until the knee clears the table.

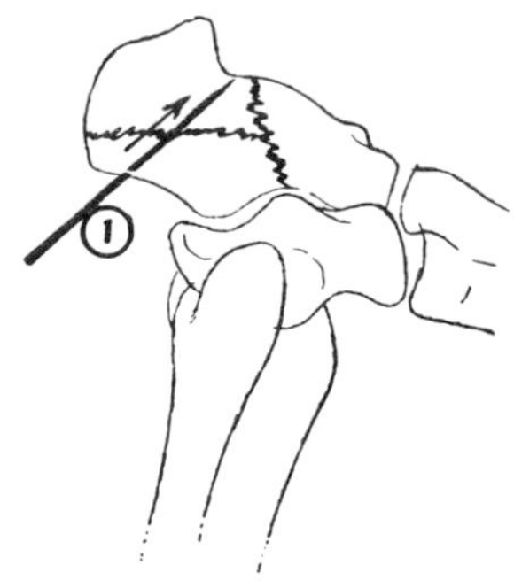

1. Tongue fragment may reduce with a palpable click as the leg is lifted off the table. After this occurs, mold the calcaneus to decrease the width of the heel using the previously described technique of Omoto et al.
2. Drill the pin across the fracture site and into the anterior calcaneal fragment.

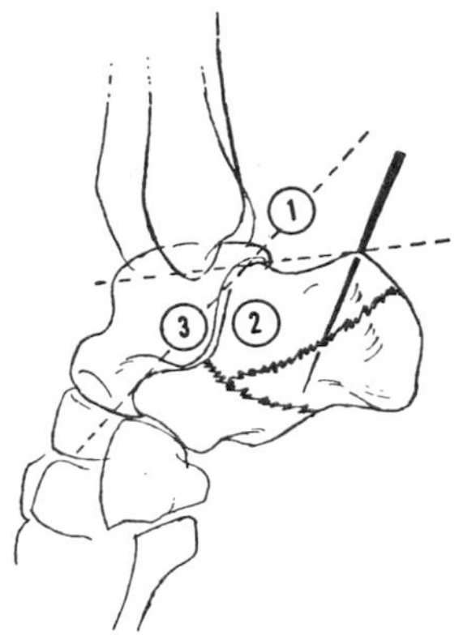

Postreduction X-Ray

1. Tuber angle has been restored.
2. Tongue fragment is elevated into normal position.
3. Articular surfaces of the subtalar joint are congruous.

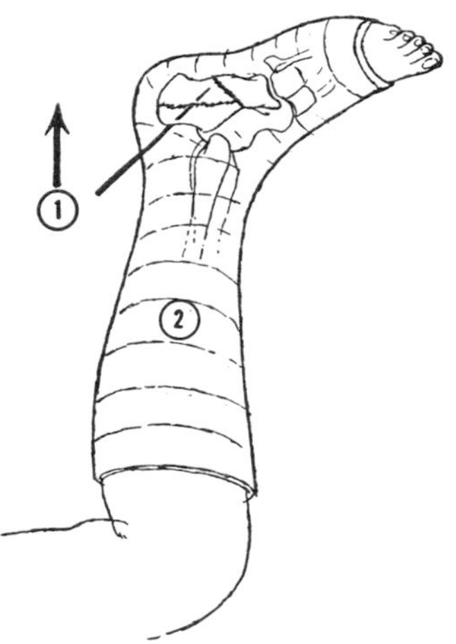

Immobilization

1. While the position is maintained by downward pressure on the pin,
2. Apply a below-knee plaster cast that incorporates the pin.

Subsequent Management

The foot is elevated for 2–4 days. Ice is applied to diminish swelling.

The pin is removed from the cast when the plaster is hardened, at the end of 2 days. Leaving the pin in longer than this is unnecessary to maintain reduction and may contribute to stiffening of the foot.

Note: It is important to use a smooth pin to allow easy removal through the plaster.

The patient may be up on crutches but should not bear weight on the fractured side.

The patient should continue to exercise the toes actively while in the plaster cast.

Remove the cast on the average by 2–3 weeks to allow active mobilization of the foot. This type of fracture is usually stable once reduced, and prolonged immobilization contributes to stiffening of the hindfoot and forefoot.

However, continue the patient on crutches for a period of 6–8 weeks until consolidation of the fracture site is evident on x-ray.

Indications for Operative Treatment (After Crosby and Fitzgibbons) Based on Computed Tomographic Findings

REMARKS

Crosby and Fitzgibbons classified calcaneal fractures into three types based on computed tomographic findings of the posterior facet joint.

In type I, the fracture fragments are small and not displaced. In type II, they are displaced, and in type III, they are comminuted.

These authors showed that type I fractures can do well with closed treatment.

Types II and III tend to have poor results with closed treatment. They therefore advocate operative treatment of type II.

The management of type III fractures tends to be poor with either operative or nonoperative treatment.

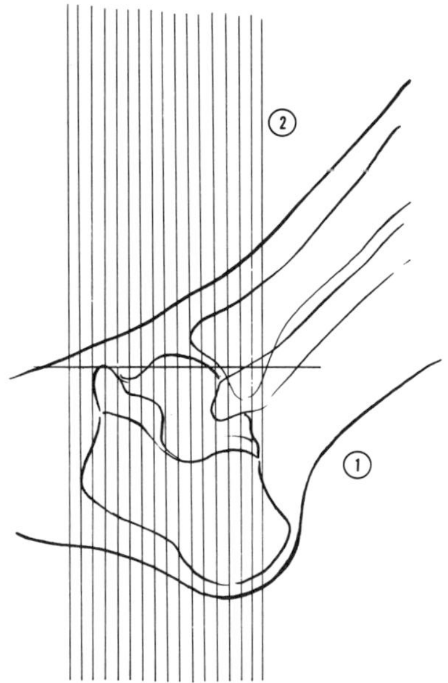

Technique

1. A computed tomographic scan is taken with the foot positioned as illustrated.
2. Multiple coronal sections are taken from the anterior to the posterior aspect of the talus.

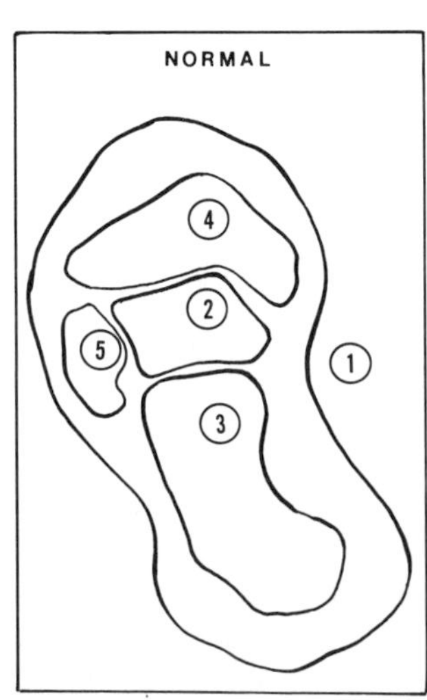

1. Coronal section shows the normal posterior facet joint.

This is formed by

2. Talus.
3. Calcaneus,
4. Tibia, and
5. Fibula form the ankle mortise.

Type I

1. Coronal section shows that the fracture of the posterior facet is absent or minimal, and the weight-bearing surface is therefore not involved.
2. Calcaneus may be slightly widened, but there is less than 2 mm of depression of the fragment.
3. There is no or minimal lateral displacement or impingement on the peroneal tendons.
4. Calcaneus is shortened, but the posterior facet joint is not involved.

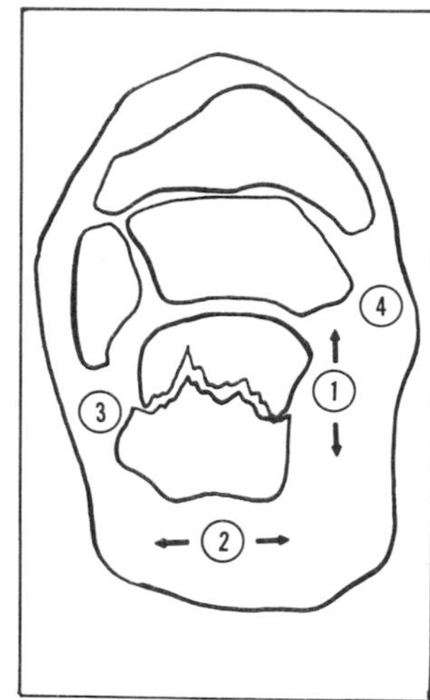

Type II

1. Coronal section shows the extent of the fracture in the posterior facet joint.
2. Articular surface of the calcaneus is disrupted, and there is 2 mm or more of depression or diastasis of the fragment.
3. Fragments are large and comminuted.

Note: This appears to be the most suitable type of fracture for open reduction and internal fixation because the fragments are large enough to fix adequately.

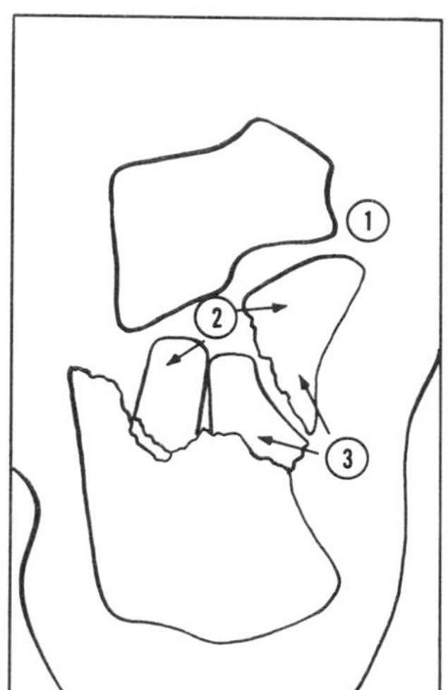

Type III

1. Coronal section is taken through a severely comminuted intra-articular fracture.
2. There is severe comminution of the posterior facet.
3. Fragments are multiple and small.

Note: This type of fracture is probably not suitable for open reduction and internal fixation and stabilization.

It may be treated by the manipulative techniques previously described to decrease the widening of the heel followed by early mobilization exercises.

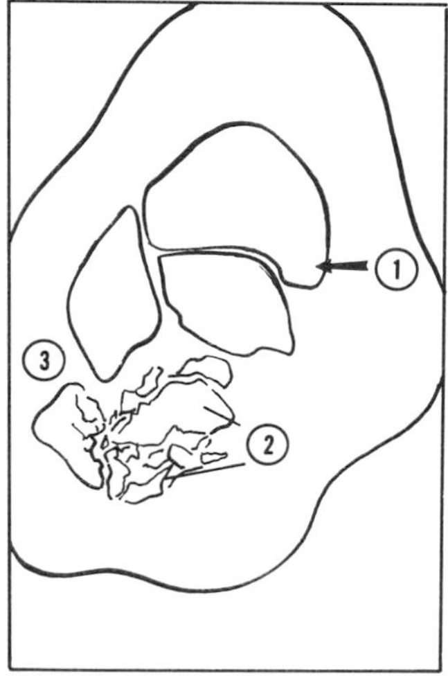

Methods of Reduction by Open Techniques (After Burdeaux)

1. Burdeaux and McReynolds developed a medial approach to the calcaneal fracture that allows realignment of the sustentaculum fragment and tuberosity fragment with open reduction technique.
2. Fixation is then achieved by a threaded Steinmann pin from the tuberosity to the sustentaculum.

Note: This minimally invasive method offers numerous advantages over more extensive open reduction techniques.

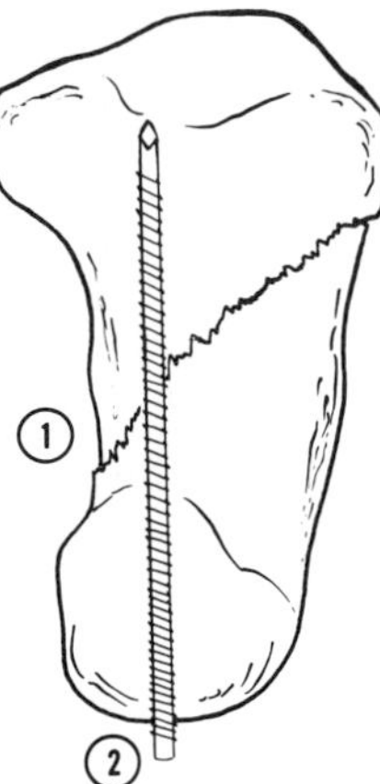

■ Dislocation of the Calcaneus

REMARKS

Any bone in the foot may be dislocated, including the calcaneus. However, this is an extremely rare injury, with only a few reported cases in literature.

The injury results from a violent twisting force on the heel, usually in a motor vehicle accident.

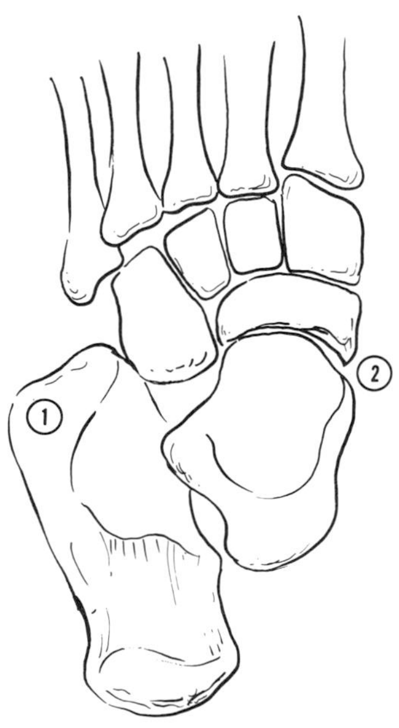

1. Calcaneus is found to lie lateral to the talus.
2. Talonavicular and distal articulations usually remain intact.

Management

The calcaneus can be reduced, in general, by closed manipulation using longitudinal traction and inversion. The reduction is usually stable but may require internal stabilization.

Alternately a Kirschner wire may be passed from the calcaneus into the cuboid.

The foot is immobilized in a short-leg cast for 6 weeks. After this, the cast and Kirschner wire can be removed.

Late Complications of Calcaneal Fractures

REMARKS

Most extra-articular and Crosby-Fitzgibbons type I intra-articular calcaneal fractures heal promptly and with satisfactory functional results. This is particularly likely when the fracture is treated by early mobilization and not by prolonged cast treatment.

The common intra-articular fractures that are displaced or comminuted (Crosby-Fitzgibbons type II or III) are the more problematic and more prone to complications.

Management should be based on an appreciation and anticipation of complications and, particularly, on the needs of the patient and the nature of the fracture. The usual elderly patient with a minimally displaced fracture does best with minimal treatment.

A laborer with a displaced fracture or fracture-dislocation or the individual with bilateral calcaneal fractures is likely to benefit from as near-anatomic reduction as possible.

If closed reduction is not successful, operative intervention is indicated to restore the normal contour (length and width) to the heel.

In most instances, heel pain gradually diminishes in the year or two after the calcaneal fracture. However, if there are structural abnormalities evident as a source of pain after the fracture heals, these should be promptly corrected.

The most common long-term complaint is

1. Lateral pain from the calcaneofibular abutment causing peroneal tenosynovitis.

Note: McLaughlin pointed out that this pain is aggravated by flexion and extension of the ankle, in contrast to the uncommon pain from the subtalar joint, which is aggravated by inversion and eversion of the foot.

2. Release of the peroneal tendon sheath and removal of the bony prominences can relieve these most common lateral pain symptoms after a calcaneal fracture.

Note: A free fat graft surrounding the tendon sheath can prevent recurrence of the bony mass and tendonitis.

3. Sural nerve may also be trapped and, therefore, require decompression or removal.

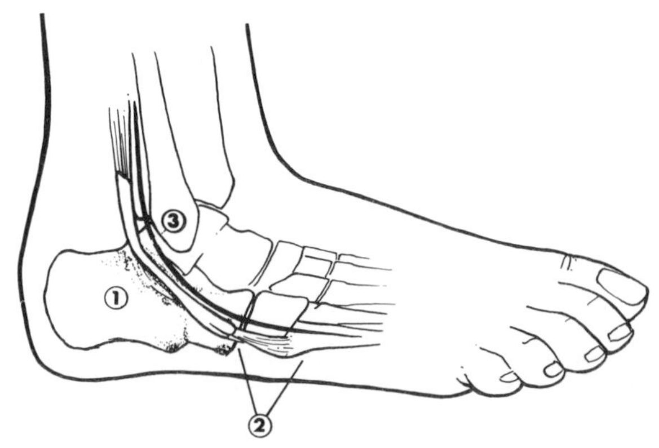

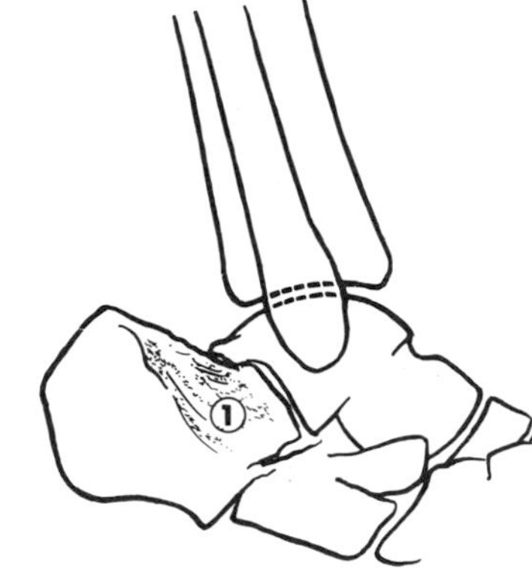

1. Distortion of the plantar surface as a result of upward displacement of the tuberosity fragment can produce a painful rocker-bottom prominence of the heel.

2. This can be relieved by soft heel cups that protect the tender heel from pressure, or

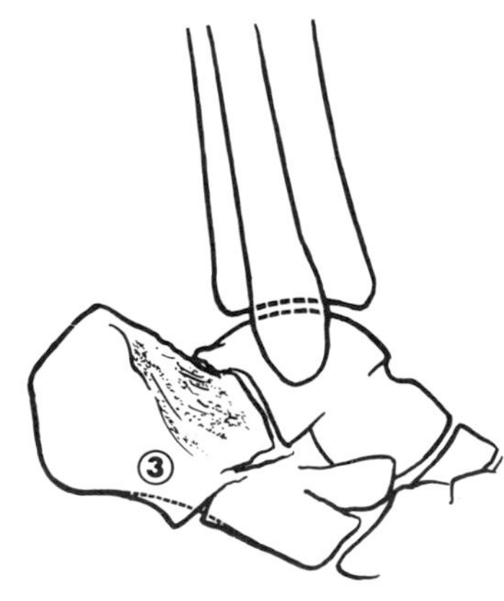

3. Surgical excision of the bony prominence may be required.

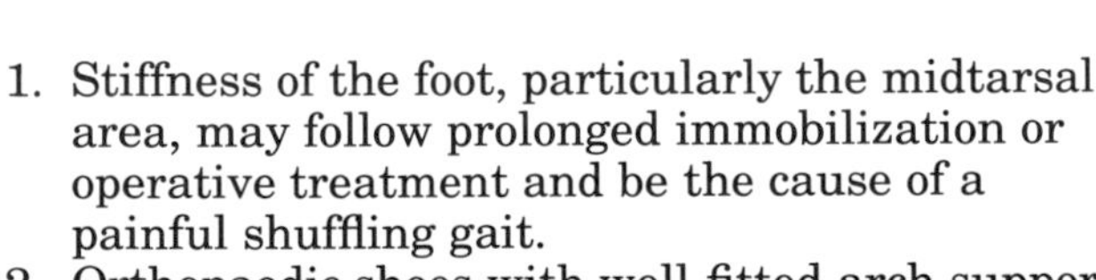

1. Stiffness of the foot, particularly the midtarsal area, may follow prolonged immobilization or operative treatment and be the cause of a painful shuffling gait.
2. Orthopaedic shoes with well-fitted arch supports and cushioned soles may relieve this generalized foot discomfort.

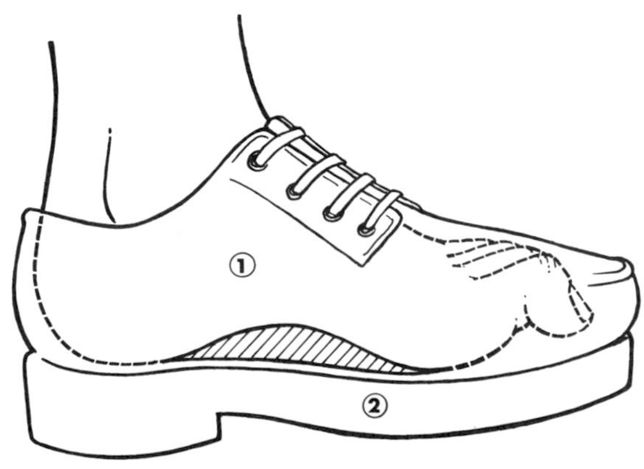

Subtalar and Triple Arthrodesis

Severely displaced, crush fractures of the calcaneus can cause considerable painful disability, particularly for patients who must earn their living by walking, standing, or climbing.

Arthrodesis of the subtalar joint or a triple arthrodesis of the subtalar, talonavicular, and calcaneal-cuboid joint may be necessary for chronic pain.

Before considering arthrodesis of either the subtalar joint or triple arthrodesis, determine whether or not most of the symptoms are due to lateral impingement rather than subtalar arthritis.

Subtalar arthrodesis by itself is frequently ineffective to relieve this pain problem. Arthrodesis of all three joints of the hindfoot should be done if the

1. Patient has pain on inversion and eversion of the foot from the joints of the hindfoot and the
2. Pain produced by impingement on the lateral peroneal tendons and the sural nerve tends to be aggravated mostly by flexion and extension of the hindfoot.
3. Triple arthrodesis may be necessary if there is no lateral impingement and the fracture involves the calcaneal cuboid and the subtalar joint. Avoid excising excessive amounts of bone to perform the arthrodesis because this can decrease the height of the heel and hindfoot and actually increase lateral impingement as a result of a loss of heel height.

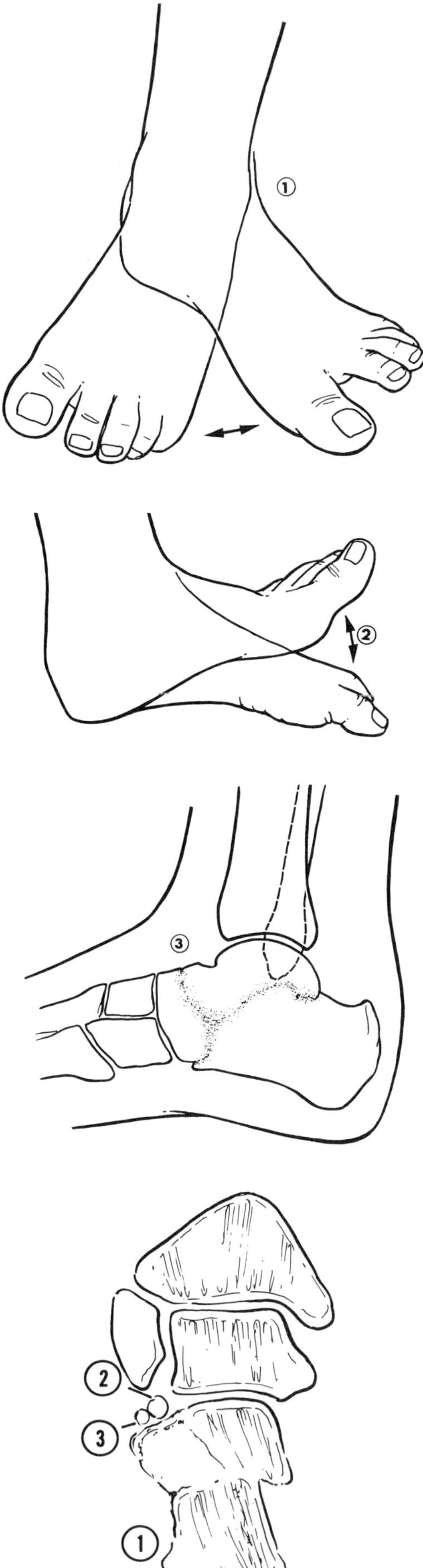

1. Before arthrodesis, evaluate the source of pain by computed tomography, which can show displacement of the tuberosity fragment laterally. This commonly causes persistent pain as a result of impingement on the
2. Peroneal tendons or the
3. Sural nerve.

Note: This lateral impingement may be relieved surgically by excising the bony prominence and releasing the peroneal tendons rather than carrying out an arthrodesis. Arthrodesis tends to shorten down the height of the heel and increase the lateral impingement.

FRACTURES AND FRACTURE-DISLOCATIONS OF THE TARSAL NAVICULA

REMARKS

The tarsal navicula is the keystone of the medial longitudinal arch of the foot.

Although fractures of the navicula are uncommon, they are among the most commonly unrecognized injuries to the foot.

Minor fractures of the tarsal navicula can become symptomatic if they displace and leave the patient with a painful flat foot.

Types of Fractures

There are four basic mechanisms that can produce fractures of the tarsal navicula.

The first occurs from inversion injury, which produces an avulsion fracture of the cortical surface of the bone. This represents the most common injury and occurs most often in women who wear high-heeled shoes.

Alternatively, an abduction twist can avulse the tuberosity of the navicula medially.

Forceful plantar flexion of the midfoot as a result of a fall or a direct blow causes the third type of fracture. The naviculocuneiform ligaments tear, and this permits a compression fracture of the navicula, which is wedged between the cuneiform and the talus. Commonly, the fracture occurs on the plantar surface of the bone.

A fourth type of navicular fracture is a stress injury. Stress fractures of the tarsal navicula have been seen commonly in racing greyhounds. They are also seen occasionally in long-distance runners who subject the foot to repetitive stress.

1. Commonly there is an avulsion of the bone's cortex produced by its ligamentous attachment.

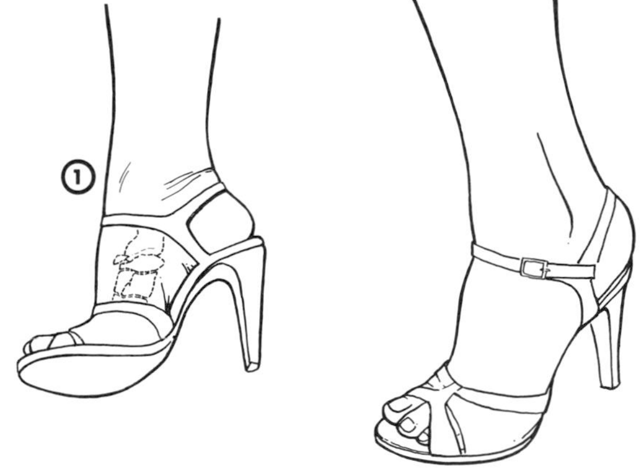

2. A second common fracture results from avulsion of the tuberosity of the navicula by the posterior tibial tendon or the deltoid and spring ligament complex.

Note: This may be mistaken for a sesamoid bone unless the x-ray is correlated with the clinical symptoms, which localize pain.

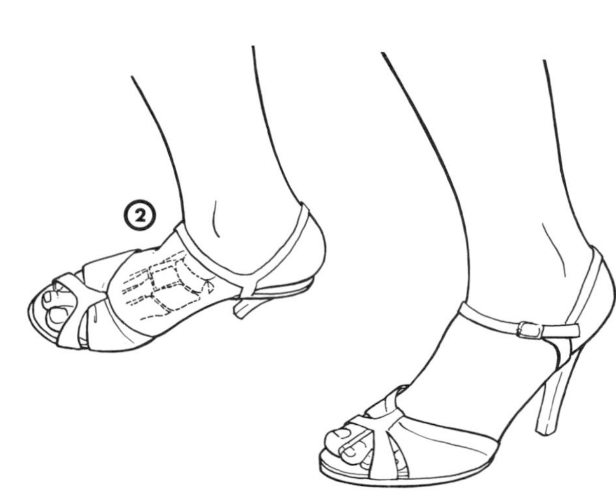

The third type of fracture results from forceful plantar flexion of the midfoot.

The naviculocuneiform ligaments tear first, producing a

1. Compression of the navicula by the medial cuneiform and fracture of the plantar surface.
2. If the talonavicular ligament fails, the bone will then dislocate dorsally.

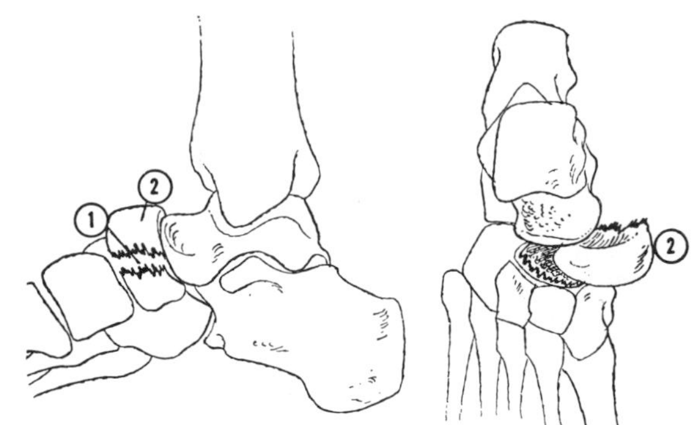

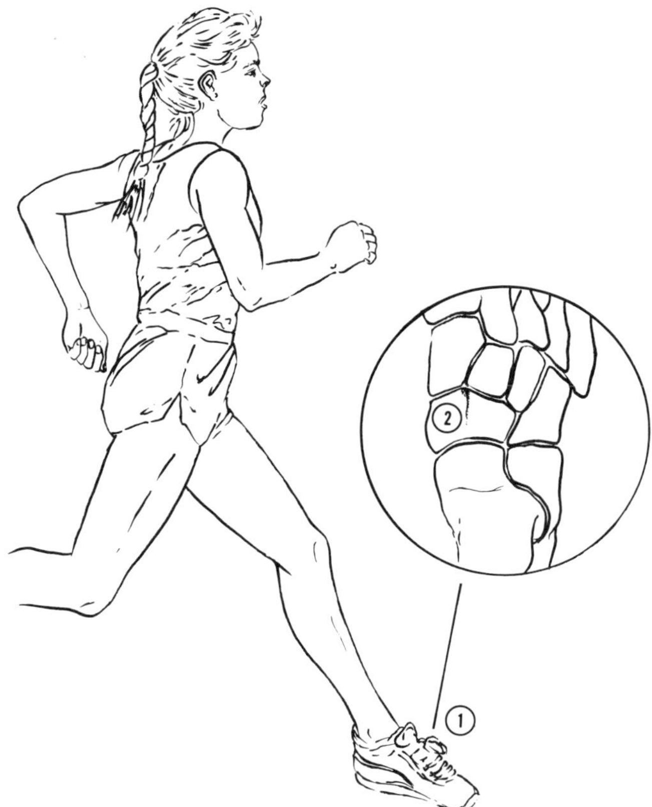

Stress Fractures

1. Rare stress fracture of the tarsal navicula is produced by a running athlete who runs on the toes or pushes off, loading the midfoot.
2. Prolonged downward pressure while standing on the toes causes gradual fatigue of the tarsal navicula, which is the keystone of the longitudinal arch of the foot.

Assessment

REMARKS

Approximately one in four navicular fractures either will not be recognized on admitting x-rays or will not be x-rayed at all because of confusion with an ankle sprain.

In many patients, the symptoms are fairly mild and are only aggravated during vigorous running or jumping. This is particularly true with a stress type of navicular fracture.

Other sources of confusion are with sesamoids in the posterior tibial tendon, which may look similar to an avulsion fracture of the navicula.

True anterior, posterior, lateral, and oblique x-rays are necessary to visualize the entire tarsal navicula. Pay careful attention to the lateral x-ray, which may be the only view that shows the fracture.

For undisplaced tarsal navicular or stress fractures, bone scan may be essential for the diagnosis.

Clinical Diagnosis

1. Patient with an undisplaced tarsal navicula gives a general vague sensation of pain on the dorsum of the foot or the
2. Medial aspect of the longitudinal arch.
3. There is usually little swelling evident.
4. When the patient stands on the toes and exerts pressure on the metatarsal heads, symptoms of pain are reproduced in the area of the navicula.

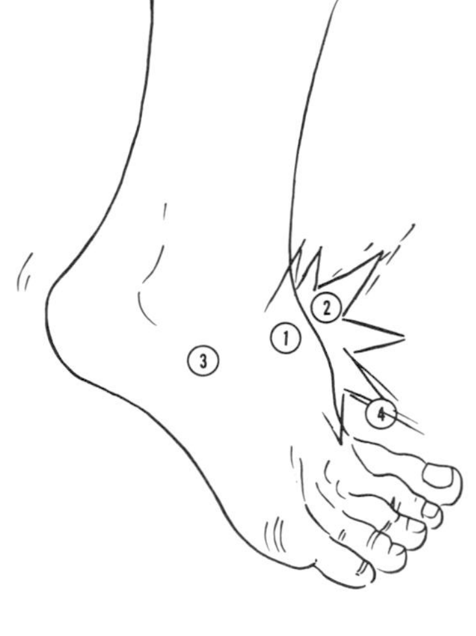

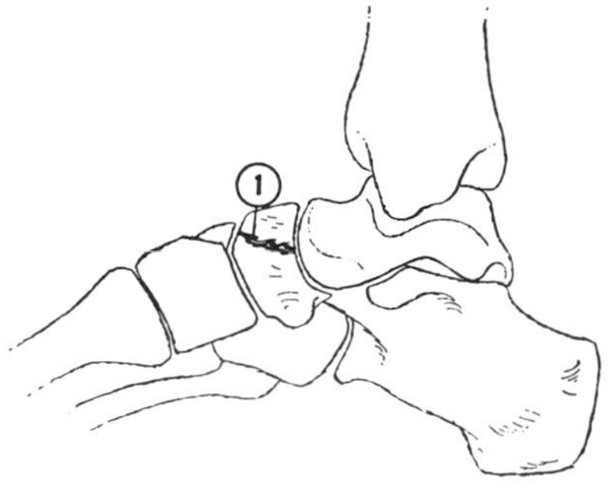

1. Frequently, the fracture may only be visualized on a lateral projection. This view should always be included in any radiographic study of the injured foot.

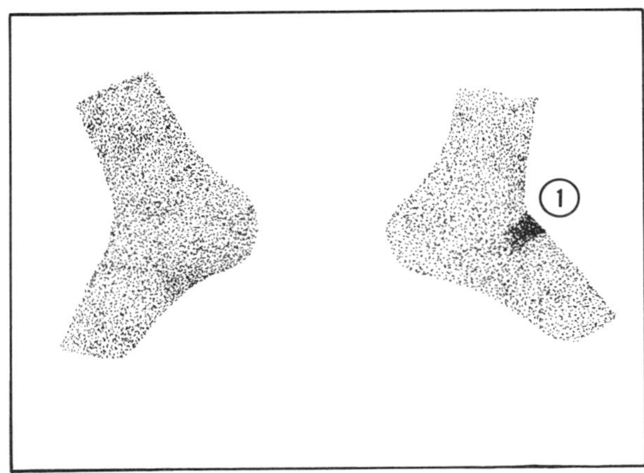

Bone Scanning

1. When the diagnosis cannot be made from plain films, bone scans can be helpful to localize the vague findings to the tarsal navicula or differentiate fractures of other tarsal bones.

■ Management

Avulsion fractures of the cortex or tuberosity and undisplaced fractures of the body of the navicula can be treated symptomatically with a walking cast.

Caution: Avulsion fractures of the navicula associated with compression fractures of the cuboid result from midtarsal dislocation caused by forceful abduction. This may require fusion of the midtarsal joint to restabilize the longitudinal arch.

Displaced fractures in the navicula or fracture-dislocations generally require open reduction and internal fixation. Closed treatment may be attempted, but the reduction should be anatomic to restore the keystone of the longitudinal arch.

If the navicular fracture is comminuted or a fracture-dislocation has gone unrecognized, fusion of the talonavicular and naviculocuneiform joints is generally necessary.

Undisplaced Fracture

Appearance on Lateral X-Ray

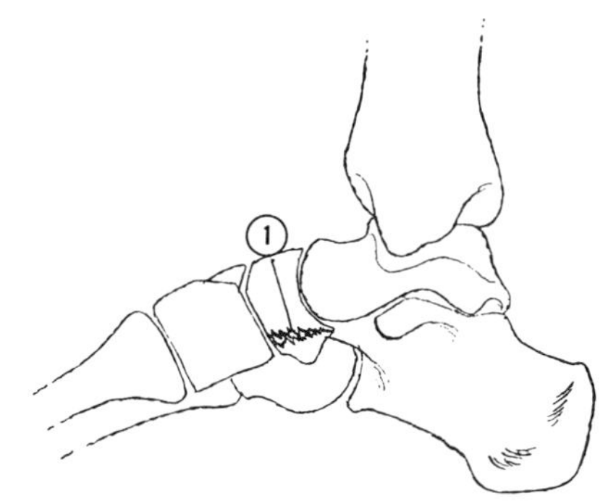

1. Fracture of the tuberosity of the navicula with minimal displacement.

Note: Distinguish this lesion from an accessory center of ossification frequently encountered at this site.

Immobilization With Non–Weight-Bearing Cast

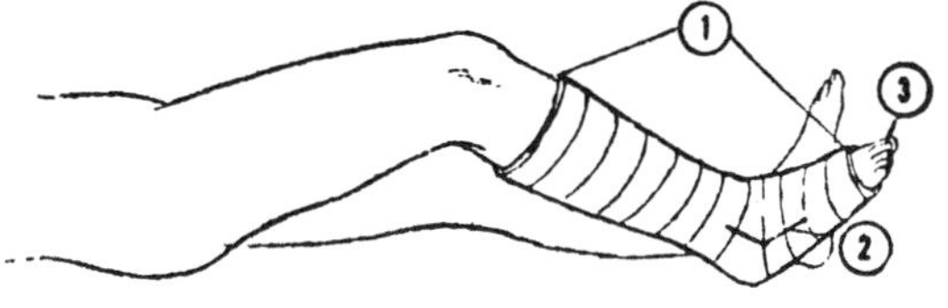

1. Apply a circular cast from behind the metatarsal heads to the tibial tubercle.
2. Foot is slightly plantar-flexed.
3. Foot is in a neutral position in regard to inversion and eversion.

■ Subsequent Management

The non–weight-bearing cast is maintained for 3–5 weeks until the patient's acute symptoms have subsided.

At this time, the foot may be wrapped with a compressive dressing or similar type of supportive dressing to allow the patient to begin partial weight-bearing with crutches.

In most instances, the symptoms should subside and function returns to normal by 5–6 weeks.

Note: Frequently, the avulsion fracture may appear to remain ununited but usually causes no symptoms.

If an ununited fracture does produce persistent symptoms, it may be removed surgically.

Displaced Fractures

Prereduction X-Ray

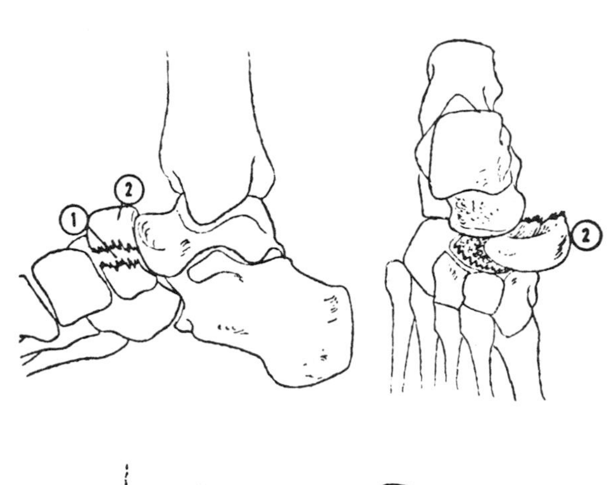

1. Fracture of the body of the navicula.
2. The dorsal fragment is displaced upward and medially.

Note: Closed reduction of the fracture-dislocation should be anatomic to restore the keystone function of the navicula to the longitudinal arch. In most instances, this is impossible to accomplish by closed means, and open reduction is necessary.

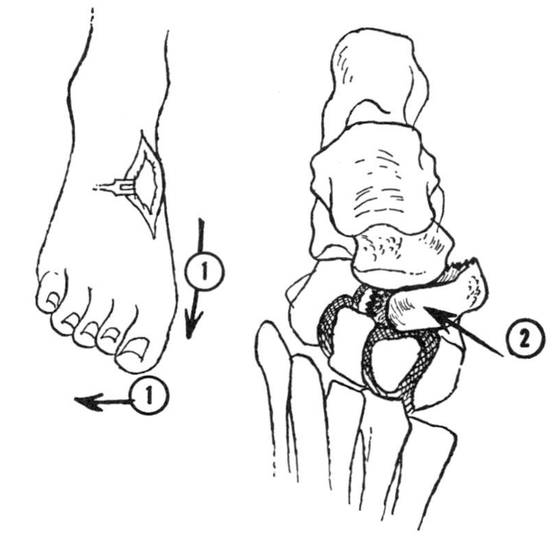

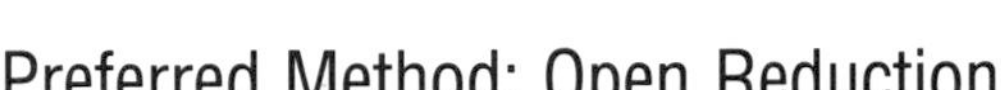

Preferred Method: Open Reduction

Most displaced fractures and fracture-dislocations of the navicula are best treated by open and anatomic reduction with internal fixation using screws or Kirschner wires.

1. Dorsal medial approach is carried out to expose the fracture.
2. Fracture is reduced by eversion and plantar flexion.

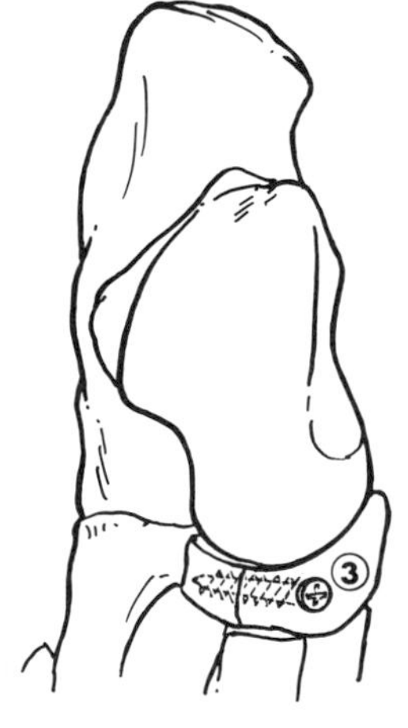

3. Fracture fragments are fixed with a cancellous screw.

Alternative Technique

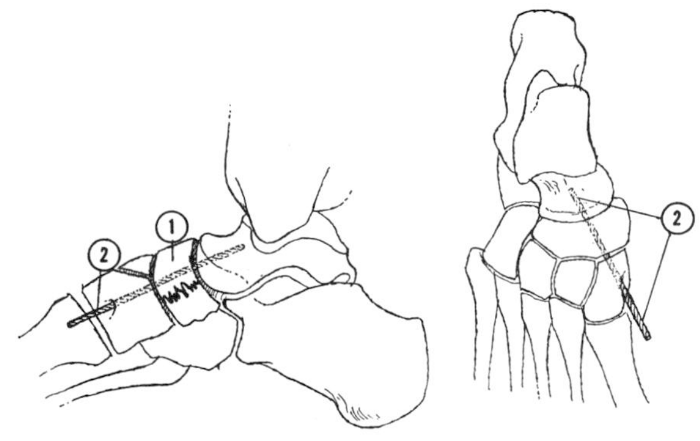

1. If the longitudinal arch is unstable or the fracture is comminuted, excision of the navicula to the talus and cuneiforms may be necessary.
2. This can be accomplished with a Steinmann pin or cannulated screw technique to stabilize the longitudinal arch.

Stress Fractures of the Navicula

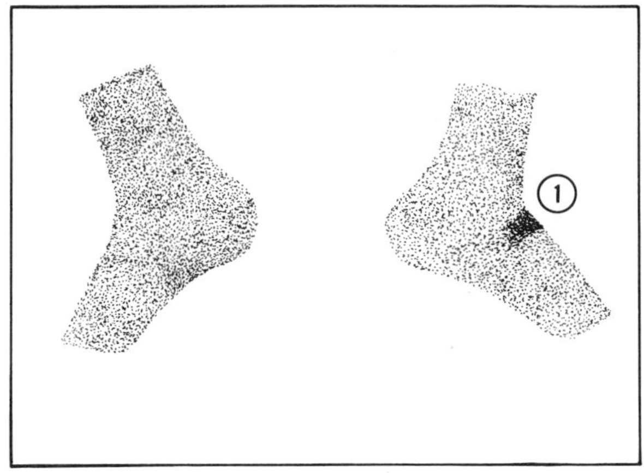

The early diagnosis of stress fractures of the navicula is important to minimize long-term symptoms.

In the athlete or long-distance runner with vague pain in the dorsum or medial longitudinal arch, the stress process should be highly suspected. The tarsal navicula is less subject to fracture than are the metatarsals but still should be carefully evaluated.

Diagnosis of Stress Fractures

1. Diagnosis is made frequently by bone scan, as previously described and confirmed by tomograms of the tarsal navicula.

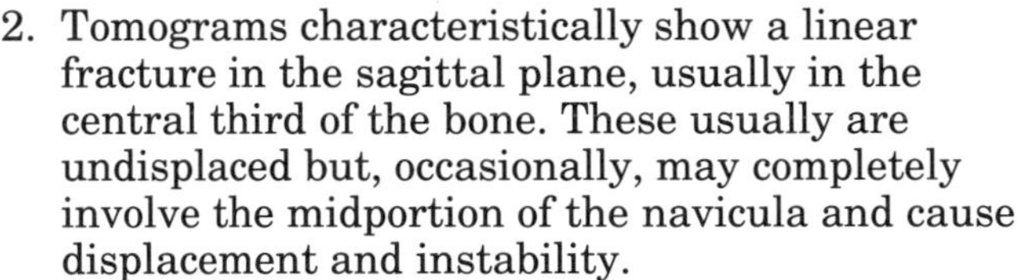

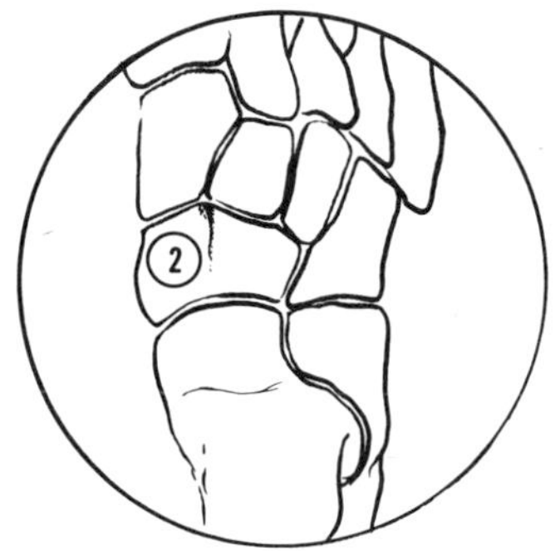

2. Tomograms characteristically show a linear fracture in the sagittal plane, usually in the central third of the bone. These usually are undisplaced but, occasionally, may completely involve the midportion of the navicula and cause displacement and instability.

Management of Stress Fractures

For undisplaced fractures, the treatment method should be a short-leg non–weight-bearing cast for 6–8 weeks, as shown previously for other navicular fractures.

It should be emphasized that, because of the importance of the tarsal navicula as the keystone of the arch, fractures of this bone should be treated by non–weight-bearing techniques. Torg et al. demonstrated a definite correlation between outcome from stress fractures and non–weight-bearing treatment.

If the stress fracture displaces or develops a nonunion, open reduction and internal fixation are necessary.

In most instances, stress fractures of the navicula considerably diminish the ability of athletes to run at a competitive level, and they should be so informed.

Management of a Chronic, Unrecognized Fracture-Dislocation

Approximately one in four fractures of the navicula may go unrecognized.

When the patient's symptoms of pain and swelling persist, the fracture or fracture-dislocation may be recognized only by means of x-rays taken several months after the injury.

The patient's painful limp from a chronic navicular injury can be relieved by fusion of the talonavicular joint and/or naviculocuneiform joint. If the subtalar joint is involved, triple arthrodesis may be necessary.

1. Nonunion with fracture-dislocation of the tarsal navicula 8 months after the original injury.
2. The keystone of the longitudinal arch is restored by fusion of the talonavicular and naviculocuneiform joints.

Note: The subtalar and calcaneocuboid joints are normal.

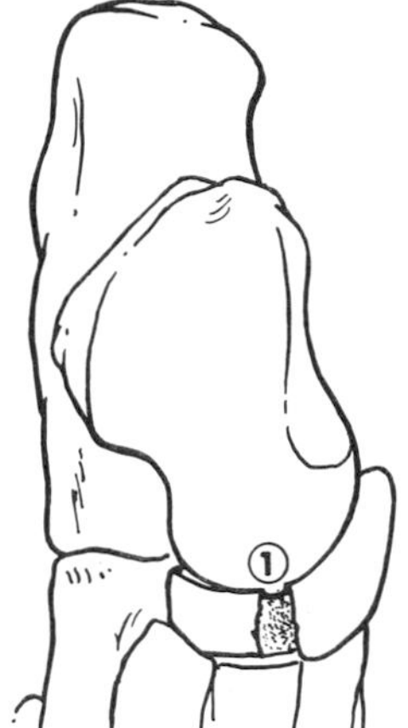

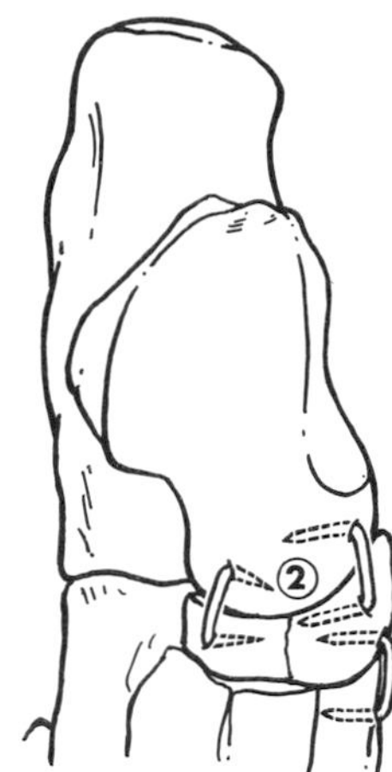

FRACTURES OF THE CUBOID AND CUNEIFORM BONES

REMARKS

Isolated injuries of the cuboid and cuneiform bones are rare and generally the result of direct injury, such as a fall with the foot in plantar flexion or having a heavy object fall directly on the foot.

In most instances, a fracture of these bones is not displaced, and reduction is usually not required.

Occasionally, fractures of the cuboid, when associated with the cuneiform or metatarsals, result from tarsometatarsal or midtarsal dislocation or subluxation. These are significantly more serious injuries than the usual fracture because they can lead to progressive symptomatic flattening of the weight-bearing arch of the foot.

Undisplaced Fractures From Direct Injury

Appearance on X-Ray

CUBOID FRACTURE

1. Comminuted fracture of the cuboid with minimal displacement.

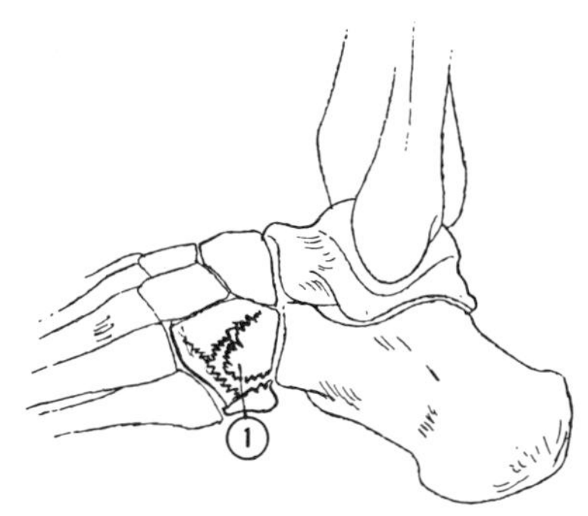

CUNEIFORM FRACTURE

1. Fracture of the second and third cuneiform bones with no displacement.

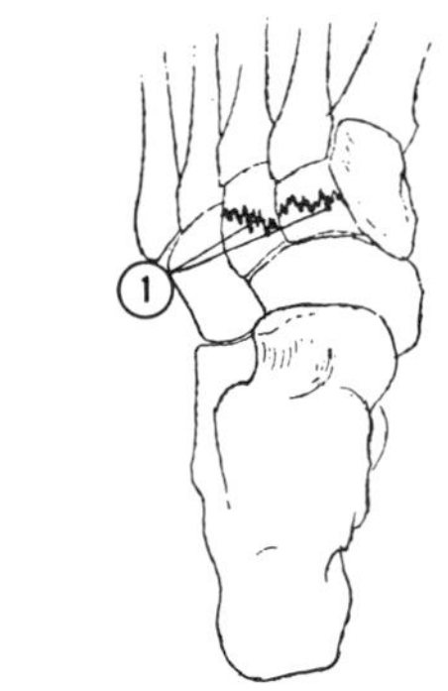

Immobilization

1. Circular plaster cast is applied from behind the metatarsal heads to the tibial tubercle.
2. Foot is in 90° of dorsiflexion.
3. Foot is in a neutral position in regard to inversion and eversion.
4. Plaster is molded well under the longitudinal arch.

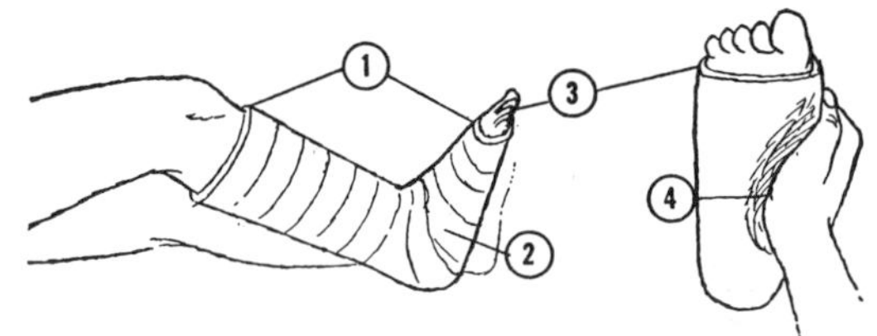

Subsequent Management

The cast may be removed by 4–6 weeks if the patient is pain free. Partial weight-bearing with crutches is continued for 2–3 weeks, after which full weight-bearing is possible.

Cuboid Fractures Associated With Occult Subluxation of the Midtarsal Joint

Appearance on X-Ray

Note: These x-rays were originally interpreted as normal.

1. Small avulsion fracture of the navicular bone is evident. (This may be confused with a sesamoid bone.)
2. Oblique x-rays show a fracture of the cuboid, including the calcaneocuboid joint.

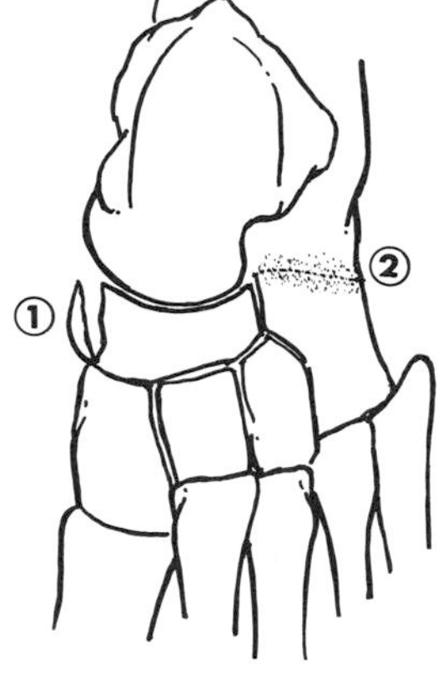

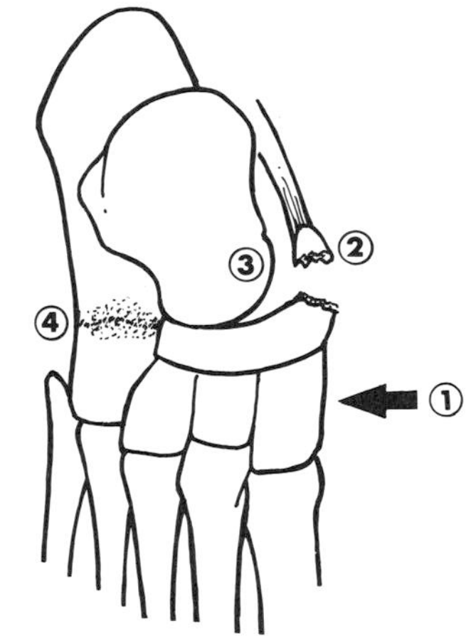

The mechanism is
1. Forced abduction.
2. Avulsion of the tuberosity of the navicula.
3. Subluxation of the talonavicular joint.
4. Compression fracture of the calcaneocuboid.

Clinical Appearance

1. Deformity of the midtarsal subluxation produces pronation of the foot and
2. Abduction of the forefoot.

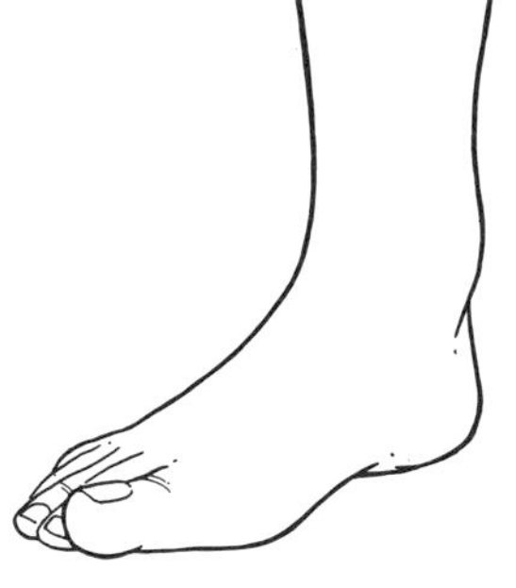

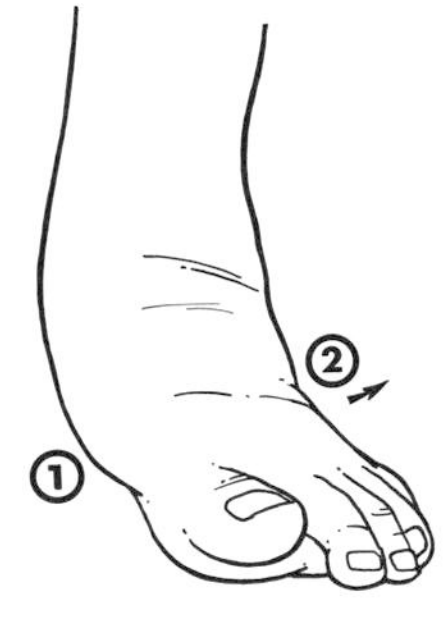

Management of Occult Fracture-Subluxation of the Midtarsal Joint

Treatment of these unstable injuries by plaster alone has resulted in persistent disability, as reported by Dewar and Evans. For fracture-subluxation, treatment should include
1. Reattachment of the avulsed navicular fragment, repair of the talonavicular joint, and
2. Fusion of the calcaneocuboid joint.

Note: For a chronic subluxed talonavicular joint, medial stabilization is also indicated.

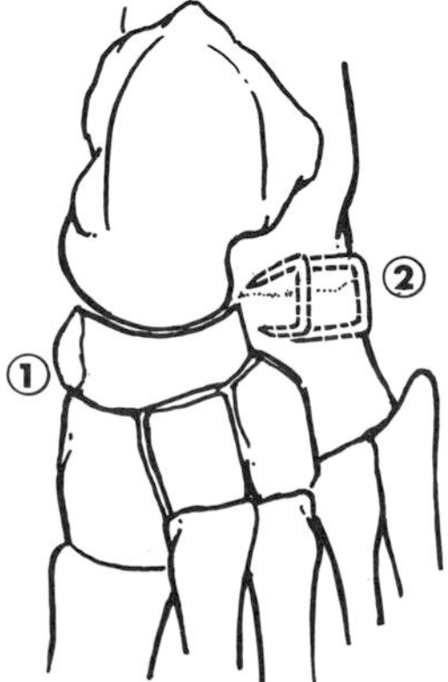

■ Other Injuries to the Midtarsal Joint

Total Dislocation of the Cuboid Without Fracture

Drummond and Hastings reported that complete dislocation of the cuboid is possible from forceful abduction of the foot.

This is an uncommon injury and may be missed on superficial clinical and radiographic examination.

Appearance on X-Ray

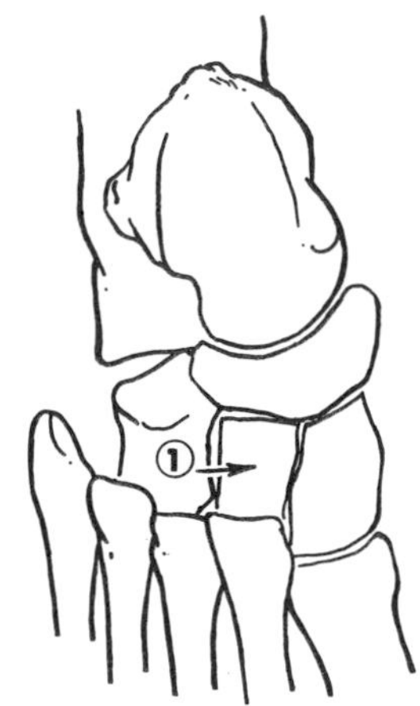

1. After a fall in which the victim lands on the inner side of the foot, the cuboid is displaced medially and

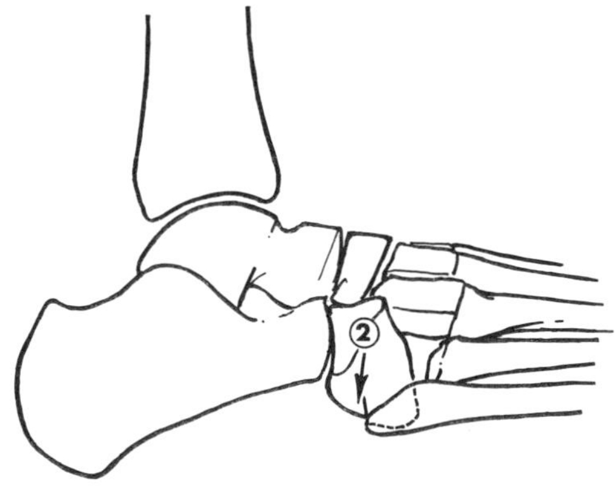

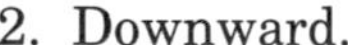

2. Downward.

Management

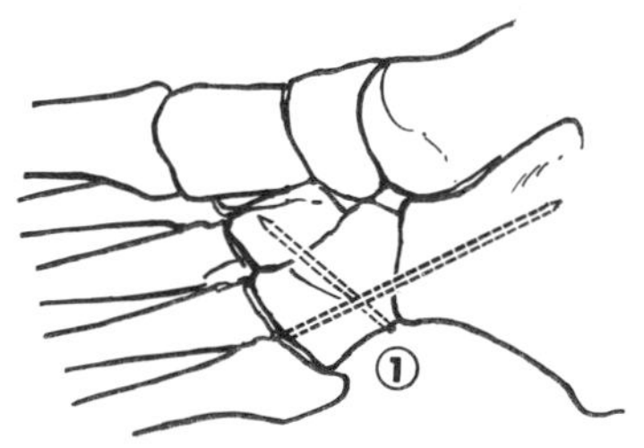

Operative reduction is necessary; it is achieved by inverting the foot to visualize and open the space normally occupied by the cuboid and then pushing the cuboid laterally back into the space.

1. Kirschner wire fixation is usually necessary to maintain reduction because the ligaments that surround the cuboid have been disrupted.

Subsequent Management

The foot is immobilized in a below-knee, non–weight-bearing cast for 6 weeks.

The cast and Kirschner wires are removed at the end of this time, and the patient is gradually allowed to resume weight-bearing on crutches.

Isolated Dislocation of the Cuneiform Bone

Schiller and Ray reported that this rare injury, isolated dislocation of the cuneiform bone, is readily missed because of its deceptive radiographic appearance.

The injury is sustained from direct violence to the foot, and the edema of the injury will mask any bony swelling or tenderness.

Careful assessment of a lateral x-ray is essential to detect the dislocation.

Prereduction X-Ray

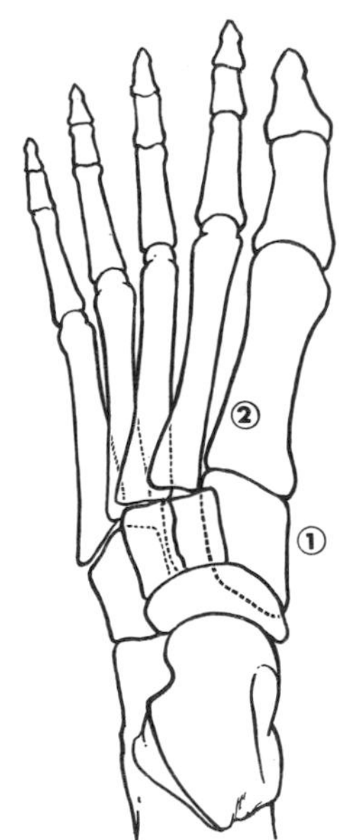

1. Except for overlapping of the navicular bone and medial cuneiform and
2. Rotation of the first metatarsal, the dislocation is not apparent on either the anteroposterior or the oblique x-ray.

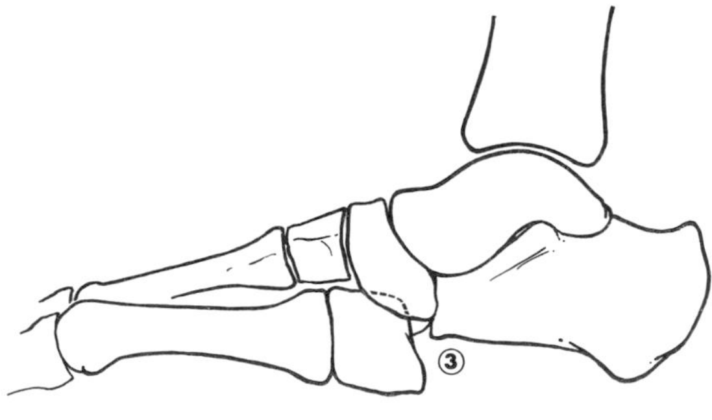

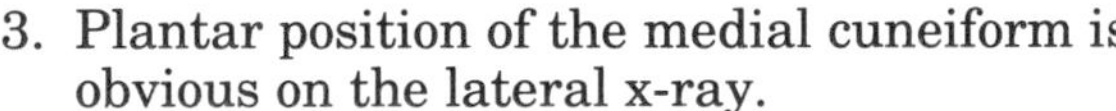

3. Plantar position of the medial cuneiform is obvious on the lateral x-ray.

Management

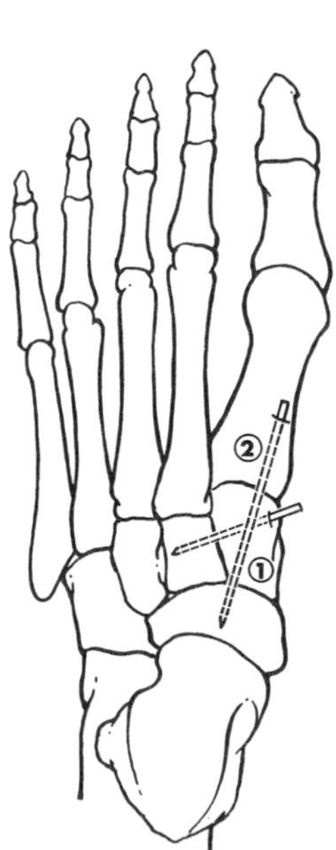

In most instances, the treatment is delayed either because of extreme swelling of the foot or because the diagnosis is not evident on initial x-rays.

The subsequent disruption to the medial longitudinal arch from this injury requires open reduction and arthrodesis of the reduced cuneiform to provide stability.

Postoperative X-Ray

1. Dislocated cuneiform has been surgically reduced under direct vision.
2. Crossed Kirschner wires are used to stabilize the naviculocuneiform and first and second cuneiform joints.

DISLOCATIONS AND FRACTURE-DISLOCATIONS OF THE MIDTARSAL JOINT

REMARKS

The midtarsal joint consists of the talonavicular and calcaneocuboid joints.

Dislocation is most often medial and is associated with a fracture of the navicular or cuboid bone. Fractures of these bones should not be treated without evaluation of the entire midfoot. Avulsion fractures may occur as isolated injuries, but they may also mask significant injury and instability of the midtarsus.

Main and Jowett described a medial midtarsal dislocation without fracture, which is considered to be a swivel dislocation of the calcaneus under the talus. This is the result of an inversion mechanism that leaves the talocalcaneal ligament intact and, therefore, does not produce the usual complete subtalar dislocation with tilting of the calcaneus. The force is sufficient to dislocate the navicular bone medial to the talus but leaves the calcaneocuboid joint intact.

The midtarsal joint can also be dislocated as a result of a force applied to the plantar-flexed foot. The injury may cause a fracture-dislocation of the navicular bone or a plantar dislocation of both the talonavicular and calcaneocuboid components of the midtarsus. A plantar dislocation of the midtarsus is distinguished from a plantar-subtalar dislocation by the maintenance of the normal subtalar joint space owing to the intact talocalcaneal ligament.

Lateral midtarsal dislocation results from forceful abduction, which causes an avulsion fracture of the navicular tuberosity and an impaction fracture of the lateral margins of the calcaneus or cuboid, as described on page 1007.

A lateral swivel dislocation may also occur at the midtarsal joint without a fracture.

Recurrent or persistent unrecognized instability of the midtarsus can follow from these injuries and requires arthrodesis of the talonavicular and calcaneocuboid joints. Hooper and McMaster reported bilateral recurrences that responded to midtarsal fusion.

Neurotrophic problems in the diabetic patient may also cause recurrent fractures and instability of the midfoot, but fusion may be difficult in this situation.

Prereduction X-Rays

MEDIAL MIDTARSAL DORSAL DISLOCATION WITH FRACTURED CUBOID

1. Inward displacement of the navicular and cuboid bones on the talus and calcaneus.
2. Tarsal bones at the level of the midtarsal joint are displaced upward.
3. Fracture of the cuboid bone with minimal displacement.

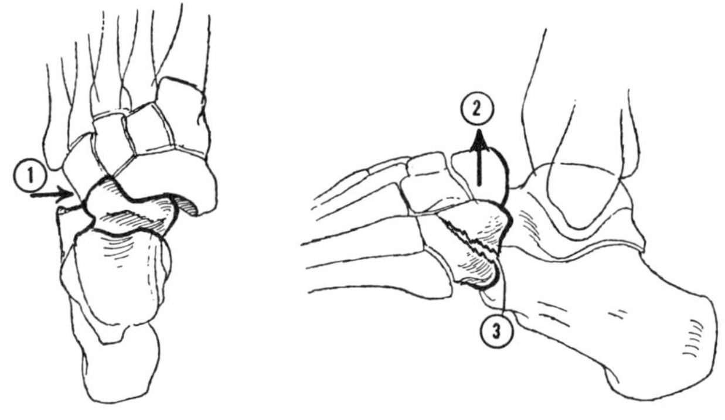

PLANTAR DISLOCATION

1. Lateral view shows dislocation of both the talonavicular and the calcaneocuboid components of the midtarsus.
2. Subtalar joint maintains its normal space because the talocalcaneal ligament remains intact.

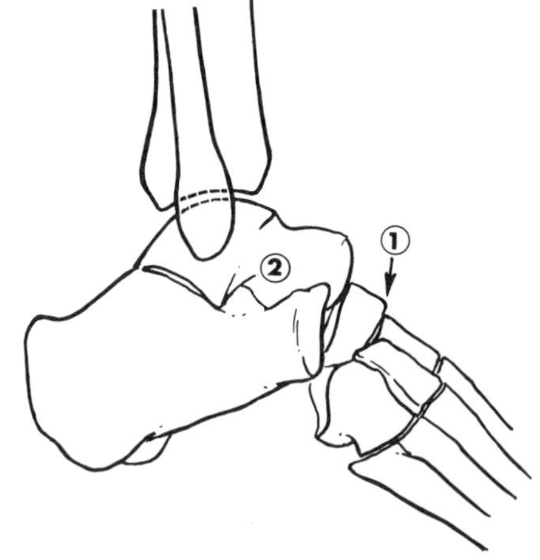

MEDIAL SWIVEL DISLOCATION

1. Anteroposterior view shows dislocation of the talonavicular component.
2. Calcaneus swivels beneath the talus, maintaining articulation with the cuboid.

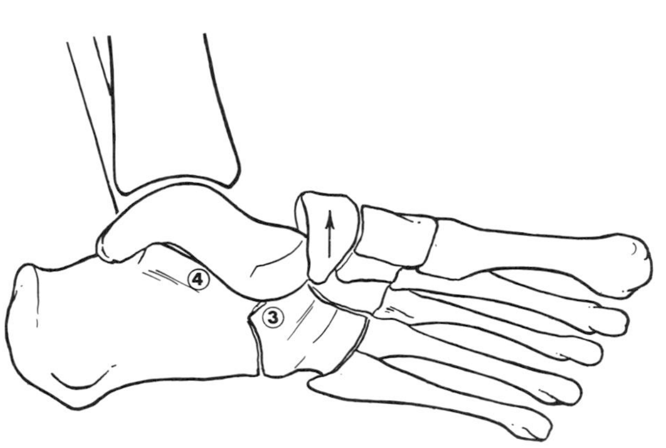

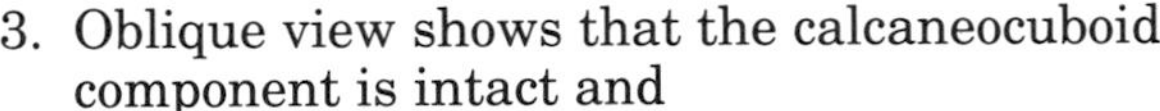

3. Oblique view shows that the calcaneocuboid component is intact and
4. Calcaneus is not tilted as it would be in a subtalar dislocation because the talocalcaneal ligament remains intact.

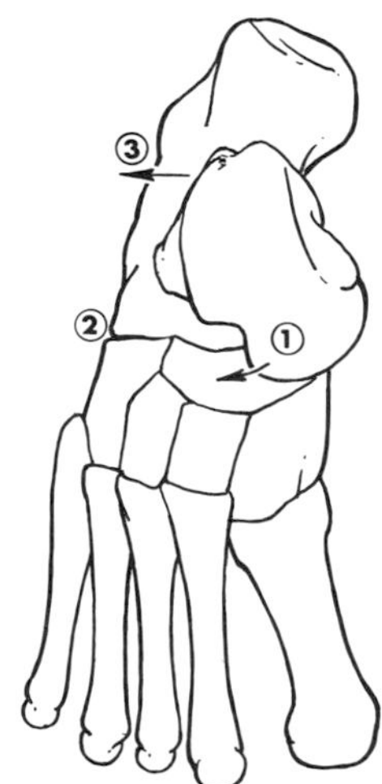

LATERAL SWIVEL DISLOCATION

1. Anteroposterior view shows that the talonavicular joint has dislocated laterally.
2. Calcaneocuboid joint remains intact.
3. Hindfoot does not evert, but the os calcis has swiveled laterally owing to the intact talocalcaneal ligament.

Management

Closed reduction is possible, but it should restore the joint to an anatomically normal position. If there is any question about the adequacy of reduction, direct surgical exploration of the joint should be carried out.

Frequently, the injury is unstable and should be stabilized by percutaneous Steinmann pin fixation of the midtarsus after reduction.

Fractures of the navicular or cuboid bone, particularly after abduction-type injuries, require internal fixation.

After reduction, test the stability of the midtarsus by abduction and adduction. If the joint is unstable, use percutaneous pin fixation.

Manipulative Reduction

1. One assistant fixes the ankle.
2. Another assistant grasps the forefoot and makes strong forward traction.
3. With the heels of the hands, the surgeon pushes the forefoot outward and the calcaneus inward; this reduces the inward displacement.

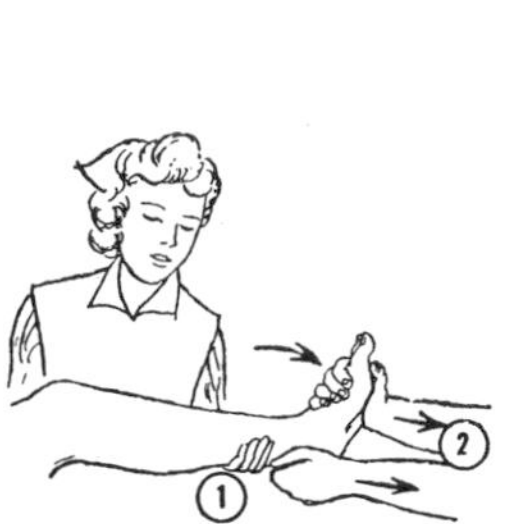

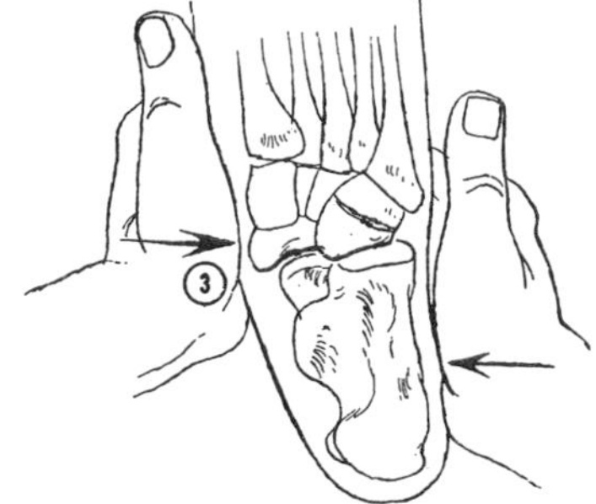

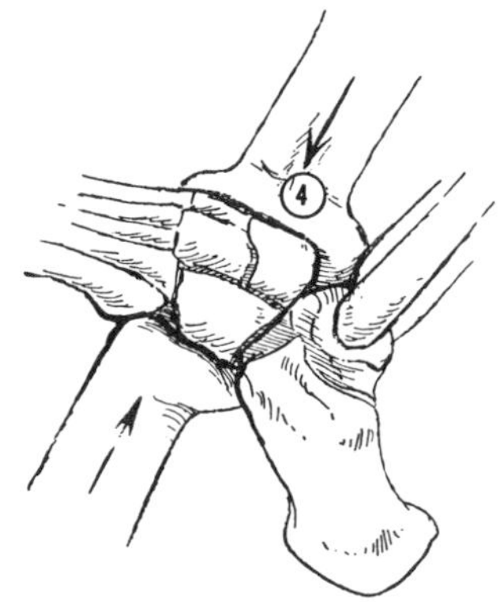

4. With the heels of both hands, direct downward pressure is made on the anterior tarsal bone; this reduces the upward displacement.

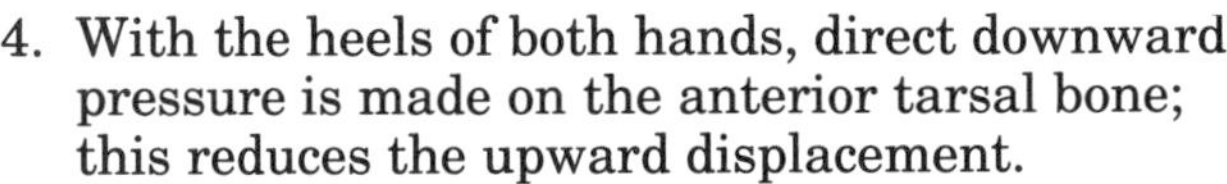

Note: This same general pattern of manipulation is used regardless of the direction of displacement.

Postreduction X-Ray

1. Navicular and cuboid bones are in a normal relationship to the talus and calcaneus.
2. Fracture of the cuboid bone.

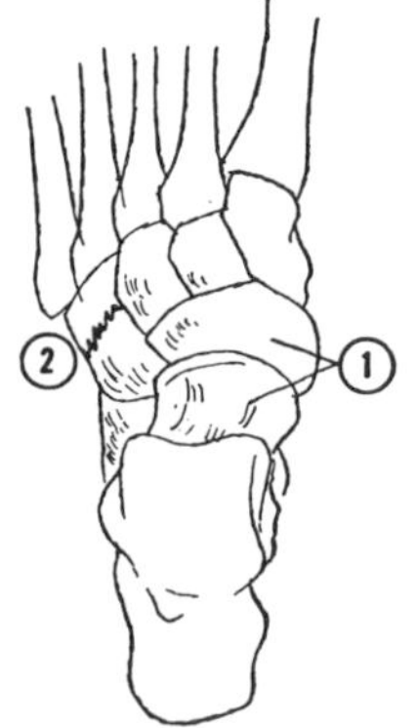

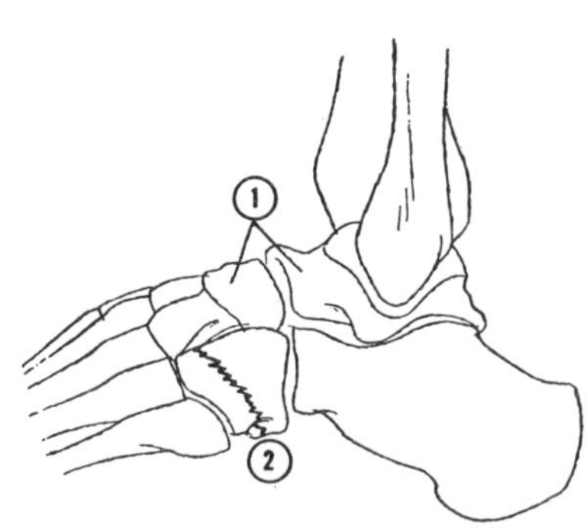

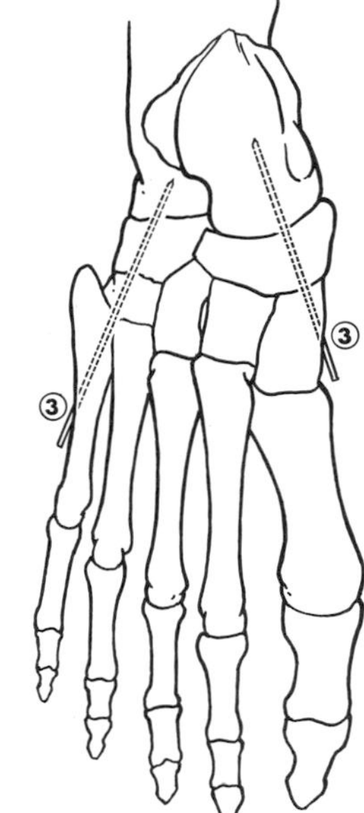

3. If the midtarsus is at all unstable, it should be fixed with percutaneous Steinmann pins.

Immobilization

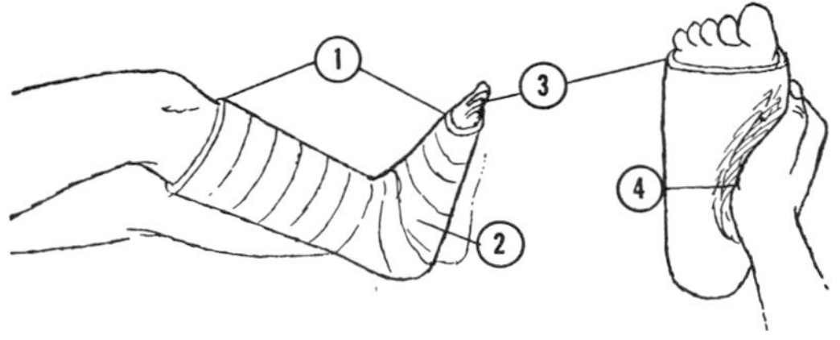

1. Circular plaster cast is applied from behind the metatarsal heads to the tibial tubercle.
2. Foot is in 90° of dorsiflexion.
3. Foot is in a neutral position in regard to inversion and eversion.
4. Plaster is molded well under the longitudinal arch.

Note: If the foot is swollen, the cast is split immediately and the foot elevated.

Postreduction Management

Allow the patient up on crutches without bearing weight on the affected foot.

Remove the cast and any percutaneous pins at the end of 6 weeks.

Fit the patient with a shoe with a longitudinal arch support.

Recurrent or Persistent Subluxation of the Midtarsus

REMARKS

Because of the relative infrequency of injuries to the midtarsal joint, persistent symptoms may occur.

This is particularly common in middle-aged women who slip or fall a short distance. The injury tends to be treated as a minor sprain, and the subtle disruption of the midtarsal region is frequently missed clinically and by x-ray.

The consequences are that these patients have prolonged symptoms, particularly if the injury involves the calcaneal cuboid and the talonavicular joint.

The more serious acute injury is evident clinically if the patient has tenderness on both the medial and lateral side of the metatarsus. With this finding, the foot is best immobilized in a cast and kept without weight-bearing for 3–4 weeks until the soft tissues stabilize the joint.

If the joints develop persistent arthritis, stabilization may be necessary to relieve the symptomatic occult midtarsal subluxation.

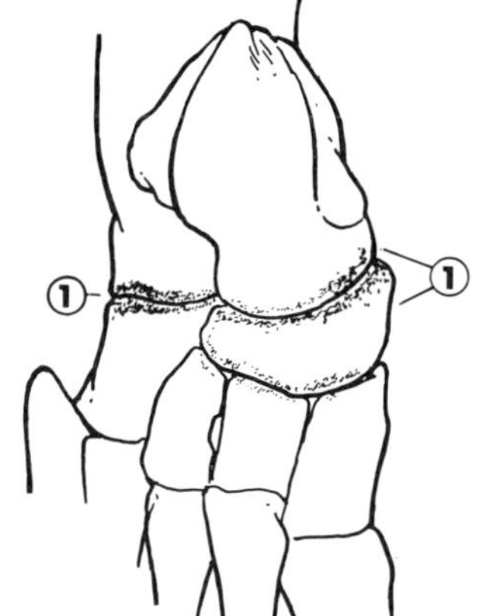

1. A subtle injury to the midtarsal joint has involved both the talonavicular and calcaneal cuboid joint. The result is an acquired flat foot and symptomatic residual arthritis.

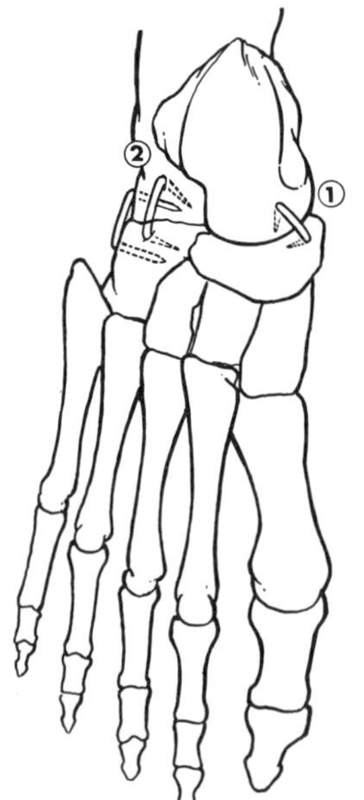

X-Ray After Fusion

1. Foot is stabilized by a fusion of the talonavicular and calcaneocuboid joints.
2. Triple arthrodesis is not necessary if the subtalar joint shows no arthritic changes.

DISLOCATIONS AND FRACTURE-DISLOCATIONS OF THE TARSOMETATARSAL JOINT

REMARKS

Fractures and dislocations of the tarsometatarsal region are uncommon injuries and, unfortunately, are commonly unrecognized.

The classic mechanism dates back to the Napoleonic era when, in a cavalry accident, a rider suffered the misfortune of his horse falling on his plantar-flexed foot. It was for this injury that Lisfranc developed his amputation through the tarsometatarsal region.

Wiley described both direct and indirect mechanisms of injury. The indirect mechanism is more common and less understood than the direct mechanism.

Visualizing the anatomy of this region is helpful to appreciate the mechanisms of injury.

Anatomy of the Tarsometatarsal Region

1. Ligamentous and bony articulations around the second metatarsal make this bone the keystone of the tarsometatarsal region.
2. The first metatarsal has no ligamentous attachment to the second and may be displaced in a divergent direction from the other metatarsals.

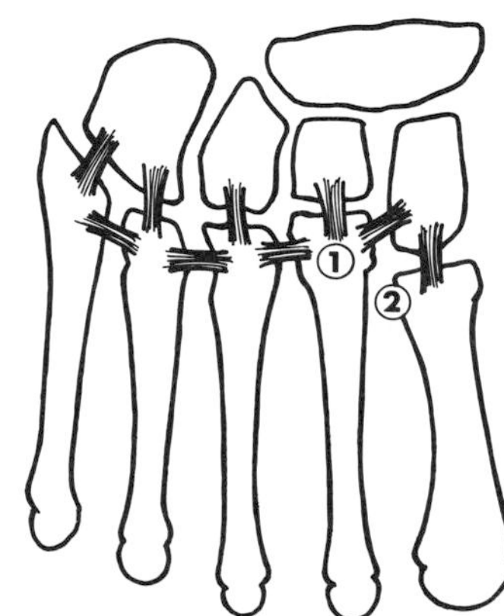

■ Direct Mechanism

The direct mechanism results from a crushing injury that can produce varying degrees of fractures and dislocations.

As with any injury to the foot, adequate anteroposterior, lateral, and oblique x-rays are necessary to appreciate the extent of damage.

Typically, the injury follows a direct blow from a heavy weight dropping on the foot. This produces the following injuries.

1. Anteroposterior and oblique x-rays show multiple fractures of the fifth and fourth metatarsals and
2. Cuboid.

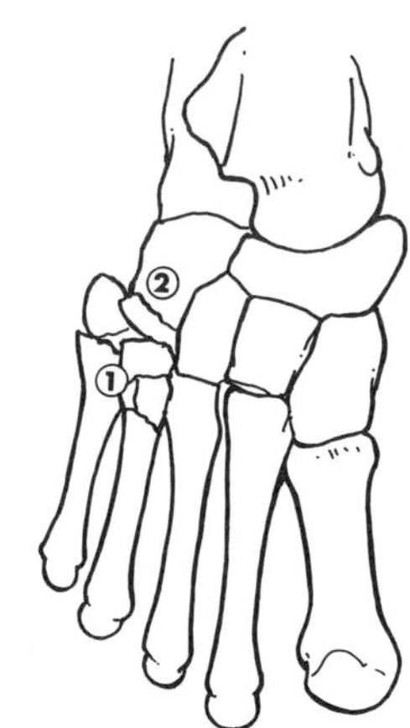

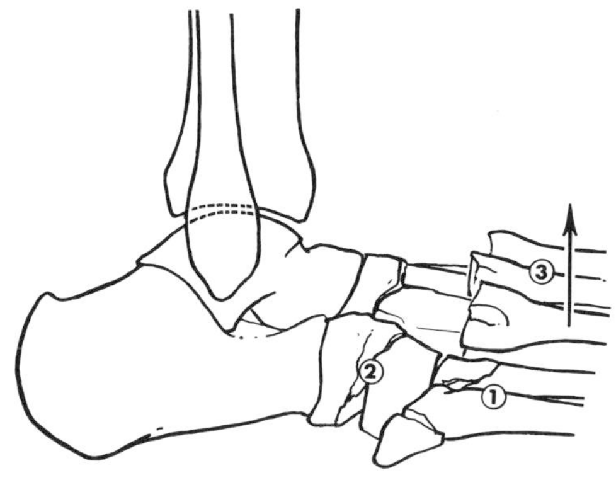

3. Lateral view shows dorsolateral dislocation not evident on the anteroposterior view.

Divergent Dislocation

Direct injury between the first and second metatarsals may cause

1. Divergent dislocation, in which the first metatarsal moves medially while the remaining metatarsals move laterally.
2. Fracture of the navicular or cuneiform bone is common.

Note: Divergent dislocations are most likely to cause extensive swelling from disruption of the dorsalis pedis vessel. The possibility of vascular insult should always be kept in mind, particularly with violent direct mechanisms.

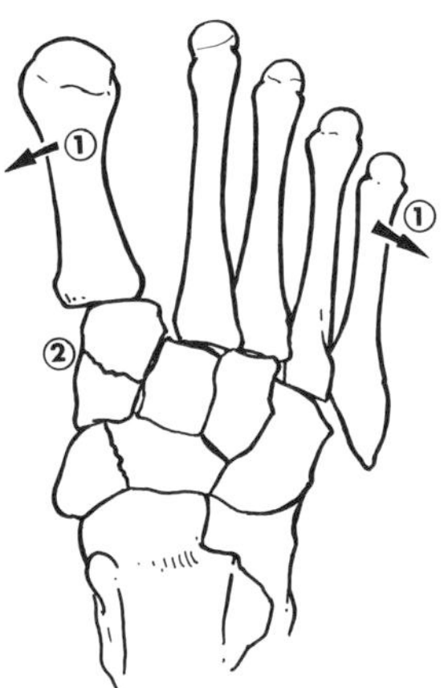

Indirect Mechanisms

Indirect mechanisms include both abduction and plantar-flexion injuries, as described by Wiley.

Abduction Mechanism

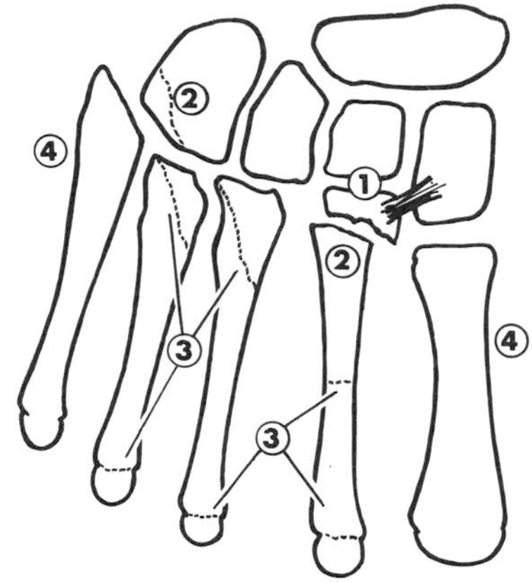

1. When the forefoot is violently abducted, the brunt of the strain is absorbed by the fixed base of the second metatarsal.
2. Fractures of the second metatarsal and of the cuboid are pathognomonic.
3. Other fractures of the metatarsal neck or bases may occur.
4. Fracture of the first or fifth metatarsal is uncommon.

Plantar-Flexion Mechanism

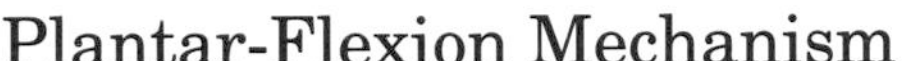

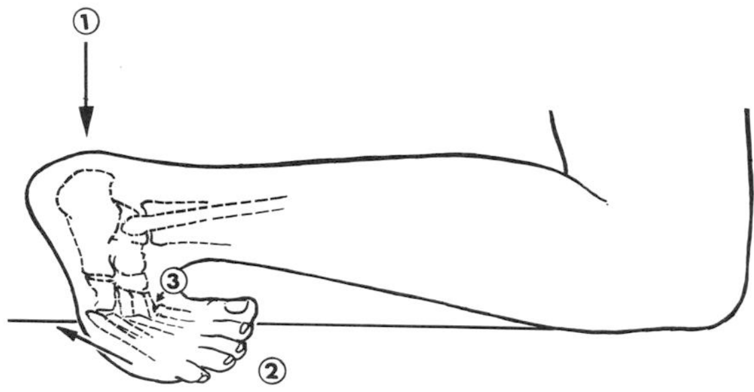

Acute plantar flexion occurs in two ways.

The least common mechanism results from a violent blow to the heel in line with the axis of the foot while the toes are fixed. This was the classic injury sustained by a Napoleonic cavalryman when his horse fell on his foot.

1. Violent force is applied to the heel in line with the axis of the foot.
2. Toes are fixed.
3. Direct heel-to-toe compression produces acute plantar flexion of the tarsometatarsal joint.

The second and more common indirect injury occurs with the ankle in acute plantar flexion or tiptoe position. This causes the foot to become a part of the entire lower leg.

The tarsometatarsal joint absorbs the brunt of forced plantar flexion and sudden deceleration.

Most commonly, this occurs in a front-end automobile collision in which the outstretched foot is violently plantar flexed and driven backward by the floorboard. Other mechanisms may be the result of trivial trauma, such as stepping off a curbstone, falling from a stepladder, or inadvertently stepping into a deep hole.

Front-End Collision

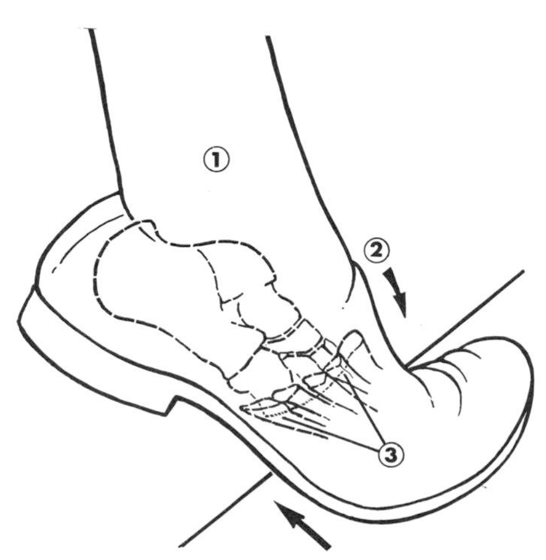

1. Foot and ankle are in maximal plantar flexion or tiptoe position at the time of injury.
2. Further plantar flexion dislocates the tarsometatarsal joint.
3. Rotation of the forefoot at the time of injury produces associated fracture of the metatarsal.

Note: The dislocated joints may reduce partially or completely after the injury. The fracture patterns of the tarsals and metatarsals then may be the only clue to the significant instability.

■ Assessment

REMARKS

Fractures produced by direct mechanisms of injury are usually quite apparent clinically because of massive swelling and pain.

A number of these tarsometatarsal injuries may be subtle and not obvious, particularly after indirect mechanisms of injury. There may be only slight widening between the bases of the first and second metatarsals, which is indicative of a significant rupture of the ligaments. Because of the subtleties of these injuries, careful clinical and radiographic evaluation are necessary.

Clinical Evaluation

1. Typically, the pain is localized to the tarsometatarsal region.
2. Pronation and abduction stress applied to the forefoot causes sharp pain in the region of the tarsometatarsal injury.

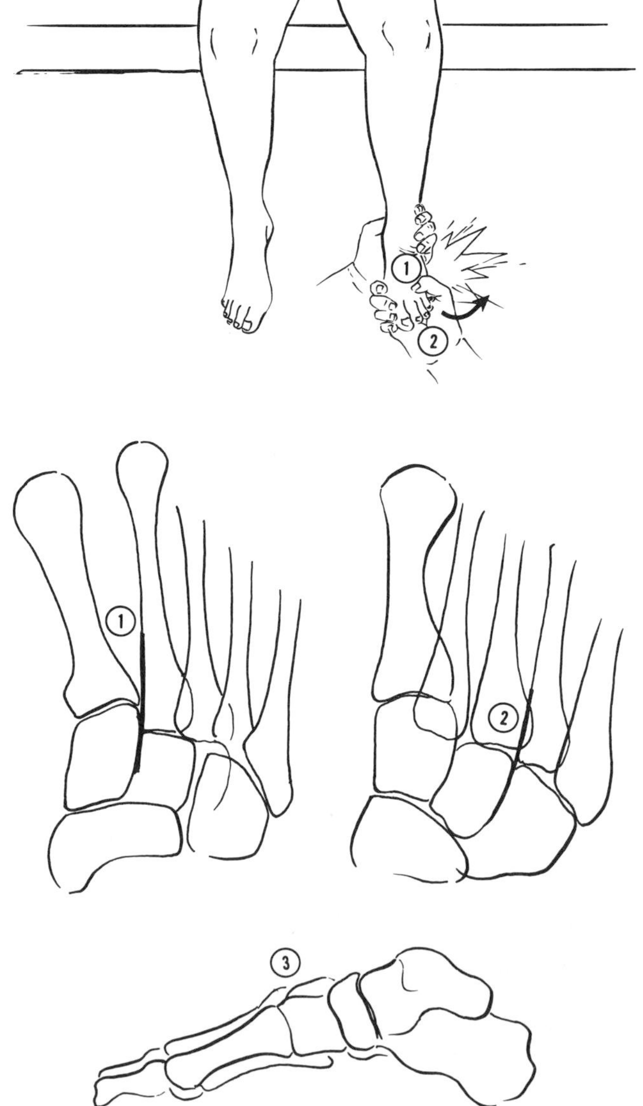

X-Ray Evaluation for Subtle Injuries of the Tarsometatarsal Joints—Normal Foot

1. On the anteroposterior view, the medial aspect of the second metatarsal and medial cuneiform lie in an unbroken line in the normal foot.
2. On an oblique view of the foot, the medial aspect of the fourth metatarsal and cuboid lies in an unbroken line normally.
3. On the lateral weight-bearing view, the dorsal aspect of the metatarsal base never lies dorsal to the medial cuneiform.

Note: In acute injuries, the first metatarsal may lie dorsally, but in the chronic disruption of this joint, it tends to sublux in a plantar direction, causing progressive flattening of the arch.

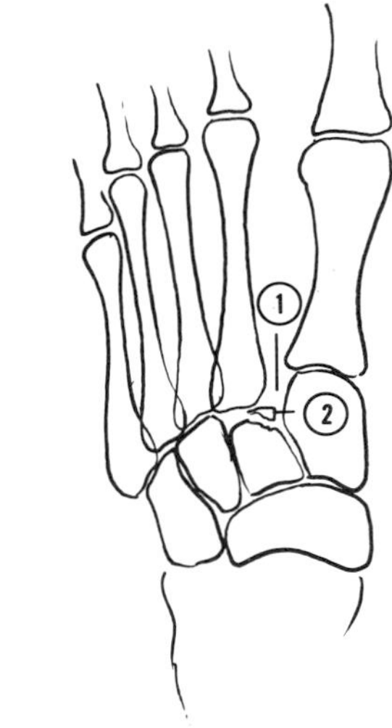

Subluxation of the Tarsometatarsal Joint

1. Subtle injury of the Lisfranc joint is evident by the 4-mm diastasis between the base of the first and second metatarsals.
2. In addition, there is slight lateral subluxation of the second metatarsal on the medial cuneiform and an avulsion in that area.

Note: Evaluation of chronic instability of the Lisfranc joint is carried out with a weight-bearing lateral x-ray.

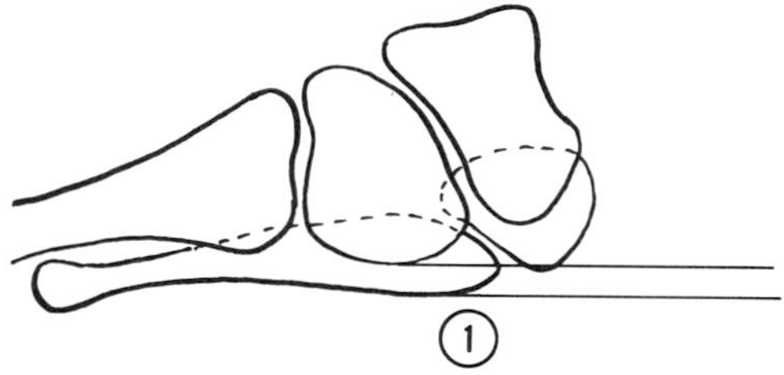

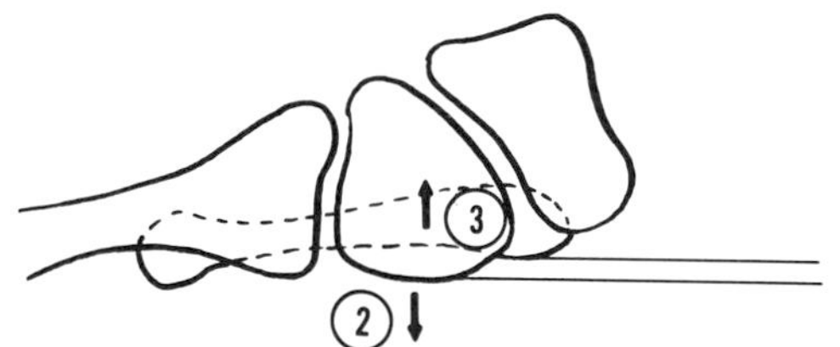

Weight-Bearing Views of Chronic Subluxation

1. Normal weight-bearing true lateral of the foot shows that the fifth metatarsal is always plantar or below the medial cuneiform.
2. If there is flattening of the foot as a result of the Lisfranc injury, the medial cuneiform is displaced plantarward to the
3. Base of the fifth metatarsal. There is a negative relationship.

Note: This acquired flat foot can be persistently symptomatic for many months and require open reduction and internal fixation of the joint. The objective in the unrecognized injury is to achieve a stable arthrodesis of the joint.

■ Significance of Subtle Injuries That Cause Chronic Subluxation of the Lisfranc Joint

When anatomic reduction is obtained by closed or open methods, satisfactory painless function is the usual result. Nevertheless, some arthritic changes may be evident even after ideal reduction of the joint.

Occasionally, some subtle tarsometatarsal injuries may lead to persistent symptoms. For example, a diastasis of as little as 2–5 mm between the first and second metatarsals can lead to persistent pain with weight-bearing.

Faciszewski et al. pointed out that injuries to this joint can lead to symptomatic flattening of the arch of the foot. On the other hand, if the longitudinal arch of the foot is maintained after these injuries, functional outcome is usually satisfactory.

Management

REMARKS

Tarsometatarsal injuries from both direct and indirect mechanisms require prompt reduction and internal stabilization of the foot.

Direct injuries to the foot frequently cause an open wound or compromised circulation, both of which need to be managed in conjunction with reduction of the injury.

Even if a closed reduction is successful, the tarsometatarsal region is so unstable that percutaneous pin fixation of the joint is wise to avoid recurrent subluxation or dislocation despite cast immobilization.

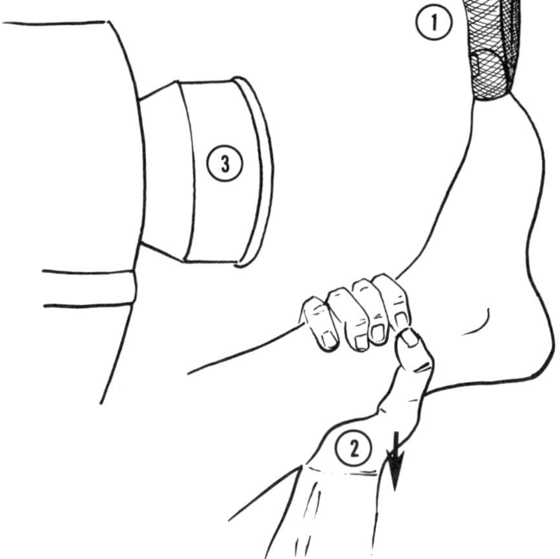

Manipulative Reduction

Technique of Reduction

1. Forefoot is suspended in Chinese finger traps.
2. Countertraction is applied to the hindfoot to bring the tarsometatarsal joint into a reduced position.
3. Positions in the anterior, posterior, and lateral planes are evaluated by careful fluoroscopic control.

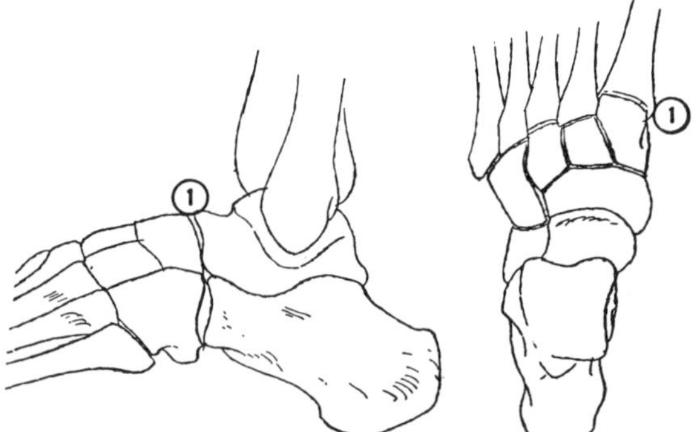

Postreduction X-Ray

1. Bases of the metatarsal bones are in a normal relationship to the tarsal bones.

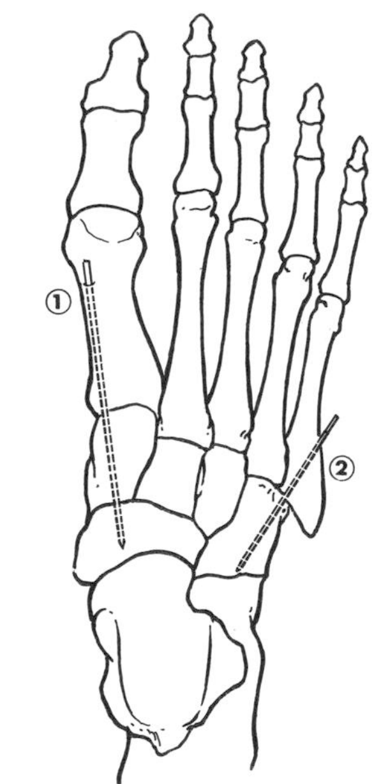

1. After reduction, the tarsometatarsal joint is stabilized by a percutaneous 2-mm Steinmann pin drilled from the first metatarsal into the navicular bone.
2. If the lateral metatarsals are not reduced, a second incision is made between the fourth and fifth metatarsals, and the reduction is accomplished under direct vision. A second smooth Steinmann pin is inserted through the fifth metatarsal into the cuboid.

Note: These two pins produce stability of all of the metatarsals; fixation of the third or fourth metatarsal is not necessary.

Immobilization

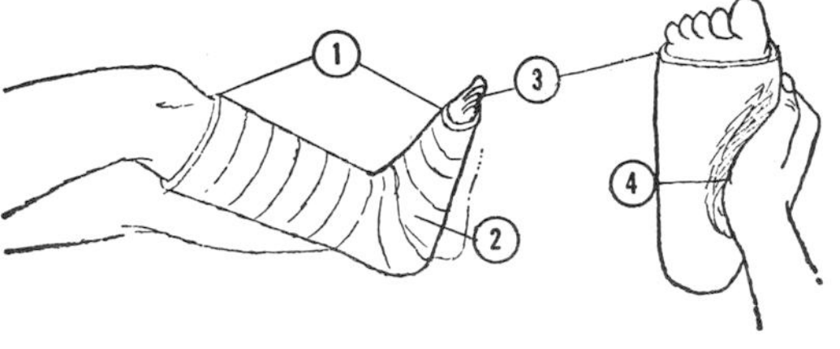

1. Padded circular cast is applied from the toes to below the knee joint.
2. Foot is at a right angle.
3. Foot is in neutral in regard to inversion and eversion.
4. Plaster is molded well under the longitudinal arch.

Postreduction Management

Elevate the limb on pillows.

Surround the foot with ice bags.

Check the circulation of the foot frequently.

After a few days, allow the patient to be up on crutches without bearing weight on the affected foot.

Remove the cast and pins at the end of 6 weeks.

The patient is then allowed partial weight-bearing on crutches for 4 weeks longer.

Subsequently, the patient is permitted full weight-bearing with the use of a longitudinal arch support.

Operative Reduction

If manipulation is not successful or if the dislocation recurs, open reduction and internal fixation should be performed.

The key to reduction is the fracture-dislocation of the second metatarsal.

Occasionally, in dislocations that cannot be reduced by closed manipulation, the anterior tibial tendon may be interposed, particularly between the navicular and first cuneiform bones. This requires replacement of the tendon and reduction and fixation of the dislocation.

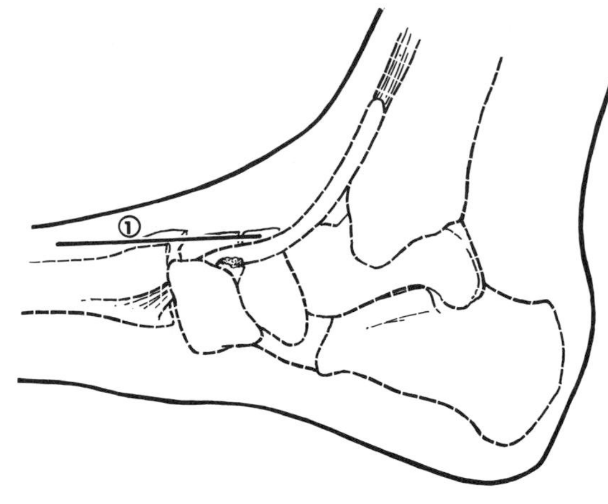

1. A longitudinal incision is made lateral to the long axis of the first metatarsal. The first and second metatarsals are reduced under direct vision.

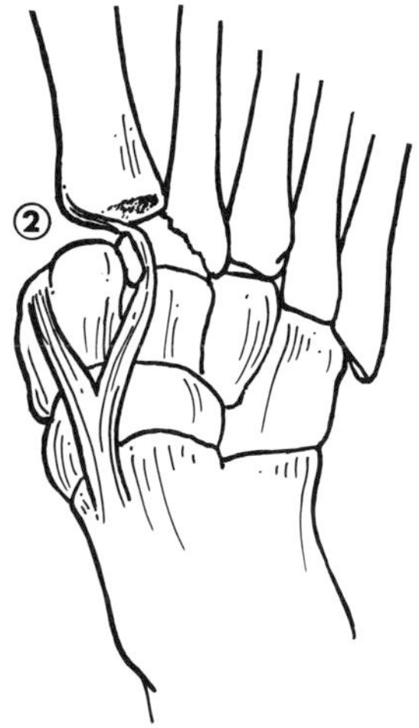

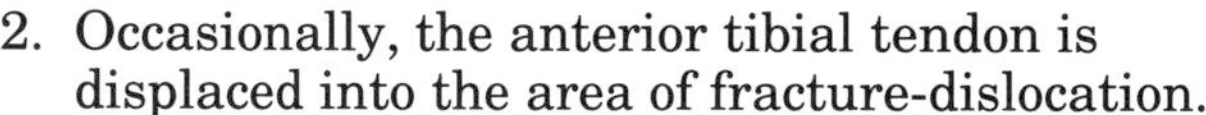

2. Occasionally, the anterior tibial tendon is displaced into the area of fracture-dislocation.

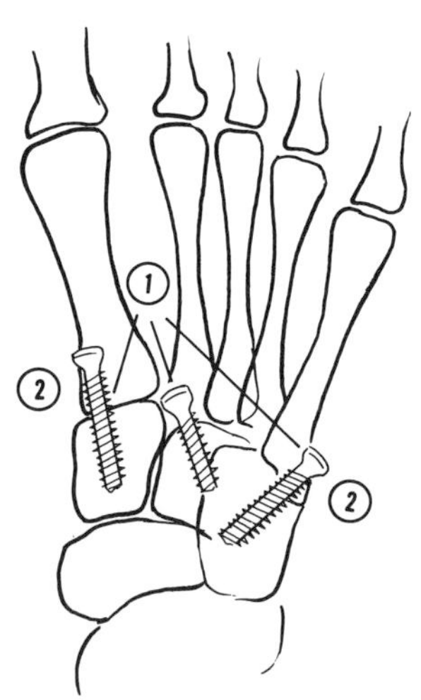

1. After reduction, the tarsometatarsal joint is stabilized by multiple screw fixation.
2. Frequently, the lateral and medial areas of the joint require stabilization.

Note: Subsequently, the screws may be removed by the end of 12–16 weeks before the patient begins full weight-bearing.

■ Special Problems: Diabetic Neurotrophic Joints (Charcot Foot), Which Cause Chronic Dislocation

REMARKS

Alterations in the autonomic blood supply to the foot as a result of long-standing diabetes produce an abnormal response to minimal injuries.

Clinically, this may present as merely a "swollen foot" in the diabetic patient with trauma.

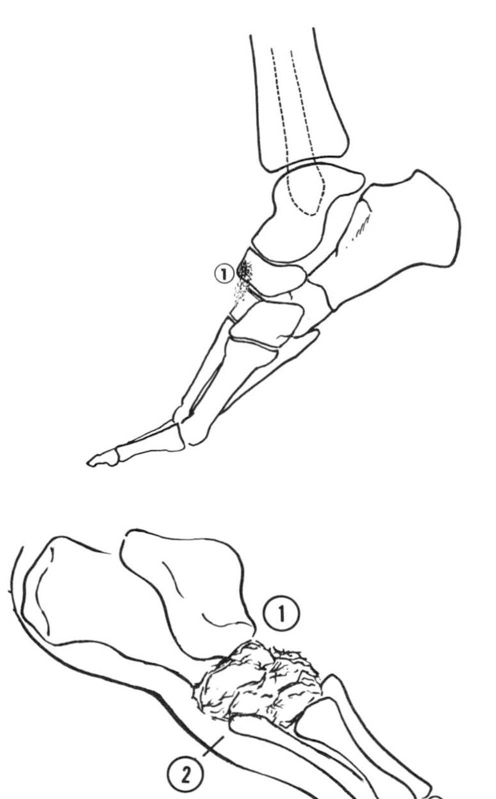

1. Repeated injuries to the diabetic foot can cause chronic disruption of the midtarsus and persistent subluxation of the joint.

Note: This is the most common cause of Charcot foot today and should be treated by fusion of the midtarsal joint, as described earlier. Fusion in the diabetic foot can be difficult, but it can be done.

Subsequent X-Ray at 4 Months

1. Abnormal blood flow to the injured foot causes bone resorption and progressive instability of the foot.
2. Rocker-bottom plantar angulation of the midfoot occurs. This results in pressure sores over the bony prominences and neurotrophic ulceration, which may lead in turn to amputation.

Management

Management of the patient with diabetes and even a minor injury to the foot requires elevation and careful observation. If the swelling can be combatted, protective cast application is indicated when the swelling goes down.

Difficulties arise when the patient is kept on crutches because frequently the opposite foot also begins to break down.

The basic underlying treatment is protective shoes and careful follow-up observation to avoid breakdown of the bony prominences.

Surgical removal of the bony prominences and internal stabilization are often indicated for progressive deformity to prevent neurotrophic ulceration.

FRACTURES OF THE METATARSAL BONES

REMARKS

Fractures of the metatarsal bones are the result of either direct, indirect, or avulsion injuries.

The fall of an object directly on the forefoot commonly fractures one or more metatarsal bones.

Avulsion fractures occur typically at the base of the metatarsals, particularly the fifth metatarsal from the pull of soft tissue attachments.

Stress fractures are also fairly common and result from prolonged running or walking. Usually, the second or third metatarsal bone is involved. These are also called march fractures because they occur commonly in army recruits on forced marches.

Most metatarsal fractures are relatively undisplaced and are best treated symptomatically.

Occasionally, some are displaced downward into the sole of the foot and need reduction and internal stabilization.

Fractures of the fifth metatarsal shaft, the so-called Jones fracture, are unique and prone to healing problems in certain active individuals. These are probably the most common metatarsal fractures that require operative stabilization.

Fractures of the Metatarsal Bones Without Displacement

Appearance on X-Ray

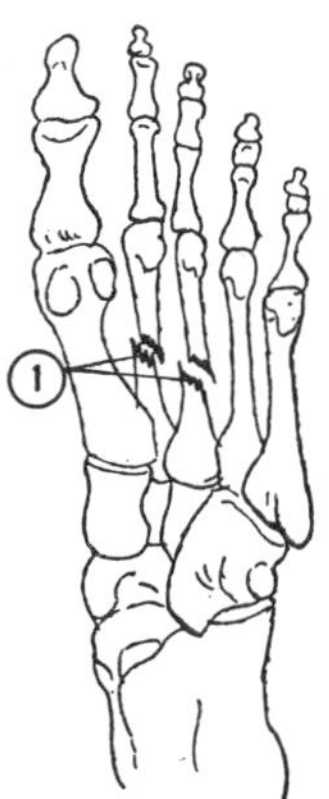

1. Fracture of the shafts of the second and third metatarsal bones with minimal displacement.

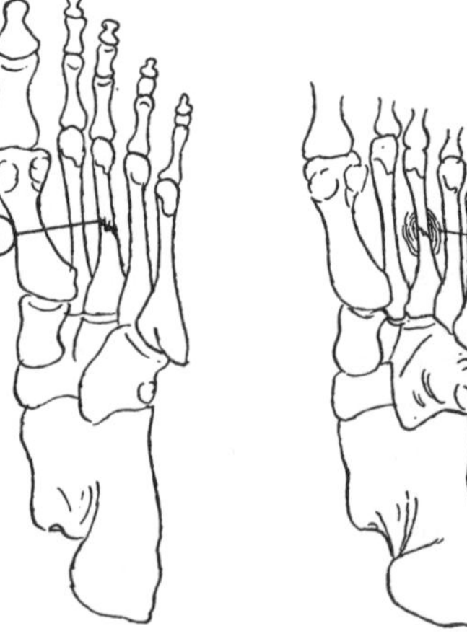

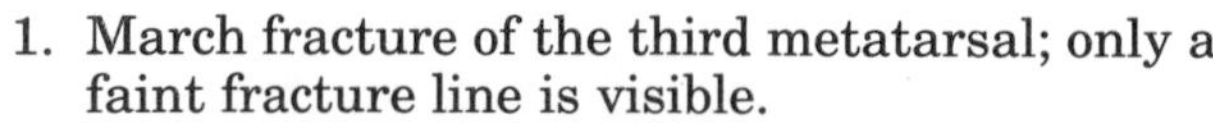

1. March fracture of the third metatarsal; only a faint fracture line is visible.
2. Same fracture 3 weeks after the onset of symptoms; note marked callus formation.

Immobilization

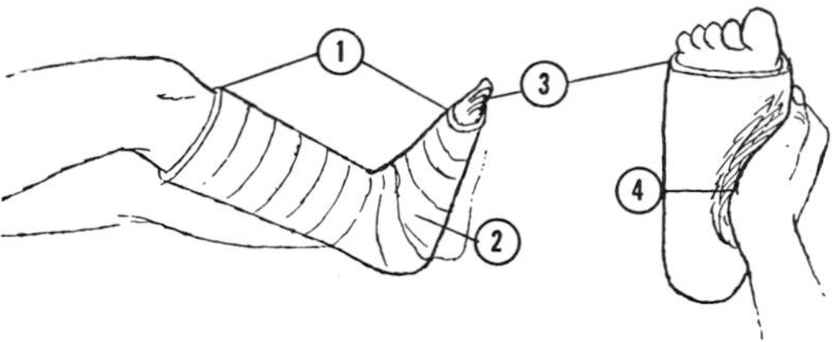

1. Circular plaster cast is applied from the toes to the tibial tubercle.
2. Foot is at a right angle.
3. Foot is neutral in regard to inversion and eversion.
4. Plaster is molded well under the longitudinal and transverse arches.

Management

Allow the patient to walk on crutches, bearing partial weight on the cast with a walking heel or cast shoe.

Three weeks of cast immobilization are adequate for most fractures of the metatarsals.

After removal of the cast, the patient should use a stiff-soled shoe with good support of the longitudinal and transverse arches.

■ Fracture of the Metatarsal Bones With Displacement

REMARKS

Displaced fractures of the metatarsals should be reduced if the displacement causes the metatarsal heads to become prominent in the sole of the foot. When the displacement is in a medial or lateral direction or dorsal, reduction need not be anatomic.

If there are multiple fractures, usually the injuries are unstable enough to warrant stabilization with Kirschner wires or some other internal fixation device.

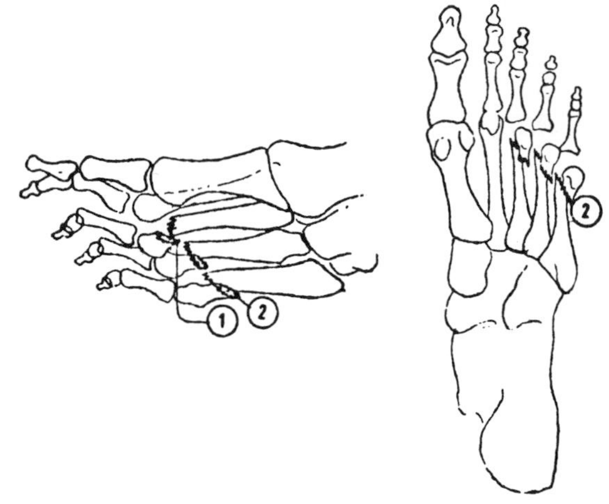

Prereduction X-Ray

1. Fracture of the neck of the third, fourth, and fifth metatarsals.
2. Distal fragments (heads of metatarsals) are displaced outward and downward.

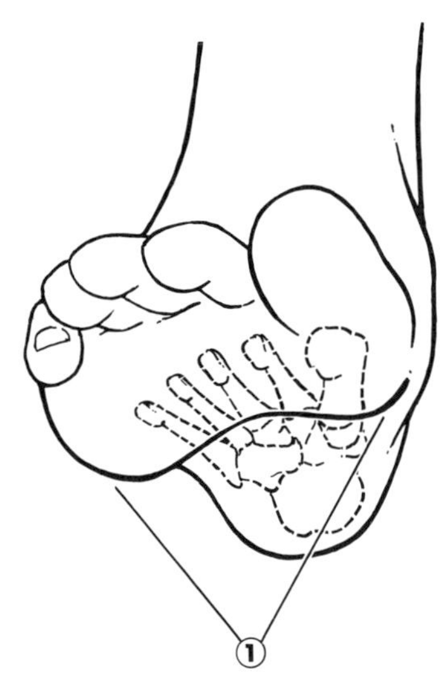

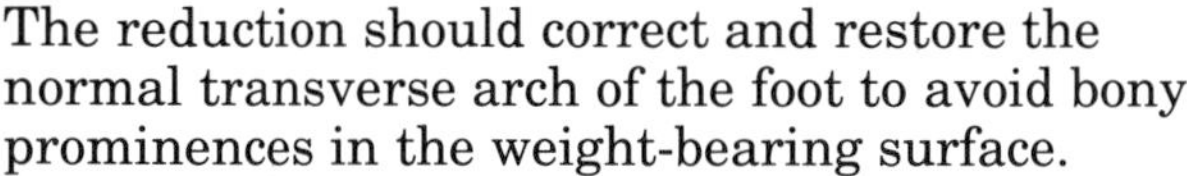

The reduction should correct and restore the normal transverse arch of the foot to avoid bony prominences in the weight-bearing surface.

1. Forefoot transverse arch is due to the architecture and relationship of the metatarsal heads, which should not be disturbed by fracture displacement.

Management

Manipulative Reduction

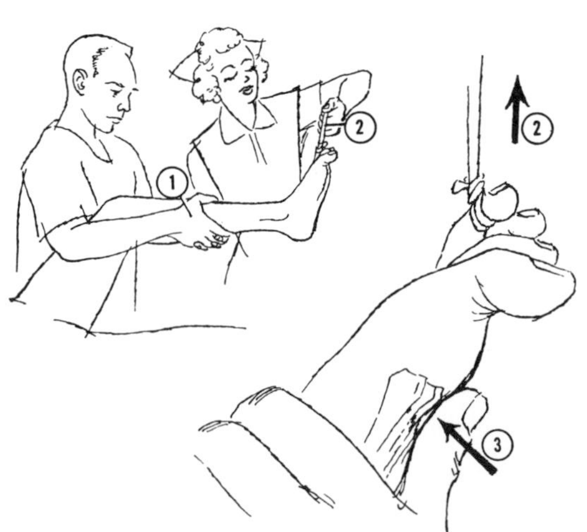

1. One assistant fixes the foot.
2. A second assistant makes steady traction on the toe by means of a loop of bandage around it.
3. By direct pressure molds, the operator reduces the fragments back into their anatomic position.

Note: This method is used for each metatarsal fracture.

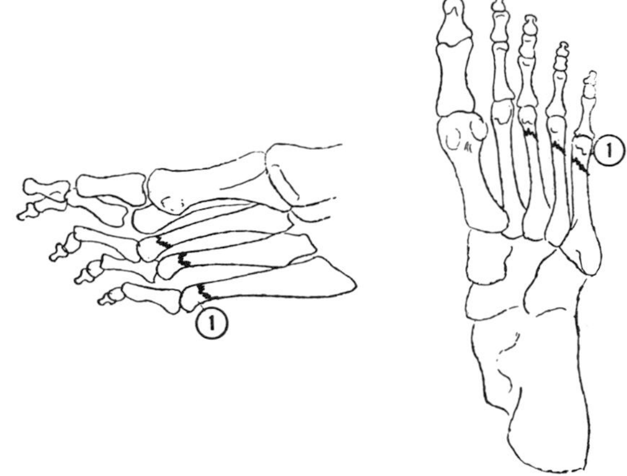

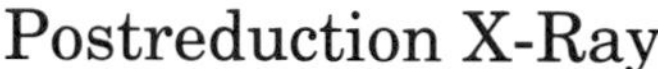

Postreduction X-Ray

1. Distal fragments of all three fractured metatarsals are in a normal relationship with the proximal fragments.

Immobilization

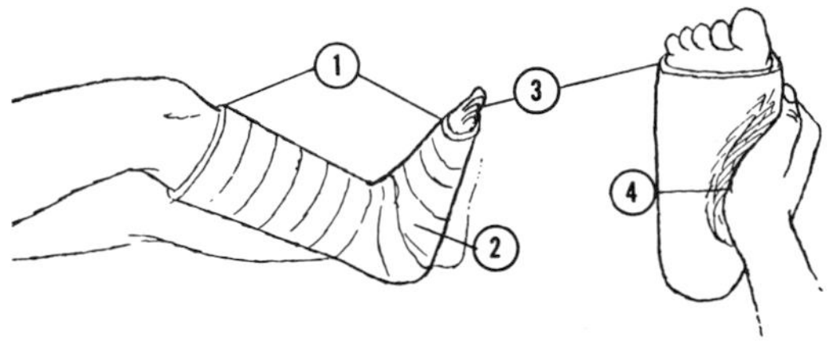

1. Circular plaster cast is applied from the toes to the tibial tubercle.
2. Foot is at a right angle.
3. Foot is in neutral in regard to inversion and eversion.
4. Plaster is molded well under the longitudinal and transverse arches.

Subsequent Management

The patient may be up on crutches without bearing weight on the fractured foot, particularly if there are multiple fractures.

Usually, by 2–3 weeks the cast may be removed, and the fracture sites may be evaluated clinically.

If the fracture remains stable and without pain, weight-bearing may be allowed in a hard-soled shoe.

If the patient remains symptomatic, reapply a cast for an additional 2 or 3 weeks.

Alternative Method: Operative Reduction

Operative intervention is indicated when manipulative methods do not achieve an accurate reduction.

Fractures just proximal to the heads are frequently difficult to maintain in normal alignment by conservative methods.

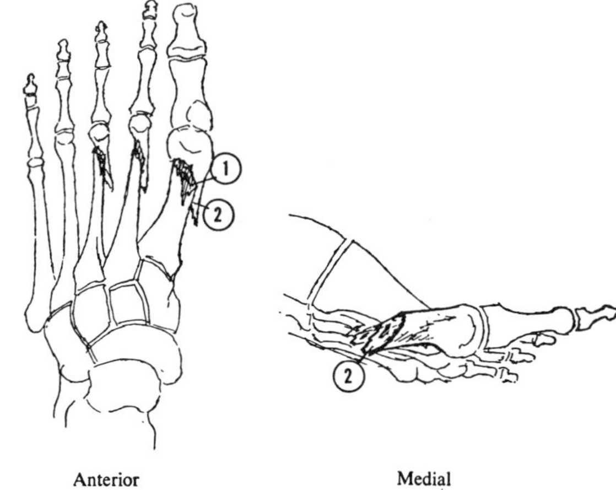

Prereduction X-Ray

1. Fractures of the shafts of the first, second, and third metatarsal bones.
2. Distal fragments are displaced downward and backward into the sole.

Note: In this instance, manipulative methods did not achieve an accurate reduction. A variety of methods of internal fixation may be used.

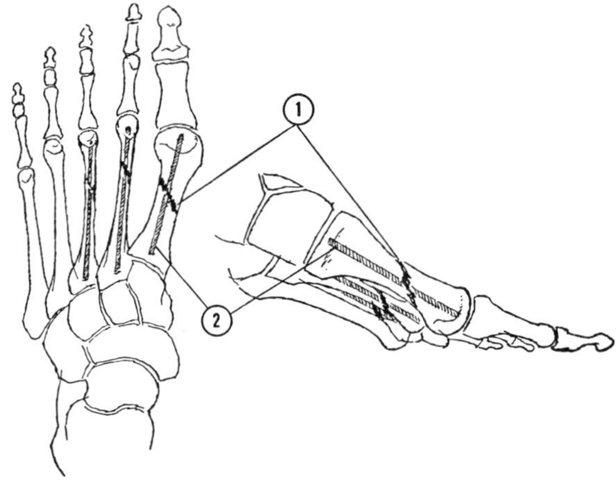

Postreduction X-Ray After Open Reduction

1. All fragments are now in anatomic position.
2. Wires transfix both fragments and maintain normal alignment of all three metatarsals.

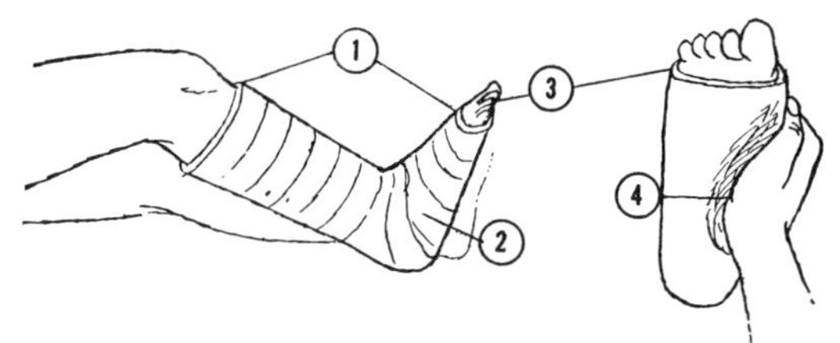

Immobilization

1. Circular plaster cast is applied from the toes to the tibial tubercle.
2. Foot is at a right angle.
3. Foot is in neutral in regard to inversion and eversion.
4. Plaster is molded well under the longitudinal and transverse arches.

Postoperative Management

Elevate the foot on pillows.

Surround the foot with ice bags.

After 3 weeks, remove the wire, and apply a short-leg plaster cast with a walking heel; again, mold the plaster well under the longitudinal and transverse arches.

Four to 6 weeks after the operation, remove the plaster cast, and allow walking in a stiff-soled shoe with an arch support for the longitudinal and transverse arches.

Tuberosity and Proximal Shaft (Jones) Fractures of the Base of the Fifth Metatarsal

REMARKS

Dameron pointed out that there are two types of fractures that occur in the proximal end of the fifth metatarsal.

The first and more common type is a fracture through the tuberosity, which is produced by inversion injury of the plantar-flexed foot. These invariably heal with minimal treatment and without complication.

The tuberosity fracture must be distinguished from the less common fracture through the proximal portion of the shaft, which has been called the Jones fracture. Sir Robert Jones reported sustaining such an injury himself while dancing around a maypole. Kavanaugh et al. demonstrated this to be a stress fracture that occurs characteristically in basketball players and other young athletes. These have a much less favorable prognosis than do tuberosity fractures.

Tuberosity fracture must also be distinguished from normal variations, particularly apophyses of the metatarsal. Dameron found apophyses radiographically visible in at least 22 per cent of children's feet. Most commonly, this is seen between 9 and 11 years of age in girls and between 11 and 14 years of age in boys.

Other structures sometimes confused with tuberosity fractures are sesamoid bones in the peroneus longus or brevis tendon, found in approximately 15 per cent of foot x-rays. The smooth, sclerotic apposing surfaces of the sesamoid bone and the proximal portion of the base of the fifth metatarsal distinguish it from a fracture. (See Chapter 10 with regard to fractures of the os peroneum.)

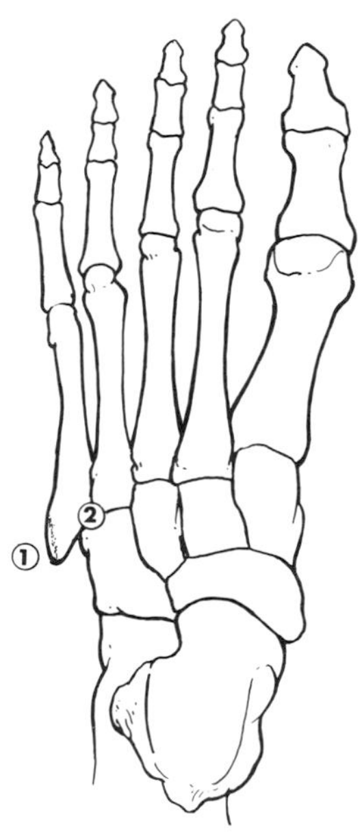

Tuberosity fracture must be differentiated from a normal apophysis.

1. Apophyseal line traverses the tubercle in a direction almost parallel to the long axis of the metatarsal.
2. It does not extend proximally into the metatarsal joint or medially into the joint between the fourth and fifth metatarsals.

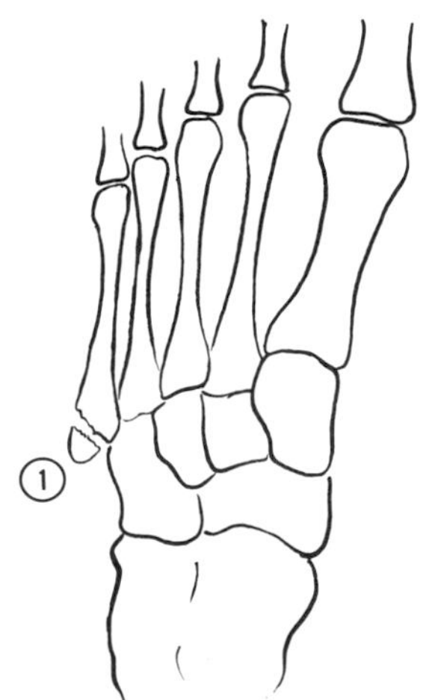

Tuberosity Fracture

APPEARANCE ON X-RAY

1. Avulsion fracture of the tuberosity is typically oblique in the region of the peroneus brevis insertion and results from inversion injury.

MANAGEMENT

The more common tuberosity fracture can be treated symptomatically, usually with a walking cast to relieve discomfort.

1. Circular plaster cast is applied from the toes to the tibial tubercle.
2. Foot is at a right angle.
3. Foot is in a neutral position as to inversion and eversion.
4. Plaster is molded well under the longitudinal and transverse arches.

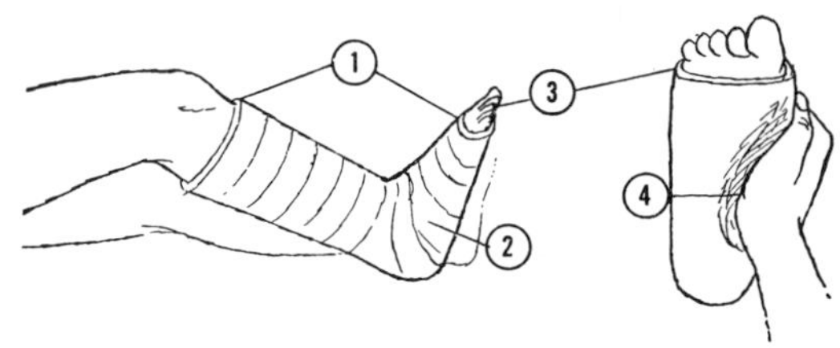

Note: Many patients are not sufficiently symptomatic with this fracture to require cast application. These may be treated with a hard-soled shoe to allow them to continue working or other activities without the restriction from the cast. In essence then, this fracture can be treated symptomatically.

Subsequent Management

The patient may bear weight on the cast as tolerated.

After 14 days, the cast may be removed, and the patient may begin walking with a hard-soled shoe.

In general, the patient need not be followed longer than 3–4 weeks because radiographic and clinical union is almost inevitable.

Even if bone union is not evident on the x-ray, the patient usually becomes pain free by 3–4 weeks. Fibrous union of these fractures therefore is an acceptable union.

Jones Fracture

APPEARANCE ON X-RAY

1. A Jones fracture is a transverse fracture that occurs 0.5 cm distal to the splayed insertion of the peroneus brevis.
2. It has the characteristic of a stress fracture in that it appears to involve only the lateral cortex on the initial x-ray but later traverses the bone completely.

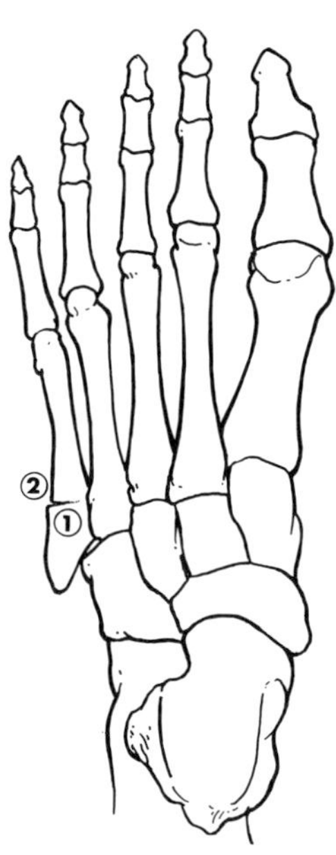

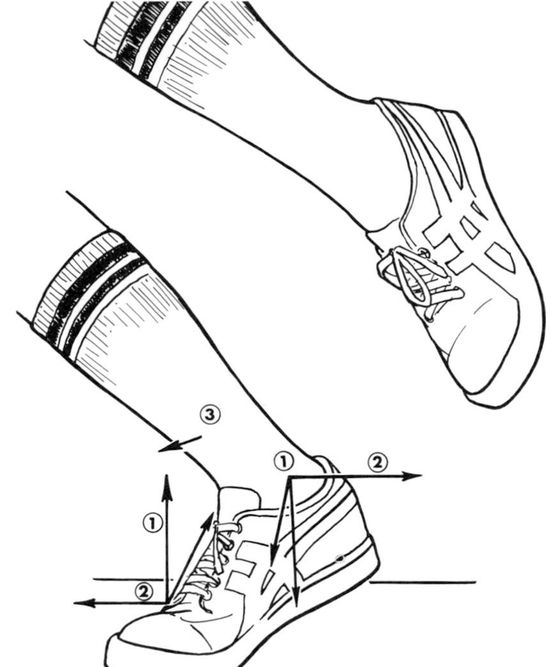

MECHANISM

Kavanaugh et al. demonstrated this injury to be a fatigue or stress fracture that results from a combination of

1. Vertical loading and
2. Mediolateral loading that is
3. Commonly sustained by a basketball player, who must constantly pivot or shift the direction of loading on the lateral border of the foot.

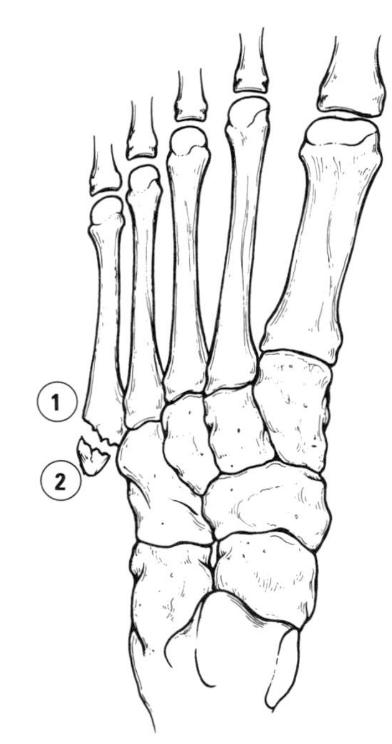

ALTERNATIVE MECHANISM IN THE NONATHLETE

1. A direct blow to the lateral aspect of the metatarsal may produce a transverse fracture.
2. This is usually more proximal than the stress fracture and also tends to be more comminuted.

Note: This type of fracture in the nonathlete is usually easier to treat and more likely to heal without refracture than is the stress fracture.

Management of a Jones Fracture in the Nonathlete or Recreational Athlete

A walking cast is applied as described for tuberosity fracture.

The cast should be continued for approximately 4–6 weeks, after which the patient may resume weight-bearing with a hard-soled shoe.

The patient should be informed that delayed union is a possibility and that sports activities should be avoided until union is secure.

On average, this may take 4 months from the time of injury.

Management of Jones Fracture in an Active Athlete or Delayed Union or Nonunion

The Jones fracture can be disabling in the athlete who is eager to return to competitive sports.

Immediate screw fixation, as advocated by Kavanaugh et al., is the most effective method to manage this select group of patients.

Conservative treatment is likely to cause prolonged disability and recurrent fatigue fracture in individuals who are unwilling or unable to refrain from vigorous activities.

Screw fixation is also recommended for patients with recurrent fracture or nonunion.

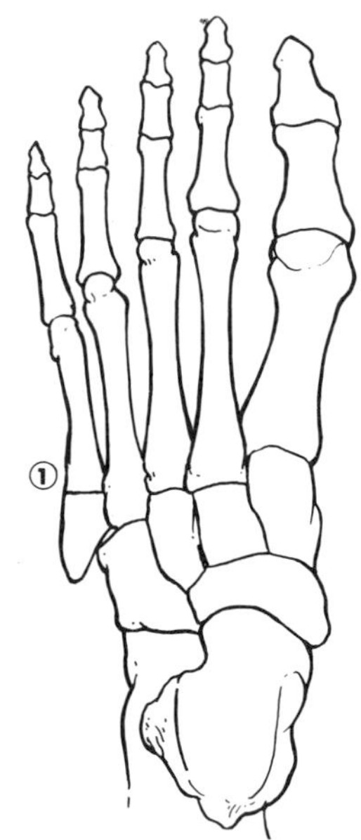

Preoperative X-Ray

1. Typical transverse stress fracture in a basketball player.

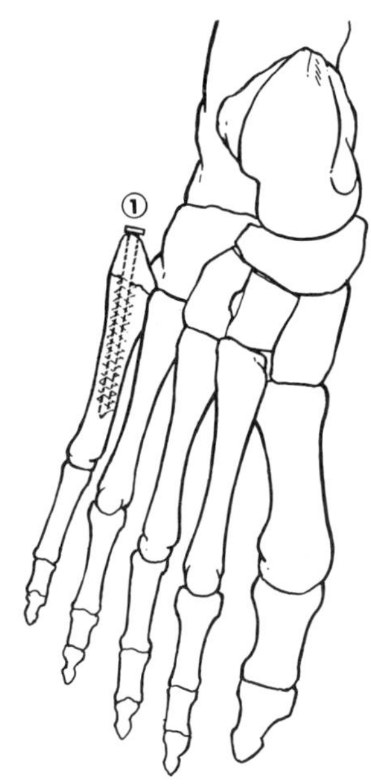

Postoperative X-Ray

1. Fracture has been stabilized by intramedullary screw fixation.

Postoperative Treatment

A compressive bandage is applied to the foot, and the foot is kept without weight-bearing with crutches for 10 days.

Subsequently, the dressing is removed, and the foot is allowed to bear weight as tolerated in a hard-soled shoe.

Return to athletic competition is usually allowed 6–8 weeks postoperatively.

DISLOCATIONS OF THE METATARSOPHALANGEAL JOINTS

REMARKS

Dislocations of the metatarsophalangeal joints are rare lesions; the great toe is most commonly involved.

Many are open lesions.

Immediate reduction is mandatory; a delay of several days may make it impossible to reduce the dislocation by closed methods.

These injuries are analogous to dislocations of the metatarsophalangeal joints of the hand and are subject to similar obstacles to reduction.

Typical Deformity

1. Proximal phalanx is displaced upward and backward in the vertical position.
2. Head of the metatarsal is prominent.
3. Distal phalanx is flexed.

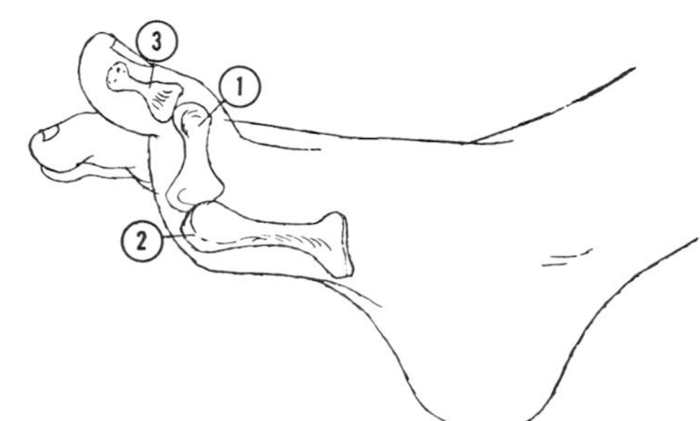

Manipulative Reduction

1. Pass a loop of bandage around the toe to make traction.
2. Make strong traction upward and backward (hyperextending the toe); this disengages the metatarsal head from the flexor tendons.

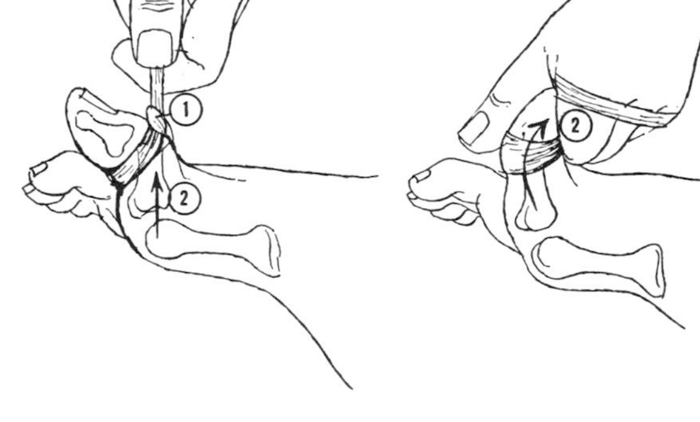

1. Now make traction upward and forward.
2. Place the thumb of the other hand behind the proximal end of the first phalanx, and force the phalanx distally and downward over the metatarsal head.

Note: The key to reduction is to push, not pull, the proximal phalanx over the metatarsal head.

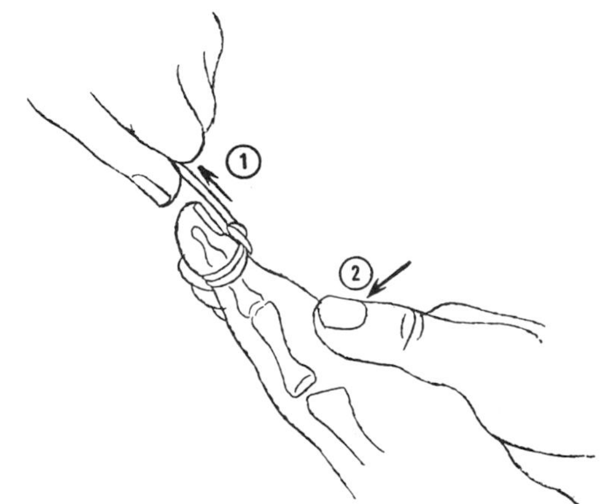

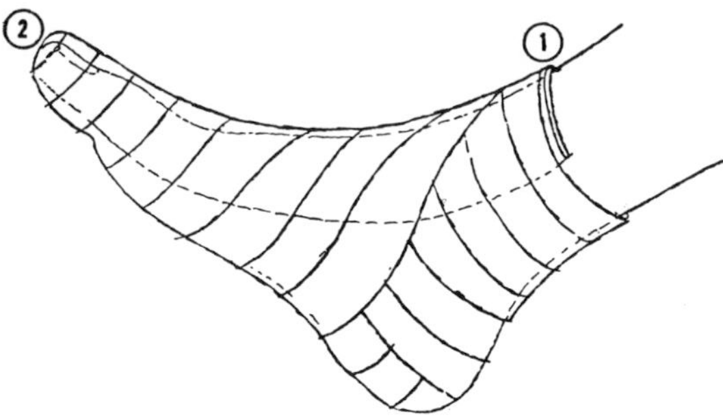

Immobilization

1. Apply a padded splint to the dorsum of the foot to prevent recurrent hyperextension of the metatarsophalangeal joint.
2. Toe is in a neutral position.

■ Management

Allow the patient up on crutches with no weight-bearing on the affected foot.

Remove the plaster splint at the end of 2 weeks.

Provide the patient with a stiff-soled shoe.

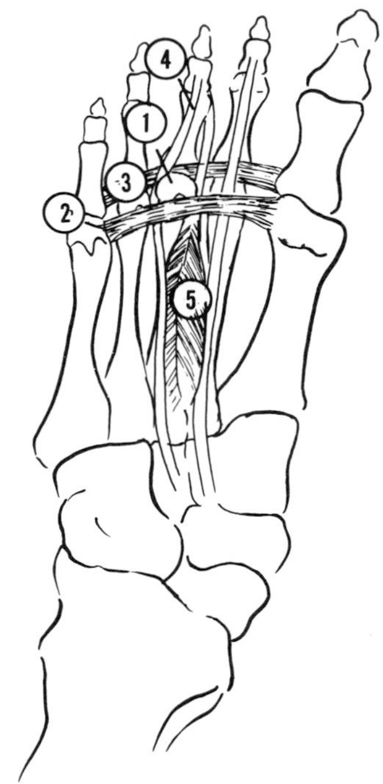

Irreducible Dislocation of the Metatarsophalangeal Joints

1. Dislocation occurs when the metatarsal head is forced through the weak point of the capsule.
2. Fibrocartilaginous plate remains on the plantar side.
3. Transverse metatarsal ligament displaces dorsally with the proximal phalanx.
4. Flexor tendons displace to the lateral side.
5. Lumbrical tendon displaces to the medial side and also contributes to the fixation of the dislocated metatarsal head.

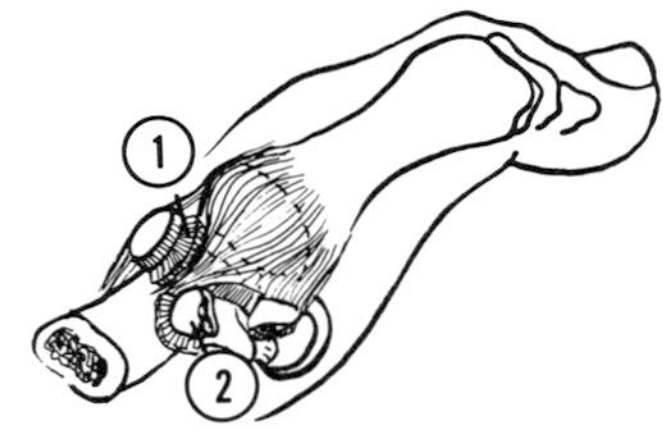

1. If the intersesamoid ligament tears or the
2. Sesamoid fractures, the resistance to reduction is less than if the ligament is attached and locks the metatarsal head in the plantar position.

Obstacles to Reduction

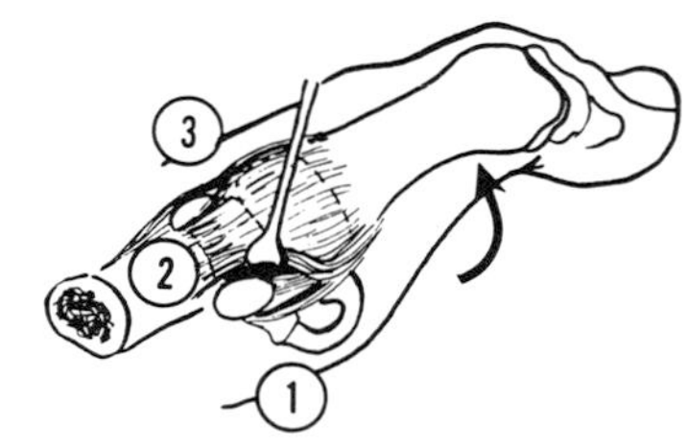

1. Dislocation occurs by rupture of the capsule attachment to the metatarsal neck.
2. This causes the hallux to dislocate with a sesamoid attached to the base of the proximal phalanx.
3. These override the dorsum of the metatarsal neck and lock the metatarsal head in the plantar position. This requires open release of the ligament to permit reduction.

Open Reduction

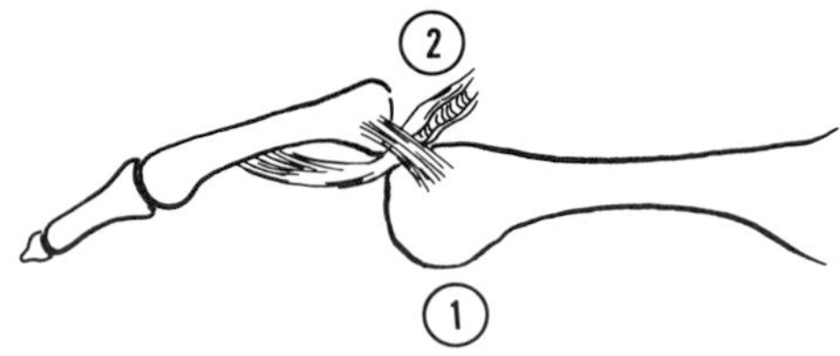

Closed reduction may not be possible, particularly if multiple metatarsophalangeal joints are dislocated.

Operative reduction should be carried out promptly to relieve the obstruction, which is usually from the

1. Capsule being detached from the metatarsal head and the
2. Fibrocartilaginous plate being flipped into the joint.

Note: A volar approach to the metatarsophalangeal joint allows visualization of these obstructions and permits release of the fibrocartilaginous plate and capsule, which form the main obstacles to reduction.

After reduction, the joints are stable and do not require longer than 2–3 weeks of immobilization.

FRACTURES OF THE TOES

REMARKS

These lesions are usually the result of crushing injuries; the great toe is most often affected.

Comminution of the phalanx occurs relatively frequently.

Many fractures are of the open type.

As a rule, displacement of the fragments is minimal.

Fractures of the Toes With Minimal or No Displacement

Appearance on X-Ray

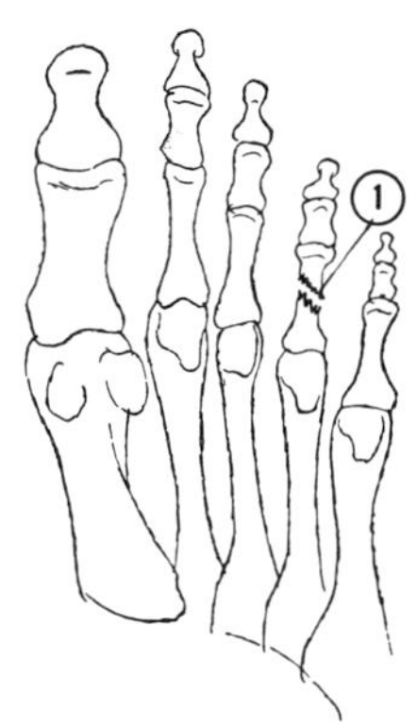

PROXIMAL PHALANX OF FOURTH TOE

1. Oblique fracture of the proximal phalanx of the fourth toe with minimal displacement. (No reduction required.)

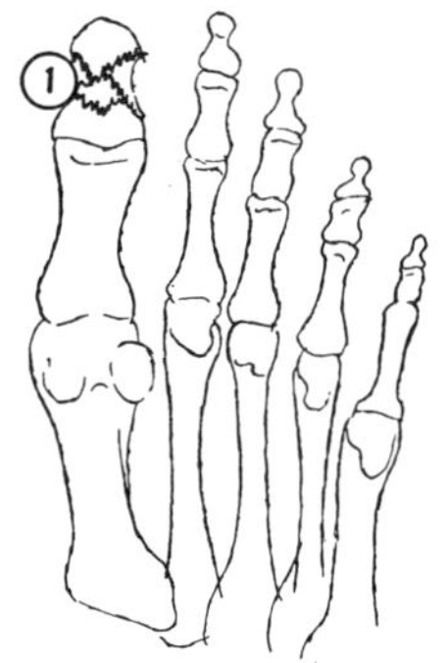

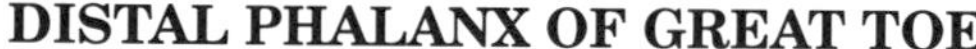

DISTAL PHALANX OF GREAT TOE

1. Comminuted fracture of the distal phalanx of the great toe.

Immobilization for Fractures of the Outer Four Toes

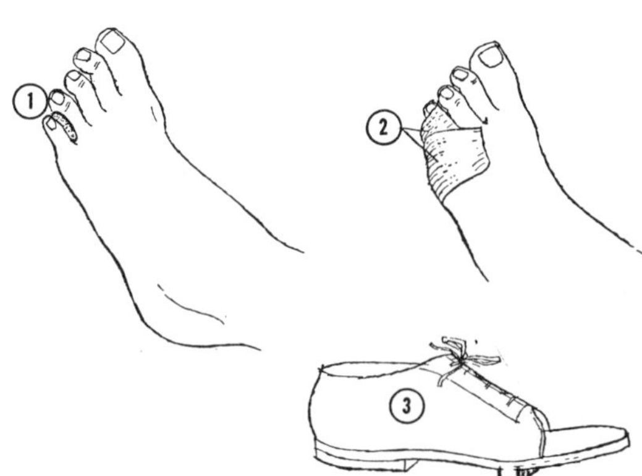

1. Place a piece of felt between the toes.
2. Fix the fractured toe to the adjacent toe with strips of adhesive.
3. Shoe with top cut out and a bar on the sole placed behind the metatarsal heads allows full weight-bearing.

Immobilization for Fractures of the Great Toe

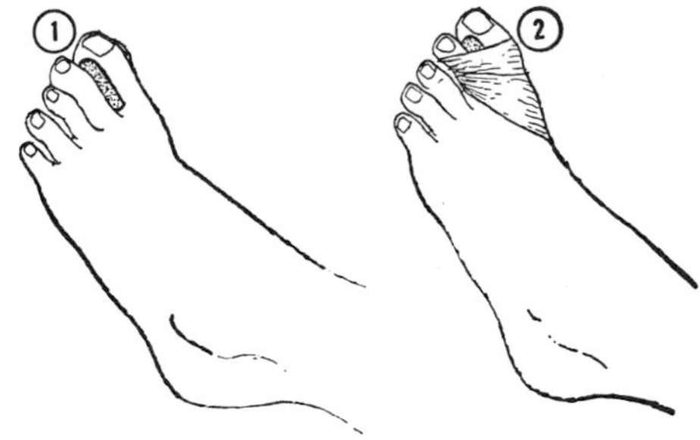

1. Place a piece of felt between the great toe and the second toe.
2. Bind the great toe to the second toe with strips of adhesive.

Management

For fractures of any of the toes, allow the patient to bear weight in a cast shoe or a shoe with a toe cap cut out and a metatarsal bar 1 cm high placed on the sole just behind the metatarsal heads.

In cases of severe swelling, elevate the foot for 2–3 days before permitting weight-bearing.

Remove the adhesive strapping after 2–3 weeks and provide the patient with a stiff-soled shoe.

■ Fractures of the Toes With Displacement

REMARKS

Generally, displacement can be corrected by simple traction on the toe.

Fractures of the proximal phalanges may exhibit forward angulation of the fragments.

If reduction is not stable and the deformity recurs after traction is released, longitudinal pin fixation may be indicated.

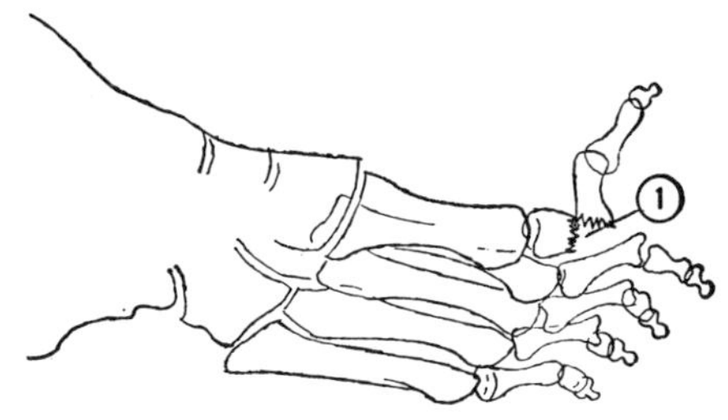

Prereduction X-Ray

1. Fracture of the proximal phalanx of the great toe with forward angulation of the fragments.

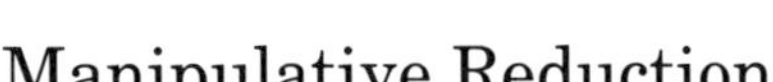

Manipulative Reduction

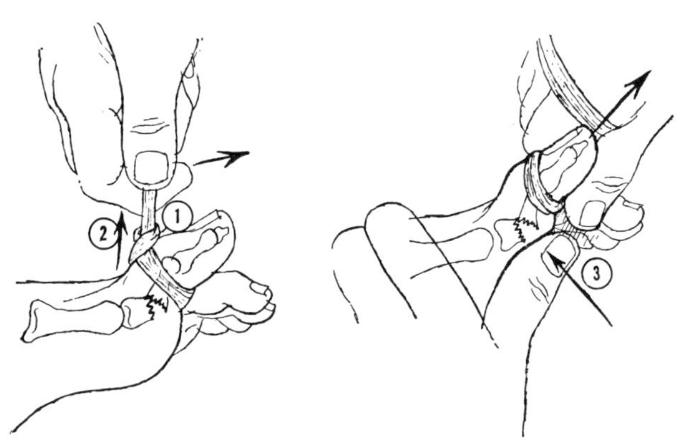

1. Pass a loop of gauze bandage around the toe.
2. Make direct traction upward and forward.
3. Place the thumb of the other hand over the apex of the angulation on the plantar aspect of the toe, and make upward pressure.

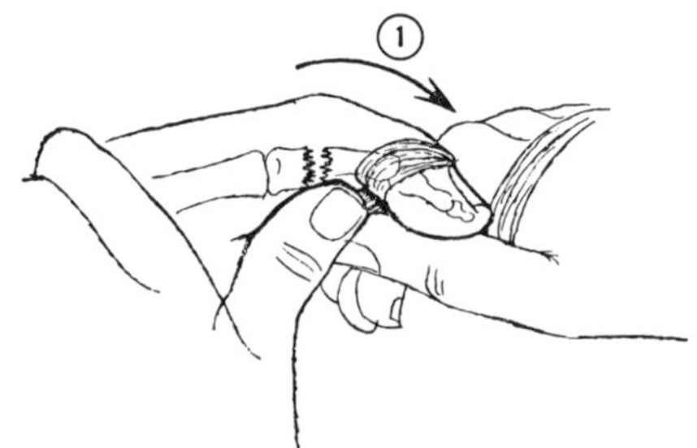

1. While traction is maintained, flex the toe.

Immobilization

1. Place a piece of felt between the toes.
2. Bind the first toe to the second toe with strips of adhesive.

Note: If reduction is lost, insert a smooth Steinmann pin percutaneously through the long axis of the toe.

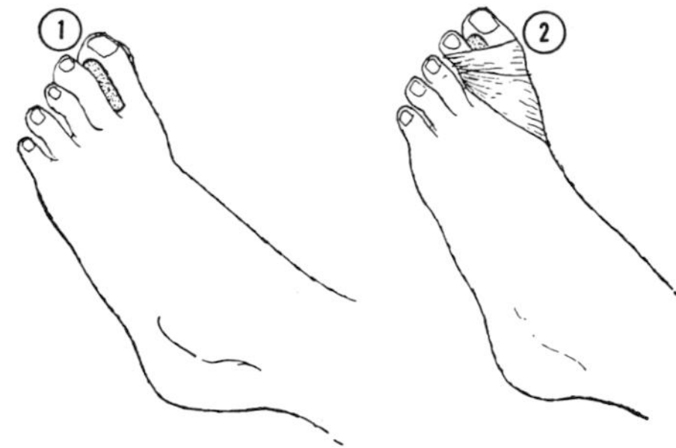

Subsequent Management

Maintain the splint immobilization for at least 3 weeks. After this time, it may be discarded.

Subsequently, the patient should protect the foot with a hard-soled shoe and bar under the metatarsal heads.

Fractures of the Sesamoid Bones of the Great Toe

REMARKS

These lesions are rare and usually are the result of repetitive direct trauma applied to the foot, which causes a stress fracture of the sesamoid between the head of the metatarsal and the ground.

The inner sesamoid is involved more often than the outer.

Fracture must be distinguished from a bipartite or tripartite sesamoid. In the former, the line of division is sharp and irregular. In the latter, it is smooth and regular, and the fragments are of equal size.

If pain and dysfunction persist after a period of immobilization and proper padding of the shoe, excision of the sesamoid is indicated.

Note: Because frequently the medial sesamoid is bipartite, the diagnosis may depend on persistent painful symptoms or even necessitate a bone scan to distinguish a fracture from a bipartite sesamoid.

Appearance on X-Ray

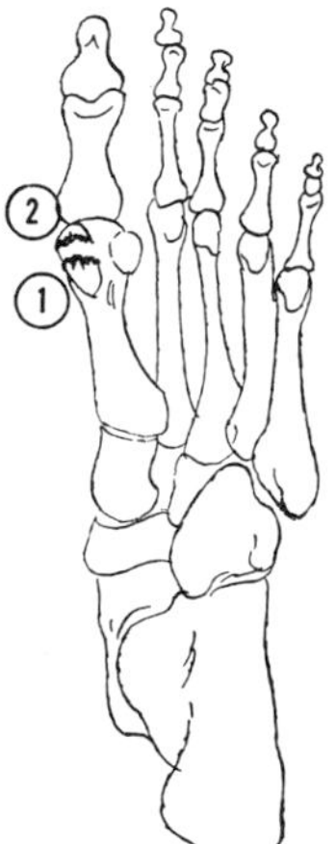

1. Fracture of the internal sesamoid.
2. Fragments are of unequal size.

Immobilization

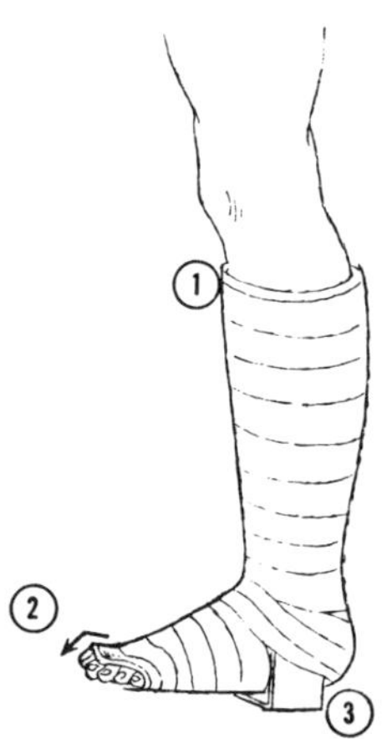

1. Apply a circular plaster cast from the toes to the tibial tubercle.
2. Great toe is moderately flexed.
3. Walking heel is incorporated in the cast.

Management

Remove the cast at the end of 4 weeks.

Permit weight-bearing in a shoe with a 1-cm bar placed on the sole of the shoe just behind the metatarsal heads.

If pain persists after several months of adequate treatment, excision of the sesamoid is indicated.

Excision is also indicated in cases of old untreated fractures that cause pain and dysfunction.

BIBLIOGRAPHY

Talus Fractures

Alexander AH, Lichtman DM: Surgical treatment of transchondral talar-dome fractures (osteochondritis dissecans). J Bone Joint Surg Am 62:646, 1980.

Berndt AL, Harty M: Transchondral fractures (osteochondritis dissecans) of the talus. J Bone Joint Surg Am 41:988, 1959.

Birt D, Townsend R: Major talar fractures. J Bone Joint Surg Am 58:733, 1976.

Black K, Ehlert K: A stress fracture of the lateral process of the talus in a runner. J Bone Joint Surg Am 76:441, 1994.

Canale ST, Belding RH: Osteochondral lesions of the talus. J Bone Joint Surg Am 62A:97, 1980.

Canale ST, Kelly FB Jr: Fractures of the neck of the talus. J Bone Joint Surg Am 60:143, 1978.

Chrisman OJ, Snook GA: Reconstruction of lateral ligament tears of the ankle. J Bone Joint Surg Am 51:904, 1969.

Court-Brown C, Boot D, Kellam J: Fracture-dislocation of the calcaneus. Clin Orthop 213:201, 1986.

Davis FJ, Fry LR, Lippert FG, et al. The patellar tendon-bearing brace: Report of 16 patients. J Trauma 14:216, 1974.

DeLee JC, Curtis R: Subtalar dislocation of the foot. J Bone Joint Surg Am 64:433, 1982.

Dennis JC, Curtis R: Blair tibiotalar arthrodesis for injuries of the talus. J Bone Joint Surg Am 62:103, 1980.

Dimon JH: Isolated displaced fracture of the posterior facet of the talus. J Bone Joint Surg Am 43:275, 1961.

Hawkins LG: Fracture of the lateral process of the talus. J Bone Joint Surg Am 47:1170, 1965.

Hawkins LG: Fractures of the neck of the talus. J Bone Joint Surg Am 52:991, 1970.

Heckman JD, McLean MR, DeLee JC: Fracture of the lateral process of the talus. Orthop Trans 5:465, 1981.

Ihle CL, Cochran RM: Fracture of the fused os trigonum. Am J Sports Med 10:47, 1982.

Kelly PJ, Sullivan CR: Blood supply of the talus. Clin Orthop 30:37, 1963.

Lemaire RG, Bustin W: Screw fixation of fractures of the neck of the talus using a posterior approach. J Trauma 20:669, 1980.

Lieberg OU, Henke JA, Bailey RW: Avascular necrosis of the head of the talus without death of the body: Report of an unusual case. J Trauma 15:926, 1975.

Lorentzen JE, Christensen SB, Krogsoe O, et al. Fractures of the neck of the talus. Acta Orthop Scand 48:115, 1977.

Morris HD, Hand WL, Dunn AW: The modified Blair fusion for fractures of the talus. J Bone Joint Surg Am 53:1289, 1971.

Mukherjee SK, Pringle RM, Baxter AD: Fracture of the lateral process of the talus: A report of thirteen cases. J Bone Joint Surg Br 56:263, 1974.

Paulos LE, Johnson CL, Noyes FR: Posterior compartment fractures of the ankle: A commonly missed athletic injury. Am J Sports Med 11:439, 1983.

Penny JN, Davis LA: Fractures and fracture-dislocations of the neck of the talus. J Trauma 20:1029, 1980.

Peterson L, Romanus B, Dahlberg E: Fracture of the column tali: An experimental study. J Biomechanics 9:277, 1974.

Pringle RM, Mukherjee SK: Fracture of the lateral process of the talus. J Bone Joint Surg Br 56:201, 1974.

Reckling FW: Early tibiocalcaneal fusion in the treatment of severe injuries of the talus. J Trauma 12:390, 1972.

Zemmer T, Johnson K: Subtalar dislocations. Clin Orthop 238:190, 1989.

Calcaneus Fractures

Braly WB, Bishop JO, Tullos HS: Lateral decompression for malunited os calcis fractures. Foot Ankle 6:90, 1985.

Buckley R, Meek R: Comparison of open versus closed reduction of intra-articular calcaneal fractures: A matched cohort in workmen. J Orthop Trauma 8:216, 1992.

Burdeaux BD: Reduction of calcaneal fractures by the McReynold's medial approach technique and its experimental basis. Clin Orthop 177:87, 1983.

Burdeaux B: The medial approach for calcaneal fractures. Clin Orthop 290:96, 1993.

Connolly JF: Persistent heel pain 20 years after calcaneal fracture and triple arthrodesis relieved by lateral decompression. J Trauma 27:809, 1987.

Court-Brown CM, Boot DA, Kellam JF: Fracture dislocation of the calcaneus. Clin Orthop 213:201, 1986.

Crosby LA, Fitzgibbons T: Computerized tomography scanning of acute intra-articular fractures of the calcaneus. A new classification system. J Bone Joint Surg Am 72:852, 1990.

Degan TJ, Morrey BF, Braun DP: Surgical excision for anterior-process fractures of the calcaneus. J Bone Joint Surg Am 64:519, 1982.

DeLee JC: Fractures and dislocations of the foot. *In* Mann RA (ed): *Surgery of the Foot.* Mosby-Year Book, St. Louis, 1986.

Deyerle WM: Long term follow-up of fractures of the os calcis. Orthop Clin North Am 4:213, 1973.

Essex-Lopresti P: The mechanism, reduction technique and results in fractures of the os calcis. Br J Surg 39:395, 1952.

Giachino AA, Uhthoff HK: Current concepts review—Intra-articular fractures of the calcaneus. J Bone Joint Surg Am 71:784, 1989.

Isbister JF: Calcaneofibular abutment following crush fractures of the calcaneus. J Bone Joint Surg Br 56:274, 1974.

James ETR, Hunter GA: The dilemma of painful old os calcis fracture. Clin Orthop 177:112, 1983.

Kitaoka H, Schaap E, Chao E, et al: Displaced intra-articular fractures of the calcaneus treated non-operatively. J Bone Joint Surg Am 76:1531, 1994.

Lance EM, Carey EJ Jr, Wade PA: Fractures of the os calcis: Treatment by early mobilization. Clin Orthop 30:76, 1963.

Lance EM, Carey EJ, Wade PA: Fractures of the os calcis: A follow-up study. J Trauma 4:15, 1964.

Leung K-S, Chan W-S, Shen WJ, et al: Operative treatment of intra-articular fractures of the os calcis—The role of rigid internal fixation and primary bone grafting: Preliminary results. J Orthop Trauma 3:232, 1989.

McLaughlin HL: Treatment of late complications after os calcis fractures. Clin Orthop 30:111, 1963.

Miller WE: Pain and impairment considerations following treatment of disruptive os calcis fractures. Clin Orthop 177:82, 1982.

Omoto H, Sakurada K, Sugi M, et al: A new method of intra-articular fracture of the calcaneus. Clin Orthop 177:104, 1983.

Paley D, Hall H: Calcaneal fractures controversies. Orthop Clin North Am 20:665, 1989.

Parkes JC II: Injuries of the hindfoot. Clin Orthop 122:28, 1977.

Parmar H, Triffett P, Gregg P: Intra-articular fractures of the calcaneus treated operatively or conservatively. J Bone Joint Surg Br 75:932, 1993.

Pozo JL, Kirwan EO, Jackson AM: The long term results of conservative management of severely displaced fractures of the calcaneus. J Bone Joint Surg Br 66:386, 1984.

Salama R, Benamara A, Weissman SL: Functional treatment of intra-articular fractures of the calcaneus. Clin Orthop 115:236, 1976.

Stephenson JR: Treatment of displaced intra-articular fractures of the calcaneus using medial and lateral approaches, internal fixation and early motion. J Bone Joint Surg Am 69:115, 1987.

Navicular and Other Midtarsal Injuries

Clohesy D, Thompson R: Fractures associated with neuropathic arthropathy in adults who have juvenile-onset diabetes. J Bone Joint Surg Am 70:1192, 1988.

Dewar FP, Evans DC: Occult fracture-subluxation of the midtarsal joint. J Bone Joint Surg Br 50:386, 1968.

Drummond DS, Hastings DE: Total dislocation of the cuboid. J Bone Joint Surg Br 57:716, 1969.

Eichenholtz SN, Levine DB: Fractures of the tarsal navicular bone. Clin Orthop 34:142, 1964.

Holstein A, Joldersma RD: Dislocation of the first cuneiform in tarsometatarsal fracture-dislocation. J Bone Joint Surg Am 32:419, 1950.

Hooper G, McMaster M: Recurrent bilateral midtarsal subluxations. J Bone Joint Surg Am 61:617, 1979.

Howie CR, Hooper G, Hughes SPF: Occult midtarsal subluxation. Clin Orthop 209:206, 1988.
Hulkko A, Orava S, Peltokallio P: Stress fractures of the navicular bone. Acta Orthop Scand 56:503, 1985.
Jacobsen FS: Dislocation of the cuboid. Orthopaedics 13:1387, 1990.
Leitner B: Obstacles to reduction in subtalar dislocations. J Bone Joint Surg Am 36:299, 1954.
Main BJ, Jowett RL: Injuries of the midtarsal joint. J Bone Joint Surg Br 57:89, 1975.
Sangeorzan BJ, Benirschke SK, Mosca V, et al: Displaced intra-articular fractures of the tarsal navicular. J Bone Joint Surg Am 71:1504, 1989.
Sangeorzan BJ, Swiontkowski MF: Displaced fractures of the cuboid. J Bone Joint Surg Br 72:376, 1990.
Schiller M, Ray R: Isolated dislocation of the medial cuneiform. J Bone Joint Surg Am 52:1632, 1970.
Torg JS, Pavlov H, Cooley LH, et al: Stress fractures of the tarsal navicular. J Bone Joint Surg Am 64:700, 1982.
Tountas AA: Occult fracture-subluxation of the midtarsal joint. Clin Orthop 243:195, 1989.

Tarsometatarsal Injuries

Anderson LD: Injuries of the forefoot. Clin Orthop 122:18, 1977.
Arntz CT, Veith RG, Hansen ST: Fractures and fracture-dislocations of the tarsometatarsal joint. J Bone Joint Surg Am 70:173, 1988.
Brunet JA, Wiley JJ: The late results of tarsometatarsal joint injuries. J Bone Joint Surg Br 69:347, 1987.
Caputo G, Cavanogh P, Ulbrecht J, et al: Assessment and management of foot disease in patients with diabetes. N Engl J Med 331:854, 1994.
Cofield R, Morrison M, Besbout J: Diabetic neuroarthropathy in the foot. Foot Ankle 4:15, 1983.
Dameron T: Fractures and anatomic variations of the proximal portion of the fifth metatarsal. J Bone Joint Surg Am 57:788, 1975.
DeBendetti JB, Evanski PM, Waugh TR: The irreducible Lisfranc fracture. Case report and literature review. Clin Orthop 136:238, 1978.
Faciszewski T, Burks RT, Manaster BJ: Subtle injuries of the Lisfranc joint. J Bone Joint Surg Am 72:1519, 1990.
Goossens MD, DeSloop N: Lisfranc's fracture-dislocations: Etiology, radiology and results of treatment. Clin Orthop 176:154, 1983.
Hardcastle PH, Reschaner R, Kutscha-Lissberg E, et al: Injuries to the tarsometatarsal joint. Incidence, classification and treatment. J Bone Joint Surg Br 64:349, 1982.
Kavanaugh J, Brauer T, Mann R: The Jones fracture revisited. J Bone Joint Surg Am 60:776, 1978.
Kristiansen B: Ankle and foot fractures in diabetes-provoking neuropathic joint changes. Acta Orthop Scand 51:973, 1980.
Myerson J: The diagnosis and treatment of injuries to the Lisfranc joint complex. Orthop Clin North Am 20:655, 1989.
Sangeorzan BJ, Veith RG, Hansen ST: Salvage of Lisfranc's tarsometatarsal joint by arthrodesis. Foot Ankle 10:193, 1990.
Vuori J, Aro H: Lisfranc joint injuries: Trauma mechanisms and associated injuries. J Trauma 35:40, 1993.
Wiley JJ: The mechanism of tarsometatarsal joint injuries. J Bone Joint Surg Br 53:474, 1971.

Toe Dislocations and Fractures

Brown TIS: Avulsion fracture of the fibular sesamoid in association with dorsal dislocation of the metatarsophalangeal joint of the hallux. Clin Orthop 149:229, 1980.
DeLuca FN, Kenmore PI: Bilateral dorsal dislocations of the metatarsophalangeal joints of the great toes with a loose body in one of the metatarsophalangeal joints. J Trauma 15:737, 1975.
Eibel P: Dislocation of the interphalangeal joint of the big toe with interposition of a sesamoid bone. J Bone Joint Surg Am 36:880, 1954.
Giannikas AC, Papachristou G, Papavasiliou N, et al.: Dorsal dislocation of the first metatarsophalangeal joint. J Bone Joint Surg Br 57B:384, 1975.
Jahss MH: Traumatic dislocations of the first metatarsophalangeal joint. Foot Ankle 1:15, 1980.
Konkel KF, Muehlstein JH: Unusual fracture-dislocation of the great toe: Case report. J Trauma 15:733, 1975.
Laurence S, Botte M: Jones' fractures and related fractures of the proximal fifth metatarsal. Foot Ankle 14:358, 1993.
Lewis AG, DeLee JC: Type I complex dislocation of the first metatarsophalangeal joint: Open reduction through a dorsal approach. J Bone Joint Surg Am 66:1120, 1984.
Orava S, Puranen J, Ala-Ketola H: Stress fractures caused by physical exercise. Acta Orthop Scand 49:19, 1978.
Rao JP, Banzon MT: Irreducible dislocation of the metatarsophalangeal joints of the foot. Clin Orthop 145:224, 1979.
Salamon PB, Gelberman RH, Huffer JM: Dorsal dislocation of the metatarsophalangeal joint of the great toe: A case report. J Bone Joint Surg Am 56:1073, 1974.

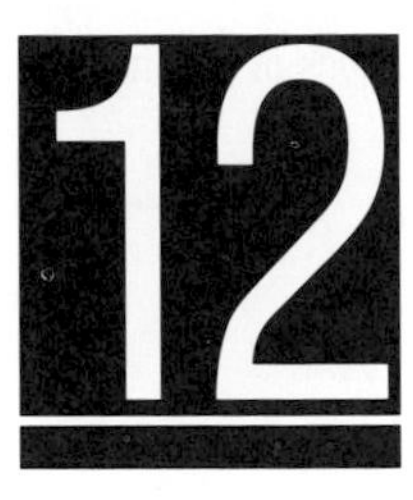

Fractures and Dislocations of the Shoulder

REMARKS

The shoulder joint includes the sternoclavicular joint, the clavicle, the acromioclavicular joint, the scapula, the scapulothoracic joint, and the glenohumeral joint.

All these structures may be injured by direct or indirect mechanisms. The result may be a fracture of the clavicle, dislocation of the acromioclavicular or sternoclavicular joint, a fracture of the scapula or glenoid, or a dislocation or fracture-dislocation of the glenohumeral joint.

FRACTURES AND DISLOCATION OF THE SHOULDER STRUCTURES

Fractures of the Clavicle

REMARKS

The clavicle is one of the most frequently fractured bones in the shoulder, especially in young children. It is usually the result of a fall directly or indirectly on the shoulder.

In children, the injury is usually uncomplicated and heals promptly.

Clavicular fractures occur in the adult as the result of more severe direct injury to the shoulder. A number of these fractures are associated with multiple injuries, including rib fractures, pneumothorax, and occasionally, neurovascular injuries to the subclavicular structures.

Although the management of the clavicular fracture in the child is relatively simple, the same injury in the adult may be more complication prone.

The clavicular fracture therefore should not be considered primarily a pediatric injury that occasionally occurs in the adult.

Mechanisms and Classification of Fractures of the Clavicle

REMARKS

Fractures of the clavicle are usually the result of a fall. The type, direction, and concentration of the force determine the type of fracture produced.

Fractures of the clavicle can be grouped into three categories: fractures of the middle third, fractures of the outer third, and fractures of the inner third.

Fractures of the Middle Third of the Clavicle

Fracture of the middle third is by far the most frequently encountered fracture of the clavicle.

It is usually produced by a direct impact; the fracture is usually segmental, at the juncture of the outer and middle thirds of the clavicle.

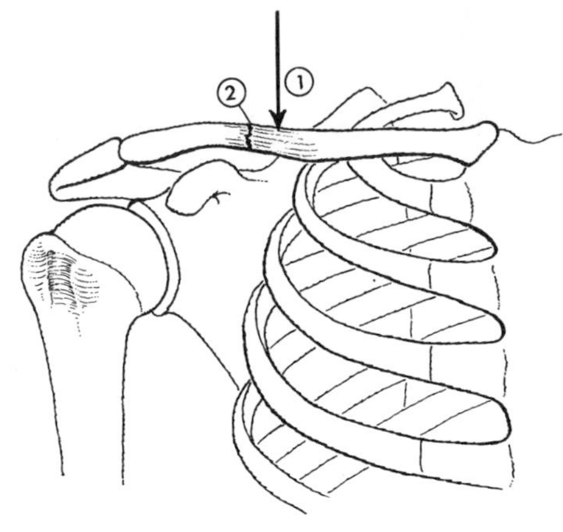

It may rarely be produced by an indirect force acting along the humerus, such as occurs when one falls on the upper extremity with the arm flexed and abducted at least 45°. The counterpoints in this mechanism are the glenohumeral and sternoclavicular joints. Usually, a spiral fracture occurs.

1. Direct force applied to middle third of the clavicle.
2. Fracture at the juncture of the middle and outer thirds.

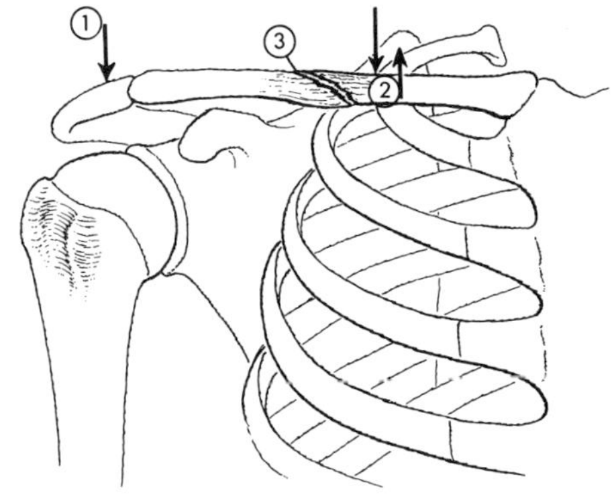

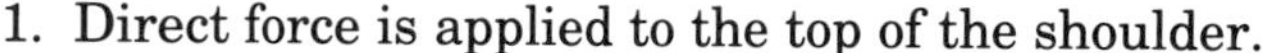

1. Direct force is applied to the top of the shoulder.
2. Clavicle is forced against the first rib. The result is a
3. Spiral fracture of the middle third of the clavicle.

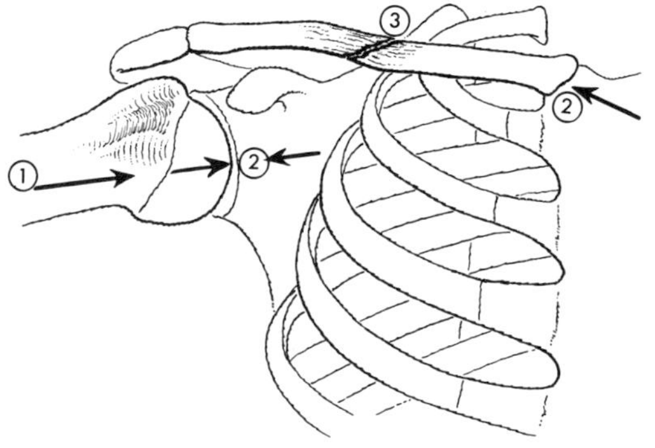

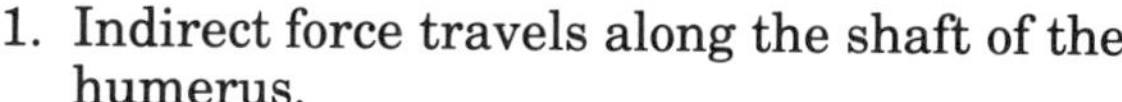

1. Indirect force travels along the shaft of the humerus.
2. Counterpoints are the glenohumeral joint and the sternoclavicular joint; the result is an
3. Oblique fracture of the middle third of the clavicle.

Fractures of the Outer Third of the Clavicle

Fractures of the outer third of the clavicle are the result of a direct force applied to the tip of the shoulder. The result may be a comminuted fracture of the distal third.

The fracture may extend into the acromioclavicular joint.

The fracture may be distal to the coracoclavicular joint.

The fracture may be associated with rupture of the capsular ligaments and the coracoclavicular ligaments.

Note: Fractures distal to the coracoclavicular ligaments may not unite if the major fragment is displaced superiorly.

1. Direct force on the distal third of the clavicle.
2. Communication of the distal third of the clavicle.

Note: All ligaments are intact, and the acromioclavicular joint is not involved.

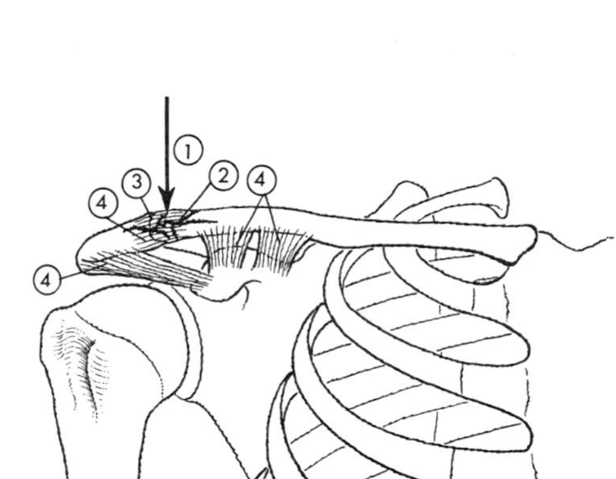

1. Direct force on the distal third of the clavicle.
2. Comminution of the distal third of the clavicle.
3. Fracture extends into the acromioclavicular joint.
4. All ligaments are intact.

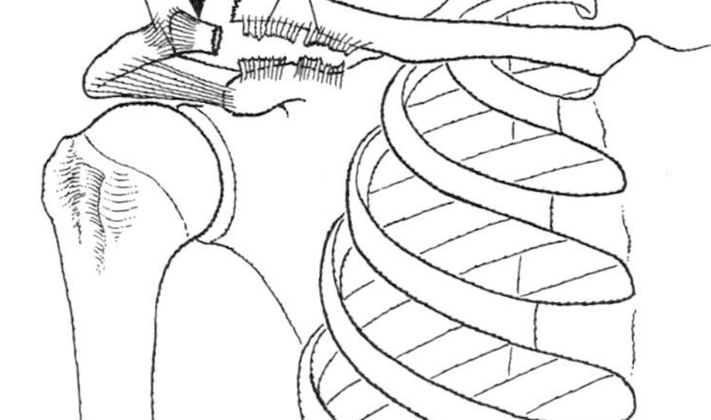

1. Direct force on the distal third of the clavicle.
2. Fracture is distal to coracoclavicular ligaments.
3. All ligaments are disrupted, and reduction of the displaced fragment may be incomplete, so that nonunion results.

Fractures of the Inner Third of the Clavicle

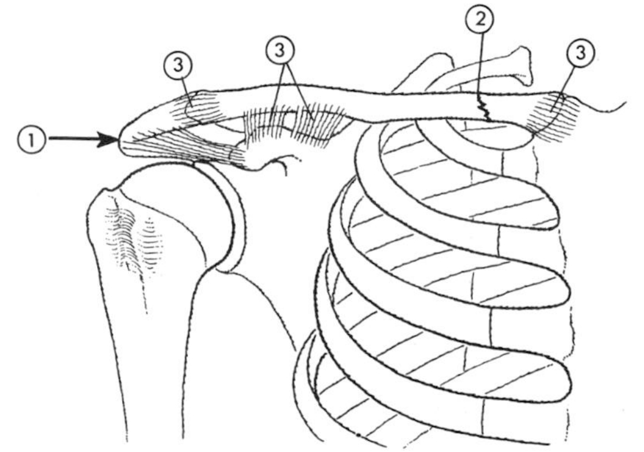

The least frequent fractures, those of the inner third, of the clavicle are the result of a direct impact applied at an angle from the lateral side.

Displacement is usually minimal, unless there is disruption of the costoclavicular ligament.

1. Direct force is applied from the side.
2. Fracture of the inner third of the clavicle occurs.
3. All ligaments are intact.

Management of Clavicular Fractures by Closed Reduction

Note: Management of this common fracture in children is discussed in Chapter 2 in the section on childhood fractures.

In Adolescents and Adults

REMARKS

The fractured clavicle in the older adolescent or the adult is the result usually of a more significant injury and causes considerably more instability and pain than in the child.

Frequently, the injury occurs in patients who have multiple injuries and who may be undergoing bed rest for pneumothorax or head injury.

As the patient is mobilized, the clavicular fracture tends to displace because of the weight of the arm, pulling the lateral fragment down while the proximal fragment displaces superiorly.

Treatment then should be directed at elevating the arm and lateral fragment to align it with the upward displaced medial fragment.

This can be accomplished by a number of methods, including a Velpeau sling and swathe, a Kenny Howard brace, a plaster yoke or a clavicular spica cast.

Mechanism of Deformity

1. Weight of the shoulder and arm pulls the lateral fragment downward.
2. Medial fragment typically displaces superiorly.
3. This causes the typical prominence under the skin, depending on the amount of displacement of the medial fragment.

Note: To achieve reduction of the clavicle fracture, it is necessary to support the weight of the arm and bring the lateral fragment up to the medial fragment.

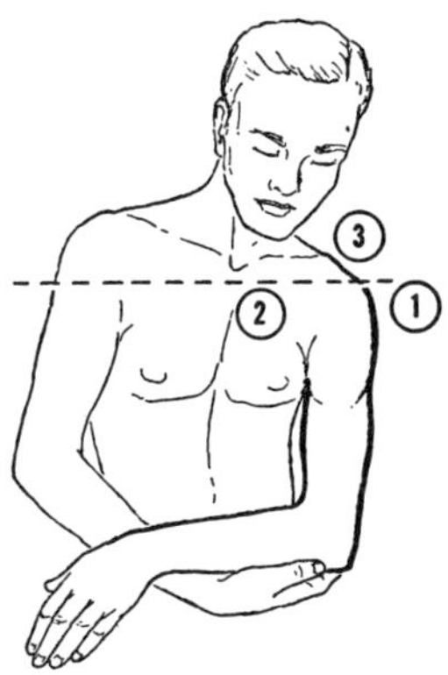

Velpeau Immobilization

1. Injured shoulder is supported in a sling, which is applied snugly enough to support and elevate the depressed lateral clavicular fragment.
2. Additional support is obtained by a bias-cut stockinette rolled around the forearm and elbow to support the extremity.
3. Tape may be applied over the bias-cut stockinette to depress the elevated medial clavicular fragment.

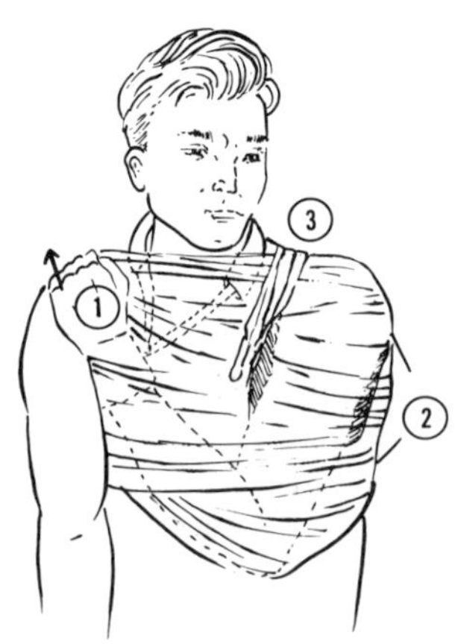

Use of a Kenny Howard Acromioclavicular Support

1. Shoulder strap applied over a piece of felt holds the clavicle down.
2. Sling supports the forearm and keeps the acromion in an elevated position.
3. Halter pulls both the shoulder strap and the sling inward.

After 3 weeks, allow free use of the arm.
Caution: This device has been noted to cause pressure sores, and the patient should be advised to report any persistent irritation or pressure problems. It also has been reported rarely to compress the anterior branch of the median nerve if the arm is held rigidly in pronation. Therefore, the patient should be allowed to rotate the forearm freely.

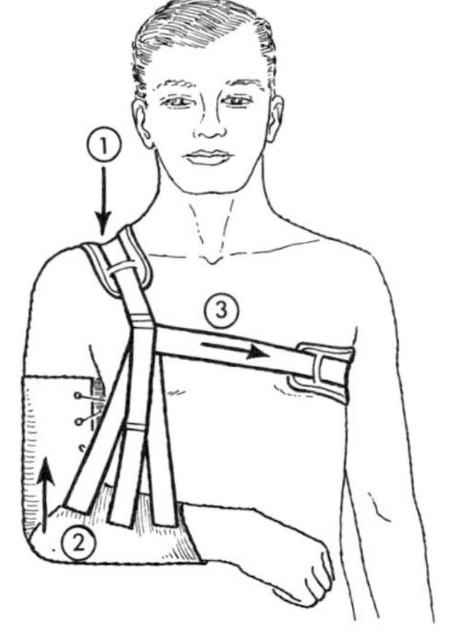

Application of Plaster Yoke for Unstable Fractures

1. Patient sits on a stool.
2. A well-padded figure-of-eight bandage is wrapped over the shoulders and through the axilla.
3. Four or five rolls of 3-in plaster are rolled over the padding.
4. Fracture is reduced by retracting the shoulders back and supporting the position with the surgeon's knee until the plaster hardens.

Note: This plaster yoke tends to be uncomfortable in the axilla and may cause compression on the axillary neurovascular structures. An alternative method is to immobilize the fracture with a clavicular spica cast.

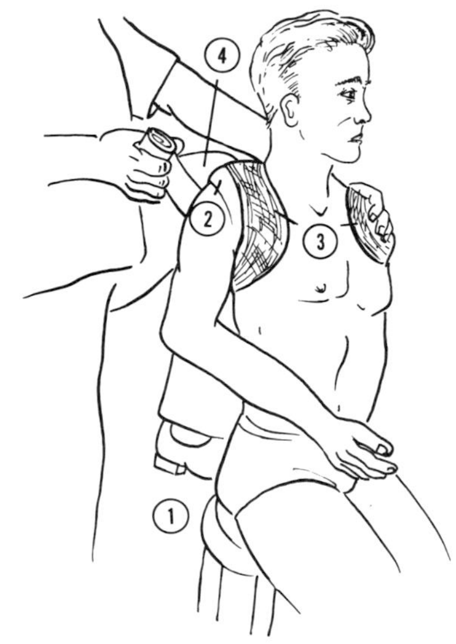

Application of Clavicular Spica Cast for Grossly Unstable Fractures in the Adult

1. Patient sits on a stool.
2. Using a body stockinette and light pads over the fracture, the operator applies the shoulder spica while pushing the shoulder superiorly and posteriorly.
3. Arm on the fracture side is incorporated in the plaster.

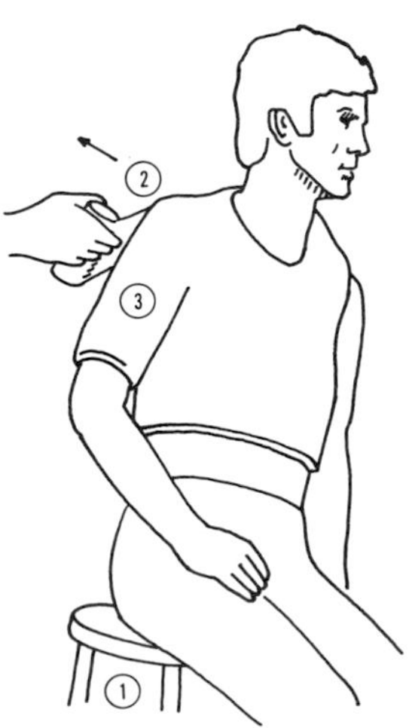

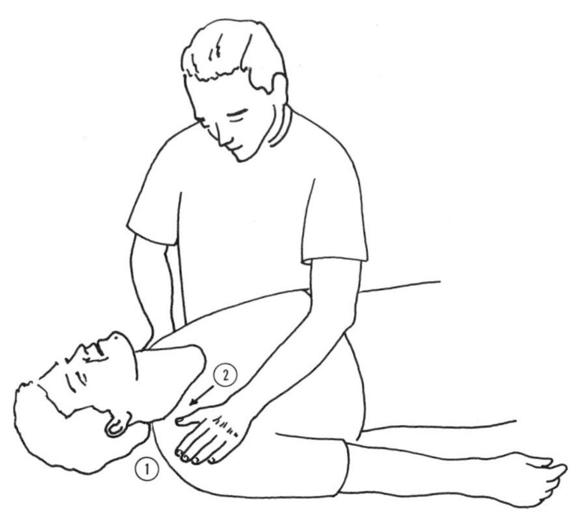

Application of Clavicular Spica Cast

Before the plaster sets,

1. Have the patient lie supine with a sandbag between the scapulae and the arms at the sides.
2. Hold the patient's shoulders back by molding upward in the deltoid region.

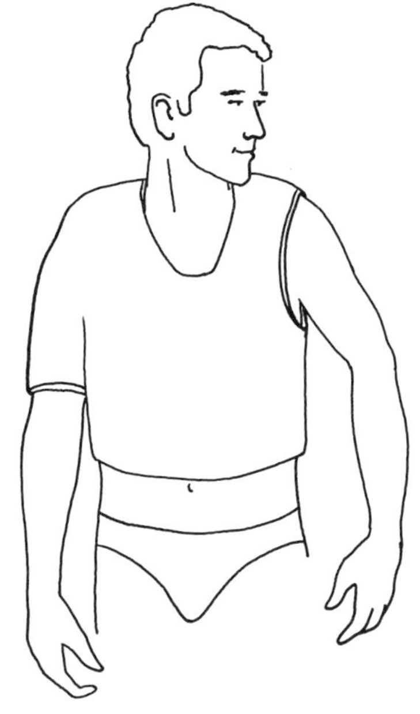

Front View of Clavicular Spica Cast

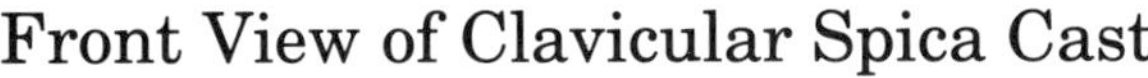

Note: Support the arm on the fractured side with a sling until pain subsides.

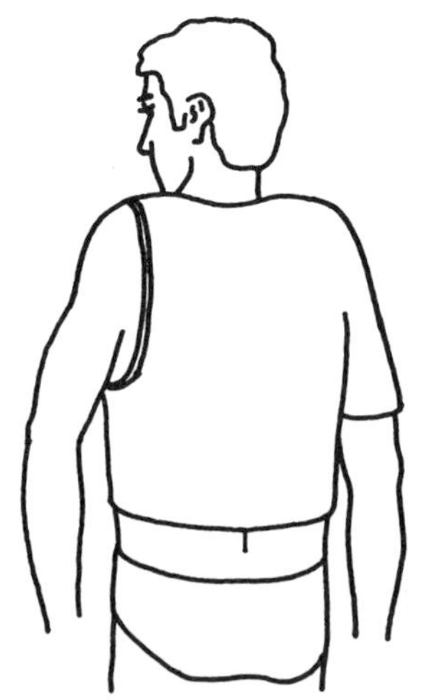

Back View of Clavicular Spica Cast

Postreduction Care

A child's fracture usually heals in 2–3 weeks of immobilization with a figure-of-eight harness.

The adult's fracture takes considerably longer and sometimes may require 6–8 weeks of immobilization in either a Velpeau sling or the clavicular spica.

Healing is best determined clinically by the fracture's stability and absence of pain. Radiographic signs lag considerably behind clinical evidence of union.

Encourage the free use of the arm and hand on the affected side during the period of immobilization. Particularly, emphasize rotation of the forearm to avoid nerve irritation from prolonged immobilization and pronation.

Alternative Method of Immobilization: Bed Rest for Patients With Multiple Injuries

For the patient who has multiple problems associated with the clavicular fractures, including pneumothorax or head injury, the clavicular fracture may be treated simply with bed rest. The elimination of gravity pull on the lateral fragment tends to provide satisfactory alignment until the patient gets out of bed. Occasionally, simple sling immobilization is all that is necessary, but this may be dispensed with if it interferes with chest tubes or nursing care.

Once the patient with multiple injuries begins to become ambulatory, the fractured clavicle should be supported by one of the methods described previously to avoid gross displacement.

Open Reduction of Fractures of the Adult's Clavicle

REMARKS

Despite the fact that approximately 1 of every 20 fractures occurs in the clavicle, healing problems are rare. Yet the clavicle is not invincible.

In the past, operative treatment of clavicular fractures has been condemned as more likely to produce nonunion than does closed treatment.

Unfortunately, closed treatment with a commercially available figure-of-eight harness, the standard treatment for children's fractures of the clavicle, has resulted in healing problems in adults that might be avoided by more complete initial immobilization. Any displaced clavicular fracture in the adult is best supported by either the Velpeau sling or a shoulder spica cast, as previously described, rather than the convenient but ineffective off-the-shelf figure-of-eight harness.

If a displaced or comminuted clavicular fracture cannot be reduced, particularly in patients with multiple fractures or head injuries, internal fixation might be considered.

Other indications for internal fixation include fractures that produce acute or persistent symptoms of thoracic outlet impingement, which has not been relieved by closed reduction.

In addition, fractures that are distal to the coracoclavicular ligament with upward displacement of the medial clavicular fracture fragment tend to require stabilization.

Because most clavicular fractures heal clinically in adults by 8–10 weeks, persistent mobility, pain, or an absence of union after this time should prompt consideration for operative fixation.

Problems of Internal Fixation

Internal fixation of the clavicle has gained a bad reputation in the past because of attempts to fix the clavicle fractures with intramedullary pins. The shape of the clavicle, which is sigmoid, virtually eliminates the possibility of inserting a straight intramedullary pin.

A consequence of misdirected pin insertion has been a number of severe complications as a result of pin migration into the mediastinum or other vital structures.

To avoid these complications and achieve adequate fixation, we have used simple fixation with a Knowles pin inserted from the medial cortex into the lateral fragment.

In the fracture with bone loss or atrophic nonunion, fixation by semitubular plate is preferable.

Problem of Internal Fixation of the Clavicle

1. Pins inserted from the lateral fragment into the medial fragment have been commonly used in the past.

   The problem is that the clavicle is a curved structure and the pins are straight.

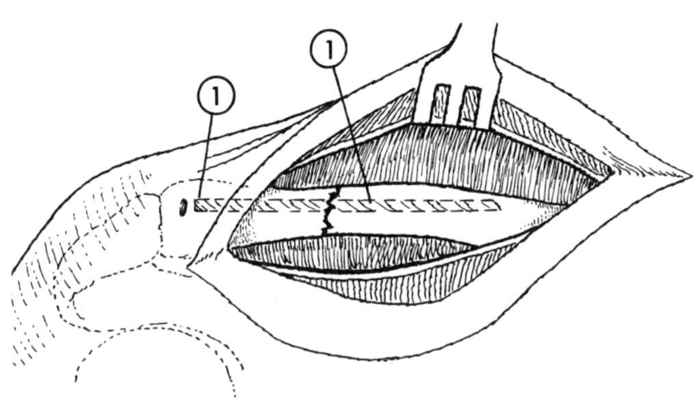

2. Result of inserting a straight pin from the lateral fragment is that the posterior cortex of the clavicle is usually penetrated. This may lead to impingement or migration into the mediastinum, with sometimes disastrous complications.

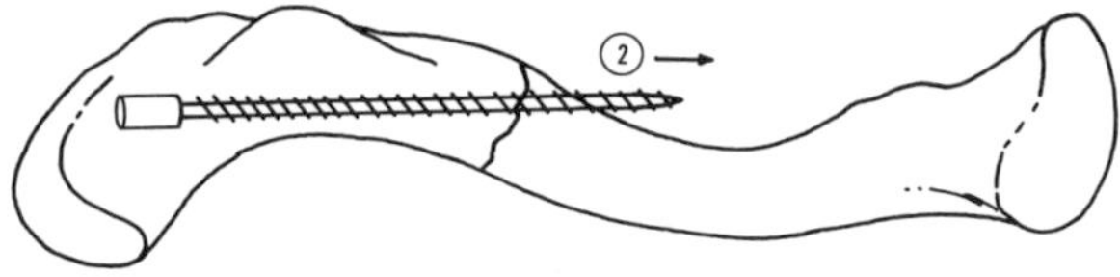

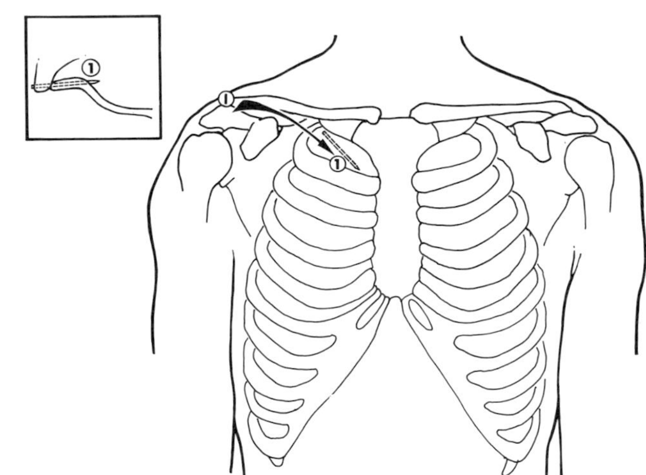

Caution: Avoid transarticular fixation of the acromioclavicular joint with pins. Too often, this leads to symptomatic degenerative arthritis of the joint or

1. Migration of the pin into the mediastinum from the acromioclavicular joint "fixation."

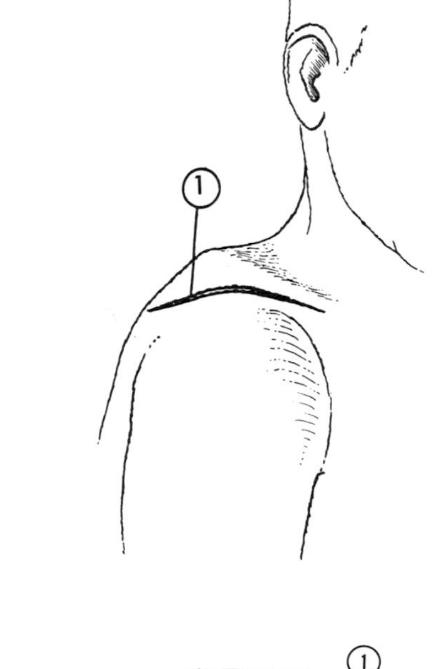

Indication for Internal Fixation

1. The most common indication for internal fixation is a failure of reduction or immobilization with previously described slings or harnesses. The prominence of the medial fragment and displacement of the lateral fragment can lead to nonunion or thoracic outlet impingement. Under these circumstances, in approximately 5 per cent of cases of adult clavicular fractures, internal stabilization may be indicated.

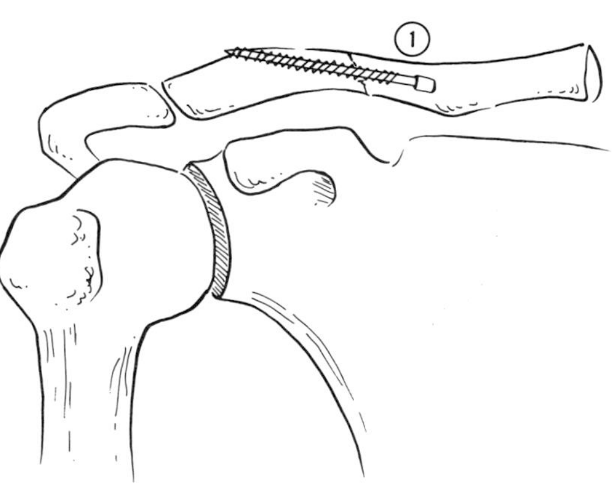

Knowles Pinning

1. The simplest method to stabilize the acutely unstable clavicular fracture is with one or two Knowles pins inserted from the medial fragment laterally across the cortices into the lateral fragment.

Note: **The combination of the hub on the Knowles pin and the direction of the pin laterally avoids the risk of damaging structures in the mediastinum. This has been a problem with pins inserted from the lateral fragment into the medial fragment, a technique that should be avoided.**

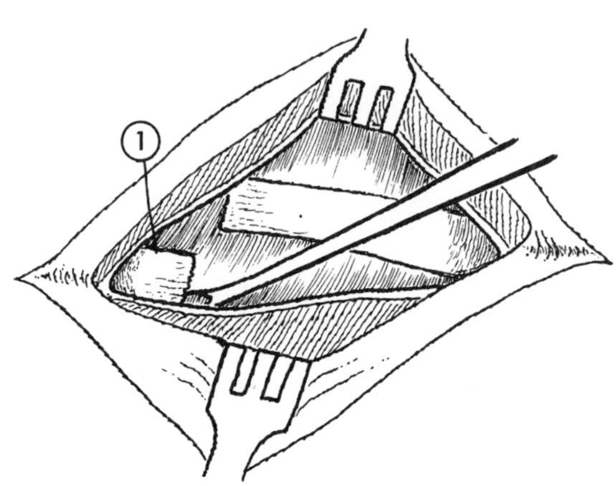

Alternative Method of Open Reduction: Plate Fixation

1. If the fracture fragments are comminuted or cannot be stabilized adequately with Knowles pins, more extensive dissection may be needed.

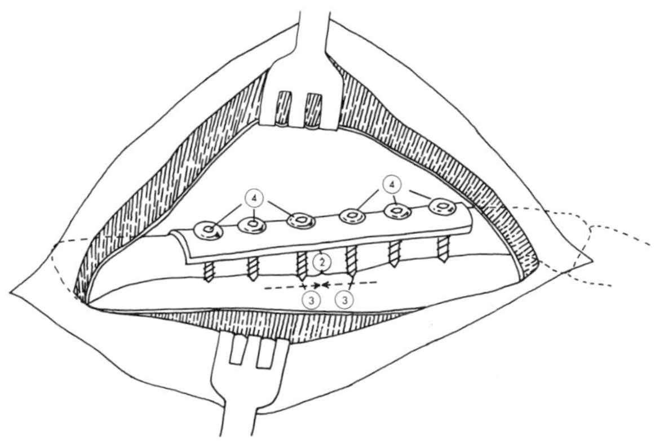

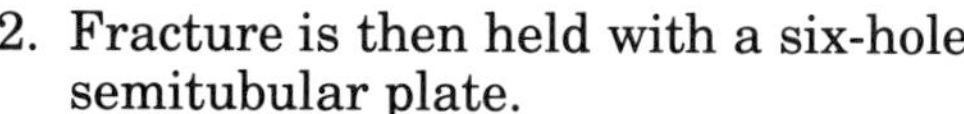

2. Fracture is then held with a six-hole semitubular plate.
3. The screws are inserted on the lateral fragment, which is then brought to the medial fragment.
4. At least two, and preferably three, screws should fix each fragment.

Other Indications for Operative Fixation

Fractures of the Lateral Third of the Clavicle With Displacement

REMARKS

Fractures of the lateral third of the clavicle may disrupt the coracoclavicular attachment to the clavicle and, thereby, produce a very unstable fracture.

These have been found to have a higher incidence of healing problems as a result of the difficulty in reducing and holding the unstable fracture.

Operative stabilization may be indicated more often with this type of fracture than with the more common fractures of the middle third of the clavicle.

1. Fracture of the lateral third of the clavicle with an
2. Intact coracoclavicular ligament is usually stable and can be treated nonoperatively with a sling and swathe.

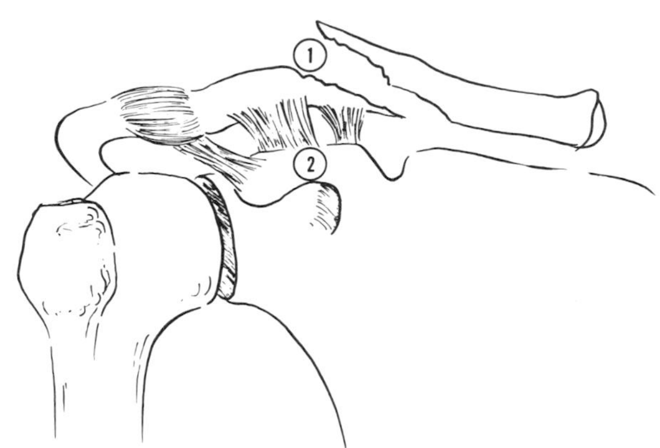

Unstable Lateral Third Fracture

1. Fracture of the lateral third of the clavicle with a
2. Disruption of the coracoclavicular ligament structure can be unstable and may require internal stabilization to avoid painful nonunion.

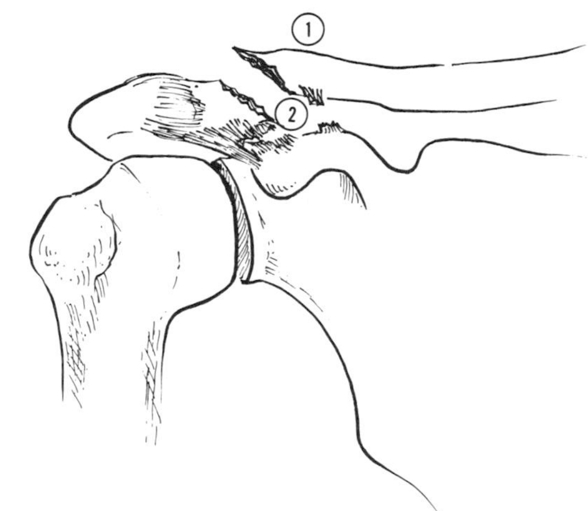

Management of Unstable Fractures of the Lateral Third

1. Lateral fragment may be resected out to the acromioclavicular joint.
2. Medial fragment may be reduced and held with a screw from the clavicle into the coracoid process.
3. This is reinforced by repair of the coracoacromial and coracoclavicular ligaments.

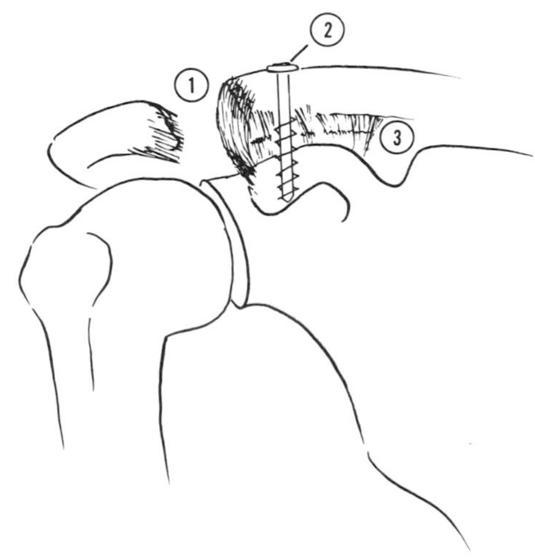

Complications of Fractures of the Clavicle

REMARKS

Although rare, complications associated with fractures of the clavicle do occur. These are most likely to follow clavicular fractures in adults.

The most common complications include nonunion; excessive callus formation at the fracture site, producing thoracic outlet syndrome; and direct injuries to neurovascular structures in the thoracic outlet.

Surgical misadventures may occur, primarily from the use of "intramedullary pin" fixation that migrates into the mediastinum.

Nonunion of Fractures of the Clavicle

REMARKS

In the past, the most common cause of nonunion of the clavicle was open surgery for fractures in the middle third. Recently, as internal fixation has been shunned, however, ununited fractures occur more frequently after immobilization with a figure-of-eight harness for the adult displaced fracture.

Any displaced clavicular fracture in the adult should be reduced and supported by devices that support the arm and immobilize the shoulder, such as the Velpeau sling or shoulder spica cast, as previously described.

If the displaced or comminuted clavicular fracture cannot be reduced, internal fixation with the Knowles pin technique should be considered.

Although the common clavicular fracture in the child heals uneventfully, the frequency of nonunion in the adult clavicular fracture approaches 3 per cent.

Nonunion of the clavicle may be hypertrophic, with excess callus, or atrophic, with little or no callus.

The hypertrophic nonunion usually causes pain, cosmetic deformity, and sometimes thoracic outlet syndrome that is sufficient to require operative treatment.

The atrophic nonunion may be associated with little or no pain, particularly in the elderly patient. Therefore, operative treatment of these nonunions should be based on the patient's symptoms and not merely on the radiographic signs.

Management of Nonunions of the Clavicle

Hypertrophic nonunions can be managed effectively by internal fixation. We have found Knowles pins to be adequate to achieve this fixation.

Bone grafting is unnecessary for the hypertrophic nonunion because there is plenty of callus already available at the fracture site.

Atrophic nonunion usually requires plate fixation and sometimes bone grafting.

Nonunion of the lateral third of the clavicle is managed by resection of the fracture fragment and repair of coracoacromial and coracoclavicular ligaments, as described previously.

Preoperative X-Ray

1. Hypertrophic nonunion of the clavicle with shortening and overriding can be treated with Knowles pins or plates.

2. Atrophic nonunion with a true pseudoarthrosis and gap of the clavicle in the elderly patient may not be sufficiently symptomatic to warrant treatment.

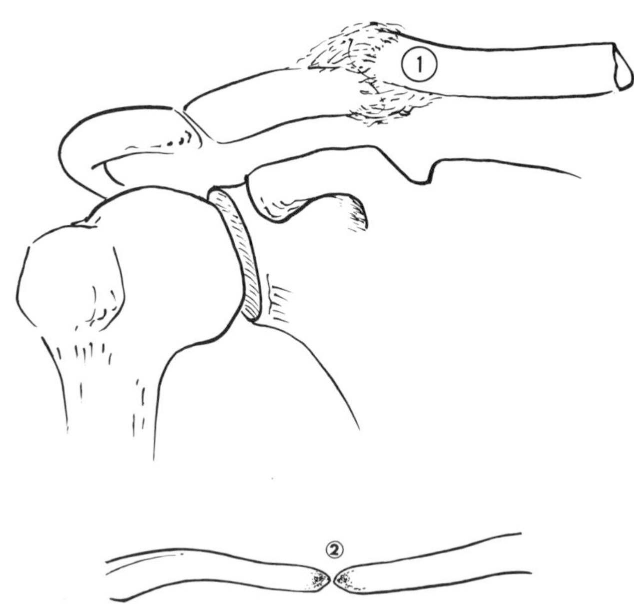

Operative Fixation of Hypertrophic Nonunion

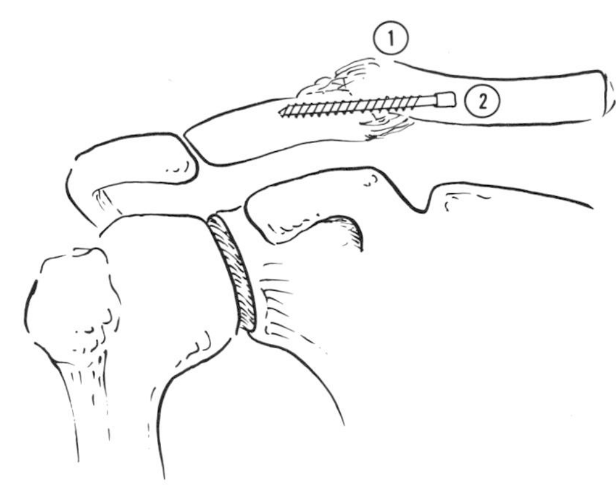

1. Fracture is left in bayonet apposition.
2. It can be stabilized simply with a Knowles pin inserted under fluoroscopic control from the medial to the lateral cortex.

Note: Additional support may be achieved with a Velpeau sling or shoulder spica cast.

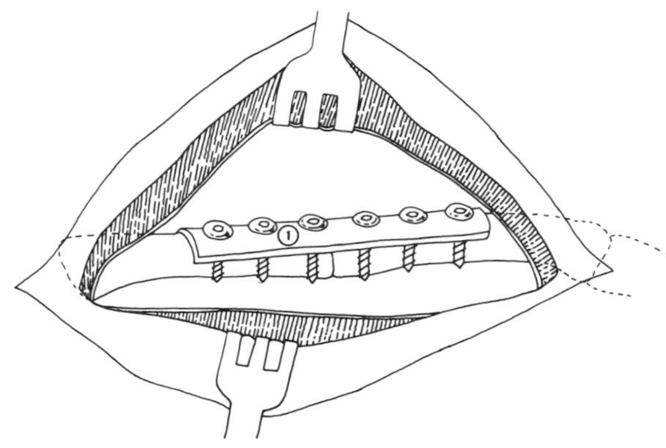

Operative Fixation of Atrophic Nonunion

1. Atrophic nonunion can best be stabilized by a semitubular plate.

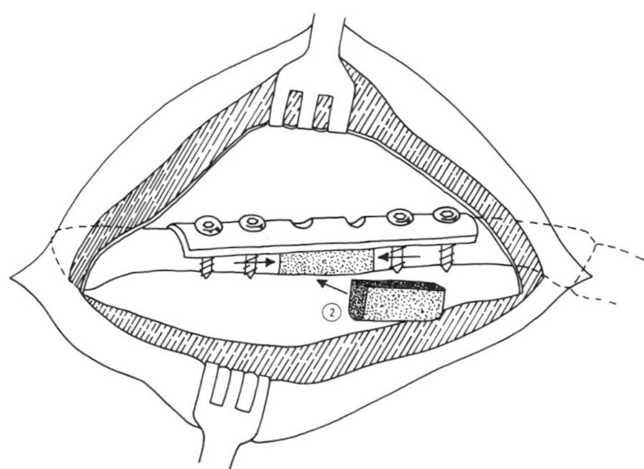

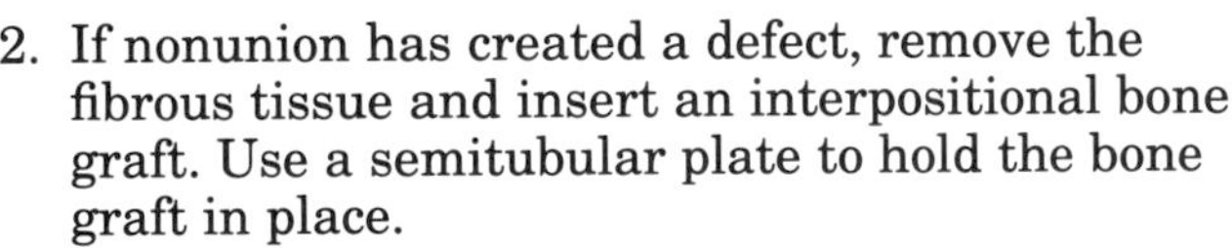

2. If nonunion has created a defect, remove the fibrous tissue and insert an interpositional bone graft. Use a semitubular plate to hold the bone graft in place.

Neurovascular Injuries From Displaced Fractures or Excess Callus at the Fracture Site

REMARKS

The neurovascular injury from clavicular fractures may be acute or chronic. Displaced fragments may injure subclavian vessels and the brachial plexus at the time of fracture. Chronic obstruction or thoracic outlet syndrome may follow repetitive trauma to the neurovascular structures, which are chronically caught between the large callus mass and the underlying first rib.

Many varieties of injuries are possible from simple compression to acute lacerations of the structures. The most common injuries are compression or angulation of the subclavian vessels and brachial plexus.

Acute symptoms of neurovascular injury should be recognized promptly because major hemorrhage can occur. The classic example of this was the death of Sir Robert Peel, the founder of the British "bobbies," who died of hemorrhage after a fracture of his clavicle.

After a severely displaced fracture of the clavicle, check the vascular and neurologic function of the limb carefully. Use arteriograms, venograms, and computed tomography (CT) as indicated to determine the site of injury.

Chronic impingement on the thoracic outlet and neurovascular structures may not be recognized as readily. The symptoms may be less dramatic and occur only with forward elevation of the arm.

Acute Neurovascular Impingement From Displaced Fractures

1. Fracture of the clavicle.
2. Lateral fragment displaces downward, especially on forward flexion of the arm.
3. Neurovascular structures are compressed against the first rib.

Note: If closed reduction does not relieve neurovascular impingement, open reduction and internal fixation are indicated.

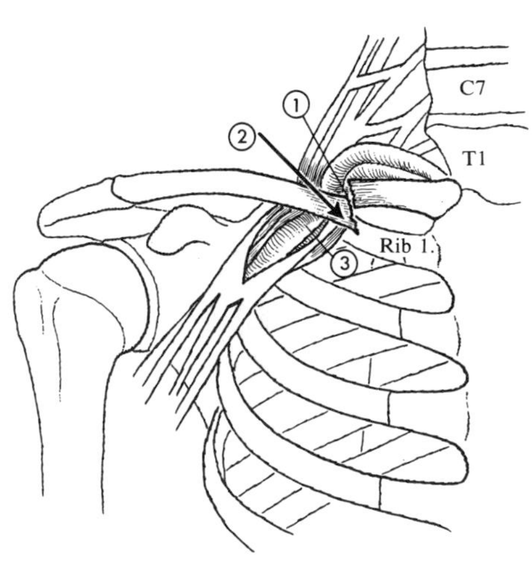

Chronic Neurovascular Impingement From Excess Callus

1. Comminuted fracture of the middle third of the clavicle.
2. Massive callus formation.
3. Compression of the neurovascular structures.
4. Interval between the clavicle and the first rib is severely reduced.

Note: Chronic impingement may only cause intermittent symptoms, depending on the position of the arm. For this reason, recognition of the problem may be delayed or confused with conditions such as a cervical disc.

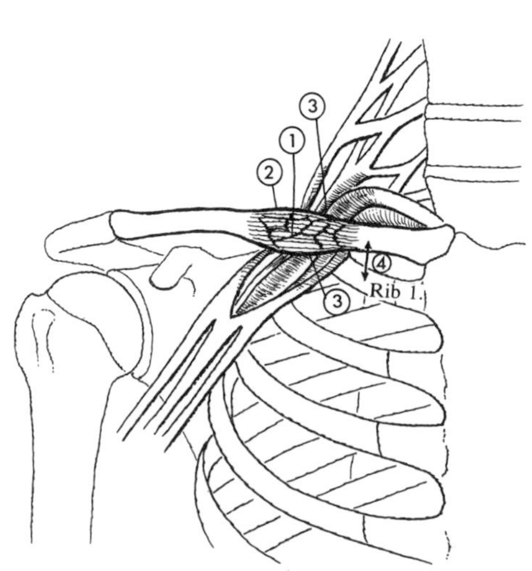

Management of Neurovascular Complications

REMARKS

Neurovascular injuries associated with displaced fractures should be recognized immediately. As a rule, they respond to simple closed reduction and adequate immobilization of the fracture.

If the symptoms of neurovascular compression are not relieved by closed reduction, open reduction and internal fixation are indicated.

In cases of long-standing compression, as excessive callus develops in the ununited or malunited fracture, neurovascular symptoms may gradually worsen. Characteristically, they are produced by positioning of the arms in a forward and elevated direction.

Chronic impingement on the thoracic outlet produced by hypertrophic nonunion is best managed by internal stabilization of the fracture site.

Excision of a Portion of the Clavicle

REMARKS

In the past, the clavicle was considered expendable or at least partially expendable. Certain segments of the clavicle can be excised with little or no dysfunction.

It has now been recognized that, if a portion of the clavicle is excised, the remaining clavicle should be stabilized somehow to either the coracoid process or the underlying rib structure.

Excision of the middle half of the clavicle has been used to expose the brachial plexus and, particularly, the subclavian vessel after an injury from a penetrating wound.

We have found that, if the medial third or half of the clavicle is excised, the lateral portion tends to re-form bone, which can impinge later on the neurovascular structures. To avoid this, the middle third of the clavicle is replaced with bone graft and with plate stabilization.

1. Excision of the clavicle distal to the coracoclavicular ligament should be stablized and the ligament repaired.
2. Sternal end of the clavicle can also sometimes be excised for chronic sternoclavicular dislocations. However, here the clavicle should be stabilized to the underlying rib.
3. Excision of the entire clavicle has been done occasionally for tumors; however, the clavicle does have a protective and functional role and should be retained whenever possible.

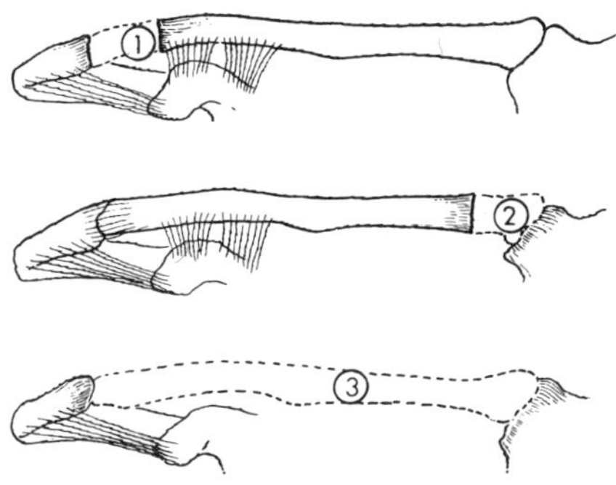

1. If the middle portion of the clavicle is completely resected to decompress the underlying neurovascular structures, the
2. Lateral portion of the clavicle frequently regenerates or forms a bone spike that impinges on the vessels and brachial plexus whenever the patient flexes and adducts the shoulder.

Note: To avoid complications from resection of the middle clavicle, we have used plate stabilization or bone fragmentation and bone grafting, as described by Shumacker.

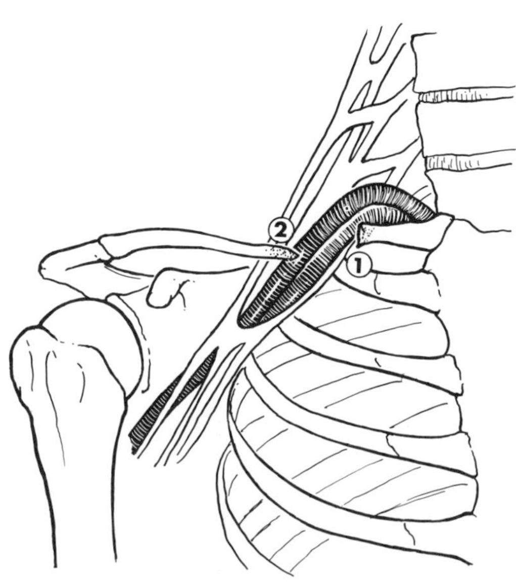

Technique of Clavicular Fragmentation (After Shumacker)

Preoperative X-Ray

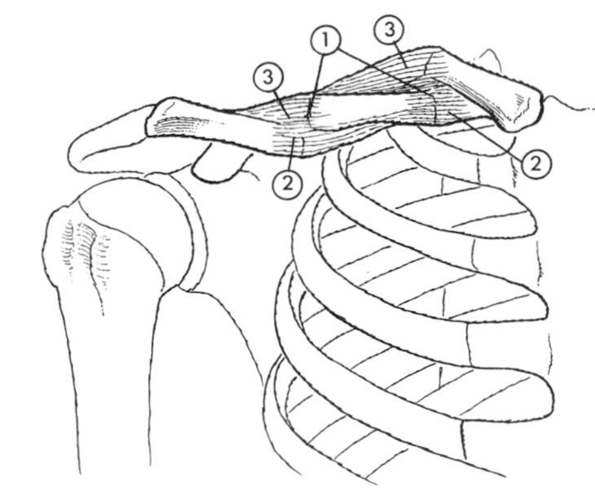

1. Segmental fracture of the middle third of the clavicle.
2. Wide separation and malalignment of the fragments.
3. Massive callus formation impinging on the thoracic outlet.

Excision of Hypertrophic Nonunion

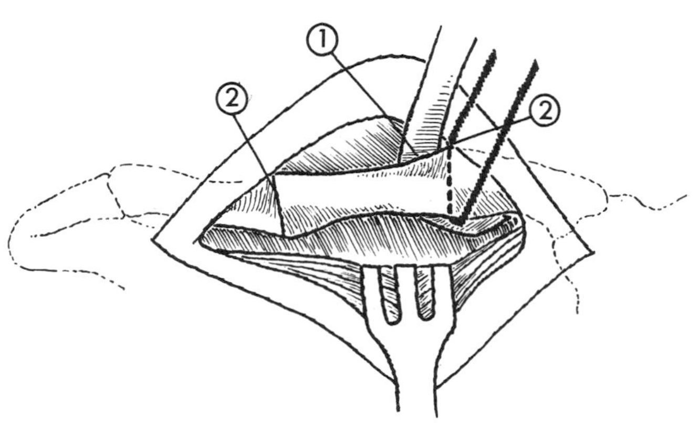

1. Hypertrophic mass is carefully dissected and the underlying neurovascular structures protected with an elevator.
2. Fragments are removed with a Gigli saw at the medial and lateral portions of the nonunion.

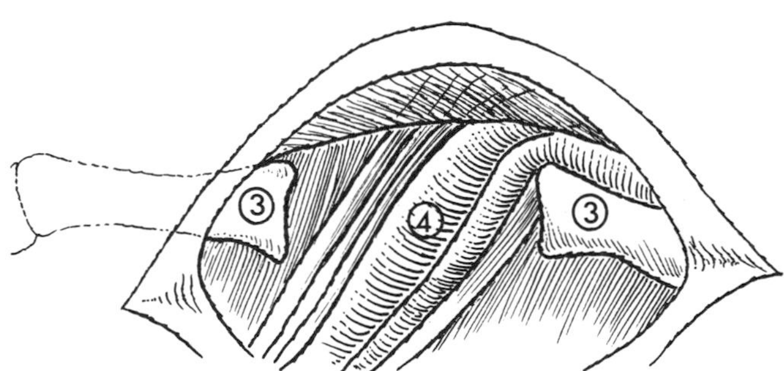

3. Middle third of the clavicle has been excised.
4. Underlying structures are free.

Fragmentation

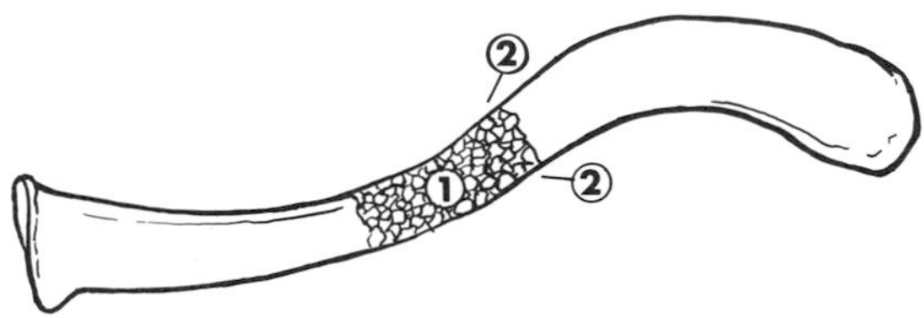

1. Callus is rongeured and milled into 2–3-mm fragments. These are repacked into the periosteal bed, which is well vascularized.
2. Periosteous sleeve is closed over these bone chips.

Note: Further stabilization is then achieved with a semitubular plate, as previously described.

Ligamentous Injuries of the Articulations of the Clavicle

Lesions of the Ligaments of the Acromioclavicular Joint

REMARKS

Although injuries to the ligaments of the acromioclavicular joint may occur in any age group, they most frequently are seen in young athletic adults.

The typical mechanism of injury is a direct blow to the tip of the shoulder, e.g., when the quarterback in football lands on his throwing shoulder after being tackled from the "blind side."

Involvement of the ligaments varies from a minor sprain, in which only a few fibers tear, to complete disruption of all fibers.

Complete disruption of the acromioclavicular joint is still compatible with normal shoulder function, but pronounced displacement may be painful or may cause an unsightly prominence.

An incompletely reduced acromioclavicular dislocation is likely to produce traumatic arthritis and painful shoulder function.

Management of these injuries requires an intelligent assessment of the patient's need rather than rote use of a set approach.

Muscular individuals who are most anxious to return to work or competitive sports may be treated symptomatically with sling support, ice applications, and exercises to strengthen the injured trapezius and deltoid muscles.

Corrective surgery may be done electively if patients decide it is necessary for their functional needs.

Thin individuals who are likely to be bothered by the prominently displaced lateral end of the clavicle may be offered early surgical correction.

Mechanisms of Injury

Most injuries result from a direct fall on the shoulder.

Occasionally, an indirectly applied force injures the acromioclavicular joint.

Depending on the intensity of the forces acting, one of several lesions may result.

Direct Mechanism

This is usually the result of a fall on the point of the shoulder, with the arm at the side or adducted slightly.

1. Direct force is applied to the point of the shoulder.
2. Scapula and the attached clavicle are forced downward and medially. The clavicle approaches the first rib. If the force continues, the

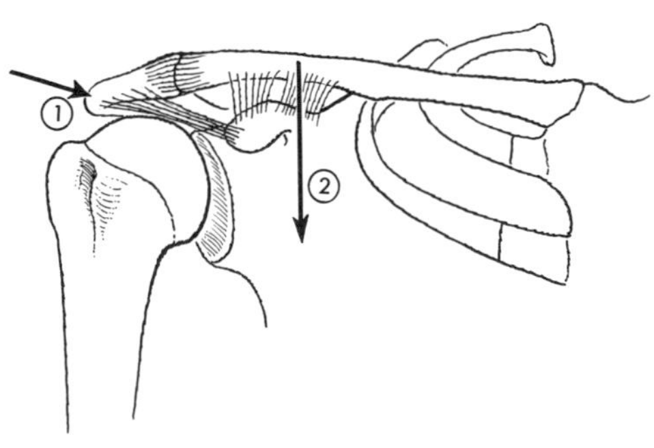

3. First rib abuts against the clavicle, producing a counterforce that may cause
4. Rupture of the acromioclavicular ligaments and the coracoclavicular ligaments and
5. Tearing of the insertions of the deltoid and trapezius muscles.

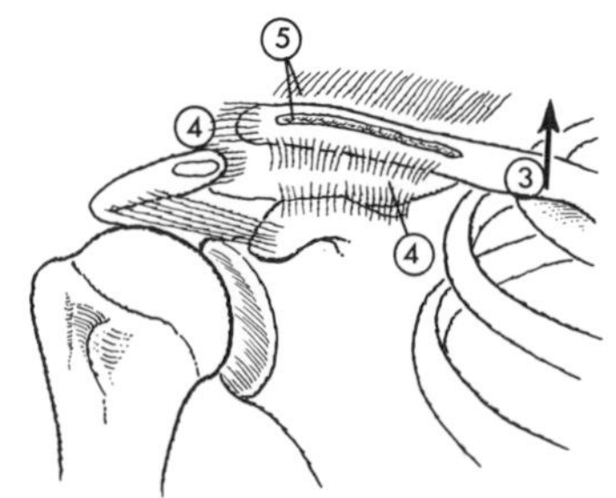

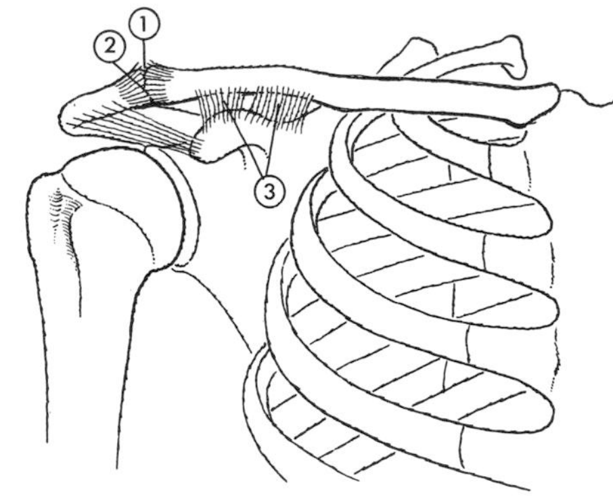

SPRAIN

1. Few fibers of the acromioclavicular ligaments stretch or even tear.
2. Acromioclavicular joint is stable; there is no laxity.
3. Coracoclavicular ligaments are intact.

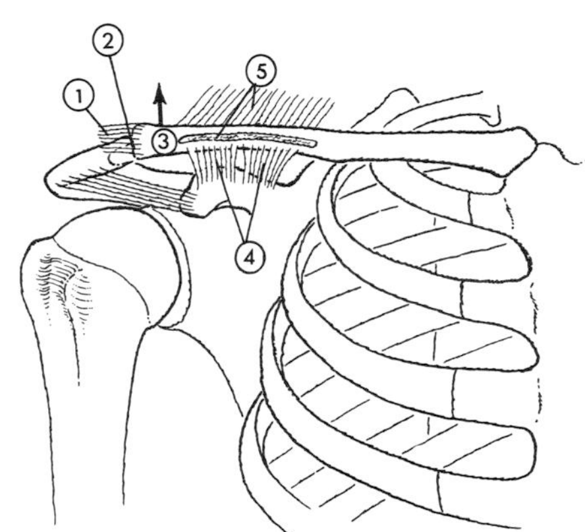

SUBLUXATION

1. Rupture of the capsule and acromioclavicular ligaments.
2. Acromioclavicular joint is unstable; there is obvious laxity.
3. End of the clavicle is displaced upward, usually by less than half the width of the end of the clavicle.
4. Coracoclavicular ligaments are intact.
5. Attachments of the trapezius and deltoid muscles to the clavicle are intact.

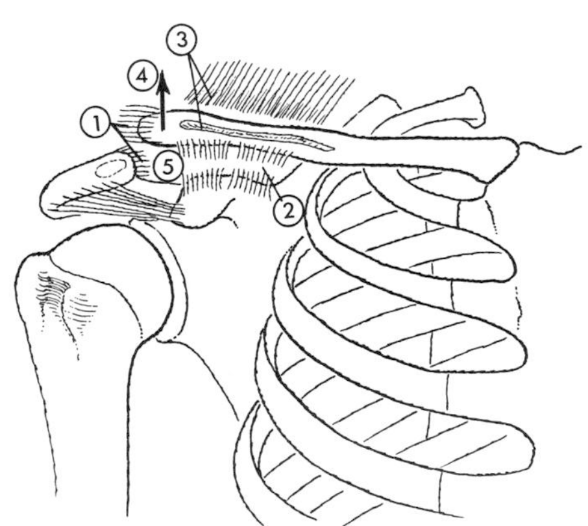

DISLOCATION

1. Rupture of the capsule and acromioclavicular ligaments.
2. Rupture of the coracoclavicular ligaments.
3. Avulsion of the attachments of the trapezius and deltoid muscles.
4. Upward displacement of the clavicle.
5. Wide separation between the clavicle and the coracoid process.

Other Injuries

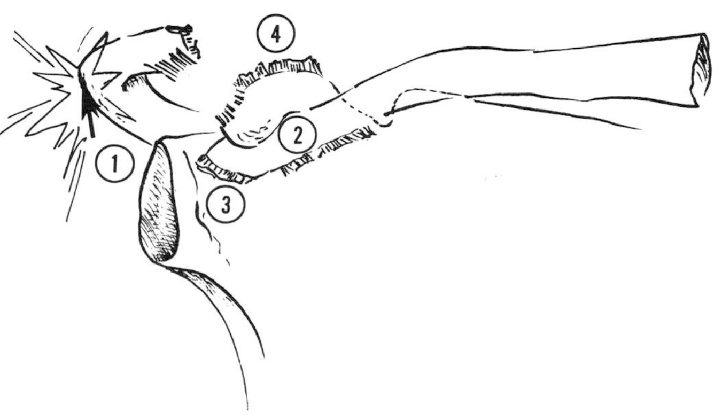

SUBCORACOID DISLOCATION

1. This occurs usually as the result of significant traumatic abduction injury to the upper shoulder.
2. Distal end of the clavicle dislocates under the coracoid process.
3. Acromioclavicular and
4. Coracoclavicular ligaments are completely disrupted.

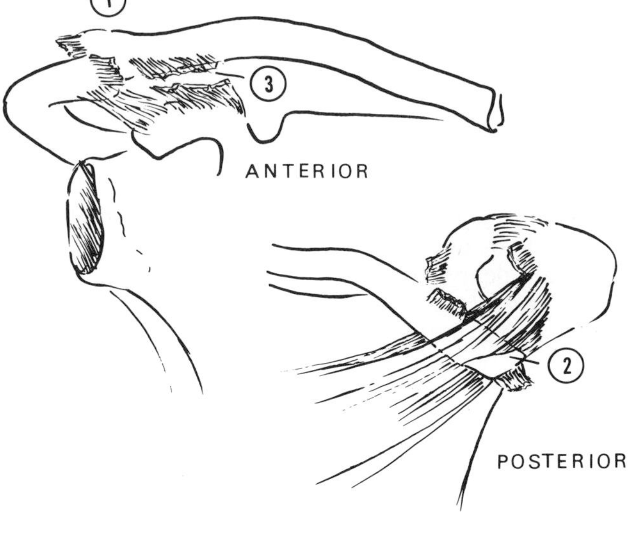

POSTERIOR DISLOCATION

1. Mechanism of this injury is similar to other types, except that the clavicle is displaced posteriorly.
2. Frequently, the displaced distal clavicle is locked within the fibers of the trapezius muscle.
3. Coracoclavicular ligaments are completely disrupted.

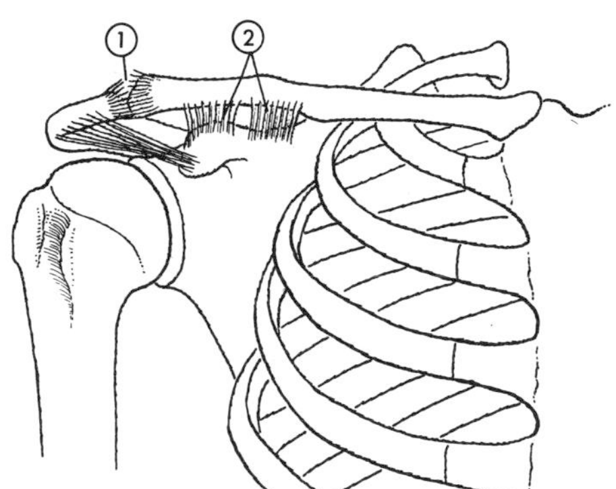

Management of Injuries of the Acromioclavicular Ligaments

Sprain

1. Minor stretching and tearing of the capsule and ligaments of the acromioclavicular joint occur.
2. Coracoclavicular ligaments are intact.

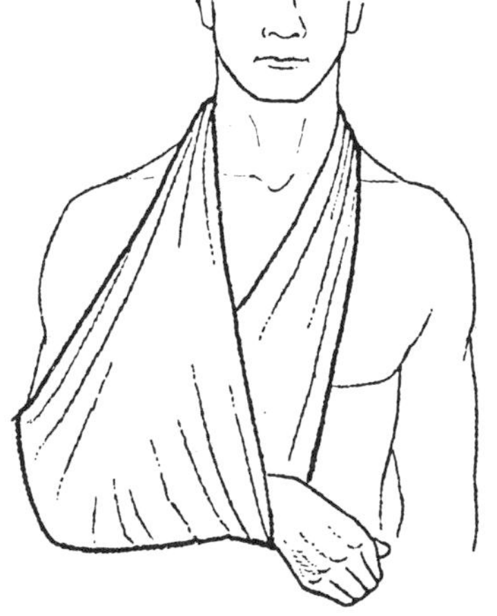

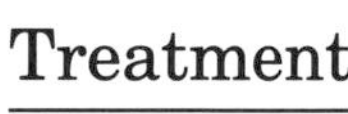

Treatment

Initially, apply ice.

After 3 days, wet heat may be applied.

Rest the limb in a sling for 3–5 days.

Begin active exercises to strengthen deltoid and trapezius muscles when the initial pain subsides.

Recovery should be complete in 7–10 days.

Subluxation

REMARKS

The subluxation responds adequately to nonoperative methods.

Depending on the needs of the patient, the subluxation may be treated symptomatically, as described for the sprain earlier, or by attempted closed reduction with acromioclavicular strapping.

Avoid the use of adhesive straps.

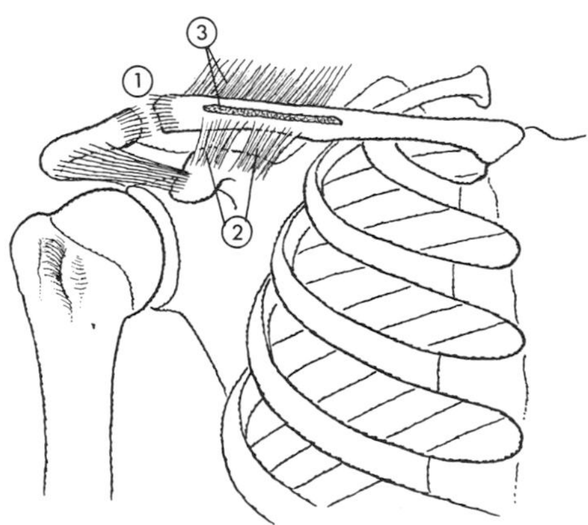

1. Capsule and the acromioclavicular ligaments are ruptured.
2. Coracoclavicular ligaments are intact.
3. Attachments of the trapezius and deltoid to the clavicle are intact.

Prereduction X-Ray

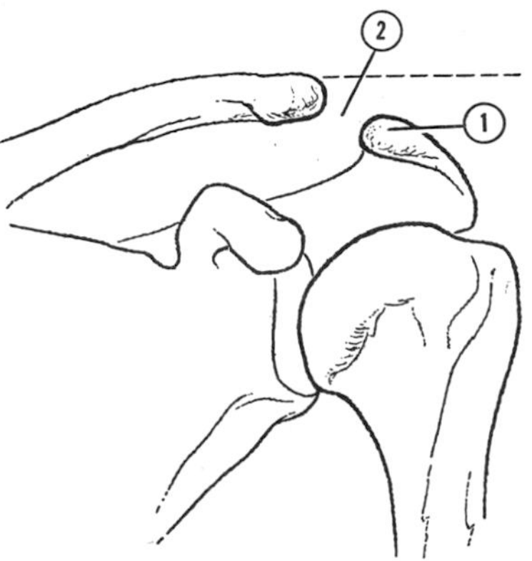

1. Acromion is slightly below the level of the clavicle.
2. Acromioclavicular joint space is widened.

Attempted reduction must be tailored to the needs of the patient.

If the patient must return to work or athletic competition promptly, symptomatic treatment for a few days with sling support is probably the wisest choice.

Otherwise, use a commercially available acromioclavicular support (e.g., a Kenny Howard sling).

Dislocation

REMARKS

Numerous methods, both closed and open, have been designed to treat dislocations.

The treatment for acromioclavicular dislocation should be tailored to the needs of the patient because normal shoulder function is possible despite a chronically dislocated acromioclavicular joint.

The injury is not a surgical emergency but one that can be treated promptly by simple shoulder support and early active range-of-motion exercises, depending on the needs of the patient. This allows most individuals to return to work or to participation in sports within 1–2 weeks, much earlier than with surgical treatment.

Typical Deformity

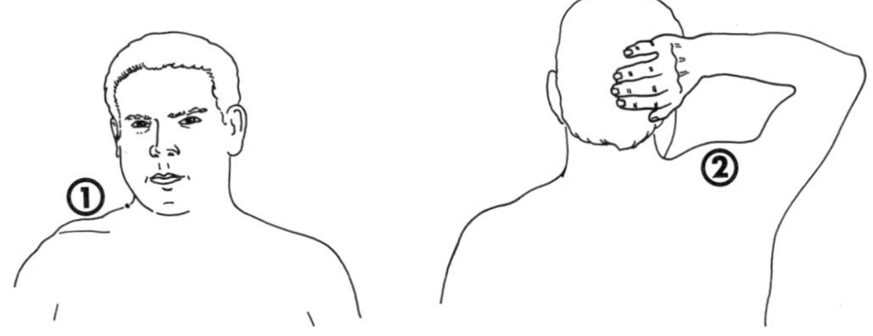

1. In a well-muscled man, a complete acromioclavicular dislocation is barely perceptible.
2. Injury was treated symptomatically with early active exercise, and at 2 weeks, the patient had returned to full activities.

Use of a Kenny Howard Acromioclavicular Support

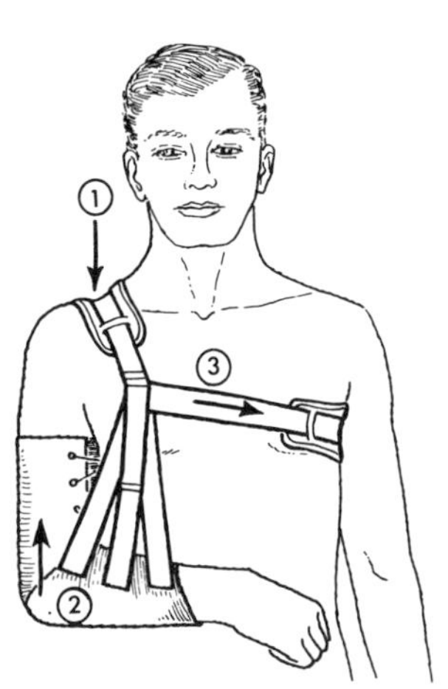

1. Shoulder strap applied over a piece of felt holds the clavicle down.
2. Sling supports the forearm and keeps the acromion in an elevated position.
3. Halter pulls both the shoulder strap and the sling inward.

After 3 weeks, allow free use of the arm.

Should surgical treatment be decided on, the procedure should avoid the following:

- The use of fixation pins across the acromioclavicular joint, which migrate all too frequently.
- The use of fixation devices likely to erode bone or to fail.
- Incomplete reduction of the acromioclavicular joint, which leads to arthritis.
- A secondary operation necessary to remove fixation.

For an excessively prominent acromioclavicular dislocation that produces discomfort, the disrupted coracoclavicular ligament can be repaired and the outer 2 cm of the clavicle can be resected so as to avoid later development of acromioclavicular arthritis.

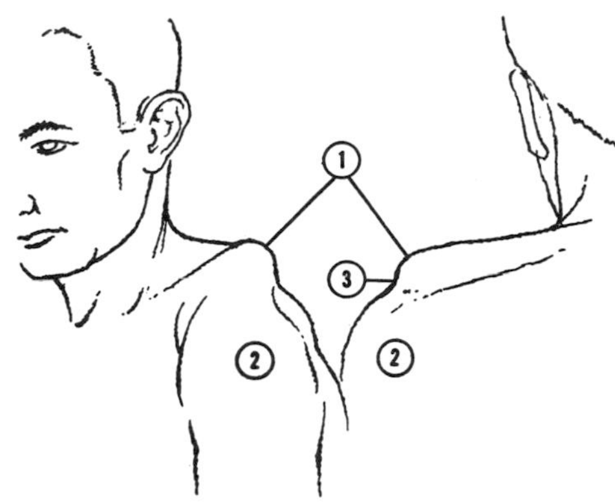

1. In this thin person, the acromioclavicular dislocation completely disrupted muscles and became very prominent under the skin.
2. Shoulder drooped downward and forward.
3. Sulcus was present between the outer end of the clavicle and the acromion.

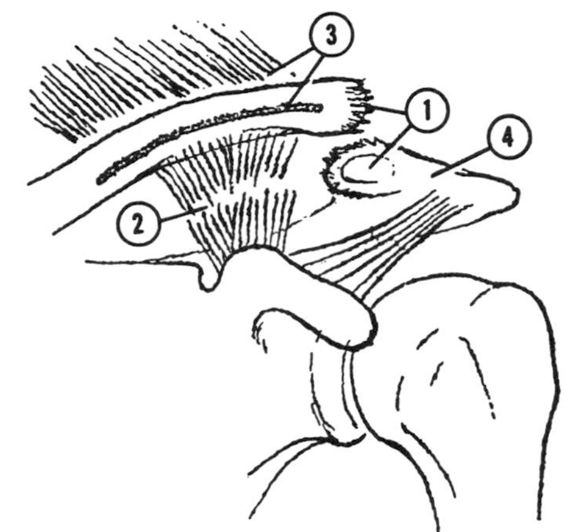

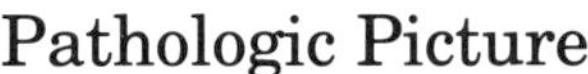

Pathologic Picture

1. Rupture of the acromioclavicular ligaments.
2. Rupture of the coracoclavicular ligaments.
3. Avulsion from the clavicle of attachments of the trapezius and deltoid muscles.
4. Acromion process is below and is widely separated from the clavicle.

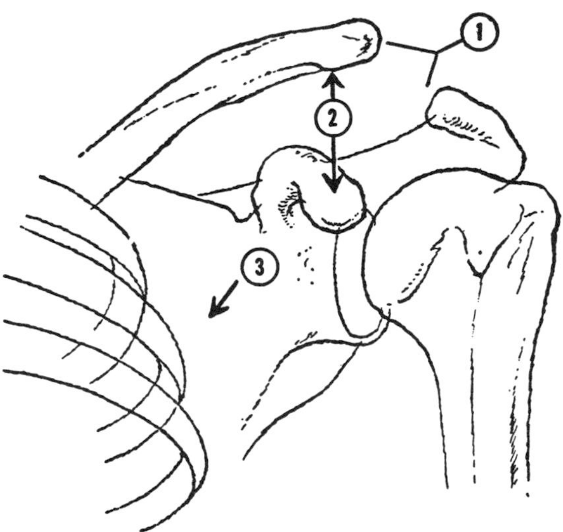

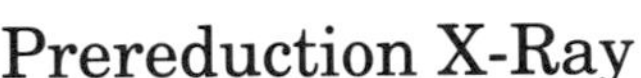

Prereduction X-Ray

1. Complete displacement of the articular surfaces of the clavicle and the acromion process occurred.
2. Interval between the clavicle and the coracoid is greatly increased.
3. Scapula is displaced downward and forward.

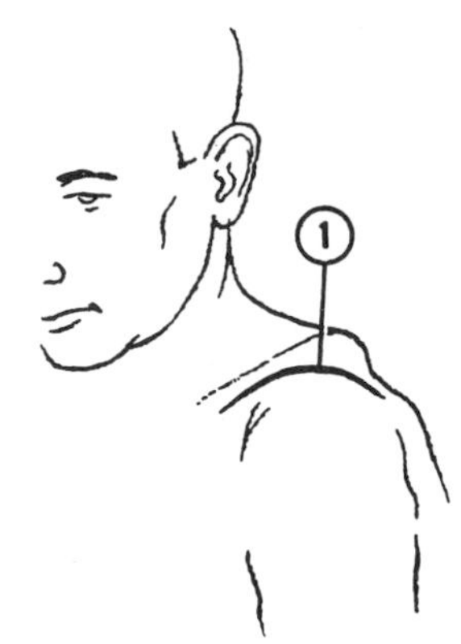

Preferred Operative Treatment (Weaver-Dunn Procedure)

1. Dislocated acromioclavicular joint is approached through the area of prominence.

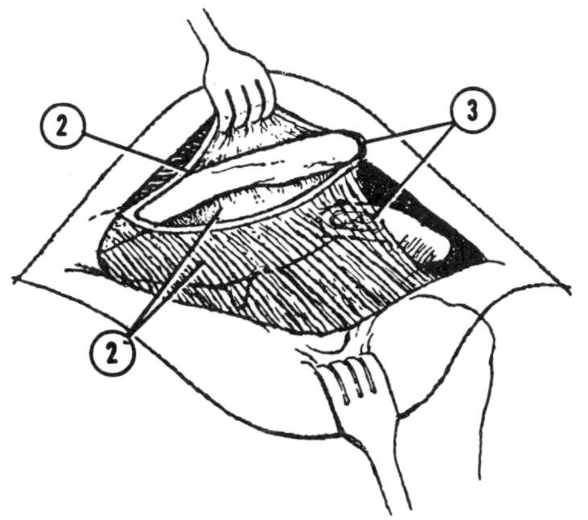

2. Clavicle is seen to be displaced upward.
3. Distal 1–2 cm of the clavicle can be resected.

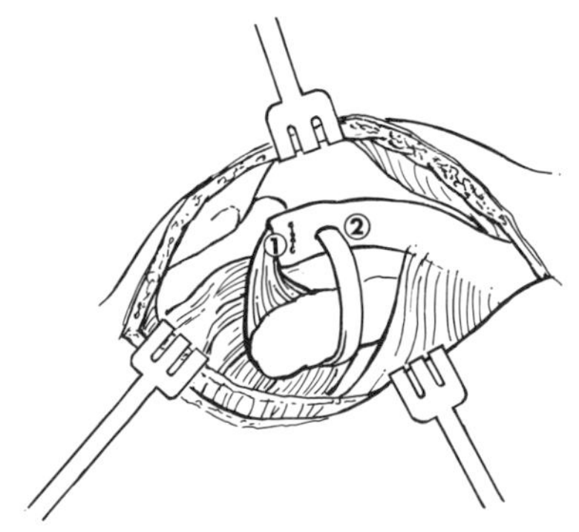

1. Coracoacromial ligament is freed and inserted into the distal end of the resected clavicle.
2. Repair is reinforced with heavy Dacron or Mersilene suture passed under the coracoid and into the clavicle.

Caution: The Weaver-Dunn repair of the coracoacromial attachment with resection of the distal clavicle is preferred to the traditional method of fixing the acromioclavicular dislocation with transarticular pins. In the past, this transarticular fixation has led to many complications because of penetration and migration into the mediastinum or other vital structures. This method should be abandoned.

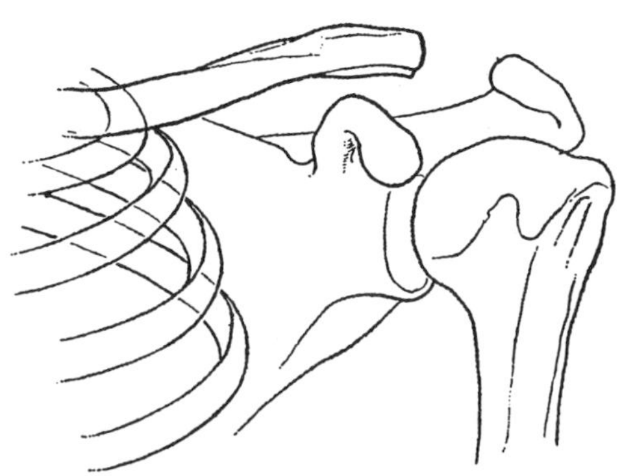

Postoperative X-Ray

The distal clavicle has been resected, and the coracoclavicular relationship has been restored.

Alternative Method of Fixation

1. Lateral portion of the clavicle is resected to avoid traumatic arthritis.
2. Medial clavicular fragment is stabilized to the coracoid process with a cortical screw. The coracoclavicular and acromioclavicular ligaments are also repaired to add to the stability.

Note: The screw may be removed at 3–4 months after the ligaments have healed.

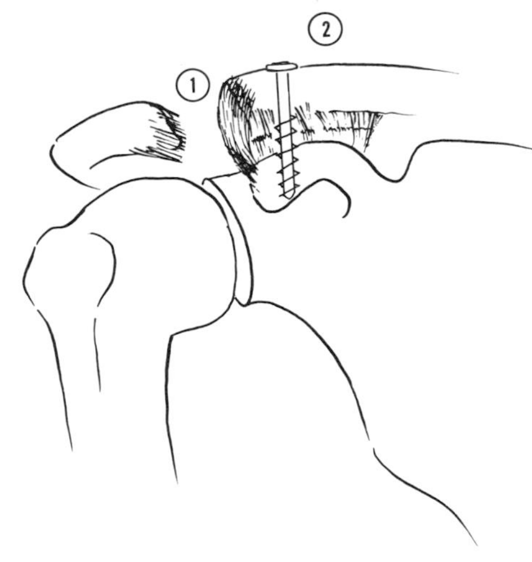

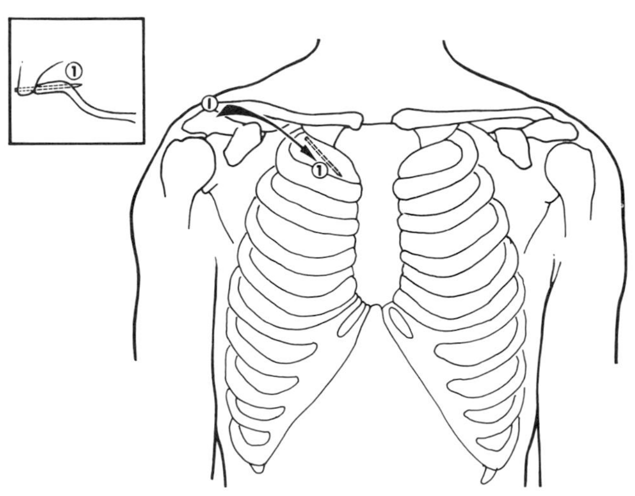

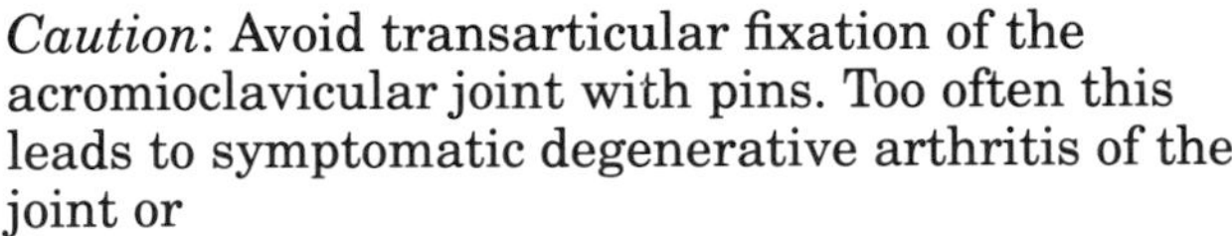
Caution: Avoid transarticular fixation of the acromioclavicular joint with pins. Too often this leads to symptomatic degenerative arthritis of the joint or

1. Migration of the pin into the mediastinum from the acromioclavicular joint "fixation."

Management of Old Acromioclavicular Dislocations

REMARKS

Many chronically dislocated acromioclavicular joints are not painful and cause no dysfunction. These lesions generally do not require surgical repair.

Occasionally, in a thin patient, a chronic dislocation becomes painful and interferes with complete elevation and abduction of the arm.

For some patients with subluxation or incompletely reduced dislocations, subsequent acromioclavicular arthritis becomes sufficiently painful to warrant treatment.

In both of these categories, resection of the outer 2 cm of the clavicle with or without repair of the coracoclavicular ligamentous supports is the procedure of choice.

Typical Deformity

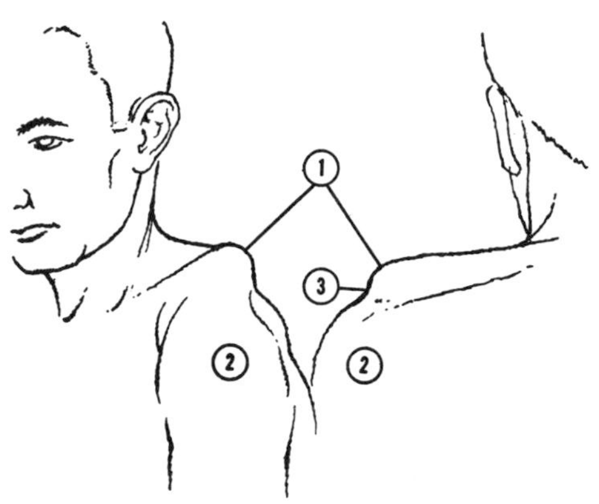

1. Clavicle is unduly prominent.
2. Shoulder droops forward and downward.
3. Wide sulcus is apparent between the acromion process and clavicle.

X-Ray of Acromioclavicular Arthritis

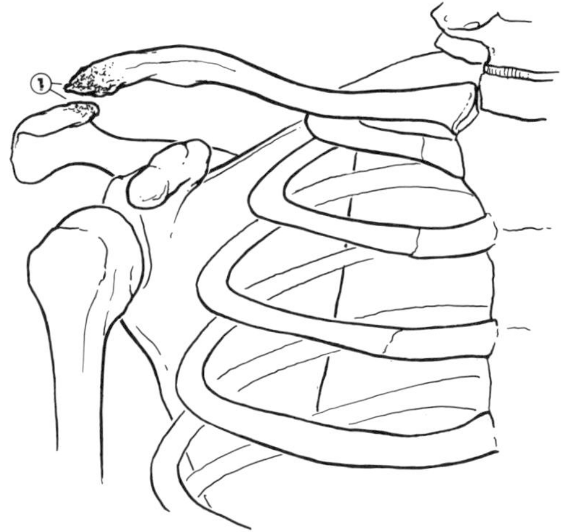

1. Partially reduced clavicle has developed symptomatic traumatic arthritis.

Postoperative X-Ray (After Resection of the Lateral Clavicle)

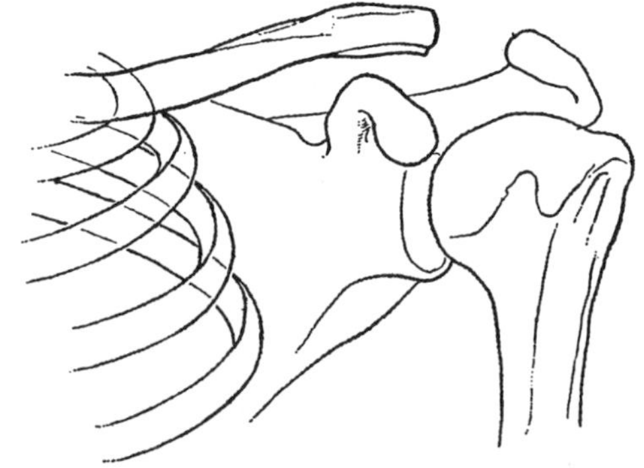

Approximately 2 cm of the outer end of the clavicle has been resected.

If the remaining portion of the clavicle is prominent, the coracoclavicular ligament can be repaired, as previously described with the Weaver-Dunn procedure.

■ Dislocations of the Medial Clavicle Growth Plate or Sternoclavicular Joint

REMARKS

The sternoclavicular joint is one of the least frequently dislocated joints in the body. This is due to the fact that the ligament supports are so strong that it takes a considerable force from either direct or indirect mechanisms to disrupt this protected joint.

These injuries are mainly injuries of the immature skeletal system; therefore, they are discussed more completely in the chapter on childhood epiphyseal plate injuries (see Chapter 2).

In adults, the sternoclavicular joint can be occasionally subject either to traumatic or atraumatic problems.

Arthritis either from trauma or other causes may also occasionally locate in this joint.

Most sternoclavicular dislocations are anterior, but a few are posterior. Posterior dislocations are of the greatest concern because they are likely to compromise the structures of the mediastinum beneath the joint.

Because most of these injuries in younger individuals are epiphyseal injuries, the medial prominence from the epiphyseal separation usually remodels, and normal alignment is restored.

In the adult (older than 25 years of age), anterior dislocation usually recurs or persists because it is not an epiphyseal injury. Consequently, the prominence of the medial clavicle may not remodel. However, this is rarely a functional or cosmetic problem.

Clinical Presentation

1. Typical appearance of the anterior sternoclavicular dislocation in the adult is a lump on the medial portion of the clavicle. In most instances, this results from a significant direct or indirect injury to the shoulder. Occasionally, it may be mistaken for a tumor if the patient cannot recall any injury to this area.

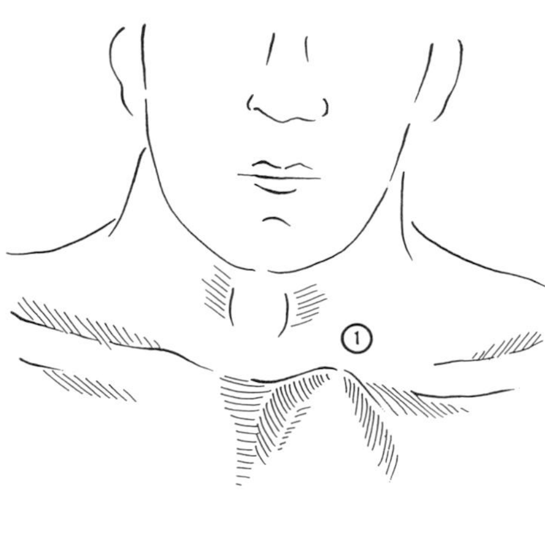

Diagnosis

1. Diagnosis with chronic dislocation is confirmed by CT. It is particularly important to determine whether mediastinal structures have been involved in the dislocation.
2. Posterior dislocation can cause significant involvement of mediastinal structures.

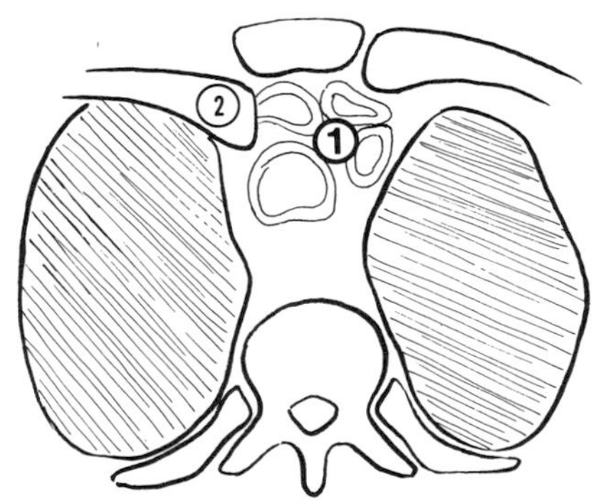

3. Anterior dislocation causes the anterior prominence but does not put the mediastinal structures at risk.

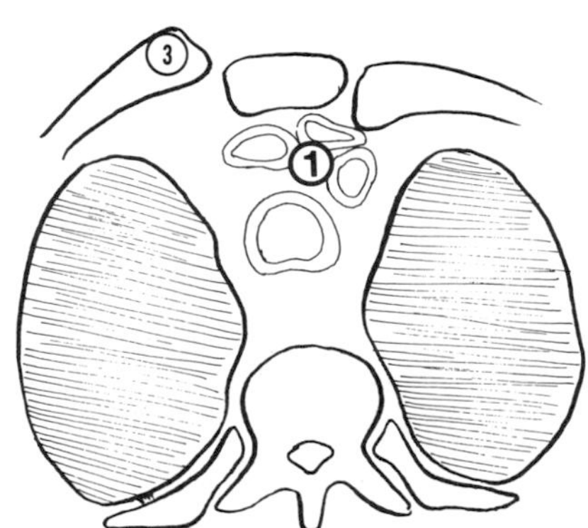

Unreduced Anterior Dislocation

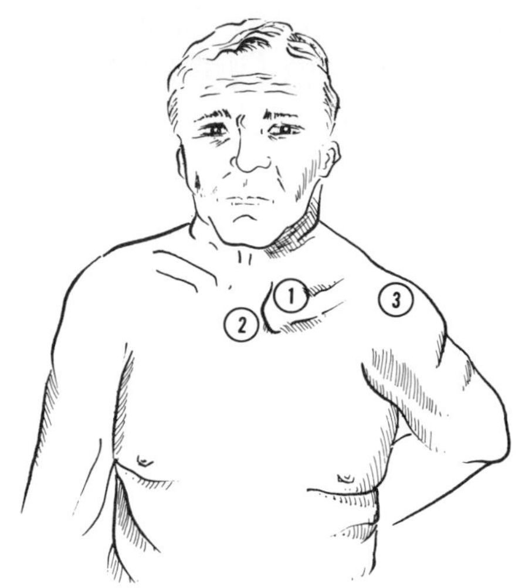

1. Patient had an anterior dislocation of the left sternoclavicular joint, which cannot be adequately reduced.
2. He has persistent excessively prominent medial clavicle, which is essentially asymptomatic.
3. He has full range of motion of the shoulder and no functional impairment in spite of the medial prominence of the clavicle.

Note: Most patients who sustain this injury are laborers or individuals subject to shoulder trauma and probably are best treated by functional exercises in spite of failure of reduction or recurrence of the dislocation.

If the patient is sufficiently symptomatic, the medial portion of the clavicle may be excised, and the clavicle may be stabilized to the underlying first rib.

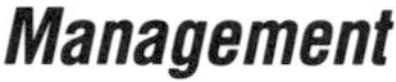

Management

An acute fracture or dislocation is reduced by the techniques described previously in Chapter 2.

In chronic dislocations, the patient is best treated symptomatically with range-of-motion exercises. Resection or reconstruction of the clavicle is likely to cause more symptoms than is the dislocation.

If the patient experiences chronic pain symptoms, the treatment of choice is resection rather than attempted reconstruction of the joint.

Resection is particularly indicated for the rare posterior dislocation that cannot be reduced by closed manipulative techniques.

Resection and Stabilization for Unreduced Anterior or Posterior Dislocations

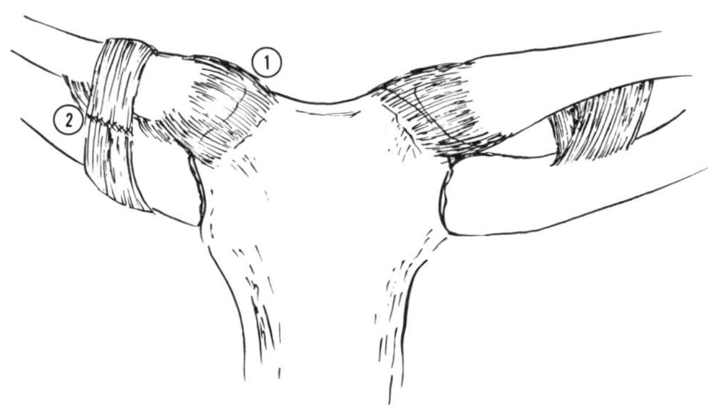

1. Medial 2 cm of the clavicle is resected with beveling of the anterior corner of the clavicle.
2. Remaining portion of the clavicle is stabilized to the first rib with heavy Dacron tape to reinforce the costoclavicular ligaments.

Caution: Avoid any internal fixation of the sternoclavicular joint with transarticular pins. These are notoriously likely to migrate and involve great vessels or other structures within the mediastinum.

Fractures of the Scapula

REMARKS

Fractures of the scapula are usually the result of severe direct injury to the posterior aspect of the shoulder.

The most common mechanism is a motor vehicle–pedestrian accident or a fall on the shoulder.

Close to 100 per cent of these injuries are associated with rib fractures, pulmonary contusions, pneumothorax, or hemopneumothorax. Head injury is also fairly common.

Ipsilateral clavicle fractures and cervical fractures or cord injuries are also associated with scapular fractures.

Because of the frequency of other associated injuries, the treatment of the scapular fracture is frequently only a secondary consideration. Fortunately, most of these injuries can be treated symptomatically with minimal residual long-term problems.

Common Types of Fractures of Scapula

1. Fracture of the body.
2. Fracture of the spine.
3. Fracture of the acromion.
4. Fracture of the base of the coracoid process.

Note: Fractures of the acromion are frequently associated with underlying injuries to the rotator cuff. If shoulder weakness persists for 6 weeks or longer after these fractures, evaluate the rotator cuff mechanism by means of a shoulder arthrogram.

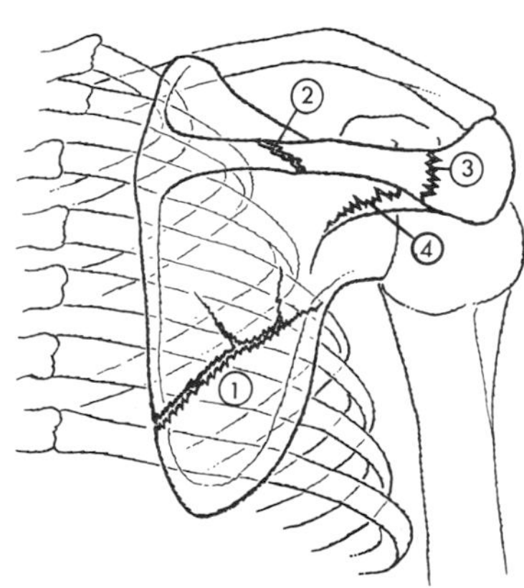

Normal Variance That May Be Mistaken for Fractures of the Scapula: Os Acromiale

1. Occasionally, a normal variant may be seen in the acromion, which may be mistaken for a fracture.
2. Varying patterns exist, which result from separation of the ossification center and are known as os acromiale. This normal variant is considerably more common than a fracture of the acromion and should be suspected before the diagnosis of fracture of the acromion is made. The patient may be tender in the region from a direct blow to the shoulder, but the typical sclerosis of the bone edges on the x-ray differentiates this abnormality of ossification from a fracture.

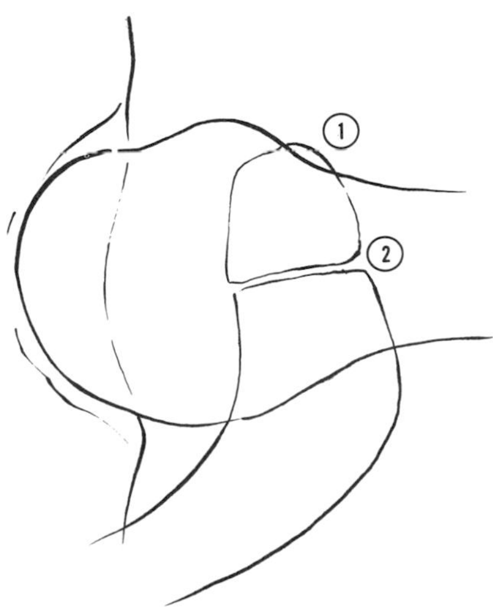

Management

By far, most scapular fractures can be treated symptomatically.

Because many of these patients have other injuries, such as rib fractures or hemothorax, the scapular fracture is initially treated with bed rest, ice applications, and analgesics.

When the patient becomes ambulatory, a compression bandage can be used to hold the scapula firmly against the chest wall. The arm is suspended in a sling.

1. Firm compression bandage using stockinette or moleskin to fix the scapula against the chest wall.
2. Suspend the arm in a sling.

Note: An alternate might also be a Velpeau sling.

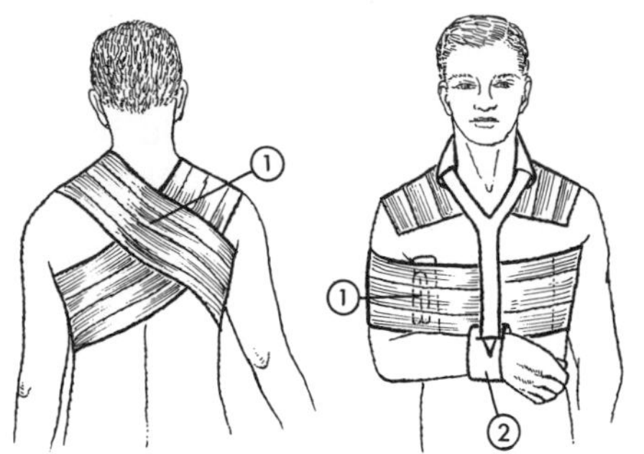

Subsequent Management

By 10–14 days, the shoulder wrap can be removed, and the patient is encouraged to use the shoulder actively to regain motion.

A program of pendulum exercises is begun and increased in range and frequency until the full range of motion is achieved.

Occasionally, there is persistent weakness of abduction as a result of hemorrhage into the deltoid or rotator cuff muscles. For the most part, these problems of weakness subside by 2–3 months as the swelling and hemorrhage are resorbed. However, some discomfort and residual weakness may be evident for a number of months with more severe fractures.

Fractures of the Neck of the Scapula

REMARKS

Fractures of the neck of the scapula usually are undisplaced. The articular surface of the glenoid is usually not disturbed, and the glenohumeral joint is intact.

For most of these fractures, anatomic reduction is not essential to obtain a good functional result.

Occasionally, if the fracture of the neck of the scapula displaces sufficiently, the rotator cuff muscles may lose their leverage and result in weakening of the shoulder.

This is especially likely if the fracture of the neck of the scapula is associated with a fracture of the clavicle. The consequence of this combination is that the fractures displace inferiorly, causing a drooped shoulder appearance. This represents a rare indication for operative treatment of a scapular fracture.

With Minimal Displacement

Appearance on X-Ray

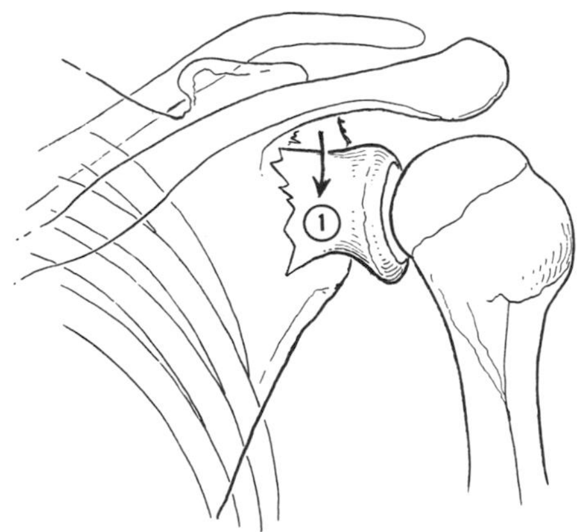

1. Glenoid fracture is displaced inward and slightly downward. The clavicle is intact and is supporting the shoulder.

Management

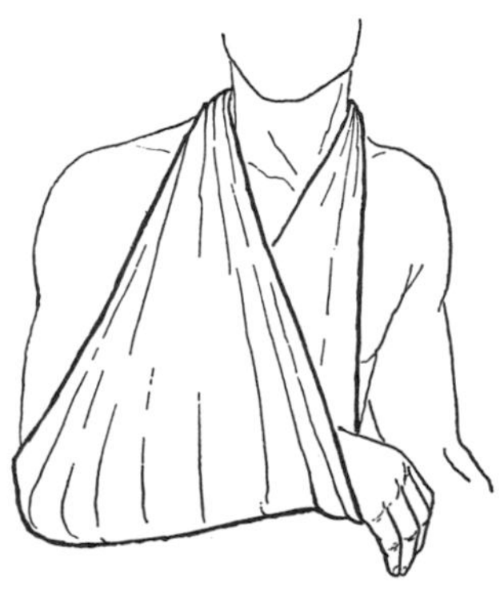

Apply ice for the first 24–36 hours; then apply heat.

Apply a triangular sling.

After 10–14 days, begin graduated active exercises of the shoulder within the tolerance of pain.

Institute daily heat application and gentle massage to all the soft tissues of the shoulder girdle.

Discard the sling after 3 or 4 weeks, and gradually increase the range and frequency of the pendulum exercises.

With Marked Displacement

These scapular fractures more often require treatment by traction or operative fixation.

The displaced scapular fracture may cause impairment of shoulder function, either as a result of dislocation or subluxation. Because of these potential problems, operative fixation may be necessary.

Marked Displacement

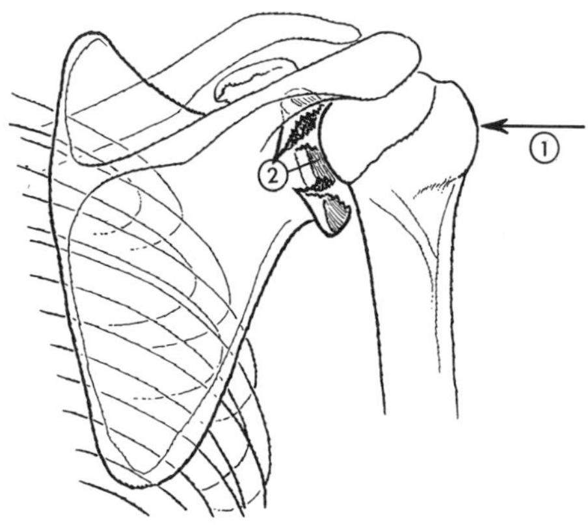

1. Direct force applied to the lateral side of the shoulder produces
2. Stellate fracture of the glenoid with severe comminution and separation of the fragments.

Note: Because of the comminution of the glenoid, the shoulder is likely to be unstable and dislocate. Operative fixation is necessary to repair fractures of the glenoid of this type and restore shoulder stability.

Management of Scapular Neck Fractures With Marked Displacement Associated With a Fractured Clavicle

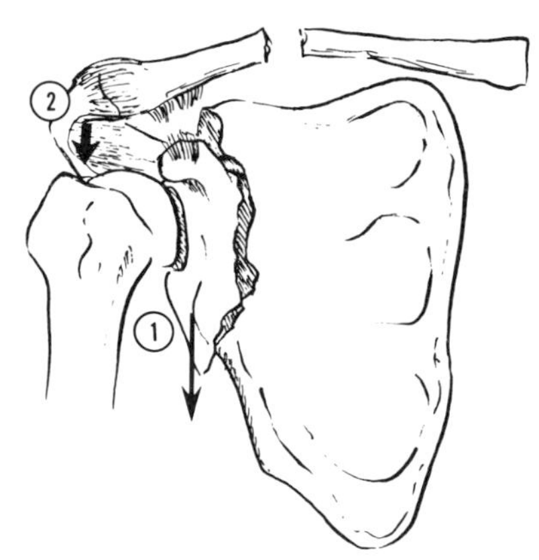

1. Fracture of the scapular neck is displaced downward and medially.
2. Fracture of the clavicle also displaces downward, allowing the shoulder to droop.

Note: Drooping of the shoulder may be permanent and also be associated with some residual weakness of the rotator cuff. For this reason, treatment with a period of traction or, occasionally, operative intervention may be necessary.

Reduction by Lateral Traction

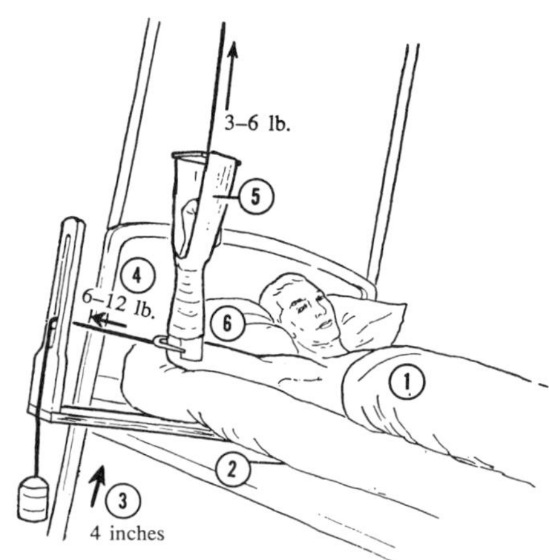

1. Patient assumes the supine position.
2. Place a board under the mattress.
3. Elevate the side of the bed 10 cm.
4. Apply skeletal traction through the base of the olecranon and add 6–12 lb (2.7–5.4 kg).
5. Apply traction to the forearm and add 3–6 lb (1.4–2.7 kg).
6. Traction is made with the arm abducted 90° and the forearm flexed 90°.

Note: Maintain traction for 2–3 weeks.

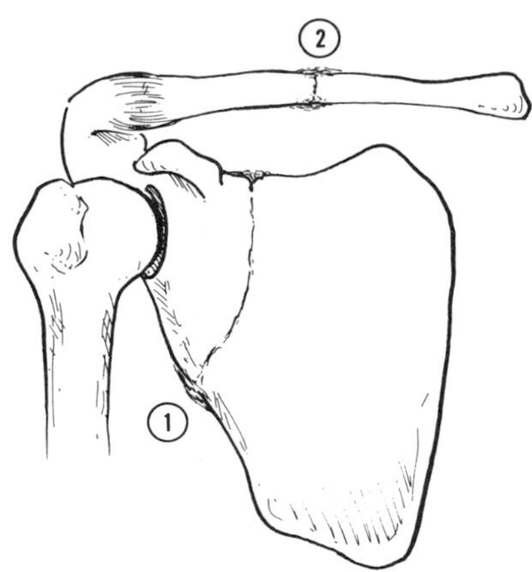

Postreduction X-Ray

1. Downward displacement of the arm and scapular neck have been corrected with early callus evident.
2. Fractured clavicle is also healing with callus sufficient to prevent progressive drooping of the shoulder.

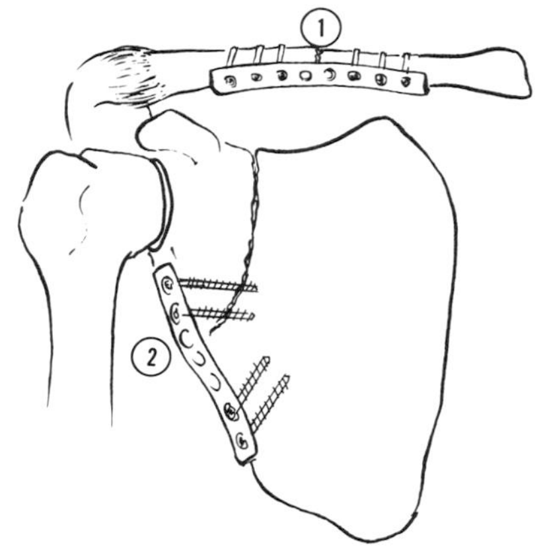

Alternative Method: Surgical Fixation

1. Unstable drooping of the shoulder can be treated by plate fixation of the clavicle and
2. Plate fixation of the scapular neck fracture.

Note: This fixation of the scapula is a fairly difficult approach and is best reserved for surgeons familiar with the anatomy of the posterior aspect of the shoulder and its relationship to the brachial plexus. In most cases, the displaced scapular neck fracture can be adequately treated by other nonoperative methods.

■ Fractures of the Glenoid

Mechanisms of Injury

REMARKS

Fractures of the glenoid are produced by either a direct or an indirect mechanism.

Direct Mechanism: Stellate Fracture

A direct force applied to the lateral side of the shoulder produces a stellate type of fracture; the degree of displacement of the fragments depends on the intensity of the force.

Most stellate fractures require no reduction because the glenoid articular surface can tolerate much incongruity and still function normally; the glenohumeral joint is not a weight-bearing joint.

In severely displaced stellate fractures, an attempt should be made to reduce the deformity.

Minimal Displacement

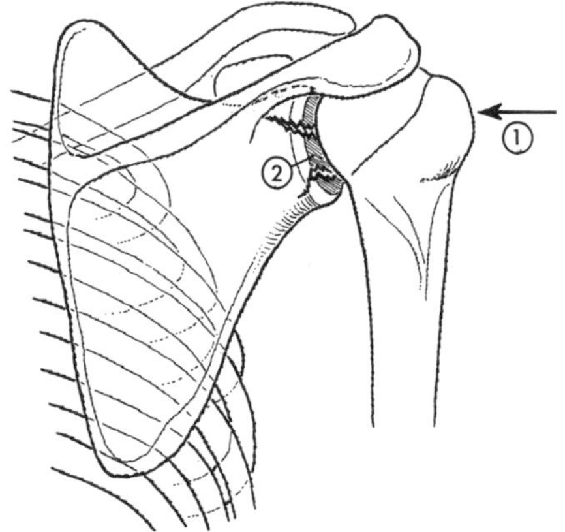

1. Direct force is applied to the lateral side of the shoulder, and
2. Stellate fracture of the glenoid with minimal displacement of the fragments occurs.

Indirect Mechanism

An indirect mechanism acts when the victim falls on the outstretched arm or flexed elbow.

An alternative mechanism is a fracture associated with an anterior or posterior dislocation of the shoulder.

The site at which the glenoid fracture is sheared off depends on the direction in which the humeral head is displaced. If it is displaced forward, a segment of the anterior aspect of the glenoid is sheared off.

If the humeral head is displaced backward, a portion of the posterior rim of the glenoid is displaced.

Management may be nonoperative if the glenoid rim fracture is not displaced. However, most displaced glenoid rim fractures require operative fixation because there is usually soft tissue disruption and subsequent shoulder instability.

Posterior Glenoid Fracture

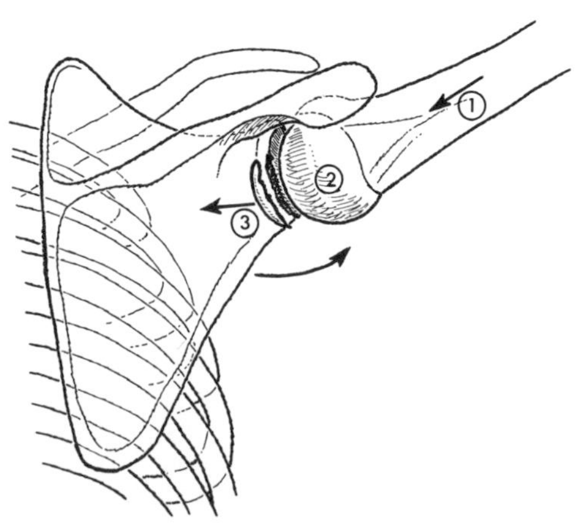

1. Force travels along the shaft of the humerus, which is flexed and abducted.
2. Head of the humerus abuts against the posterior portion of the glenoid.
3. Segment of the glenoid is driven backward.

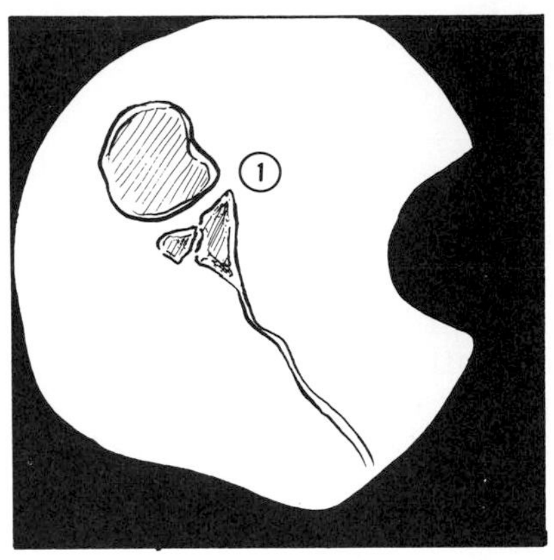

Computed Tomographic View

1. A CT scan of the shoulder is frequently helpful to demonstrate the amount of fracture displacement and irregularity of the glenoid surface not evident from the plain x-ray.

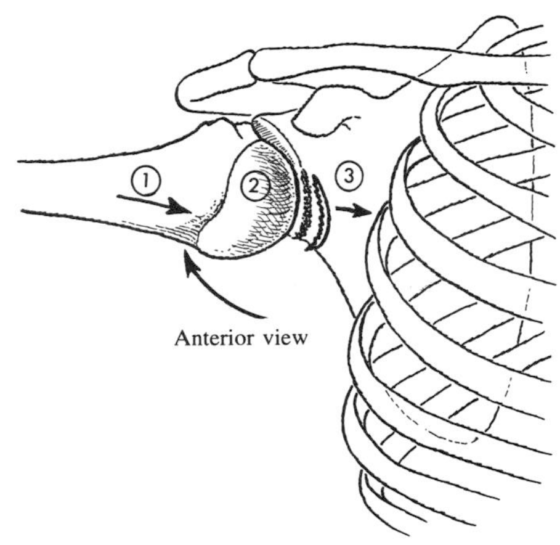

Anterior Glenoid Rim Fracture

1. Humeral head is forcibly abducted and externally rotated, producing an anterior subluxation or dislocation.
2. Head of the humerus shears off the anterior portion of the glenoid.
3. Segment of the glenoid with the capsular attachment is displaced forward.

Management of Fractures of the Glenoid

Stellate Fractures

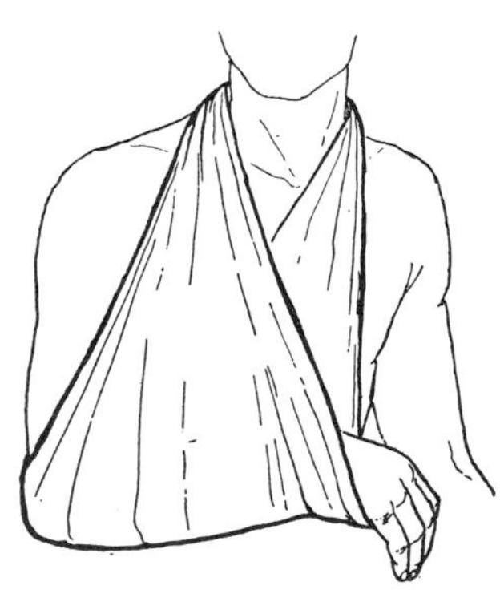

Apply a triangular sling for 2 weeks.

Institute progressive shoulder exercises on a regulated program (5 or 10 minutes every hour).

Note: If the patient has signs of shoulder instability, i.e., either subluxation or recurrent dislocation, operative repair of the capsule and bone fragments or Bankart lesion may be necessary subsequently.

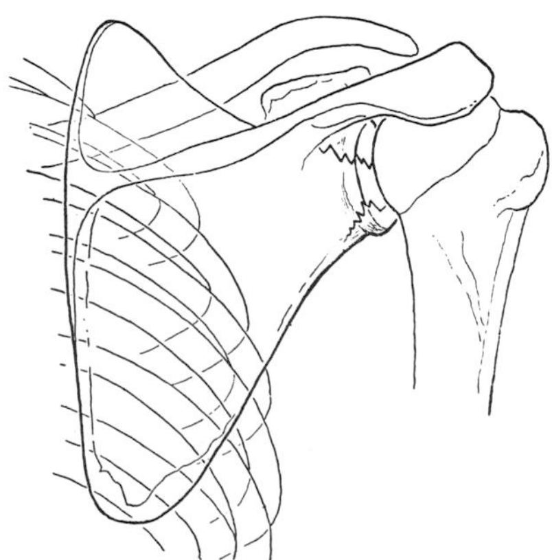

Postreduction X-Ray

Normal configuration of the glenoid fossa is restored.

Operative Management of Specific Glenoid Rim Fractures

Fractures of the glenoid rim can lead to shoulder instability, which requires operative repair. This is true even for minimally displaced fractures.

Fractures of the anterior or posterior portion of the glenoid result from dislocations of the shoulder and are frequently associated with recurrent instability and pain in the shoulder.

Even "minor," barely perceptible fractures of the inferior glenoid may produce symptoms of recurrent pain and subluxation, particularly in young, active individuals.

The larger fracture results most often from the humeral head impacting violently against the anterior glenoid rim at the time of the dislocation. The same mechanism produces the Hill-Sachs lesion, or a compression fracture of the posterolateral aspect of the humeral head.

A small inferior glenoid fracture may result from an avulsion mechanism that occurs when the shoulder is forcefully externally rotated and abducted, stretching the capsular attachment to the glenoid labrum.

Symptoms of shoulder pain and clicking or subluxation after such an avulsion injury can be confusing because the shoulder may never completely dislocate. The physician should search carefully on the x-ray for inferior glenoid rim fractures that would indicate the nature of the patient's problem.

Examples of Fractures

1. Fractures of the anterior portion of the glenoid with minimal displacement.
2. Fractures of the posterior portion of the glenoid with minimal displacement.
3. Avulsion fractures of the glenoid rim (associated with dislocations of the glenohumeral joint).
4. Avulsion fractures of the inferior glenoid rim caused by severe contracture of the triceps. This occurs most often in athletes who throw.

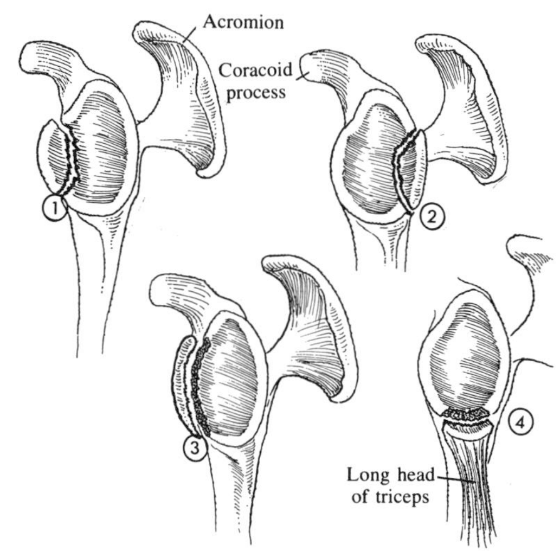

Anterior Glenoid Fracture Associated With Recurrent Dislocation

1. Fracture of the anterior portion of the glenoid.
2. Fragment is displaced forward more than 1 cm.

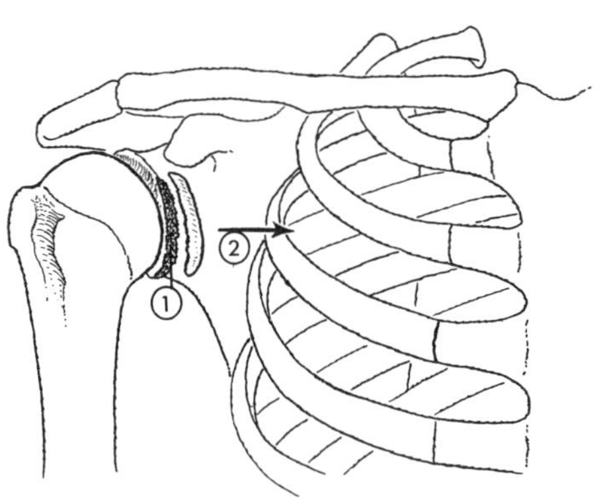

Avulsion Fracture Associated With Recurrent Shoulder Subluxation

1. Oblique axillary view is necessary to see the anterior inferior glenoid fracture.
2. Subtle fracture indicates the location of the avulsion injury that is producing the symptoms of pain and instability on external rotation and abduction of the shoulder.

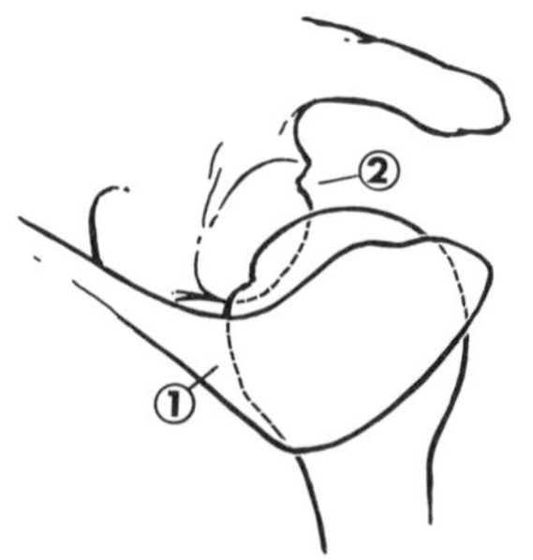

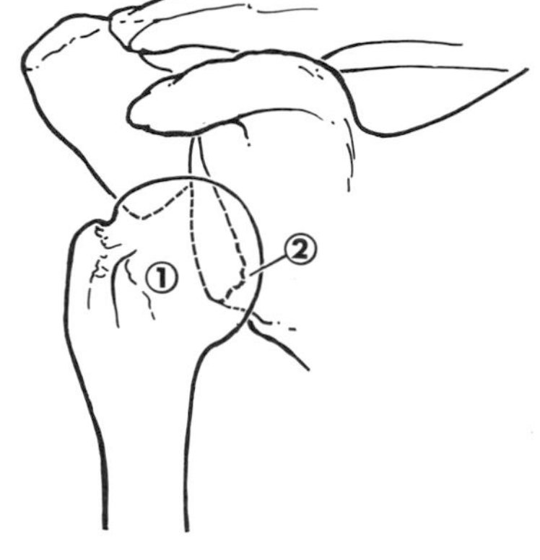

Anteroposterior View of Subluxation

1. Anterior subluxation of the humeral head produces a
2. Subtle small avulsion fracture of the inferior glenoid.

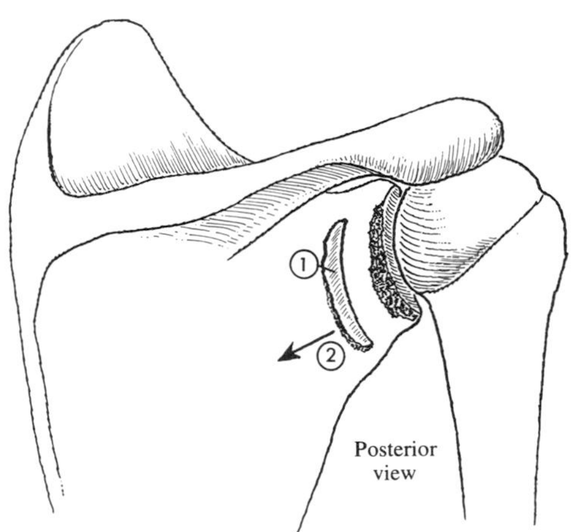

Posterior Avulsion Fracture

1. Fracture of the posterior portion of the glenoid.
2. Fragment is separated more than 1 cm.

Note: Frequently, this injury is associated with recurrent posterior instability and usually should be repaired.

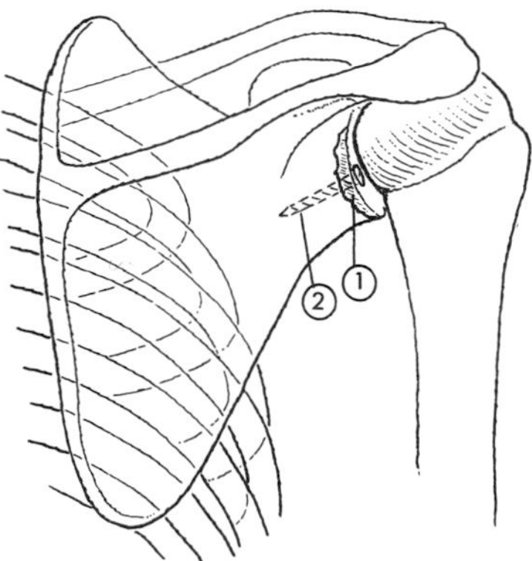

Operative Management

1. Fragment that is displaced is best reduced operatively and fixed along with the torn capsule or Bankart lesion.
2. Although a screw may be used for fixation, it is preferable to use sutures into the bone, which are less likely to loosen or migrate.

■ Dislocation of the Scapula

REMARKS

Although rare, dislocation of the scapula occasionally is encountered.

Manipulative maneuvers will reduce the displaced scapula.

Open reduction is usually not necessary.

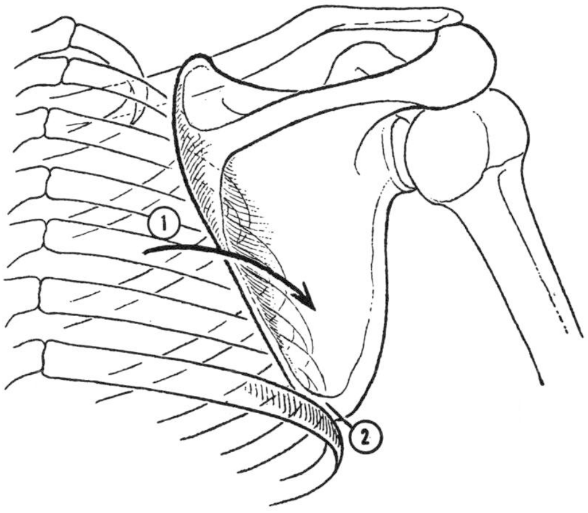

Prereduction X-Ray

1. Entire body of scapula is displaced outward and rotated outward.
2. Lower angle is wedged between the ribs.

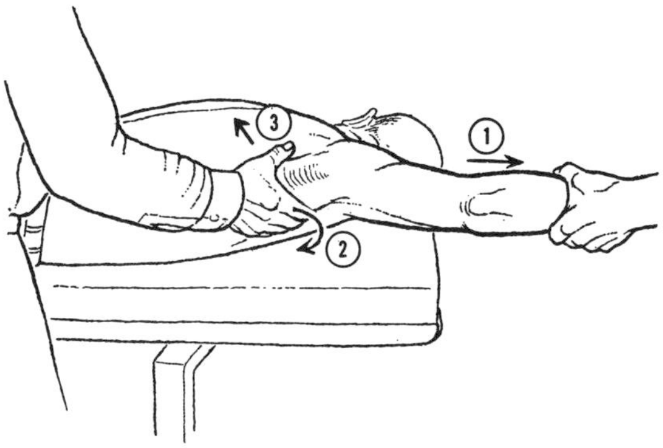

Manipulative Reduction

1. Assistant makes steady traction on the hyperabducted arm.
2. Surgeon grasps axillary border of scapula and, by the same movement, rotates the bone forward and
3. Pushes the scapula directly backward.

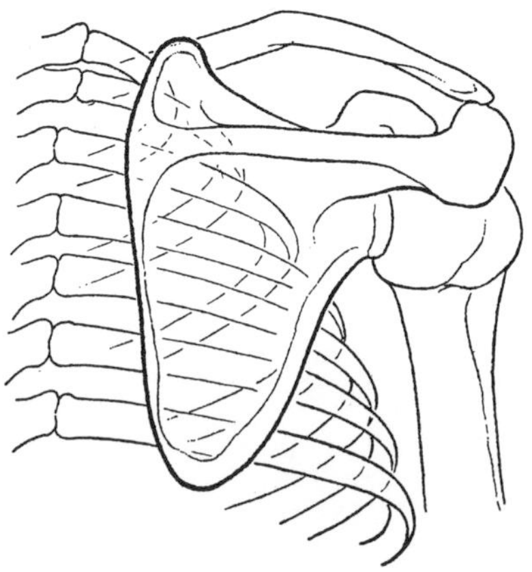

Postreduction X-Ray

Scapula has returned to its normal anatomic position.

Strapping and Immobilization

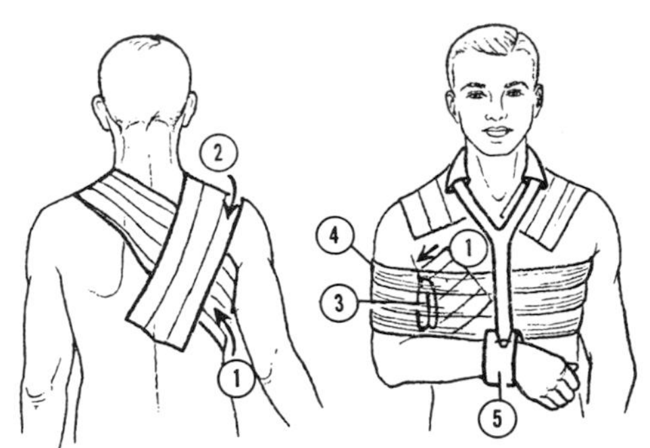

Use 8 or 10 long strips of 7.5-cm adhesive.

1. Beginning in front of the chest, pass the strips under the arm, over the scapula, and around the chest to the top of the opposite shoulder.
2. Apply three strips over the affected shoulder from front to back.
3. Place a large cotton pad in the axilla.
4. Bind the arm to the side with a 10-cm bias-cut stockinette encircling the body.
5. Support the forearm with a collar-and-cuff sling.

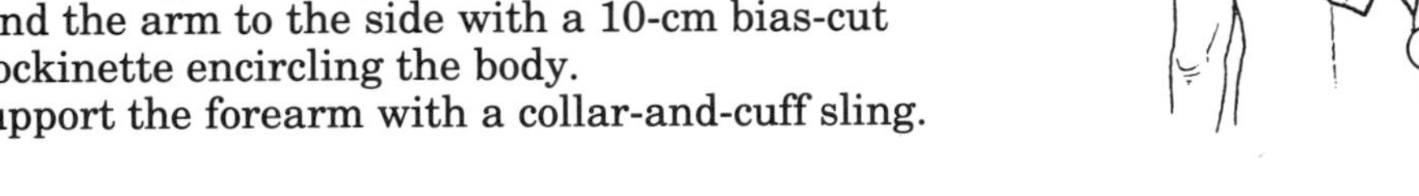

Postreduction Care

Reinforce the dressing after 7–10 days.

Discard the dressing after 2 weeks.

Encourage active free use of shoulder within the patient's tolerance of pain.

Institute a regulated program of active exercises for the shoulder, hand, and fingers.

Normal function usually is achieved in 4–6 weeks.

Traumatic Lateral Scapula Displacement: Scapulothoracic Dissociation

REMARKS

This severe traumatic injury, the scapulothoracic dissociation, has also been called a closed forequarter amputation.

It results from a highly violent wrenching injury to the shoulder, which is characterized by massive muscle disruption, and results in lateral displacement of the scapula on the chest wall.

A typical mechanism is severe direct trauma to the shoulder as a result of a fall off a speeding motorcycle.

These patients frequently have multiple injuries, and the essential nature of the scapular injury may not be recognized at first.

Because of the complete separation of the scapula and upper extremity from the thoracic attachments, i.e., scapulothoracic dissociation, serious neurovascular injury almost invariably is present.

Frequently, the only external sign of this serious injury is massive swelling and ecchymosis of the anterior and posterior aspects of the shoulder.

Diagnosis

1. Radiographic diagnosis depends on a nonrotated chest film that allows accurate measurement of the distance of the scapular border from the spinous processes in the midline.
2. Greater than 1 cm of lateral displacement of the scapula compared with the uninjured side usually indicates significant soft tissue disruption consistent with a scapulothoracic dissociation.
3. Associated injuries also include clavicular fractures or
4. Acromioclavicular or sternoclavicular dislocations.

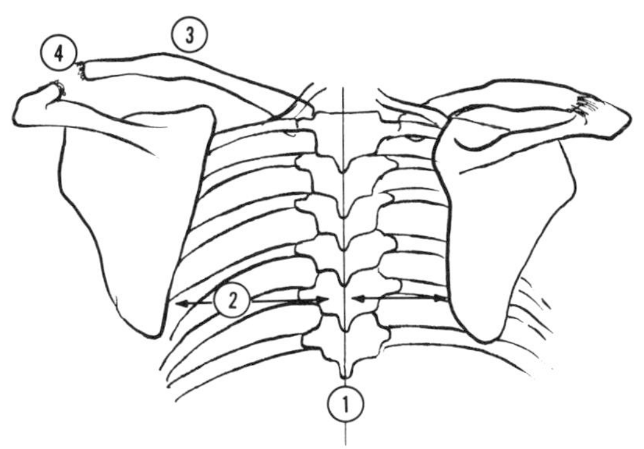

Management

If scapulothoracic displacement or dissociation is recognized, it is important to evaluate carefully for neurovascular injury.

Most of these injuries produce significant avulsion of the deltoid, pectoral, or other muscles and the brachial plexus and axillary vessels.

When limb ischemia is evident, emergent revascularization is indicated.

Above-elbow amputation has been recommended if complete anatomic disruption of the brachial plexus has occurred; however, this is rarely done in practice.

A few case reports have been published of scapulothoracic dissociation without neurovascular compromise. However, for most, management of this injury is primarily directed at restoration or correction of the vascular injury to prevent exsanguination or complete ischemia of the limb.

If there is complete avulsion of the brachial plexus at the nerve root level, surgical repair has not been possible in most reported cases.

GLENOHUMERAL DISLOCATIONS AND SUBLUXATIONS

REMARKS

The glenohumeral joint is the most mobile and unstable joint in the body.

Only 25–30 per cent of the humeral head is covered by the glenoid in any position.

The capsule of the shoulder is a relatively lax and redundant structure to allow the wide mobility required of the glenohumeral articulation.

The chief question is not why the glenohumeral joint is subject to frequent dislocations but why it does not dislocate all the time.

The answer to these questions appears to be due to the intrinsic architecture and pressure within the joint as well as the ligaments and muscles about the joint.

Stabilizing Mechanisms of the Shoulder

REMARKS

The usual structures considered to be the important stabilizers of the shoulder include the capsular ligament and muscles about the joint.

The capsule is particularly important in resisting anterior or posterior dislocation of the humeral head out of the relatively shallow glenoid. The important stabilizers of the shoulder joint that prevent anterior or posterior displacement are the capsular ligaments, particularly the middle and inferior glenohumeral ligaments.

The evidence is that a major force preventing downward dislocation of the glenohumeral joint is atmospheric pressure. The difference in colloid osmotic pressure of normal synovial fluid within the joint and the pressure outside the joint creates a negative intra-articular pressure of approximately −4 mm Hg. The consequence is that the humeral head is maintained in the glenoid by a suction effect, which is eliminated by puncturing the capsule.

Anatomic studies point out that the capsule looseness is so great inferiorly and superiorly that the arm should fall about 2.5 cm from the scapula if the muscles were dissected. However, this occurs only if the capsule is punctured to allow atmospheric air to gain access into the joint and eliminate the negative suction effect.

The muscles about the shoulder contribute minimally to shoulder stability, except for the rare patient with involuntary instability who can subluxate the shoulder by unbalanced muscle activity. For most patients with shoulder instability, the major defect is caused by the capsular ligaments and attachments of these ligaments to the glenoid and the glenoid labrum.

Glenohumeral Structures

1. Capsule is extremely loose and redundant superiorly and inferiorly to allow full range of motion of the shoulder joint.
2. Only about 30 per cent of the humeral head is covered by or articulates with the glenoid. This is slightly increased by the labrum, which deepens the glenoid.
3. Biceps tendon is an intra-articular structure, which passes through the capsule. However, this is carefully sealed off to prevent communication with the extra-articular structures. Because of this normally tightly sealed capsule, the intra-articular pressure is below atmospheric pressure. This is the major mechanism preventing downward subluxation of the joint.

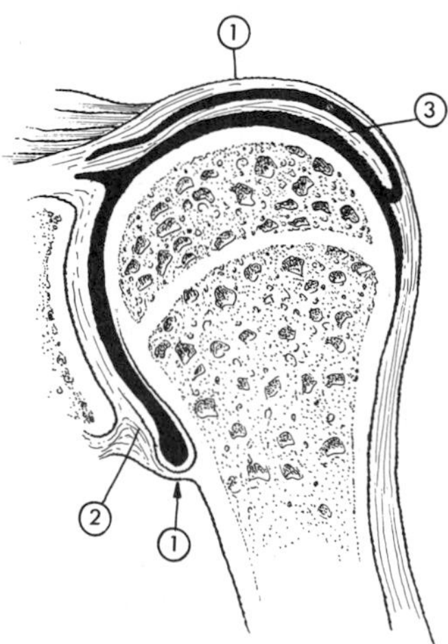

Redundancy of the Glenohumeral Capsule

1. Glenohumeral capsule is redundant to allow for the great mobility of the shoulder.
2. Glenohumeral joint space communicates with the subscapularis recess.
3. Additional communication with the bicipital sheath occurs.
4. This seals off generally around the region of the transverse humeral ligament. This sealing off of the redundant capsule permits the capsule to maintain a negative intra-articular pressure relative to atmospheric pressure.

Note: The glenohumeral joint does not communicate with the subacromial space.

■ Stabilizing Structures

Glenohumeral Ligaments

Glenohumeral Ligaments (From Behind)

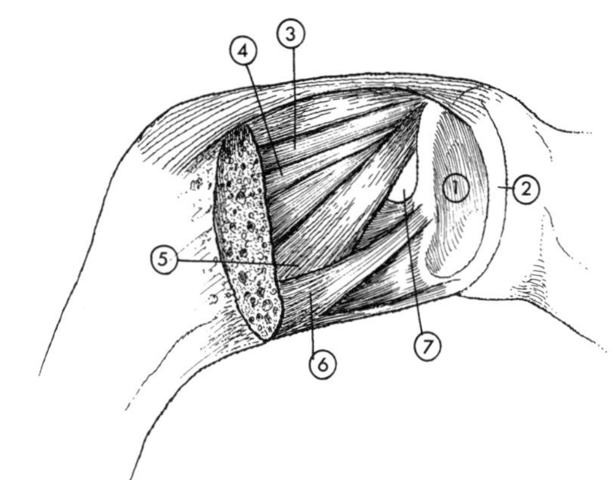

1. Glenoid fossa.
2. Glenoid labrum.
3. Biceps (long head).
4. Superior glenohumeral ligament.
5. Middle glenohumeral ligament.
6. Inferior glenohumeral ligament.
7. Subscapularis recess.

Note: Observe that all three ligaments are directed toward the superior aspect of the glenoid fossa.

The subscapularis recess communicates with the inside of the joint cavity.

Stabilizing Mechanism of the Shoulder Against Gravity

NEGATIVE INTRA-ARTICULAR HYDROSTATIC PRESSURE

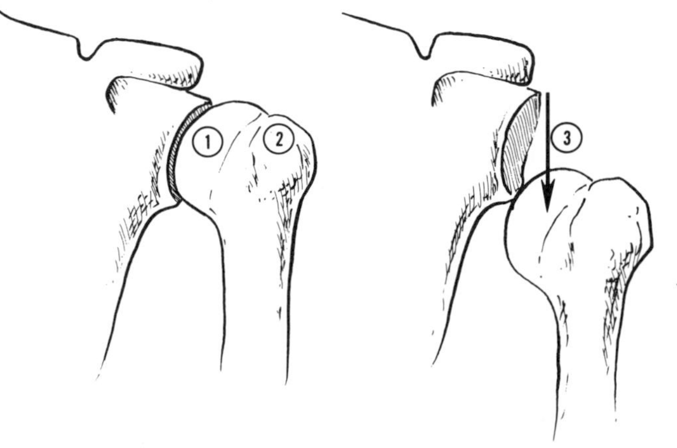

1. Normally, the humeral head remains articulating with the glenoid in spite of forces of gravity pulling it downward or the application of heavy weights to the arm.
2. Even if the muscles about the shoulder are completely anesthetized, this relationship is normally maintained.
3. If the glenohumeral joint is merely punctured with a needle, the negative intra-articular hydrostatic pressure can be lost, and the humeral head can be demonstrated to sublux inferiorly within the redundant axillary fold of the capsule. This indicates that atmospheric pressure is important to stabilize the shoulder against downward displacement.

Muscles

REMARKS

The important muscles that envelop the glenohumeral joint consist of two muscular sleeves, an inner sleeve made up of the rotator cuff muscles and an outer sleeve consisting of the deltoid, the teres major, and the pectoralis major.

These two groups of muscles operate one within the other and are separated by an efficient gliding mechanism consisting of the subacromial bursa and fine, filmy areolar tissue.

The function of the muscular groups or sleeves is mainly active range of motion. The muscle contribution to stability of the shoulder is relatively insignificant.

Imbalance of the muscles about the shoulder may occasionally produce voluntary subluxation. Except for these individuals, the importance of muscle strengthening or reconditioning exercises is relatively minimal for the unstable shoulder.

A number of procedures have been developed to transfer muscles about the shoulders to correct instability, but these may not address the underlying problem, which is damage to the capsule ligaments that are the important stabilizers of the shoulder.

Because of the arrangement of the rotator cuff muscles about the shoulder, these are frequently injured at the time of either acute dislocation or chronic repetitive impingement. The subscapularis tendon is particularly at risk from acute anterior dislocation.

The supraspinatus tendon is also commonly avulsed in acute anterior dislocation, particularly in the elderly patient with relatively weak bone structure.

Shoulder Musculature (Superior View)

Note: The contribution of muscles to shoulder stability is minimal. However, the rotator cuff muscles, particularly the supraspinatus and subscapularis, are commonly injured at the time of acute dislocation. This may cause some residual weakness of the shoulder after the dislocation is reduced.

1. Supraspinatus.
2. Subscapularis.
3. Infraspinatus.
4. Musculotendinous cuff.
5. Acromion.
6. Coracoacromial ligament.
7. Deltoid.
8. Coracoid process.
9. Coracohumeral ligament.
10. Pectoralis minor.

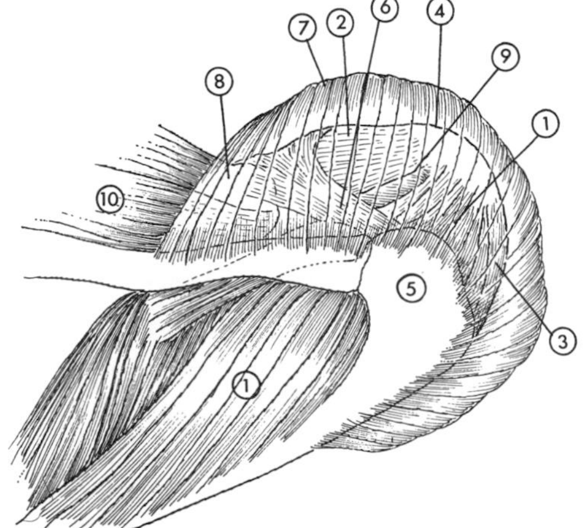

Functional Mechanism of Muscles of the Glenohumeral Joint

REMARKS

Abduction and flexion of the humerus are achieved by the synchronous action of two groups of muscles. The first group includes the deltoid, supraspinatus, and pectoralis major. The second group consists of the infraspinatus, teres minor, and subscapularis.

The latter group constitutes a functional unit that depresses the humeral head and fixes it firmly against the glenoid so that the former group can abduct and flex the arm. Without the stabilizing effect of the rotator muscles, the deltoid would pull the humerus vertically under the acromion.

The rotator muscles pass from the scapula posteriorly, superiorly, and anteriorly and blend with one another and the fibrous capsule to form a tough musculotendinous cuff around the head of the humerus before inserting into the humerus. Together, they hold the head of the humerus snugly against the glenoid while the deltoid elevates the arm.

Neurovascular Structures Near the Joint

REMARKS

Neurovascular structures may be injured during a dislocation or the reduction of a dislocation of the glenohumeral joint.

Large Neurovascular Structures Most Often Injured

1. Axillary artery and brachial plexus.
2. Musculocutaneous nerve.
3. Clavicle.
4. Deltoid.
5. Pectoralis minor.
6. Biceps.
7. Pectoralis major.
8. Subscapularis.
9. Teres major.
10. Coracobrachialis.

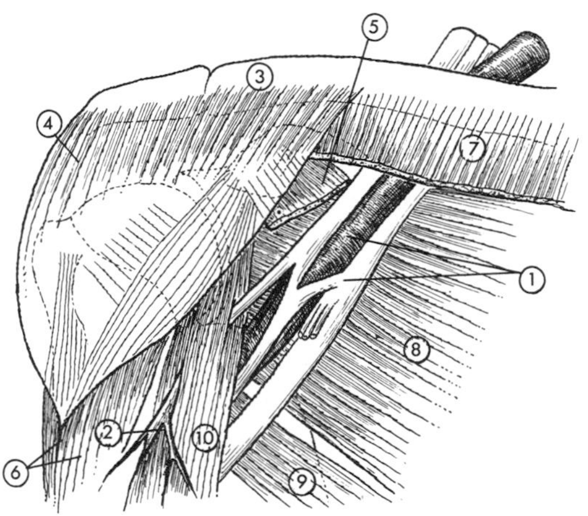

Axillary Nerve

1. Infraspinatus.
2. Teres minor.
3. Teres major.
4. Triceps muscle.
5. Quadrangular space.
6. Axillary nerve.
7. Anterior branch of axillary nerve.
8. Posterior branch of axillary nerve.
9. Cutaneous branch of posterior branch of axillary nerve.
10. Nerve to teres minor.

Note: The axillary nerve is by far the most common nerve injured at the time of acute dislocation. Careful electromyographic studies have shown there may be some damage to as many as 30 per cent of shoulder dislocations. The nerve also must be carefully protected during surgical procedures to repair recurrent dislocations.

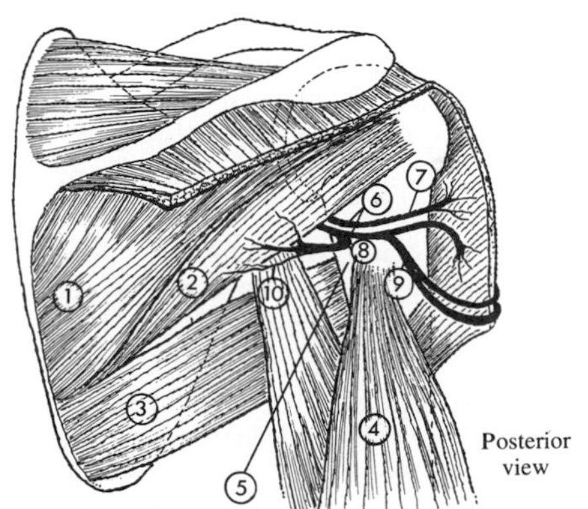

Normal Motions of the Shoulder and Causes of Dislocations

REMARKS

The upper arm possesses a global range of motion (almost 360°). This consists of the summation of the ranges of motion possible in four articulations, i.e., the glenohumeral, sternoclavicular, acromioclavicular, and thoracoscapular joints.

Although the relationships of these structures vary from individual to individual, in general, for every 15° of motion, 10° occurs at the glenohumeral joint and 5° at the scapulothoracic joint.

If the glenohumeral joint is fused, scapulothoracic motion can increase considerably.

Sternoclavicular and acromioclavicular joints also contribute to shoulder elevation. However, the sternoclavicular joint is more important because it contributes approximately 40° while the acromioclavicular joint contributes no more than 20° to the total range of elevation.

1. Scapula has moved upward and forward on the chest wall 60°.
2. Humerus has reached 180° elevation, having moved 120° in relation to the glenoid.
3. Scapulohumeral ratio is 1 to 2.
4. Elevation of the clavicle at the sternoclavicular joint and at the acromioclavicular joint permits 60° of scapular motion (40° at the sternoclavicular joint and 20° at the acromioclavicular joint).

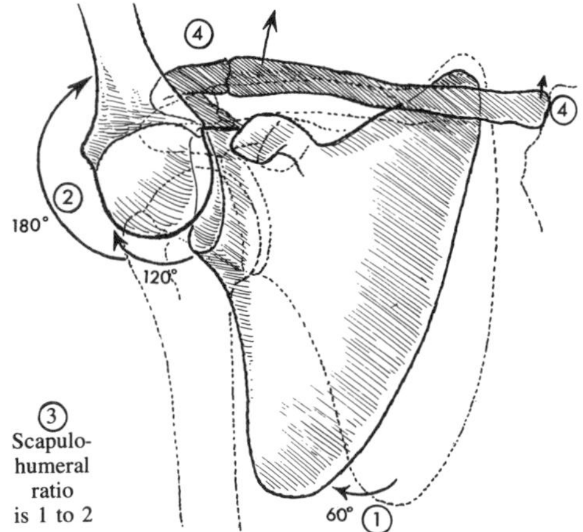

Normally, to reach the overhead position in the sagittal plane, the arm must be rotated internally. In the coronal plane, it must be rotated externally.

During elevation, if rotation of the humerus is in the correct plane, the greater tuberosity slips under the acromion, and motion is smooth and rhythmic from beginning to end.

If rotation of the humerus is obstructed, the greater tuberosity impinges against the acromion and becomes locked in this position. Forcing the humerus beyond the locked position results in either a dislocation or a fracture of the humerus. A typical mechanism is football tackling in which the runner does not stop but drives the tackler's arm backward in forceful abduction and external rotation.

Most individuals sustain an anterior dislocation from vigorous activities, particularly participation in sports. Consequently, most patients with an anterior dislocation are young adults.

Forceful abduction and external shoulder rotation may also be produced by a fall on the outstretched arm in which the humerus is in a fixed position but the glenoid moves away from it. Dislocations in older individuals are usually sustained by this mechanism.

Five per cent of glenohumeral dislocations are posterior and are produced by forceful internal rotation and adduction. The most common cause of this is a seizure from epilepsy or alcohol withdrawal.

Direct impact on the anterior aspect of the humerus during a fall may also produce posterior glenohumeral dislocation or fracture-dislocation.

Direct impact to the posterior aspect of the shoulder, e.g., in a fall from a horse, may cause anterior dislocation, but more often a fracture-dislocation results from direct violence to the shoulder.

For the humerus to be displaced out of the glenoid, the soft tissue support structures must be torn and stretched. The structures most often injured anteriorly are the glenoid labrum, the glenohumeral ligaments of the capsule, and the subscapularis. The structures most often injured posteriorly are the glenoid labrum, the capsule, and the infraspinatus.

Anterior Sprains and Subluxations of the Shoulder

REMARKS

As with any joint, the shoulder may be subject to sprain, subluxation, and dislocation.

Sprains and subluxations are most frequently the result of indirect minor injury in activities such as weight lifting, throwing, or other repetitive external rotation and abduction shoulder motions.

Acute shoulder dislocations are usually the result of more forceful injury, which disrupts areas of capsular attachment to the glenoid, allowing the humeral head to displace anteriorly.

The usual site of sprain or dislocation is the attachment of the capsule to the glenoid, particularly through the inferior glenohumeral ligament.

In contrast to the dislocation, which is usually obvious, the individual with a sprain or subluxation of the shoulder may have a less apparent diagnosis. Typically, the symptoms are aching in the shoulder, particularly in the posterior aspect.

Occasionally, the individual with a subluxating shoulder will experience "a drop arm sensation." The shoulder suddenly becomes weak when held in an externally rotated, extended position, as in serving in tennis or throwing.

1. Mechanism of sprain or subluxation of the shoulder is usually repetitive forceful external rotation and abduction, such as in weight lifting or
2. Repetitive throwing.

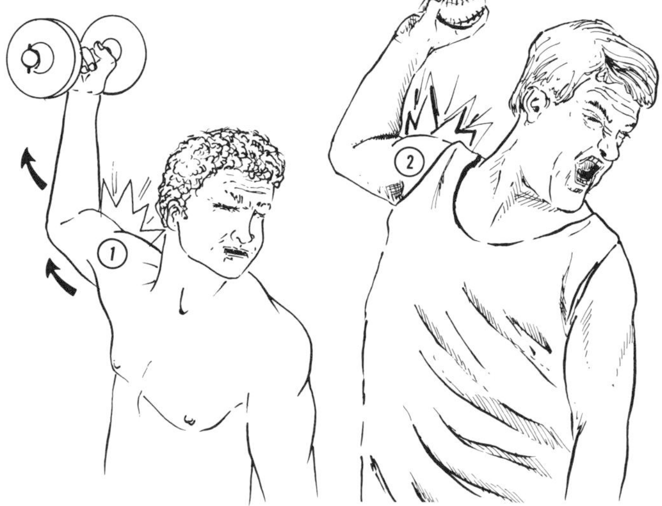

Mechanism of Sprain or Subluxation

1. Humeral head is in the locked position.
2. Arm is abducted and externally rotated.
3. Acromion impinges against the greater tuberosity.
4. Anterior ligaments and capsule are severely stretched—some fibers tear, but the continuity of the structures remains intact.

Note: The defect in the anterior capsule may lead to recurrent anterior subluxation.

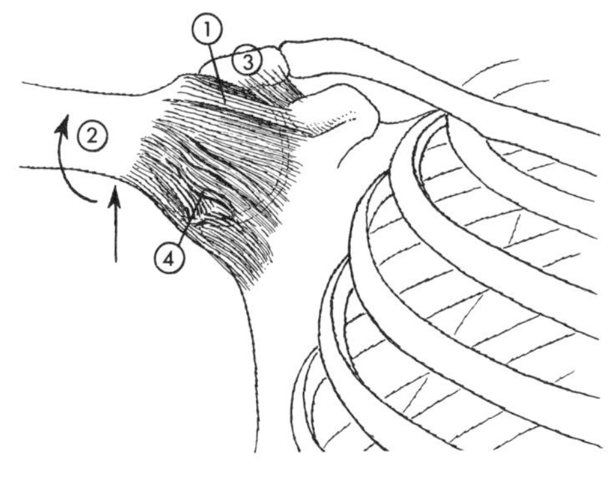

Mechanism of Anterior Dislocation

1. Acromion impinges against the greater tuberosity and levers it out of the joint anteriorly.
2. Anterior ligaments and capsule are severely stretched and torn, thus permitting a dislocation.

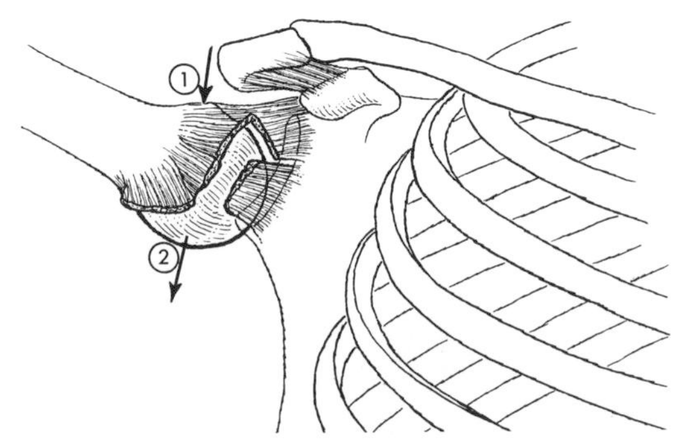

Diagnosis of Anterior Instability of the Shoulder

REMARKS

At one time, it was believed that the only instability problem occurring in the shoulder was a dislocation. However, Rowe, Protzman, and others showed that there is a wide range of instability problems that cause symptoms, ranging from subluxation to gross dislocation.

The patient may experience subluxation of the shoulder without any history of prior dislocation.

In addition, recurrent dislocation may be associated with interval symptoms of subluxation.

Finally, recurrent dislocation occurs without symptoms of subluxation in most patients.

It is important to distinguish the symptoms from sprain or subluxation of the shoulder and contrast them with symptoms from rotator cuff tendinitis, which can also be associated with sports such as throwing, repetitive lifting, or swimming.

The symptoms of shoulder instability characteristically are associated with a positive apprehension test with anterior subluxation of the shoulder.

Symptoms of rotator cuff tendinitis are usually diagnosed by a positive impingement test.

Apprehension Test for Subluxation and Dislocation

1. Patient's arm is placed in approximately 90° of abduction.
2. Elbow is flexed 90° and the forearm supinated 60°.
3. Examiner's opposite hand is placed across the patient's acromion.

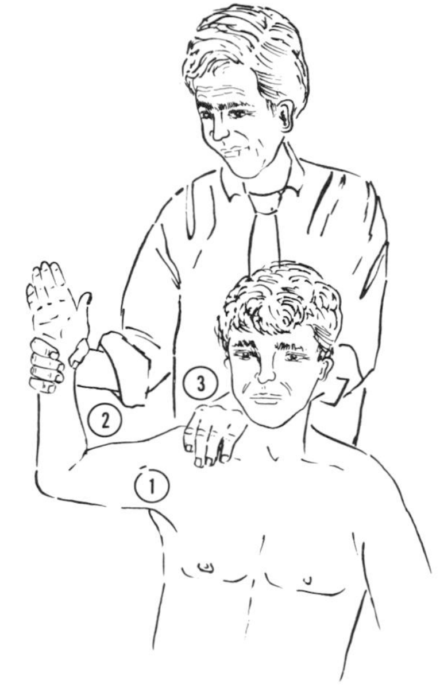

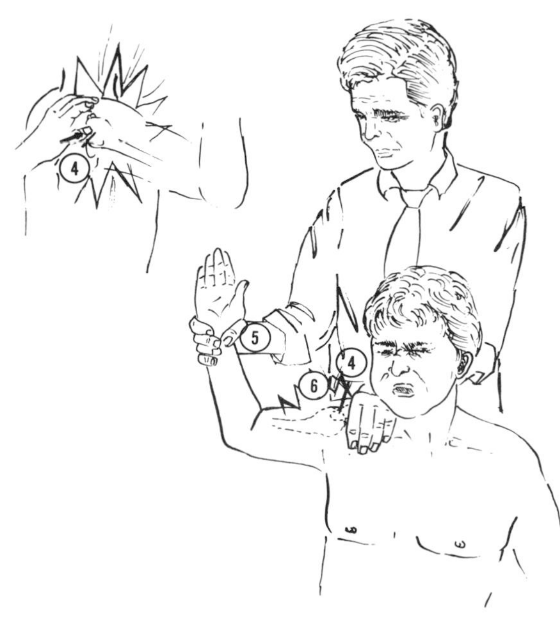

4. Examiner's thumb pushes the humeral head downward and forward while the
5. Hand supporting the limb moves the arm into slightly greater abduction.
6. When an anterior subluxation or dislocation is present, patients complain that they have an apprehension that the shoulder is slipping out of place.

Note: Pain in the posterior aspect of the shoulder frequently occurs with anterior subluxation, probably as a result of a pull on the posterior capsular structures. It must be distinguished from rotator cuff problems by tests for impingement.

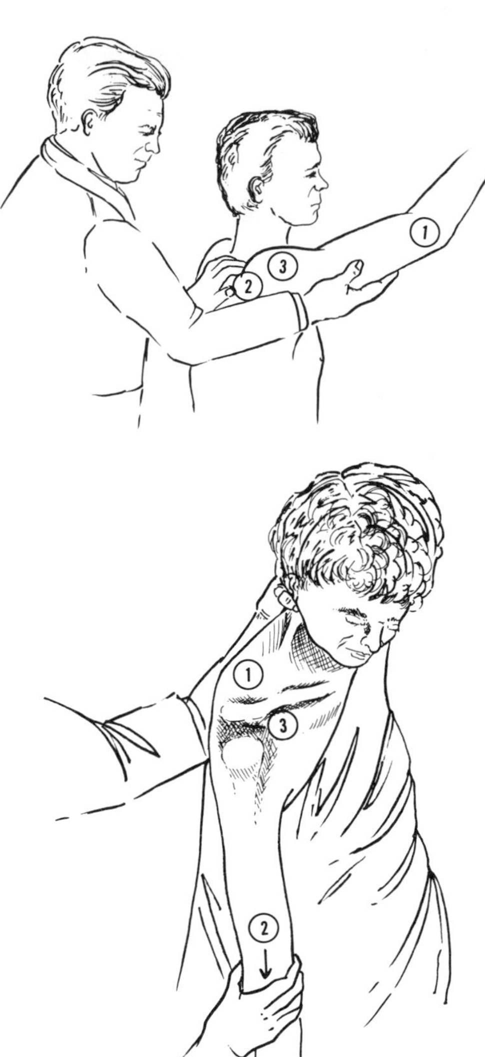

Neer's Impingement Test for Rotator Cuff Injury

1. Patient's pain is reproduced when the arm is forced into elevation.
2. Greater tuberosity is jammed against the anterior inferior surface of the acromion.
3. In this position, the acromion is pushed down against the tuberosity to elicit the symptoms from impingement of the rotator cuff caught between the tuberosity of the humerus and the undersurface of the acromion.

Sulcus Sign of Inferior Displacement

1. With a few individuals, negative pressure is not apparently sufficient to hold the humeral head in the glenoid.
2. If the humerus is pulled down inferiorly, subluxation into the axillary fold may occur, either passively or actively.
3. Result is a sulcus that becomes evident in the subacromial space between the acromion and the humeral head.

Note: Most of these patients with inferior subluxation are asymptomatic.

X-Ray Diagnosis of the Unstable Shoulder

REMARKS

Diagnosis of the grossly unstable dislocated shoulder is usually straightforward and readily apparent.

The diagnosis of the subtle anterior or posterior subluxation may not be so easily made. Frequently, the episodes of instability are brief, and there may be no obvious dislocation. The patient may be unaware that the shoulder is subluxed.

After an adequate history and physical examination, if the diagnosis is uncertain, roentgenographic evaluation may be helpful.

X-rays should include an anterior view of the true glenohumeral joint and an axillary view to show any defects of the glenoid labrum.

1. Anteroposterior view of the shoulder should be perpendicular to the plane of the scapula rather than the standard anteroposterior view of the shoulder.
2. This permits adequate visualization of the entire glenoid rim where small fractures may indicate avulsion injuries of the capsule.
3. In addition, small defects of the humeral head are consistent with a diagnosis of recurrent instability or dislocation.

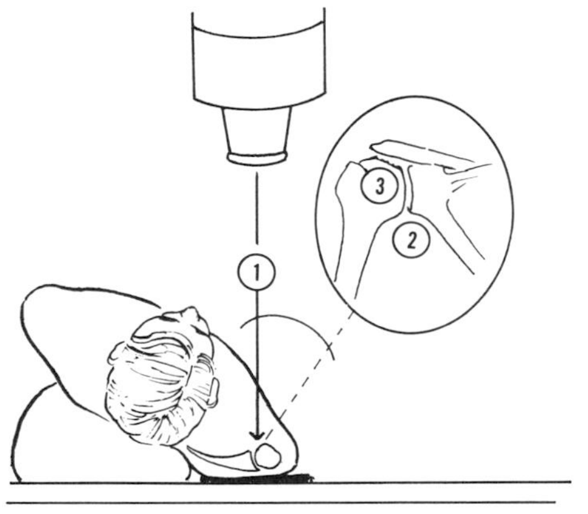

1. Careful axillary views may also show avulsion fractures of the anterior rim consistent with anterior subluxation or,
2. Rarely, avulsion fractures of the posterior rim, which indicate a posterior instability.

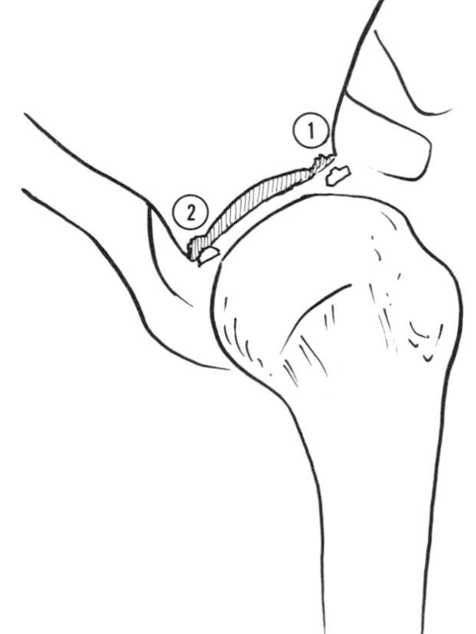

Management of Anterior Sprains and Subluxations of the Glenohumeral Joint

REMARKS

Once the diagnosis of an acute sprain or subluxation is made, the individual should be advised to avoid any activity or exercise that displaces the shoulder in the "at-risk" position.

If the episode is an initial one, it is worthwhile to immobilize the shoulder for 1–2 weeks; however, in most instances, this does not prevent recurrence of the problem unless the patient avoids the activities that cause the instability.

The athlete or weight lifter should avoid maneuvers that produce forced abduction, extension, and external rotation of the shoulder.

In addition, exercises should be recommended that promote the stabilizers of the scapula and modify the forces that put the shoulder at risk.

If the problem is a relatively atraumatic one, exercises may be helpful. However, exercises are usually not effective if the problem results from a significant initial injury that disrupts the glenohumeral ligament.

Management for Acute Subluxation

Apply ice for the first 24–36 hours.

Apply a triangular sling.

After 5–7 days, when the pain subsides, begin active range-of-motion exercises. Subsequently, the patient should be instructed in specific exercises to avoid recurrence of the problem.

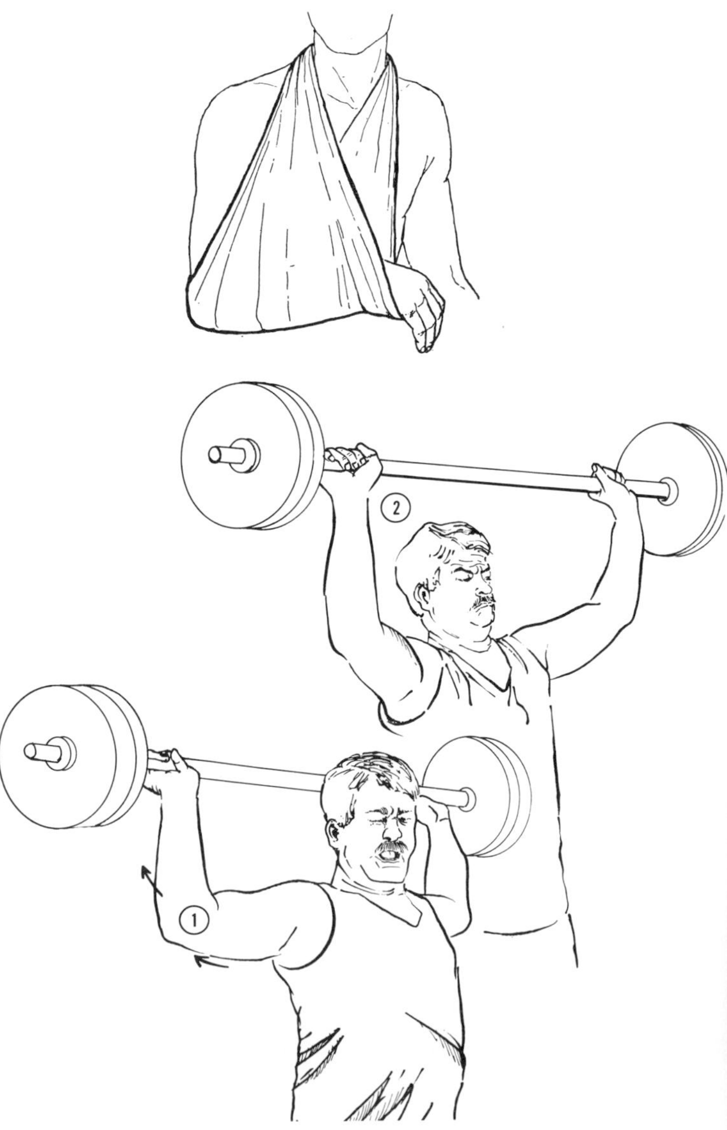

Conditioning Exercises to Avoid Subsequent Subluxations

1. Patient should avoid activities that require extremes of external rotation, abduction, and extension of the shoulder.
2. Exercises can be used that strengthen muscles but avoid strain on the ligamentous structures of the shoulder.

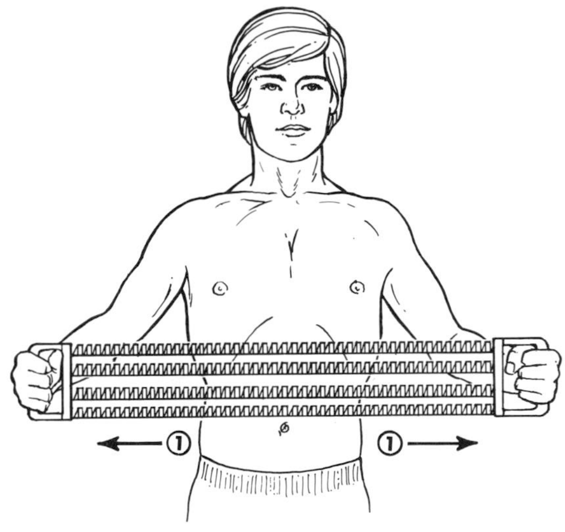

Management

Exercises to strengthen shoulder control may be helpful and should include

1. Abduction,

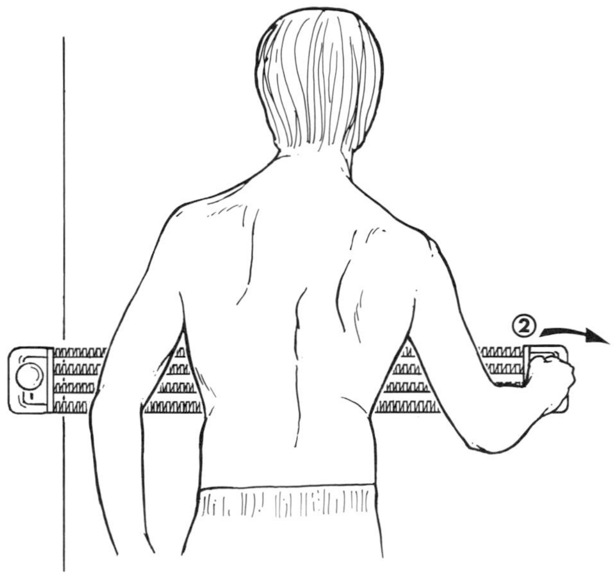

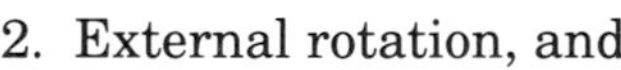

2. External rotation, and

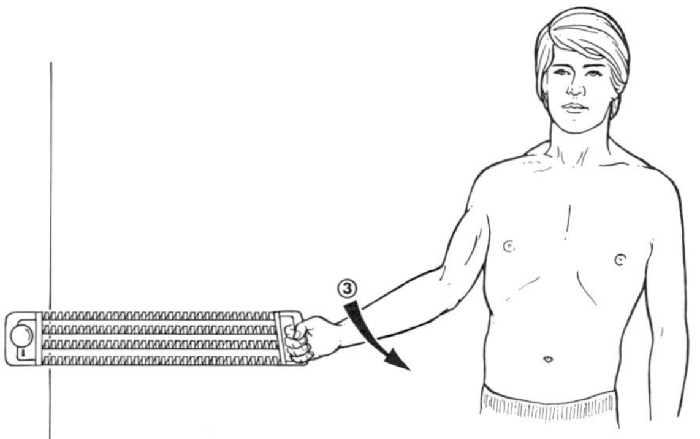

3. Internal rotation.

■ Inferior Subluxation

REMARKS

Inferior subluxation of the glenohumeral joint is most often a transitory complication of trauma to the shoulder. It resolves spontaneously in most instances and does not require open reduction of the joint.

The most common injury associated with inferior displacement is a humeral surgical neck fracture in an elderly patient. Fractures of the greater tuberosity may also result in inferior displacement of the humeral head.

The probable explanation for this transitory displacement of the humeral head inferior to the glenoid is loss of the intra-articular negative pressure or suction that ordinarily maintains the humeral head in the glenoid socket against gravity forces.

Occasionally, inferior subluxation is associated with paralysis of the shoulder muscles or hemiplegia, which may become a permanent problem.

However, the usual cause is a transitory loss of support of the humeral head in the glenoid, which can be corrected by a period of sling support of the arm and rapid exercises to restore normal range of motion to the shoulder.

Most Common Cause of Inferior Subluxation: Humeral Surgical Neck Fracture

1. Fracture of the humeral surgical neck may cause loss of intra-articular negative pressure.
2. If the fracture is treated by prolonged immobilization, progressive inferior displacement of the humeral head becomes evident.

Note: To avoid this complication, it is best to begin active range-of-motion exercises for these fractures as soon as the pain subsides.

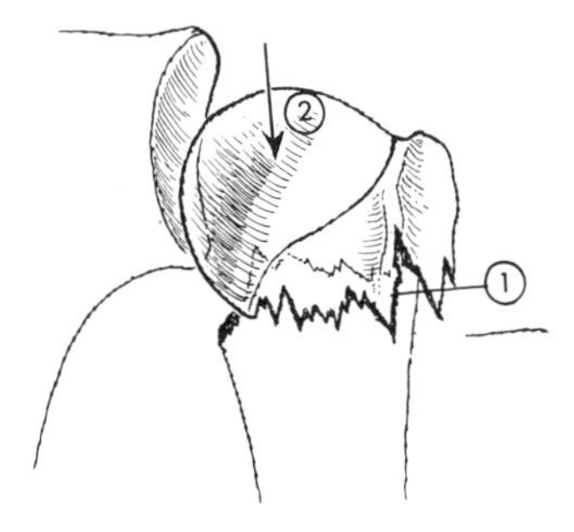

Other Types of Inferior Subluxation: Rotator Cuff Injury

1. If the rotator cuff has been acutely avulsed, the negative intra-articular pressure and the superior support structures or "roof of the shoulder" are lost.
2. Humeral head displaces inferiorly, and the space beneath the acromion is considerably wider.

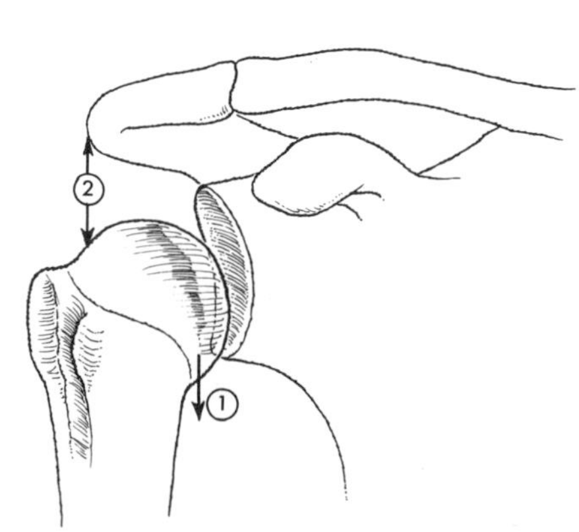

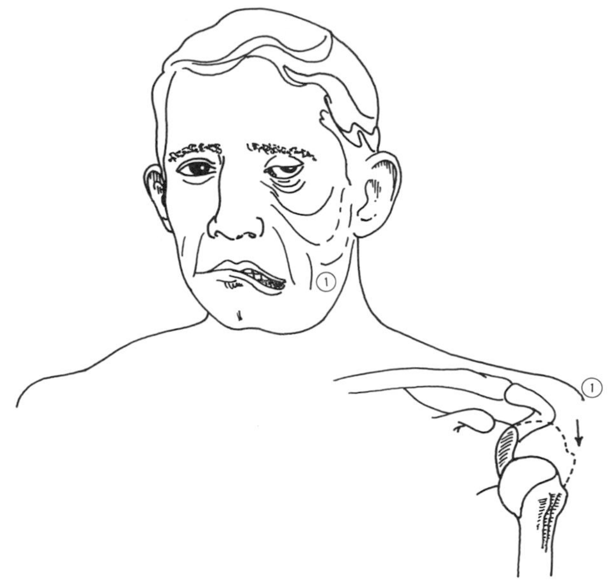

Nontraumatic Causes of Inferior Subluxation From Hemiplegia

1. Inferior subluxation from neurologic involvement after cerebral vascular accident can cause persistent shoulder pain from inferior subluxation. Rarely, other neurologic causes include axillary or suprascapular nerve palsy, but these are usually transitory.

Management

The incidence of inferior subluxation after a fracture of the proximal humerus is approximately 20 per cent.

A transitory inferior subluxation of the humeral head occurs in all patients after open reduction of fracture of the shoulder.

The treatment therefore should be sling support and early range-of-motion exercises to restore normal intra-articular pressure.

Rapid spontaneous recovery is seen in most patients with inferior subluxation, although it may take a few months in the more severely injured.

Patients with obvious weakness of the deltoid from axillary nerve or other injuries also take longer until the nerve injury recovers.

The prognosis for quick resolution of the subluxation after an injury to the shoulder or fracture of the proximal part of the humerus is excellent. However, patients with neurologic causes of subluxation, such as hemiplegia, require prolonged sling or brace support to avoid progressive downward subluxation until some neurologic recovery takes place.

If the inferior subluxation is due to rotator cuff tear, operative repair is indicated.

Superior Subluxation of the Humeral Head

REMARKS

Superior displacement or subluxation of the humeral head under the acromion can occur gradually after a shoulder dislocation if the rotator cuff is completely torn.

Hyperabduction injuries with an extremely violent wrenching load on the shoulder may cause this complication.

The resultant rotator cuff avulsion may initially cause an inferior subluxation during the period of immobilization.

However, as the deltoid muscle abducts the arm without the rotator cuff functioning to hold the humeral head in the glenoid, the humeral head displaces superiorly.

Superior migration or subluxation is a classic sign of chronic rotator cuff disruption.

This complication is also discussed later in this chapter in the section on the complications of dislocations.

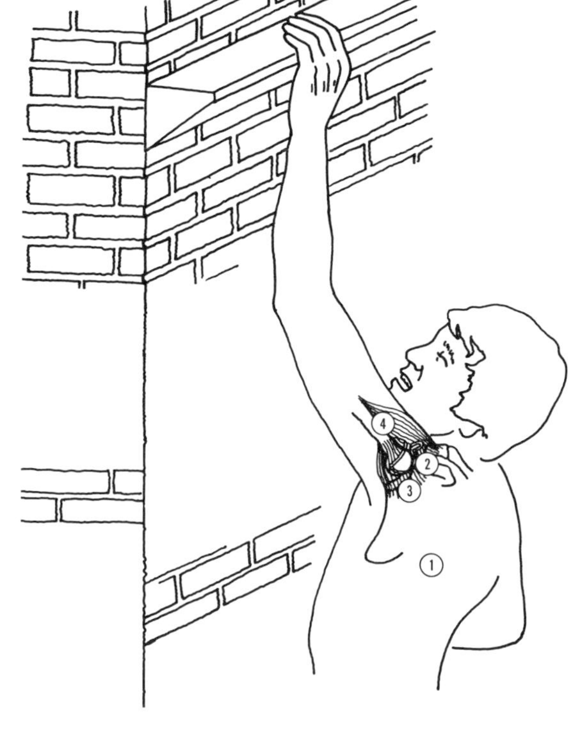

Mechanism of Rotator Cuff Disruption

1. Hyperabduction injury and forceful avulsion of the rotator cuff occur when individuals fall and catch their body weight with one shoulder.
2. Rotator cuff insertion is avulsed from the greater tuberosity.
3. Capsule may also be avulsed superiorly from the glenoid.
4. Humeral head may dislocate inferiorly, producing a luxatio erecta.

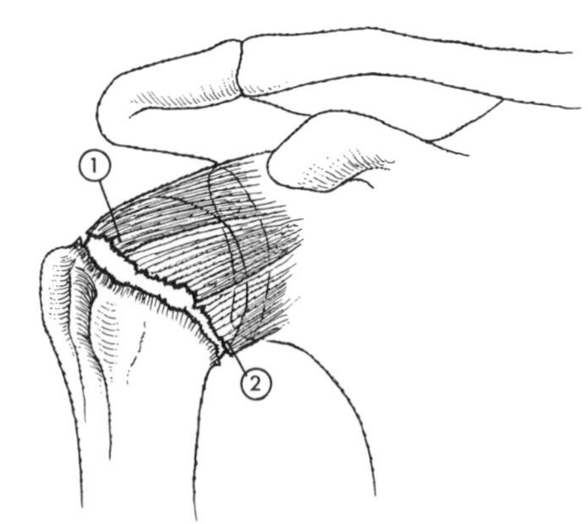

Initial Picture of Subluxation After Rotator Cuff Disruption

1. Cuff is avulsed from its attachment, and the intra-articular negative pressure is lost in the joint.
2. Humeral head tends to displace inferiorly.

Subsequent Cause of Superior Subluxation

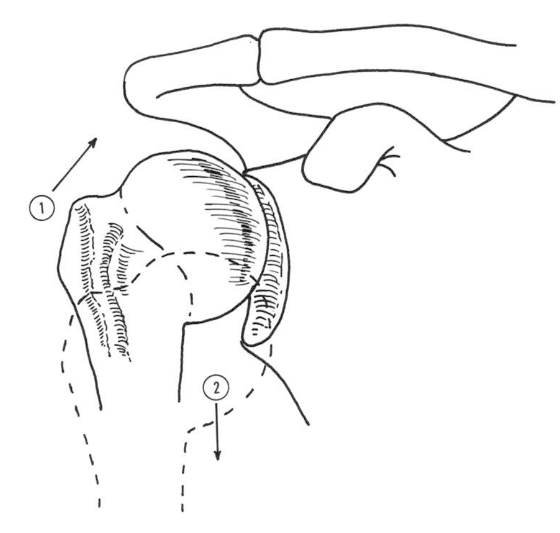

1. Torn rotator cuff no longer stabilizes the humeral head in the glenoid as the deltoid abducts the shoulder. The result is a classic upward migration consistent with rotator cuff tear.
2. If traction is applied or if the patient holds a weight in the involved arm, the humeral head will displace inferiorly as a result of the loss of rotator cuff support.

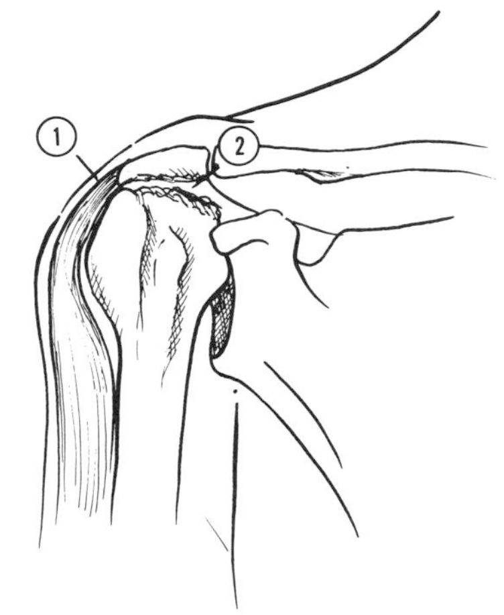

Rotator Cuff Arthropathy From Chronic Subluxation

1. Deltoid unopposed by the rotator cuff pulls the humeral head upward to abduct the arm.
2. Result can lead to chronic wearing down of the superior aspect of the humeral head underneath the acromion (rotator cuff arthropathy).

Pathologic Findings in Rotator Cuff Tear

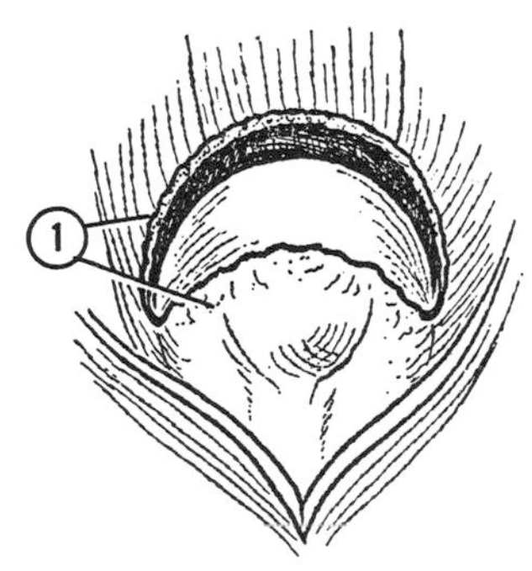

1. Rotator cuff tears associated with dislocations can be of significant size and cause complete detachment of the supraspinatus tendon and other tendons of the rotator cuff. This is best corrected surgically to avoid long-term weakness at shoulder abduction.

Repair of Torn Rotator Cuff

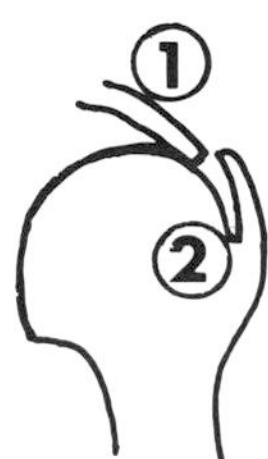

1. Torn tendon must be mobilized to restore it to its normal insertion on the humeral head.
2. It should be sutured directly to bone for a firm repair.

Posterior Sprains, Subluxation, and Dislocations From Adduction and Internal Rotational Injuries

REMARKS

Posterior sprains, subluxations, and dislocations are injuries that disrupt the posterior capsule or glenoid as a result of less frequent mechanisms.

The severity of the injury is determined by the degree of the applied forces.

Subluxation results from forces greater than those that cause a sprain and less than those that produce a posterior dislocation.

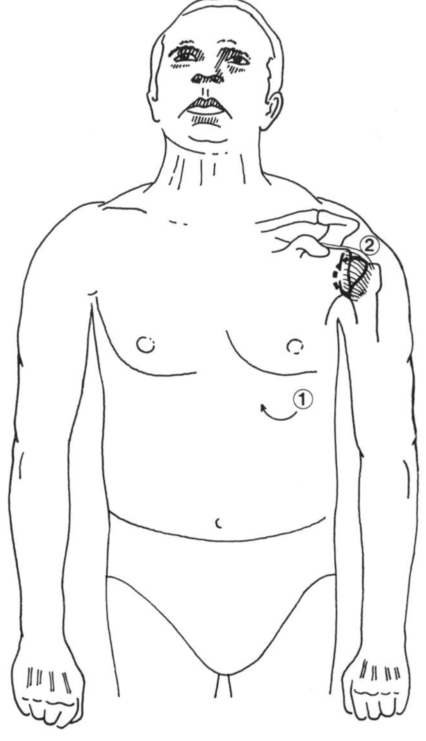

Sprain

1. During an epileptic seizure, the shoulder is forcefully adducted and internally rotated.
2. Posterior capsule is stretched—some fibers are torn, but its continuity is intact.

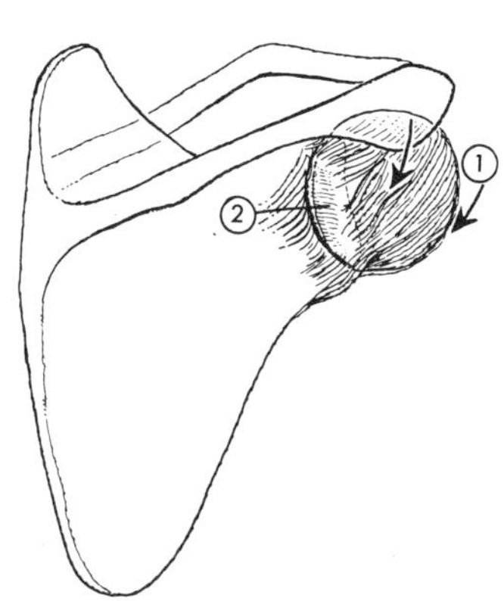

Subluxation

1. Violent internal rotation levers the head backward and outward, partially out of the glenoid fossa.
2. Posterior capsule is partially torn, thus permitting a subluxation.

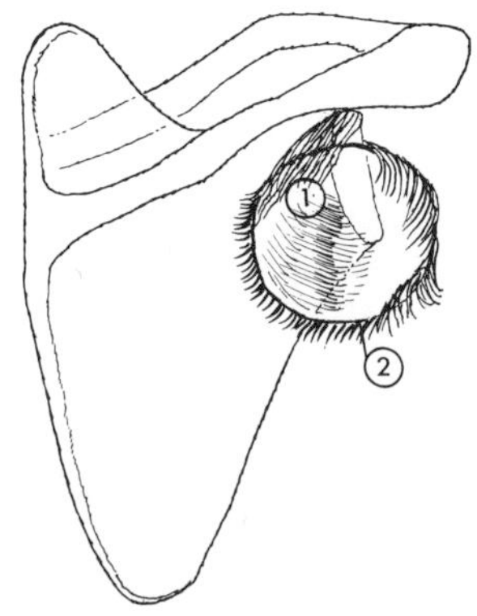

Posterior Dislocation

1. Violent internal rotation levers the humerus completely out of the glenoid fossa.
2. Posterior capsule is severely torn, thus permitting a posterior dislocation.

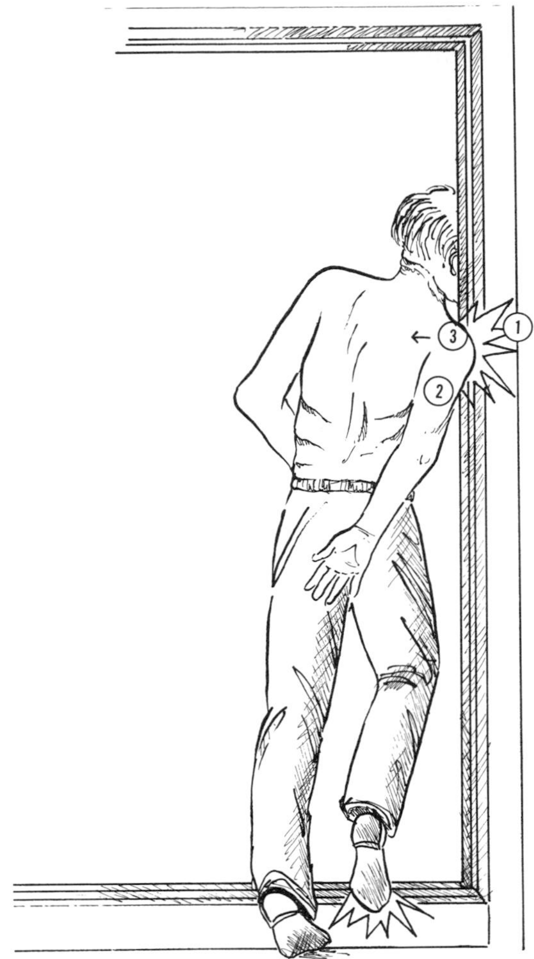

Posterior Sprain, Subluxation, or Dislocation From Direct Impact on the Shoulders

1. Direct blow to the anterior aspect of the shoulder is sustained in a fall.
2. Arm may be internally rotated at the time of the injury.
3. Forces from the anterior blow direct the internally rotated humeral head posteriorly over the rim of the glenoid. The extent of the injury to the posterior capsule and glenoid labrum determines whether the result is a sprain, subluxation, or dislocation.

Symptoms of Posterior Sprain or Subluxation

Posterior sprain, subluxation, or even recurrent dislocation can be confused with anterior shoulder instability. Shoulder pain is localized frequently to the posterior aspect of the joint. Typically, the symptoms from posterior instability are produced by internal rotation and abduction. (Symptoms of anterior instability occur with external rotation and abduction.)

1. Characteristically, the symptoms of shoulder instability or pain occur with the arm placed in a position of forward elevation and internal rotation (as in the pushup position).
2. Fractures of the lesser tuberosity or anteromedial head of the humerus may occur, which are consistent with a posterior displacement of the head over the rim of the glenoid.

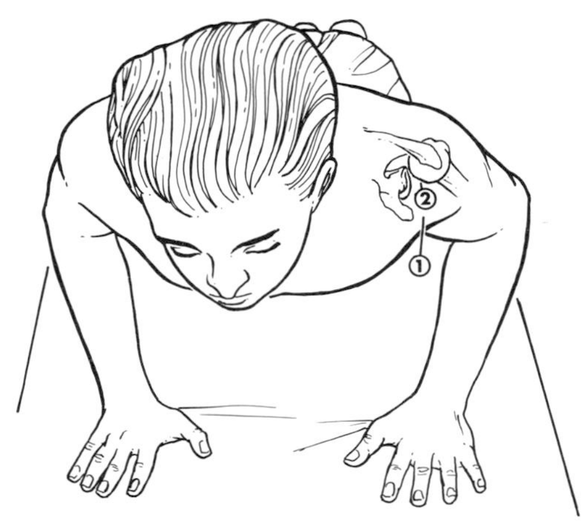

Management of Acute Posterior Subluxations

Careful assessment is necessary to determine that the shoulder is not dislocated posteriorly, because this may not be evident on standard x-rays of the shoulder.

If a diagnosis of posterior sprain or subluxation is made, a brief period of immobilization for 7–10 days is indicated to relieve the acute symptoms.

After this, the patient is started on a program of exercises to strengthen the external rotator muscles of the shoulder and avoid activity that produces the posterior subluxation.

(Management of the acute posterior dislocation is discussed in the section on reducing shoulder dislocations.)

1. Apply a pad of cotton in the axilla.
2. Wrap a 15-cm cotton bandage around the arm and chest to maintain the shoulder in extension and neutral rotation.
3. *Do not* use a sling, which necessitates adduction and internal rotation.

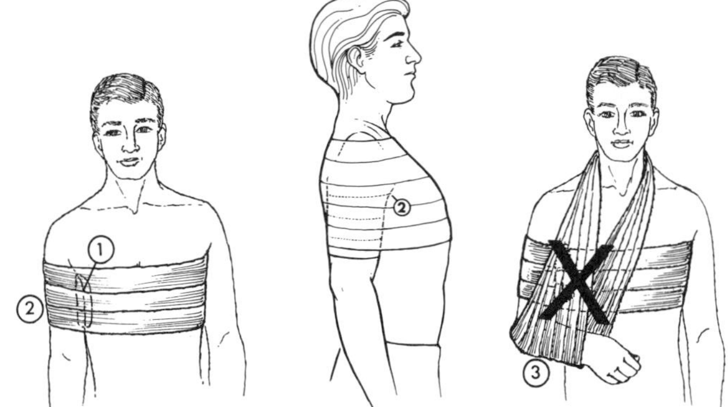

Subsequent Management

Maintain external immobilization for 1–2 weeks.

During this period, encourage motion of the wrist and fingers.

After this period, institute an active program of exercises.

Begin with pendulum exercises every waking hour for 5 to 10 minutes.

Progressively increase the exercises in range and frequency.

Allow free use of the arm within the tolerance of pain.

Strenuous activity is permissible after 4–6 weeks.

■ Management of Acute Glenohumeral Dislocations

REMARKS

Acute dislocations may be either anterior or posterior relative to the glenoid cavity. Approximately 95 per cent are anterior, and 5 per cent are posterior.

Acute dislocations can occur in any age group after the first decade. However, the most common age is from 15–30 years. The most common patient is a young teenage male athlete who subjects the shoulder to a violent external rotation–abduction injury.

Bilateral acute dislocations may occasionally occur but are most often associated with epileptic seizures.

Other injuries about the shoulder can be associated with the dislocation and should be looked for during the initial evaluation.

Approximately 25 per cent of acute dislocations may have a fracture of either the greater tuberosity or the glenoid rim.

In addition, neurovascular structures, particularly the axillary nerve or other components of the brachial plexus, may be injured.

Always check for impairment of nerve or circulatory disruption of the extremity before and after reduction.

Additional commonly associated injuries are rotator cuff ruptures. This is particularly to be suspected in the older patient who has either superior or inferior subluxation of the humeral head, which persists after reduction.

Types of Anterior Dislocations

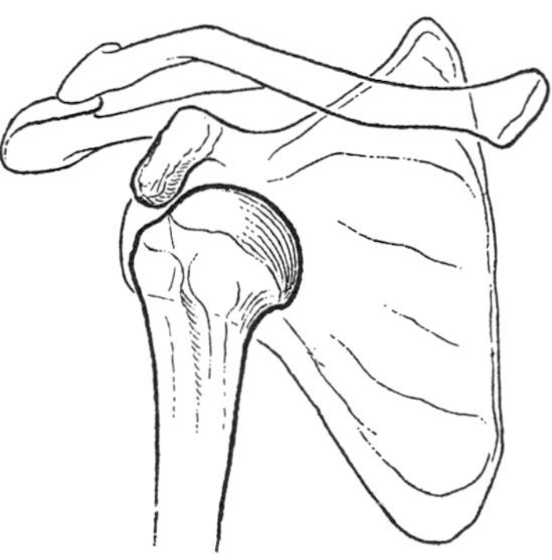

Subcoracoid dislocation (most common type).

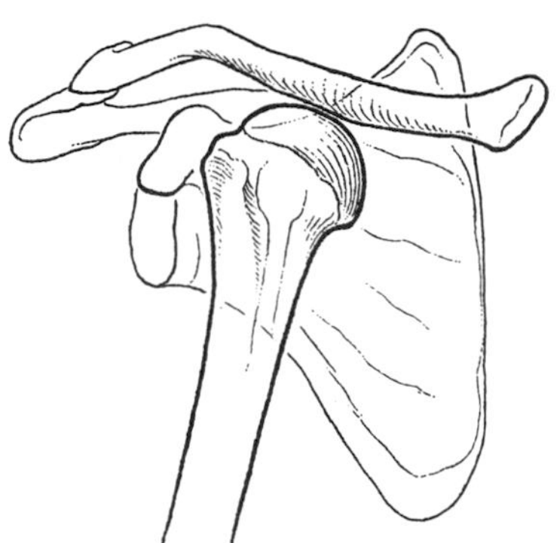

Subclavicular dislocation (rare type).

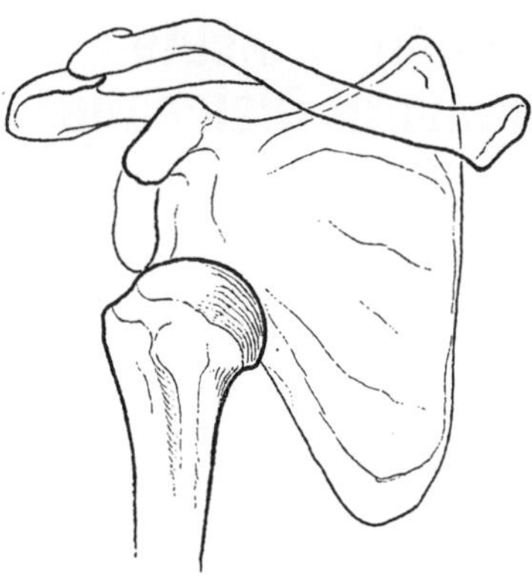

Types of Anterior Dislocations

All types of anterior dislocation should be reduced promptly.

Subglenoid dislocation (rare type).

Typical Deformity of Subcoracoid Dislocation

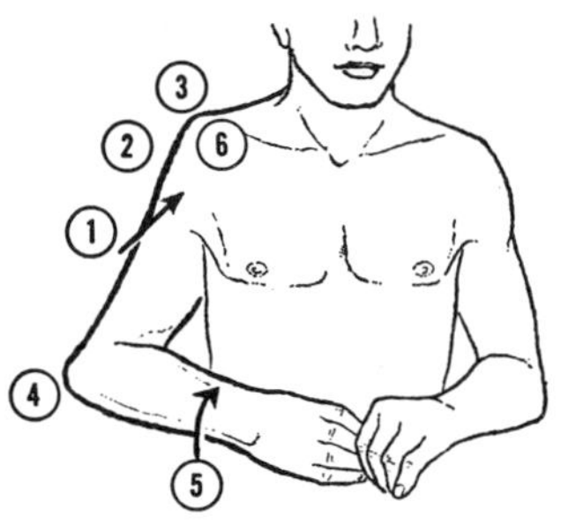

1. Arm is fixed in slight abduction and directed upward and inward.
2. Shoulder is flattened.
3. Acromion process is unduly prominent.
4. Elbow is flexed.
5. Forearm is rotated internally.
6. Abnormal prominence exists in the subcoracoid region.

Reduction of Anterior Dislocations

REMARKS

Anesthesia is usually not necessary if the dislocation is less than a few hours old.

It is important to gain the patient's confidence before any manipulation is attempted. Ask the patient to rotate externally the dislocated arm actively to feel that motion is possible without pain.

All techniques should require minimal force to achieve the reduction. Extreme force is likely to produce a fracture or cause further injury to the shoulder. If the reduction cannot be achieved without anesthesia, occasionally general anesthesia is indicated; rarely, open reduction may be necessary.

The common methods of reduction include Stimson's technique, the Hippocratic method, and Kocher's maneuver.

Stimson's Technique

This should be tried first because it is the least traumatic if patients can relax their shoulder muscles.

1. Patient is prone on the edge of the table.
2. Then 10-kg weights are attached to the arm, and the patient maintains this position for 10–15 minutes, if necessary.
3. Occasionally, gentle external and internal rotation of the shoulder aids in the reduction.

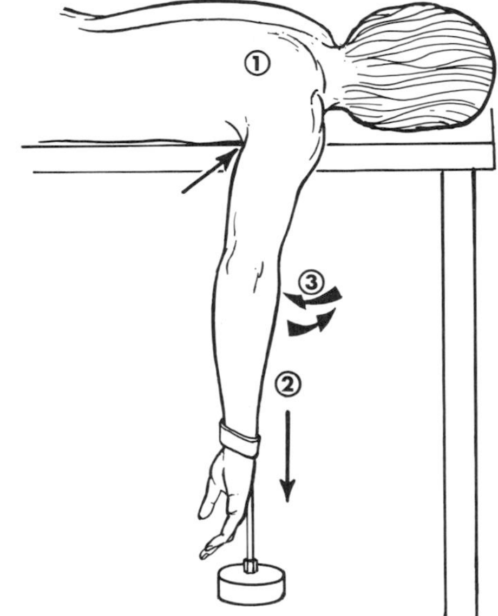

Hippocratic Method

1. Physician's stockinged foot is placed between the patient's chest wall and axillary folds but not in the axilla.
2. Steady traction is maintained while the patient gradually relaxes.
3. Shoulder is slowly rotated externally and adducted.
4. Gentle internal rotation reduces the humeral head.

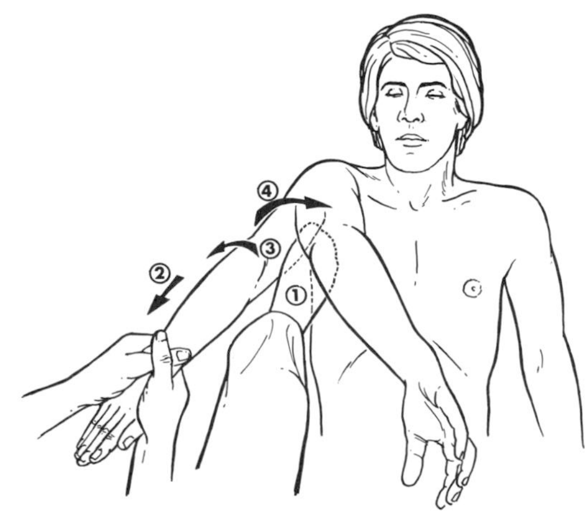

Kocher's Maneuver

Kocher's method should be painless and gentle with gradual correction of the deformity.

The surgeon should always tell the patient what is going to happen and obtain the patient's confidence.

1. Affected elbow is flexed to 90°.
2. Wrist and point of the elbow are gently grasped by the surgeon as the patient relaxes. At all times, the arm is kept pressed against the body.
3. Arm is slowly externally rotated up to about 80° where resistance is felt.

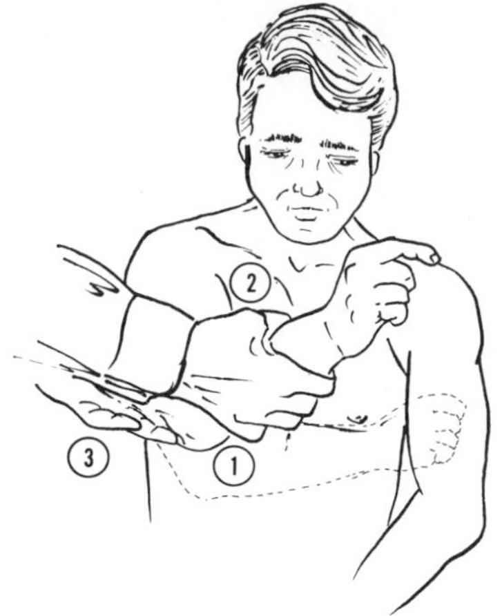

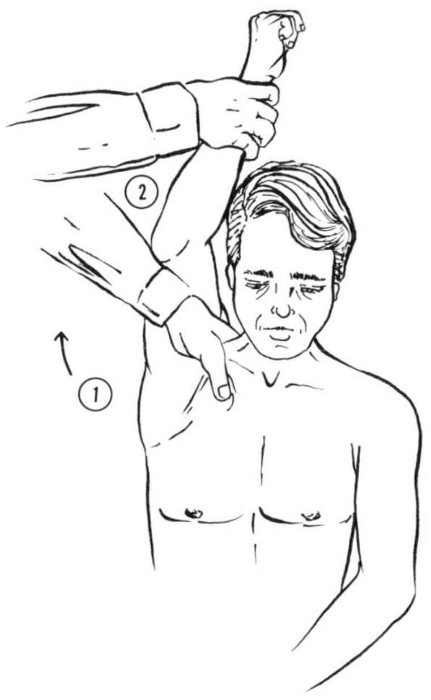

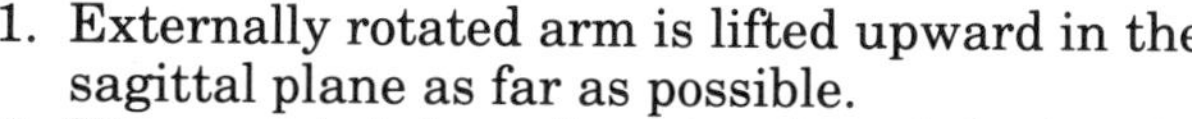

1. Externally rotated arm is lifted upward in the sagittal plane as far as possible.
2. Humerus is internally rotated, and the head gently pops into the joint as reduction is achieved.

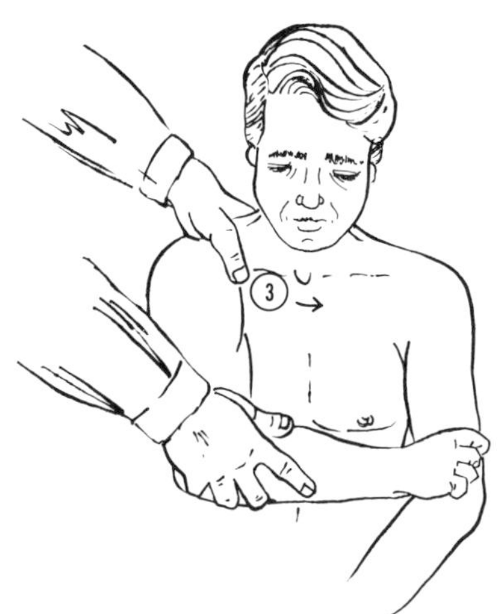

3. Internally rotated arm is then brought down against the chest with the shoulder reduced.

Caution: With Kocher's or any maneuver to reduce the shoulder, avoid heavy, forceful rotation, which can produce a fracture. If the dislocation cannot be reduced by these methods, general anesthesia is necessary to achieve adequate muscle relaxation. Particularly, be gentle and careful in reducing the dislocated shoulder in the elderly patient with osteoporotic bones because the humeral head is easily fractured in this age group.

Alternative Method: Traction and Countertraction

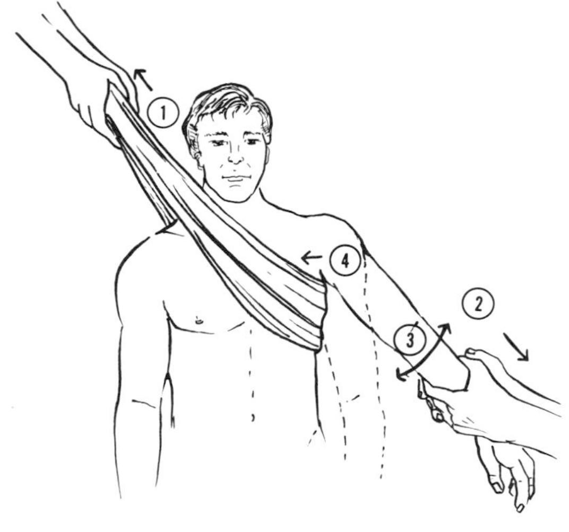

1. For larger patients and if help is available, countertraction may be necessary using a swathe wrapped through the axilla to stabilize the chest.
2. After the patient is sedated, gentle traction is applied for 5–10 minutes at the arm in the line of the deformity.
3. As the traction is increased gradually, internal or external rotation is used to disengage the head of the humerus over the glenoid rim.
4. With a very gentle maneuver, the reduction can usually be accomplished and the head slipped into the socket with relief of the patient's symptoms.

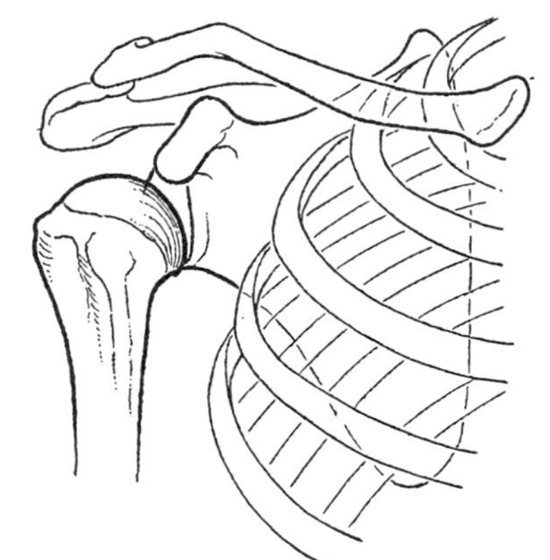

Postreduction X-Ray

The head of the humerus is in a normal relationship to the glenoid cavity, and no fracture has occurred.

After reduction, check for

- Neurologic deficits.
- Vascular embarrassment of the extremity.
- Rupture of the rotator cuff.

Note: Suspect rotator cuff tear if there is superior or inferior subluxation of the reduced humeral head on x-ray.

- Sensory loss in lesions of axillary nerve. Hypoesthesia or sensory loss in the area of distribution of the sensory branch of the axillary nerve.
- Sensory loss in lesions of musculocutaneous nerve. Impaired sensation along the lateral border of the forearm.

Note: Paralyses of the biceps brachii, the coracobrachialis, and the brachialis may be associated lesions.

Postreduction Immobilization for Young Patients

Apply a shoulder immobilizer that

- Restricts abduction.
- Restricts all rotatory motions.
- Restricts extension.
- Allows motion at the elbow, wrist, and fingers.
- Permits healing of soft tissue structures and minimizes the incidence of recurrence.

Velpeau Bandage Immobilization

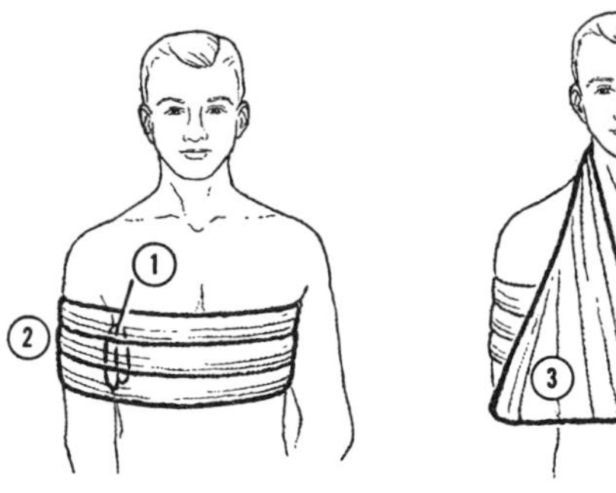

1. Place cotton pad in axilla.
2. Encircle arm and chest with a 15-cm cotton bandage.
3. Apply a triangular sling.

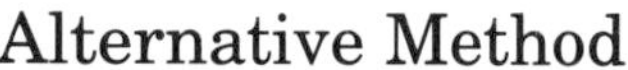

Alternative Method

STOCKINETTE-VELPEAU IMMOBILIZATION (AFTER GILCHRIST)

A relatively simple and comfortable means of immobilizing the shoulder is by the use of a long stockinette.

Take a 10-cm stockinette 3 m in length, and

1. Cut a 15-cm slot along one folded crease approximately one third from the end. Pass the patient's hand into the slot and down into the long end of the stockinette so that the slot fits in the axilla.

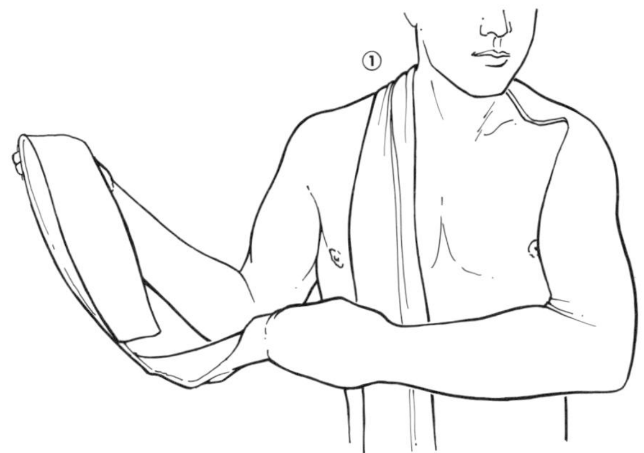

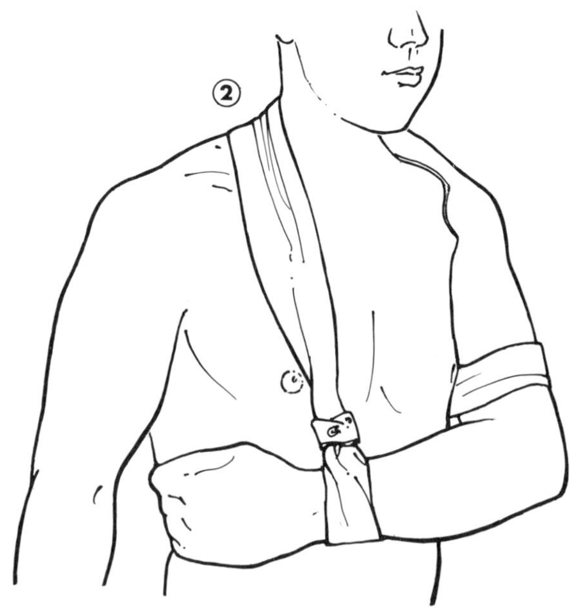

2. With the patient's arm in internal rotation and the forearm across the waist, the long end of the stockinette is passed around the opposite end of the abdomen and across the back. The short end is passed around the patient's neck, looped about the wrist, and secured with a safety pin.

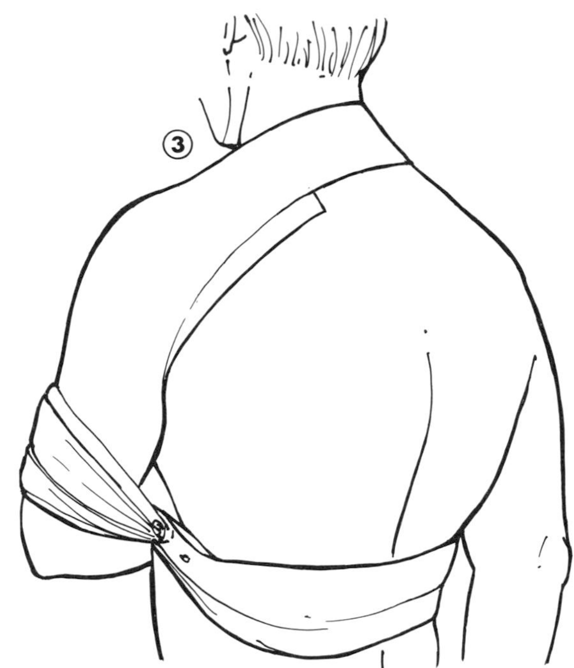

3. End of the stockinette that has been passed across the back is pulled tightly, wrapped around the affected arm, and secured with a safety pin. The flap created by the axillary slot may be taped over the deltoid region to prevent the stockinette from slipping forward or backward off the shoulder.

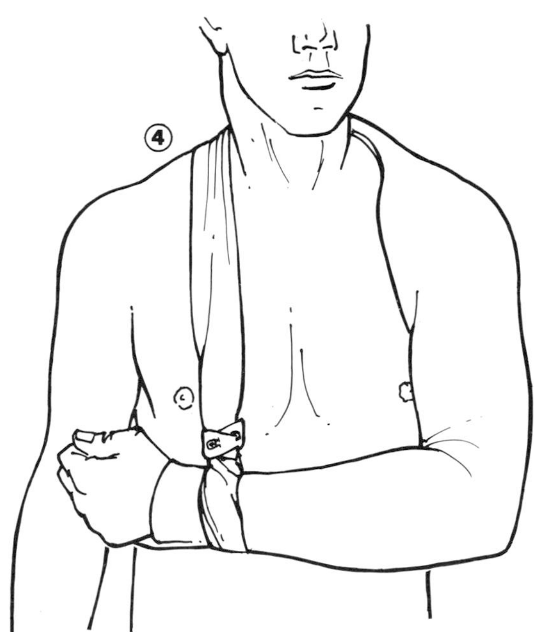

4. A 2.5-cm transverse cut is made in the stockinette to free the patient's hand. This slot may be reinforced with a tape applied loosely around the wrist.

Postreduction Immobilization for Middle-Aged and Elderly Patients

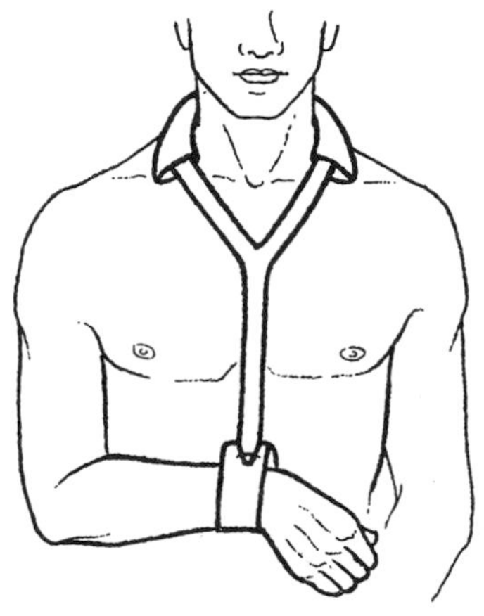

Apply collar and cuff that

Allow sufficient motion to prevent a frozen shoulder.

Limit abduction and external rotation sufficiently to prevent redislocation.

Permit free active motion at elbow, wrist, and fingers.

Discontinue immobilization 1–2 weeks after the injury.

Postreduction Management

Encourage the patient to move the elbow, wrist, and fingers on the injured side.

There is no evidence that prolonging immobilization of the shoulder prevents recurrences of the dislocation.

Recurrences of the dislocation are primarily dependent on the age and activity of the individual. The active young athlete under the age of 25 years is highly likely to have recurrent dislocation of varying frequency despite immobilization.

In general, it is adequate to immobilize the shoulder for approximately 1 week until the acute swelling and symptoms subside.

Encourage the patient to avoid strenuous sports for approximately 6–8 weeks after the shoulder has dislocated, but advise the patient that repeated injury to the shoulder is likely to cause recurrence of the dislocation and may require operative repair.

Particularly, avoid prolonged immobilization in the older patient (more than 30 years of age) who is more likely to develop a stiff shoulder than an unstable shoulder after these injuries.

Luxatio Erecta

REMARKS

This lesion is the result of a severe hyperabduction mechanism (see illustration for the section "Mechanism of Rotator Cuff Injury").

It frequently is associated with significant injury to the rotator cuff.

After reduction, if there is evidence on the x-ray of inferior subluxation or superior displacement of the humeral head, surgical reattachment of the tendons, particularly of the supraspinatus tendon, should be considered.

Rotator Cuff Disruption

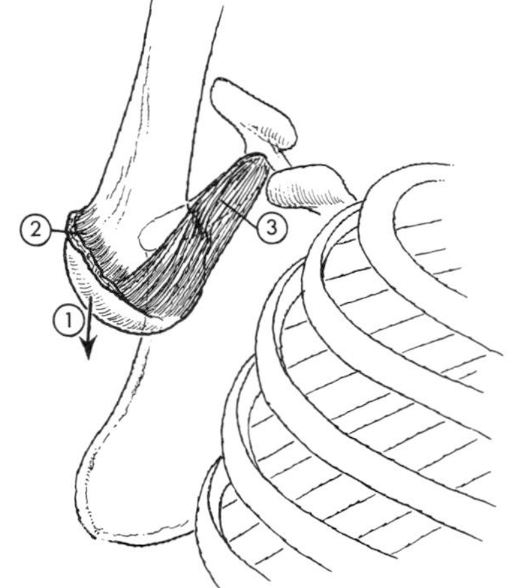

1. As the humeral head leaves the glenoid cavity, it may become locked with the shoulder abnormally elevated.
2. Soft tissues that attach to the humeral head, particularly the rotator cuff, are completely torn.
3. Anterior capsule and other tendons are stretched considerably, causing subsequent instability.

Note: Frequently, the head of the humerus may move from this markedly abducted position to an inferior subcoracoid position.

Luxatio Erecta

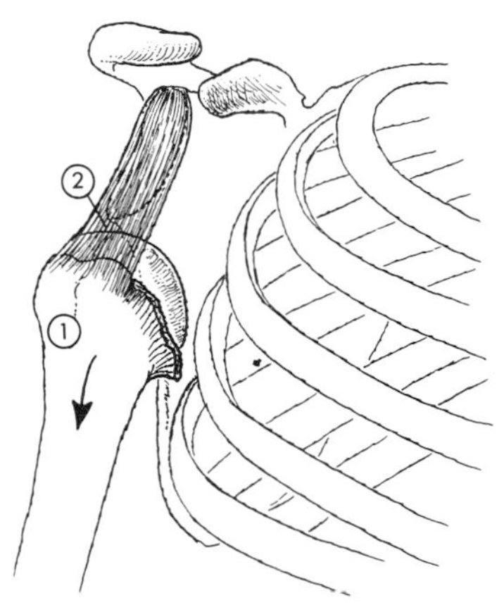

1. Arm may droop to the side.
2. Humeral head then displaces to a subglenoid position.

Note: From this position, it may also move to a subcoracoid position. The shoulder may be reduced readily, but the rotator cuff injury requires operative repair.

Prereduction X-Ray

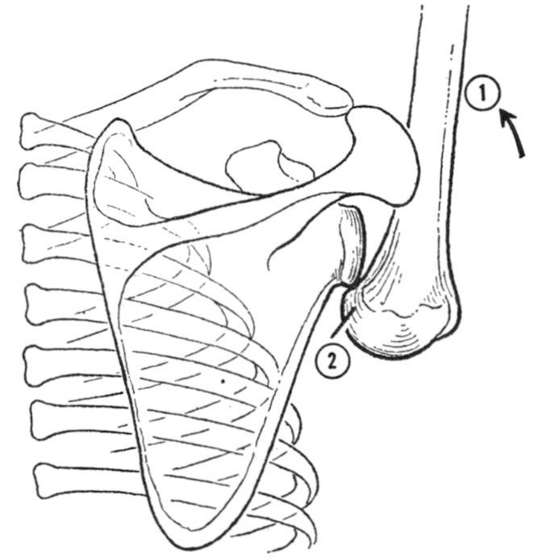

1. Arm is in full abduction.
2. Humeral head lies inferior to the glenoid fossa.

Manipulative Reduction

1. Surgeon makes steady traction upward and outward on the abducted arm.
2. Assistant makes countertraction downward.

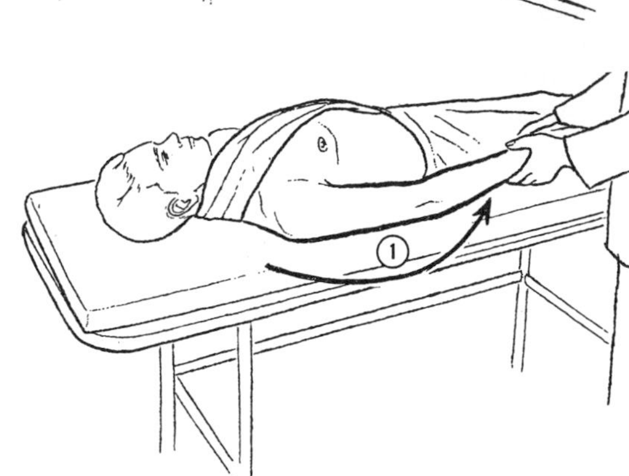

Reduction is indicated by an audible clunk.
1. Arm is then brought to the side.

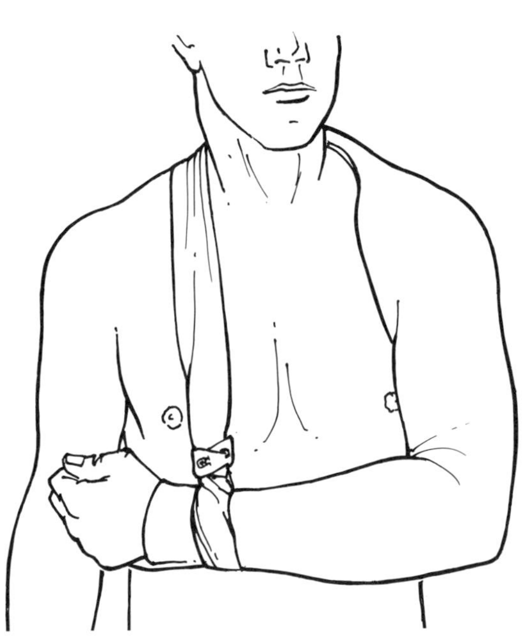

Immobilization

Apply a shoulder immobilizer.

Postreduction Management

Encourage motion at the elbow, wrist, and fingers.

Discard the apparatus after 1–2 weeks.

Institute a program of graduated motions within the limits of pain.

Begin with motions in stooped position every waking hour for 5 or 10 minutes.

Later, add abduction and external rotation exercises.

Allow free use of arm within the limits of pain and fatigue, but do not permit strenuous sports activities for 2–3 months after reduction.

Rotator cuff injury is commonly associated with this unusual dislocation and should be repaired surgically.

Irreducible Fresh Dislocations

REMARKS

By far, most dislocations are reduced by one of the maneuvers previously described.

If the patient is heavily muscled or overly anxious and cannot relax, avoid repetitive manipulation, and use a general anesthetic to relax the muscles.

In most instances, the dislocated shoulder that cannot be reduced in the emergency room with the patient awake is readily reducible once the patient is asleep and the muscles are relaxed.

Rarely, there are structures interposed between the humeral head and the glenoid that completely block reduction and require open repair. These may include a portion of the rotator cuff, the capsule, or the long head of the biceps tendon.

An occasional cause of an irreducible dislocation is an unrecognized chronic dislocation. This chronic dislocation can be mistaken to be acute, particularly in the inebriated or confused patient seen in the emergency room.

For the chronic dislocation, closed reduction under anesthesia may be effective if the dislocation is not older than 4–6 weeks.

If the dislocation is older than 4–6 weeks, open reduction is needed to reduce the humeral head into the glenoid without inflicting further damage on the joint.

Occasional Causes of Failure of Closed Reduction

1. Reduction is not possible because the ruptured rotator cuff lies in front of the glenoid fossa like a curtain.
2. Reduction is not possible because the inferior capsule is interposed between the humeral head and the glenoid fossa.
3. Reduction is not possible because the biceps tendon is displaced posteriorly and prevents apposition of the humeral head to the glenoid fossa.

Note: A carefully obtained history should distinguish a chronic dislocation from an irreducible fresh dislocation.

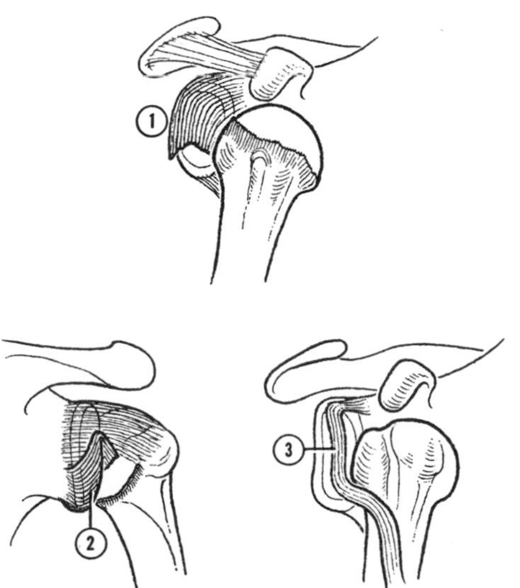

Old Anterior Dislocation as a Cause of Irreducible Injury

REMARKS

Old anterior dislocations are serious lesions and may be complicated further by treatment.

Closed reduction under general anesthesia is usually possible in dislocations less than 4 weeks old.

The results are better with closed than with open methods of reduction.

Open reduction is usually necessary if the dislocation is more than 6 weeks old or if closed methods have failed. However, old dislocations are in some instances painless and permit a fair degree of function. In elderly patients, such a lesion can be left undisturbed. If the age of the injury is uncertain or the patient's shoulder is relatively pain free, operative treatment should be avoided.

Closed methods may be complicated by fracture of the humerus, rupture of the axillary artery, or injury to the brachial plexus. These disasters may also occur in operative reduction of a chronic dislocation.

In young patients and in patients with pain or vascular embarrassment, reduction is necessary.

Regardless of the method of reduction used, complete restoration of function is rarely achieved.

The primary obstruction to reduction is the capsule, which folds over the glenoid and becomes scarred sufficiently to obstruct repositioning of the humeral head. For this reason, a posterior surgical approach to the shoulder is the most effective way to achieve reduction for chronic anterior dislocation, provided that reduction is indicated.

Prereduction X-Ray

Anterior dislocation less than 4 weeks old.

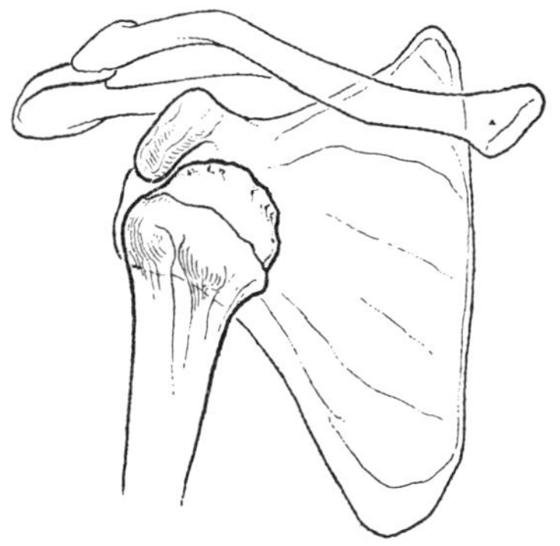

Closed Reduction

The Hippocratic method is preferred.

Use a general anesthetic. *Complete relaxation is essential.*

1. Physician's stockinged foot or a sling is applied between the patient's chest wall and axillary folds but not in the axilla.
2. Steady traction is maintained while the muscles are relaxed.
3. Shoulder is gently rotated externally and adducted.
4. Gentle internal rotation reduces the humeral head.

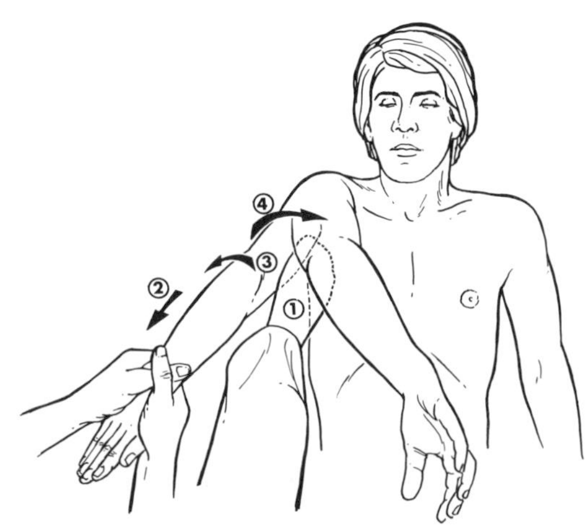

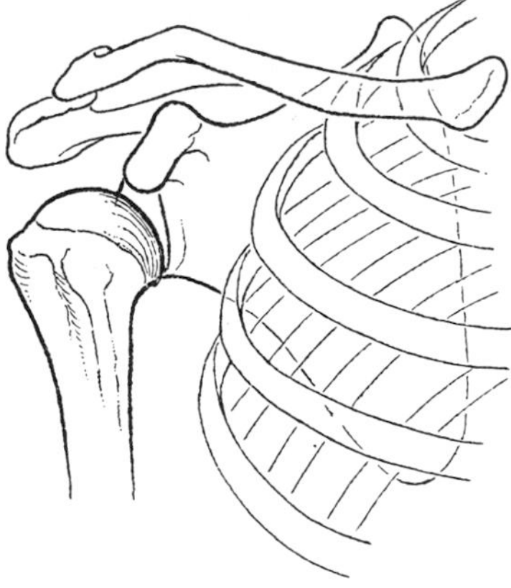

Postreduction X-Ray

The humeral head has returned to its normal anatomic position. No fracture has occurred. *Caution*: In cases of failure, try the maneuver once more. *Repeated attempts are dangerous*. Failure of closed reduction after two attempts indicates that surgical reduction is required.

Infraspinatus Repair for Chronic Anterior Dislocation by the "Back Door" Approach

REMARKS

Although operative reduction is rarely indicated, to deal with the lesions of chronic anterior dislocation, the author uses a back door approach to the shoulder.

The objectives of this posterior or back door approach are

- To remove the posterior capsule, which has become scarred down in the glenoid and prevents reduction, and
- To avoid extensive dissection of the anterior muscles and capsule, which causes gross instability after the reduction.

Obstruction to Closed Reduction (After 4–6 Weeks)

Failure to accomplish a closed reduction is due to

1. Bowstring of the posterior capsule, forming an intra-articular scar.
2. Posterolateral fracture of humeral head, which is impacted against the glenoid.
3. Anterior avulsion of the glenoid labrum or fracture of the glenoid from impaction of the humeral head.
4. Stripping of the anterior capsule and subscapularis from the neck of the scapula.

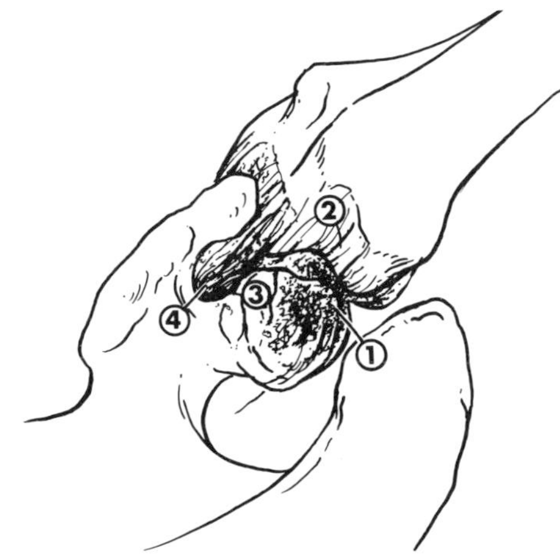

Infraspinatus Repair for Chronic Anterior Dislocation

1. The back door approach is made beneath the spine of the scapula, extending out beyond the glenohumeral joint.

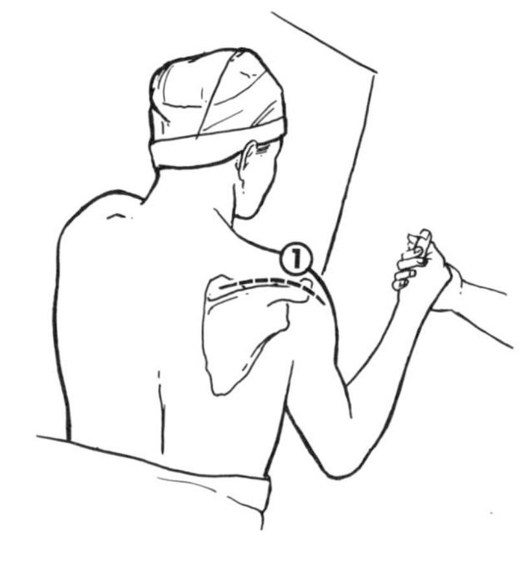

Repair

1. Interval between the infraspinatus and the teres minor is identified, and the infraspinatus tendon and capsule are detached from the greater tuberosity.

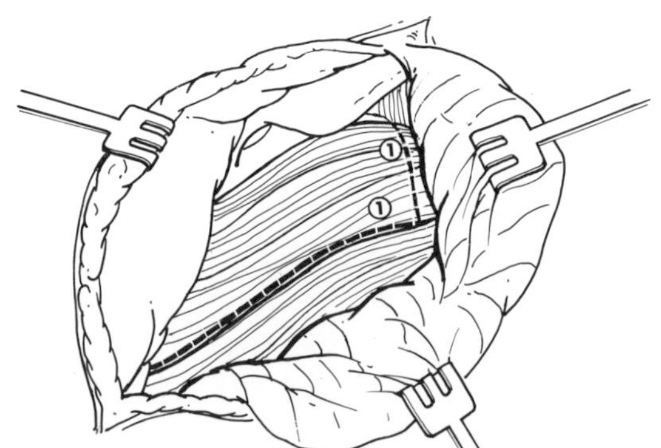

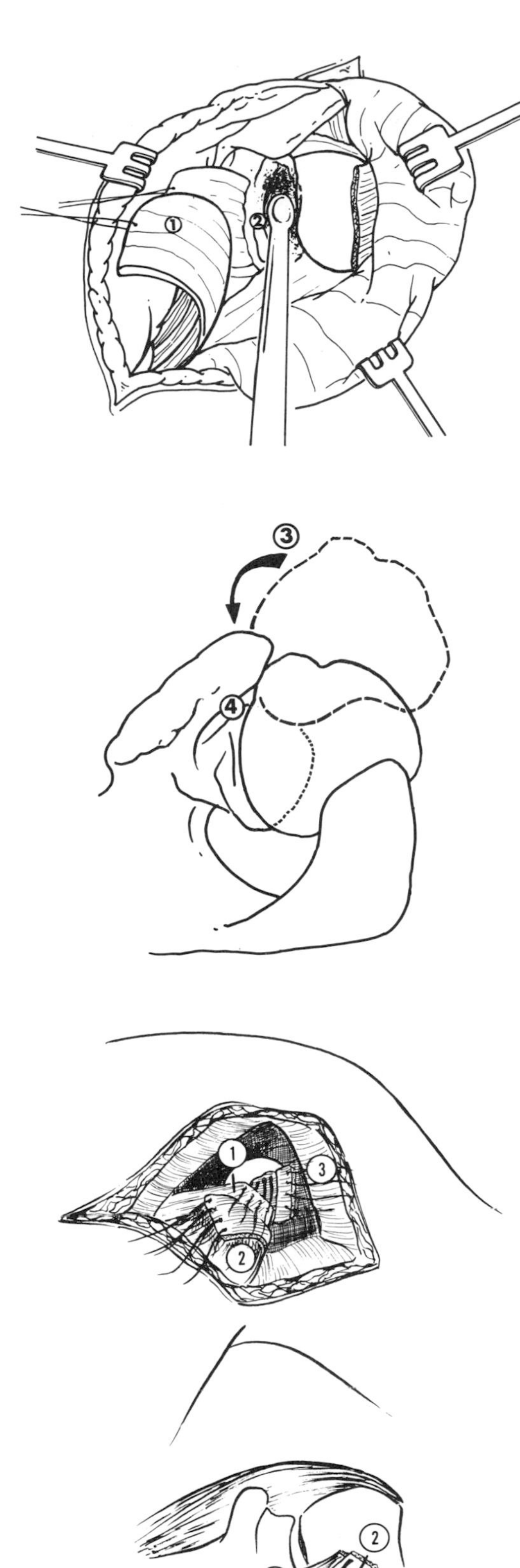

1. The infraspinatous tendon is tagged with a suture and retracted along with the capsule.
2. Scarred intra-articular capsule is excised from the glenoid cavity and freed anteriorly.

3. Humeral head is gently elevated back into the glenoid cavity while an assistant applies traction on the elbow.
4. Anterior capsule may have to be peeled off the humeral head, but the subscapularis usually can be left undisturbed.

1. After reduction of the head of the humerus into the glenoid, the posterior capsule is attached to the defect.
2. The infraspinatus is also attached into the defect using implanted sutures.
3. Lateral capsule is imbricated over the medial capsule and reinforces the posterior repair.

Note: Postoperative immobilization in a Velpeau shoulder immobilizer is continued for 3–6 weeks, depending on the degree of stability achieved by the repair.

Acute Posterior Dislocation

REMARKS

Acute posterior dislocation is often overlooked and occurs more frequently than generally realized. Of all acute dislocations, posterior dislocation occurs in 4–5 per cent.

It frequently follows epileptic seizures or occurs during electroconvulsive therapy or may result from a direct blow to the front of the shoulder during a fall.

The x-rays are usually misleading because the anteroposterior view can be misinterpreted as normal. Axillary views, which are essential to make the diagnosis, may not be obtained because of the patient's pain, unless the physician personally supervises the positioning.

Careful clinical assessment of any patient with a painful stiff shoulder after an injury is essential to make the diagnosis of posterior dislocation.

The key to diagnosis is finding the shoulder locked in internal rotation and adduction.

It is essential that the shoulder motion be evaluated from the neutral position, i.e., with the elbow flexed rather than the elbow extended. Otherwise, rotation of the forearm may mask the locked internally rotated position of the shoulder.

Mechanism of Injury

Characteristically, the acute posterior dislocation occurs from a direct blow to the anterior shoulder or from forceful internal rotation and adduction.

1. Patient with a posterior dislocation is frequently an individual with a seizure disorder or an elderly patient who falls and strikes the anterior aspect of the shoulder.
2. Characteristically, the arm is in internal rotation and adduction at the time of injury.
3. Direct blow to the anterior aspect of the internally rotated and adducted shoulder produces the posterior dislocation.

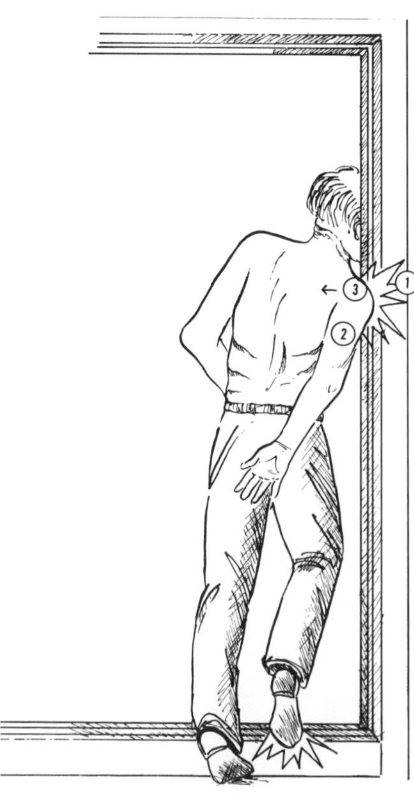

1. Classic and most reliable physical finding of a posterior shoulder dislocation is a locked internally rotated and adducted shoulder. This can be detected only with the shoulder in the neutral position, i.e., with the elbows flexed and held against the trunk.
2. In the neutral (anatomic) position, the shoulder should be capable of approximately 30° of external rotation. In the dislocated shoulder, external rotation is impossible because of the locked position of the humeral head posterior to the glenoid.

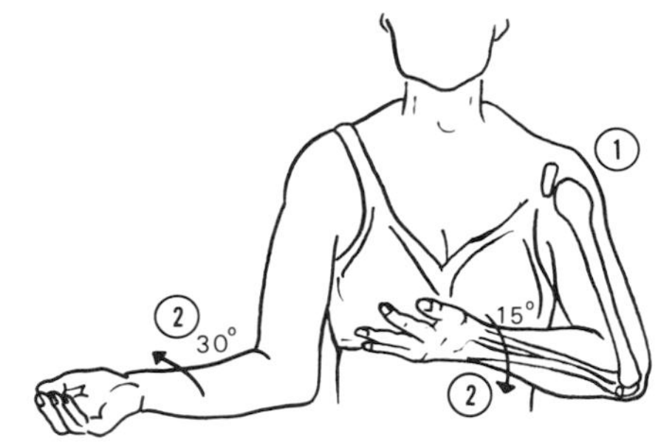

3. If the elbow is extended and the forearm is rotated, the locked internally rotated position of the shoulder may not be evident, and the clinical diagnosis may be missed. Note that, although the patient may appear to have external shoulder rotation with the elbow extended, she still is unable to turn her palm up on the dislocated side.

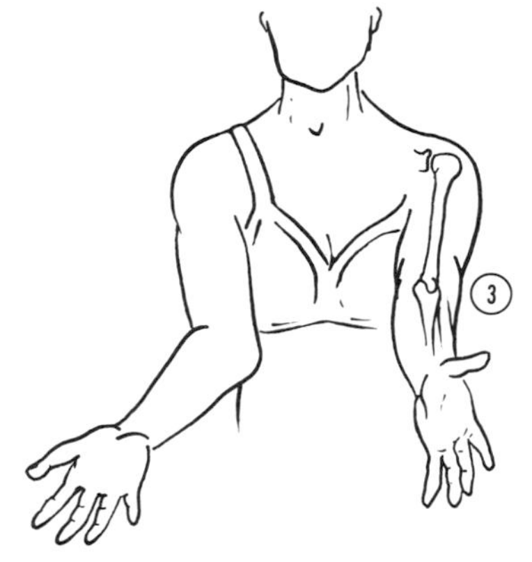

Other Clinical Findings With Posterior Dislocation

1. Anterior fullness of the shoulder is lost.
2. Shoulder is more prominent in the posterior deltoid region.

Note: These subtle physical findings may not be evident if the shoulder is acutely swollen, but the locked internally rotated, adducted position is specific for posterior dislocation.

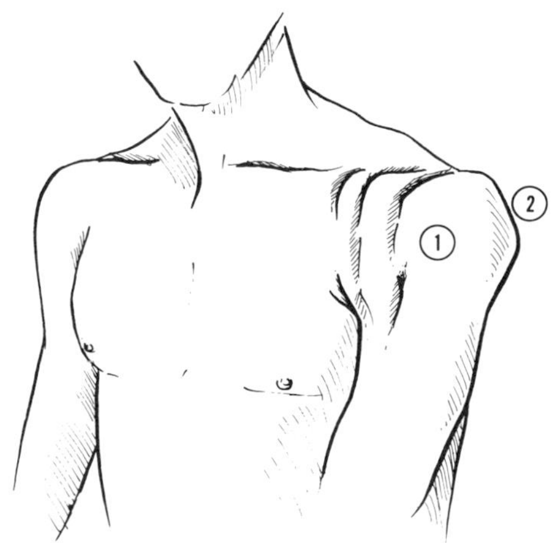

X-Ray Assessment

REMARKS

X-rays are often misleading because the usual anteroposterior and oblique views may not show the correct relationship between the humeral head and the glenoid.

Axillary views, which are essential to make the diagnosis, may not be obtained because of the patient's pain. However, axillary views can always be obtained with the upshot technique.

Upshot X-Ray Technique for Axillary View

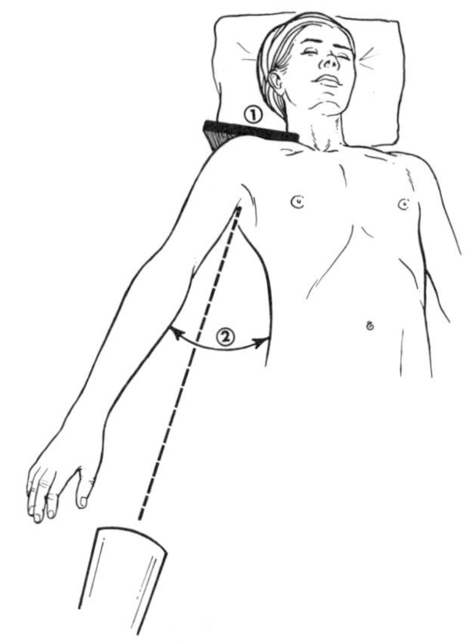

To make the diagnosis of a posterior dislocation, an axillary view is essential. The difficulty of obtaining this view, caused by the patient's pain, can be overcome by using the following procedure.

1. Cassette is placed above the shoulder while the x-ray beam shoots upward through the axilla.
2. Gentle abduction to 40° allows visualization of the posterior dislocation.

Variable X-Ray Appearance

Marked Internal Rotation of Humerus

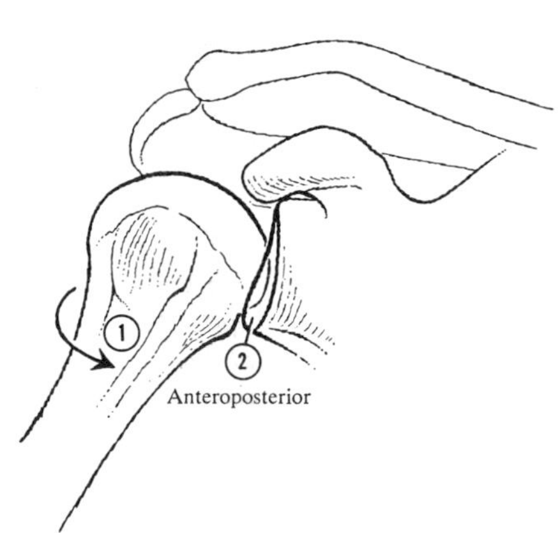

ANTEROPOSTERIOR VIEW

1. Marked internal rotation of the shaft of the humerus occurs.
2. Inferior portion of the glenoid fossa is exposed and is not overlapped by the spherical articular surface of the head.

Minimal Internal Rotation of Humerus

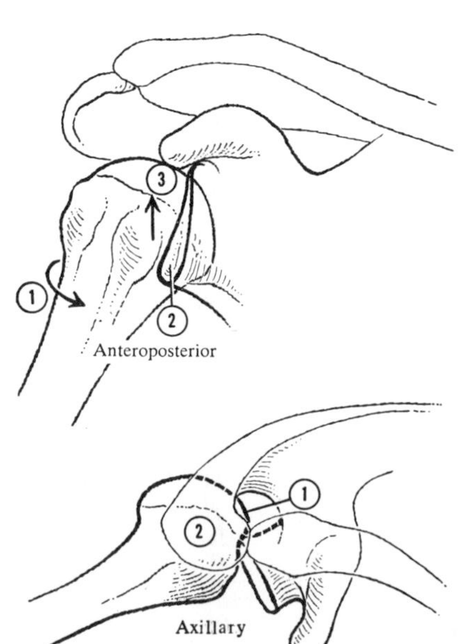

ANTEROPOSTERIOR VIEW

1. Shaft of the humerus is rotated internally.
2. Shadow of the glenoid overlaps that of the humeral articular surface, but this may be interpreted as normal.
3. Humeral head is displaced upward in relation to the glenoid.

Note: The subtle posterior displacement and overlap of the humeral head on the glenoid may not be recognized and the posterior dislocation may not be diagnosed unless adequate axillary views are also obtained.

AXILLARY VIEW

This view is critical for proper diagnosis.

1. Humeral head is behind the glenoid.
2. Humeral head is displaced upward.

Reduction Technique

Reduction of the acute posterior dislocation is usually readily accomplished with the patient sedated or under general anesthesia.

If there is any question about the duration of the dislocation (more than a few days), reduction should be done under general anesthesia with gentle manipulation.

Caution: Attempted vigorous reduction of a chronic dislocation with the patient awake may cause complete fracture of the humeral head and result in disruption of the blood supply to the proximal humerus.

1. Apply gentle, steady traction on the dislocated arm in the direction of the deformity. The elbow is flexed approximately 90°.
2. Assistant reduces the posterior dislocated humeral head by pressing downward on the posterior prominence.
3. Adduct arm with traction maintained.

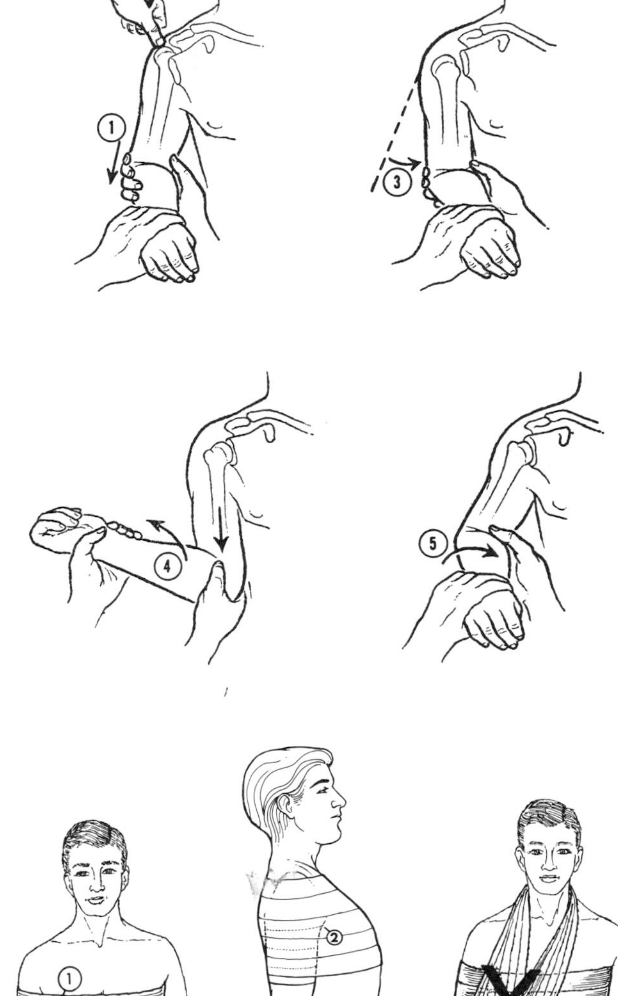

When the head reaches the glenoid rim, effect reduction with a movement that

4. Rotates the arm externally and then
5. Gently rotates the arm internally.

Postreduction Immobilization

1. Pad the axilla.
2. Wrap a 15-cm bias-cut bandage around the arm and forearm so that the humerus is extended and in neutral rotation.
3. Avoid the use of a sling, which adducts and internally rotates the shoulder.

Alternative Method

SPICA CAST IMMOBILIZATION

This method is used for very unstable reductions of posterior dislocation.

Apply the plaster spica that holds arm so that the arm is

Abducted 30°–35°,

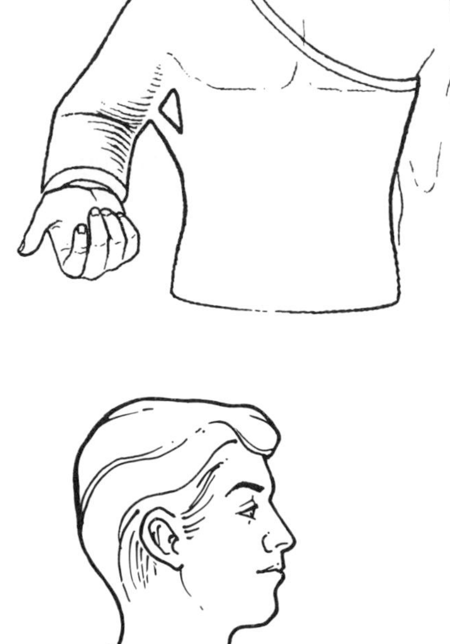

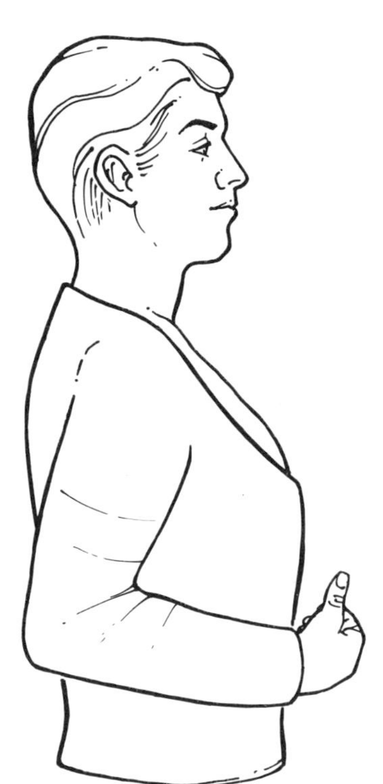

Slightly rotated externally, and

Slightly behind the plane of the trunk.

Postreduction Management

Encourage motion at the wrist and fingers.

Discard the apparatus after 2–3 weeks.

Institute a program of graduated motions within the limits of pain.

Begin with pendulum motions in a stooped position every waking hour for 5 or 10 minutes.

Add abduction and external rotation exercises.

Allow free use of arm within limits of pain and fatigue.

Do not permit strenuous sports activities for a minimum of 3 months.

Old Posterior Dislocations

REMARKS

Posterior shoulder dislocation remains one of the most frequently unrecognized serious orthopaedic injuries.

The delay in recognition may range from a day to several months or even years.

Like unrecognized anterior dislocations, unrecognized posterior dislocations occur most often in elderly persons or in the patient with a seizure disorder or alcoholism.

The diagnosis goes unrecognized, either because the patient does not seek medical advice for a number of days or the medical evaluation is incomplete and the condition is treated as a painful stiff or frozen shoulder.

Occasionally, the dislocation is bilateral, particularly in patients with seizure disorders.

The clinical examination is reliable to make the diagnosis if the locked internally rotated and adducted position of the shoulder is recognized. However, this finding may be confused if the condition is bilateral.

Anteroposterior x-rays are often interpreted as normal with posterior dislocation, but the axillary view shows the dislocation and is diagnostic.

Dislocations of more than 2–3 weeks are difficult if not impossible to reduce. Adequate and safe reduction demands muscle relaxation under general anesthesia. Vigorous manipulation should be avoided because the humeral head can be readily fractured, particularly in the elderly patient who is subject to this problem.

In most instances, if the dislocation is more than 1–2 weeks old, open reduction is the wisest choice.

Unrecognized posterior dislocation is one of the most common identifiable causes of arthropathy, leading to the need for arthroplasty or total shoulder replacement.

The dislocated humeral head quickly erodes against the glenoid and articular cartilage and may be irreversibly damaged. For this reason, many investigators believe that primary shoulder arthroplasty is indicated for the dislocation that goes unrecognized for more than a few weeks.

Characteristic Presentation

1. Patient is frequently an elderly individual or someone subject to a seizure disorder.
2. Dislocation may be bilateral.
3. Typically, the patient is unable to supinate the hand and forearm because of marked internal rotation and adduction at the shoulder joint.

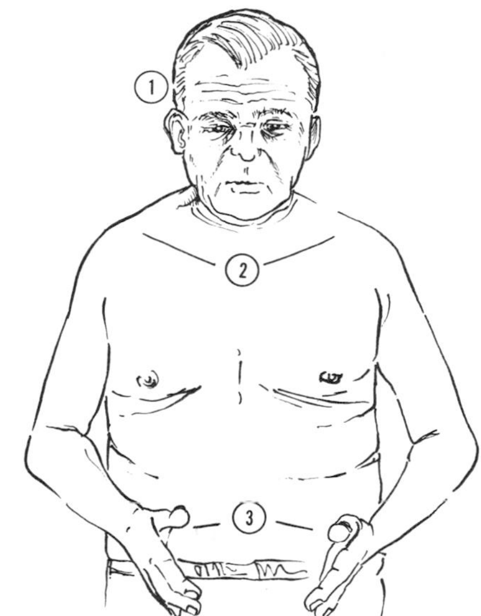

Chronic Posterior Dislocation of 6 Weeks' Duration

1. Humeral head has developed erosive changes from being locked against the posterior aspect of the glenoid.
2. Large wedge-shaped anteromedial defect occurs from the humeral head being locked against the glenoid.
3. Locked position and defect on the anteromedial head is best seen on the axillary view. There may also be a fracture of the glenoid rim.

Note: This locked position of the humeral head on the glenoid makes reduction difficult after more than 2–3 weeks. Frequently, the shoulder may remain locked for several months and go on to rapid degenerative arthritis, requiring a total shoulder replacement.

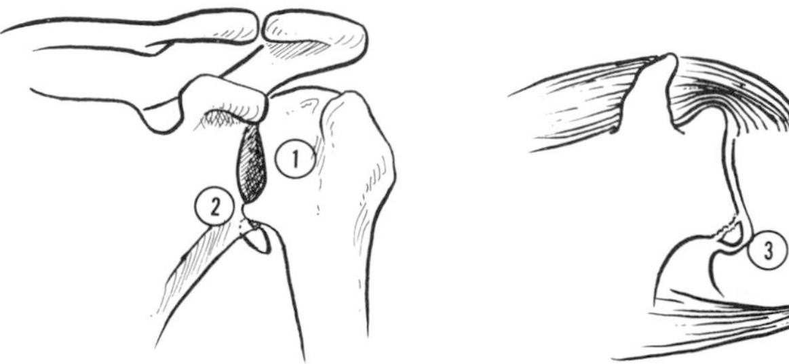

Management

REMARKS

Posterior dislocations that go unrecognized for a few days may be reduced by gentle closed manipulation under adequate general anesthesia.

For chronic dislocation of more than 2–3 weeks, open reduction is usually wisest.

Occasionally, it has been recommended that elderly patients with chronically dislocated shoulders may be insufficiently symptomatic to warrant open operative treatment. However, for most, chronic dislocation does cause pain and shoulder arthropathy sufficient to indicate the need for operation.

If the shoulder joint is found to be destroyed as a result of the chronic dislocation, a shoulder joint replacement may be necessary.

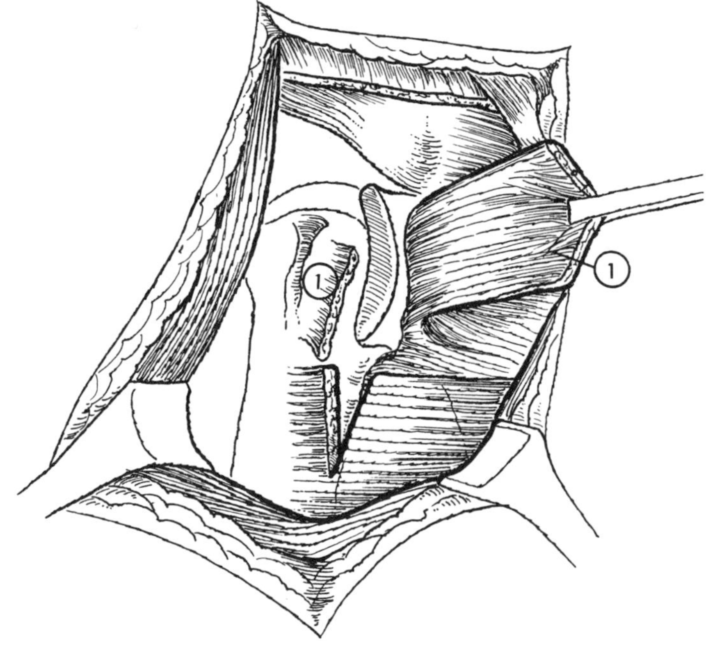

Obstacles to Reduction

1. If the recently dislocated shoulder cannot be reduced with gentle manipulation, as previously described, open exploration of the joint is indicated. Usually, the subscapularis tendon and capsule are found wedged between the head of the humerus and the glenoid head posteriorly.

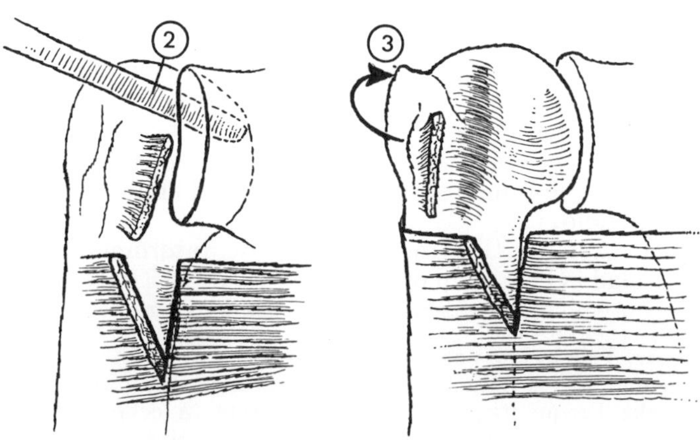

2. After the subscapularis tendon is divided, the humeral head can be reduced by placing a skid between the dislocated head and the glenoid. This disengages the defect of the humeral head from the posterior glenoid rim.
3. Arm is externally rotated to complete the reduction.

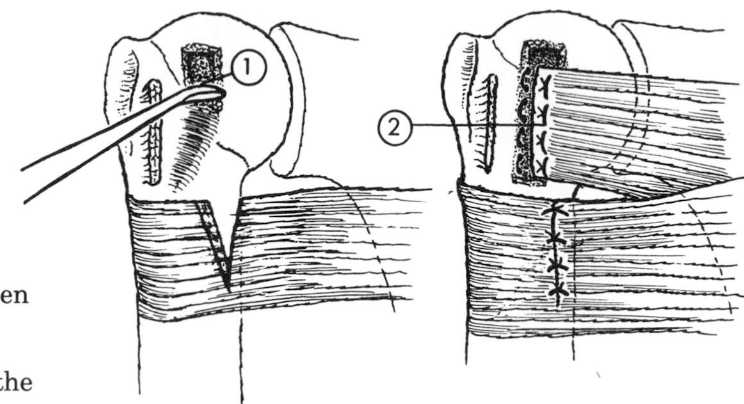

1. Area of the humeral head medial defect is then curetted to prepare a surface for tendon transfer.
2. Subscapularis tendon is then transferred to the defect and fixed by sutures into the bone.

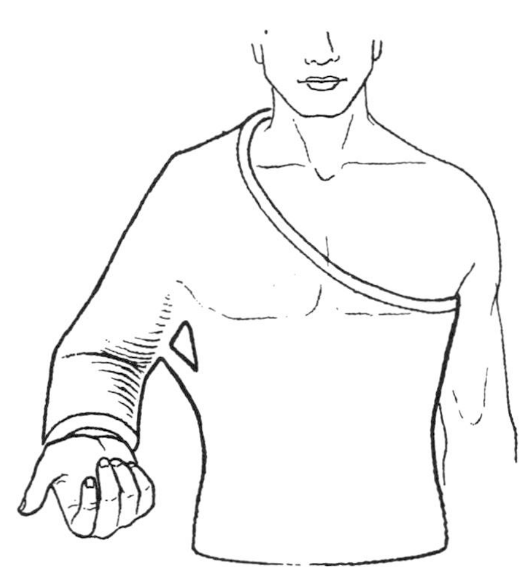

Postoperative Management

In the postoperative period, apply a plaster spica cast that holds the arm abducted 30°–35°, slightly rotated externally, and slightly behind the plane of the trunk.

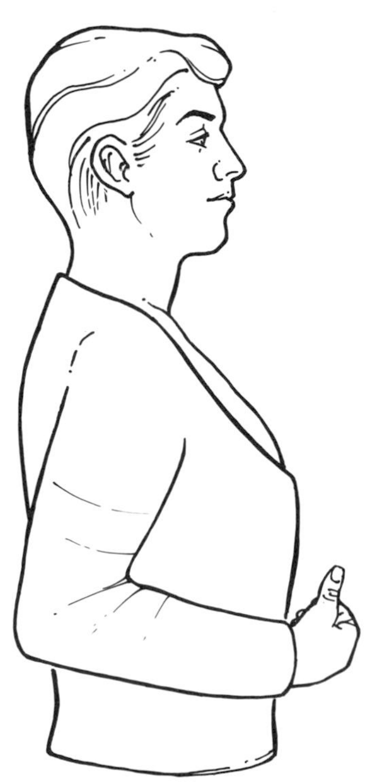

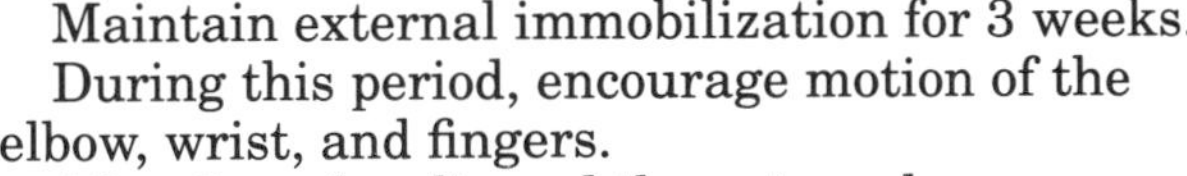

Maintain external immobilization for 3 weeks.

During this period, encourage motion of the elbow, wrist, and fingers.

After 3 weeks, discard the external immobilization.

Institute pendulum exercises on a regulated program of 5 to 10 minutes every waking hour.

Increase gradually the range and frequency of the exercises, always within the tolerance of pain.

Add external rotation and abduction exercises.

The return to a maximum level of painless function depends on the duration of the dislocation prior to reduction and the degree of secondary joint changes.

Note: If the joint is severely affected, primary arthroplasty is preferable.

Management of Complications of Glenohumeral Dislocation

REMARKS

Acute traumatic dislocation may be associated with one or more of numerous complications.

Awareness of this possibility is most important in the detection of these lesions because early detection and treatment may prevent an unfavorable result.

The most significant complications are

- Injury to the axillary artery.
- Injury to the brachial plexus or the peripheral nerves.
- Tear of the rotator cuff.
- Fractures—these may involve the glenoid, humeral head, acromion, tuberosities, and neck and shaft of the humerus.
- Recurrent dislocation.

Injury to the Axillary Artery

REMARKS

Injury to the axillary artery is most likely to occur in elderly patients with arteriosclerotic vessels or in patients whose shoulders are scarred by recurrent dislocation. It is not so rare that it should not be checked for and recognized promptly.

Characteristically, the shoulder swells rapidly, the patient has severe pain and paralysis of the arm, and the radial pulse is no longer palpable.

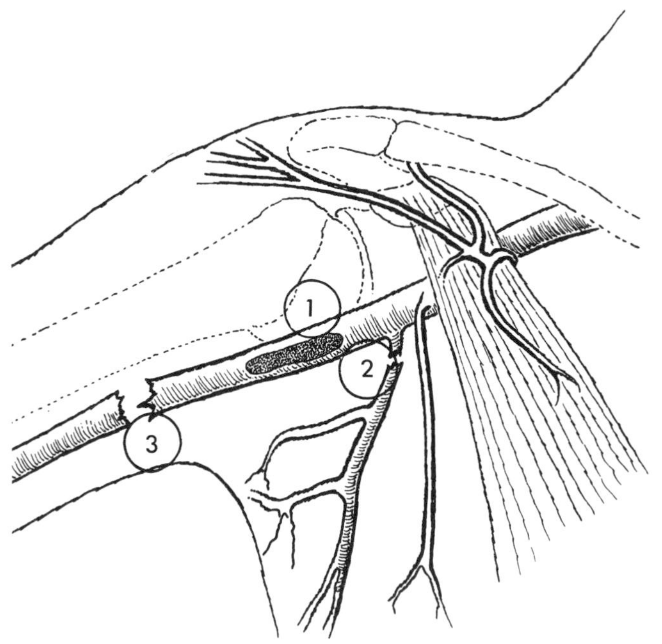

The types of arterial damage that may occur are

1. Intimal damage followed by thrombosis;
2. Avulsion of a large branch from the artery, usually, the subscapular or circumflex artery; and
3. Rupture of the main trunk of the axillary artery.

Any dislocated shoulder should be reduced by gentle manipulation, but this is especially true in elderly patients, in whom the reduction is done most safely with general anesthesia.

If an old, chronically dislocated shoulder is not recognized as such and manipulation is attempted too forcefully, vascular disruption may occur. Do not try to reduce a dislocation that is known or suspected to be chronic by repeated closed manipulation, especially without anesthesia.

When the arterial rupture is recognized, the bleeding may be slowed by digital pressure, which compresses the axillary artery against the first rib. Prompt surgical exploration should then be carried out through a subclavian-axillary approach with resection of the damaged artery and vascular anastomosis or graft.

Ligation should be avoided in the elderly patient because arteriosclerotic vessels have poor collateral circulation and gangrene inevitably follows.

Management

If vascular impairment occurs, the shoulder should be reduced promptly and gently. If vascular impairment is not relieved, explore the vessels through a subclavian-axillary approach.

Prior to surgical exploration, the hemorrhage can be controlled by compressing the subclavian artery against the first rib.

The damaged vessel should be resected in its entirety; graft replacement may be necessary.

Subclavian Approach

1. With the arm abducted, an incision is made from the lower border of the clavicle, down the arm, and along the deltopectoral groove.
2. Pectoralis major is released and is retracted inferiorly to expose the axillary vessels.
3. Pectoralis minor is detached from the coracoid for greater exposure.
4. Bleeding vessel is clamped.

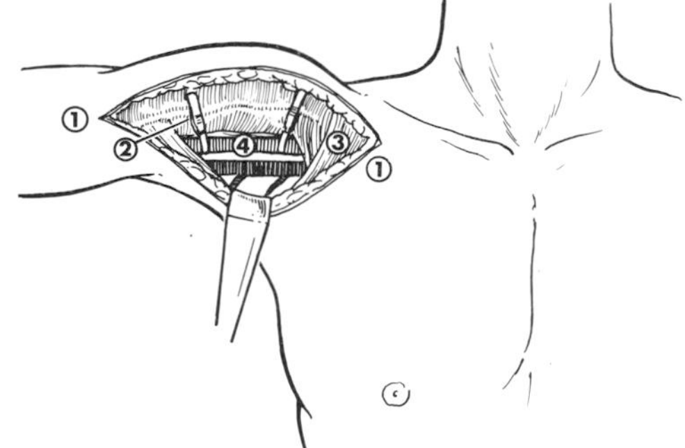

After exposure and control of the bleeding vessel, the

1. Frayed ends of the artery are resected.
2. End-to-end anastomosis is performed, or a saphenous vein graft is inserted.

Note: Ligation of the vessels under these circumstances should be avoided because collateral circulation in the elderly patient is inadequate.

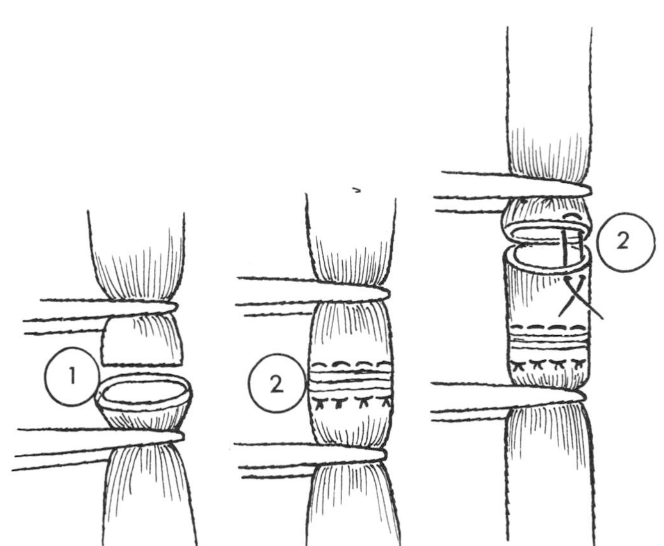

Injury to Nerves

REMARKS

Injury to peripheral nerves and the brachial plexus may occur with acute dislocations of the shoulder.

The occurrence rate of nerve injury in dislocation varies in frequency from 5–30 per cent of cases, depending on the thoroughness of the examination.

Because the axillary nerve runs along the subscapularis, it is exposed to injury from an anterior dislocation. Electromyography demonstrates damage to the axillary nerve in more than 30 per cent of dislocations. This is most often transitory and, frequently, is not associated with sensory loss.

Axillary nerve damage should be suspected in a patient who regains shoulder abduction slowly after reduction.

Occasionally, the brachial plexus, particularly the medial cord, which includes the ulnar and median nerves, is damaged. Recovery from the stretch injury to the plexus is usually spontaneous but may cause painful paresthesias for several months after the injury.

The prognosis for recovery is good with single nerve lesions because, as a rule, the nerve deficit is temporary. The prognosis is less favorable with multiple nerve injuries; in some cases, the nerve deficit may be permanent.

The diagnosis of nerve damage may be recognized by sensory deficit, but frequently electromyography is necessary to confirm or recognize occult nerve injuries.

The chief differential diagnosis is to distinguish weakness in the shoulder after reduction caused by axillary nerve injury from rotator cuff disruption. Weakness is considerably greater with the tendon disruption, which generally requires operative repair, in contrast to axillary nerve palsy, which frequently recovers spontaneously.

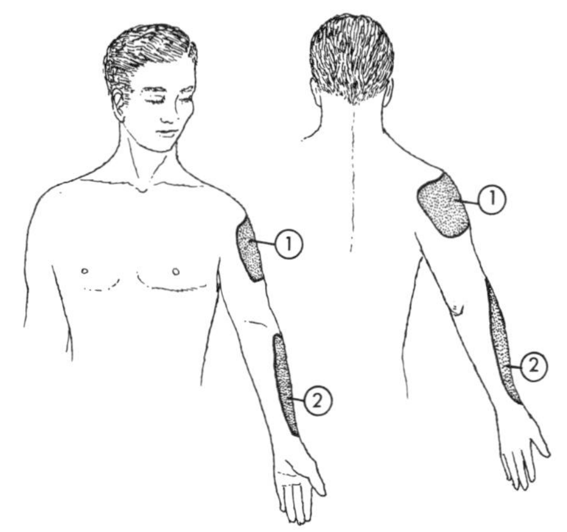

1. Area of hypoesthesia or sensory loss associated with injury to the axillary nerve.
2. Area of sensory loss associated with injury to musculocutaneous nerve.

Note: If there is significant weakness of elevation of the arm persisting for several weeks after reduction, tear of the rotator cuff should be suspected rather than isolated axillary nerve palsy.

Management

For most intraclavicular and axillary nerve lesions associated with dislocation, treatment is supportive.

The return of deep sensation is the first evidence of an incomplete lesion.

While motor function is coming back, muscle tone should be maintained by active and assisted range-of-motion exercises.

Joint stiffness should be avoided by a program of therapy to the elbow, wrist, and fingers.

Frequently, as the nerve function returns, painful paresthesias may cause discomfort to the patient. However, the patient should be advised that this is generally a good sign and responsive to mild analgesics.

If no clinical or electromyographic evidence of return exists after 3 months and the motor deficit warrants it, surgical exploration of the nerves may be considered.

Rupture of the Rotator Cuff

REMARKS

Rupture of the rotator cuff is rare in young adults but fairly common in older patients.

Rotator cuff disruption is common with dislocations produced by hyperabduction or in luxatio erecta in any age group.

Initially, rotator cuff rupture may not be recognized when the arm is immobilized after reduction.

Suspect a rotator cuff tear if there is persistent superior or inferior subluxation, especially if the patient is unable to abduct the shoulder.

Check the abduction power of the shoulder after the shoulder immobilizer is discarded. Should abduction remain limited for more than 2 weeks, suspect a rotator cuff injury.

The principal differential diagnosis to be made for patients with these symptoms is between rotator cuff injury and axillary nerve damage. Electromyography establishes axillary nerve damage; shoulder arthrography or magnetic resonance imaging (MRI) demonstrates the rotator cuff tear.

When the diagnosis of a cuff tear is established, surgical repair should be prompt to relieve the pain and decreased shoulder strength these patients usually experience.

Typical Deformity Associated With Large Tear of Cuff

1. In attempting to abduct the arm, the patient shrugs the shoulder; the deltoid contracts forcefully.
2. No abduction or weak abduction is present in the glenohumeral joint.
3. Few degrees of abduction are possible by fixing the humeral head in the glenoid cavity and rotating the scapula outward.
4. Abduction is usually weak against any resistance.

Note: In some patients, the only significant manifestation of rotator cuff injury is persistent pain in the shoulder several weeks or months after reduction. (See impingement syndrome.)

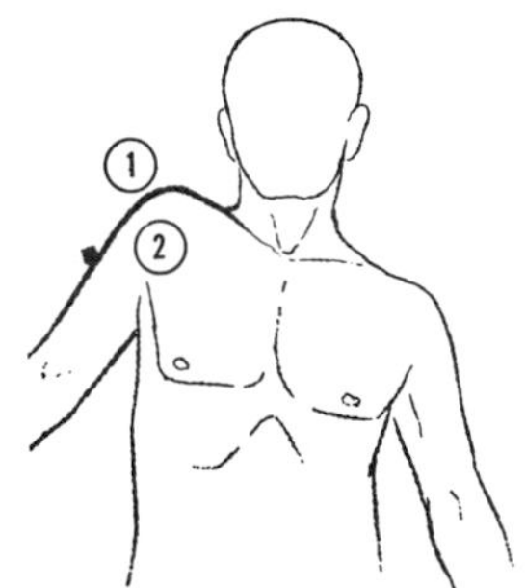

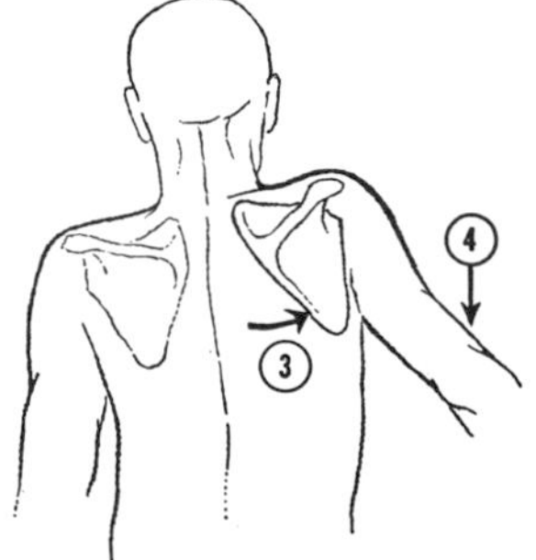

Technique of Shoulder Arthrography

1. Patient lies supine with arm by the side and internally rotated.
2. After sterile preparation, the area below and slightly lateral to the coracoid is injected with 10 mL of a local anesthetic down to the neck of the scapula.
3. Then a 20-gauge short-beveled needle, 6-cm long, is inserted and is directed toward the glenoid.
4. Needle should enter the joint space above the axillary folds, and the position should be confirmed by means of image-intensified fluoroscopy.

Note: Longitudinal traction on the arm helps to open up the joint space.

5. Use 12 mL of contrast solution mixed with 4 mL of lidocaine. Inject 2 mL first, and then determine by fluoroscopy that the dye is in the joint. Then inject the remaining dye.

Note: X-rays should be taken promptly after the injection and should include axillary views. If the suspected tear is a chronic one, the leak may be seen only after the patient has abducted and elevated the arm.

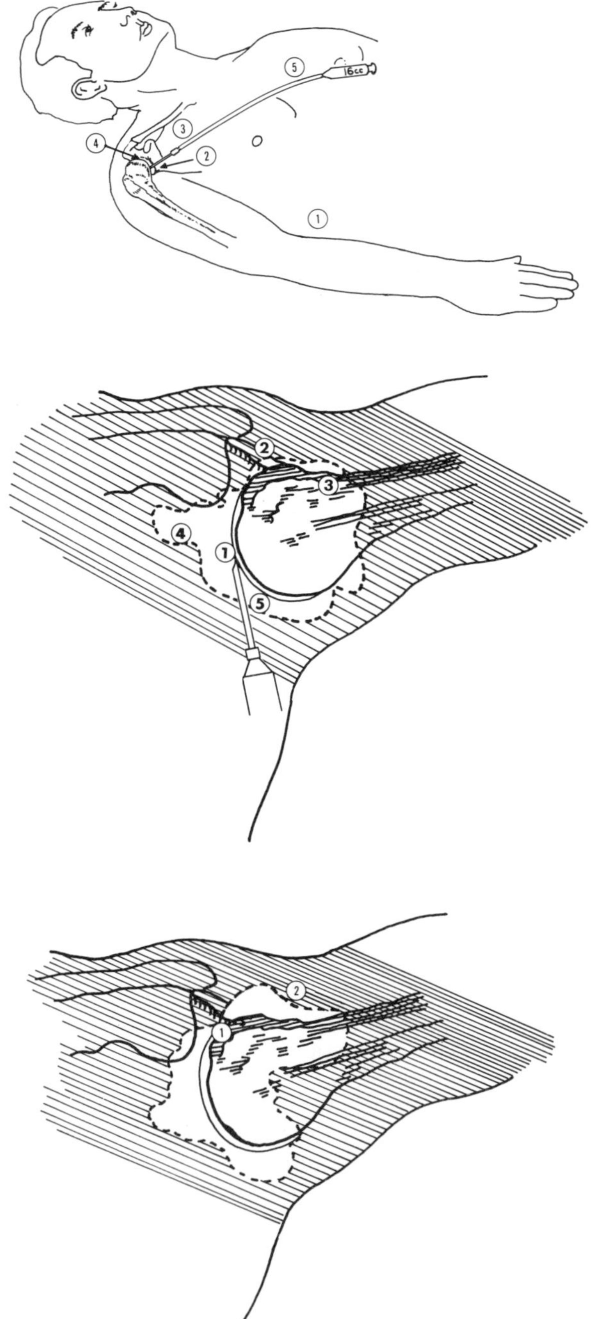

NORMAL ARTHROGRAM

1. Glenohumeral joint does not communicate with the
2. Subacromial bursa.
3. Bicipital tendon sheath is filled with dye.
4. Subscapularis bursa and the
5. Axillary pouch fill with the solution.

Note: MRI, when available, may also be useful for diagnosing rotator cuff rupture.

ARTHROGRAM AFTER SUPRASPINATUS TENDON RUPTURE

1. Subacromial bursa fills with dye.
2. On 100° abduction, the dye-filled bursa “sticks out like a sore thumb.”

Management

When a primary acute dislocation occurs in an older patient, there should be a high index of suspicion that the rotator cuff has also been torn because most patients in the age group older than 40 years have some weakness of this structure.

Frequently, once the dislocation is reduced, the rotator cuff tear is small enough that it does not cause any significant residual weakness problems.

However, if the patient demonstrates a persistent weakness of abduction and external rotation, this is most often due to a rupture of the rotator cuff rather than to a nerve injury.

If surgical repair is indicated to provide stability in the older patient, initial attention should be directed to the torn rotator cuff as well as to the anterior capsule or subscapularis.

1. Operative repair should be done promptly when a diagnosis of rotator cuff disruption is made in association with dislocated shoulder.

A delay in repair makes it difficult to reattach the rotator cuff to the humeral head and may compromise the results.

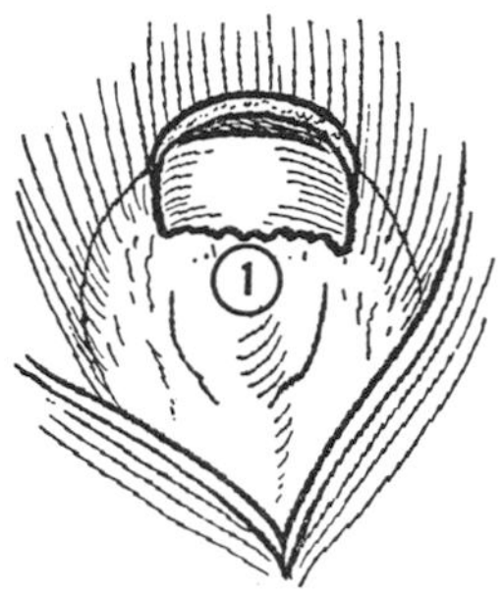

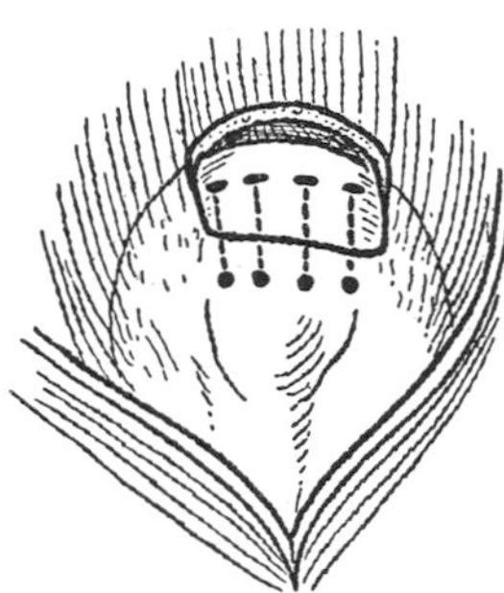

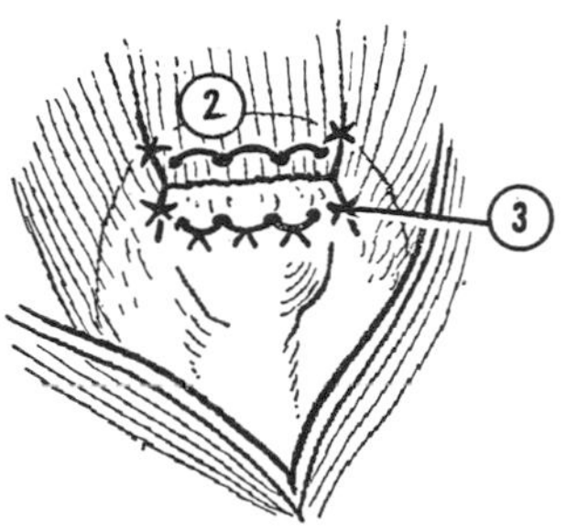

2. Rotator cuff should be brought down directly to bony attachment for best restoration of function.
3. Various implantable suture techniques are available to achieve good reattachment of the tendon to the bone if the rotator cuff problem is not a chronic one.

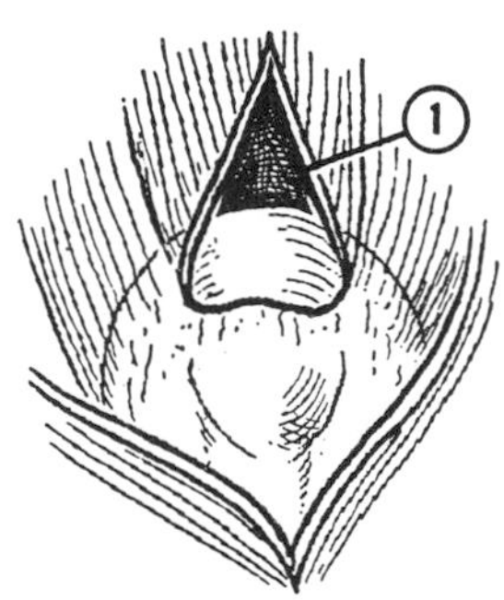

1. If the rotator cuff disruption is chronic, particularly in the elderly patient, adequate repair may not be possible because of the size of the defect. In this instance, decompression of the subacromial space may be carried out by resection of a portion of the acromion to relieve the painful impingement problem. This will not restore normal shoulder strength but is preferable to more extensive attempts at tendon grafting or reconstruction.

Fractures That Complicate Dislocations

REMARKS

All shoulder dislocations impact the humeral head against the glenoid labrum. This fractures the glenoid or tears the labrum, producing the Bankart lesion, which is thought to be the primary cause of recurrent shoulder dislocation.

In addition, as the shoulder dislocates anteriorly, a violent response of the muscles can cause an impaction fracture of the posterolateral aspect of the humeral head. This defect can be large, especially with recurrent dislocations in patients with seizure disorders.

In the older patient, impaction of the humeral head causes a complete fracture or avulsion of the greater tuberosity and rotator cuff attachment. This fracture of the greater tuberosity may spare the anterior capsule and glenoid labrum so that redislocation is less common in the older than in the younger patient. However, the avulsion fracture of the greater tuberosity often produces residual rotator cuff weakness and painful limitation of active motion.

It is also possible that, as the shoulder dislocates, particularly in the elderly patient, an undisplaced fracture through the anatomic or surgical neck may occur, in addition to the fracture of the tuberosity. Overvigorous manipulation in an attempt to reduce this fracture-dislocation can produce a completely displaced head fragment and a much more difficult problem to resolve for the patient.

Keep in mind the possibility of worsening the displacement of the fracture while attempting to reduce a dislocation with a fracture, particularly in an older patient with osteoporotic bone.

Mechanism of Injury

1. Humeral head dislocates anteriorly and impacts against the anterior aspect of the glenoid.
2. This results in a fracture of the glenoid or avulsion of the glenoid labrum.
3. Humeral head develops an impaction fracture in the younger patient, but in the older individual, an
4. Avulsion of the greater tuberosity or fracture of the head of the humerus occurs.

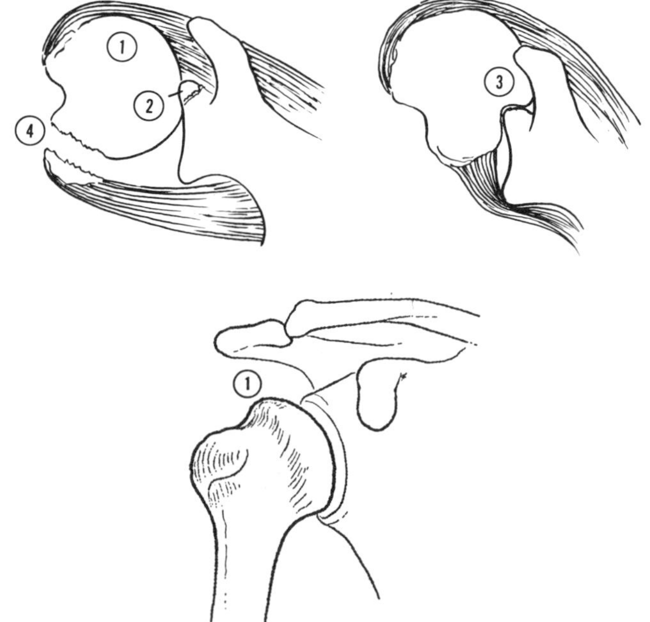

Notch Defect (Hill-Sachs Defect) in a Patient With Recurrent Dislocations From Seizure Disorders

1. The largest posterolateral defects in fractures are associated with the recurrent dislocations in patients with severe seizure problems. These can involve almost the entire third of the posterolateral head and may contribute to the instability problem.

Anteromedial Defect With Recurrent Posterior Dislocation

1. Acute or recurrent posterior dislocation is considerably less frequent than anterior dislocation but also produces a fracture of the head of the humerus.
2. This is typically located in the anteromedial aspect of the head and is a mirror image of the posterolateral defect or Hill-Sachs lesion produced by an anterior dislocation.
3. Impaction of the posterior dislocated head against the glenoid produces a fracture of the lesser tuberosity or anteromedial notching of the head. There is frequently an avulsion of the posterior labrum.

Note: Any fracture of the lesser tuberosity should alert the physician to the probability that the shoulder has dislocated posteriorly.

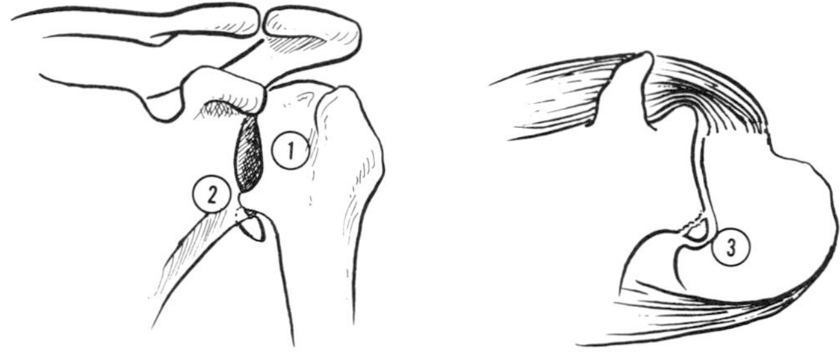

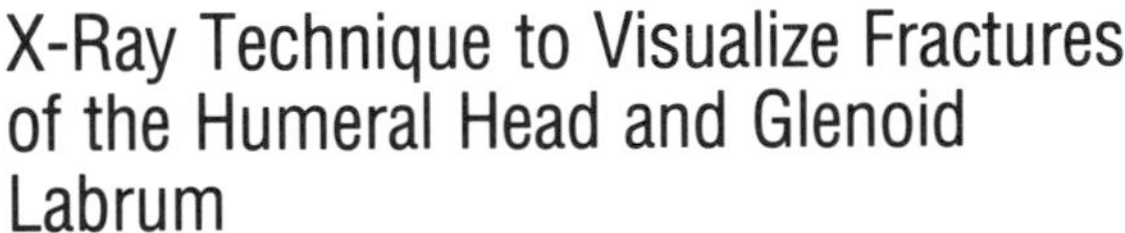

X-Ray Technique to Visualize Fractures of the Humeral Head and Glenoid Labrum

In addition to the standard anteroposterior and axillary views previously described, oblique views are necessary to see both the posterolateral aspect of the humeral head and the glenoid labrum.

The bony structures of the humerus frequently are obscured in the posterolateral aspect of the head. Therefore, many defects or fractures posteriorly may not be seen on routine x-rays. Because of this, the x-ray should be tangential to the superior surface of the head to show the posterolateral fracture.

In addition, to show the glenoid fractures adequately, an angled or West Point view may be needed.

View for Hill-Sachs Posterolateral Fracture

1. Tube is angled 30° from the perpendicular.
2. Patient's shoulder is abducted slightly and is internally rotated so that the arm rests on the chest.

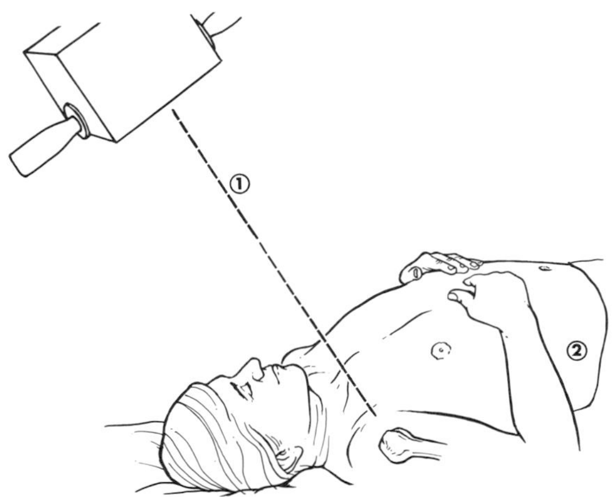

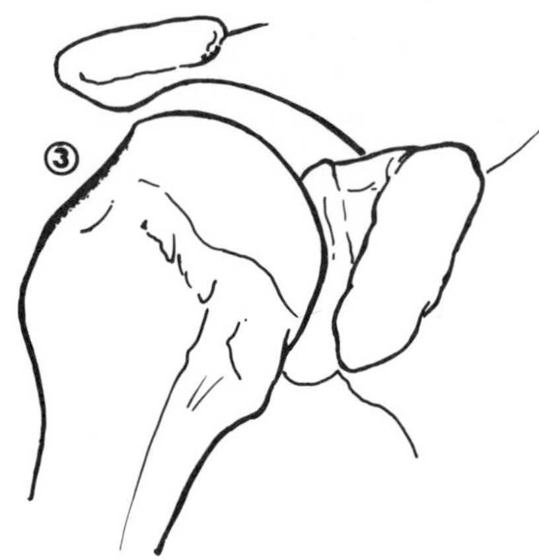

3. Posterolateral defect may vary from a subtle flattening to a deep compression fracture of the humeral head.

Note: Humeral head impaction fractures require no treatment other than that necessary for the dislocation.

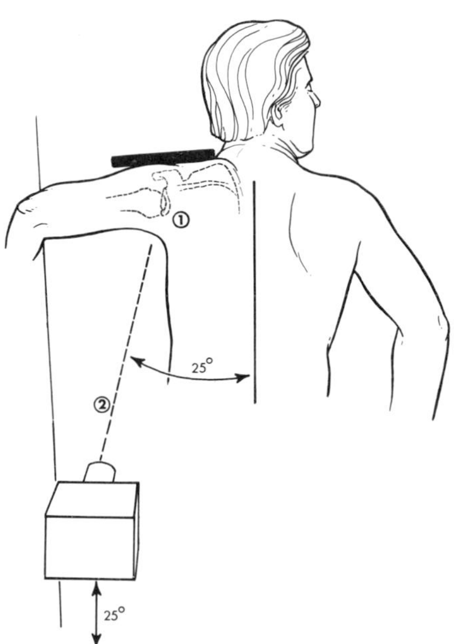

West Point View for Glenoid Fracture With Anterior Dislocation

TECHNIQUE

1. Patient is prone with the involved shoulder raised by pads.
2. X-ray beam is angled 25° downward and 25° medially toward the axilla.

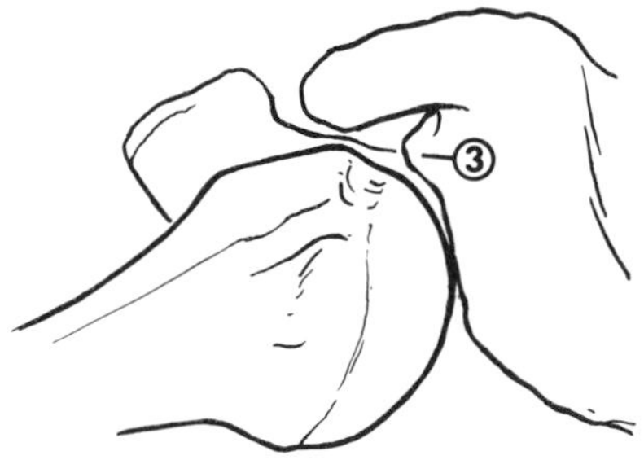

APPEARANCE ON X-RAY

3. Resultant tangential axillary view of the glenoid may show small anterior fragmentation associated with subluxation.

Displaced Fractures of the Greater Tuberosity Associated With Dislocations

REMARKS

These fractures occur characteristically in the dislocated shoulder in the patient older than 40 years of age.

As the humeral head dislocates over the glenoid, the injury to the osteoporotic bone causes a complete fracture through the greater tuberosity, which displaces. The amount of displacement may vary from minimal to wide displacement with retraction of the tuberosity under the acromion.

In general, the dislocation with fracture may be one of three types:

- Type I. The tuberosity follows the humeral head.
- Type II. The tuberosity retains its normal relationship to the scapula.
- Type III. The tuberosity is retracted under the acromion.

Severe damage to the rotator cuff may accompany all three of these fractures. Therefore, if anatomic reduction is not achieved by closed reduction, surgical repair of the fracture and the rotator cuff is indicated.

Prereduction X-Rays

TYPE I

1. Greater tuberosity has followed the humeral head.
2. Humeral head occupies a position at a distance from the glenoid fossa.

   In this fracture-dislocation, the cuff is severely stretched or may be ruptured. Check for rupture.

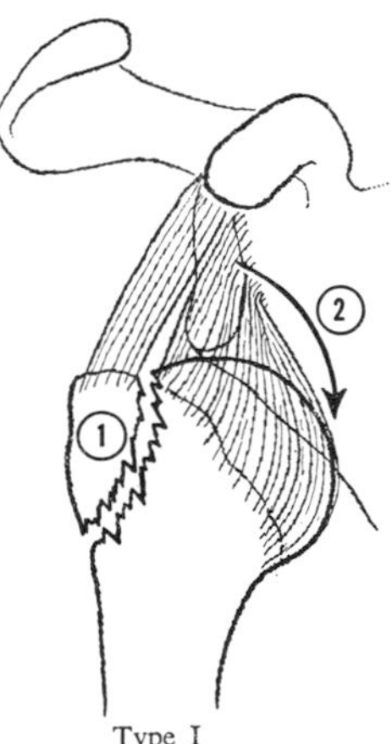

Type I

TYPE II

3. Greater tuberosity is in its normal position in relation to the glenoid fossa.
4. Humeral head is displaced from the glenoid cavity.

   If reduction fails, suspect posterior displacement of the biceps tendon or interposition of the cuff and the tuberosities in front of the head. Closed reduction is usually possible, provided that the greater tuberosity has not retracted under the acromion (type III fracture).

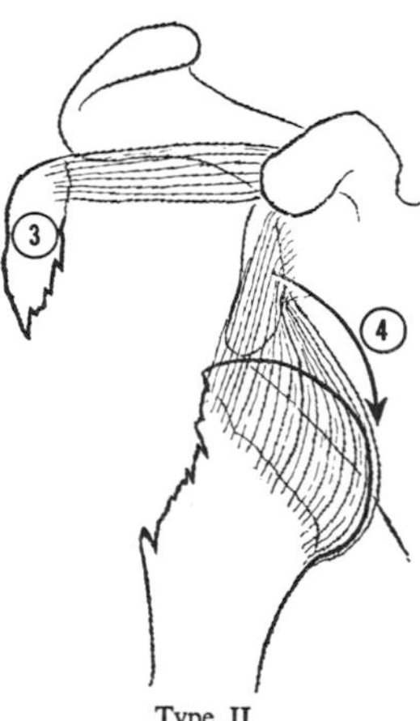

Type II

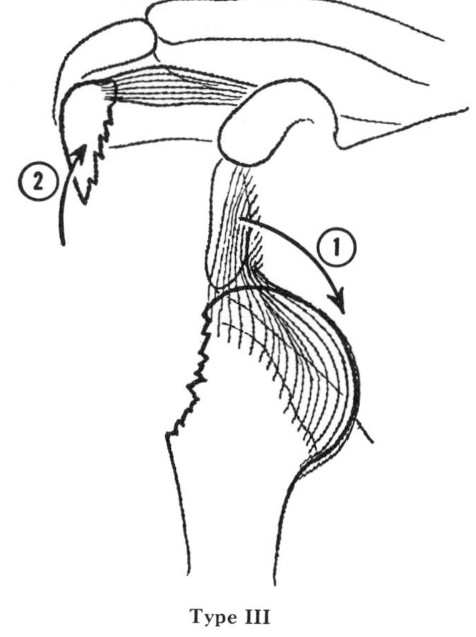

Type III

TYPE III

1. Humeral head is dislocated anteriorly.
2. Greater tuberosity is retracted under the acromion process.

Note: Because of the gross disruption of the rotator cuff in this type of injury, open reduction should be the primary method of reduction.

Management of Greater Tuberosity Fractures With Dislocated Shoulders

Manipulative Reduction

HIPPOCRATIC TECHNIQUE

Caution: It is best with any fracture in the older patient with osteoporotic bone to carry out this reduction under general anesthesia. Avoid any kind of violent or vigorous manipulation because there may be an unrecognized extension of the fracture into the surgical neck region, which can completely displace and cause loss of circulation to the dislocated humeral head.

At all times, the manipulation should be done slowly, steadily, and with adequate muscle relaxation.

1. Physician's stockinged foot is placed between the patient's chest wall and axillary folds but not in the axilla.
2. Steady traction is maintained while the patient gradually relaxes.
3. Shoulder is slowly rotated externally and adducted.
4. Gentle internal rotation reduces the humeral head.

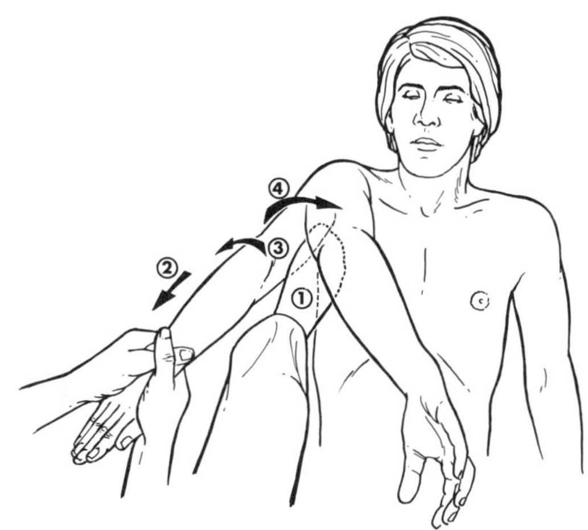

POSTREDUCTION X-RAY

1. Head is reduced.
2. Tuberosity is in its normal position.

Note: Displacement of the tuberosity more than 3–5 mm is likely to cause impingement against the acromion.

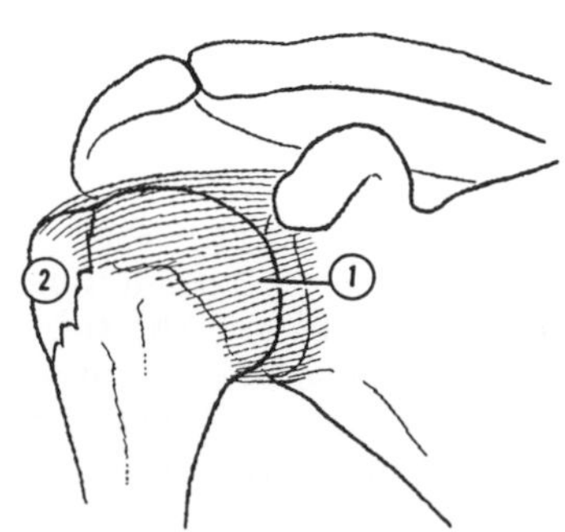

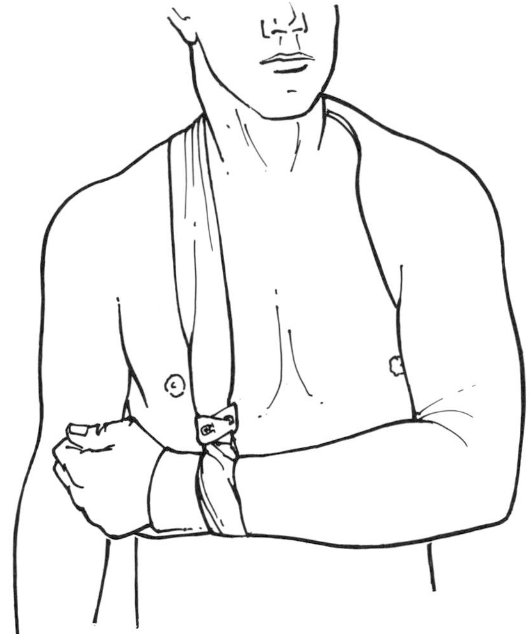

IMMOBILIZATION

Apply a shoulder immobilizer.

Postreduction Management

Follow the patient with repeated x-rays during the first week or two after reduction.

Frequently, the tuberosity that was initially thought to be adequately reduced may be displaced as a result of avulsion from the rotator cuff muscles.

It is not uncommon to see the tuberosity displaced beneath the acromion after what was considered to be an adequate reduction.

If the tuberosity remains in anatomic alignment, the patient should begin motion at the elbow, wrist, and fingers after the first week.

Discard the shoulder immobilizer after 3–4 weeks, and begin a program of graduated range-of-motion exercise.

Begin with motions in the stooped position every hour for 5–10 minutes, and later advance to abduction and external rotation exercises.

Allow use of the arm within the limits of pain and fatigue.

Do not permit strenuous sports for a minimal of 3–4 months.

Indications for Operative Repair

Although some of the tuberosity fracture fragments heal adequately, it is generally best to repair operatively any that are not anatomically reduced.

Even minimal displacement of the tuberosity of 5 mm can cause problems as the fracture callus develops and narrows down the subacromial space. This leads to significant impingement problems on attempted elevation of the arm.

Because of this problem, which can cause significant limitation and persistent weakness, it is often best to repair the avulsed bone fragment operatively.

Indication for Surgery

1. Commonly, a minimally displaced tuberosity fracture after reduction is found to displace further in the first week or so during immobilization because of the continued pull of the attached tendons and rotator cuff structures.
2. If the displaced fracture of the tuberosity heals in a displaced position, the callus and bony formation frequently cause impingement on the acromion and result in painful limitation of shoulder motion.

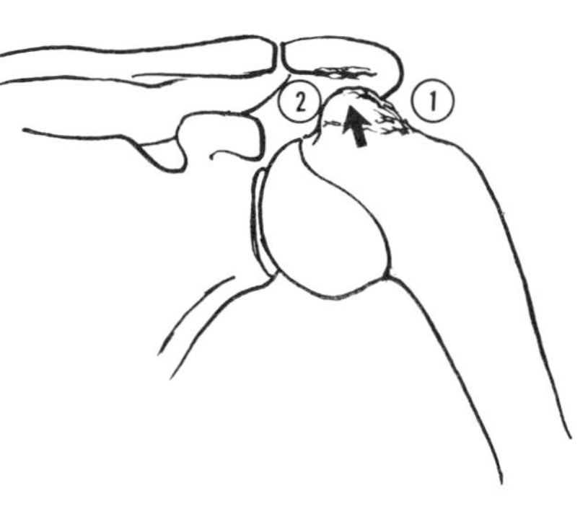

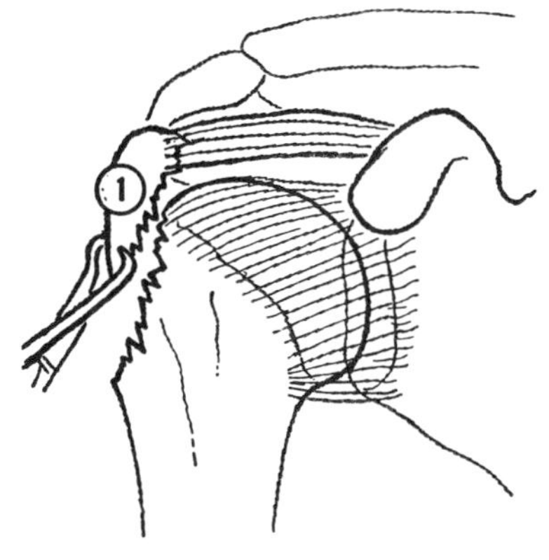

1. Frequently, the tuberosity is displaced further after reduction and requires direct open repair to reattach it back to its proper position on the humeral head.

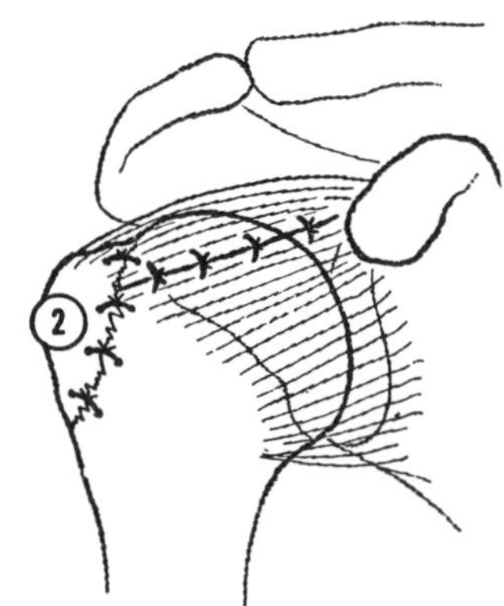

2. Tuberosity fragment can be sutured directly to bone, and the rotator cuff tear, which is always associated with these fractures, is also repaired. This allows the optimal recovery of shoulder function.

Other Indications: Type III Completely Displaced Tuberosity Fragments

1. Dislocation of the humeral head with
2. Wide displacement of the tuberosity fracture indicates complete disruption of rotator cuff. This is an acute severe injury, which is best treated by open repair because, usually, a large number of major structures are injured.

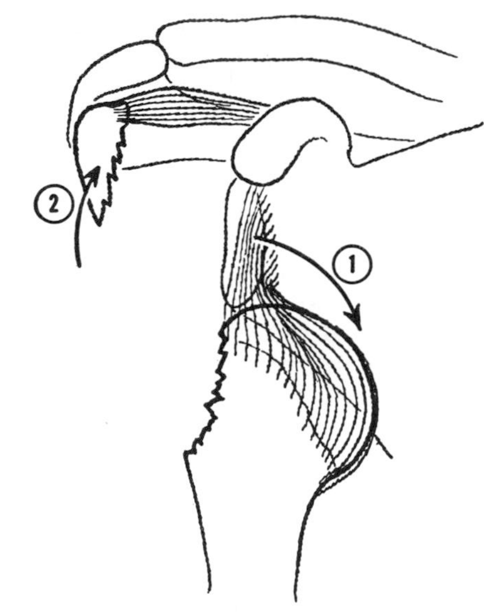

Type III

Reduction and Repair of Acute Type III Injuries

1. Biceps tendon is frequently found obstructing the reduction because it is caught between the tuberosity and the humeral head.
2. Rotator cuff is often found in the glenoid cavity between the glenoid and the humeral head.
3. Shoulder is reduced after the soft tissue obstructions are cleared.
4. Tuberosity fragment is fixed with sutures to the bone.
5. Biceps tendon is stabilized to the humerus.
6. Tuberosity fragment may also be fixed with a screw.
7. Rotator cuff can then be completely repaired.

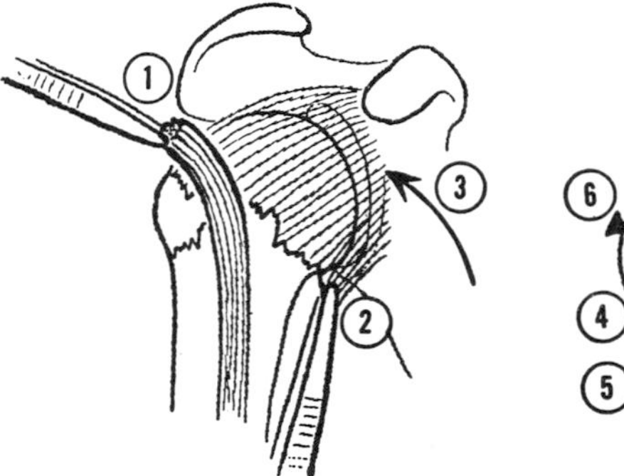

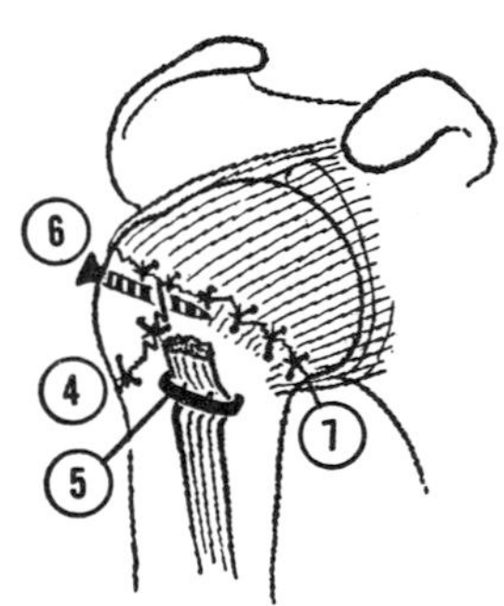

Fractures of the Head and Neck of the Humerus With Dislocation

REMARKS

Fracture-dislocations of the head and neck of the humerus are serious injuries that occur usually from severe direct violence to the shoulder.

In contrast to the usual dislocation, these injuries result from a fall or direct blow on the shoulder.

The result of the injury produces a variety of combinations of fractures. These include fractures of the greater or lesser tuberosity, fractures through the anatomic neck, or fractures through the surgical neck in addition to the dislocation.

This more severe injury is discussed further in the chapter on fractures of the humerus (see Chapter 13).

Occasionally, overvigorous attempted reduction of a dislocation in a patient without adequate muscle relaxation produces a complete fracture of the head and neck of the humerus with dislocation. This is particularly likely in the patient who has an unrecognized or undisplaced fracture through the surgical neck in addition to dislocation.

A displaced fracture created at the time of manipulation is much more difficult to manage than is the usual fracture of the tuberosity that is associated with dislocation.

Complete displacement of the dislocated humeral head fragment frequently deprives the humeral head of its blood supply and can lead to avascular necrosis and long-term loss of joint function.

Iatrogenic Injury

1. Occasionally, overvigorous manipulation by the surgeon may produce a complete fracture-dislocation of the humeral head.
2. This is particularly likely in the elderly patient with an unrecognized undisplaced surgical neck fracture in association with a fracture of the greater tuberosity.

Note: Any suspicion of a fracture in an elderly osteoporotic patient with a dislocation warrants the use of general anesthesia for gentle manipulation to achieve reduction rather than reduction without adequate anesthesia, which may risk displacement of the fracture.

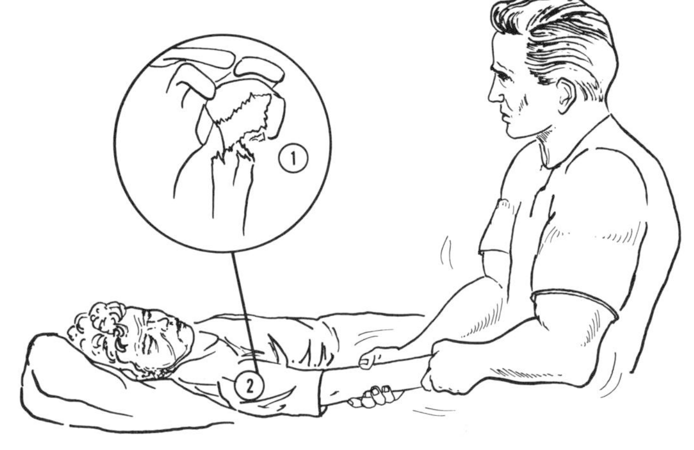

Arterial Vascularization of the Humeral Head

1. Humeral head has been shown to be perfused primarily by branches from the anterior circumflex artery.
2. Anterolateral artery runs parallel to the lateral aspect of the long head of the biceps.
3. Blood supply enters the humeral head where the proximal end of the intertubercular groove meets the greater tuberosity.

Note: With complete displacement through the anatomic neck, this important blood supply is usually lost, and avascularity of the humeral head becomes a problem.

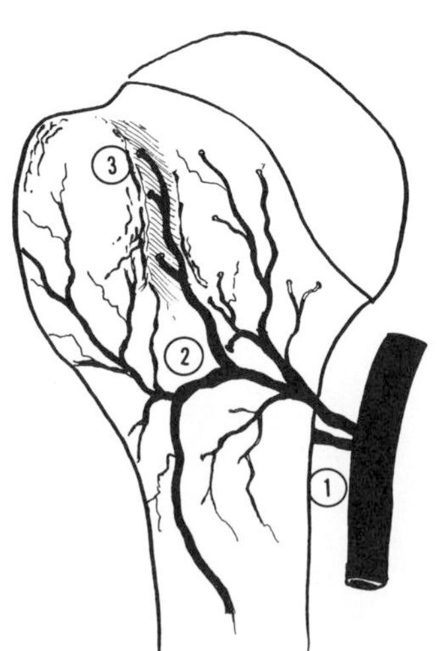

Closed Reduction of Fracture-Dislocation of the Shoulder (After Dingley and Denham)

REMARKS

Fracture dislocations of the shoulder are extremely difficult to reduce closed and generally require open reduction.

They may occur in patients with other serious injuries who are not candidates immediately for open reduction. Under these circumstances, a closed reduction may be worth attempting.

If conventional reduction methods using the Hippocratic technique of traction and direct pressure on the humeral head do not reduce the acute injury, a threaded Steinmann pin may be used to achieve reduction of the dislocated head.

Prereduction X-Ray

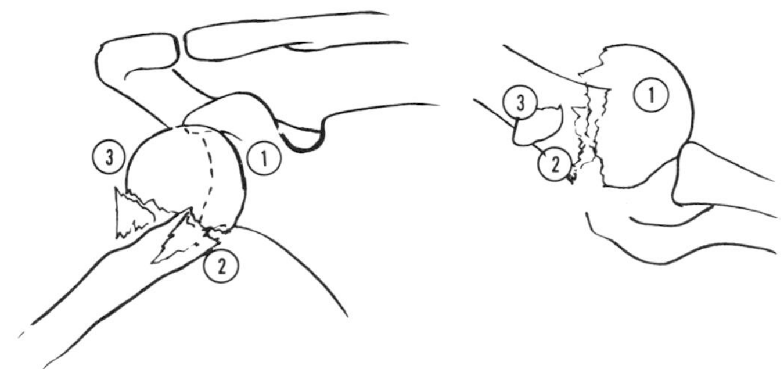

1. Anteroposterior and lateral x-rays show the dislocated right humeral head.
2. There is a fracture of the surgical neck and a
3. Fracture of the superolateral aspect of the head.

Closed Reduction Technique (After Dingley and Denham)

This method is preferred for patients who cannot undergo immediate open reduction. The technique reduces the humeral head but does not adequately stabilize a fracture or repair a rotator cuff disruption.

1. With general anesthesia, an 8-mm Steinmann pin is inserted 2–3 cm distal to the acromion under x-ray control.
2. Steinmann pin is advanced by pressure until contact is made with the humeral head, at which time the pin is drilled into the humeral head to obtain good purchase on the bone.
3. Assistant stabilizes the displaced humeral head while the pin is inserted.

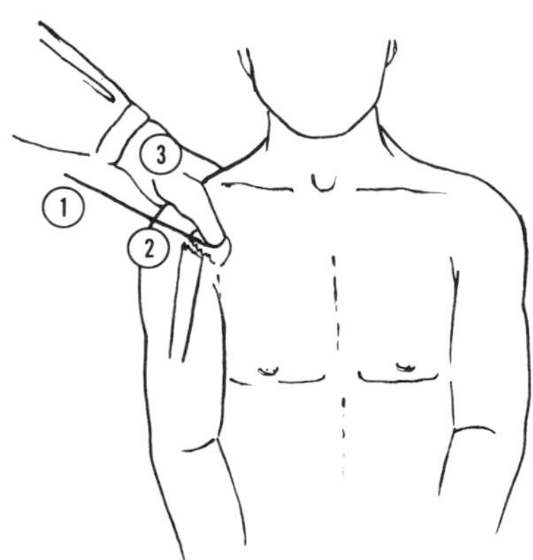

1. Lateral traction is then applied to the Steinmann pin while
2. Gentle downward traction is placed on the arm.
3. Reduction is accomplished with an audible click.

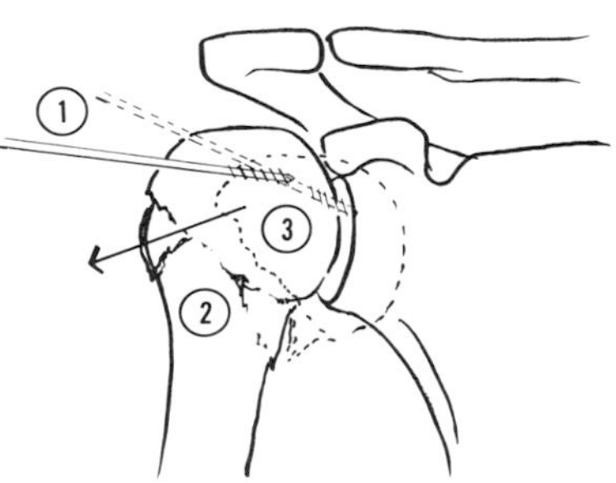

Subsequent Management

Remove the Steinmann pin as soon as the x-ray confirms adequate reduction.

If the technique does not achieve reduction, it should not be repeated with overvigorous manipulation, which may add further damage or fracture the humeral head.

If the tuberosity fragments or other associated fractures are persistently displaced, subsequent open reduction and internal fixation or prosthetic replacement are indicated.

Open Reduction (Preferred Technique)

REMARKS

Most fracture-dislocations of the humerus require open reduction with internal fixation to restore stability to the joint and repair rotator cuff disruption.

Occasionally, the fracture may be so comminuted that primary prosthetic replacement is necessary. However, most of these injuries can be restored by techniques that retain the normal humeral head.

The key problems are to achieve adequate stability of the fracture, repair the rotator cuff, and avoid devascularization of the humeral head.

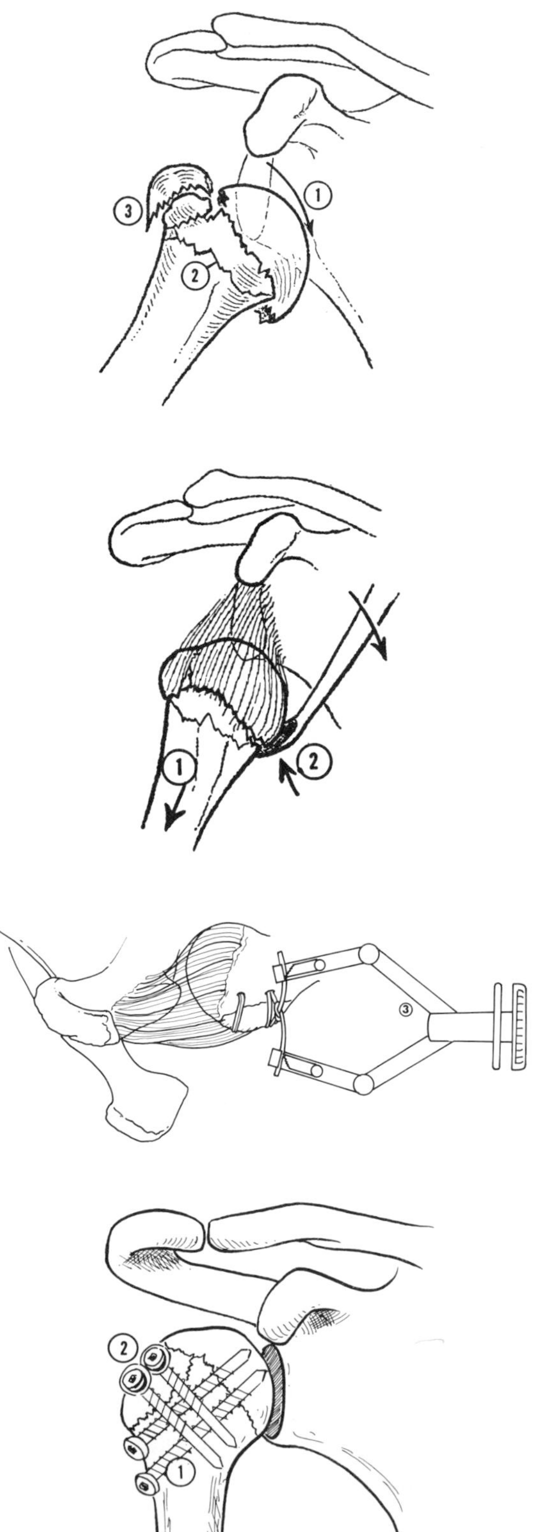

Prereduction X-Ray

1. Dislocation of the humeral head.
2. Fracture of the humeral neck.
3. Fracture of the tuberosities.

Preferred Technique of Open Reduction and Repair

1. After surgical exposure, the dislocation is surgically reduced by leverage and traction.
2. Displaced humeral head is gently levered back into the glenoid cavity, taking care to preserve whatever soft tissue attachment remains. Gentle rotation may be necessary to reduce the head fragment.
3. If the soft tissues and blood supplies are partially or completely intact, it is best to repair the rotator cuff and tuberosity fragments with heavy wire sutures.

Alternative Method

1. Anatomic neck fracture may be fixed with multiple cannulated screws.
2. Tuberosity fragment may also be stabilized with screws.

Alternative Methods: Resectional or Prosthetic Arthroplasty for Fracture-Dislocation

The dislocated and fractured humeral head, in rare instances, may not be amenable to operative restoration of normal anatomy. This is particularly likely in the osteoporotic patient or in the fracture that actually splits the head into multiple fragments.

In these circumstances, an arthroplasty of some type is indicated. This includes resection of the humeral articular surfaces and reattachment of the rotator cuff to the surgical neck.

In most instances, the procedure of choice is replacement with a shoulder arthroplasty. However, if a prosthetic joint is not available, resectional arthroplasty is a reasonable alternative because shoulder function can be restored and pain can be relieved if the rotator cuff attachments are carefully repaired.

Example of Resectional Arthroplasty

1. Displaced fragment of the anatomic neck is found at surgery not to be amenable to internal fixation. Multiple fragments exist, and splitting of the head against the glenoid has occurred. This can be treated by resection of the head fragments and repair of the rotator cuff tendon.
2. Rotator cuff fragments are reattached to the surgical neck by heavy wire sutures.
3. Neck is reduced into the glenoid, and the capsule is reattached to stabilize the neck fragment in a near-normal relationship.

Note: Prosthetic arthroplasty is presently the preferred method to manage the severely displaced fracture-dislocation if removal of the head fragment is necessary.

4. Fragments of the tuberosity are reattached to each other with wire sutures passed through drill holes in the proximal humerus.
5. Neer prosthesis is inserted to replace the resected humeral head. The medullary canal should be drilled to accommodate a tight-fitting stem. The articular surface of the prosthesis should be 30° retrograde for stability, and overvigorous bone resection should be avoided because this may cause inferior subluxation of the prosthesis.

Note: It is critical that the rotator cuff and deltoid be maintained in close physiologic tension to avoid complications of inferior subluxation or dislocation and impairment of shoulder motion with prosthetic replacement of acute fractures.

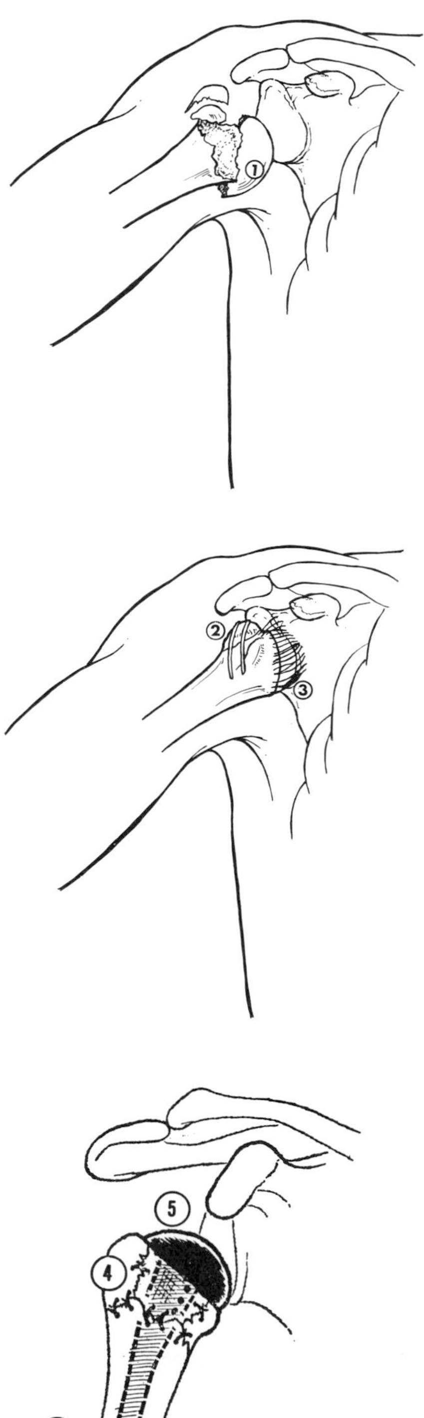

Other Fractures That Complicate Dislocation

REMARKS

The fractures discussed here are rare but may be a cause of pain or disability after reduction.

In general, the fracture component can be disregarded, and the patient can be treated in the same manner as with an uncomplicated dislocation.

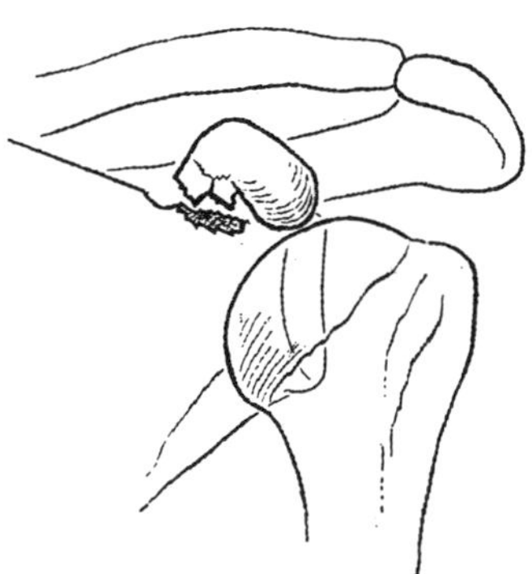

Fracture of the Coracoid Process and Subcoracoid Dislocation

Fracture of the Acromion and Subcoracoid Dislocation

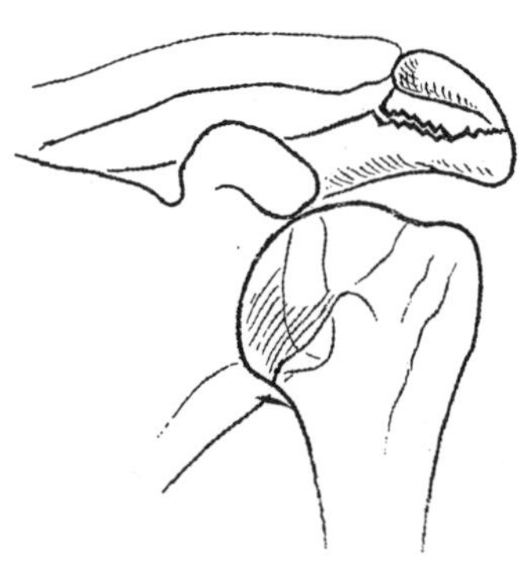

Note: This may be associated with rotator cuff disruption. Suspect tendon rupture if there is persistent weakness of abduction after recovery from the initial injury.

Also distinguish a fracture of the acromion with an irregular fracture line from os acromiale, which is a normal variant (see Chapter 11).

Management

These injuries may be treated as uncomplicated anterior dislocations.

The fracture component may generally be disregarded if tendon rupture is not associated.

Recurrent Dislocation of the Shoulder

REMARKS

The major factor that determines whether a shoulder dislocation will recur is the age of the patient at the time of the initial dislocation. The degree or duration of postreduction immobilization has little bearing on the recurrence rate.

The common dislocation in a teen-aged male athlete has an 80–90 per cent probability of recurring within 2 years.

Dislocation with a fracture of the glenoid has an equally high chance of recurrence.

Dislocation in a 45-year-old man, which is usually associated with a fracture of the greater tuberosity, has only a 15 per cent chance of recurrence. Recurrent dislocation in older patients is infrequent, except in naturally "loose-jointed" individuals.

Disruption of the anterior capsule and subscapularis support may not be sufficient to allow recurrent dislocation but will permit sudden episodes of subluxation and pain that significantly disable the individual. This is especially likely in a young athlete who has "wrenched" a shoulder and subsequently experiences episodes of subluxation. These transient recurrent subluxations should be recognized as real problems for the patient and should be treated appropriately.

Primary Anatomic Causes of Recurrent Dislocation

1. The most common findings in association with recurrent dislocation relate to the distortion of the capsule and ligament structures. The middle humeral ligament is stretched out or completely avulsed.
2. A large redundant subscapularis recess exists, allowing displacement of the humeral head anteriorly.
3. Major support of the inferior glenohumeral ligament is lost or stretched out. In addition, the ligamentous attachment to the glenoid has been avulsed.
4. Only a small portion of the glenoid labrum is continuous with the capsule inferiorly. The avulsion of this attachment anteriorly and inferiorly is the primary cause of the recurrent dislocation, which should be repaired (Bankart lesion).

Note: The anterior tendon of the subscapularis also is stretched out and requires repair, but the major defect that allows recurrent dislocation is the Bankart lesion, which must be repaired for restoration of stability.

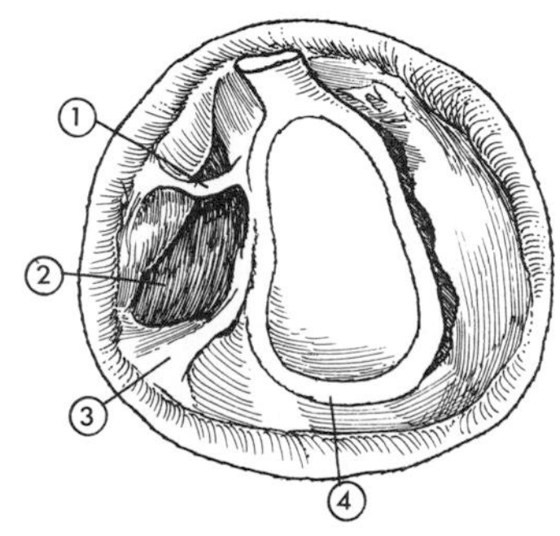

Surgical Repair for Recurrent Anterior Dislocation

REMARKS

Shoulder stability can be restored by a variety of operations.

The objective, however, should be to repair the basic underlying defect, which is in the capsule and glenoid labrum.

In addition, the stretched out subscapularis tendon should also be tightened.

The preferred operation should be done expeditiously and should not require screw or staple fixation, which can cause future problems. The repair should decrease the external rotation and abduction range of shoulder motion as little as possible.

In most instances, the preferred method of repair is a Bankart operation.

Bankart's Procedure

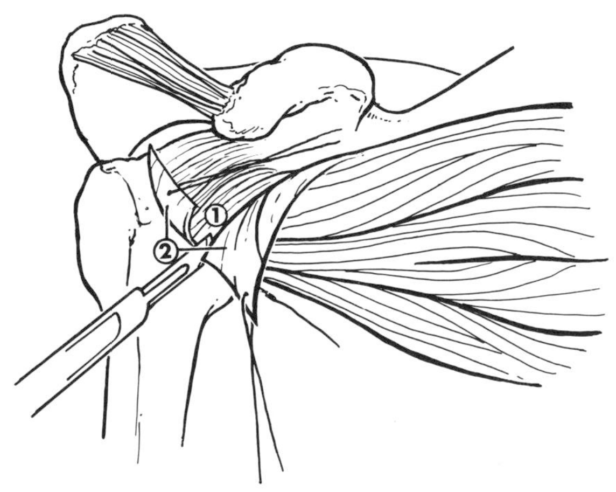

1. Capsule and subscapularis tendon are exposed and detached from their insertion on the lesser tuberosity simultaneously.
2. Subscapularis tendon is then dissected and freed from the capsule to allow dissection back to the glenoid labrum. The joint is then opened and inspected for loose bodies or other defects.

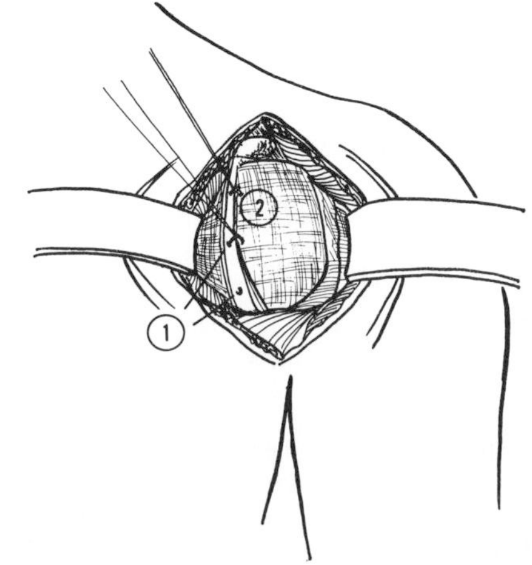

1. Defects in the capsular attachment or glenoid labrum are identified. Drill holes are then made through the edge of the glenoid.
2. Capsule and glenoid labrum are then reattached to the normal attachments with sufficient tension to restrict external rotation of the shoulder to approximately 15°.

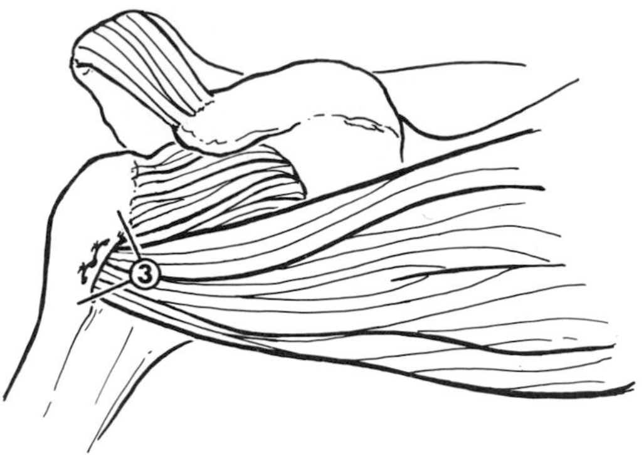

3. After repair of the Bankart lesion is accomplished, the subscapularis tendon is reattached laterally. This also should restrict external rotation to slightly beyond the neutral position of the shoulder.

Postoperative Management

Postoperatively, the shoulder is immobilized in a sing and swathe until the soft tissues have healed for approximately 2 weeks.

The patient is then gradually started on a range-of-motion exercise program to restore external rotation and abduction to the shoulder.

This may take several months to accomplish, and the patient should be encouraged to persist with the exercises to restore shoulder range of motion to close to normal.

External rotation and abduction is particularly important to young athletes who use the shoulder for throwing motions.

Other Problems of Stability: Recurrent Voluntary and Involuntary Posterior Dislocations, Subluxations, and Multidirectional Instability Problems

REMARKS

Posterior dislocation and subluxation are frequently voluntary. That is, young, loose-jointed individuals may be able to dislocate the shoulder posteriorly at will by fixing the scapula.

The humeral head may be atraumatically retracted posteriorly over the glenoid using voluntary muscle action.

Intra-articular injury to the glenoid labrum or humeral head is not found in this group.

Psychological and psychiatric problems may be superimposed on the shoulder instability and may defeat the best therapy.

In most instances, a deconditioning exercise program will diminish the patient's tendency to demonstrate the instability and avoid inordinate problems from attempted surgical reconstruction.

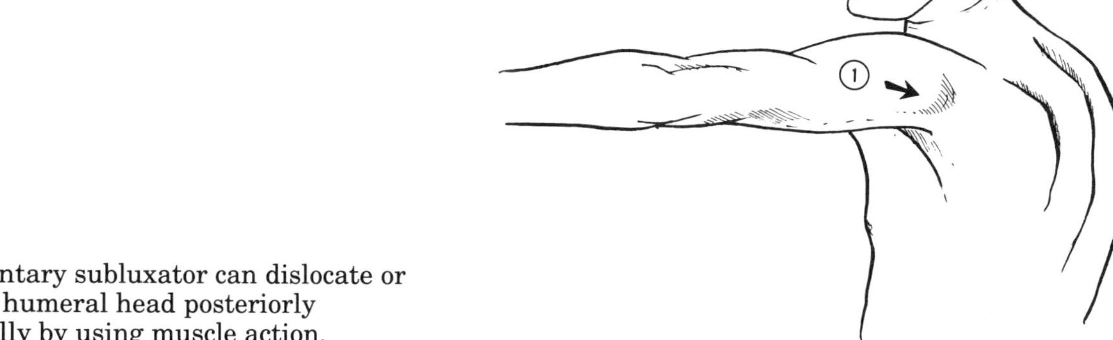

1. Typical voluntary subluxator can dislocate or displace the humeral head posteriorly atraumatically by using muscle action.

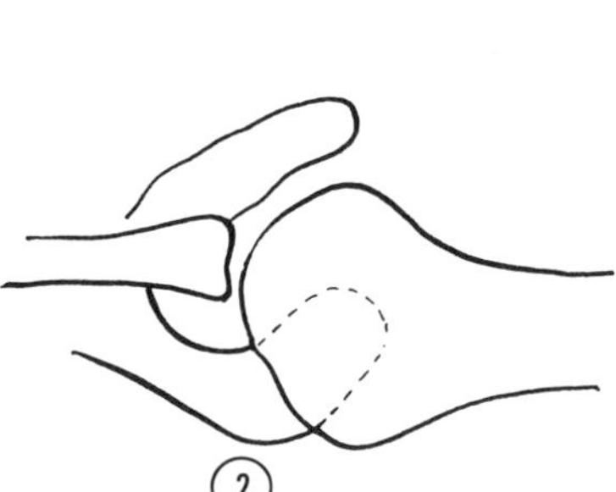

2. X-ray shows the humeral head located and

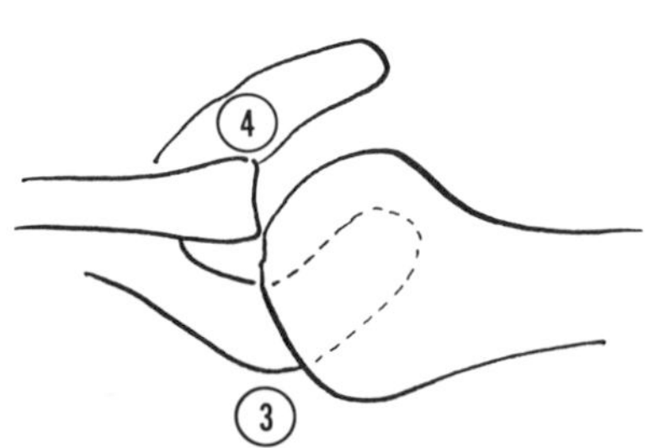

3. Subluxated posteriorly by voluntary muscle action.
4. No lesions on the labrum or humeral head are evident.

Note: These individuals do not require aggressive surgical treatment but benefit most by counseling against using this subluxation as "a party trick" and also by working on exercises to strengthen the stabilizing shoulder muscles.

Involuntary Multidirectional Instability

REMARKS

It is important to distinguish the unique disorder of shoulder laxity and instability due to involuntary posterior recurrent dislocation from the voluntary dislocation.

These patients may have generalized capsular laxity and are frequently very athletic individuals.

There may be symptomatic complaints of discomfort and fatigue.

Typically, these shoulders may be unstable in multiple directions and are not responsive to the usual surgical procedure.

The finding of involuntary inferior dislocation or posterior dislocation or the sulcus sign may be a warning that this multidirectional instability is present.

These patients are usually psychologically normal and may give a history of significant trauma precipitating the problem.

They are best evaluated by careful roentgenograms and stress, preferably under anesthesia, to assess the multidirectional instability.

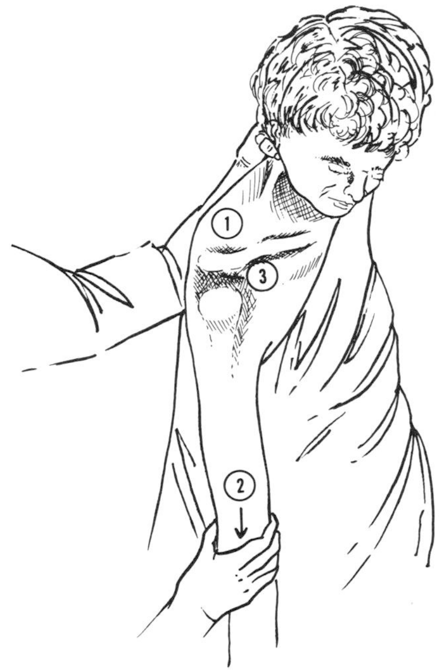

1. Typical patient with multidirectional instability is an active, athletic young person who may complain of discomfort with certain activities, such as carrying heavy loads.
2. Inferior displacement of the humerus is evident with traction on the distal arm.
3. Sulcus sign develops as a result of inferior displacement of the humeral head.

Other Signs

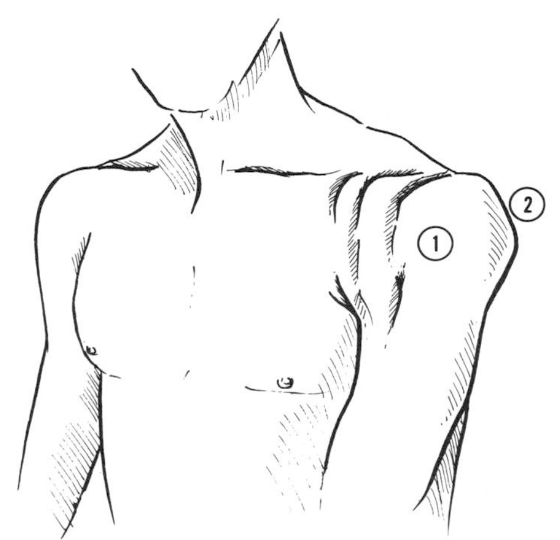

1. Active muscular individual with capsular laxity may initially be thought to be dislocating anteriorly or,
2. At times, posteriorly.

Note: Recognition of multidirectional instability in these rare patients is important, as described previously in this chapter in the section on subluxation.

Management

The main thing to keep in mind is that, occasionally, some shoulders may be dislocating in multiple directions, particularly if there is gross laxity and a sulcus sign present.

It is important to recognize this unique disorder and to start the patient on a vigorous nonoperative program of exercise and strengthening to relieve the symptoms.

If the symptoms do not respond to a supervised exercise program, a procedure, such as that described by Neer involving multiple shifting of the capsule structures, may be indicated. However, this is best done by a surgeon specifically familiar with the procedure, because it is considerably more complex than the standard repairs for shoulder dislocations.

Hawkins and others pointed out that many patients with multidirectional or posterior shoulder instability can accept the disability and can be treated conservatively. In contrast, operative procedures for this condition are prone at times to more than the usual amount of complications.

Other Problems: Posttraumatic Frozen Shoulder

REMARKS

Most of this chapter has been devoted to the subject of shoulder instability after injury. A converse problem in the shoulder is stiffening as a result of usually minor injury.

The shoulder, which is the most mobile joint in the body, demands considerable flexibility to maintain its near-global range of motion.

Management of fractures about the shoulder should incorporate a program of early exercises to restore motion, which is critical to shoulder function.

In certain patients, particularly in the middle-aged group, the shoulder can stiffen after minimal injury or no injury at all.

The stiffening becomes progressively worse and has been termed the "frozen shoulder."

Typically, the patient is a middle-aged woman who had a minor injury from a fall or repetitive stress on the shoulder. The shoulder becomes painful and progressively stiff.

The important differentials of this condition include a posterior dislocation, an infection, and a tumor, either primary or metastatic to the shoulder.

Clinical Presentation

1. Typical patient with a frozen shoulder is a middle-aged woman with a minor injury or repetitive strain on the shoulder. Frequently, there is history of "overuse" rather than acute trauma.
2. Shoulder is characteristically painful with or without motion. It is particularly painful in abduction and external rotation.

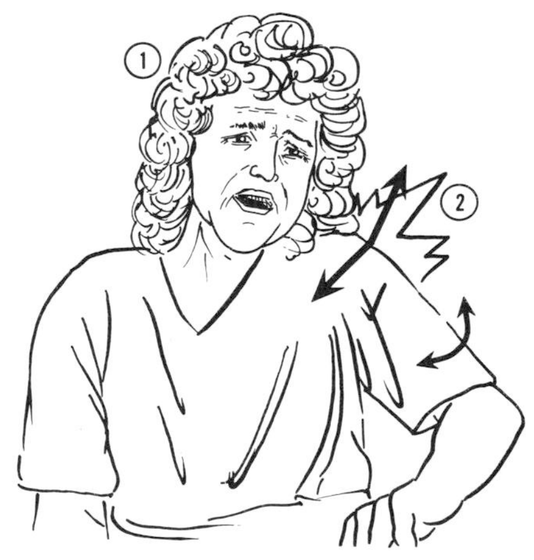

3. In addition, the patient complains of pain with the shoulder in extension and internal rotation, as required to get to the back or hook a bra strap.

Note: This global limitation of motion in all directions contrasts with the specific limitation of motion found with a posterior dislocation or a rotator cuff disruption. Posterior dislocations stiffen in internal rotation and adduction. The rotator cuff disruption is painful on shoulder elevation.

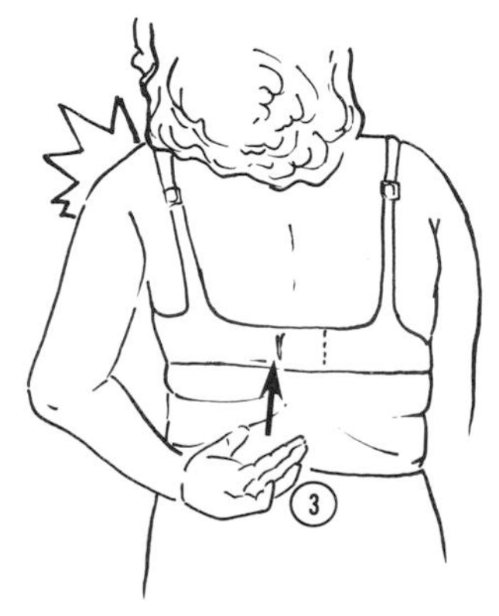

Pathologic Findings of the Frozen Shoulder

REMARKS

The underlying pathogenesis of this condition is an alteration in the usually redundant axillary fold of the capsule. This is evident on arthrogram of the shoulder, which shows obliteration of the axillary fold of the capsule.

Lundberg showed that there is an alteration in the matrix of the shoulder capsule that occurs with middle age. This causes fibroplasia of the collagen of the capsule, which creates a "checkrein" effect, restricting motion of the capsule and, therefore, the shoulder in all directions.

The clinical manifestation of a frozen shoulder is limitation of motion of the shoulder in all directions. This contrasts with the rotator cuff problem, which causes limitation of motion mainly on elevation or abduction and external rotation.

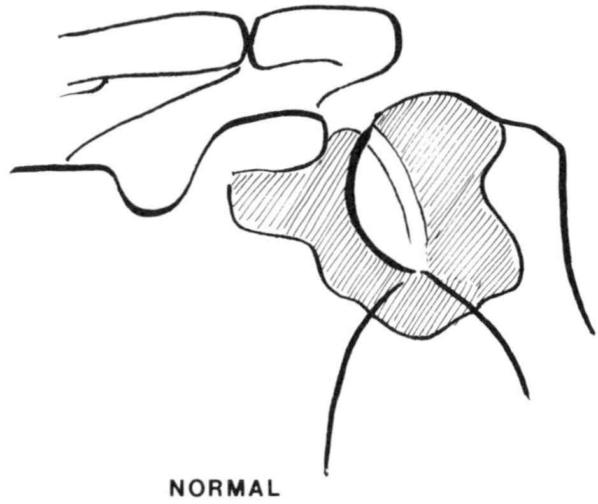

Arthrogram

1. Frozen shoulder results from chemical alteration in the capsule of the shoulder. This causes a checkrein effect in the axillary region and loss of motion of the shoulder in all directions. The arthrogram shows decreased filling of the altered joint capsule, particularly in the usually spacious axillary region, compared with the normal arthrogram.
2. Rotator cuff is not torn, and there is no leakage of dye through the roof of the shoulder.

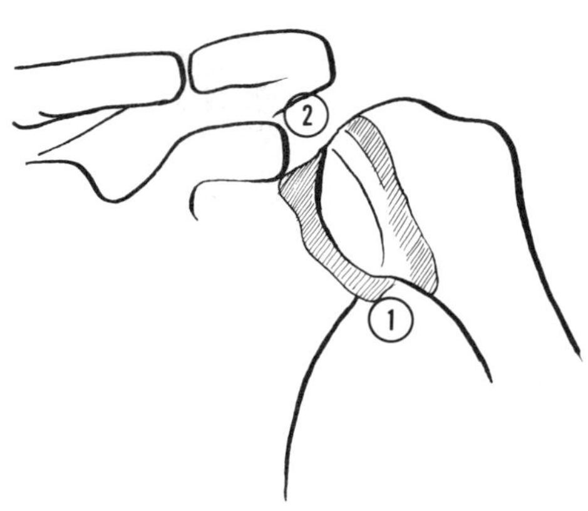

Management

Management of the frozen shoulder is directed at restoring mobility of the capsule of the shoulder, particularly in the axillary region.

Active motion of the shoulder is not usually beneficial in overcoming the checkrein effect. This is resistant to active motion and requires the assistance of gravity or a passive stretching release of the restricting checkrein in the capsule.

Usually, the exercise therapy should be self-administered with the help of a family member and not just dependent on a professional therapist.

The patient should be advised that, with 6 weeks of these passive stretching exercises, symptoms of pain in the shoulder and the restriction of motion should be improved.

If motion does not improve in 6–8 weeks, manipulation of the shoulder may be necessary.

Gravity-Assisted and Passive Exercises for the Painful, Stiff Shoulder

Gravity Exercises

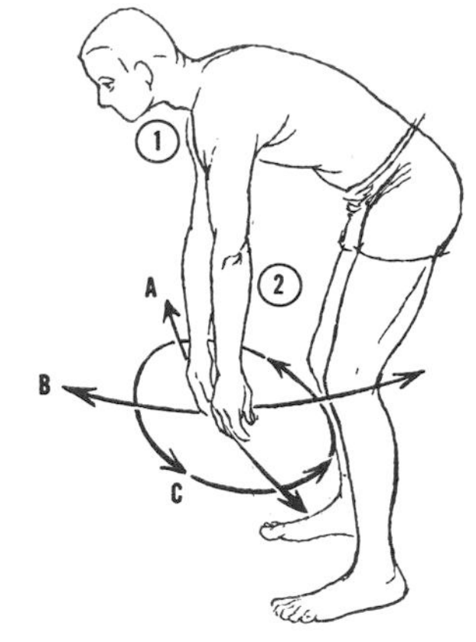

First start with gravity exercises.

1. Patient bends far forward, holding shoulders and trunk immobile.
2. Arms hang loosely and swing like a pendulum (A) across the front of the body, (B) backward and forward, and (C) in a circle.

Note: The arc at first is small and then is gradually increased.

Passive Stretching Shoulder Exercises

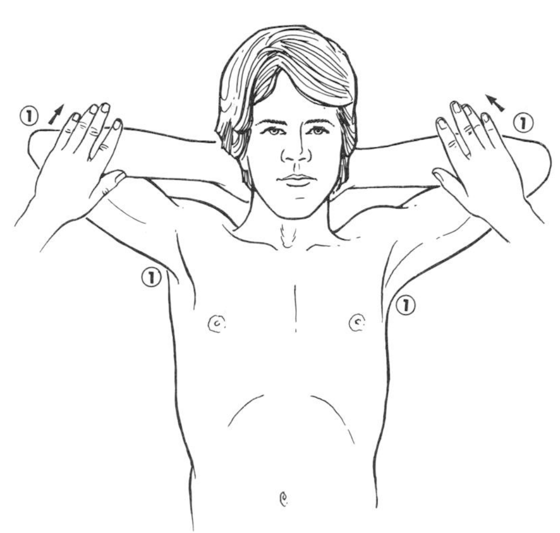

These are most valuable for the painful stiffening of the shoulder that can occur after very minor injury and can persist for many months or years. The patient must work to regain motion in all planes, including external rotation and abduction as well as extension and flexion.

1. Patient stands with scapulae against the wall and hands clasped behind the head. The patient abducts and externally rotates the shoulder rapidly to touch elbows to wall. This may require assistance to get full external rotation and abduction.

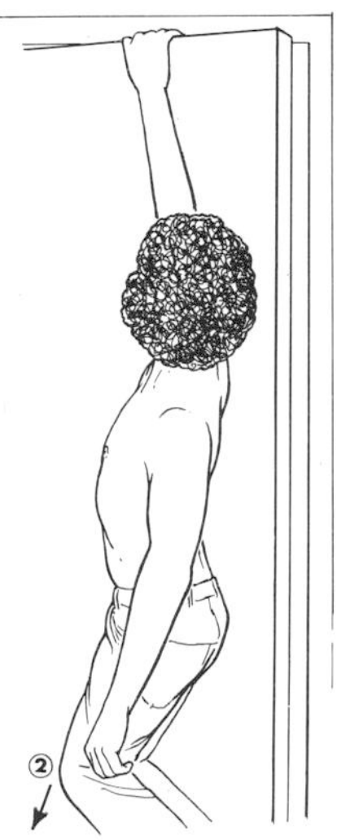

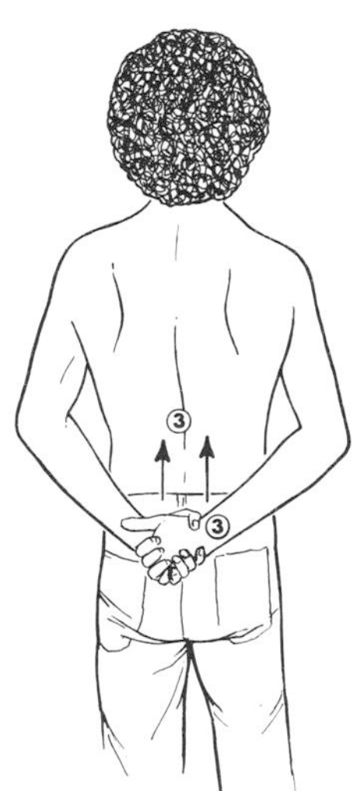

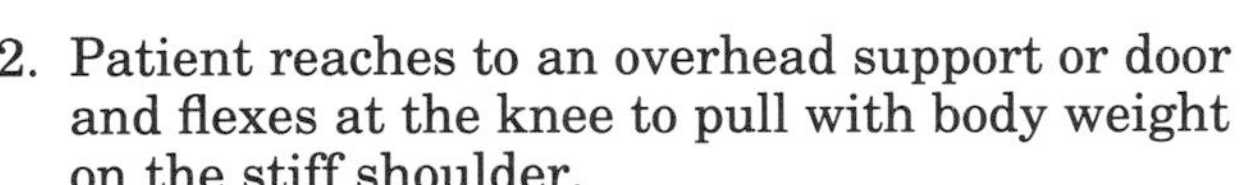

2. Patient reaches to an overhead support or door and flexes at the knee to pull with body weight on the stiff shoulder.
3. Patient reaches behind the back, grasps the wrist on the side of the stiff shoulder, and pulls upward toward the opposite scapula.

Technique of Shoulder Manipulation

REMARKS

If the patient has persistent painful limitation of motion after 6–8 weeks of the previously described exercise program, manipulation of the shoulder can be helpful.

It is important to rule out other conditions that cause painful stiff shoulder, including a locked posterior dislocated shoulder, infection, tumors, or pulmonary lesions before advising manipulation.

Shoulder manipulation should always be done under a general anesthetic with complete muscle relaxation and adequate assistance.

The shoulder should not be manipulated vigorously but with a firm maneuver that should overcome the checkrein effect of the adherent capsular fold in the axillary region.

In most instances, the manipulation achieves prompt release of the adherent capsular axillary fold. However, it should not be pushed with overvigorous rotational maneuvers.

Once the release of the capsule is achieved, the shoulder should be maintained in an elevated position in the plane of the scapula until the patient can resume the exercises to maintain the motion achieved.

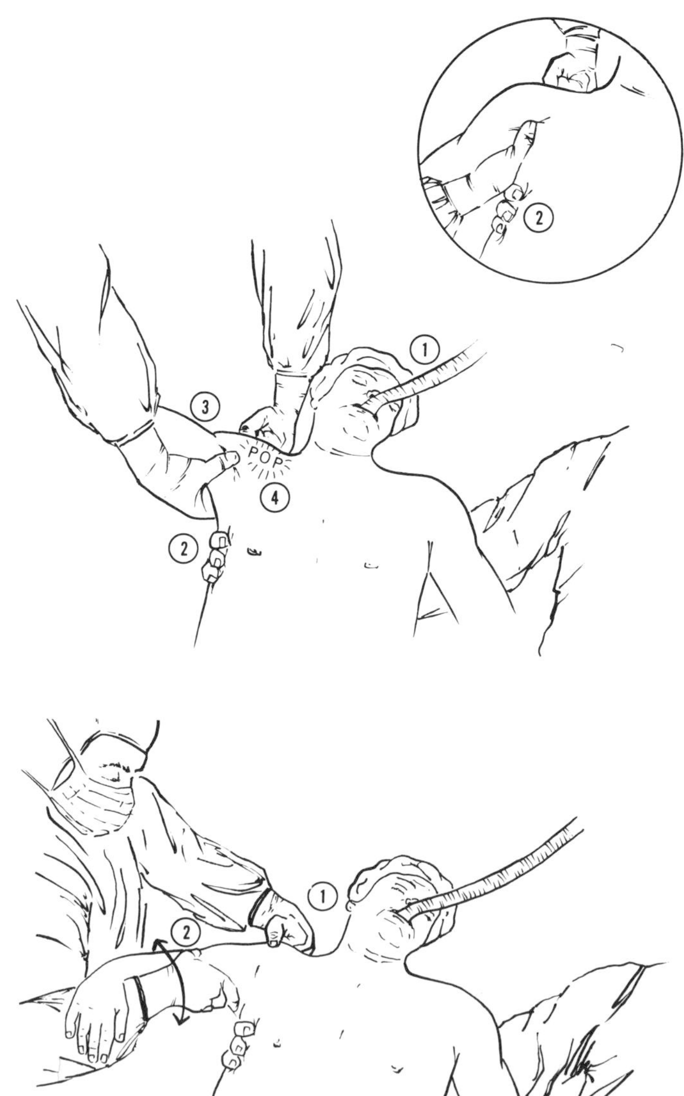

1. With the patient under general anesthesia and with complete muscle relaxation, an assistant reaches behind the back of the patient to grasp the axillary border of the scapula.
2. Surgeon grasps the humerus in the region of the surgical neck while stabilizing the scapula with the opposite hand.

Note: Do not use long leverage on the humerus because this can cause further damage and actually fracture the humerus if overvigorous manipulation is applied.

3. Arm is abducted away from the body in the plane of the scapula. It is important to use the plane of the scapula, which is the position in which the capsule is most loose.
4. At the point of restricted motion, usually about 60° of elevation, release is felt and heard like a dry twig breaking up adhesions.

1. Subsequently, motion of the shoulder is freer, and the arm can be raised to 80° or 90° of elevation.
2. It is gently externally and internally rotated in approximately 80° of elevation.

Caution: Avoid vigorous internal rotation, which can cause a fracture of the tuberosity of the humerus if it is done with overleverage.

Postmanipulation Management

After manipulation is achieved, the patient is transferred back to bed with the arm in an elevated position and supported by pillows.

The arm is secured to an overhead frame with the shoulder abducted and externally rotated until the patient is awake and passive exercises can be resumed by the patient.

It is useful to inject a long-acting local anesthetic into the joint to relieve the acute symptoms subsequent to manipulation. Adequate pain medicine should be prescribed for the first 24 hours after manipulation because the shoulder can be painful and pain may prevent the patient from resuming the important postoperative exercises.

BIBLIOGRAPHY

Clavical Fractures

Anderson K, Jensen PO, Lauritzen J: Treatment of clavicular fractures. Acta Orthop Scand 57:71, 1987.
Ballmer FT, Gerber C: Coracoclavicular screw fixation for unstable fractures of the distal clavicle. J Bone Joint Surg Br 73:291, 1991.
Boehme D, Curtis RJ, Dehaan JT, et al.: Nonunion of fractures of the mid-shaft of the clavicle. J Bone Joint Surg Am 73:1219, 1991.
Connolly JF, Dehne R: Nonunion of the clavicle and thoracic outlet syndrome. J Trauma 29:1127, 1989.
Howard FM, Shaffer SJ: Injuries to the clavicle with neurovascular complications. A study of 14 cases. J Bone Joint Surg Am 47:1335, 1965.
Jupiter JB, Leffert RD: Non-union of the clavicle. J Bone Joint Surg Am 69:753, 1987.
Kona J, Bosse MJ, Staeheli JW, et al.: Type II distal clavicle fractures: A retrospective review of surgical treatment. J Orthop Trauma 4:115, 1990.
Lyons F, Rockwood C: Migration of pins used in operations on the shoulder. J Bone Joint Surg Am 72:1262, 1990.
Manske DJ, Szabo RM: The operative treatment of mid-shaft clavicular nonunions. J Bone Joint Surg Am 67:1367, 1985.
Neer CS: Fractures of the distal third of the clavicle. Clin Orthop 58:43, 1968.
Neer CS: *Shoulder Reconstruction.* WB Saunders, Philadelphia, 1990.
Neviaser RJ, Neviaser TS, Neviaser JT, et al.: A simple technique for internal fixation of the clavicle. Clin Orthop 109:103, 1975.
Nordback I, Markkula H: Migration of Kirschner pin from clavicle into ascending aorta. Acta Chir Scand 151:177, 1985.
Penn I: The vascular complications of fracture of the clavicle. J Trauma 4:819, 1964.
Shumacker H, Resection of the clavicle with particular reference to the use of bone chips in the periosteal bed. Surg. Gyn Otol 84:245, 1947.
Spar I: Total claviculectomy for pathological fractures. Clin Orthop 129:236, 1977.
Stanley D, Trowbridge EA, Norris SH: The mechanism of clavicular fracture. J Bone Joint Surg Br 70:461, 1988.
Weaver J, Dunn H: Treatment of acromuclavicular injuries. J Bone Joint Surg Am 54:1187, 1972.
Wilkins RM, Johnston RM: Ununited fractures of the clavicle. J Bone Joint Surg Am 65:773, 1983.
Wood VE: The results of total claviculectomy. Clin Orthop 207:186, 1986.
Zenni EJ, Krieg JK, Rosen MJ: Open reduction and internal fixation of clavicular fractures. J Bone Joint Surg Am 63:147, 1981.

Acromioclavicular Injuries

Bannister GC, Wallace WA, Stableforth PG, et al.: The management of acute acromioclavicular dislocation. J Bone Joint Surg Br 71:848, 1989.
Dias JJ, Steingold RA, Richardson RA, et al.: The conservative treatment of acromioclavicular dislocations: Review after 5 years. J Bone Joint Surg Br 69:719, 1987.
Eskola A, Vainionpaa S, Korkala O, et al.: Four-year outcome of operative treatment of acute acromioclavicular dislocation. J Orthop Trauma 5:9, 1991.
Inman VT, Saunders JB, Abbott LC: Observation on the function of the shoulder joint. J Bone Joint Surg Am 26:1, 1944.
Larsen E, Bjerg-Nielson A, Christiansen P: Conservative or surgical treatment of acromioclavicular dislocation: A prospective, controlled, randomized study. J Bone Joint Surg Am 68:552, 1986.
O'Neill D, Zarins B, Gelberman R, et al: Compression of the anterior interosseous nerve after use of a sling for dislocation of the acromioclavicular joint. J Bone Joint Surg Am 72:1100, 1992.
Rockwood CA, Matsen FA: *The Shoulder.* WB Saunders, Philadelphia, 1990.
Smith DW: Coracoid fracture associated with acromioclavicular separations. Am J Sports Med 7:62, 1979.

Sternoclavicular Joint Injuries

Buckerfield CT, Castle ME: Acute traumatic retrosternal dislocations of the clavicle. J Bone Joint Surg Am 66:379, 1984.
deJong KP, Sukol DMKS: Anterior sternoclavicular dislocation: A long term follow up study. J Orthop Trauma 4:420, 1990.
Eskola A, Vainionpaa S, Vastamaki M, et al.: Operation for old sternoclavicular dislocation. Results in 12 cases. J Bone Joint Surg Br 71:63, 1989.
Levinsohn EM: Computed tomography in the diagnosis of posterior dislocation of the sternoclavicular joint. Clin Orthop 140:12, 1979.
Lewonowski M, Bassett G: Complete posterior sternoclavicular epiphysis separation. Clin Orthop 881:84, 1992.

Scapular Fractures

Ada JR, Miller ME: Scapular fractures. Clin Orthop 269:174, 1991.
Ebraheim NA, Pearlstein SR, Savolaine ER, et al.: Scapulothoracic dissociation (closed avulsion of the scapula, subclavian artery, and brachial plexus): A newly recognized variant, a new classification, and a review of the literature and treatment options. J Orthop Trauma 1:18, 1987.
Hardegger FH, Simpson LA, Weber BG: The operative treatment of scapular fractures. J Bone Joint Surg Br 66:725, 1984.
Ideberg R: Unusual glenoid fractures: A report on 92 cases. Acta Orthop Scand 58:191, 1987.
Kavanagh B, Cofield R: Open reduction and internal fixation of displaced intra-articular fractures of the glenoid fossa. J Bone Joint Surg Am 75:479, 1993.
McGinnis M, Denton JR: Fractures of the scapula: A retrospective study of 40 fractured scapulae. J Trauma 29:1488, 1989.
Mick CA, Weiland AJ: Pseudoarthrosis of a fracture of the acromion. J Trauma 23:248, 1983.
Oreck SL, Burgess A, Levine AM: Traumatic lateral displacement of the scapula: A radiographic sign of neurovascular disruption. J Bone Joint Surg Am 66:758, 1984.
Rubenstein JD, Ebraheim NA, Kellam JF: Traumatic scapulothoracic dissociation. Radiology 157:297, 1985.
Thompson DA, Flynn TC, Miller PW, et al.: The significance of scapular fractures. J Trauma 25:974, 1985.
Wilber MC, Evans EB: Fractures of the scapula. J Bone Joint Surg Am 59:358, 1977.

Glenohumeral Dislocations and Subluxations and Their Complications

Alnot JY: Traumatic brachial plexus palsy in the adult. Retro- and infraclavicular lesions. Clin Orthop 237:9, 1988.
Bhan S, Mehara AK: A simple and universal method for reduction of dislocation of the shoulder. Int Orthop 18:14, 1993.
Blom S, Dahlback LO: Nerve injuries in dislocations of the shoulder joint and fractures of the neck of the humerus. A clinical and electromyographic study. Acta Chir Scand 136:461, 1970.
Burstein AH: "Fracture classification systems: Do they work and are they useful?" (editorial). J Bone Joint Surg Am 75:1743, 1993.
Cofield RH: Comminuted fractures of the proximal humerus. Clin Orthop 230:49, 1988.
Connolly J: Humeral head defects associated with shoulder dislocations—their diagnostic and surgical significance. Instr Course Lect 21:42, 1972.
Connolly J, Regen E, Evans OB: The management of the painful, stiff shoulder. Clin Orthop 84:97, 1972.
Craig EV: The posterior mechanisms of acute anterior shoulder dislocation. Clin Orthop 190:212, 1984.

Din KM, Meggitt BF: Bilateral four-part fractures with posterior dislocation of the shoulder. J Bone Joint Surg Br 65:176, 1983.
Dingley A, Denham R: Fracture-dislocation of the humeral head: A method of reduction. J Bone Joint Surg Am 55:1299, 1973.
Einarsson F: Fractures of the upper end of the humerus: Discussion based on follow-up of 302 cases. Acta Orthop Scand 32(suppl):10, 1958.
Ferkel RD, Hedley AK, Eckardt JJ: Anterior fracture-dislocations of the shoulder: Pitfalls in treatment. J Trauma 24:363, 1984.
Gilchrist DK: A stockinette-Velpeau for immobilization of the shoulder girdle. J Bone Joint Surg Am 49:750, 1967.
Goldman A, Sherman O, Price A, et al.: Posterior fracture dislocation of the shoulder with biceps tendon interposition. J Trauma 27:1083, 1987.
Hall RH, Isaac F, Booth CR: Dislocations of the shoulder with special reference to accompanying small fractures. J Bone Joint Surg 41:489, 1959.
Hawkins RJ, Bell RH, Gurr K: The three-part fracture of the proximal part of the humerus. J Bone Joint Surg Am 68:1410, 1986.
Hawkins RJ, Koppert G, Johnson G: Recurrent posterior instability (subluxation) of the shoulder. J Bone Joint Surg Am 66:169, 1984.
Hawkins RJ, Neer CS II, Pianta RM, et al.: Locked posterior dislocation of the shoulder. J Bone Joint Surg Am 69:9, 1987.
Hawkins RJ, Switlyk P: Acute prosthetic replacement for severe fractures of the proximal humerus. Clin Orthop 289:156, 1993.
Hersche O, Gerber C: Iatrogenic displacement of fracture-dislocations of the shoulder. J Bone Joint Surg Br 76:30, 1994.
Howell SM, Imobersteg AM, Seger DH, et al.: Clarification of the role of the supraspinatus muscle in shoulder function. J Bone Joint Surg Am 68:398, 1986.
Jardon OM, Hood LT, Lynch RD: Complete avulsion of the axillary artery as a complication of shoulder dislocation. J Bone Joint Surg Am 55:189, 1973.
Kay SP, Amstutz HC: Shoulder hemiarthroplasty at UCLA. Clin Orthop 228:42, 1988.
Kinnett JG, Warren RF, Jacobs B: Recurrent dislocation of the shoulder after age fifty. Clin Orthop 149:164, 1980.
Kofoed H: Revascularization of the humeral head. A report of two cases of fracture-dislocation of the shoulder. Clin Orthop 179:175, 1983.
Lee CK, Hansen HR: Post-traumatic avascular necrosis of the humeral head in displaced proximal humeral fractures. J Trauma 21:788, 1981.
Leffert RD, Seddon H: Infraclavicular brachial plexus injuries. J Bone Joint Surg Br 47:9, 1965.
Lundberg BJ: The frozen shoulder. Acta Orthop Scand (suppl 119), 1969.
McLaughlin HL: Posterior dislocation of the shoulder. J Bone Joint Surg Am 34:584, 1952.
Mink JH, Harris E, Rappaport M: Rotator cuff tears: Evaluation using double-contrast shoulder arthrography. Radiology 157:621, 1985.
Morrey BF, Janes JM: Recurrent anterior dislocation of the shoulder. J Bone Joint Surg Am 88:252, 1976.
Neer CS II: *Shoulder Reconstruction.* WB Saunders, Philadelphia, 1990.
Neviaser FJ: Painful conditions affecting the shoulder. Clin Orthop 173:63, 1983.
Pasila M, Faroma H, Kiviluoto O, et al.: Early complication of primary shoulder dislocation. Acta Orthop Scand 49:260, 1978.
Protzman R: Anterior instability of the shoulder. J Bone Joint Surg Am 62:909, 1980.
Rokous JR, Feagin JA, Abbott HG: Modified axillary roentgenogram. A useful adjunct in the diagnosis of recurrent instability of the shoulder. Clin Orthop 82:84, 1972.
Rowe CR: Prognosis in dislocations of the shoulder. J Bone Joint Surg Am 38:957, 1956.
Rowe CR, Pierce DS, Clark JG: Voluntary dislocation of the shoulder. J Bone Joint Surg Am 55:445, 1973.
Rowe CR, Zarins B, Ciullo JV: Recurrent anterior dislocations of the shoulder after surgical repair. J Bone Joint Surg Am 66:159, 1984.
Schulz TJ, Jacobs B, Patterson RL: Unrecognized dislocations of the shoulder. J Trauma 9:1009, 1969.
Sidor ML, Zuckerman JD, Lyon T, et al: The Neer classification system of proximal humeral fractures. J Bone Joint Surg Am 75:1745, 1993.
Siebenrock KA, Gerber C: The reproducibility of classification of fractures of the proximal end of the humerus. J Bone Joint Surg Am 75:1751, 1993.
Stableforth PG: Four-part fractures of the neck of the humerus. J Bone Joint Surg Br 66:104, 1984.
Tanner MW, Cofield RH: Prosthetic arthroplasty for fracture-dislocations of the proximal humerus. Clin Orthop 179:116, 1982.
Thakur AJ, Narayan R: Painless reduction of shoulder dislocation by Kocher's method. J Bone Joint Surg Br 72:524, 1990.
Toolanen G, Hildingsson C, Hedlund T, et al: Early complications after anterior dislocation of the shoulder in patients over 40 years. Acta Orthop Scand 64:549, 1993.
Yosipovitch Z, Tikkva P, Goldberg I: Inferior subluxation of the humeral head after injury to the shoulder. J Bone Joint Surg Am 71:751, 1989.
Young TB, Wallace WA: Conservative treatment of fractures and fracture-dislocations of the upper end of the humerus. J Bone Joint Surg Br 67:373, 1985.
Zuckerman JD, Matsen FA: Complications about the glenohumeral joint related to the use of the screws and staples. J Bone Joint Surg Am 66:175, 1984.

13 Fractures of the Humerus

MECHANISMS PRODUCING HUMERAL FRACTURES

REMARKS

For the most part, fractures of the upper end of the humerus occur from indirect mechanisms in the same age group as femoral neck fractures and Colles' fractures, that is, the elderly. They are "fragile bone" types of fracture. Most proximal humeral fractures (80 per cent) occur in osteoporotic patients who fall on the outstretched hand with the elbow extended. The resultant axial and torsional loading is transmitted up to the humerus and shoulder and produces characteristic fractures.

Bone is weakest in torsional strength and is most likely to fail from the indirect force of twisting. Yamada has shown, in evaluating mechanics of torsional failure, that the direction of the fracture line consistently is determined by the direction of the twist. Fractures produced by external twisting of the arm run in an oblique or spiral fashion from the distal medial cortex to the superior lateral cortex. Fractures produced by internal torsion run in a distal lateral to proximal medial direction.

The mechanisms of fracture also determine the displacement. Internal torsion characteristically causes medial displacement of the distal fragment. External torsion produces superolateral displacement of the distal fragment and sometimes anterior dislocation of the head fragment.

Fractures that are produced by direct loading tend to occur in younger, more active patients. Direct bending can produce a typical transverse fracture of the midshaft of the humerus. This can occur from a fall directly on the abducting distal humerus that locks the proximal humerus in the glenoid. The bending moment is then applied to the midshaft and produces a characteristic transverse fracture.

Another common direct mechanism is a fall on the upper arm. A direct blow to the shoulder, as in a fall from a height, may cause a severe comminution or a fracture-dislocation of the proximal humerus. The prognosis for satisfactory healing after severe direct injuries to the humerus is significantly worse than after moderate indirect injuries.

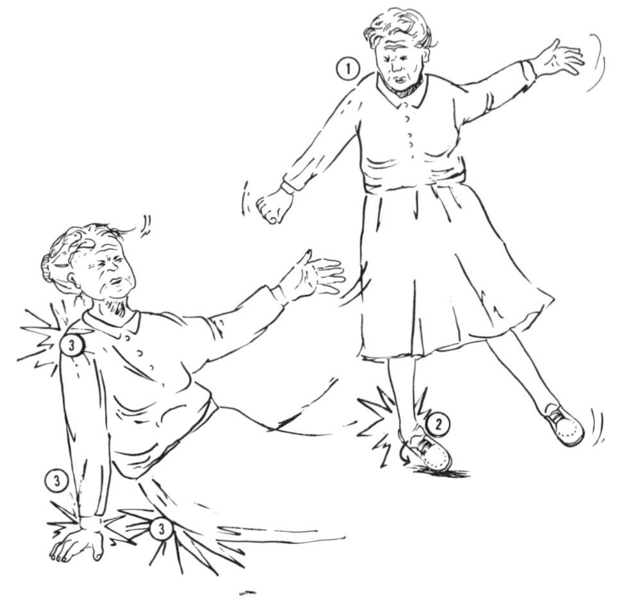

■ Indirect Mechanisms Producing Axial and Torsional Loading

Mechanisms of Injury

1. This is typically a fracture of osteoporotic bone in an elderly patient that results from a fall on the outstretched arm.
2. Other similar types of osteoporotic bone occur in the wrist,
3. In the hip, and
4. Sometimes in the ankle.

External Torsional Fracture

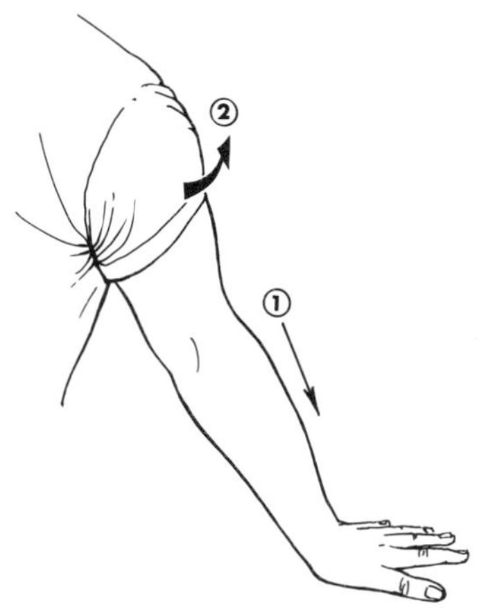

1. A fall on the outstretched arm with the elbow extended applies a heavy axial load directly onto the proximal humerus.

Note: If the elbow were flexed at the time of the fall, a different structure, such as the elbow or the wrist, would be injured.

2. In addition to pure axial loading, these injuries always combine a rotational loading. In this instance the rotational load is in the external direction. This produces a specific type of fracture, which differs from the internal rotation.

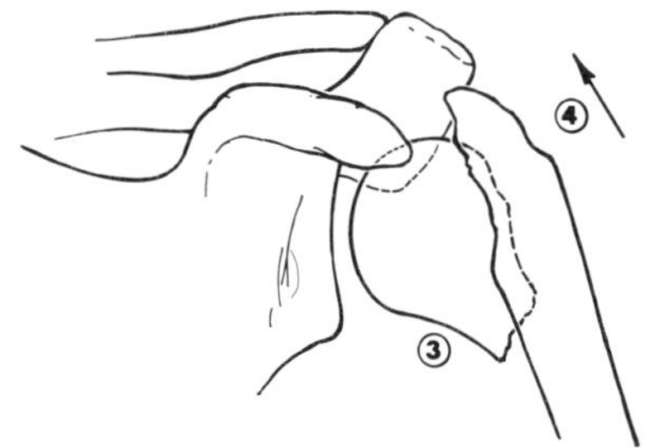

3. A typical fracture from external torsion results from failure that begins in the distal medial cortex and runs to the proximal lateral cortex.
4. The distal fragment is displaced superiorly and laterally by the force vectors.

Note: In the past these have been called *abduction fractures* but should more correctly be called *external rotational fractures.*

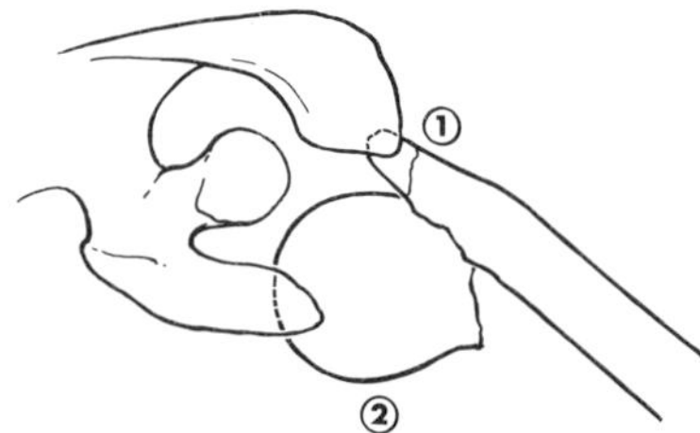

1. Extreme external torsion may produce a three-fragment or four-fragment fracture and
2. Anterior dislocation of the humeral head.

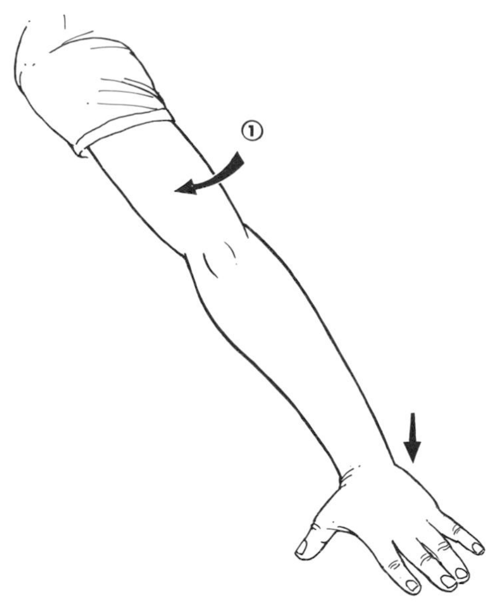

1. A fall on the outstretched arm may combine axial loading with internal rotation at the shoulder.

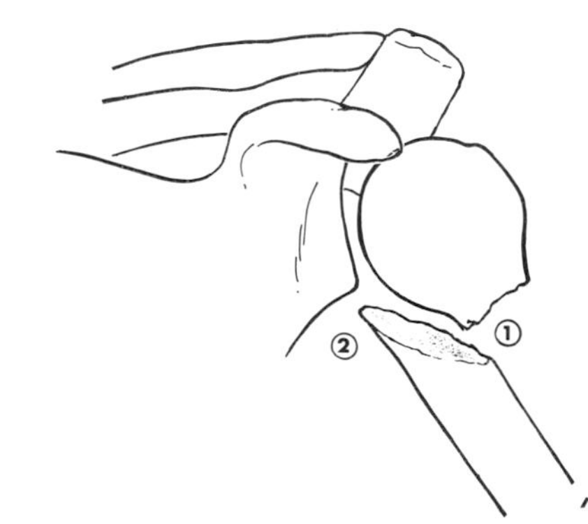

Internal Torsional Fractures

1. Failure resulting from internal torsion runs from the distal lateral to the proximal medial cortex of the humerus.
2. The force vectors displace the distal fragment medially.

Note: In the past this has been called an *adduction fracture,* but the true mechanism is an internal rotational force displacing the shaft fragment medially.

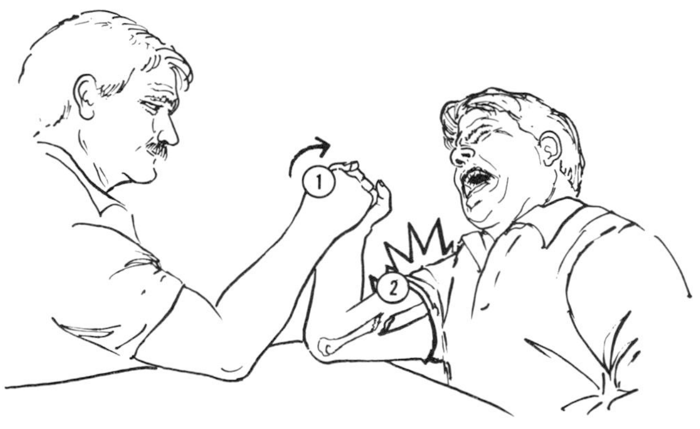

External Torsional Fracture

1. A rotational injury may occur with vigorous sports such as arm wrestling.
2. The forceful external rotation of the elbow causes the spiral oblique fracture with a typical external rotational pattern.

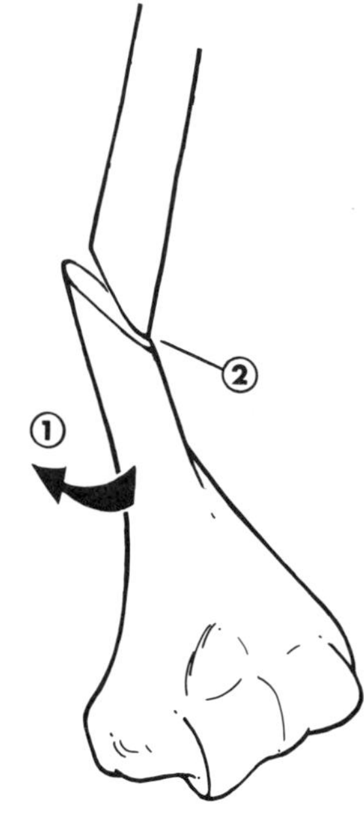

1. External torsion in the younger patient causes a fracture of the distal humerus.
2. Characteristically the failure line runs from the distal medial cortex to the proximal lateral cortex.

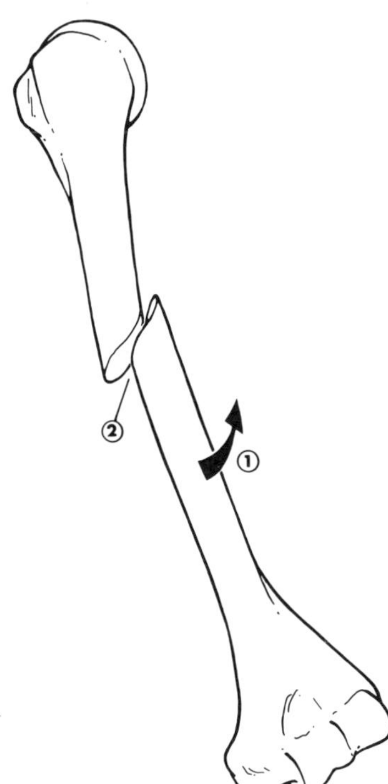

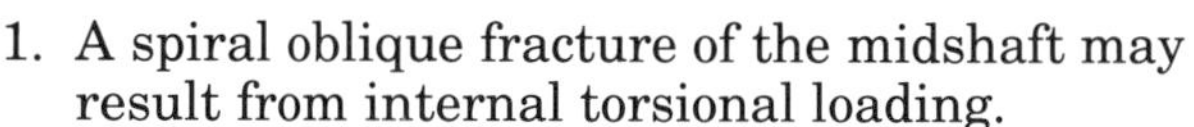

1. A spiral oblique fracture of the midshaft may result from internal torsional loading.
2. The failure line begins in the distal lateral cortex and runs to the proximal medial cortex.

Direct Mechanisms Producing Humeral Fractures

Bending Fractures

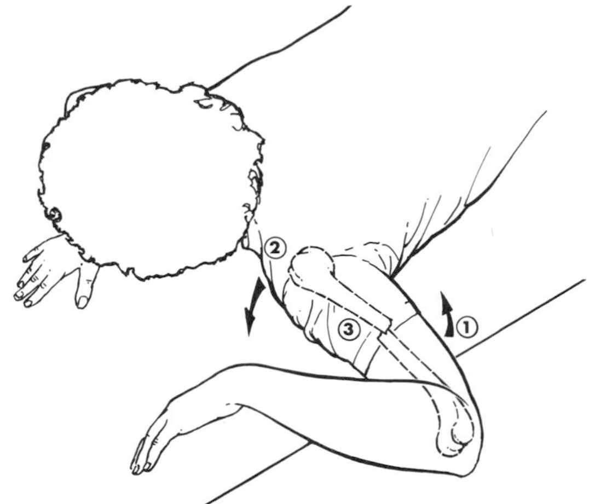

1. The person falls on the distal humerus and forcefully abducts the arm.
2. The proximal humerus is locked in the glenoid.
3. The bending moment produces a typical transverse fracture of the midshaft of the humerus.

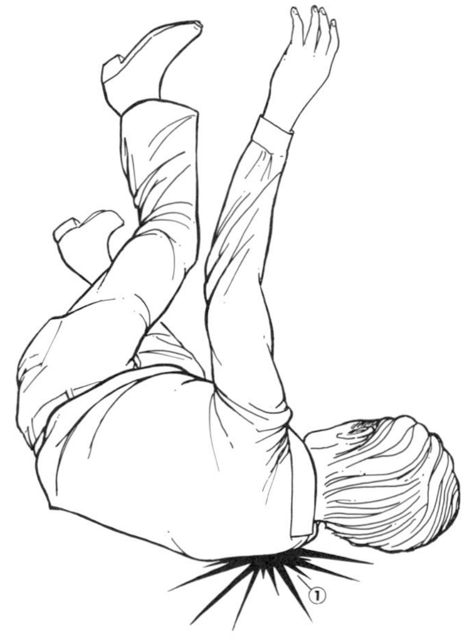

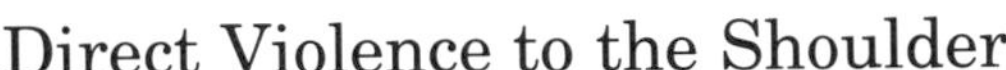

Direct Violence to the Shoulder

1. A direct blow on the shoulder, as in a fall from a horse, may violently fracture one or all of the four major anatomic structures in this region. These include

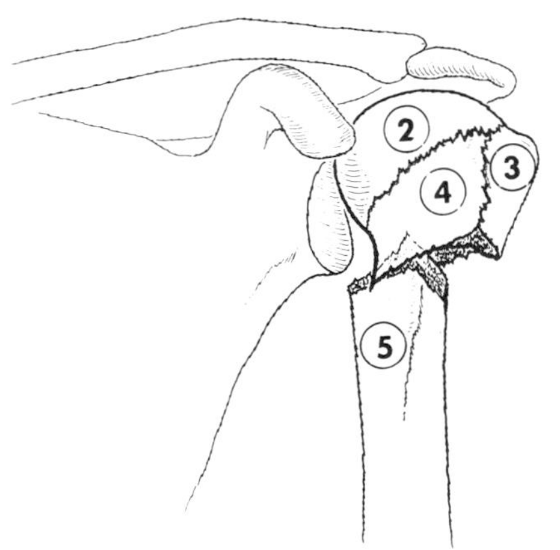

2. The anatomic neck,
3. The greater tuberosity,
4. The lesser tuberosity, and
5. The surgical neck.

Note: With fractures of the greater tuberosity from direct injury to the shoulder, always check carefully for anterior dislocation of the shoulder. When the lesser tuberosity has been fractured from a direct injury, check thoroughly for posterior shoulder dislocation.

■ Types of Displaced Fractures

Humeral Head–Splitting Fractures

A. The first type usually consists of two parts:
   1. Dislocation of the head of the humerus and
   2. Fracture of the greater tuberosity.

B. A three-part fracture frequently consists of
   1. A fracture-dislocation of the head,
   2. A fracture of the greater tuberosity, and
   3. A fracture through the shaft.

C. A four-part fracture frequently consists of
   1. A dislocation of the head,
   2. A fracture of the greater tuberosity,
   3. A fracture through the lesser tuberosity, and
   4. A fracture of the shaft.

Note: The more severely displaced and the greater number of fractures that are present, the more likely is the need for open reduction of these injuries.

D. A humeral head–splitting fracture slices through the articular surface of the humeral head.
   1. This direct impact on the articular surface of the humeral head inflicts significant damage.
   2. The head splits into multiple fragments. This usually requires some type of reconstructive arthroplasty or total joint replacement.

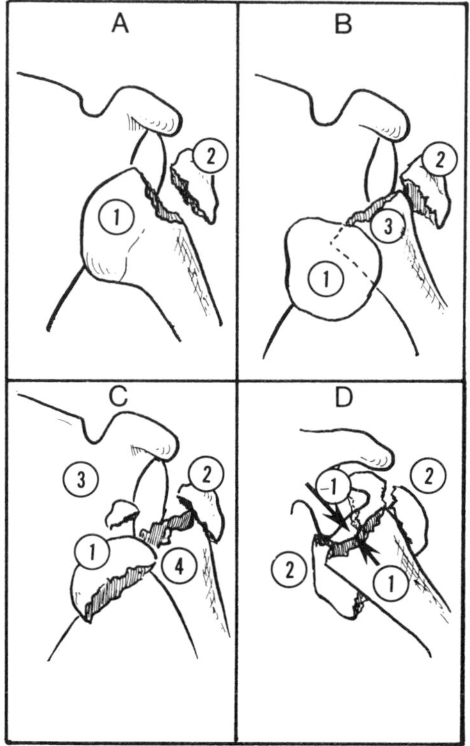

Evaluation

REMARKS

A chief goal in evaluating the patient with a fractured humerus is to detect any associated injuries. With fractures of the proximal humerus, look carefully for associated dislocation of the humeral head.

Fractures of the greater tuberosity are associated with anterior dislocations. Fractures of the lesser tuberosity are most consistently associated with posterior dislocation. The presence or absence of dislocation associated with a fracture can be best evaluated by an adequate axillary x-ray.

Rotator cuff disruptions are also commonly associated with proximal humeral fractures. This is particularly true if there is a displaced fracture of the greater tuberosity.

CT or magnetic resonance imaging (MRI) can be quite helpful for evaluating rotator cuff involvement. However, not every fracture of the proximal humerus warrants such extensive and expensive x-ray study. Only those with possible evidence of rotator cuff disruption on the plain films (i.e., tuberosity fracture) should be considered for such studies.

Fractures of the humerus are occasionally associated with neurovascular injury. Vascular injury should be suspected with grossly displaced internally rotated fractures of the proximal humerus, which may impinge on the brachial artery. Radial nerve injury is quite common with humeral shaft fractures but usually heals spontaneously. The neurovascular status should be carefully assessed before and after reducing the humeral fracture.

X-Ray Technique

1. The most important x-ray for evaluating the fracture of the proximal humerus is an axillary view to ascertain the relationship of the humeral head to the glenoid. This can always be obtained, even when the arm is immobilized in a sling.
2. The fractured arm may be gently abducted 20–30° to allow the x-ray tube to project up through the axilla.
3. A cassette is placed on the superior aspect of the shoulder to permit adequate visualization of the relationship between the humeral head and the glenoid.
4. The patient may support the arm by holding on to an intravenous (IV) pole, or the arm may be supported by an assistant.

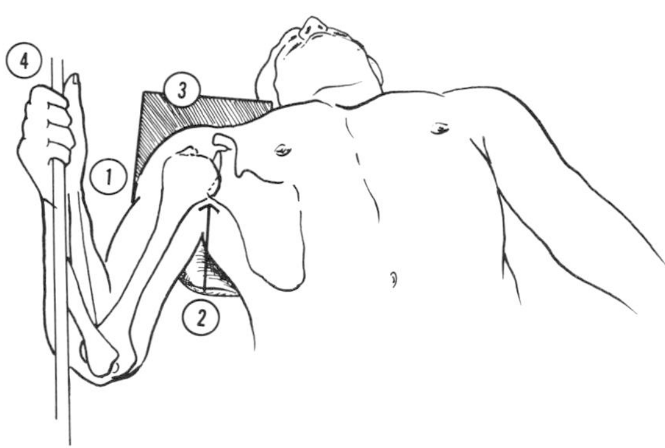

Computed Tomographic Evaluation

1. Most dislocations and fractures of the proximal humerus can be adequately evaluated by standard plain x-rays, including an axillary view. In fracture-dislocations computed tomography (CT) may be necessary to assess the extent of injury.
2. CT is very helpful in determining the amount of displacement of the tuberosity fracture and the potential for rotator cuff disruption.

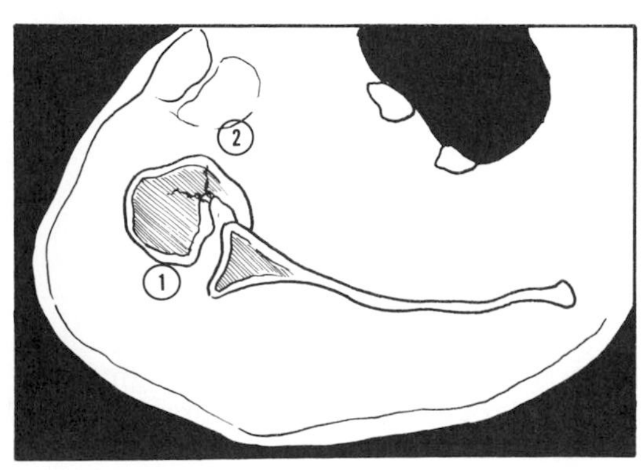

Management of Fracture of the Upper End of the Humerus

REMARKS

Fractures of the upper humerus, with very few exceptions, can and should be treated by closed methods in which early functional range-of-shoulder motion is used to stimulate healing. The deltoid and rotator cuff muscles provide intrinsic stability to most of these fractures in the elderly patient. Early functional exercises utilizing these muscles help align the fracture and promote callus.

Attempted closed reduction by manipulating the fracture is unnecessary unless there is evidence of neurovascular compromise from the displaced fracture. An exception to this rule of closed reduction is the occasional dislocation of the head of the humerus or rotator cuff disruption, which necessitates prompt open reduction and operative repair.

Although there is sometimes a tendency to try to establish arbitrary x-ray criteria of fracture angulation or displacement as indications for closed or open reduction, the usual two-part fracture of the surgical neck can be treated very effectively with an early functional exercise program. The main criteria are that the humeral head has not dislocated and that the rotator cuff is not disrupted.

In contrast to the usual fracture sustained by indirect loading on osteoporotic bone, the proximal humerus fractured by a severe direct blow to the shoulder usually sustains multiple displaced fractures and requires operative reduction and internal fixation.

Types of Fractures That Can Be Treated Without Reduction and by Early Functional Exercises

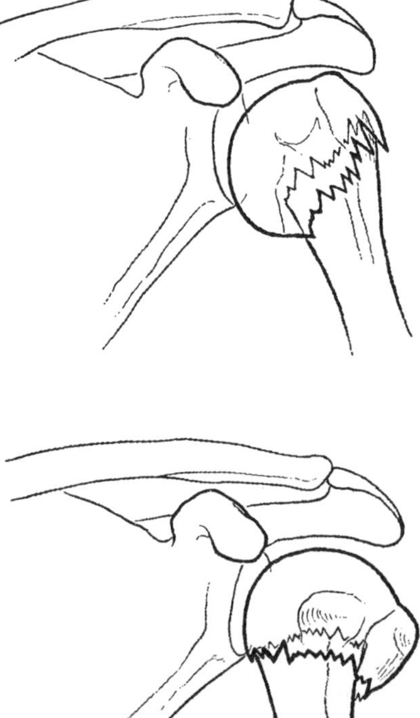

An impacted external torsional fracture of the surgical neck of the humerus is a typical fracture in osteoporotic bone. Although there is a varus and internal torsion displacement as a result of this fracture, this angulation does not preclude good restoration of function. The main concern is that the humeral head is articulating with the glenoid and that the rotator cuff is intact.

Impacted internal torsional fracture of the surgical neck of the humerus; the proximal fragment is in the externally rotated valgus position, which will not affect shoulder function.

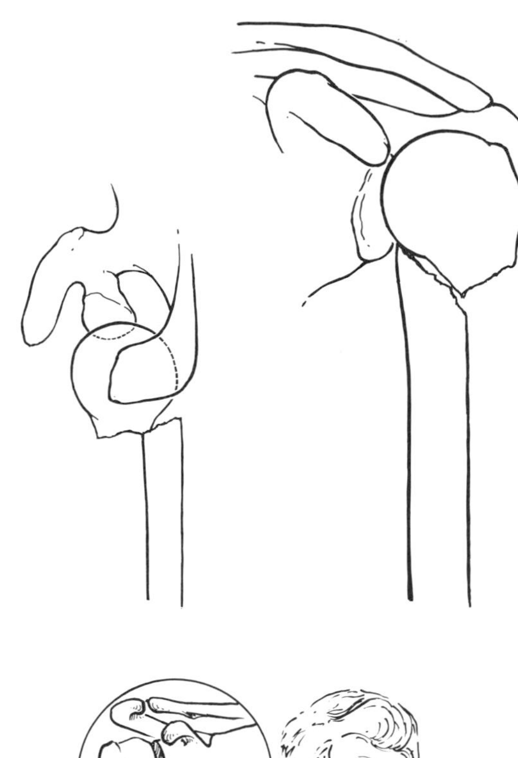

A displaced surgical neck fracture produced by internal torsion is impacted with displacement. The medial and posterior displacement of the distal fragment does not require disimpaction because shoulder function will not be impaired by healing in this position.

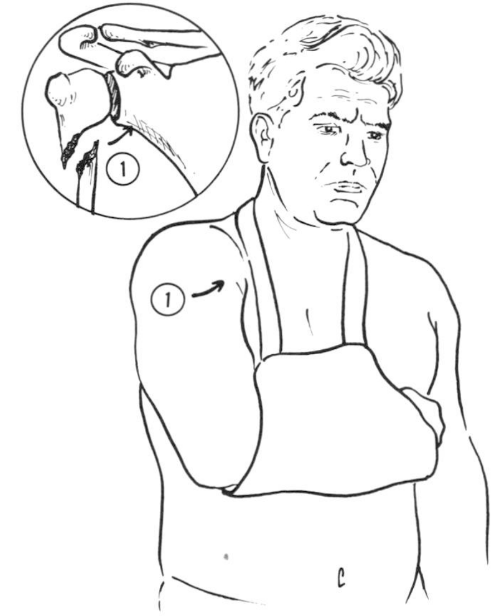

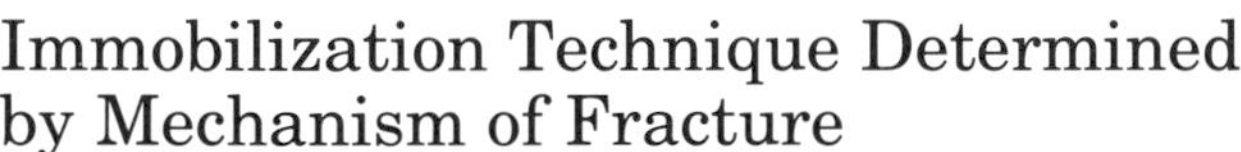

Immobilization Technique Determined by Mechanism of Fracture

1. Internally rotating a surgical neck fracture originally produced by internal rotation—that is, in a sling—does not improve position and, in fact, may make it worse.

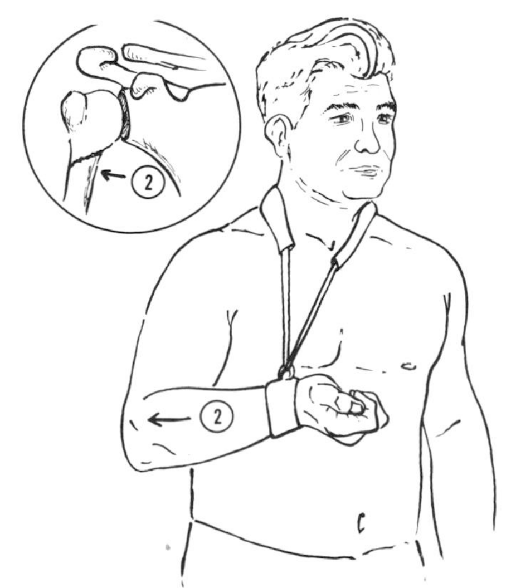

2. The treatment preferred for the internally rotated fracture with medial displacement is to allow the shoulder to externally rotate, with functional exercises to restore alignment.

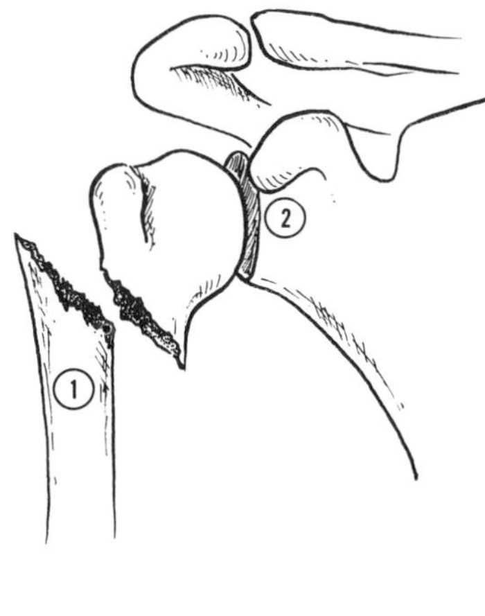

1. This fracture resulted from external torsion of the surgical neck with upward and outward displacement of the shaft.
2. The humeral head is articulating with the glenoid and is not dislocated.

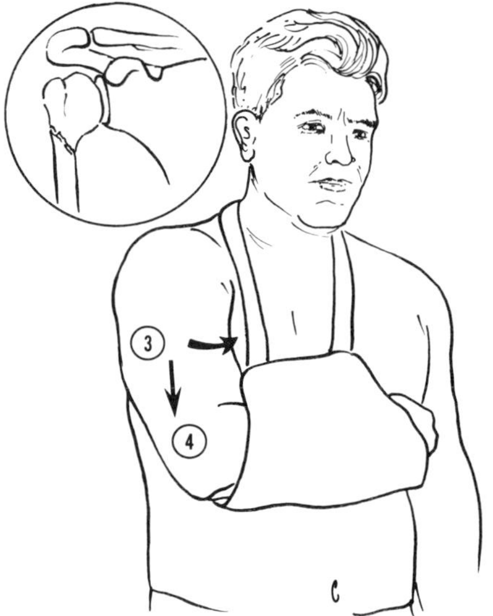

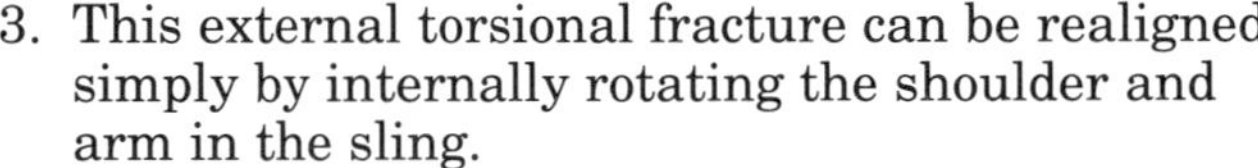

3. This external torsional fracture can be realigned simply by internally rotating the shoulder and arm in the sling.
4. The downward weight of the arm usually will correct the superior displacement of the shaft fragment without the need for manipulation.

Management of Proximal Humeral Fractures by Early Functional Exercise

REMARKS

The fracture is immobilized in a sling and swathe for 3–5 days until the initial swelling and pain subside. Within the first week, the patient can be encouraged to remove the arm from the sling and begin extending the elbow. Gravity and the shoulder musculature are thus used to align the fracture.

For fractures resulting from external torsional injuries, internal rotational exercises should be emphasized. Conversely, for those resulting from internal torsional injury with medial displacement, external rotation exercises should be emphasized.

Exercise Program

REMARKS

Within the first 1 or 2 weeks after fracture when the swelling subsides, begin a gravity-assisted circumduction exercise program. Three to 5 weeks after injury, passive stretching exercises may be instituted to regain external rotation and abduction motion. This program should continue for at least 3–4 months to achieve full range of motion after a fracture of the proximal humerus.

Gravity Exercises

First start with gravity exercises.

1. The patient bends far forward, holding the shoulders and trunk immobile.
2. The arms hang loosely and swing like a pendulum (A) across the front of the body, (B) backward and forward, and (C) in a circle.

Note: The arc at first is small, then is gradually increased.

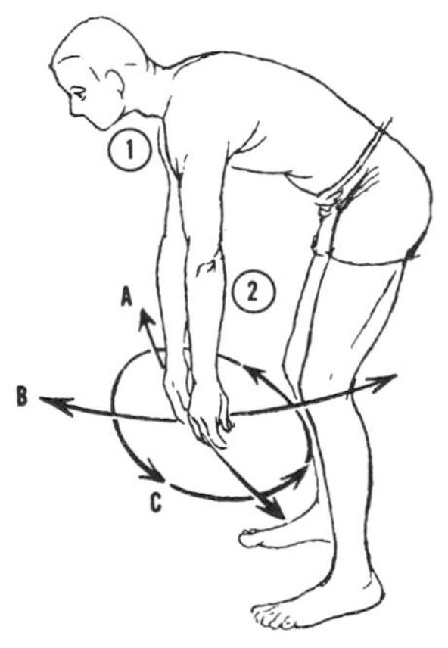

Passive Stretching Shoulder Exercises

These are most valuable for the painful stiffening of the shoulder that can occur after very minor injury and can persist for many months or years. The patient must work to regain motion in all planes, including external rotation and abduction, as well as extension and flexion.

1. The patient stands with scapulae against the wall and hands clasped behind the head. The patient abducts and externally rotates the shoulder rapidly in order to touch the elbows to the wall. This may require assistance to get full external rotation and abduction.

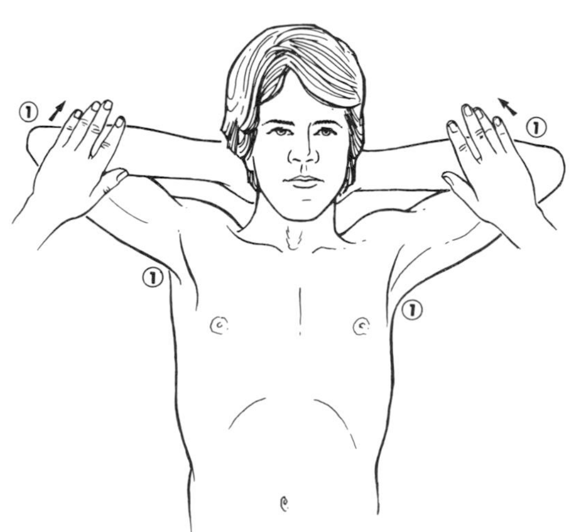

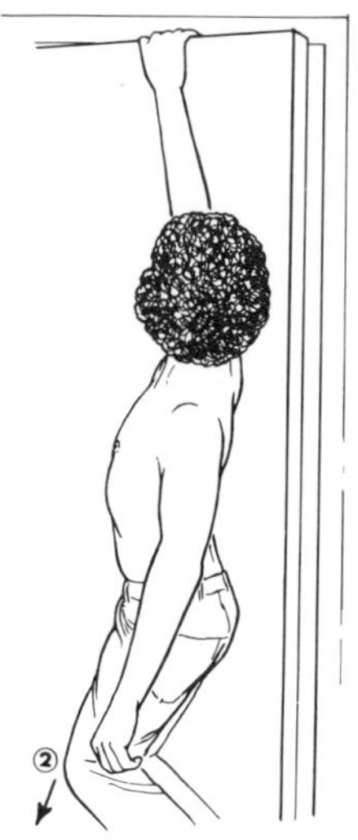

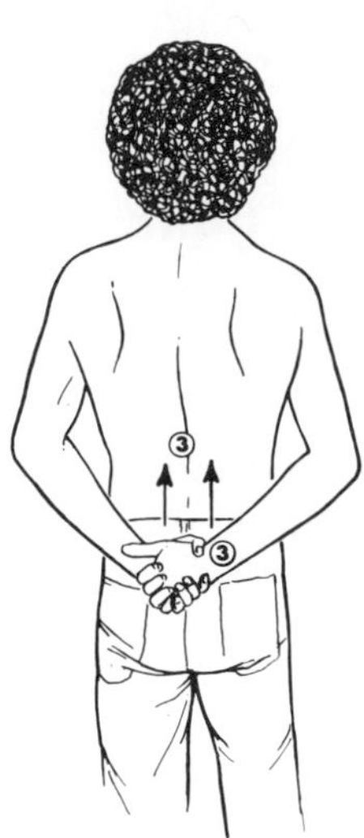

2. The patient reaches to an overhead support or door and flexes at the knee to pull with body weight on the stiff shoulder.
3. The patient reaches behind the back, grasps the wrist on the side of the stiff shoulder, and pulls upward toward the opposite scapula.

■ Subsequent Management

By 3–5 weeks the initial pain and discomfort have generally subsided and the patient can start external rotational and abduction exercises. Return of full range of motion may take several months but can be expedited by a program of passive-stretching shoulder exercises at 4–6 weeks.

It is important to not wait for radiographic signs of fracture union to be evident before commencing with the range-of-motion exercise program. These injuries are treated with emphasis on the soft tissue damage as well as the bony damage.

In particular, the patient should work on pendulum exercises hourly rather than relying on an occasional visit to a professional therapist. Professional therapists are helpful for the more complex rehabilitation problems but should not be utilized for the routine proximal humeral fracture. For this type of fracture, the best therapy is that in which the patient and the family members work to regain function of the shoulder.

Closed Management—Surgical Neck Fracture With Marked Displacement

REMARKS

Almost without exception, surgical neck fractures may be treated by an early functional exercise program. This entails not anatomic reduction but, rather, early restoration of muscle function as soon as the initial pain subsides. Even fractures in this area with considerable displacement can be treated by a functional method, provided the humeral head is not dislocated or the rotator cuff system is not disrupted.

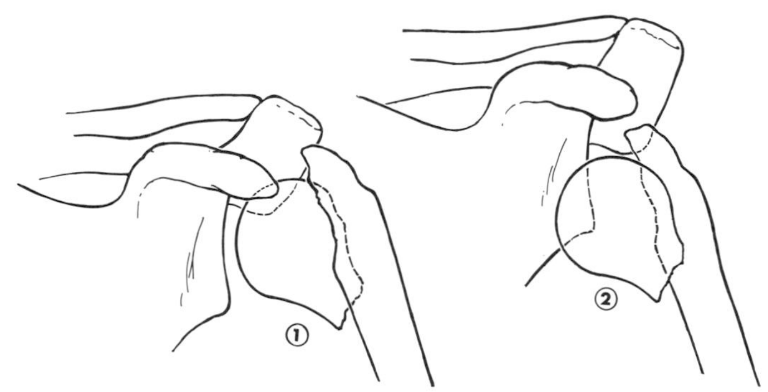

1. A comminuted external torsional fracture. The distal fragment displaces superiorly and laterally.
2. These external torsional fractures should be evaluated carefully with axillary views to determine whether the head fragment has dislocated anteriorly.

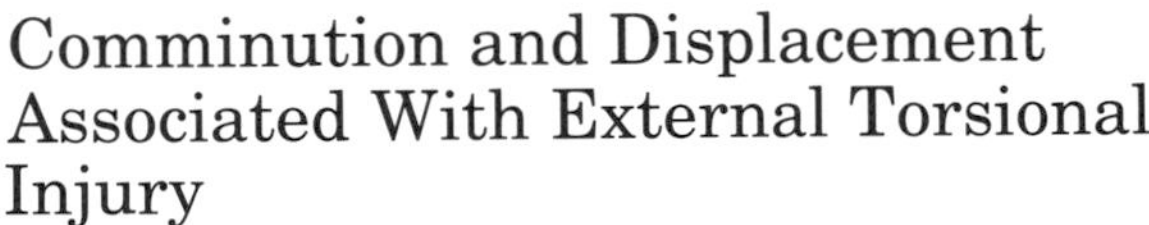

Comminution and Displacement Associated With External Torsional Injury

In most instances these two fragment fractures are not dislocated and may be treated by early functional exercises. A hanging cast may be useful temporarily to pull down the shaft fragment to align with the head-and-neck fragment.

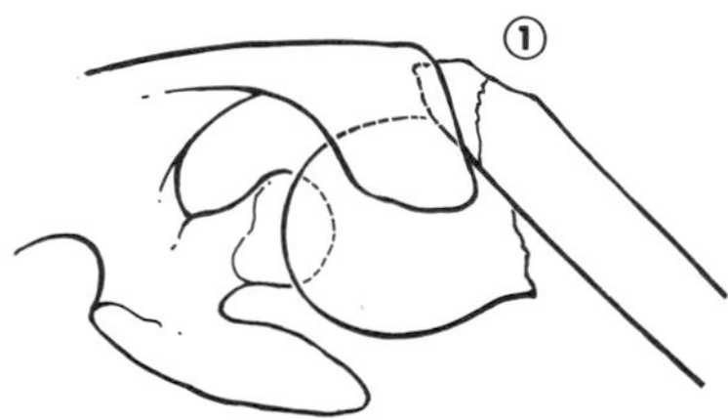

1. The axillary view shows that the humeral head is articulating with the glenoid; however, posterior displacement of the shaft fragment is evident. This may be corrected by manipulation or traction with a hanging cast.

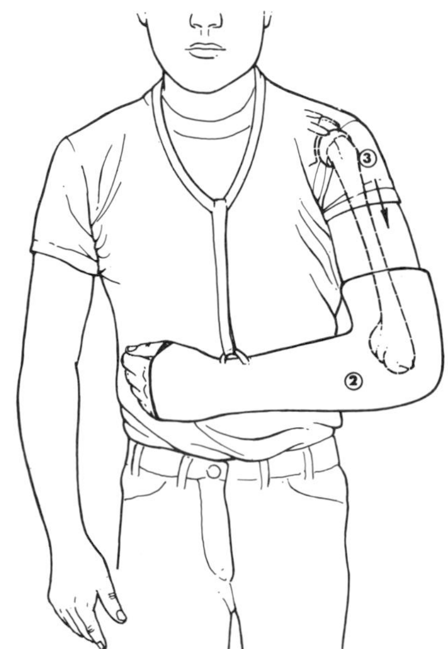

2. A lightweight hanging cast is used to pull the distal fragment inferiorly.
3. Some medial displacement of the distal fragment is acceptable, as it will not impinge on the acromion during shoulder motion.

Subsequent Management

The hanging cast can be removed by 2–3 weeks as the fracture reduces with the pull of gravity. Subsequently the patient can be started on circumduction and range-of-motion exercises, as illustrated previously.

Healing at Eight to Ten Weeks After Fracture Treated by Functional Exercise Program

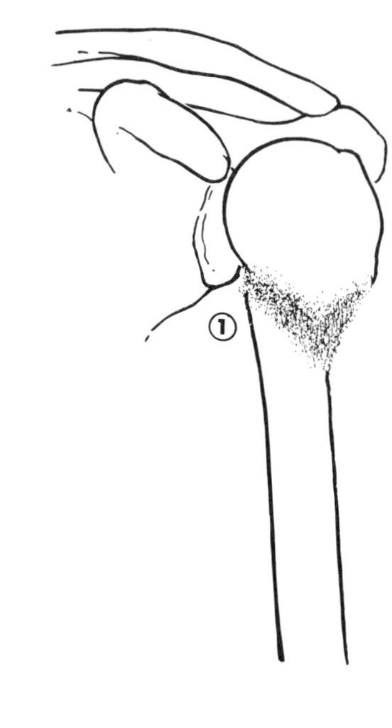

1. Perfect anatomic reduction is not essential for fractures of the surgical or anatomic neck, provided that the rotator cuff function is not impaired. Bayonet apposition may be quite satisfactory.

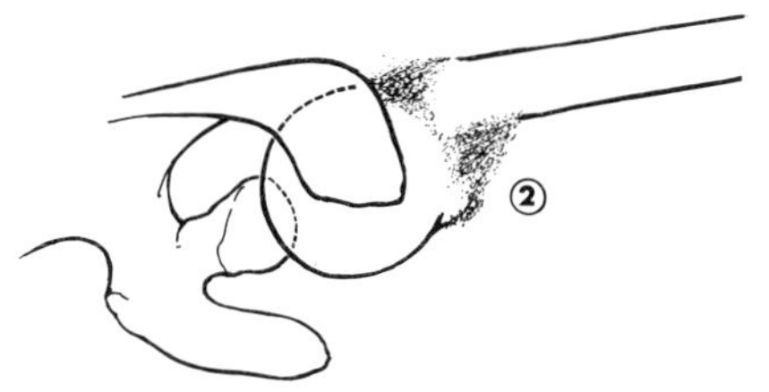

2. Axillary view of a surgical neck fracture healed in bayonet apposition demonstrates excellent functional range of motion without impingement on the acromion.

Closed Management—Comminuted Fracture of the Surgical Neck From an Internal Rotational Injury

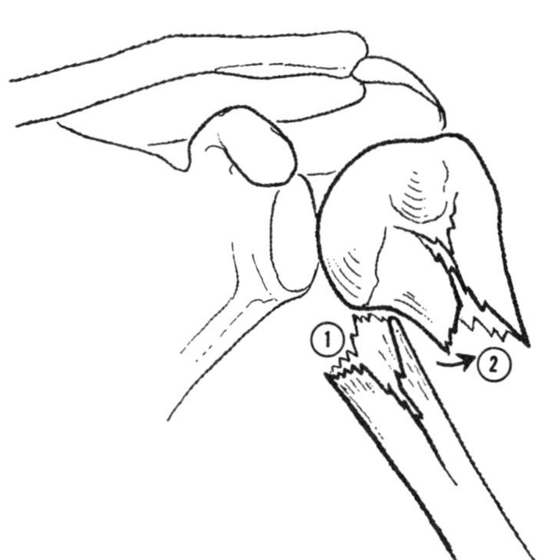

1. The internal rotation of the shaft on the proximal humerus has caused humeral displacement.
2. The proximal fragment and the head remain articulating with the glenoid, although varus angulation has occurred at the fracture.

Manipulative Reduction

REMARKS

Attempts at manipulation of the displaced surgical neck fracture usually are unnecessary and futile. Displacement of the fracture usually recurs and, as previously illustrated, does not cause any functional impairment if it heals in a displaced position.

Occasionally the shaft fracture may be sufficiently displaced that symptoms of neurovascular compromise develop. In this rare instance, manipulative reduction or even internal fixation may be necessary.

Complete muscle relaxation is essential. This is best attained by general anesthesia.

1. With the patient recumbent, the operator makes steady traction on the arm in line with the long axis of the body.
2. While traction is maintained, the arm is adducted across the anterior surface of the thorax and is flexed in relation to the frontal plane of the body. This restores the length of the humerus.
3. The operator then places the other hand in the axilla, and while firm pressure is made on the head fragment with the thumb, the shaft fragment is pushed outward.
4. After the fragments are aligned, traction is released, gradually engaging the fragments.

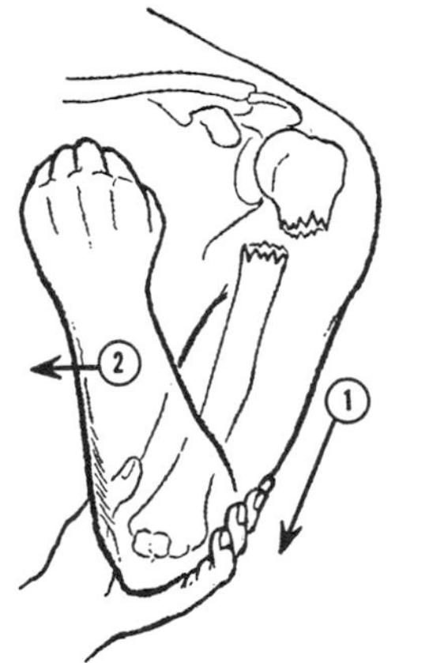

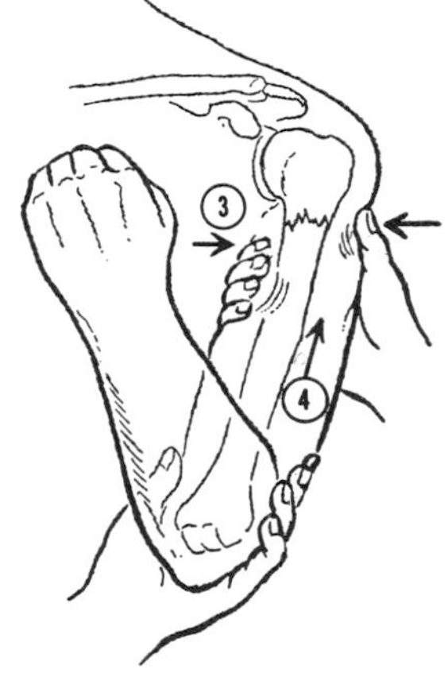

Alternative Method: Skeletal Traction

Gentle manipulation and gravity traction from the arm weight are sufficient to reduce and hold most humeral fractures. Occasionally, if the patient must be kept in bed for reasons other than the fracture, traction may be employed; as a general rule, however, skeletal traction should be avoided.

1. Traction is made by use of a threaded pin or wire through the base of the olecranon. Drill from the ulnar aspect to the radial side to avoid impaling the ulnar nerve.
2. Begin traction with the arm in a flexed, adducted position to disimpact the fracture and gradually abduct to no more than 60° so as to align the distal fragments with the proximal fragments.
3. Apply sufficient traction to maintain alignment.

Caution: Avoid too much traction. The fracture must not be distracted.

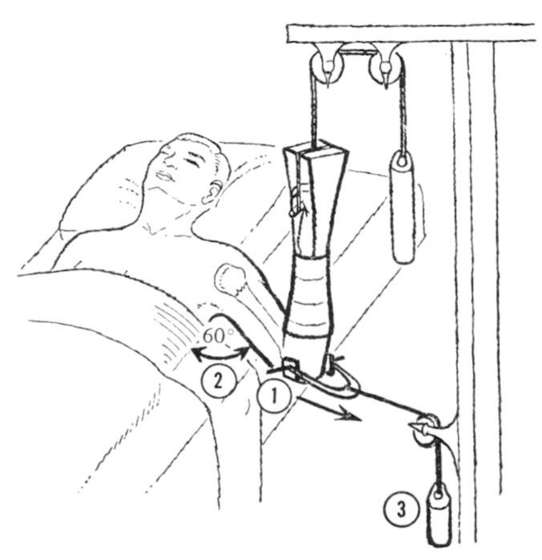

Fractures of the Proximal Humerus That Frequently Necessitate Open Reduction and Internal Fixation

REMARKS

The main indications for open reduction of proximal humerus fractures are dislocations of the humeral head and disruptions of the rotator cuff. A rare injury that may necessitate internal fixation is a fracture through the anatomic neck rather than the surgical neck. This can be an unstable injury with a high risk of avascular necrosis, which may be best stabilized much as a fracture of the neck of the proximal femur would be stabilized.

Indication for Operative Fixation: Rotator Cuff Disruption

Any displacement of the greater tuberosity fracture should be viewed with suspicion and careful analysis for rotator cuff disruption. In the past some displacement of these fragments has been accepted, but quite often this can lead to permanent weakness from either associated rotator cuff disruption or impingement from displacement of the fracture and the fracture callus beneath the acromion. This illustration shows a fairly undisplaced fracture that was initially treated closed.

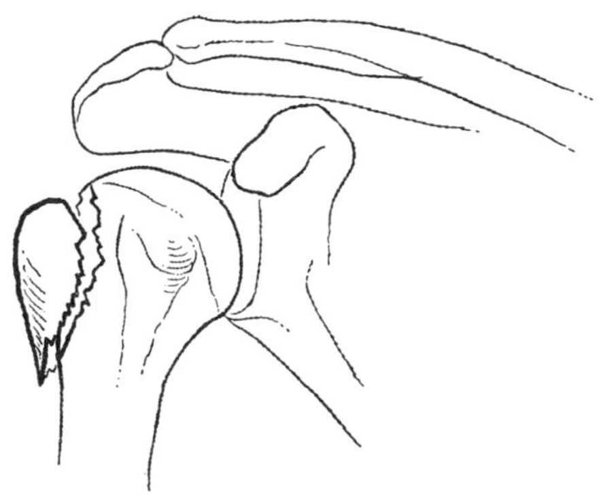

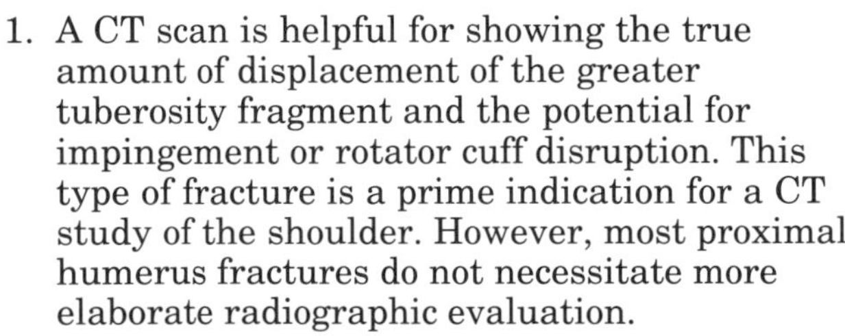

1. A CT scan is helpful for showing the true amount of displacement of the greater tuberosity fragment and the potential for impingement or rotator cuff disruption. This type of fracture is a prime indication for a CT study of the shoulder. However, most proximal humerus fractures do not necessitate more elaborate radiographic evaluation.

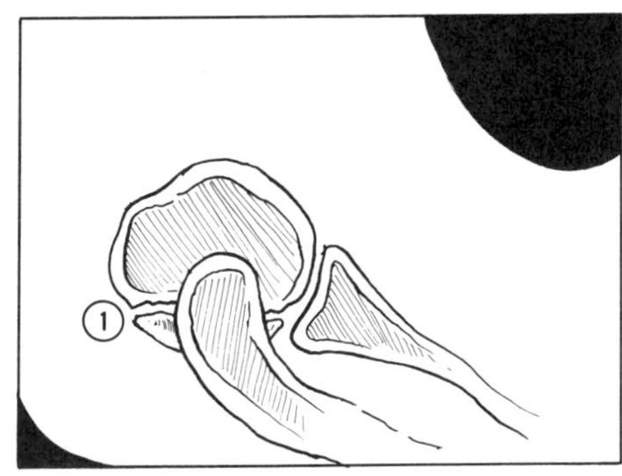

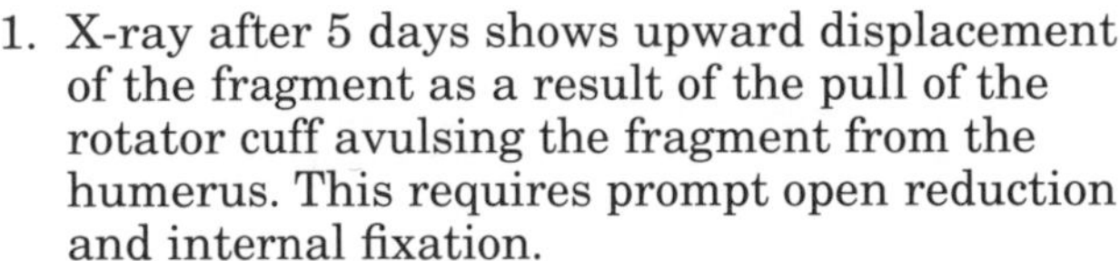

1. X-ray after 5 days shows upward displacement of the fragment as a result of the pull of the rotator cuff avulsing the fragment from the humerus. This requires prompt open reduction and internal fixation.

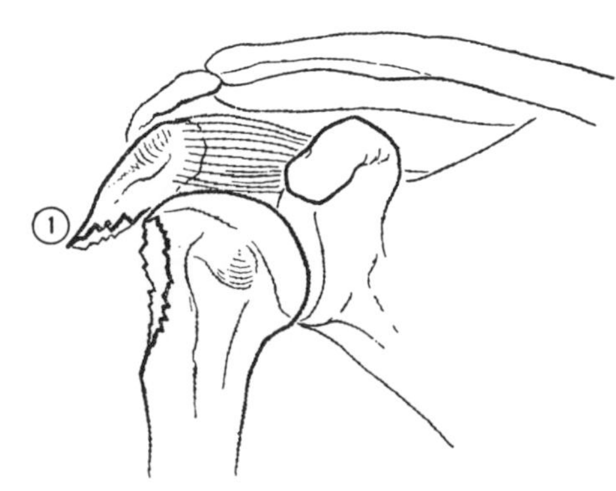

Reduction of a Displaced Greater Tuberosity Fracture

1. The displaced fragment with its rotator cuff attachment necessitates open reduction under direct visualization to reattach the tuberosity to its proper position.
2. The tuberosity fragment can be fixed with cannulated screws into the humeral head, and
3. The rotator cuff is repaired at the same time.
4. Frequently a resection of the anterior acromion and acromial coracoid ligament is necessary to prevent impingement of the tendon and tuberosity fragment on the undersurface of the acromion overlying the acromial coracoid ligament.

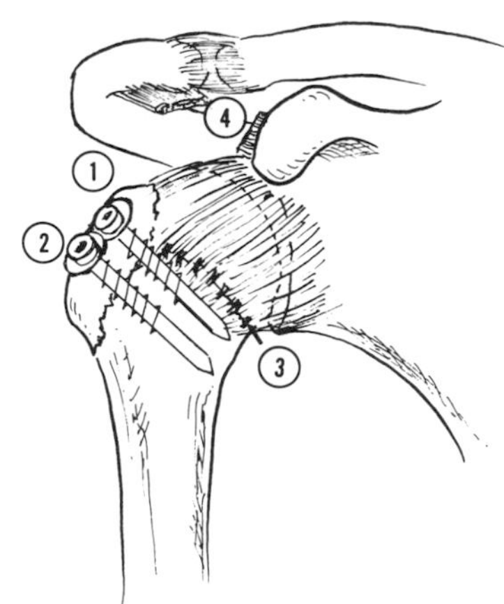

Other Indications for Operative Reduction

Fractures of the Lesser Tuberosity

REMARKS

The avulsion fracture of the lesser tuberosity hardly ever occurs as an isolated injury. Most frequently it is associated with a posterior dislocation of the humeral head or a four-part comminuted fracture-dislocation.

The rare isolated avulsion fracture may displace as a result of the pull of the subscapularis tendon. The result is that it can lie between the coracoid process and the head of the humerus and may block shoulder motion. The displaced fracture fragment of the lesser tuberosity is best restored to its normal position by operative methods; however, the injury is most likely to be associated with an acute or chronic posterior instability of the humerus. (See also section on recurrent posterior dislocation of the shoulder.)

Preoperative X-Ray

Fractures of this type are quite commonly associated with acute posterior or recurrent posterior dislocation of the humeral head; therefore, the axillary view is always necessary to look for this problem in the typical notching of the anteromedial aspect of the humeral head from recurrent dislocation.

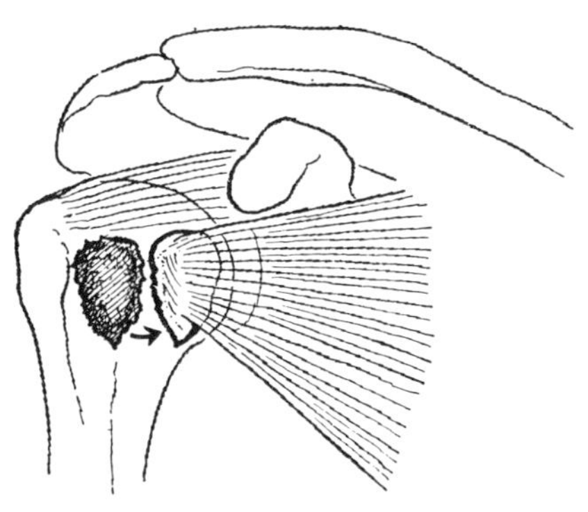

Operative Reduction

1. The defect is visualized quite commonly in the anteromedial aspect of the humeral head.
2. The avulsed fragment and subscapularis tendon should be buried into the defect to stabilize the humeral head and to prevent recurrent posterior dislocation.

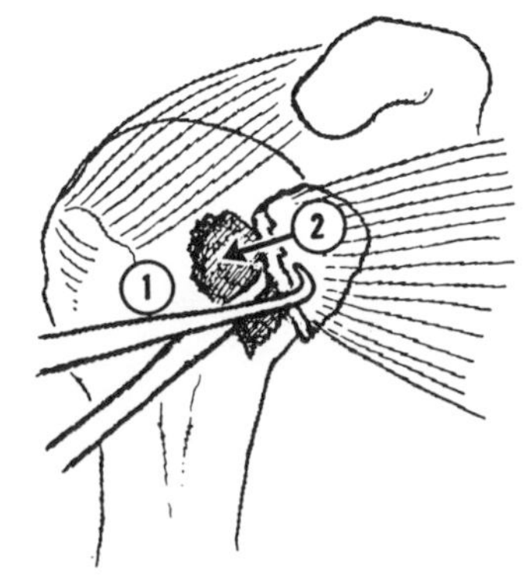

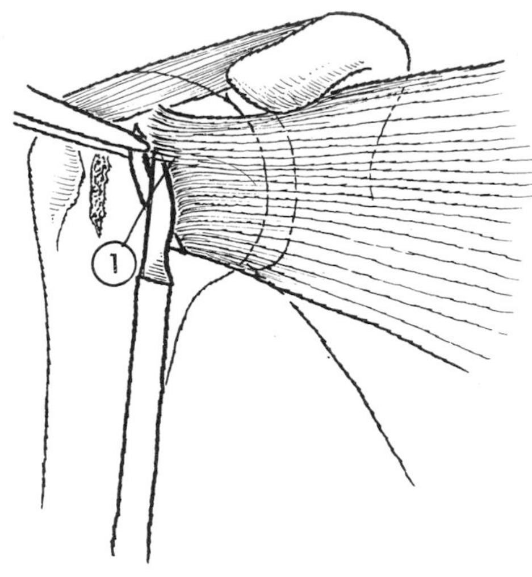

1. If the avulsion fracture is small and associated with a posterior dislocation, it is best to shorten the subscapularis tendon and reattach the tendon directly into the defect.

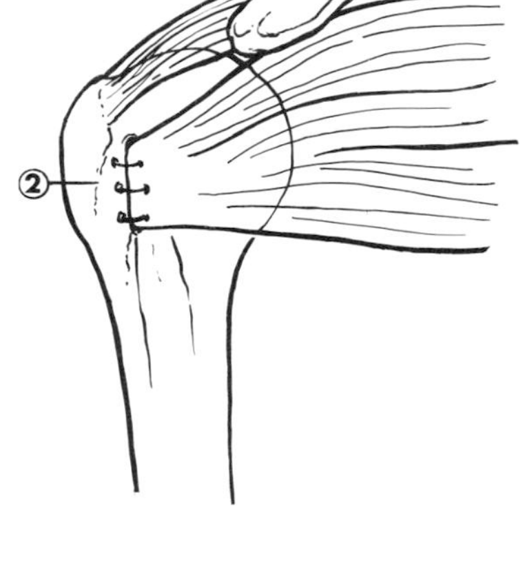

2. The tendon can be fixed to the anteromedial defect by multiple interrupted sutures buried in bone.

Anteromedial Fractures of the Head With Posterior Dislocation

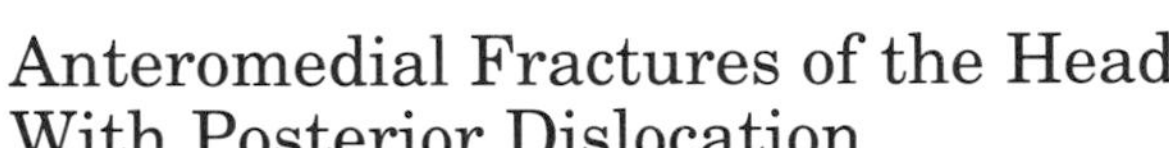

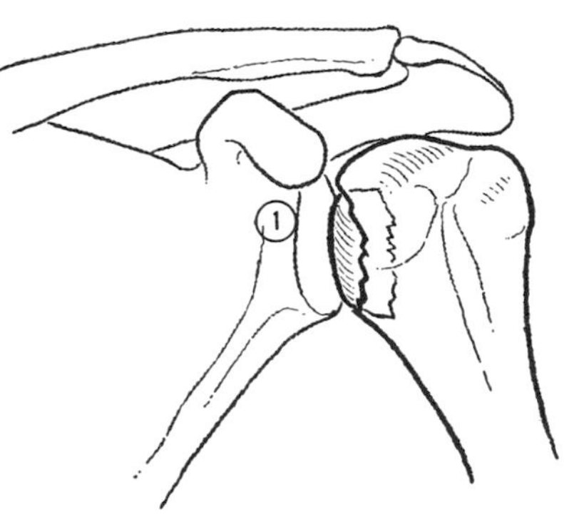

1. Another indication for operative treatment of the proximal humerus is a dislocation associated with a fracture. Look carefully, particularly when there is a fracture of the anteromedial joint surface, as illustrated here. These quite often accompany posterior dislocation.

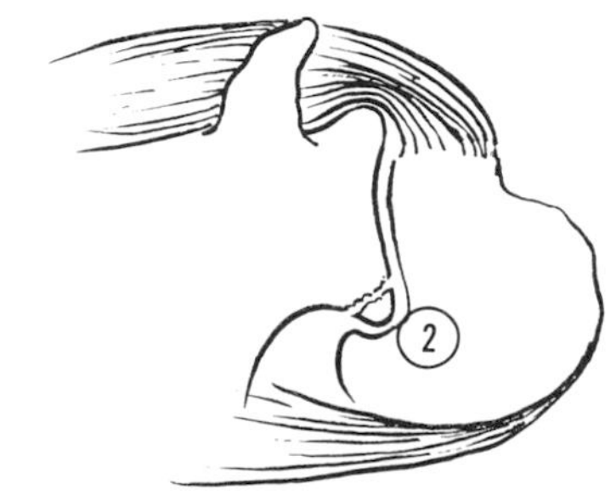

2. Axillary view shows fracture of the anteromedial aspect of the humeral head that is severely posteriorly dislocated and necessitates prompt open reduction.

Fractures of the Anatomic Neck of the Humerus

REMARKS

The anatomic neck of the humerus is the residual scar resulting from ossification of the old physeal growth plate. The area is anatomically important because it marks the site where the ascending branches of the anterior humeral circumflex penetrate into the humeral head to supply circulation to the proximal aspect of the head.

Immediately beneath the anatomic neck is the attachment of the capsule and rotator cuff muscles. Because the area is relatively protected by these structures, fractures of the proximal humerus are usually at or below the tuberosity through the surgical neck rather than through the anatomic neck. Injury to this area is more likely to occur in the immature adolescent skeleton with a partially closed growth plate. After growth plate closure, the anatomic neck is well protected and rarely fractured.

If fracture occurs, it is usually the result of a direct impact or dislocation. There is a fairly good chance that circulatory damage and avascular necrosis may result. Because of the high risk of complication from loss of blood supply, this fracture is best stabilized internally, preferably with multiple pins.

Epiphyseal Fracture in the Child

1. Type II epiphyseal fracture has occurred.
2. There is a triangular fracture of the metaphysis.
3. The shaft fragment of the humerus is displaced upward in relation to the head fragment.

Note: These fractures are reduced by the manipulative techniques described in Chapter 2.

Appearance on X-Ray

ANATOMIC NECK FRACTURE IN AN ADULT

1. The fracture line runs through the old epiphyseal line, which is also the point of vascular entry into the humeral head. The distal fragment displaces superiorly and laterally and will impinge on the acromion during shoulder abduction.

The objective of treatment is to reduce the superior displacement of the distal fragment without further impairing blood supply to the humeral head.

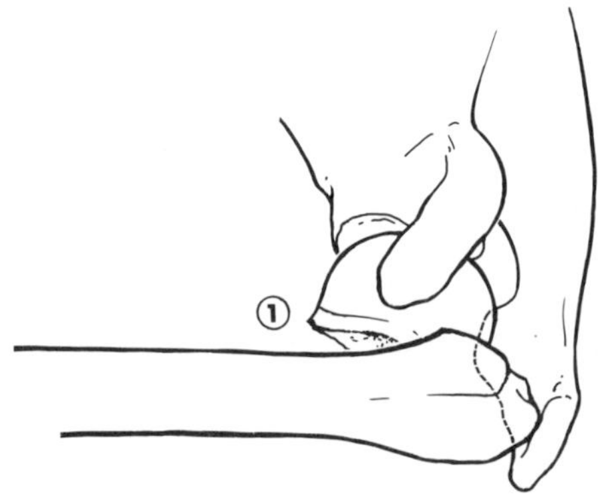

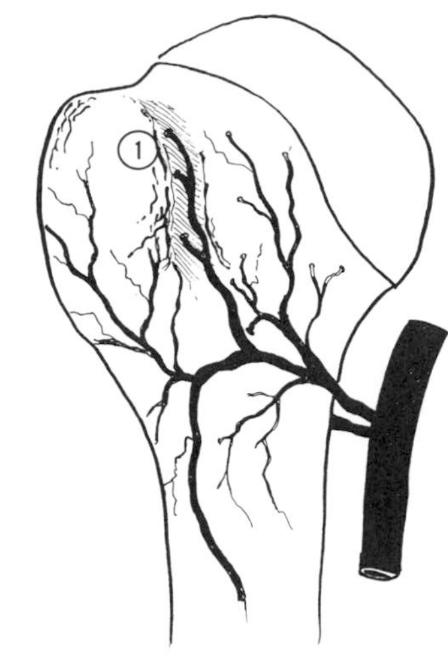

Blood Supply to the Humeral Head

1. Blood supply to the proximal humerus and the humeral head is dependent on the ascending branch of the anterior humeral circumflex artery, as shown here.

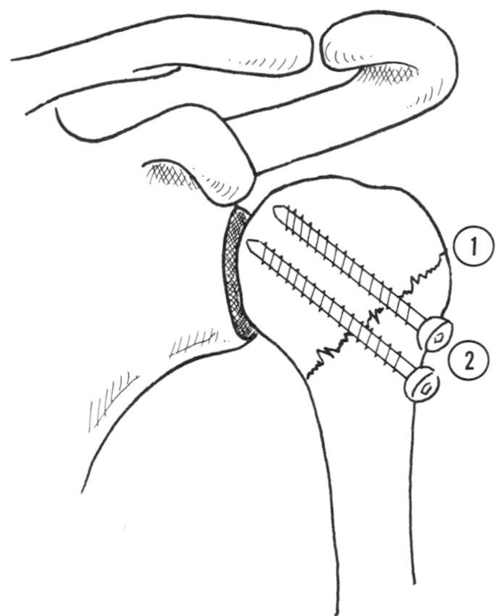

Operative Reduction and Percutaneous Pinning of a Displaced Anatomic Neck

1. The displaced shaft can be aligned to the head fragment by direct longitudinal traction.
2. The position is then held by cannulated screws inserted under image-intensified fluoroscopy to pin the shaft to the head as well as to pin the femoral neck fracture.

Note: Subsequent management with a sling and early range-of-motion exercises is then possible; however, the patient should be cautioned that damage to the blood supply is likely with this uncommon fracture and may lead to avascular necrosis of the humeral head.

Avascular Necrosis

Appearance on X-Ray

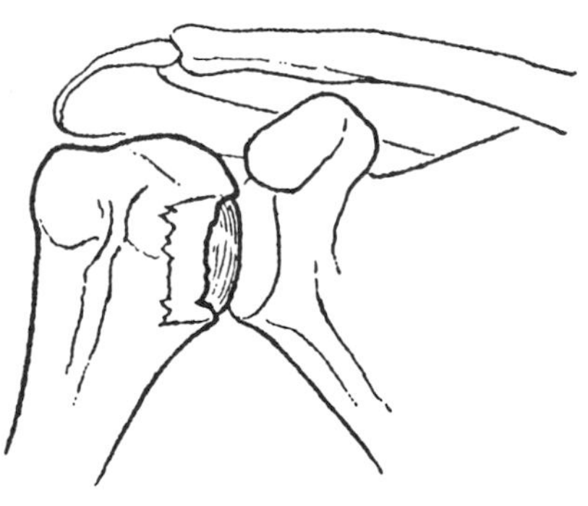

Fractures of the anatomic neck or impaction fractures of the subchondral bone can cause avascular necrosis if the blood supply is disrupted. Over the subsequent year or two after injury, this can lead to significant pain and functional impairment.

A chronic unrecognized posterior shoulder dislocation also produces an arthropathy of this type.

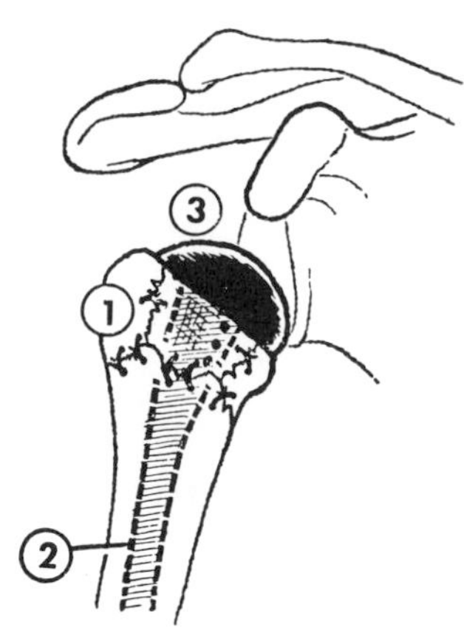

Management

1. If pain is severe, the humeral head is replaced with a Neer prosthesis.
2. The stem of the prosthesis fits snugly in the shaft.
3. The head is slightly retroverted, and the rotator cuff is reattached to its normal insertion.

Other Indications for Operative Treatment of Proximal Humeral Fractures with Rotator Cuff Disruption

Open reduction and internal fixation are indicated primarily for proximal humeral fractures in association with dislocation or rotator cuff disruption. In addition to these indications, occasionally internal fixation is warranted for the patient with multiple injuries, pathologic fractures, or nonunion. A number of methods are available to fix the proximal fracture of the humerus, but the author's preference is to use cannulated screws inserted in a manner similar to pinning of a femoral neck fracture.

A fracture of the anatomic neck or the greater tuberosity of the humerus is a good indication for internal fixation to achieve stability and prompt healing.

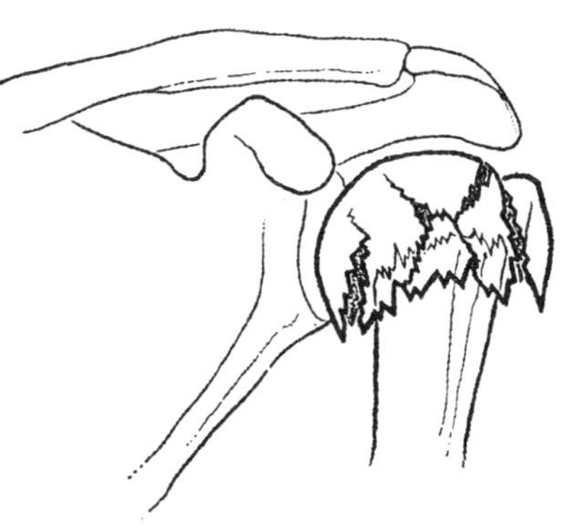

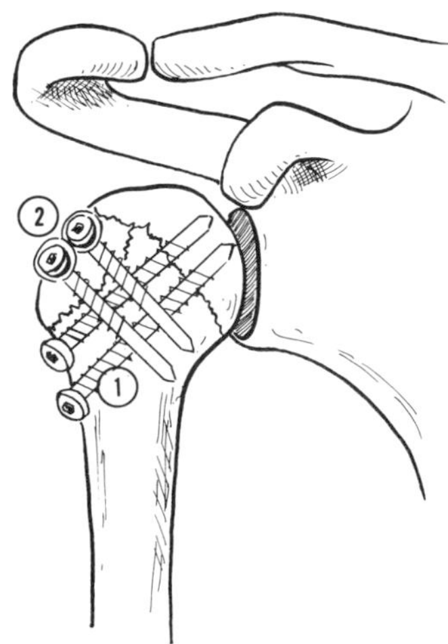

1. The humeral neck fracture can be pinned by cannulated screws.
2. The displaced tuberosity can also be fixed with cannulated screws if the bone fragment is sufficiently large. Otherwise, the tendon should be sutured directly to bone.

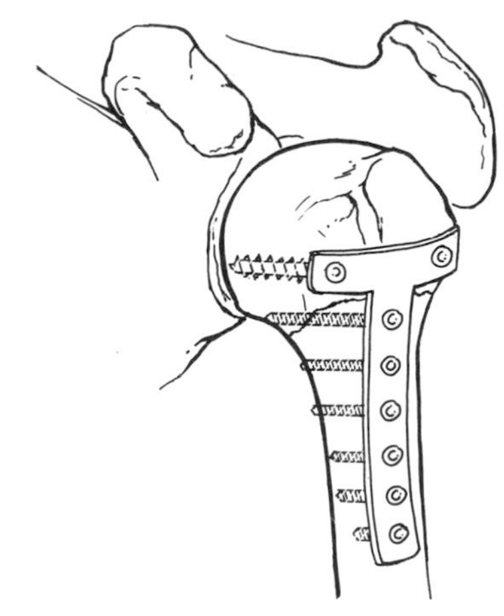

Nonunion of the Proximal Humerus

Nonunion of the proximal humerus may be fixed with a T-plate or blade plate technique to stabilize the shaft to the head fragment.

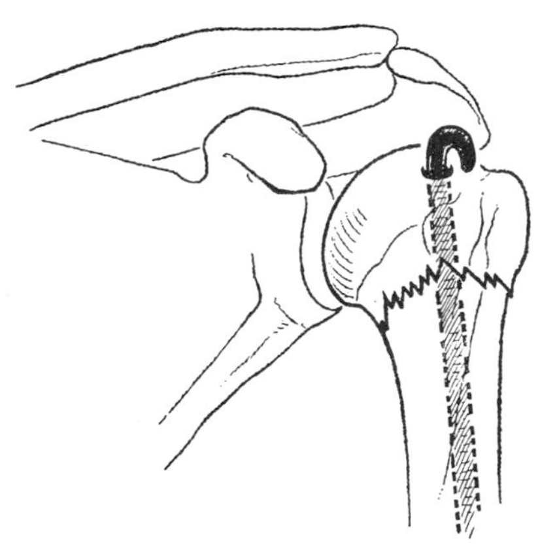

Rush pin fixation has been used to stabilize proximal humeral fractures, but the pin tends to migrate and impinge on the acromion. This may be prevented by inserting one pin closer to the tuberosity and away from the rotator cuff. In general, the author's preference now is for cannulated screws rather than Rush pin fixation, because these provide better mechanical fixation and avoid problems with the pin backing out.

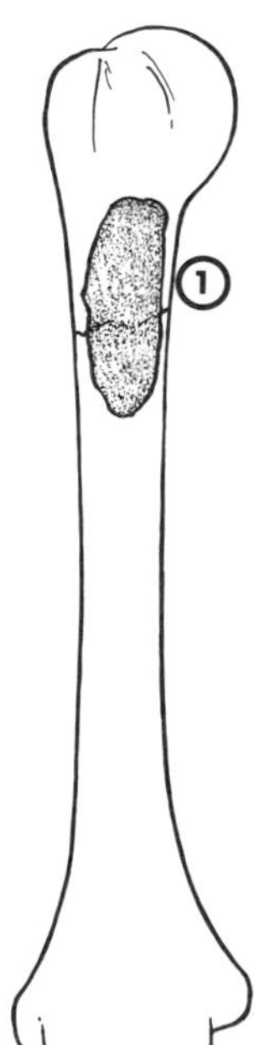

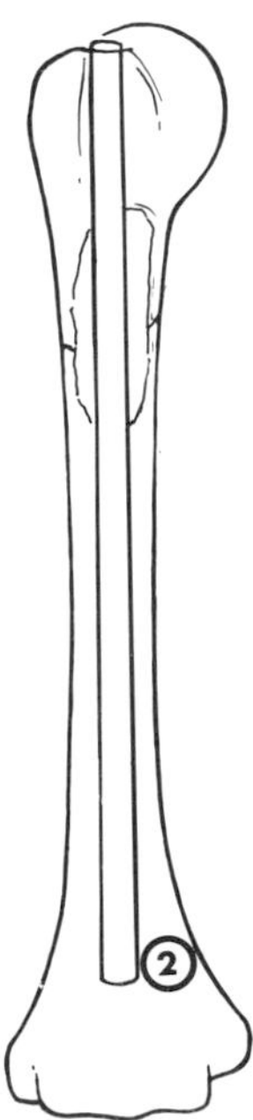

Pathologic Fractures From Metastatic Malignancy

1. The proximal humerus is a fairly common site for fracture caused by metastatic carcinoma from a primary lesion in the breast or lung.
2. Adequate fixation may be achieved with an intramedullary rod and cement. This then allows further treatment of the lesion with radiation or chemotherapy.

FRACTURES OF THE SHAFT OF THE HUMERUS

REMARKS

Most of these fractures of the humeral shaft are the result of a direct bending injury in vehicular accidents, falls, or gunshot wounds. Occasionally indirect twisting injuries following a blow or arm wrestling will produce the fracture.

A bending mechanism applied to the distal end of the humeral shaft with the proximal end locked in the glenoid is the typical mechanism of these injuries. This mechanism is more common in the active adult than in the elderly patient with osteoporotic bone, in whom the fracture occurs in the proximal humerus.

Direct Mechanisms

Bending Fractures

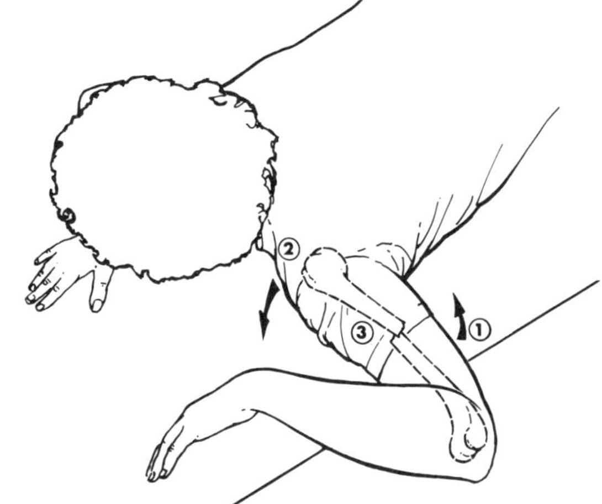

1. The victim falls on the distal humerus and forcefully abducts the arm.
2. The proximal humerus is locked in the glenoid.
3. The bending moment produces a typical transverse fracture of the midshaft of the humerus.

Indirect Torsional Mechanisms

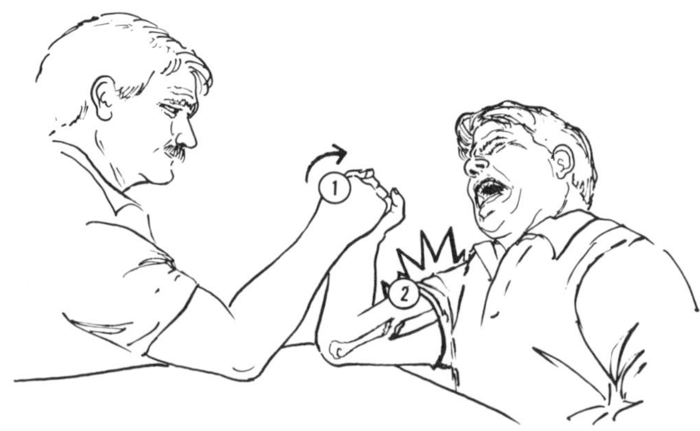

1. A rotational injury may occur with vigorous sports such as arm wrestling.
2. The forceful external rotation of the elbow causes the spiral oblique fracture with a typical external rotational pattern.

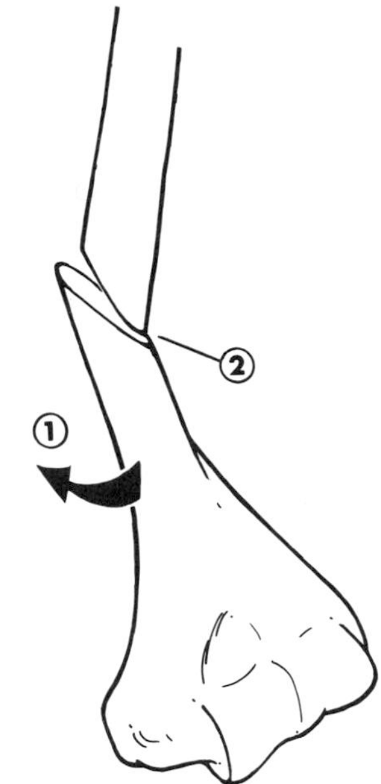

Typical External Rotational Fracture

1. External rotational torsional injury in the younger patient is characterized by a typical fracture pattern.
2. Characteristically, the fracture line runs from the distal medial cortex upward to the proximal lateral cortex.

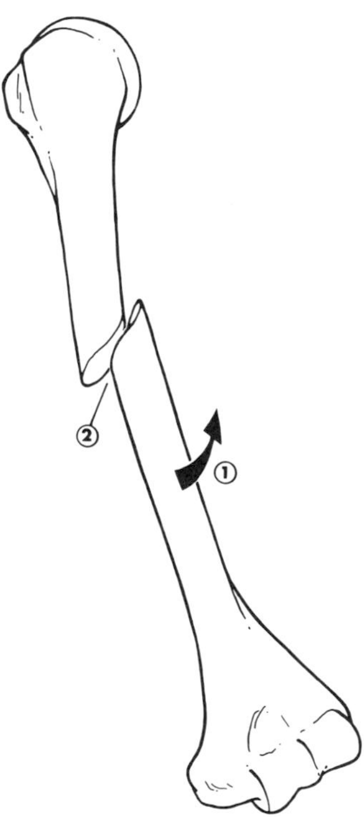

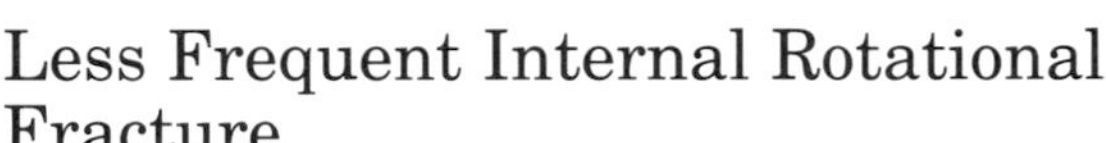

Less Frequent Internal Rotational Fracture

1. A spiral oblique fracture of the midshaft may result from internal torsional loading.
2. The failure line begins in the distal lateral cortex and runs to the proximal medial cortex.

Management

REMARKS

At one time, fractures of the humeral shaft were prime candidates for nonunion, particularly when devices such as spica casts or airplane splints were used. These attempts at reducing the fracture with external immobilization generally proved detrimental to healing. This was because they inhibited functional muscle control of the fracture.

More recently, treatment has emphasized gravity reduction and the use of functional muscle activity to control the fracture and to stimulate callus formation.

Humeral shaft fractures, like femoral shaft fractures, are surrounded by a richly vascularized envelope of muscle. Fracture reduction can be accomplished merely with the use of gravity and muscle function. Muscle function does not deform the fracture; rather, it aligns the fracture. This is in contrast to what traditionally has been taught about the deforming force of muscle pull.

The major forces causing fracture deformity are the initial injuries, either bending or torsional. These cause the fracture to deform in the direction in which it was bent or twisted initially, not in the direction of muscle pull. Most of these fractures can be aligned simply with the use of gravity and early functional muscle activity.

Appearance on X-Ray

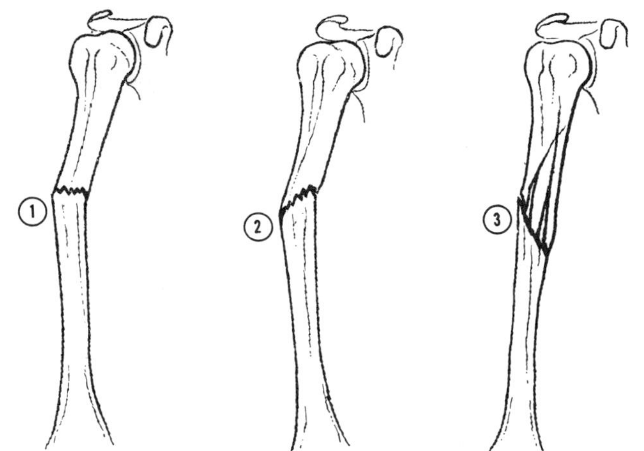

1. Transverse fracture of the shaft with minimal displacement.
2. Slight oblique fracture of the shaft with good contact of bone fragments and minimal angulation.
3. Comminution of the shaft with good alignment and minimal separation of fragments.

Initial Immobilization

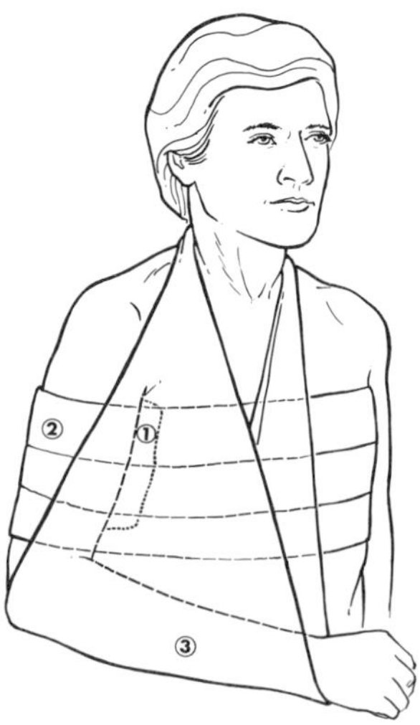

1. Pad the axilla.
2. Wrap the arm against the chest in position that maintains reduction.
3. Support the arm with a sling for angulated fractures, and encourage active elbow muscle contraction.

Alternative Method: Initial Immobilization for Angulation

1. The assistant makes mild steady downward traction.
2. Apply a long slab of plaster (10-cm wide) directly to the skin. The slab extends from the level of the acromion down the lateral aspect of the arm, around the elbow, and up the medial aspect of the arm to the axilla.
3. The slab is maintained in position by a cotton elastic bandage.
4. Place a pad of cotton in the axilla.
5. Place the arm in a triangular sling.

Caution: Avoid ending the plaster slab high in the axilla because this may cause irritation of the skin or pressure on the brachial plexus. As swelling subsides at 1–2 weeks, apply a cast sleeve.

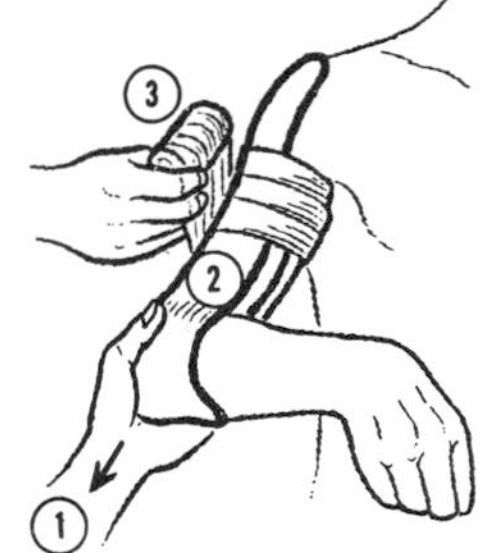

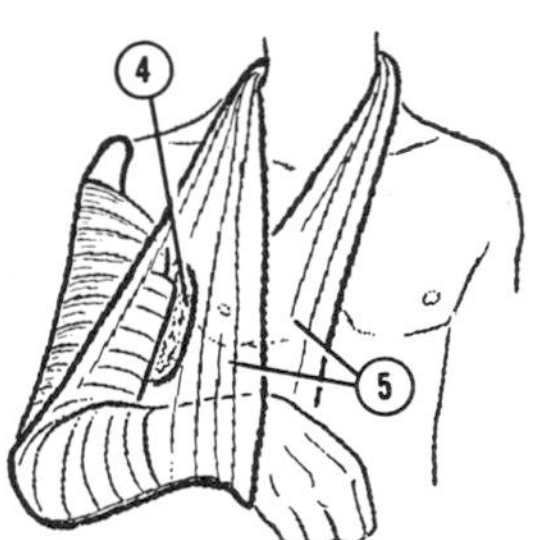

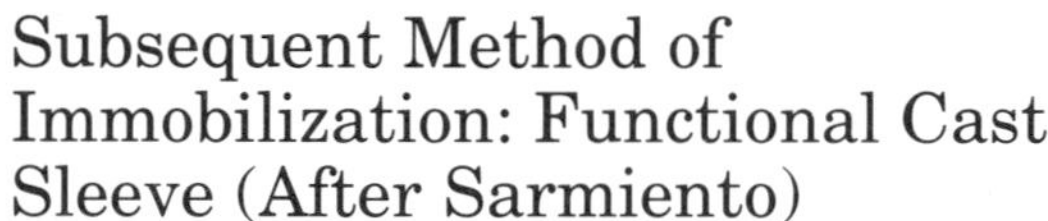

Subsequent Method of Immobilization: Functional Cast Sleeve (After Sarmiento)

1. Plaster cast or prefabricated polypropylene brace extends medially from 2.5 cm below the axilla to about 1 cm above the medial epicondyle and
2. Extends laterally from below the acromion to just above the lateral epicondyle.
3. Sleeve allows complete range of elbow and shoulder motion.
4. Velcro straps on brace permit removal for cleaning and adjustment as edema subsides.

Note: Sling support is used until the patient regains active elbow muscle control.

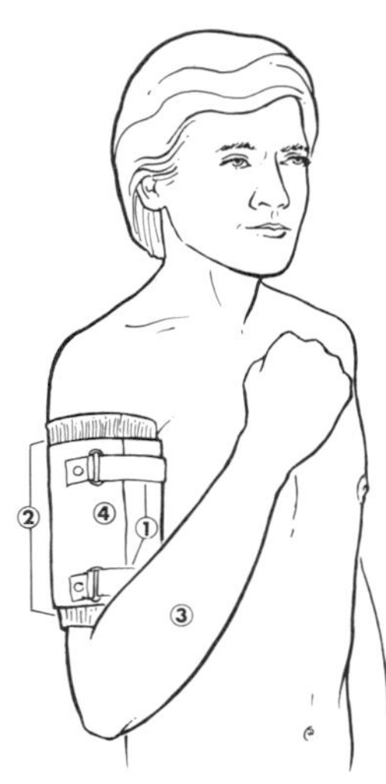

Alternative Immobilization: Simple Hand Sling (Spak Method)

To maximize the primary healing response after the initial immobilization (3–5 days), use a collar-and-hand sling, giving no support to the elbow or forearm on the fracture side.

1. With the elbow flexed at right angles, the patient grips the lower end of the sling.
2. If the patient cannot maintain the grip, fix the sling to the hand with adhesive tape but do not wind the sling around the hand.
3. Instruct the patient in circumduction shoulder exercises and allow progression to shoulder elevation.

Note: Until strength returns, a temporary support (either a pillow or a splint) for the limb may be necessary at night.

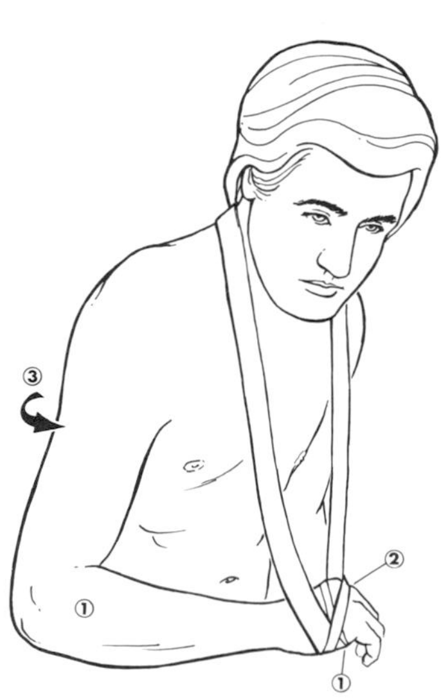

Subsequent Management

A shoulder harness may be attached to the proximal portion of the cast sleeve and may be looped around the neck to prevent slippage. Encourage the patient to exercise all joints of the fractured limb actively and passively.

Within the first week after application of the sleeve or hand sling, the patient should begin pendulum exercises with the elbow extended. This frequently corrects any residual angulation. By 6–8 weeks the sleeve or sling may be discarded, when there is clinical and radiographic evidence of union.

■ Fractures With Marked Displacement or Angulation

Appearance on X-Ray

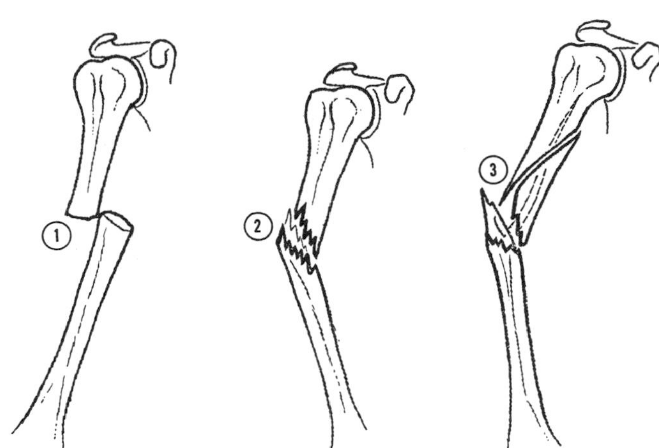

1. Transverse fracture with complete displacement and overriding of fragments.
2. Oblique fracture with serration of bone ends.
3. Comminuted fracture with marked angulation.

Management

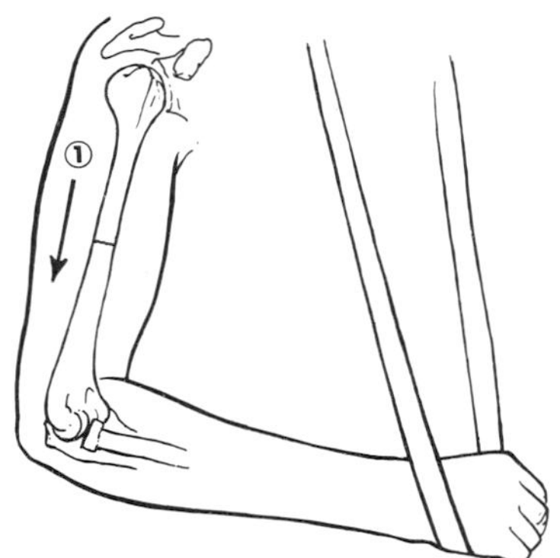

Manipulative reduction is unnecessary if
1. The weight of the arm and

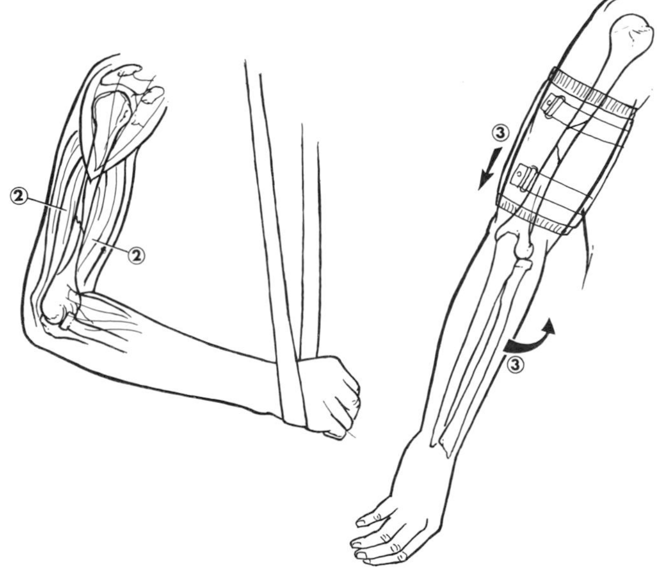

2. The surrounding muscular envelope are permitted to work for, instead of against, reduction.
3. Pendulum exercises with the elbow in extension will correct any residual deformity.

Note: The fracture sleeve stabilizes but does not completely immobilize the fracture.

X-Rays One Week After Beginning Active Elbow Extension

1. The fragments are engaged and in acceptable alignment.

Note: Any of these fractures that remain in the bayonet position may nevertheless heal with an acceptable functional result. Shortening of the humerus does not cause any impairment of muscle function in most instances.

2. The serrated ends of the fragments are engaged. Contact is good. Alignment is excellent.
3. Angulation has been corrected. Contact of the fragments is adequate.

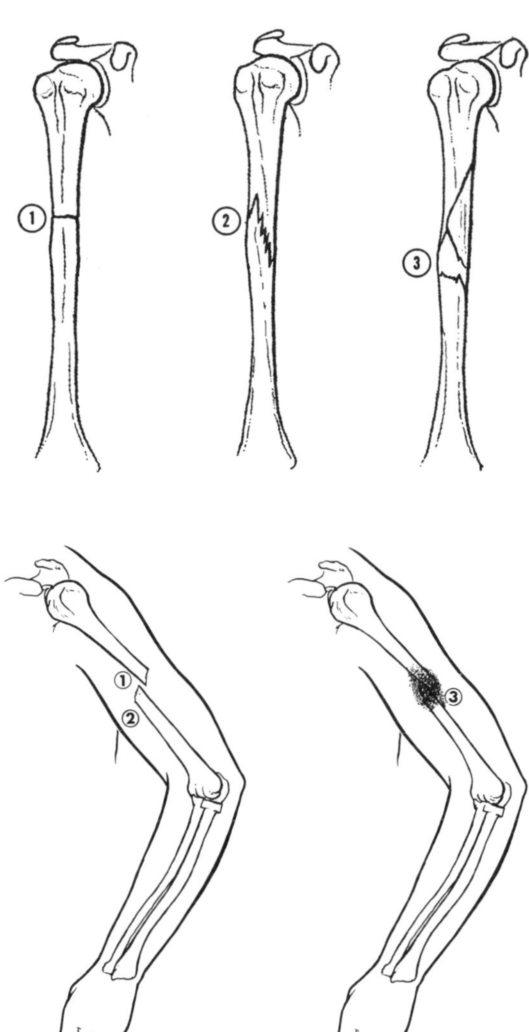

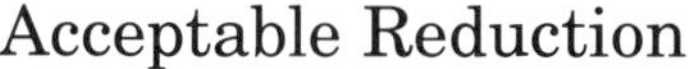

Acceptable Reduction

1. One to 2 cm of shortening or
2. Angulation of 5°–10° will
3. Heal without significant cosmetic or functional impairment.

Note: Healing by external callus is prompt when functional muscle exercises are incorporated into treatment.

COMPLICATIONS OF HUMERAL FRACTURES

Torsional-Varus Deformity of Distal Humeral Fractures

Fractures of the distal humerus may be forced into an internal torsional-varus deformity. This results from treatment with methods such as the hanging arm cast, which maintains the forearm against the patient's trunk, thereby internally rotating the distal fragment. Techniques that support the limb but encourage elbow motion alleviate the tendency of the distal fragment to rotate internally.

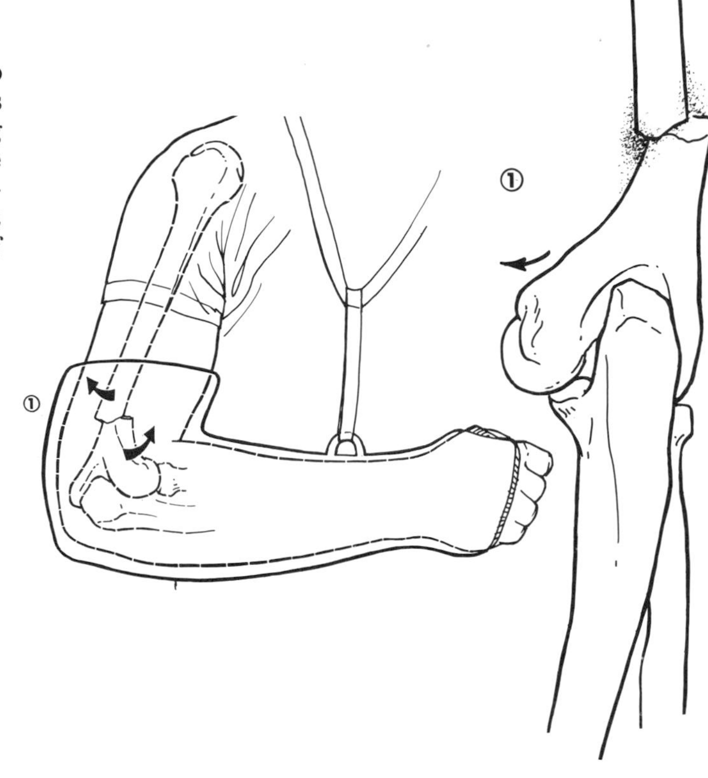

1. Internal torsion results from positioning the forearm continuously against the chest. Tilting of the internally rotated distal fragment produces a varus angulation.

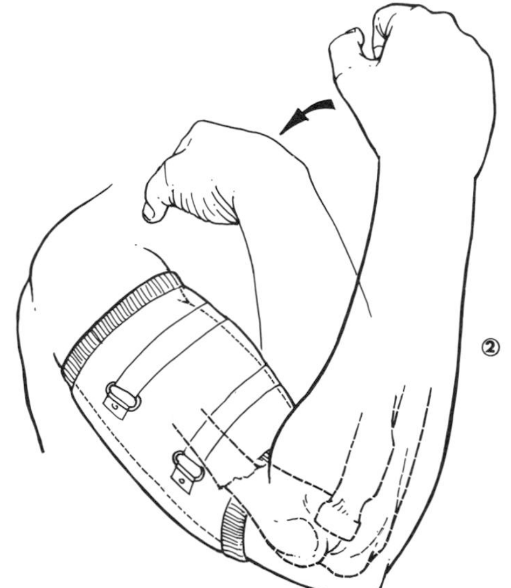

2. If the fracture is treated by allowing active elbow motion, the distal fragment becomes aligned in the axis of elbow joint motion.

Note: Torsional deformities of the distal humerus are not as functionally significant as are torsional deformities of the distal femur. Corrective osteotomy is usually not necessary.

Radial Nerve Involvement in Fractures of the Shaft of the Humerus

REMARKS

Radial nerve injuries occur most frequently in association with midshaft fractures. The nerve lesion usually is a benign neurapraxia that recovers spontaneously.

Radial nerve injury associated with a gunshot wound or an open fracture of any kind is least likely to recover spontaneously. Operative exploration of the open fracture and the nerve is warranted.

Because 15–20 per cent of humeral shaft fractures involve the radial nerve, always check for nerve injury before and after treatment, and record the findings. The clinical features of radial palsy are as follows:

- Wrist drop,
- Loss of supination of forearm,
- Loss of extension of the fingers and thumb, and
- Sensory deficits on dorsum of forearm, hand, and thumb.

The majority of radial nerve injuries from humeral fractures heal spontaneously, but approximately one in five does not heal.

In most instances, the period of observation for spontaneous recovery should be at least 12 weeks, which allows time for fracture consolidation. If there is no clinical or electromyographic indication of nerve regeneration by that time, neurolysis is indicated.

The most common indication for operative exploration is radial nerve palsy associated with an open fracture or penetrating injury. Under these circumstances the nerve can be explored primarily and, if possible, an end-to-end suture carried out. If necessary, the humerus can be shortened before internal fixation to take tension off the nerve repair. The radial nerve is primarily a motor nerve, and therefore repair of this nerve is usually quite successful.

An additional indication for operative exploration is the nerve injury that develops during treatment or reduction of the fracture.

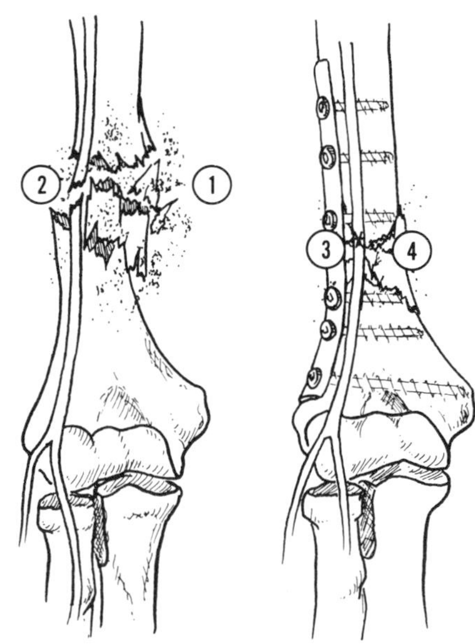

1. A gunshot wound has fractured the distal humerus and produced a radial nerve palsy.
2. The nerve has been explored and found to be completely severed.
3. It is repaired primarily.
4. The tension on the nerve repair can be eased by shortening of the humerus before internal fixation.

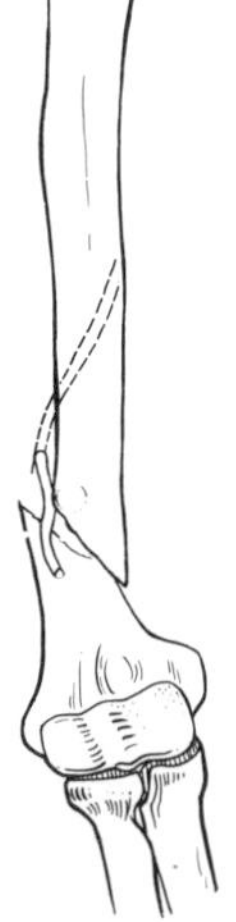

Occasionally the radial nerve is entrapped at the fracture site. This produces a characteristic angulation and overriding, which persists at the fracture. Under this rare circumstance, early exploration and open reduction of the fracture site are warranted in order to decompress the radial nerve. This is indicated especially if the palsy occurs after attempted reduction or bracing of the fracture.

■ Vascular Injuries Associated With Humeral Fractures

REMARKS

Penetrating wounds of the arm from high-velocity gunshot injuries frequently inflict damage on the vessels as well as on the humerus. This injury mandates prompt repair of the injured vessel, if at all possible, and stabilization of the humerus, preferably with external fixation or plates. When the status of the circulation is restored to normal, the external fixator may be removed and a fracture brace applied.

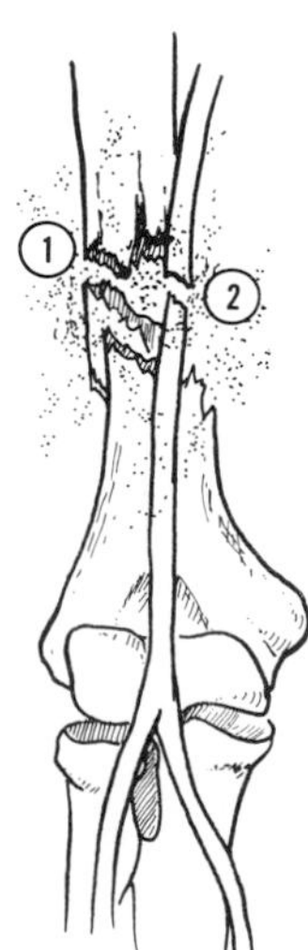

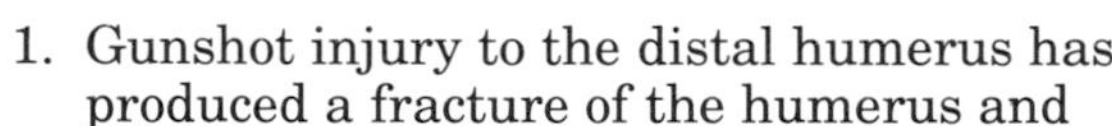

1. Gunshot injury to the distal humerus has produced a fracture of the humerus and
2. An associated injury to the brachial artery.

External Fixation Technique for Humeral Fractures With Vascular Injury

REMARKS

External fixation is usually not needed for most humeral fractures, except if there is excessive soft tissue or neurovascular damage. The major complication of external fixation is damage to neurovascular structures. Therefore, the pins should be inserted under direct visualization of the humeral cortex, with care taken to protect any underlying neurovascular structures.

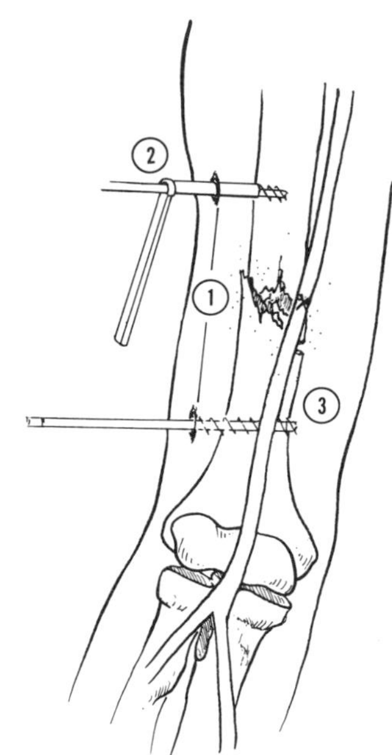

1. Two-centimeter incisions for pin placement are made down to the bone; care is taken to avoid neurovascular structures.
2. A soft tissue drill guide is placed to protect the tissues.
3. Both cortices of the humeral shaft are drilled.

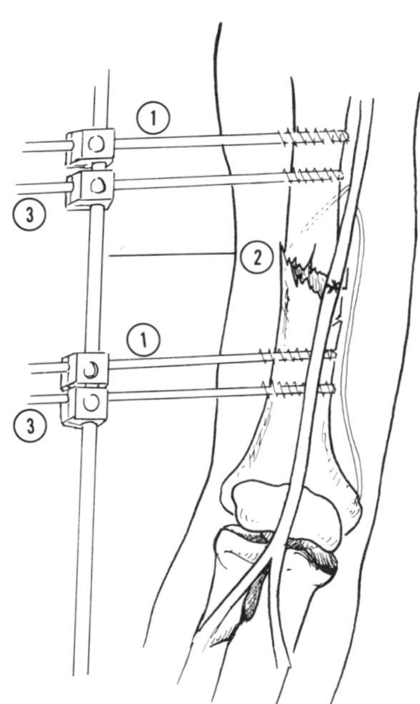

1. Two transfixing pins are inserted proximal and distal to the fracture site.
2. The fracture is reduced under fluoroscopic control, and a connecting rod is applied.
3. With the same technique, two more transfixion pins are inserted proximal and distal to the fracture site, and the connecting rod is attached to all four pins.

Note: External fixation may be applied to the fracture either before or after the vessel is repaired.

Subsequent Management

The external fixator may be removed when the distal circulation has been restored to normal. A fracture brace can then be used, usually by the second or third week, to allow stabilization of the fracture and to encourage active range of motion to the injured muscles. This should be modified according to the extent of the injury and the stability of the vascular repair.

■ Fractures of the Shaft of the Humerus in Polytrauma

REMARKS

Displaced humeral shaft fractures occur in many victims of polytrauma, including cerebral concussion, hemothorax, abdominal injuries, or multiple fractures, which prevent mobilization of the victim. Temporary skeletal traction may be necessary to align the fracture while the patient is in bed, but fracture distraction must be avoided. Traction should be discontinued as soon as the patient can be mobilized. A simple hand sling support or a humeral cuff may then be employed until the fracture heals.

Humeral shaft fractures, when combined with major fractures in other long bones such as the forearm, femur, or tibia, frequently necessitate plate fixation with other techniques to permit prompt patient mobilization and rehabilitation. Humeral fractures in severely confused, agitated, or psychotic patients may necessitate early internal fixation to prevent inadvertent penetration of the fracture ends through the skin.

Prereduction X-Ray

Oblique fracture of the humerus with angulation and overriding in a patient who suffered a hemothorax and cerebral concussion.

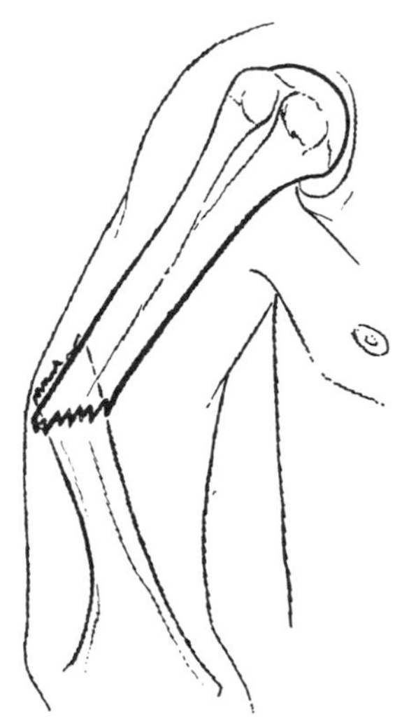

Temporary Immobilization in Skeletal Traction

1. While the patient recovers from a head injury,
2. And as long as the chest tubes are in place, to prevent immobilization of the arm against the chest,
3. A threaded Kirschner wire is used for traction and is inserted through the upper end of the ulna.
4. The forearm is suspended with the elbow flexed 90°.
5. Traction is made in line with the humerus and with the arm in slight abduction.

Caution: Start with 5 lb (2.3 kg) of weight and take a repeat x-ray within 24 hours. Adjust the amount of weight so that the alignment is maintained but the fragments are not distracted. If the patient is agitated or psychotic, internal fixation may be indicated.

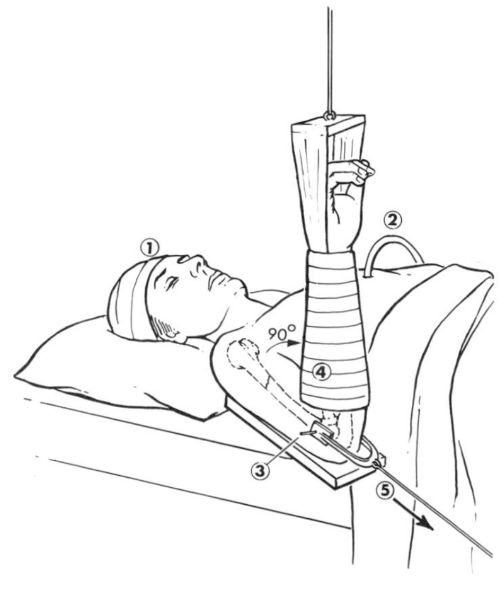

Secondary Immobilization

As soon as the head and chest injuries allow the patient to be mobilized, remove all the traction apparatus and apply a humeral sleeve cast or brace.

1. A plaster cast or prefabricated polypropylene brace extends medially from 2.5 cm below the axilla to slightly above the medial epicondyle and
2. Extends laterally from below the acromion to just above the lateral epicondyle.
3. The sleeve allows complete range of elbow and shoulder motion.
4. Velcro straps on brace permit removal for cleaning and adjustment as the edema subsides.

Note: A sling support is used until the patient regains active elbow muscle control.

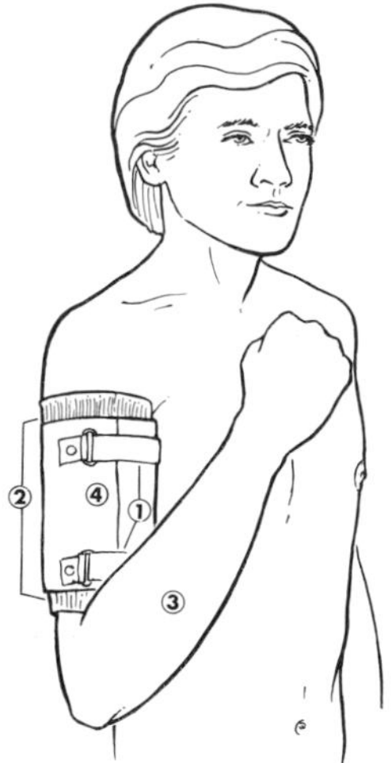

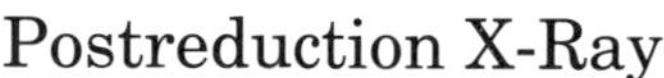

Postreduction X-Ray

1. The fragments are satisfactorily reduced and have not been distracted.
2. Union has occurred by primary external callus evident at 6 weeks.

Note: Healing by external callus occurs promptly when functional muscle exercises are incorporated into treatment.

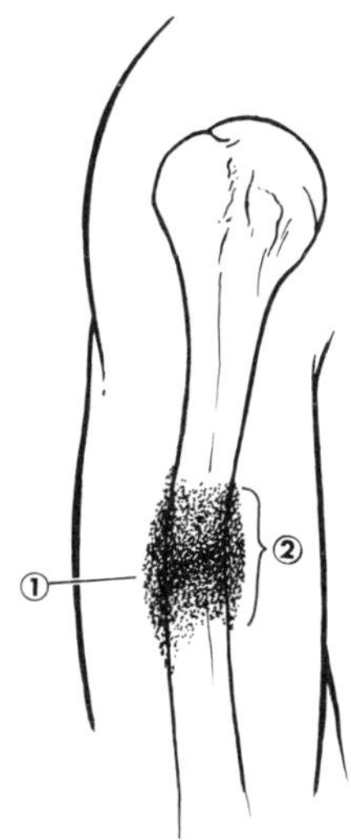

■ Fractures of the Shaft of the Humerus in Association With Multiple Long Bone Fractures or Head Injury

REMARKS

This is one of the few exceptions to the generally effective rule regarding closed treatment for most humeral shaft fractures. Internal fixation of the humeral shaft fracture in a patient with multiple long bone fractures permits prompt mobilization and functional restoration.

Open reduction and internal fixation of upper limb fractures may be combined with closed or open treatment of long bone fractures in the lower limb. Open reduction and internal fixation are also indicated for patients with head injuries associated with the humeral fracture. These patients may not be able to cooperate with closed treatment and may convert a closed fracture to an open injury during a seizure or uncontrolled thrashing. Under these circumstances it is often wiser to stabilize the fracture internally than to persist with closed treatment.

Preoperative X-Rays

1. Bilateral humeral shaft fractures combined with
2. Fracture of the left femoral shaft.
3. The angulated fracture of the distal third of the humerus caused radial nerve paralysis.

Note: Open reduction and internal fixation of both humeral fractures permit mobilization of the patient in a cast brace for femoral fracture within 4 weeks after injury.

The fracture of the midshaft of the humerus is treated by plate fixation. The angulated distal third fracture is immobilized with intramedullary pins and cerclage wiring after decompression of the radial nerve.

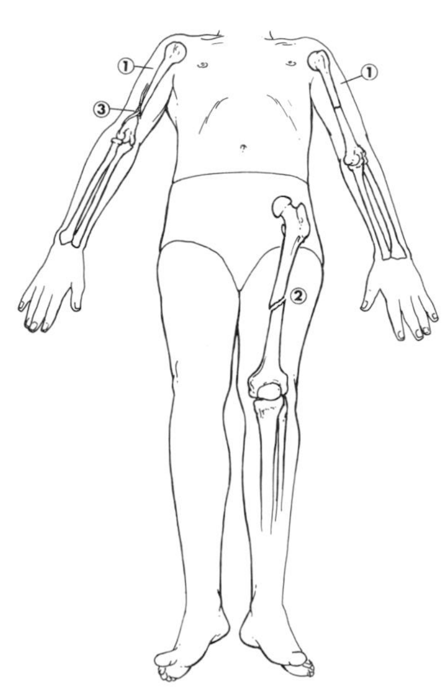

Operative Fixation

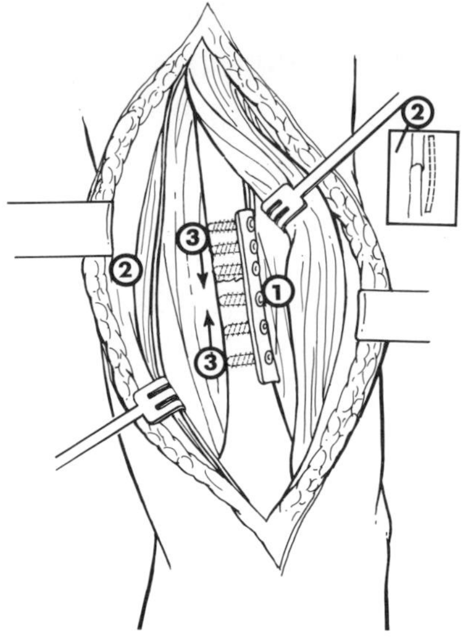

Preferred Fixation of Humeral Fractures

1. The best method of stabilizing most humeral fractures is by open reduction and plate fixation. This allows compression of the fracture and avoids distraction of the fracture, which sometimes occurs with intramedullary fixation.
2. The plate may need to be bent slightly before application to allow proper alignment of the fracture.
3. Dynamic compression technique is available to achieve stable fixation and to promote prompt healing of the fracture.

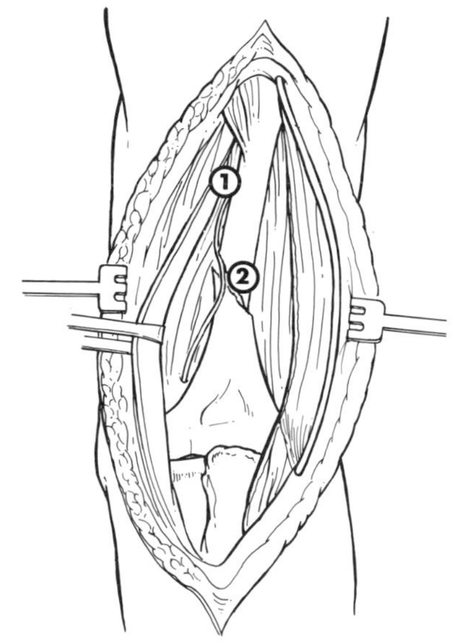

Alternative Method: Fracture of Distal Third of Humerus With Radial Nerve Involvement

1. Henry's anterolateral approach is used to expose the radial nerve proximally and
2. To follow it to the fracture site, where it is entrapped.

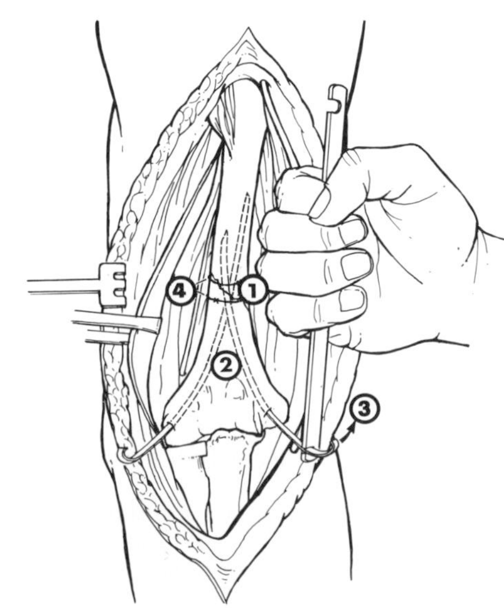

REDUCTION

1. The angulated fracture is reduced while the nerve is protected.
2. Two Rush pins are passed simultaneously through both condyles and across the fracture site, with the sled runner striking the opposite cortex.
3. Bending the pins slightly helps them conform to the contour of the lower humerus.
4. Cerclage wires may be added for additional support. The radial nerve is completely free of the fracture.

Note: Reconstruction plates might also be used to stabilize a distal humeral fracture.

■ Delayed Union or Nonunion of Fractures of the Shaft of the Humerus

REMARKS

Humeral fracture union should be evident after 8–10 weeks of closed treatment, provided that the patient has carried out the functional exercises as described. If for some reason the patient has been inhibited from using the arm and fracture motion is still evident 10 weeks after injury, internal fixation should be employed. To delay for 5–6 months a decision about inevitable operative treatment only increases the difficulty of fixation and diminishes the amount of function returned.

A compression plate or neutralization plate with screws is the most effective method of fixing the humeral fracture for nonunion. Nonunions with bone defects should also be treated by cancellous grafting. The plate is applied to the convex side of the angulated nonunion. Frequently this requires placement on the posterior cortex.

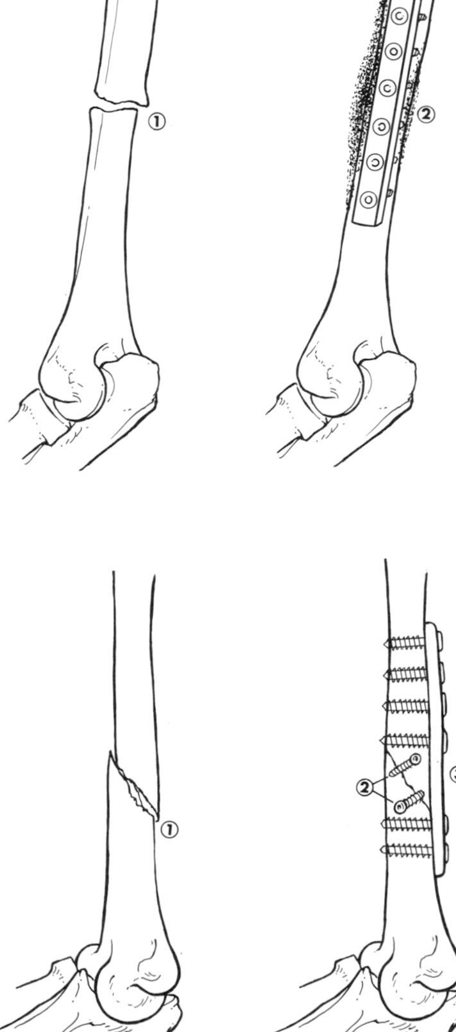

1. Nonunion of a transverse midshaft fracture at 4 months.
2. Union after compression plating and cancellous graft.

1. Nonunion of a spiral oblique fracture at 4 months.
2. Union after lag screws and
3. Neutralization plate applied posteriorly on the convex surface.

Other Problems—Fracture of the Supracondyloid Process

REMARKS

This is a rare lesion, but because of the proximity of the median nerve, symptoms of median nerve neuritis may obscure the lesion. The supracondyloid process is a bony prominence of varying size situated on the anteromedial aspect of the humerus 5–7 cm above the medial epicondyle. Between this process and the medial epicondyle stretches a fibrous band from which a portion of the pronator teres muscle arises. Through the interval between the humerus and the fibrous band pass the brachial artery and the median nerve.

Fracture of the supracondyloid process causes locking and pain, and may cause irritation of the median nerve. Fracture is usually the result of direct trauma. Treatment of fracture is by excision of the fragment.

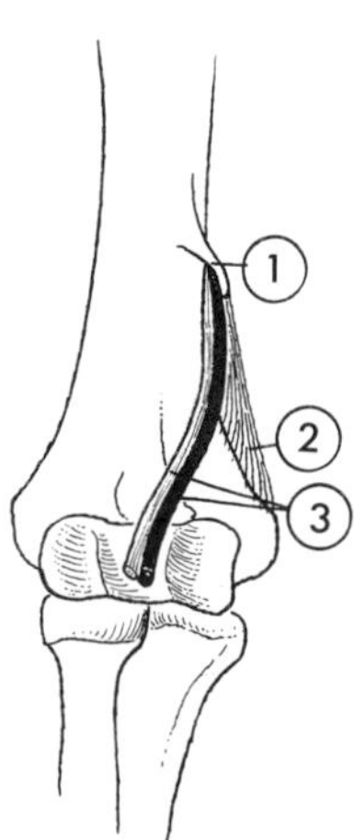

1. Supracondyloid process.
2. Fibrous band.
3. Brachial artery and median nerve.

Note: Fractures of this process may manifest with symptoms of medial neuropathy.

BIBLIOGRAPHY

Fractures of the Upper Humerus

Burstein A: Fracture classification systems: Do they work and are they useful? J Bone Joint Surg Am 75:1743, 1993.
Cofield RH: Comminuted fractures of the proximal humerus. Clin Orthop 230:49, 1988.
Din KM, Meggitt BF: Bilateral four-part fractures with posterior dislocation of the shoulder. J Bone Joint Surg Br 65:176, 1983.
Hawkins RJ, Bell RH, Gurr K: The three-part fracture of the proximal part of the humerus. J Bone Joint Surg Am 68:1410, 1986.
Horak J, Nilsson BE: Epidemiology of fracture of the upper end of the humerus. Clin Orthop 112:250, 1975.
Keene JS, Huizenga RE, Engber WD, et al.: Proximal humeral fractures. A correlation of residual deformity with long-term function. Orthopedics 6:173, 1983.
Lentz W, Meuser P: The treatment of fractures of the proximal humerus. Arch Orthop Trauma Surg 96:283, 1980.
Mills HJ, Horne G: Fractures of the proximal humerus in adult. J Trauma 25:801, 1985.
Sidor M, Zuckerman J, Lyon I, et al: The Neer classification systems for proximal humeral fractures. J Bone Joint Surg Am 75:1745, 1993.
Stableforth PG: Four-part fractures of the neck of the humerus. J Bone Joint Surg Br 66:104, 1984.
Williams DJ: The mechanism producing fracture-separation of the proximal humeral epiphysis. J Bone Joint Surg Br 63:102, 1981.
Young TB, Wallace WA: Conservative treatment of fractures and fracture-dislocation of the upper end of the humerus. J Bone Joint Surg Br 67:373, 1985.

Shaft Fractures: Closed Treatment

Balfour GW, Mooney V, Ashby ME: Diaphyseal fractures of the humerus treated with a ready made fracture brace. J Bone Joint Surg Am 64:11, 1982.
Ciernik IF, Meier L, Hollinger A: Humeral mobility after treatment with hanging cast. J Trauma 31:230, 1991.
Garth WP, Leberte MA, Cool TA: Recurrent fractures of the humerus in a baseball pitcher. J Bone Joint Surg Am 70:305, 1988.
Mast JW, Spiegel PG, Harvey JP, et al: Fractures of the humeral shaft. Clin Orthop 112:254, 1975.
Moon MS, Kim I, Han IH, et al: Arm wrestler's injury: Report of seven cases. Clin Orthop 147:219, 1980.
Sarmiento A, Kinman PB, Galvin EG, et al.: Functional bracing of fractures of the shaft of the humerus. J Bone Joint Surg Am 59:596, 1977.
Spak I: Humeral shaft fractures. Acta Orthop Scand 49:234, 1978.

Shaft Fractures: Operative Treatment

Durbin RA, Gottesman MJ, Saunders KC: Hackethal stacked nailing of the humeral shaft fractures. Experience with 30 patients. Clin Orthop 179:168, 1983.
Kunec JR, Lewis RJ: Closed intramedullary rodding of pathologic fractures with supplemental cement. Clin Orthop 188:183, 1984.
Mast JW, Spiegel PG, Harvey JP, Harrison C: Fractures of the humeral shaft. Clin Orthop 12:254, 1975.
Pierce RO, Hodurski DF: Fractures of the humerus, radius, and ulna in the same extremity. J Trauma 19:182, 1979.
Rush LV: *Atlas of Rush Pin Technics: A System of Fracture Treatment.* Berivon Co., Meridian, MS, 1955.
Stern PJ, Mattingly DA, Pomeroy DL, et al.: Intramedullary fixation of humeral shaft fractures. J Bone Joint Surg Am 66:639, 1984.
Van der Griend RA, Tomasin J, Ward EF: Open reduction and internal fixation of humeral shaft fractures. J Bone Joint Surg Am 68:430, 1986.

Plate Fixation

Bell MJ, Beauchamp CG, Kellam JK, et al.: The results of plating humeral shaft fractures in patients with multiple injuries. J Bone Joint Surg Br 67:293, 1985.
Lange RH, Foster RJ: Skeletal management of humeral shaft fractures associated with forearm fractures. Clin Orthop 195:173, 1985.
Muller ME, Allgower M, Willenegger H: *Manual of Internal Fixation.* Springer-Verlag, New York, 1970.
Rogers JF, Bennett JB, Tullos HS: Management of concomitant ipsilateral fractures of the humerus and forearm. J Bone Joint Surg Am 66:552, 1984.

External Fixation

Green SA: *Complications of External Skeletal Fixation: Causes, Prevention and Treatment.* C Thomas, Springfield, IL, 1981.
Hisenkamp M, Burny F, Andrianne Y, et al.: External fixation of the fracture of the humerus: A review of 164 cases. Orthopedics 7:1309, 1984.
Smith DK, Cooney WP: External fixation of high energy upper extremity injuries. J Orthop Trauma 4:7, 1990.

Neurovascular Injuries

Bostman O, Bakalim G, Vainionpaa S, et al.: Immediate radial nerve palsy complicating fracture of the shaft of the humerus: When is early exploration justified? Injury 16:499, 1985.
Burge P, Rushworth G, Watson N: Patterns of injury of the terminal branches of the brachial plexus. J Bone Joint Surg Br 67:630, 1985.
Gainor B, Mitzler M: Humeral shaft fracture with brachial artery injury. Clin Orthop 204:154, 1986.
Hayes MJ, Van Winkle N: Axillary artery injury with minimally displaced fracture of the neck of humerus. J Trauma 23:431, 1983.
Holstein A, Lewis GB: Fractures of the humerus with radial-nerve paralysis. J Bone Joint Surg Am 45:1382, 1963.
Kaiser TE, Sim FH, Kelly PJ: Radial nerve palsy associated with humeral fractures. Orthopedic 4:1245, 1981.
Lim EVA, Day LJ: Thrombosis of the axillary artery complicating proximal humeral fractures. J Bone Joint Surg Am 69:778, 1987.
Pollock FH, Drake D, Bovill EG, et al.: Treatment of radial neuropathy associated with fractures of the humerus. J Bone Joint Surg Am 63:239, 1981.
Smyth EHJ: Major arterial injury in closed fracture of the neck of the humerus: Report of a case. J Bone Joint Surg Am 51:508, 1969.
Zuckerman JD, Flugstad DL, Teitz CC, King HA: Axillary artery injury as a complication of proximal humeral fractures: Two case reports and a view of the literature. Clin Orthop 189:234, 1984.

Nonunion Complications

Connolly JF: Electrical treatment of nonunions. Its use and abuse in 100 consecutive fractures. Orthop Clin North Am 15:89, 1984.
Connolly JF: Common avoidable problems in nonunions. Clin Orthop 194:226, 1985.
Foster RJ, Dixon GL, Bach AW, et al.: Internal fixation of fractures and non-unions of the humeral shaft. J Bone Joint Surg Am 67:857, 1985.
Huckstep R: The intramedullary compression nail. *In* Seligson D (ed): *Concepts in Intramedullary Nailing.* Grune & Stratton, New York, 1976.
Jupiter JB: The treatment of complex nonunions of the humeral

shaft with a combination of surgical techniques. J Bone Joint Surg Am 72:701, 1990.

Pritchett JW: Delayed union of humeral shaft fractures treated by closed flexible intramedullary nailing. J Bone Joint Surg Br 67:715, 1985.

Trotter DH, Dobozi W: Nonunion in fracture of the shaft of the humerus: Rigid fixation, bone grafting, and adjunctive bone cement. Clin Orthop 240:162, 1986.

Sever JW: Nonunion in fracture of the shaft of the humerus: Report of five cases. JAMA 104:382, 1935.

Weber GB, Cech O: *Pseudarthrosis: Pathophysiology, Biomechanics, Therapy, Results*. Grune & Stratton, New York, 1976.

14 Fractures and Dislocations in the Region of the Elbow

FRACTURES OF THE LOWER END OF THE HUMERUS

REMARKS

Fractures in this region are caused most often by indirect injury to the elbow resulting from a fall on the outstretched, extended arm. Most distal humeral fractures occur in children and are classified as supracondylar fractures. These and other fractures around the child's elbow are discussed in the section on childhood fractures.

Distal humeral fractures in adults may be produced by indirect injuries but are frequently the result of direct violence, for example, side-swipe injury to the elbow resting on a car window. The adult fracture may range from a displaced supracondylar to a comminuted intercondylar or T-shaped fracture involving the articular surface. The prognosis for an elbow fracture in the adult is poorer than for children's fractures. For this reason the trend has been toward operative fixation of most elbow fractures in the adult to achieve fracture stability and to allow restoration of joint motion.

Mechanisms and Types of Fractures of the Lower End of the Humerus in Adults

REMARKS

Mechanisms producing fractures of the lower humerus are either direct or indirect. The most common mechanism is a fall on the outstretched hand and arm, which produces a fracture of the distal humerus, which usually displaces in extension. Occasionally the patient may fall directly on the flexed elbow and the result is anterior displacement. Other injuries from indirect mechanisms include condylar and epicondylar fractures of the distal humerus.

More severe fractures result from direct mechanisms, such as a side-swipe injury or blow to the posterior aspect of the humerus with the elbow flexed. These frequently involve the intercondylar region and may produce displacement and comminution of the articular surface of the elbow. These result in the most difficult fracture management problems.

Indirect Mechanism

1. A typical indirect mechanism is a fall on the outstretched arm, producing a distal humeral fracture with posterior displacement or fractures of the condyles or epicondyles.

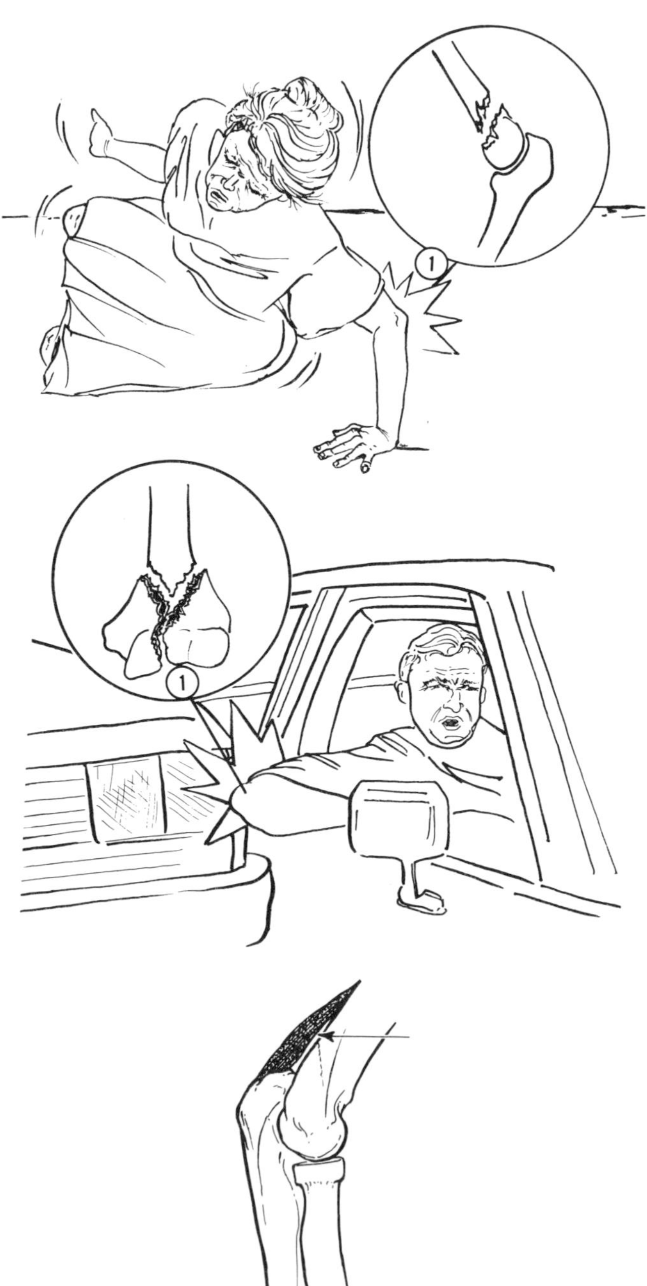

Direct Mechanism

1. An intercondylar or T-condylar fracture results from a direct blow to the posterior aspect of the olecranon or elbow with the elbow flexed. This can cause a variety of fractures of the distal humerus and humeral condyles and comminution of the articular surface.

Undisplaced Fracture

A relatively undisplaced fracture is seen occasionally in the adult elbow after injury. It is much more common to see an undisplaced fracture in a supracondylar fracture of the child's elbow. The typical fat pad sign caused by posterior hemorrhage is seen more often in the child's elbow than in the adult's.

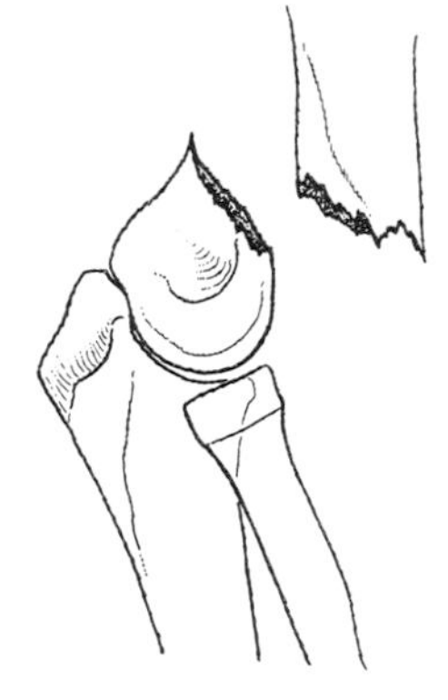

■ Distal Humeral Fracture Displaced in Extension

Commonly the distal humeral fracture results from an extension load on the elbow in the adult and characteristically displaces backward and upward.

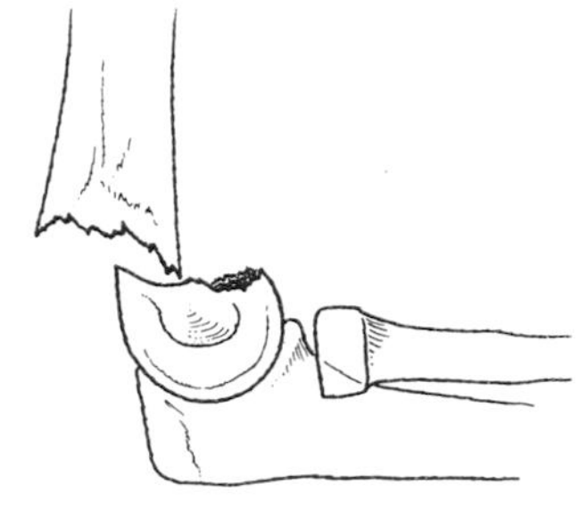

Flexion Type Fractures in the Adult

Occasionally the distal fragment may displace forward in the adult elbow. This is usually the result of a fall directly on the posterior aspect of the elbow.

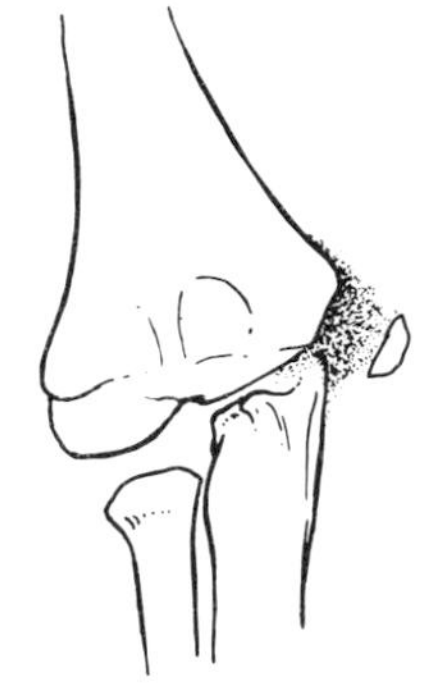

Medial Epicondylar Fractures

These avulsion fractures are less common in the adult than in the child but can occur.

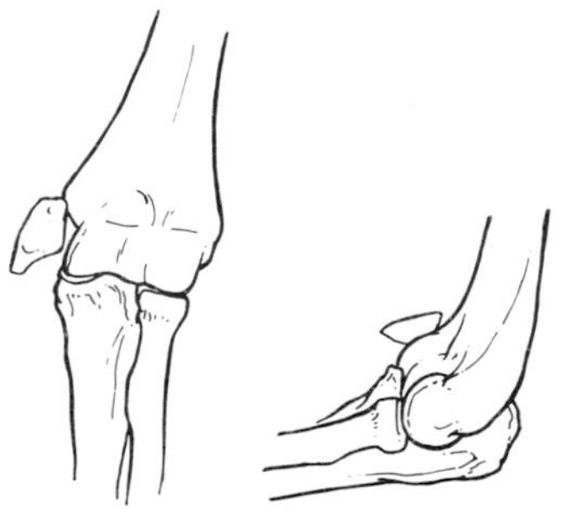

Condylar Fractures

Fractures of the medial or lateral condyles may also occur, and these sometimes displace sufficiently to require operative fixation.

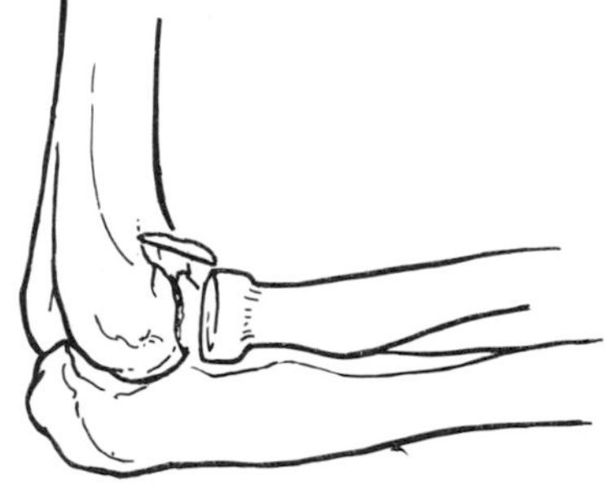

Capitellum Fractures

A shear fracture of the capitellum is also a fairly uncommon, but commonly unrecognized, injury to the adult elbow.

Assessment of Fractures in the Lower End of the Humerus

REMARKS

Fractures around the elbow carry more than their share of complications, both early and late; therefore, these injuries should be treated with anticipation of potential problems. Prompt recognition and management are most critical for the early problems that are discussed here.

Early complications include the following:

- *Vascular injuries:* Extensive antecubital swelling can produce forearm muscle compartment syndrome with subsequent ischemic contracture of the forearm muscles as well as ischemic neuropathy. Careful assessment for compartment syndrome is necessary in any swollen elbow after a fracture or dislocation. Circular cast application should be avoided in the acutely swollen elbow, particularly if the elbow is flexed beyond the right angle.
- *Nerve injuries:* Elbow fractures can produce neurapraxia of the median, ulnar, or radial nerve, most of which are temporary.
- *Late complications:* These are discussed elsewhere in the chapter and include the following:
- *Loss of elbow motion:* Particularly in flexion, this is sometimes a source of disability after an elbow fracture in an adult. For this reason, operative stabilization is preferred for most elbow fractures to restore range of motion as early as possible after injury.
- *Instability:* Instability of the elbow can occur when fractures associated with a dislocation cause recurrent subluxation or dislocation.
- *Myositis ossificans:* Myositis ossificans or soft tissue calcifications may follow these injuries or vigorous operative or nonoperative therapy.
- *Nonunion:* This is sometimes associated with fractures in the lateral and medial condyle with any displacement.
- *Malunion:* This can occur with supracondylar fractures and fractures of the lateral and medial condyle with any displacement.
- *Delayed neuropathy:* Progressive nerve palsy can result from a cubitus valgus or varus deformity, particularly after a lateral condylar fracture.

VASCULAR AND NEURAL COMPLICATIONS ASSOCIATED WITH FRACTURES AND DISLOCATIONS OF THE ELBOW JOINT

Vascular Complications

Mechanism of Injury

REMARKS

Vascular complications occur so commonly with direct and indirect injury to the elbow that the circulation should be assumed to be impaired until proven otherwise. Vascular damage is frequently associated with open fractures and dislocations, which are usually produced by direct blunt trauma, for example, gunshot wounds, or by penetrating injuries, for example, glass lacerations of the antecubital region.

The most specific signs of direct arterial injury are pulsatile bleeding from the wound or rapid swelling after injury. Direct violence to the elbow that produces these signs warrants close examination for evidence of the distal circulatory impairment and prompt exploration of the vessels if evidence is found.

Supracondylar fracture, produced by an indirect mechanism from a fall on the outstretched hand, most often causes circulatory impairment secondary to antecubital swelling rather than to direct arterial insult. Prompt elevation of the limb in traction after a distal humeral fracture permits venous drainage through the antecubital region and prevents "strangulation" of neurovascular structures.

Rarely, reduction of the fracture will cause arterial insufficiency and loss of radial pulse due to impalement of the brachial artery. Be alert to this possibility after reduction, because it indicates the need to decrease elbow flexion and possibly to explore the artery.

Elbow dislocation, particularly open dislocation, is more likely than a supracondylar fracture to lacerate the brachial artery directly. Loss of the radial pulse with signs of impending ischemia that persist after reduction of the elbow dislocation indicates the need for surgical exploration of the artery without delay.

Direct Injuries

These cause direct arterial damage:

1. Glass laceration is the most common cause of arterial injury in this area, with or without fracture.

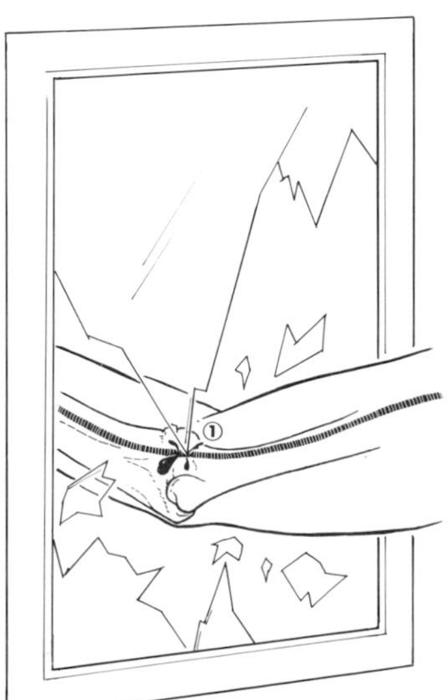

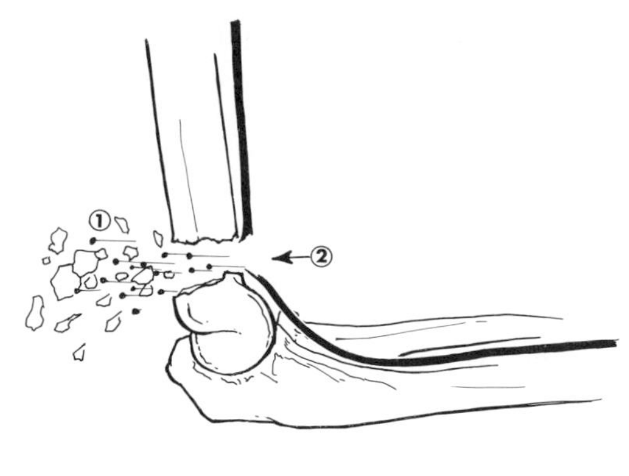

2. Direct blunt trauma to the elbow causing open fracture or dislocation commonly damages the brachial artery.

Compartment Syndrome From Supracondylar Fracture

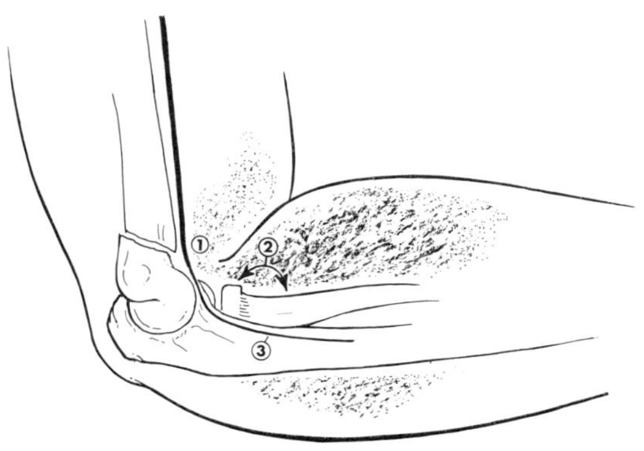

This damages the circulation indirectly through swelling.

1. The artery is usually intact.
2. Soft tissue swelling from the fracture occludes the venous return from the forearm. When venous pressure within the forearm compartment approaches the diastolic pressure,
3. Arterial flow is occluded and neuromuscular ischemia ensues.

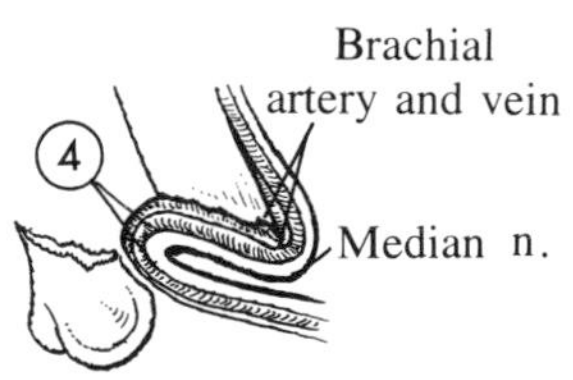

4. Rarely, neurovascular structures are actually entrapped by the fracture and circulation is worsened by reduction.

Elbow Dislocation

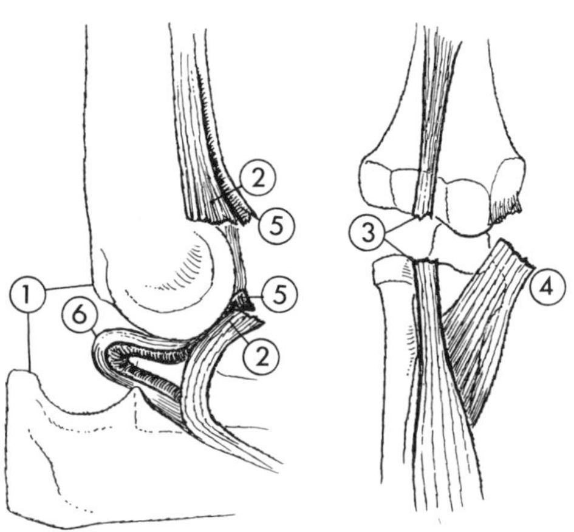

The brachial artery is most likely to be damaged with open dislocation.

1. There is wide displacement of ulna from the humerus.
2. This is usually associated with an open wound and direct injury to the antecubital region.
3. The lacertus fibrosis is torn.
4. The common flexor muscles are avulsed.
5. The extreme force of dislocation tears the artery.
6. The median nerve may also be injured or entrapped.

Diagnosis of Arterial Injuries in the Upper Limb: The "P" Signs

REMARKS

The most specific sign of arterial injury is pulsatile bleeding or rapid swelling. Even a history of pulsatile bleeding associated with an open or penetrating wound to the elbow should indicate the diagnosis.

The earliest sign of impending, progressive ischemia of the forearm muscle is pain on passive extension of the patient's fingers. Ischemic muscle causes pain, whether in the heart or in the forearm, by the accumulation of cellular breakdown products, particularly potassium, that provoke pain impulses and further muscle contraction. Passive stretching of the fingers brings the irritated, ischemic state of the muscle to clinical attention.

The absence of a radial pulse may or may not be significant, particularly after indirect injury, for example, a supracondylar fracture. Noninvasive methods of measuring blood flow, such as the Doppler flowmeter technique, give reliable, objective information and should be readily available to evaluate all questionable cases.

Invasive arteriography may occasionally be helpful in evaluating elbow injuries in the adult, but after supracondylar fracture in a child, this arterial study itself may produce sufficient vasospasm to impair the peripheral circulation.

The other P signs of arterial injury besides pulsatile bleeding, pain, and pulselessness are paresthesias and paralysis, indicative of peripheral nerve ischemia. Partial ischemia causes the nerve to be hyperirritable and produces painful paresthesias. Total ischemia causes nerve conduction to cease promptly.

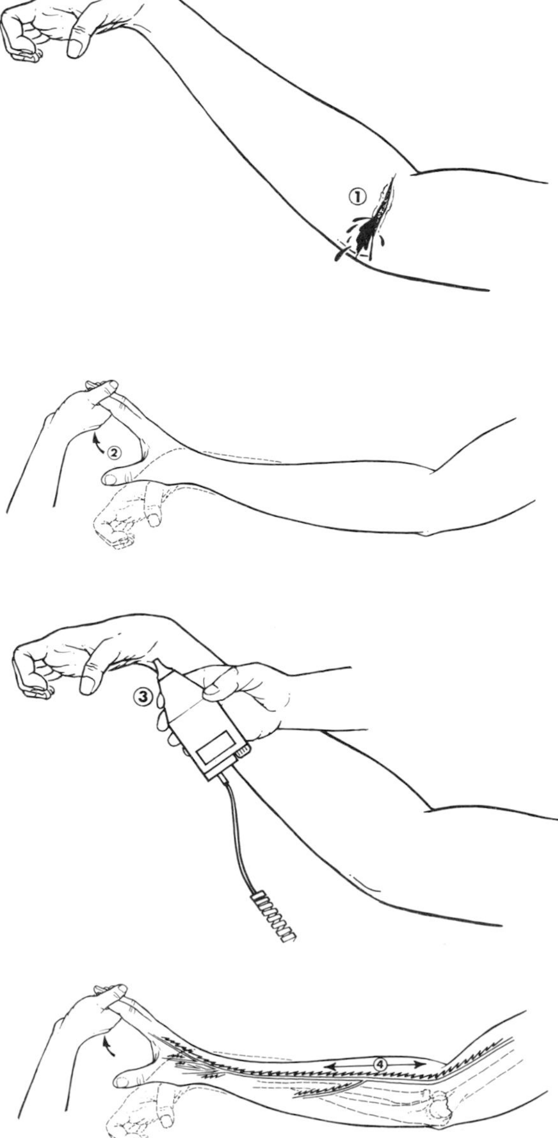

P Signs of Arterial Injury

1. Pulsatile bleeding or rapid swelling around the elbow is most specific.
2. Pain on passive extension indicates impending forearm muscle ischemia.
3. Palpation of the pulse may be difficult if the limb is swollen. In this circumstance the pulse can still be measured by a Doppler flowmeter.
4. Paresthesia and paralysis due to nerve ischemia are early signs of a sudden major arterial interruption, such as axillary artery thrombosis.

Compartment Pressure Measurements

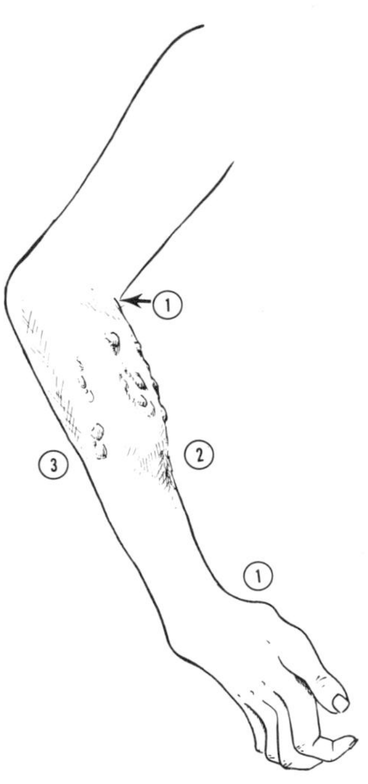

1. A classic problem that develops after a crush injury to the elbow is occlusion of flow to the forearm compartments. This may lead to progressive forearm compartment ischemia despite a palpable radial pulse.
2. The forearm is tense and swollen, and the patient has pain in the forearm muscles and with passive extension of the fingers. The ischemic injury may develop after tightly wrapping the injured elbow subsequent to a dislocation or a fracture.
3. The first concern in managing fractures of the elbows is to evaluate the swelling by the clinical signs and, if necessary, by compartment pressure measurements, as discussed elsewhere. If there are real or potential signs of forearm muscle ischemia, management of this problem takes precedence over management of the fracture.

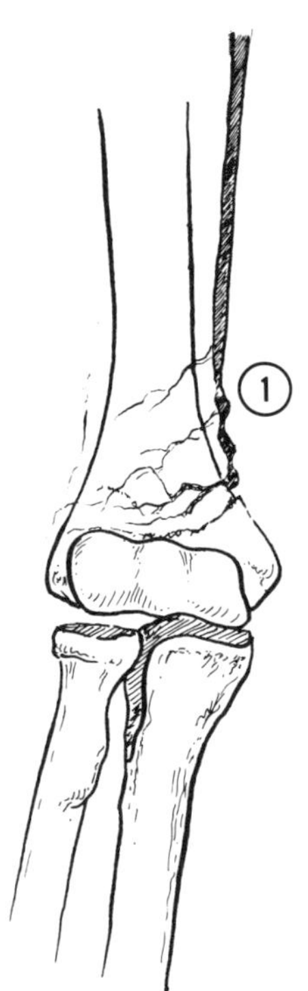

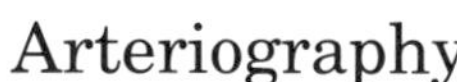

Arteriography

1. An arteriogram may be necessary to demonstrate the level of vascular interruption after an elbow injury. This allows the vascular surgeon to plan the repair or graft.

Note: Arteriograms may not be useful in the younger child with an elbow injury and in fact may sometimes inordinately delay necessary forearm fasciotomy and surgical exploration of the vessel. The use of arteriograms should then be selective.

Management

REMARKS

If the physical signs indicate potential impairment of circulation, the next step depends on the nature of the injury to the vessels. In direct injuries, lacerations, open dislocations, or penetrating wounds to the elbow, the likelihood of significant arterial injury is so high that surgical exploration should not be delayed. Arteriography is usually useful but not essential to help locate the precise level of the lesion, but it should not delay necessary surgical exploration.

Keep in mind that if there is a crush injury to the arm, distal radial flow may be normal despite progressive development of a forearm compartment syndrome. In this situation measurement of intracompartmental pressure is necessary to determine the degree of potential problem.

In the usual indirect injury, most typically a supracondylar fracture with less than 6 hours of ischemia, a period of elevation with traction for 1–2 hours will usually diminish swelling sufficiently to permit adequate flow. If elevation of the limb does not restore circulation promptly or if the signs of impending ischemia are present for 6 hours or more or compartment pressures are elevated, prompt forearm fasciotomy and exploration of the brachial artery are indicated. In approximately half the cases a dorsal fasciotomy should also be performed in addition to volar fasciotomy. Arterial repair is usually unnecessary after indirect injury, except for the rare situation of impalement of the artery by the fractured bone.

Management of Circulatory Impairment Within Six Hours After Distal Humeral Fracture

Ten to 15 per cent of distal humeral fractures will cause loss or diminution of the radial pulse and swelling of the forearm. Most cases respond to elevation and traction.

1. Use skeletal traction or

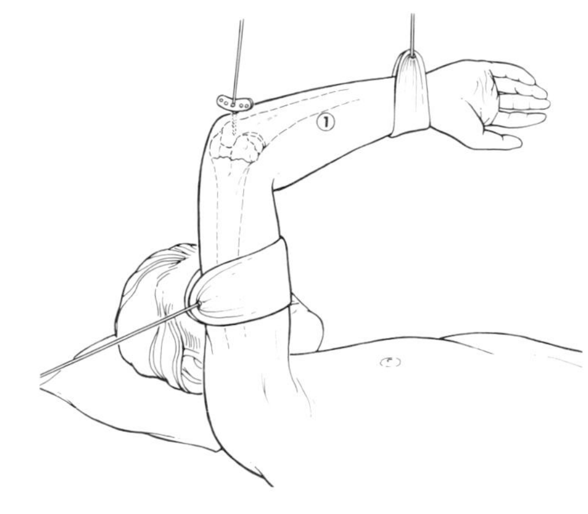

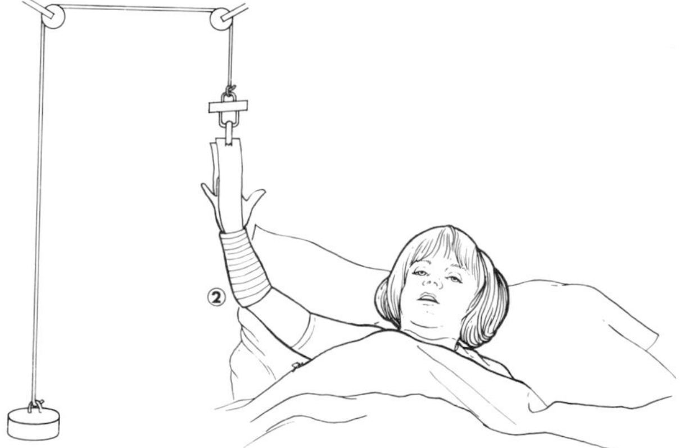

2. Side arm traction.

Subsequent Management

As the swelling subsides the pulse usually becomes palpable distally; however, if signs of muscle or nerve ischemia or other persistent evidence of compartment syndrome develop, prompt operative intervention is indicated. When the circulatory status has been restored to normal, usually by 2–3 days, traction may be discontinued and the fracture reduced by either closed or open methods.

Management of Ischemia Six Hours or More After Distal Humeral Fracture: Operative Management

REMARKS

Indications for prompt surgical intervention are loss of pulse, as demonstrated by flowmeter measurement, after direct injury, laceration, open fracture, or a gunshot wound to the elbow. Indirect injuries, such as supracondylar fracture, in which distal flow is not regained after 2 hours of elevation or in which ischemia is still manifest 6 hours after injury, should be surgically explored. The objective is to decompress the forearm by fasciotomy while exploring the brachial artery. Some degree of neuromuscular damage will ensue if the limb is completely ischemic for more than 6 hours.

Preoperative Care

Avoid direct application of ice to the ischemic forearm, because temperatures below 65°F (18.1°C) may inflict cold injury on top of the ischemic injury. Use intravenous broad-spectrum antibiotics preoperatively and postoperatively for a total of 36 hours or longer if indicated by the degree of wound contamination and muscle injury.

Life-threatening cardiorespiratory and central nervous system injuries must be cared for and shock must be treated prior to embarking on the peripheral artery exploration. Avoid systemic heparinization. Local injection of heparin (10,000 units in 100 mL saline) into the divided or traumatized artery at the time of exploration gives adequate anticoagulation.

Techniques of Fasciotomy for Indirect Injuries

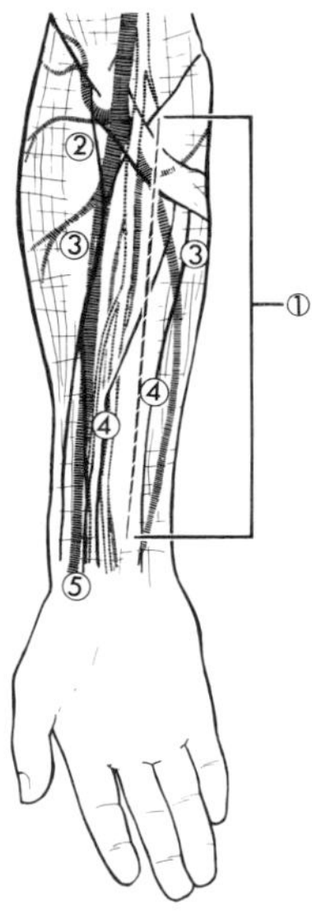

1. The incision should extend from elbow to wrist. Avoid placing the incision directly over distal tendons and nerves.
2. Incise the deep fascia as far distally as necessary to evacuate the hematoma and decompress the forearm muscles.
3. Open the epimysium if the muscles are still tight.
4. Decompress the deep muscle compartments and nerves.
5. Monitor the distal radial artery flow by palpation or a flowmeter, and explore the brachial artery if the distal flow is still inadequate.

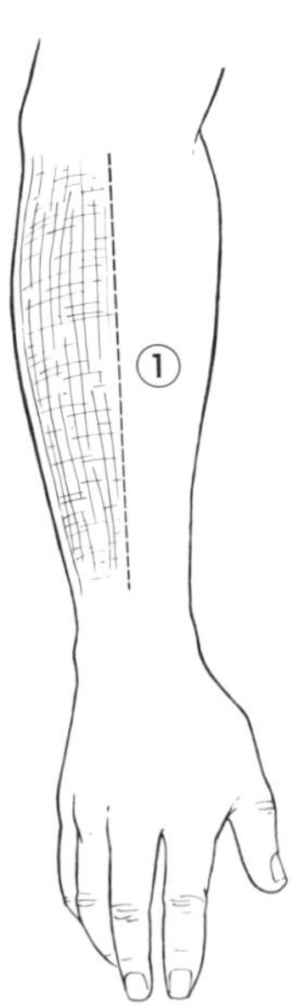

1. Dorsal fasciotomy should also be done if the volar decompression does not produce sufficient lowering of the dorsal compartment pressure.

What to Do With the Brachial Artery

Surgery of the arterial lesion should be carried out by a vascular consultant if at all possible. The findings to be expected include segmental or diffuse arteriospasm, severe contusion with thrombosis, and complete laceration of the vessel. Local arteriospasm may respond to topical 2.5–5 per cent papaverine or other antispasmodic agents.

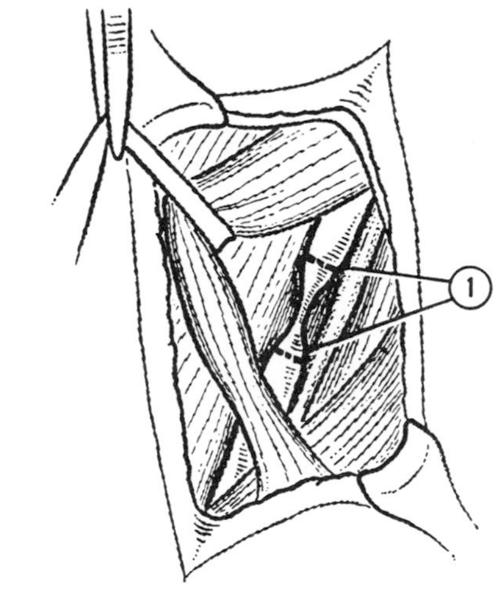

Arteriospasm

1. This segment of the brachial artery shows marked arteriospasm.

Most often the vessel should be opened by a small arteriotomy, and a Fogarty catheter should be used to dilate the area of spasm and to remove the thrombosed intima. Resection with end-to-end anastomosis may be effective for laceration or contusion of the vessel, but be certain that all of the damaged area is resected prior to repair, because the extent of vascular damage may be greater than is initially apparent. A reversed saphenous vein graft is used if there is any tension on the anastomosis.

2. A Fogarty catheter is passed across the site of spasm to dilate the vessel and
3. To remove the thrombus causing the vasoconstriction.

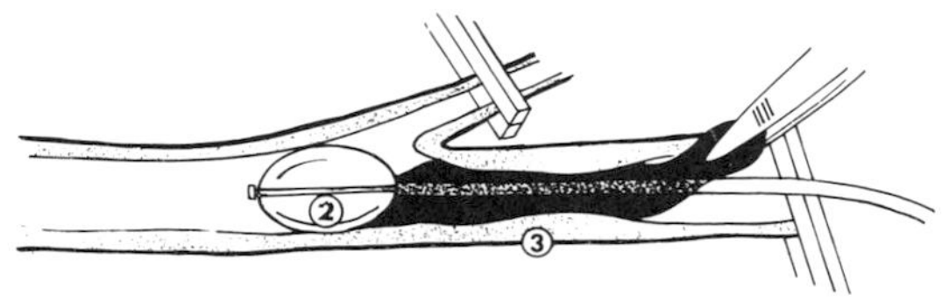

Reconstitution of the Artery by Anastomosis

1. End-to-end anastomosis.

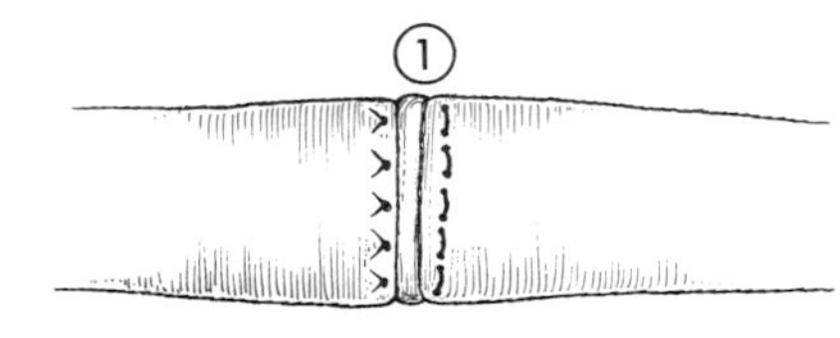

2. Another type of anastomosis suitable for small arteries.

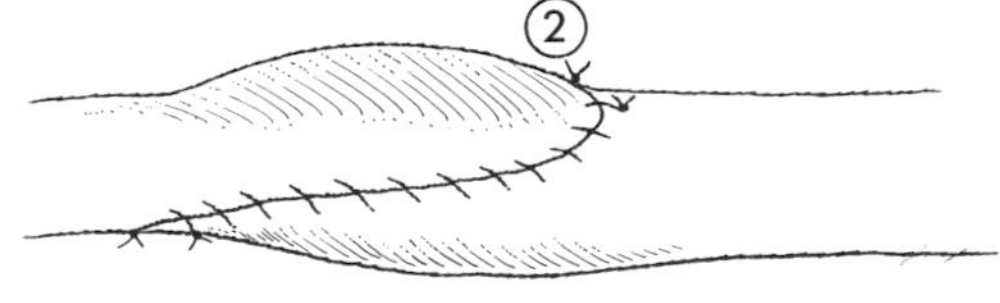

Management of the Fracture

A supracondylar fracture associated with ischemic injury may be immobilized by percutaneous Kirschner wires.

1. The Kirschner wires are introduced through the lateral epicondyle.

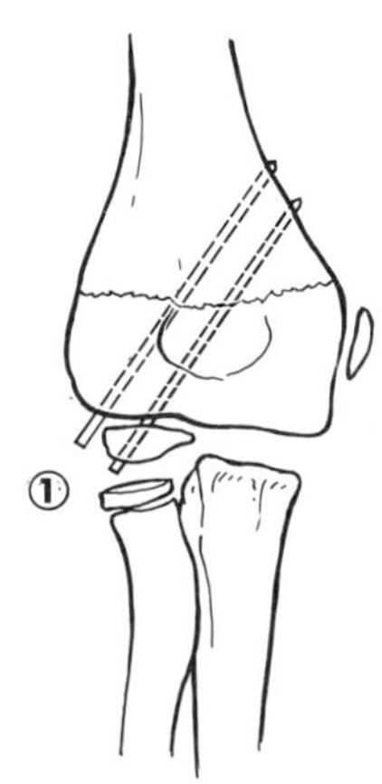

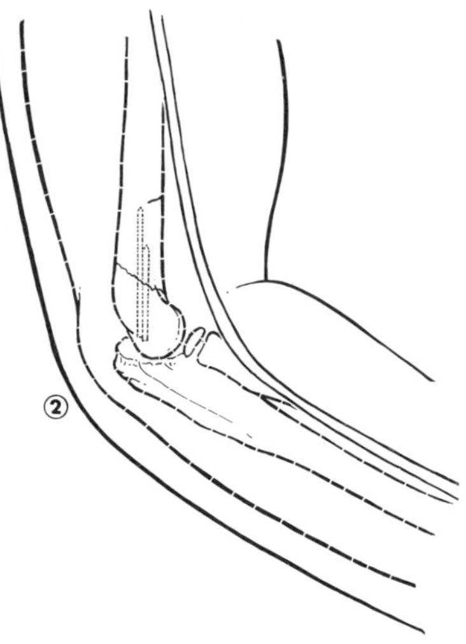

2. The limb is supported in a posterior splint with slight elbow flexion.

Postoperative Management

If the circulation has been restored by fasciotomy, elevation of the limb helps venous return. Continue to monitor distal flow with hourly flowmeter measurements for the first 24–36 hours.

The fasciotomy incision may be closed by 7 days, as soon as the swelling subsides. A secondary closure is preferable to skin grafting in the forearm. The patient may begin gentle active range-of-motion exercises after 3 weeks; the limb should be protected in a sling when not exercising. The fixation wires may be removed 6–8 weeks after the fracture.

Neural Complications

REMARKS

Neural injuries are more common complications of elbow fractures and dislocations (10–20 per cent of cases) but cause less permanent impairment than do vascular disruptions. Neural injuries are often concomitant with vascular injuries.

The nerve injury depends to a great extent on the direction and displacement of the skeletal injury. The commonest cause of ulnar nerve injury is a posterolateral dislocation of the elbow, particularly with displacement of the medial epicondyle. Entrapment of the ulnar nerve should be seriously considered with any such injury, particularly if the medial epicondyle fragment is displaced into the elbow joint.

The median nerve is injured with displaced supracondylar fractures, particularly with wide separation of the fragments. For the most part, the median nerve is known for its ability to escape injury in supracondylar fractures. The radial nerve is most at risk with fracture-dislocations of the elbow, such as the Monteggia fracture or fracture of the olecranon with dislocation of the elbow.

As a rule spontaneous recovery occurs in most nerve injuries with elbow fractures and dislocations. However, spontaneous recovery usually takes no longer than 10–12 weeks, after which time consideration should be given to operative exploration. The commonest nerve lesion requiring operative decompression is an ulnar nerve that is entrapped after posterolateral dislocation with fracture of the medial epicondyle.

The median nerve should be explored if there is evidence of progressive nerve injury after closed manipulation, particularly of a supracondylar fracture or dislocated elbow. An additional indication for operative exploration is the Matev sign, which becomes evident on x-ray at 2–3 months. This indicates that the median nerve may be entrapped in bone at the area of injury and requires surgical decompression.

Indications for Operative Exploration of Neural Injury

1. The commonest indication is a posterolateral dislocation of the elbow with
2. A displaced intra-articular medial epicondyle fracture.

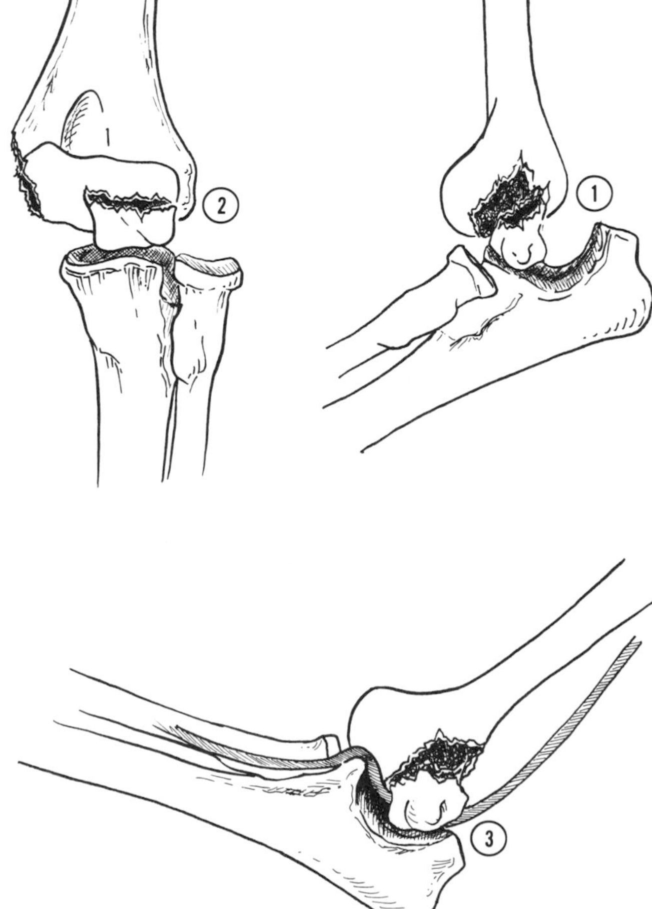

3. This is generally associated with entrapment of the ulnar nerve in the elbow joint and is an indication for acute operative exploration.

Median Nerve Entrapment

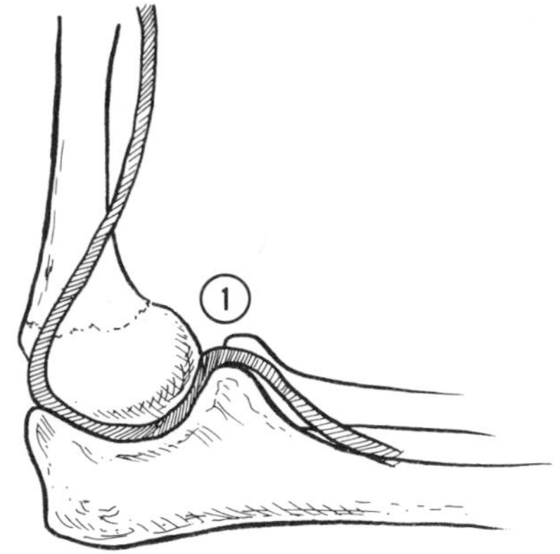

1. Median nerve entrapment is less likely to occur than ulnar nerve entrapment, although it may be evident after reduction of a supracondylar fracture or elbow dislocation. The nerve may be caught within the elbow or

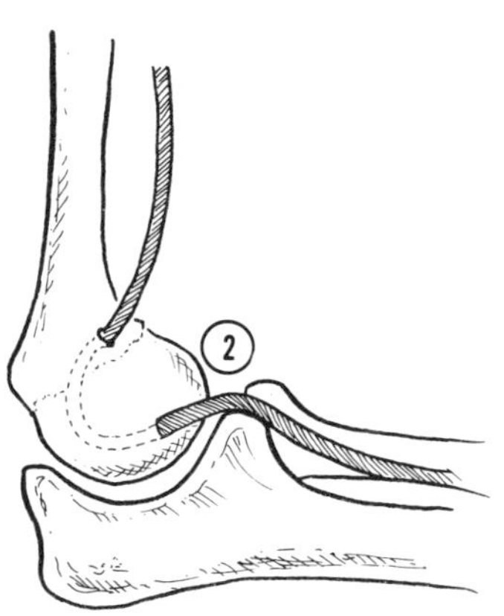

2. Trapped in the area of an epicondylar fracture or looped in front of the elbow.

Note: Although this condition is infrequent, failure to diagnose this type of entrapment may have serious functional effects. Therefore, pay special attention to assessing nerve function before and after reduction of an injury around the elbow. Particularly avoid pronating or hyperextending the dislocated elbow, because this seems to entrap the median nerve more readily. The method of reducing the dislocated elbow should always keep the forearm supinated.

Other Indications—Matev Sign

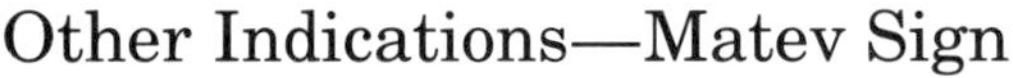

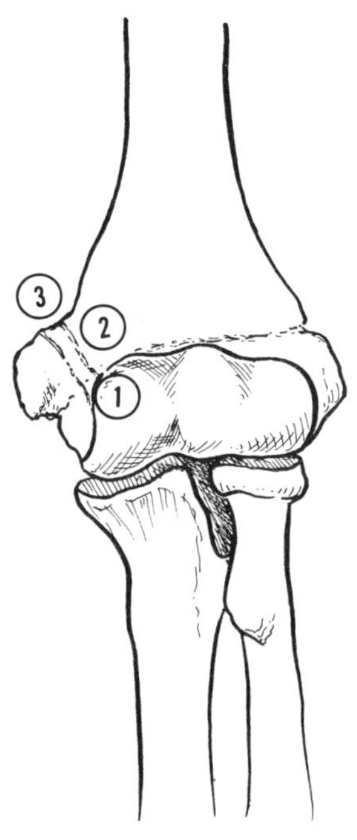

1. This is a radiographic sign of entrapment of the median nerve in bone that usually becomes evident by 2 months after injury.
2. It is characterized by sclerotic lines surrounding the area of median nerve entrapment in bone.
3. There is also a cortical disruption and interruption of the periosteum in the area where the nerve enters the bone.

Note: This x-ray finding should be correlated with clinical findings, which include sensory loss in the area of the hand innervated by the median nerve and weakness of the long flexors of the thumb and index finger. The abductor pollicis brevis is often paralyzed, and the Tinel sign may be present at the elbow. The elbow usually has a normal range of motion and, surprisingly, is pain-free despite the trapped nerve.

Management

Closed Management of Distal Humeral Metaphyseal Fractures

REMARKS

If the distal humeral metaphyseal fracture is not associated with acute neurovascular compromise, the main concern becomes reduction and stabilization to restore elbow function. Of all large joints the elbow is the most prone to stiffening after even relatively undisplaced fractures. For this reason, treatment should be designed for early restoration of joint motion, particularly flexion, the loss of which is most disabling.

Long-arm cast treatment of these fractures is best avoided. Distal metaphyseal humeral fractures not only stiffen in a long-arm cast but tend to rotate the elbow joint internally, particularly if immobilized with the cast against the chest. This internal torsion on the fracture produces a cubitus varus deformity, which is particularly unsightly in slender women.

Fractures of the distal humerus that do not involve the joint may readily be treated with the fracture-brace method described in Chapter 13. This type of fracture can be managed initially by temporary splintage followed by a fracture brace or sleeve when the swelling subsides at 5–7 days. Elbow flexion at this level may produce some angulatory displacement, but elbow function can usually be restored to close to the normal range.

An alternative treatment, particularly for distal humeral fractures involving the metaphyseal region, is with extension block splinting followed by a fracture brace or sleeve. This encourages elbow motion and prevents torsional deformity.

If the fracture is unstable, the usual tendency toward posterior displacement can be reduced by hyperflexing the elbow once the swelling has subsided. An extension block splint can be used to gradually allow the hyperflexed elbow to further flex and slowly extend. By the time the fracture consolidates at 3–4 weeks, a fracture brace or sleeve may be applied. The intent is to emphasize restoration of flexion initially and only permit elbow extension as the fracture consolidates.

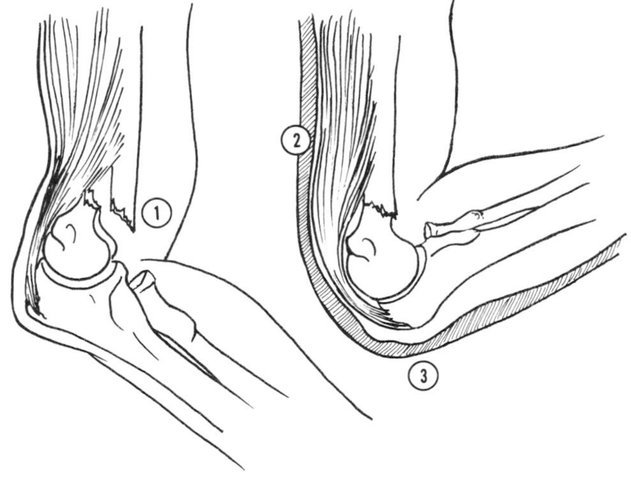

1. A distal metaphyseal fracture with posterior displacement can be reduced by hyperflexing the elbow beyond a right angle once the acute swelling subsides.
2. This uses the bulky triceps muscle and tendon posteriorly to achieve the reduced position.
3. A posterior splint can be applied loosely to allow the elbow further flexion.

Note: The patient should be encouraged to flex the elbow while in the splint to maintain flexion motion in the joint and continue to maintain fracture stability.

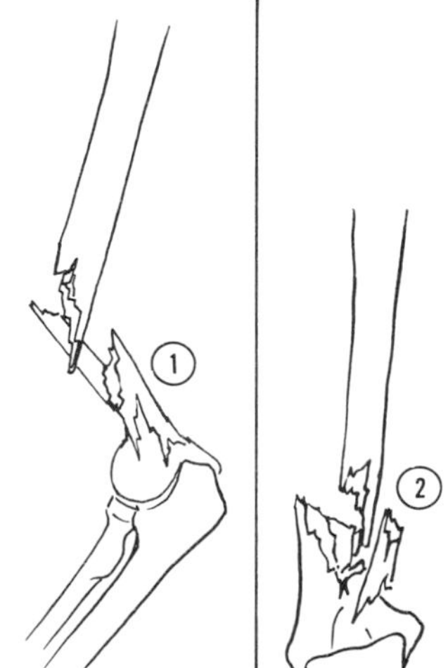

1. A severely comminuted fracture of the distal third of the humerus is associated with
2. A butterfly fragment.

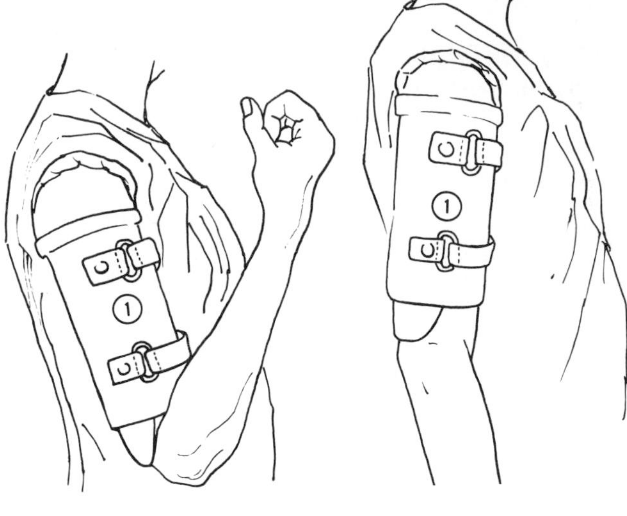

1. Fractures even at this level of the humerus can be treated with a fracture brace with a sleeve that extends posteriorly toward the distal humerus. This allows the patient to flex the elbow while still adequately supporting the fracture.

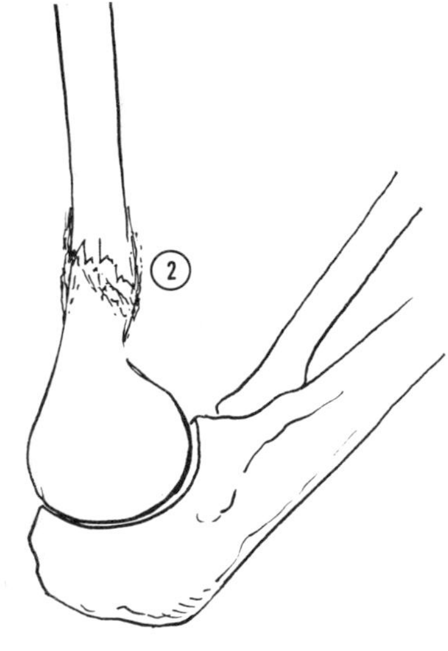

2. Treatment of a distal humeral fracture with a functional sleeve may produce some residual anterior angulation.

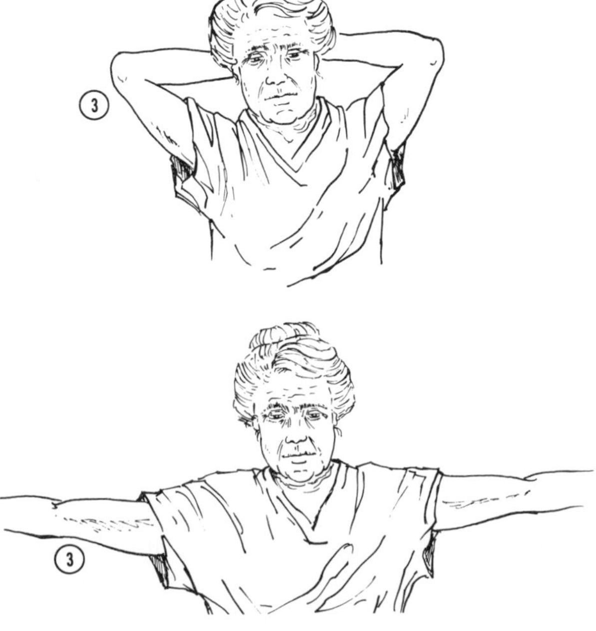

3. Functional results are usually quite good despite some residual angulation of the distal humerus after fracture-brace treatment.

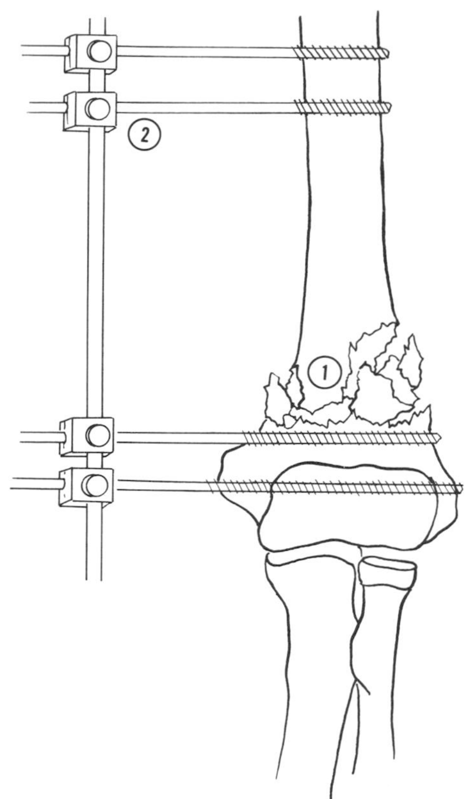

External Fixation of Distal Humeral Fractures

1. Rarely an unstable distal humeral fracture may require external fixation if the wound is open or the fracture cannot be reduced.
2. The proximal and distal pins are best inserted under direct vision of the bone to avoid entrapping the radial nerve. An orthofix or a similar device is applied as previously described (see Chapter 1). The external fixation device should be removed after 4–6 weeks, when the fracture can be supported by a fracture brace or splint. During the time the fracture is immobilized by external fixation, active elbow range-of-motion exercises should be encouraged.

Subsequent Management

As the elbow is extended, the fracture can be supported in a fracture brace. In general, a long-arm cast should be avoided with these fractures because immobilization in a long-arm cast with the arm against the chest tends to internally rotate the elbow and produce a cubitus varus deformity.

These distal humeral fractures tend to consolidate quickly in most people and by 8 weeks are clinically stable so that the fracture brace can usually be discarded. Exercises can then be used to regain extension, although full extension may not return. The emphasis of functional exercises should be to restore flexion to a maximum level but accept limitation of extension of 30° or less.

Closed Management of Distal Humeral Metaphyseal Fractures With Anterior Displacement of the Elbow

REMARKS

These rare injuries occasionally occur as a result of a blow to the posterior aspect of the distal humerus. For these fractures the usual technique of reduction with hyperflexion may not achieve a stable position.

Soltanpur has shown that the fracture can be reduced by applying a cast in two stages. This method takes advantage of the fact that the displaced fracture fragment behaves as a part of the forearm. Therefore, posterior displacement of the patient's hand and forearm also pushes the distal metaphyseal fracture posteriorly to achieve reduction.

Technique of Reduction

STAGE I

1. The surgeon grasps the condyles and pulls distally to disengage the fracture fragments.
2. The elbow is flexed to slightly less than 90°.
3. The limb is wrapped in cast padding by an assistant.
4. A circular cast is applied around the upper arm only.

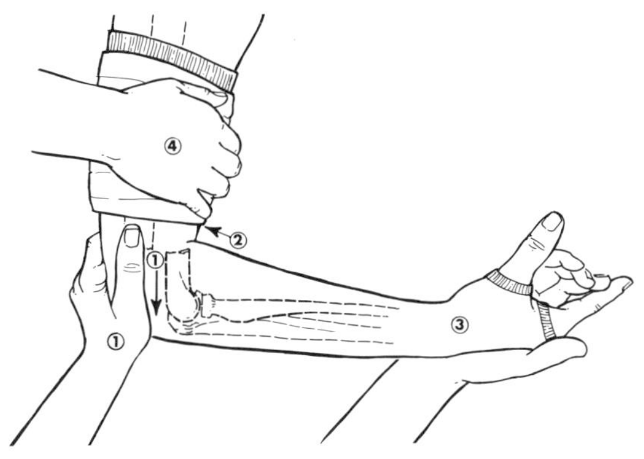

STAGE II

When the upper arm cast has set,

1. The surgeon supports the upper arm and
2. Pushes the patient's hand, forearm, and condylar mass downward to reduce the fracture with the aid of the forearm.
3. The assistant completes the long-arm plaster cast.

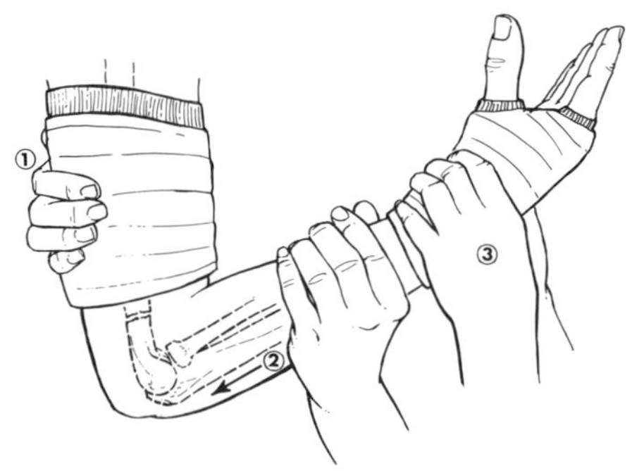

Note: If the fracture cannot be stabilized in the long-arm cast after it is reduced by this maneuver, operative intervention with plate fixation is indicated.

Postreduction Management

Confirm the position by x-ray and recheck within a week. The plaster cast may be discarded by 6 weeks, and the arm may be placed in a sling. Begin a program of active exercises. *Do not* permit passive stretching of the elbow joint.

SUPRACONDYLAR AND INTERCONDYLAR FRACTURES OF THE HUMERUS IN THE ADULT

REMARKS

These lesions are infrequent in comparison with supracondylar fractures in children. They occur most often in adults more than 40 years of age. The mechanism of injury is usually direct trauma to the elbow that drives the olecranon against the humeral articular surface and fractures or splits the distal end.

The rare minimally displaced fracture without rotational deformity may be treated by a trial of cast immobilization. For the most part, these fractures develop rotational deformity or comminution and are thus treated by operative fixation.

A second alternative in the elderly patient with a severely comminuted or "bag of bones" fracture is extension block splintage with early range of motion. A third form of treatment that has become less popular than in the past is skeletal traction. This is best restricted to the severely comminuted fracture that cannot be adequately fixed internally. Patients who must be confined to bed for other injuries are also candidates for treatment of distal humeral fractures by skeletal traction.

Types of Supracondylar and Intercondylar Fractures

Supracondylar fracture without intercondylar displacement. This is a rare injury because most supracondylar fractures in older patients are associated with split condyles.

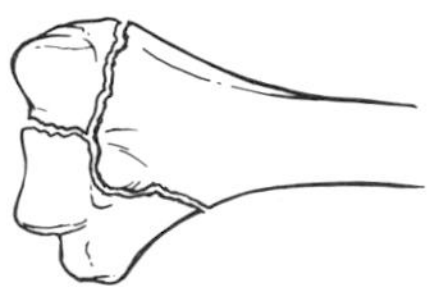

T-shaped intercondylar fractures with trochlear and capitellar fragments separated but not appreciably rotated in the frontal plane.

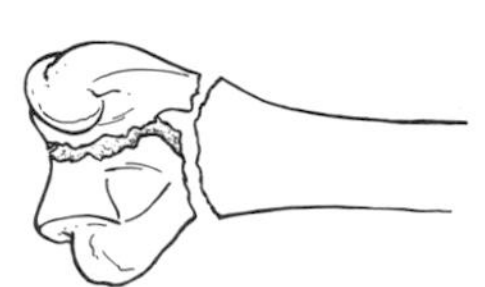

Displaced T-Condylar Fracture

Unfortunately many of the distal intercondylar and T-condylar fractures in older osteoporotic patients are displaced and comminuted. This makes internal fixation quite difficult and prone to complications.

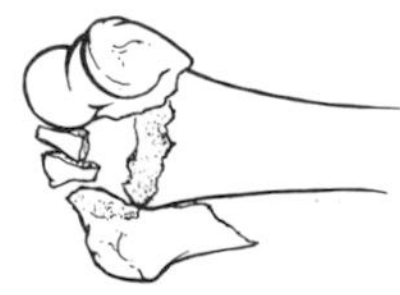

■ Management

Indications for Operative Management of Supracondylar and Intercondylar Fractures in the Adult

REMARKS

Operative treatment in the past has been associated with poor results from these fractures due to failure to achieve sufficiently adequate immobilization of the fracture to permit restoration of elbow motion. Newer techniques have allowed better methods of secure fixation to permit restoration of elbow motion, and particularly restoration of elbow flexion.

However, if the fixation cannot be made rigid, frequently a postoperative regimen of skeletal traction or extension block splintage may still be necessary for the severely comminuted fracture.

Therefore, the surgeon who selects operative fixation of the comminuted fracture must be fully experienced with the use of internal fixation techniques around the elbow. Otherwise, the treatment may make the problem worse.

Techniques of Fixation

1. Although Kirschner wires have been used in the past, these are best used only for a temporary fixation.
2. The preferred method of fixing the condyles is with a cancellous or cortical lag screw. These may be cannulated screws inserted over the Kirschner guide.

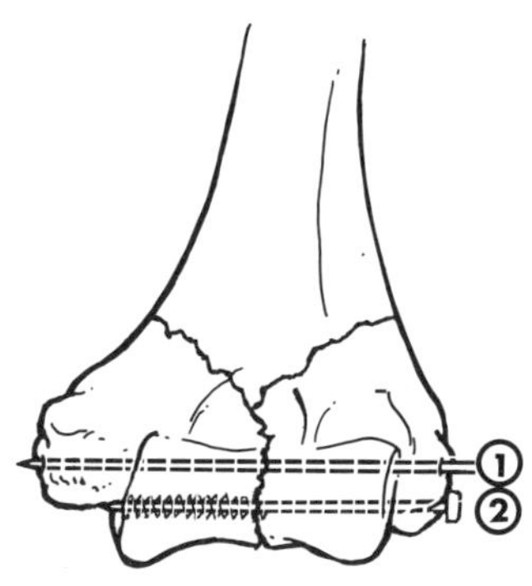

3. Once the condyles have been reduced, crossed lag screws may be inserted to fix the condyles to the metaphyseal bone.
4. A preferred method, in addition to or as a substitution for, screw fixation, is with flexible reconstruction plates, which give more rigid fixation of the condyles to the metaphyseal bone.

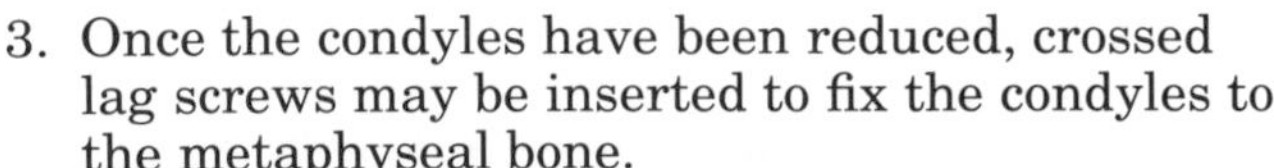

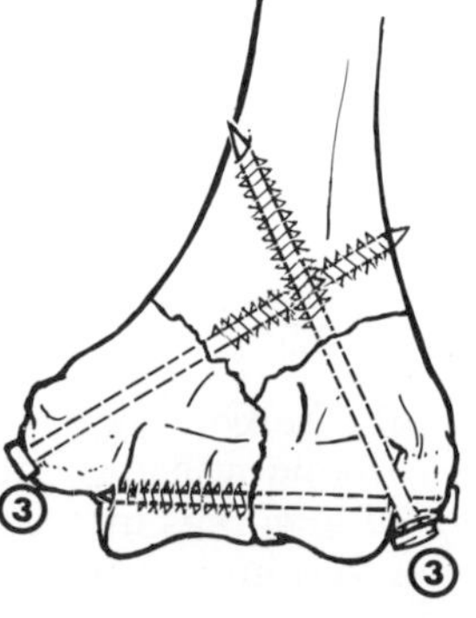

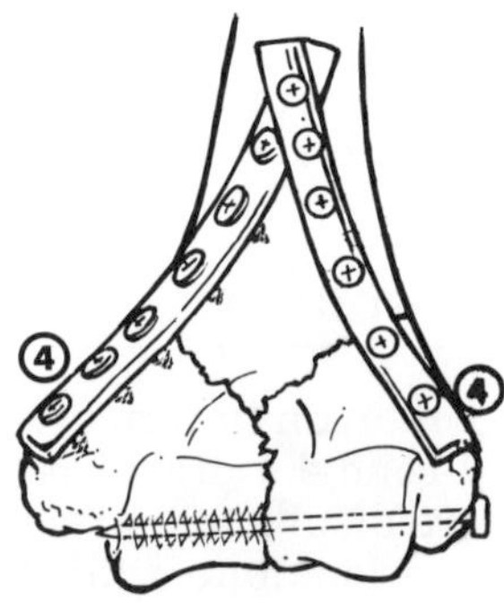

Postoperative Management

A plaster splint is applied posteriorly until the swelling subsides by 3–5 days. Following this active range-of-motion exercises of the elbow are begun, with the emphasis on flexion.

After 2 or 3 weeks the elbow may be exercised actively out of the splint to increase the range of elbow motion. Maximum restoration of motion will be slow in coming.

Note: If internal fixation is inadequate or insecure, postoperative skeletal traction may be necessary until fracture healing is evident.

Type of Fracture for Which Traction May Be Indicated

Severe comminution of articular surface with rotational displacement of the condyles.

Note: These fractures can be open injuries, which should be treated with immediate debridement followed by a Kirschner wire traction technique.

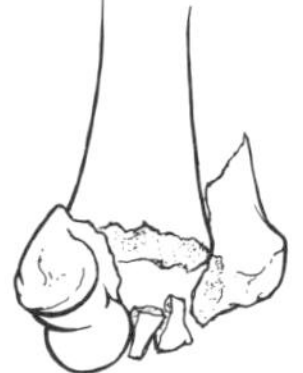

Manipulative Reduction

1. An attempt is made at reduction of the condyles by applying steady traction with the elbow extended 135°.
2. The medial and lateral condyles are compressed together by direct manipulation.

Note: Following manipulation, a pin is inserted into the olecranon to reapply skeletal traction and to allow early immobilization of the elbow.

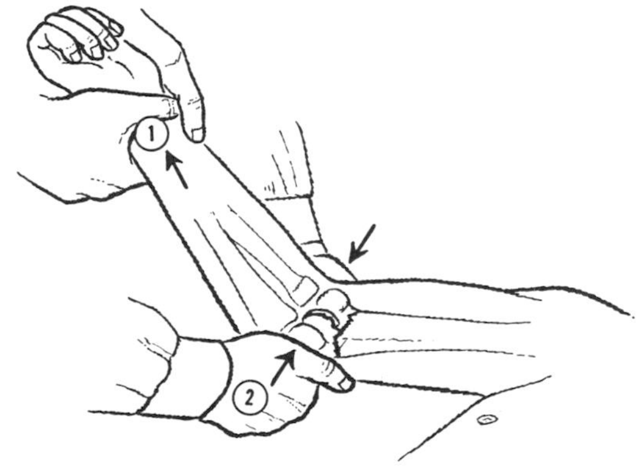

Management by Skeletal Traction

1. The patient lies on a firm bed fitted with a lateral traction apparatus.
2. Elevate the side of the bed slightly for countertraction.
3. Pass a 3-mm Kirschner wire through the olecranon from the medial to lateral sides. Be sure to avoid the ulnar nerve, and apply 5–8 lb (3–4 kg) of traction.
4. Rotational deformity of the condyles can be corrected by rotation of the forearm.
5. Abduct the shoulder approximately 70°.

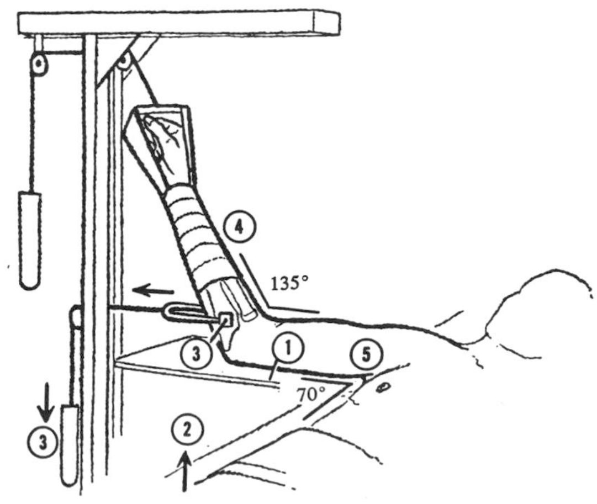

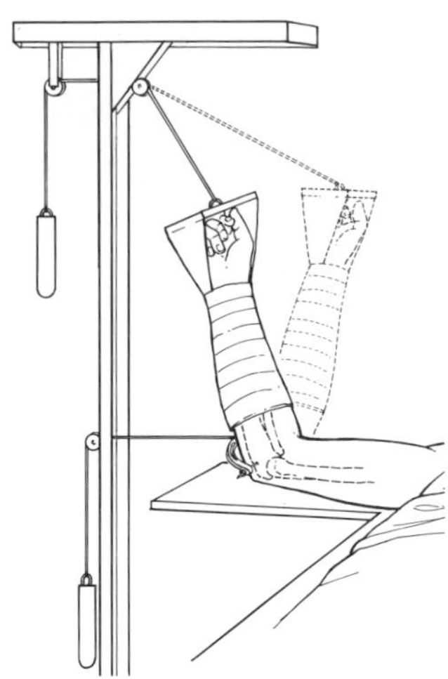

Postreduction Management

Traction is continued for at least 3 weeks. During this time the elbow is progressively flexed to maintain motion beyond 90° of elbow flexion.

X-Rays During Traction

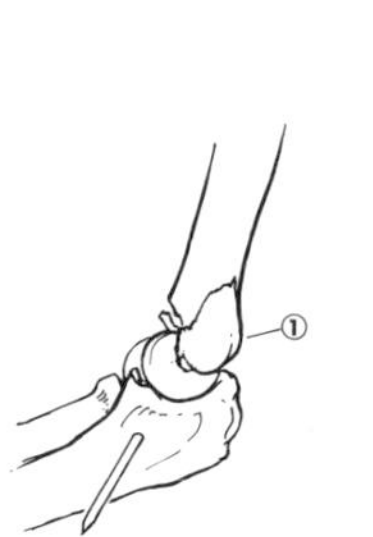

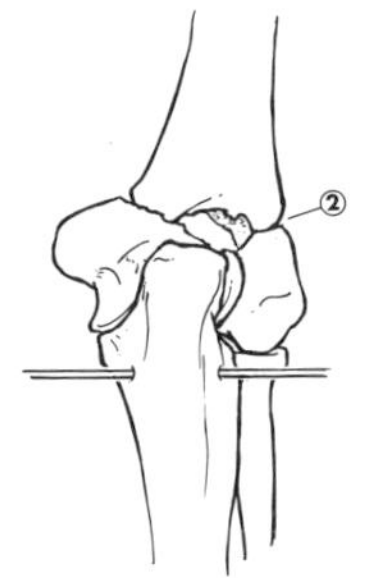

1. Condyles have been approximated and rotational malalignment has been corrected by rotation of the forearm.
2. Distraction of the fracture fragment should be avoided.

Subsequent Management

After 3 weeks of traction, the joint is supported in an extension block splint with the elbow flexed beyond the right angle. The patient is encouraged to flex the elbow as maximally as possible, and a collar and cuff is used to position the elbow in maximum flexion.

Consolidation of the fracture is usually evident by 6–8 weeks, at which time the elbow may progressively be extended. The elbow is most likely to be stiff in flexion and limited in extension, but this is the most desirable compromise, because flexion is most essential to elbow motion to allow the hand to come to the face.

Flexion Exercise and Extension Block Splinting for T-Condylar Fractures in the Elderly

REMARKS

Although anatomic reduction and adequate internal fixation are ideal to allow early mobilization, many of these fractures in osteoporotic bone may not be suitable for operative fixation. Brown and Morgan have shown that less than anatomic reduction with emphasis on early range of motion may give satisfactory results. This method has the great virtue of simplicity and provides a satisfactory functional outcome in the elderly patient.

As the swelling subsides, the fractured condyles may be manipulated to compress them together. Subsequently the elbow can be flexed to 120° using a collar and cuff and a Velcro wrap to approximate alignment. After 5–7 days the patient is encouraged to move the elbow actively.

Prereduction X-Ray in a Comminuted T-Condylar Fracture in an 80-Year-Old Patient

1. The fragments are separated and are displaced with rotational deformity.

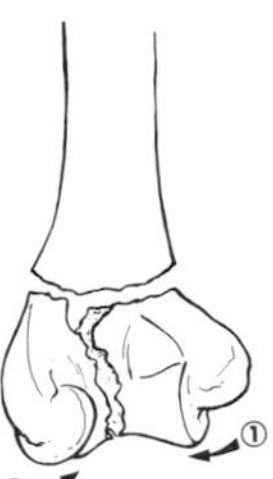

Manipulative Reduction

1. Under a general anesthetic traction is applied to the elbow in a flexed position.
2. The condyles are molded together to achieve approximation of the condyles and the metaphyseal fragment.

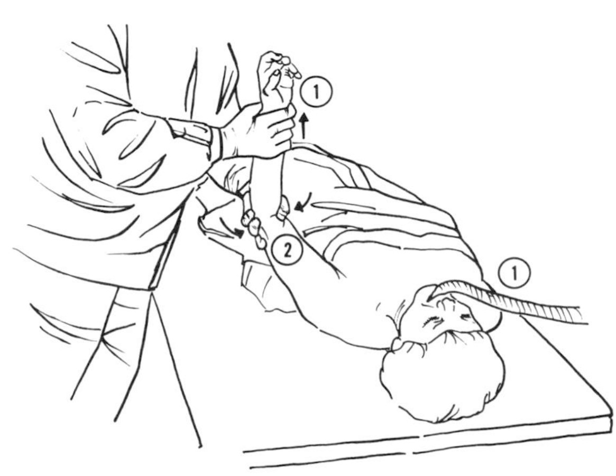

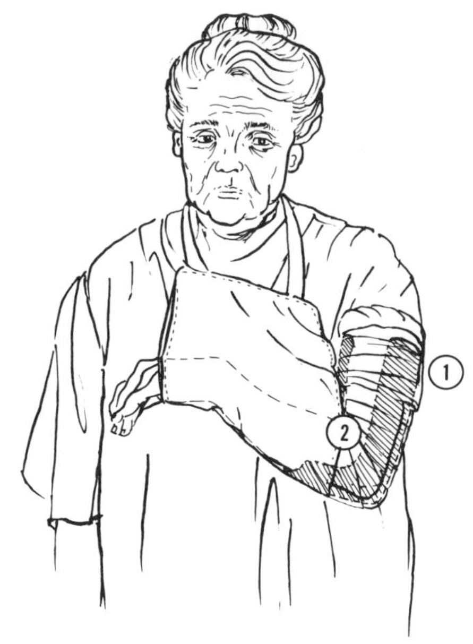

Initial Immobilization

1. Initially a posterior splint or sugar-tong splint is applied to support the elbow and fractured arm in a comfortable position.
2. The posterior splint avoids tight constriction of the arm, which tends to swell after these fractures. In addition, the arm should be elevated with a sling to diminish swelling.

Extension Block Splinting

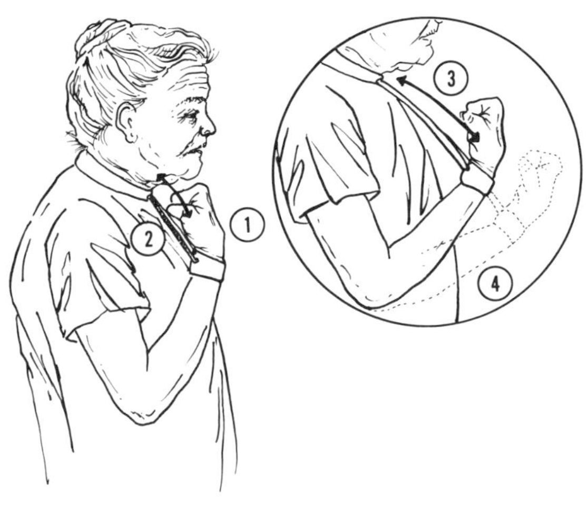

1. After the swelling subsides the elbow is flexed maximally. This can be done using a collar and cuff or Velcro straps.
2. The patient is encouraged to work at flexing the elbow, but extension beyond a right angle is prevented.
3. As the fracture consolidates by 3–4 weeks, the elbow may be gradually extended to a right angle by loosening the strap to permit elbow extension.
4. When the fracture is not actively exercised, it should be held in maximum flexion with a collar and cuff or Velcro straps. This allows the fracture to heal with maximum elbow flexion but can limit full extension of the elbow. Flexion is the more important motion to regain, and elbow extension can be sacrificed to gain flexion.

Subsequent Management

After 6 weeks the fracture is usually sufficiently united to discontinue the collar and cuff. Active exercises should be continued for 3–4 months until range of motion ceases to improve. With this technique the fracture may be reduced to an acceptable but nonanatomic position.

The usual arc of motion achieved with this method is 100° or about the range needed for most functional activities. The treatment is designed to maintain maximum flexion but lose some elbow extension. Flexion that is not gained in the first 3–5 weeks is not likely to be gained subsequently. Elbow extension may be improved, however, with several months of active exercise.

FRACTURE OF THE CAPITELLUM IN THE ADULT

REMARKS

Injuries to the capitellum occur commonly from a fall on the outstretched arm. This injury usually fractures the radial head but may damage the capitellum by direct transmission of the force through the radial head, which acts like a piston and shears off the capitellum into the radial fossa.

Injuries of this type are deceiving because they may appear minor but can cause significant limitation of elbow motion. A true lateral x-ray will demonstrate the free osteochondral fragment displaced anterosuperiorly into the radial fossa.

There are two types of injuries to the capitellum, (1) a complete anterior displacement of the capitellar fragment and (2) a partial decortication or bruising that may be associated with a radial head fracture.

Operative treatment with excision of the fragment is usually more effective than attempted closed reduction. The trochlear-ulnar articulation allows excision of the entire capitellum and radial head as well, if necessary for comminuted fractures, without causing valgus instability of the elbow. Even a portion of the anterior trochlear surface may be excised with the capitellar fragment without compromising elbow stability, provided that the posterior trochlear surface is intact.

Preoperative X-Ray—Shear Fracture of the Capitellum

1. Fracture is not evident on the anteroposterior x-ray, but the lateral x-ray, showing the capitellar fragment displaced into the radial fossa, is diagnostic.
2. The impact of the radial head "bruises" the articular cartilage of the capitellum and may form a type of osteochondritis dissecans. This may not displace and may be manifested only by a persistent block of elbow extension or symptoms of a loose body. It may also only be seen during arthrotomy for removal of the fractured radial head.

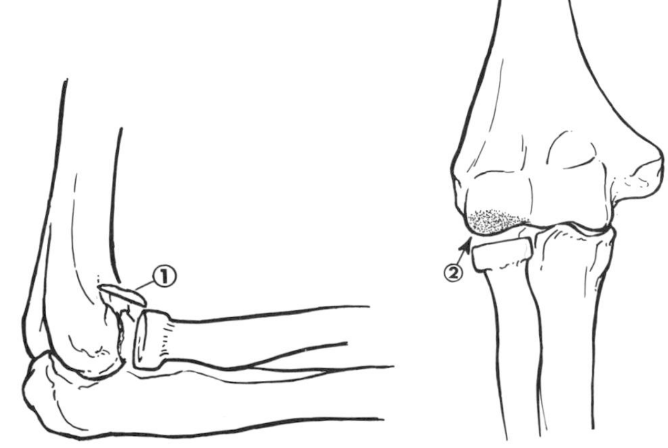

■ Management

Closed Treatment of Fractures of the Capitellum

Although, in general, operative treatment of displaced fractures is preferable, occasionally excellent results may follow closed reduction.

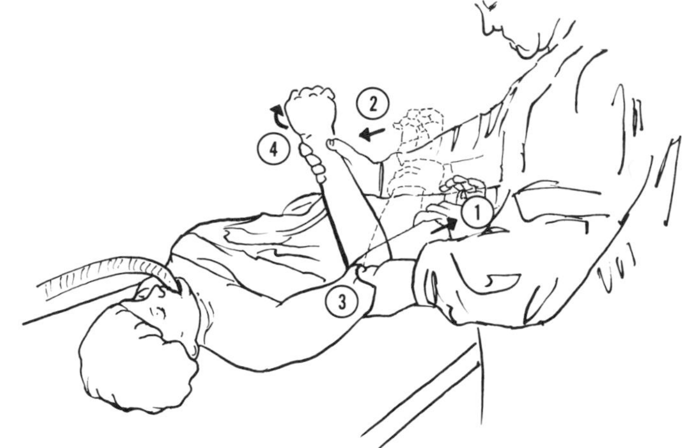

Technique of Closed Reduction (After Christopher)

1. Under general anesthetic traction is applied to the supinated forearm on the fractured side.
2. The forearm and elbow are flexed to 90° while
3. Pressure is applied simultaneously in the area of the displaced fracture fragment.
4. The forearm is pronated to stabilize the fragment with the radial head.

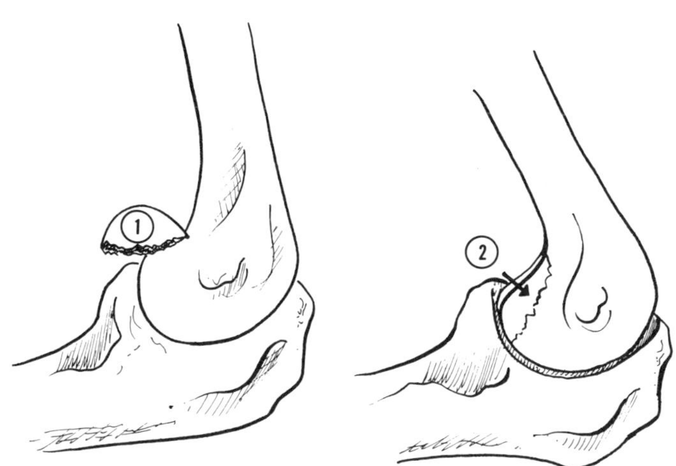

Prereduction and Postreduction X-Ray

1. Prereduction x-ray shows the fractured capitellum displaced anteriorly.
2. Postreduction x-ray shows anatomic reduction, which is maintained with the elbow flexed and the forearm pronated. This uses the radial head to maintain the reduced position of the fracture fragment.

Subsequent Management

The elbow is immobilized in a posterior splint in the hyperflexed position for no more than 3 weeks. Active extension may be allowed if the fracture remains stable at the end of 3 weeks. The main motion that must be maintained is flexion of the elbow. Extension will return gradually as the patient resumes active exercise.

Note: If the capitellar fragment displaces after the closed reduction, open reduction and excision or internal fixation is necessary to avoid a poor result or stiffening of the elbow.

Excision

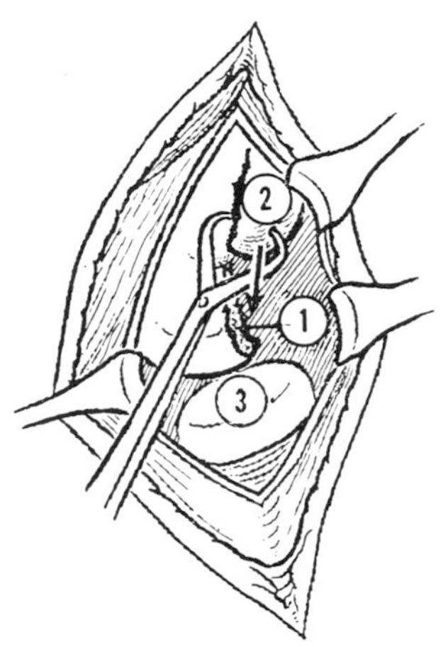

1. The radiohumeral joint is opened and all loose debris are removed from the surface of the capitellum.
2. The capitellar fragment is removed because it is not sufficiently large to repair.
3. If the radial head is fractured, it may also require excision.

Note: The stability of the elbow should be carefully checked after any procedure that removes bone from the elbow.

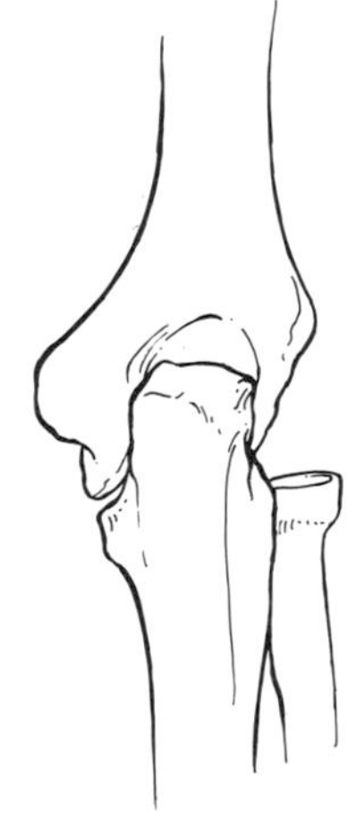

Postoperative X-Ray

A sizable capitellar fragment may be removed without impairing the stability of the elbow.

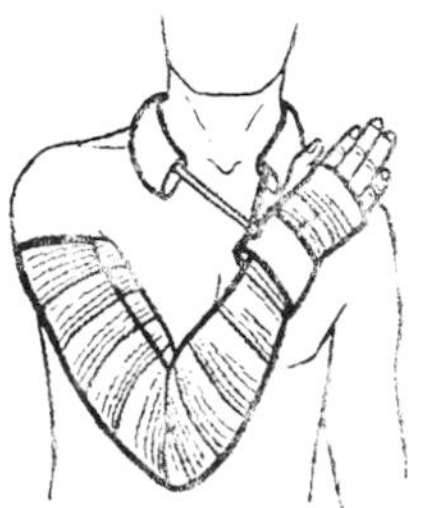

Postoperative Management

The arm is immobilized in a posterior splint with the elbow flexed 90 degrees. Active range of motion is begun at 5–7 days, when the wound edema and pain have subsided. Avoid passive stretching exercises and intensive physical therapy.

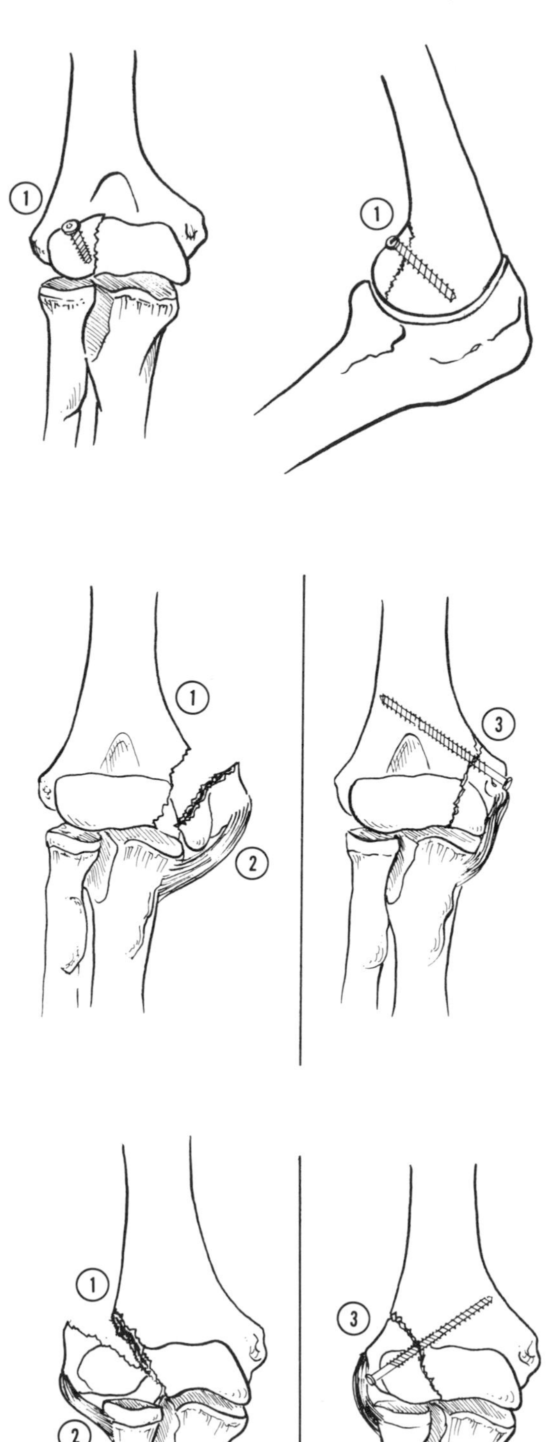

Alternative Method for Larger Capitellar Fragments

1. Screw fixation may be possible when the fragment is sufficiently large to hold the screw. The screw must be inserted obliquely in such a manner that it avoids blocking motion of the radial head on the capitellum.

Other Fractures Around the Elbow in the Adult—Fractures of the Medial and Lateral Condyles

1. Fractures of the lateral or medial condyle are infrequent in the adult elbow but do occur.
2. They tend to displace even with cast immobilization due to traction from the muscle attachment (either the flexor or extensor origin).
3. They are best managed by prompt internal fixation to achieve stability and allow early restoration of elbow flexion.

DISLOCATIONS OF THE ELBOW JOINT

Posterior Dislocations of the Elbow Joint

REMARKS

Except for the shoulder, the elbow is the joint most frequently dislocated, and in children less than 10 years of age elbow dislocation occurs more often than any other luxation. Generally the radius and the ulna, which are firmly bound together by the annular ligament and interosseous membrane, displace posteriorly as a unit. Occasionally displacement occurs laterally, medially, or anteriorly, but most dislocations are posterior.

Considerable violence is absorbed by the elbow during dislocation, and 30–40 per cent of dislocations are associated with fractures of adjacent structures. The most common associated fracture in children (less than 14 years of age) is avulsion of the medial epicondyle. In adults the associated fracture may involve the coronoid process or the radial head, the capitellum, or the olecranon.

Because elbow dislocations traumatize the anterior brachial muscle, myositis ossificans may complicate the injury, particularly if passive exercise is inflicted on the patient. Emphasis on active rather than passive range-of-motion exercises to regain elbow motion has diminished the occurrence of this complication significantly.

Dislocated elbows are always at risk of vascular injury. The frequency of vascular impairment (1–3 per cent) after dislocation is not as high as with supracondylar fractures, but the results may be equally catastrophic.

Because of the extent of trauma from elbow dislocation, simple posterior plaster slabs are preferable to circular casts for temporary immobilization after reduction. Close follow-up is essential after reduction, with the patient either remaining in the hospital or returning to the surgeon's office within 24 hours of reduction.

Nerve injury, most often a temporary neurapraxia, may also complicate management. The ulnar and median nerves are usually damaged by the same injury that disrupts the brachial artery.

Reduction of the elbow dislocation is usually quite simple. It is the management of the common complications, particularly of associated fractures and vascular and nerve injuries, that makes the difference between good and poor results.

As with any dislocation or subluxation, elbow dislocation may be subject to recurrence if bony, ligamentous, and muscular support structures are disrupted sufficiently. Most elbows are quite stable after reduction, but the degree of instability can only be evaluated by testing the range of joint motion subsequent to reduction.

Rarely, a patient will be seen with a chronically dislocated elbow that can be reduced by traction and closed technique if it is less than 4 weeks old. Dislocations older than 4 weeks require extensive open procedures, which are indicated primarily for persistent and severe pain.

Typical Mechanism of an Elbow Dislocation

1. A fall backward on the arm with the elbow in a flexed position and
2. The forearm supinated is the commonest mechanism.
3. The injury causes the radius and ulna to dislocate posterior to the humerus.
4. There may also frequently be an associated fracture of the radial head or
5. The coracoid process of the ulna.

Note: In a child with an elbow dislocation, the commonest fracture is an avulsion of the medial epicondyle.

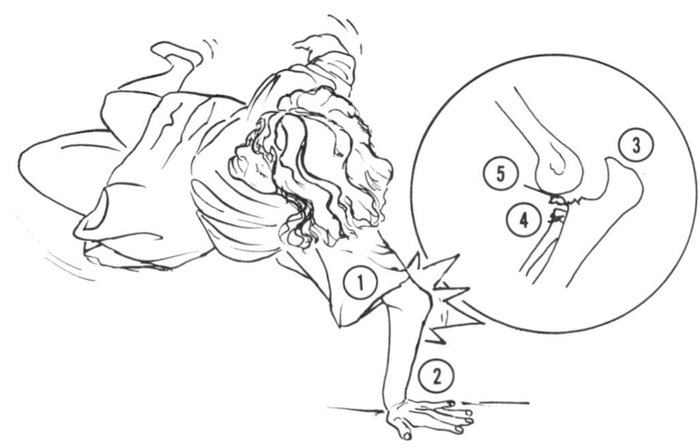

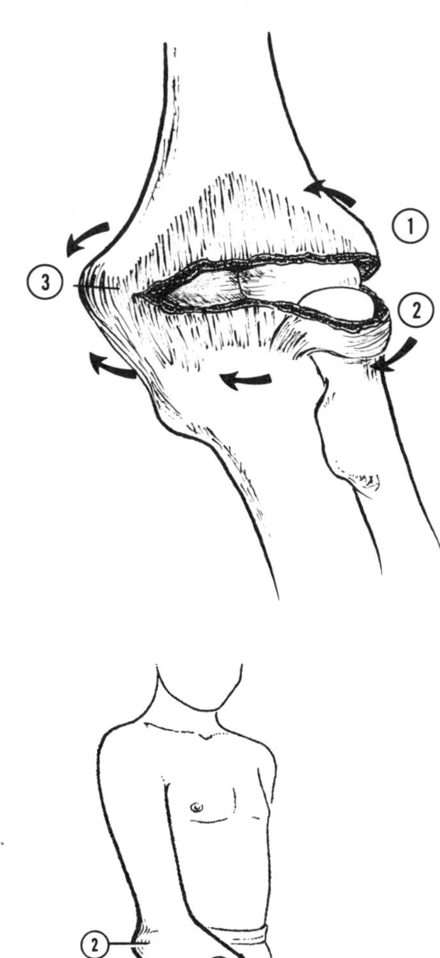

Pathophysiology

1. Soft tissue injury associated with dislocation progresses in a circle from lateral to medial in three stages.
2. The lateral capsule fails first, followed by the anterior and posterior capsule.
3. Complete or partial disruption of the medial collateral ligament may also occur with severe injury.

Note: In most instances, the major instability is due to failure of the lateral capsular ligamentous support.

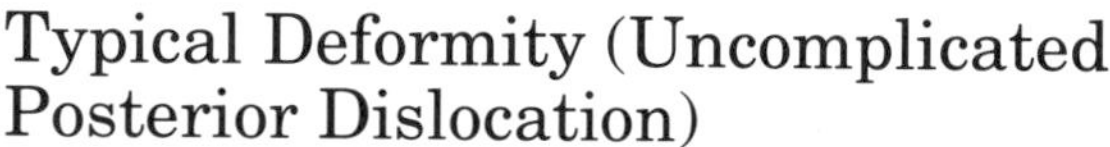

Typical Deformity (Uncomplicated Posterior Dislocation)

1. The forearm appears to be shortened.
2. The olecranon is very prominent.

Prereduction X-Ray

LATERAL VIEW

1. Both bones of the forearm are displaced backward and are behind the humerus.
2. The coronoid process of the ulna impinges on the posterior aspect of the humerus in the olecranon fossa.

ANTEROPOSTERIOR VIEW

3. In this instance both bones are displaced radially.
4. The radius and ulna maintain their normal anatomic position in relation to each other.

Note: Always check carefully prior to reduction for alteration in distal CMS (circulation, motor, sensory) function.

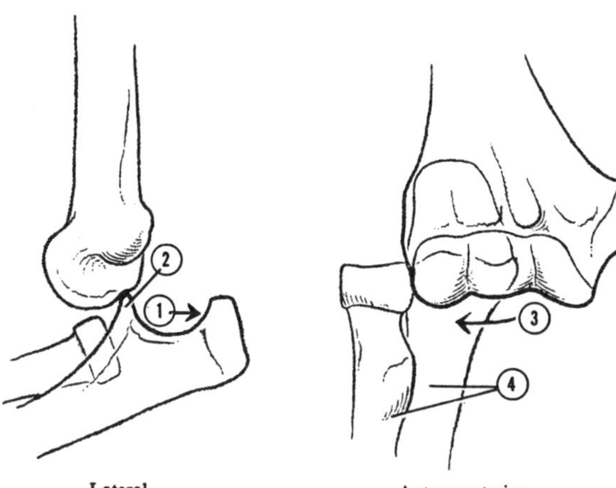

Anesthesia for Reduction

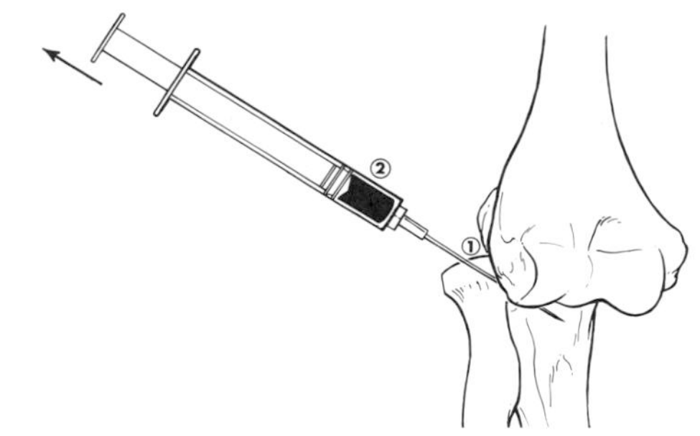

Local anesthesia may be quite effective for the usual patient with elbow dislocation. For the extremely anxious patient, use general anesthesia.

1. Insert a 20-gauge needle into the joint proximal to the dislocated radial head.
2. Aspirate hemarthrosis.

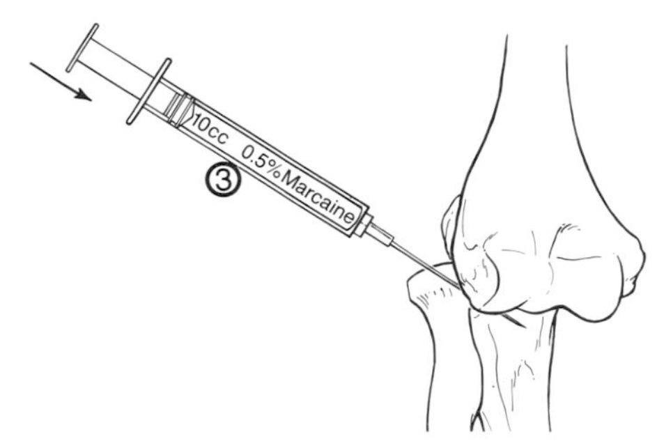

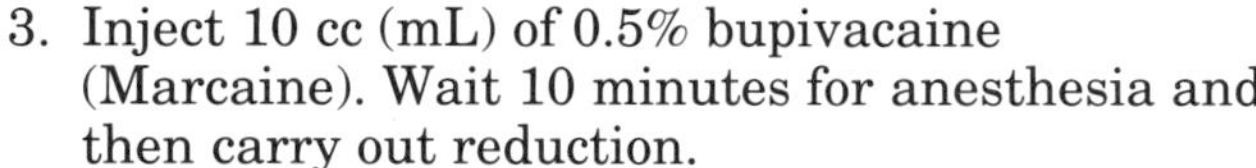

3. Inject 10 cc (mL) of 0.5% bupivacaine (Marcaine). Wait 10 minutes for anesthesia and then carry out reduction.

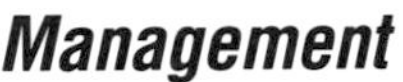

Management

Manipulative Reduction

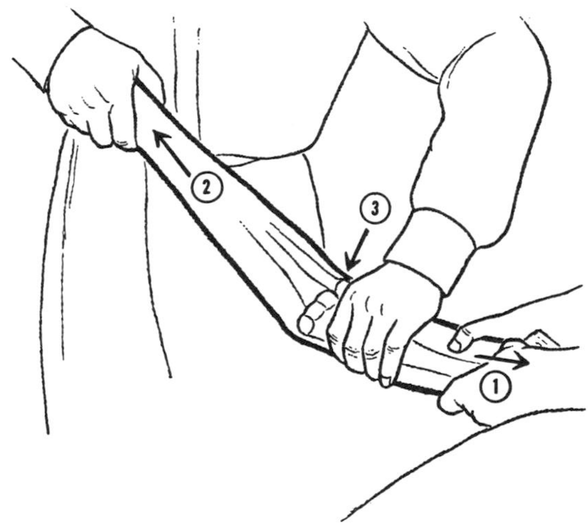

1. While an assistant holds the arm and makes steady countertraction,
2. Grasp the wrist with one hand and make steady traction on the forearm in the position in which it lies.
3. While traction is maintained, correct any lateral displacement with the other hand.

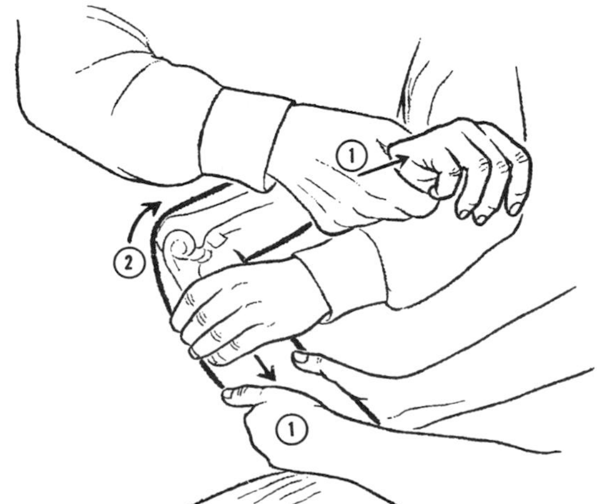

THEN

1. While traction is maintained,
2. Gently flex the forearm.

Note: With reduction a click is usually felt and heard as the olecranon engages the articular surface of the humerus.

Evaluation of Stability Following Reduction

1. Gently move the elbow through normal range of motion in flexion and extension, and
2. Medial and lateral stressing. If the elbow is unstable, several diagnoses are possible: (a) in a child, entrapment of the medial epicondyle; (b) in an adult, an unstable fracture of the radial head or olecranon; or (c) medial and lateral disruption of the capsule.

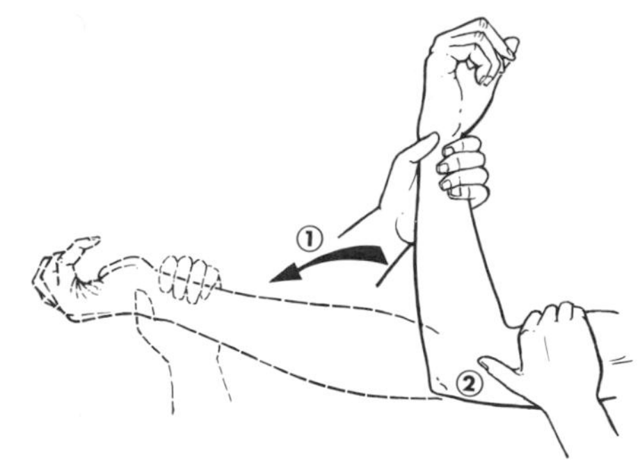

Quigley Technique of Reduction by Traction on the Dangling Arm

Usually no anesthesia is necessary as long as the movements are gentle. Reduction by this method controls the position of the olecranon, which is important if there is a medial or lateral component to the dislocation.

1. The patient is prone on an examining or x-ray table. This eliminates the tendency to nausea or vomiting and syncope if the manipulation is carried out in the upright position.
2. The forearm is allowed to dangle toward the floor and
3. The operator applies traction by grasping the wrist and slowly pulling in the direction of the long axis of the forearm. This is done gently, without sudden movement.
4. After muscle relaxation occurs, the olecranon is grasped with the operator's other hand using the thumb and index finger. The olecranon is then guided to the reduced position without force. In this way medial or lateral components of the dislocation can be controlled and corrected.

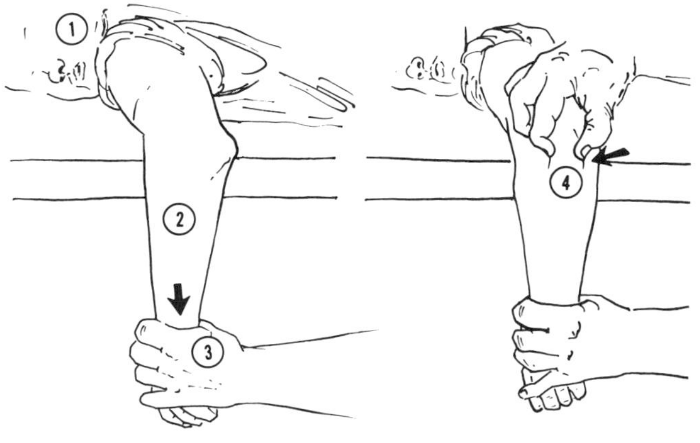

Alternative Leverage Method to Reduce Posterior Dislocation of the Elbow

Hankan has shown that posterior dislocation can be reduced using leverage of the surgeon's forearm. This can be accomplished without a skilled assistant or special equipment.

1. Under local anesthetic or light sedation, the patient's dislocated elbow is positioned with the forearm fully supinated.
2. The surgeon's forearm opposes the volar surface of the dislocated forearm.
3. The fingers are interlocked in a clasping grip.

Note: If the patient is long limbed, the surgeon may choose to grasp the wrist rather than the hand.

4. The surgeon's hand then guides the flexion of the patient's elbow, and the interposed forearm of the surgeon serves as a lever to achieve reduction.

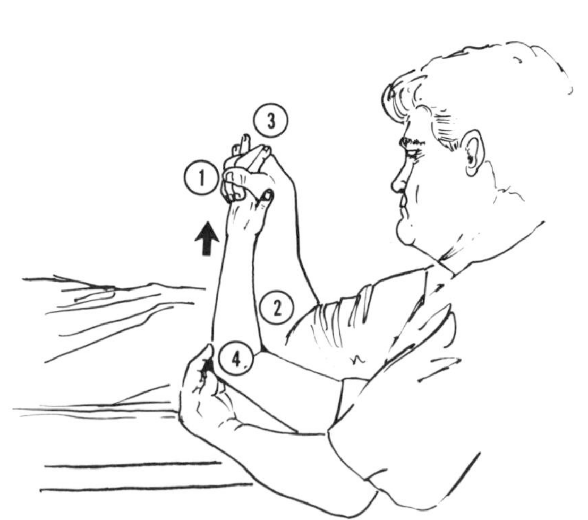

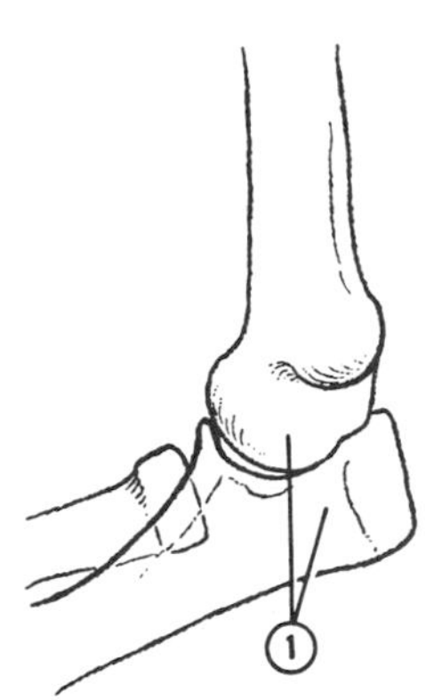

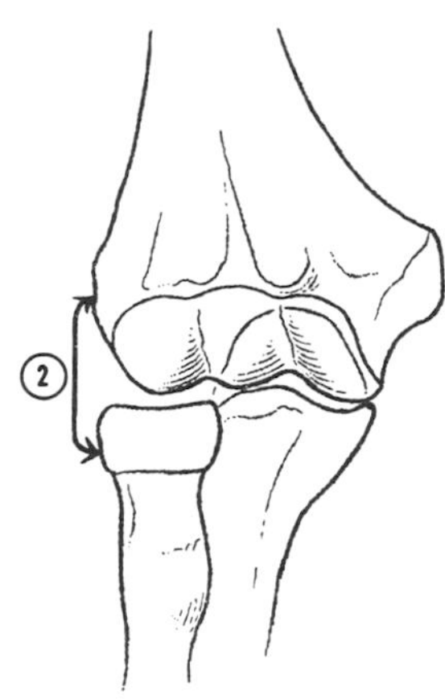

Postreduction X-Ray

1. The articular surface of the humerus is in its normal position in relation to the ulna.
2. Both bones have been restored from a lateral position to their normal positions in relation to the humerus.

Immobilization

1. Apply a posterior plaster splint from the upper arm to the base of the fingers.
2. Flex the elbow to 90° or as much as swelling will permit without embarrassing the circulation. Maintain the supinated position and avoid pronating the forearm.
3. Fix the plaster splint with a cotton elastic bandage.
4. Suspend the arm with a collar and cuff.

Note: Avoid the use of a circular cast, which would add considerably to the risk of ischemic muscle injury. Always check carefully after reduction for alteration in distal CMS (circulation, motor, sensory) function.

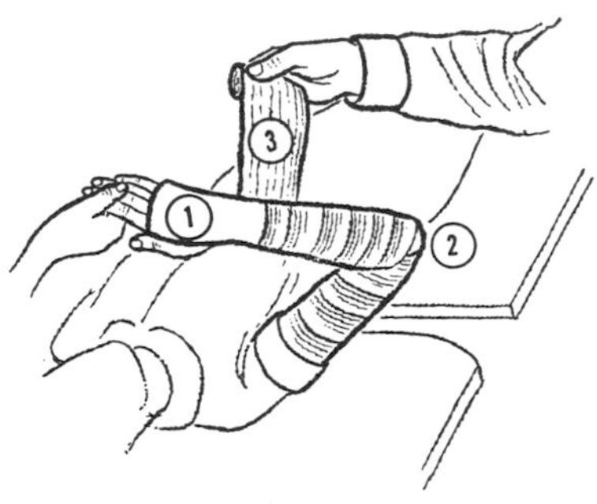

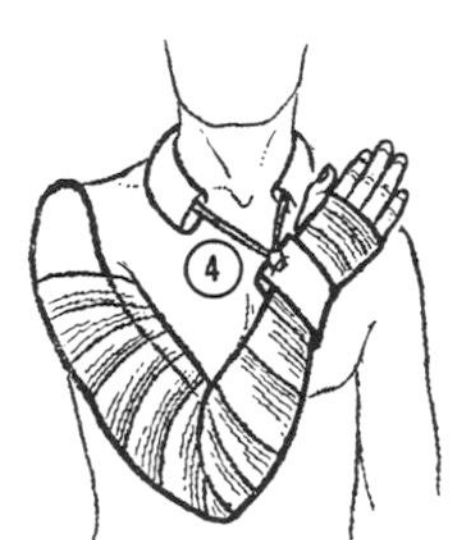

Postreduction Management

The patient and his or her injured arm should be observed carefully for the first 24–36 hours to detect any signs of circulatory embarrassment. As the swelling subsides, usually by 3–5 days, the stable elbow should be exercised actively to regain full flexion and extension.

Prolonged immobilization for more than 2 weeks after an elbow dislocation tends to leave the elbow with some permanent residual loss of motion, particularly loss of extension. In most patients this is not disabling, but for some, particularly those who play racket sports, this loss of full extension is annoying.

For the rare injury that proves to be unstable after reduction, immobilization with the elbow flexed for 2–3 weeks is usually necessary. However, if the instability was due to a fracture of the radial head or an associated olecranon fracture, operative stabilization may be necessary. Caution the patient to avoid passive stretching of the elbow because this can cause myositis ossificans to develop in the brachialis muscle.

Anterior Dislocation of the Elbow Joint

REMARKS

This lesion is very rare. It is usually associated with a fracture of the olecranon. There is severe soft tissue trauma, especially neurovascular.

Prereduction X-Ray

1. The olecranon is in front of the anterior surface of the lower end of the humerus.
2. The radial head is in front of and proximal to the external condyle.

Note: Always check carefully prior to reduction for alteration in distal CMS (circulation, motor, sensory) function.

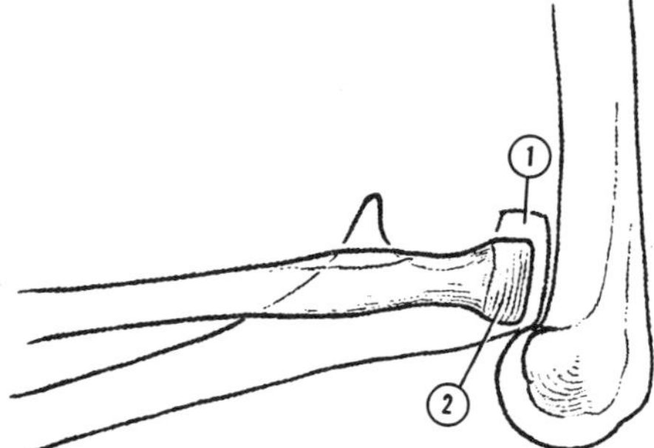

Management

Manipulative Reduction

Reduction is performed with the patient under local or general anesthesia.

1. An assistant grasps the arm and makes countertraction.
2. The operator grasps the wrist with one hand and makes traction in the line of the arm, and
3. With the other hand applies firm, steady pressure downward and backward on the upper end of the forearm. A click usually indicates that reduction is achieved.

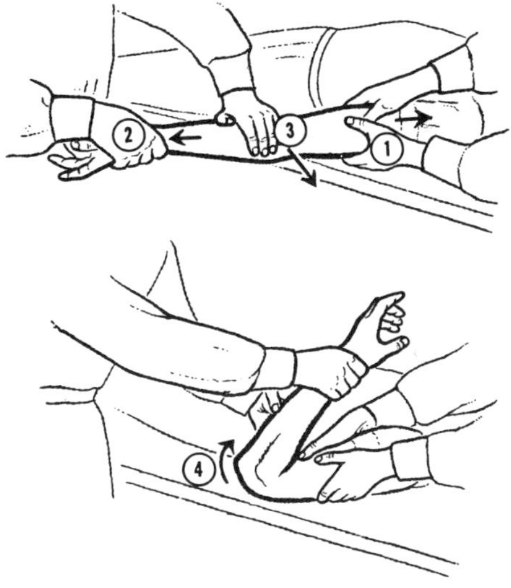

4. The arm is flexed to 45° beyond a right angle.

Evaluation of Stability

Following reduction,

1. Gently move the elbow through its normal range to check stability in extension.
2. If the elbow is unstable in extension, several diagnoses are possible: (a) in a child, entrapment of the medial epicondyle; (b) in an adult, unstable fracture of the radial head or the olecranon; or (c) posterolateral disruption of the capsule.

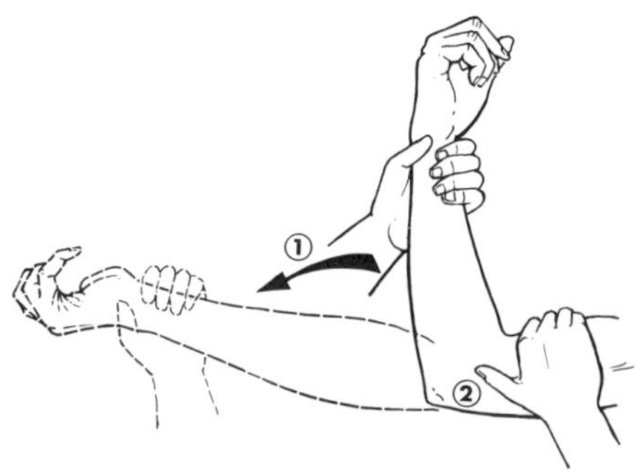

Immobilization

1. Apply a posterior plaster slab from the upper arm to the base of the fingers.
2. Hold the arm at an angle of 135°.
3. Encircle the arm and slab with a cotton elastic bandage.
4. Support the arm in a triangular sling.

Note: Avoid the use of a circular cast, which would add considerably to the risk of ischemic injury. Always check carefully after reduction for alteration in distal CMS (circulation, motor, sensory) function.

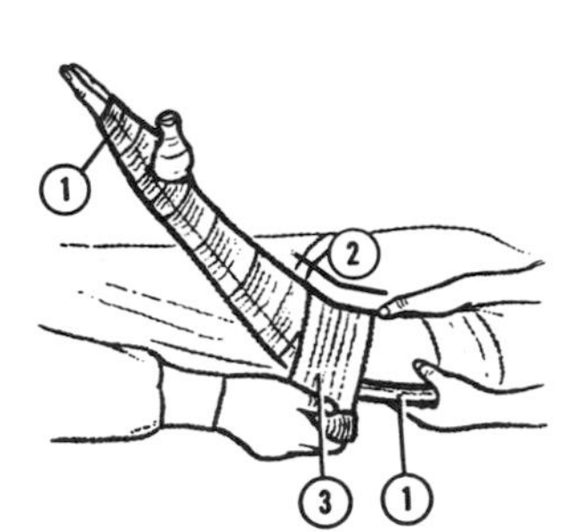

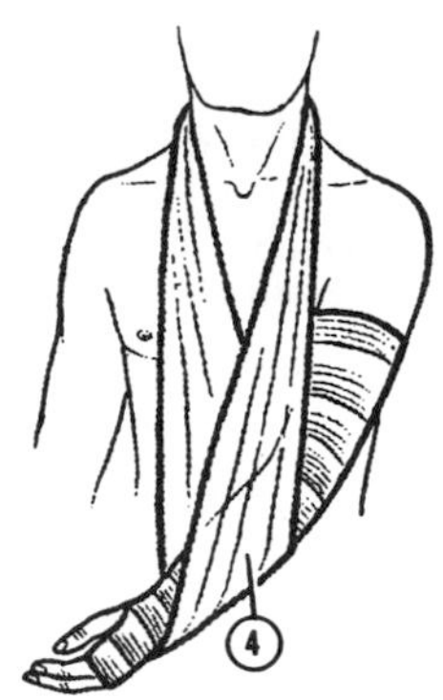

Postreduction Management

Observe the patient carefully for the first 24–36 hours for signs of circulatory impairment. If the elbow was stable immediately after reduction, allow gentle active exercises as soon as swelling subsides, usually by 3–5 days. If the elbow was unstable after reduction and no fracture was evident treat for soft tissue disruption by immobilization for 2–3 weeks.

If instability is due to fracture, open reduction may be necessary to permit early range-of-motion exercise. Emphasize the patient's need for active exercise after immobilization is discarded. Avoid passive stretching of the elbow, which has been implicated as a cause of myositis ossificans in the brachialis muscle.

■ Lateral Dislocation of the Elbow Joint

REMARKS

This lesion is rare and is usually associated with extensive soft tissue trauma. The medial ligaments are disrupted.

Typical Deformity

1. The elbow is broadened.
2. The axis of the forearm is displaced laterally in relation to the humerus.
3. The forearm is pronated.
4. The internal condyle is unduly prominent.
5. The olecranon is lateral to the external condyle.
6. The head of the radius may be prominent and readily palpable.

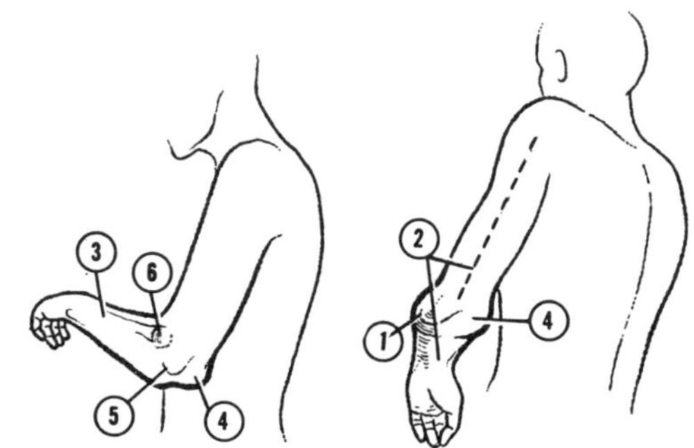

Prereduction X-Ray

1. The olecranon fossa is displaced lateral to the external condyle.
2. The forearm is pronated.
3. The radial head lies above the level of the olecranon.

Note: Always check carefully prior to reduction for alteration in distal CMS (circulation, motor, sensory) function.

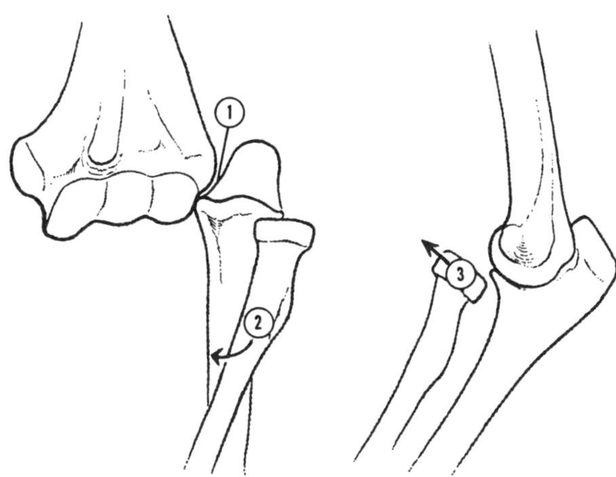

Management

Manipulative Reduction

Reduction is performed with the patient under local or general anesthesia.

1. An assistant steadies the arm.
2. The operator uses one hand to produce moderate traction at the wrist, with the elbow short of complete extension.
3. The other hand first forces the upper end of the ulna *(A)* downward, *(B)* outward, and *(C)* backward.

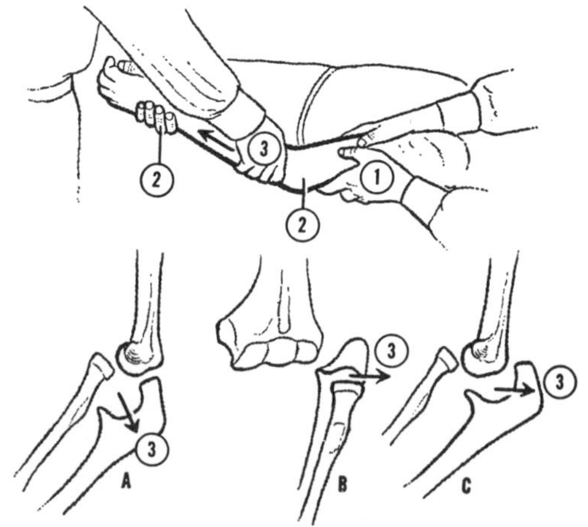

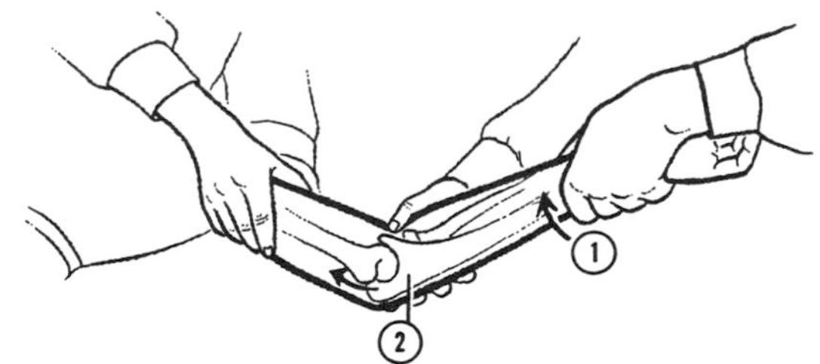

THEN

1. The operator supinates the forearm and
2. Pushes the ulna around the end of the humerus and

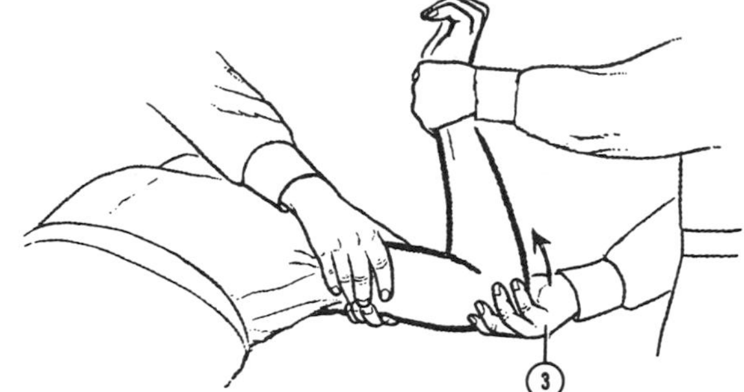

3. Flexes the elbow to a point permitted by soft tissue swelling.

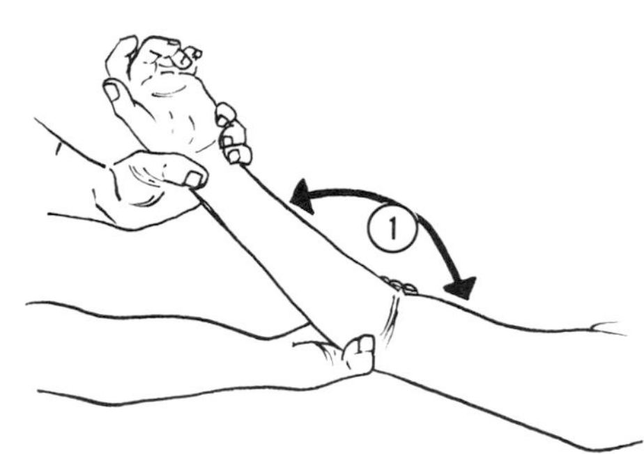

Evaluation of Stability Following Reduction

1. Gently move the elbow through normal range of motion in flexion and extension and

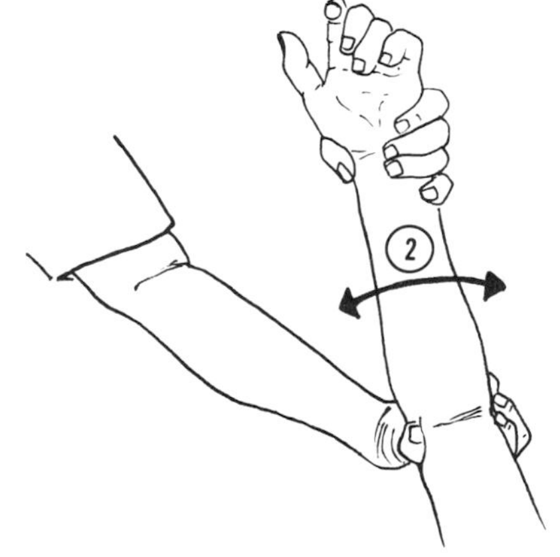

2. Medial and lateral stressing. If the elbow is unstable, several diagnoses are possible: (a) in a child, entrapment of the medial epicondyle; (b) in an adult, an unstable fracture of the radial head or olecranon; or (c) medial and lateral disruption of the capsule.

Postreduction X-Ray

1. The olecranon fossa articulates with the trochlea.
2. The radial head articulates with the capitellum.

Immobilization

1. Apply a posterior plaster slab from the upper arm to the base of the fingers.
2. Flex the elbow 90° or as much as the swelling will permit without embarrassing the circulation of the arm.
3. Fix the plaster slab with a cotton elastic bandage.
4. Suspend the arm with a collar and cuff.

Note: Avoid the use of a circular cast, which would add considerably to the risk of ischemic muscle injury. Always check carefully after reduction for alteration in distal CMS (circulation, motor, sensory) function.

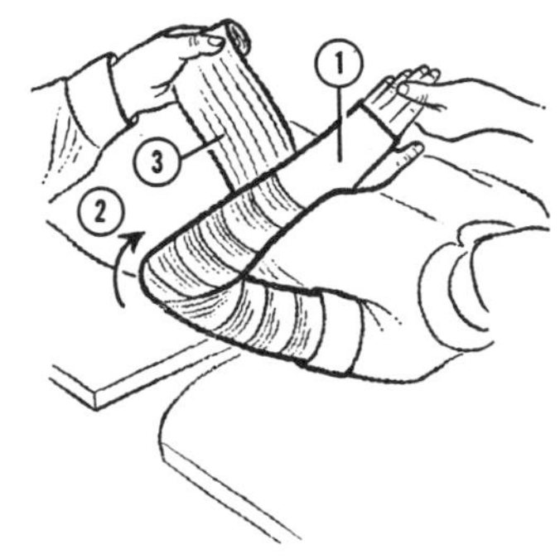

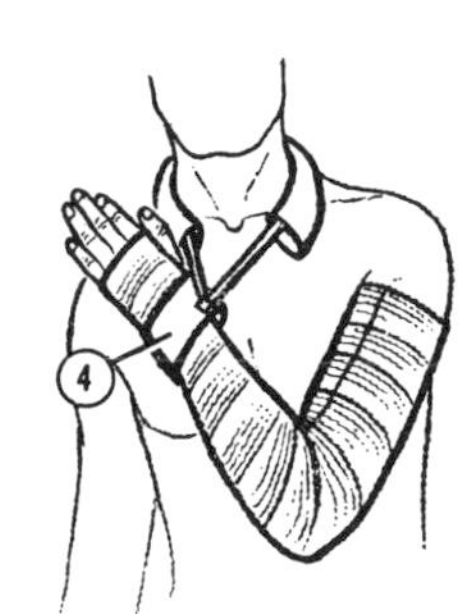

Postreduction Management

Observe the patient carefully for the first 24–36 hours for signs of circulatory impairment. If the elbow was stable immediately after reduction, allow gentle active exercises as soon as swelling subsides, usually by 3–5 days.

If the elbow was unstable after reduction and no fracture was evident, treat for soft tissue disruption by immobilization for 2–3 weeks. If instability is due to fracture, open reduction may be necessary to permit early range-of-motion exercise.

Emphasize the patient's need for active exercise after immobilization is discarded. Avoid passive stretching of the elbow, which has been implicated as a cause of myositis ossificans in the brachialis muscle.

Medial Dislocation of the Elbow Joint

REMARKS

This is a rare lesion and the amount of medial displacement of the forearm bones varies. Generally, the radial head follows the ulna; occasionally, it may maintain its normal position in relation to the capitellum. Soft tissue damage is usually severe, including rupture and tearing of the lateral ligaments.

Typical Deformity

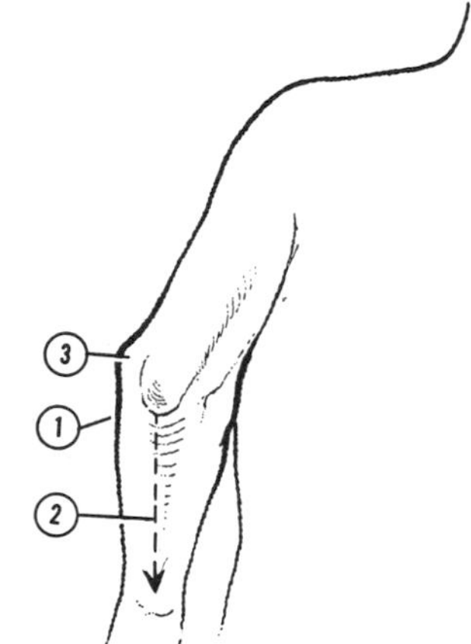

1. The elbow is broadened.
2. The long axis of the forearm is displaced inward.
3. The external condyle is unduly prominent.

Prereduction X-Ray

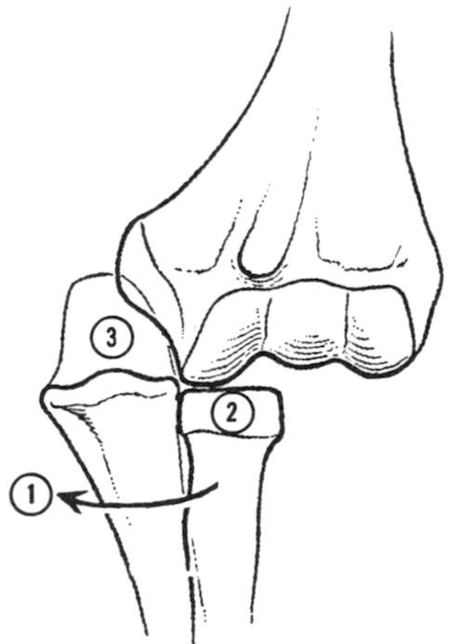

1. Both bones of the forearm have shifted medially.
2. The head of the radius rests on the trochlea.
3. The olecranon fossa is medial to the internal condyle.

Note: Always check carefully prior to reduction for alterations in distal CMS (circulation, motor, sensory) function.

Management

Manipulative Reduction

Reduction is performed with the patient under local or general anesthesia.

1. While an assistant holds the arm steady,
2. Grasp the wrist with one hand and make moderate traction in the line of the forearm with the elbow just short of complete extension.
3. While traction is maintained, with the other hand force the upper end of the ulna downward and outward; a click usually indicates complete reduction.

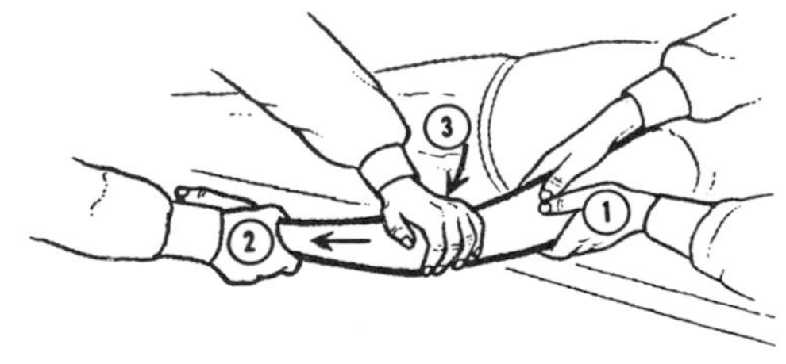

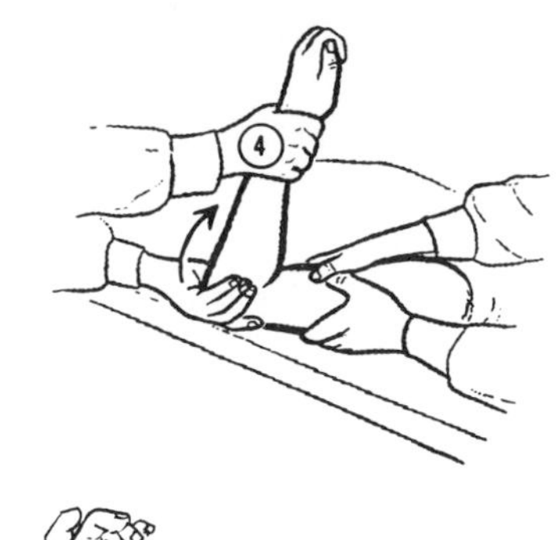

4. Release traction on the forearm and bring the forearm into as much flexion as soft tissue swelling will permit without embarrassing the circulation of the forearm and hand.

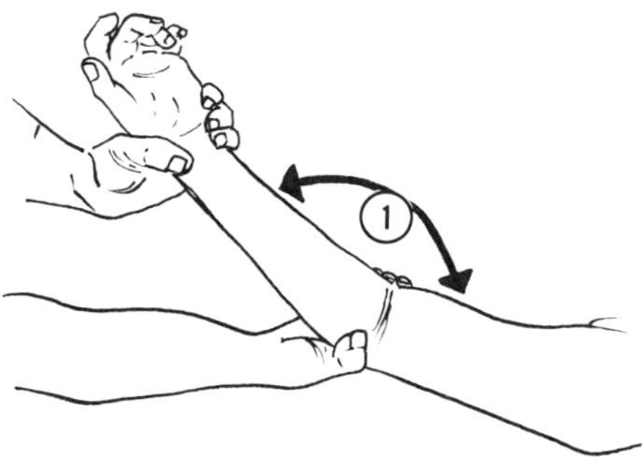

Evaluation of Stability Following Reduction

1. Gently move the elbow through normal range of motion in flexion and extension and

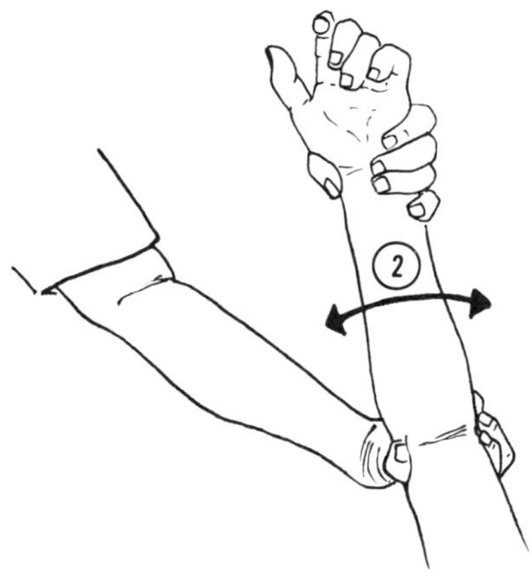

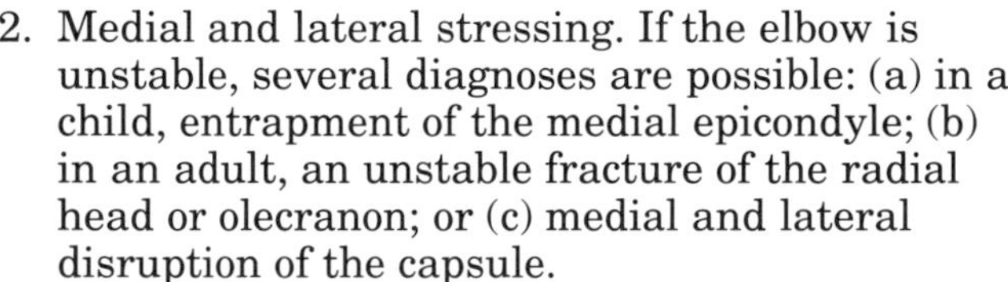

2. Medial and lateral stressing. If the elbow is unstable, several diagnoses are possible: (a) in a child, entrapment of the medial epicondyle; (b) in an adult, an unstable fracture of the radial head or olecranon; or (c) medial and lateral disruption of the capsule.

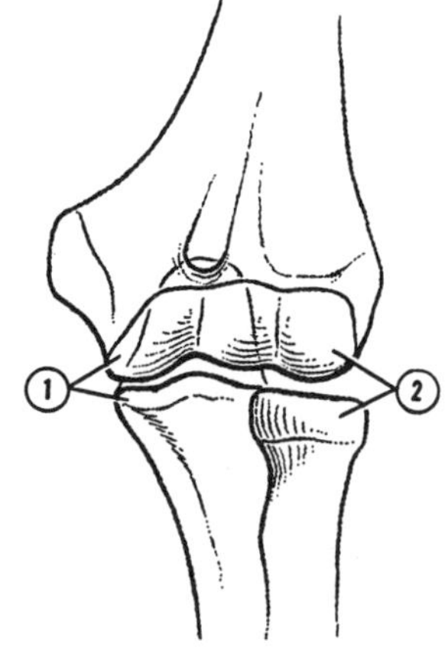

Postreduction X-Ray

1. The olecranon fossa of the ulna is in normal relation to the trochlea.
2. The radial head articulates with the capitellum.

Immobilization

1. Apply a posterior plaster slab from the upper arm to the base of the fingers with the forearm supinated.
2. Flex the elbow as much as the swelling will permit without embarrassing the circulation of the arm.
3. Fix the plaster slab with a cotton elastic bandage.
4. Suspend the arm with a collar and cuff.

Note: Avoid the use of a circular cast, which would add considerably to the risk of ischemic muscle injury. Always check carefully after reduction for alteration in distal CMS (circulation, motor, sensory) function.

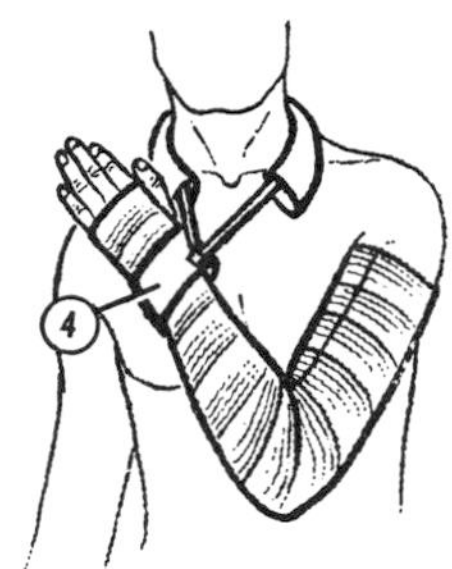

Postreduction Management

Observe the patient carefully for the first 24–36 hours for signs of circulatory impairment. If the elbow was stable immediately after reduction, then allow gentle active exercises as soon as swelling subsides, usually by 3–5 days.

If the elbow was unstable after reduction and no fracture was evident, treat for soft tissue disruption by immobilizing for 2–3 weeks. If instability is due to fracture, open reduction may be necessary to permit early range-of-motion exercise.

Emphasize the patient's need for active exercise after immobilization is discarded. Avoid passive stretching of the elbow, which has been implicated as a cause of myositis ossificans in the brachialis muscle.

Divergent Dislocation of the Elbow Joint

REMARKS

This lesion is extremely rare and occurs only if the annular and interosseous ligaments, which bind the radius and ulna, are completely disrupted. The two bones may then be displaced in an anteroposterior or a medial-lateral direction.

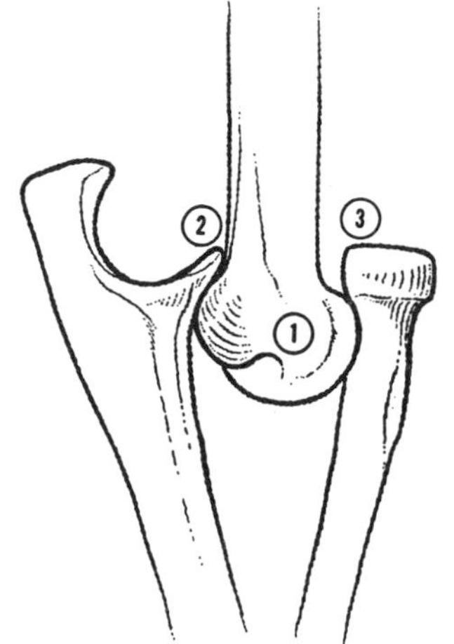

Anteroposterior Type

1. The distal end of the humerus lies between the two forearm bones.
2. The ulna is behind the humerus.
3. The radius is in front of the humerus.

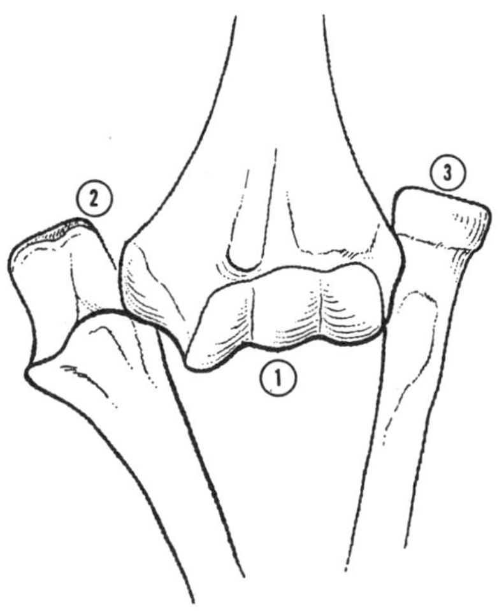

Medial-Lateral Type

1. The distal end of the humerus lies between the forearm bones.
2. The ulna is displaced medially.
3. The radius is displaced laterally.

Note: Always check carefully prior to reduction for alteration in distal CMS (circulation, motor, sensory) function.

Management

Manipulative Reduction

ANTEROPOSTERIOR TYPE

1. While an assistant steadies the arm,
2. Make steady traction on the extended forearm with one hand and
3. Backward pressure on the ulna with the other hand. When the sigmoid engages the trochlea,
4. Make firm downward pressure on the radial head and
5. Flex the arm to the limit permitted by the soft tissue swelling and the supinated forearm.

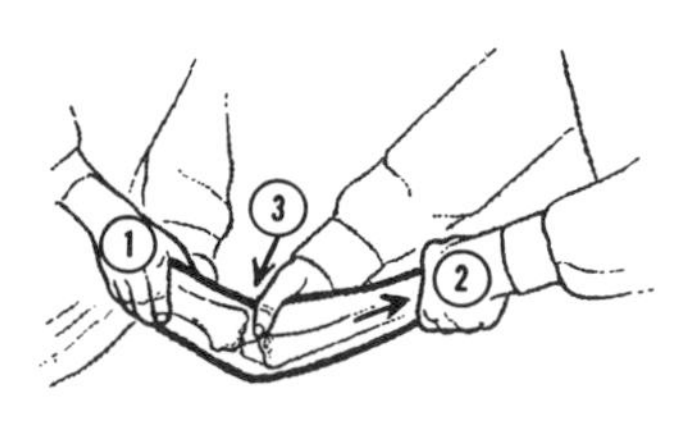

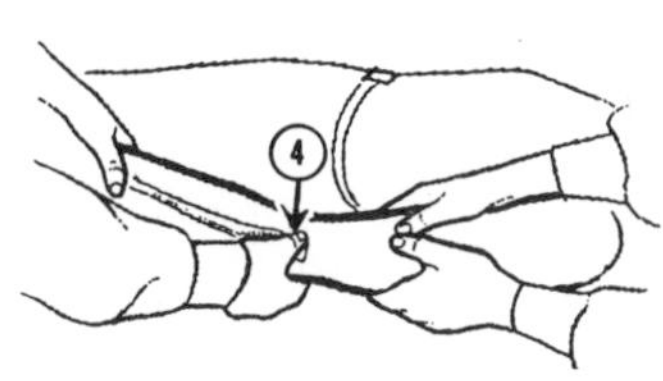

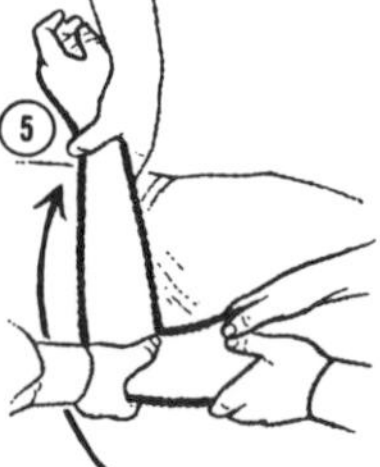

LATERAL TYPE

1. While an assistant steadies the arm,
2. Make steady traction on the extended forearm with one hand and
3. Downward pressure on the upper end of the forearm with the other hand; then,
4. Squeeze together the radius and the ulna and
5. Flex the forearm to a point permitted by the soft tissue swelling.
6. Supinate the forearm.

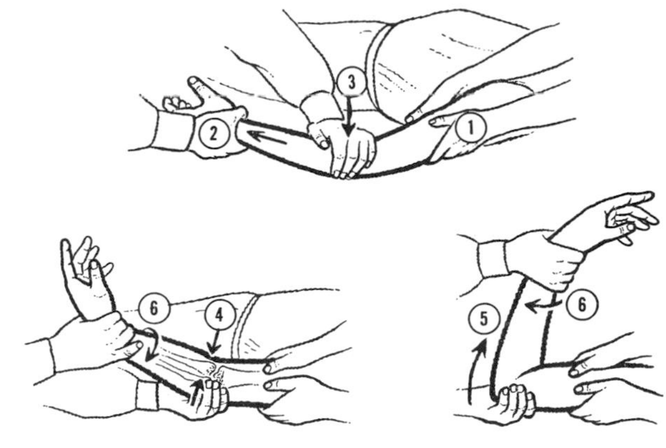

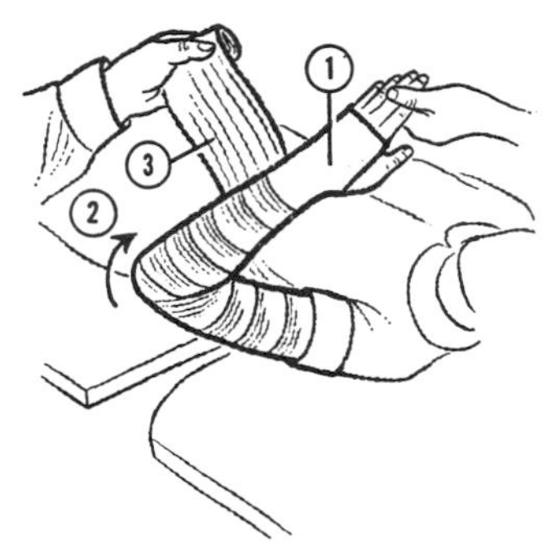

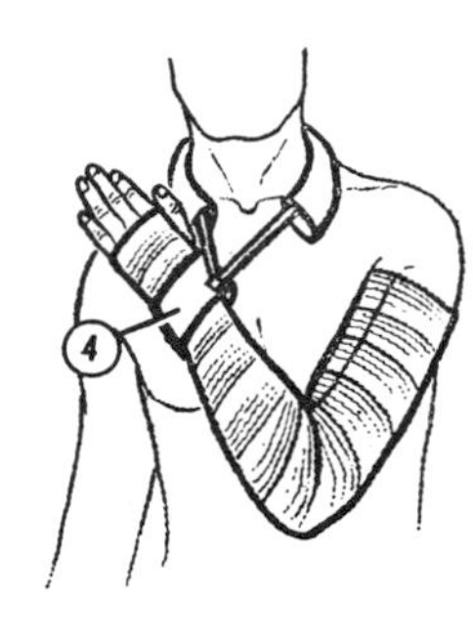

Note: Evaluate stability by passive flexion and extension of the elbow. Disruption of the soft tissues to the degree sufficient to produce this dislocation usually necessitates performing reconstructive procedures after the swelling of the acute injury has subsided. Always check carefully after reduction for alteration in distal CMS (circulation, motor, sensory) function.

Immobilization

1. Apply a posterior plaster slab from the upper arm to the base of the fingers.
2. Flex the elbow as much as swelling will permit without embarrassing the circulation of the arm.
3. Fix the plaster slab with a cotton elastic bandage.
4. Suspend the arm with a collar and cuff.

Postreduction Management

This injury can cause considerable instability of the radius and ulna depending on the extent of disruption of the annular and interosseous ligaments. Because the injury is most common in children, a trial period of immobilization in a posterior splint is indicated unless closed reduction is not possible.

If the radius and ulna are reduced at the time of elbow reduction, the arm may be immobilized in a posterior splint for 3 weeks with the elbow flexed 90°. The forearm is maintained in supination.

After this period of immobilization, the stability can be re-evaluated and the patient encouraged to start on range-of-motion exercises for the elbow. If the elbow is unstable and the radial head tends to dislocate, reconstruction of the annular ligament is necessary.

■ Proximal Radial Translocation With Dislocation

REMARKS

This is a rare injury that has only been reported in a few cases. It is most often associated with dislocation in the child. Proximal translocation may go unrecognized unless the x-rays after reduction are carefully scrutinized.

In this situation the proximal part of the radius crosses over the proximal part of the ulna to articulate with the trochlea. The ulna then articulates with the capitellum. The mechanism of this crossover is difficult to explain, although it may be a combination of a posterolateral dislocation associated with pronation of the forearm. Characteristically the young patient presents after reduction and splint removal with a painful, stiff elbow. The forearm is usually held in pronation and no supination is possible.

Any reduction of elbow dislocation should avoid pronating the forearm because this tends to displace the radius over the ulna and may be partially responsible for this rare translocation. The reduction technique should supinate the forearm to maintain the normal relationship between the radius and the ulna.

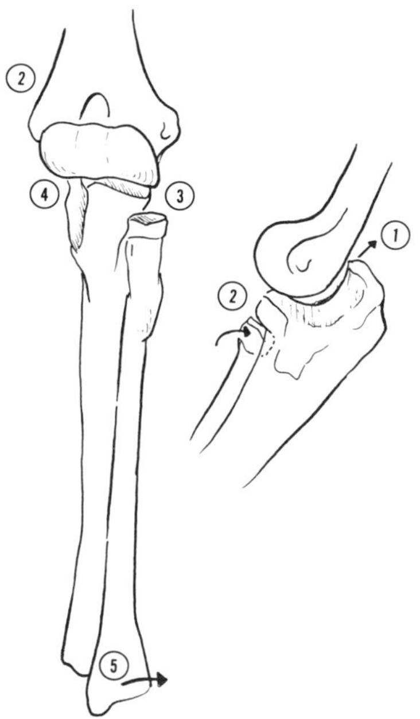

Mechanism

1. The mechanism of proximal translocation may be a posterolateral dislocation,
2. Associated with pronation of the forearm.
3. The result is that the radius is forced to articulate with the trochlea while
4. The ulna articulates with the capitellum.
5. Reduction of an elbow dislocation should avoid pronating the forearm because this may displace the radius over the ulna and occasionally produce a translocation, especially in children.

Management

This injury has not been successfully reduced by closed manipulation. It may be possible to achieve reduction in an acute injury with adequate anesthetic by gently supinating the forearm prior to reduction of the posterolateral elbow dislocation.

In all reported instances, this rare injury has required open reduction of the dislocations because it usually presents as a complication and is recognized late in the course of treatment.

Fractures Associated With Dislocation of the Elbow Joint

REMARKS

Approximately 30 per cent of elbow dislocations will sustain associated fractures, most commonly avulsion fractures of the medial epicondyle in the child or of the coronoid process in the adult. In general, these fractures can be ignored and the patient treated for the primary problem of dislocation.

Immobilization for more than 5–7 days is unnecessary; in fact, prolonged immobilization (4–6 weeks) to achieve x-ray union of minor avulsion fractures associated with dislocations may cause significant and prolonged elbow stiffness, even in young children. Results of elbow dislocation associated with fracture tend to be worse in both children and adults than are the results of dislocation alone. One reason is the severity of the initial injury. Another major factor is treatment of the fracture by prolonged external immobilization.

The major consideration in a child with an avulsion fracture of the medial epicondyle is whether the fragment has displaced into the joint or whether it includes a portion of the unossified trochlea. Gross displacement of an epicondylar fragment to the level of the elbow joint raises these possibilities as well as the need for operative repair. Minimally displaced epicondylar fractures should be treated symptomatically and should not necessitate prolonging immobilization for more than 1–2 weeks (see also Chapter 2).

In most instances an associated coronoid fracture does not contribute to instability of the elbow, and therefore range-of-motion exercises need not be delayed after reduction because of a minimally displaced coronoid process fracture. A fracture of the olecranon associated with the dislocation can cause the elbow to be unstable. This combination is a major indication for early operative intervention. For such a fracture-dislocation, internal fixation of the ulna is usually necessary to stabilize the dislocation of the elbow.

Radial head fractures associated with elbow dislocations may also be a source of elbow instability. The undisplaced radial head fracture may need nothing more than a brief period of temporary support. However, the stability of the elbow after reduction should be carefully evaluated by flexion and extension, and medial and lateral stressing. If such a test of elbow stability demonstrates that the radial head fracture causes the elbow to redislocate, operative stabilization is indicated.

Posterior Dislocation of the Elbow and Fracture of the Coronoid Process

REMARKS

Fracture of the coronoid frequently complicates posterior dislocation of the elbow. The fracture can usually be ignored. Reduction of the dislocation and immobilization in acute flexion usually result in healing of the fracture with no dysfunction.

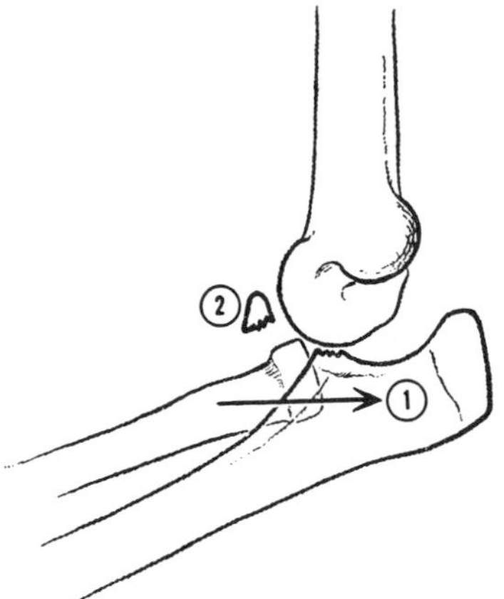

Prereduction X-Ray

1. Posterior dislocation of the ulna and radius.
2. Fracture of the coronoid process with moderate displacement due to pull of the brachialis muscle.

Management

Manipulative Reduction

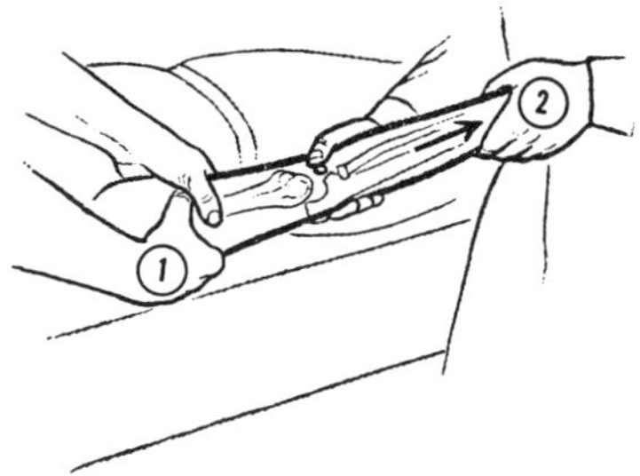

Note: Before reduction, aspiration of the elbow will relieve pain from hemarthrosis, and a local anesthetic may also be instilled.

1. An assistant steadies the arm.
2. The operator makes steady traction in the line of the elbow.

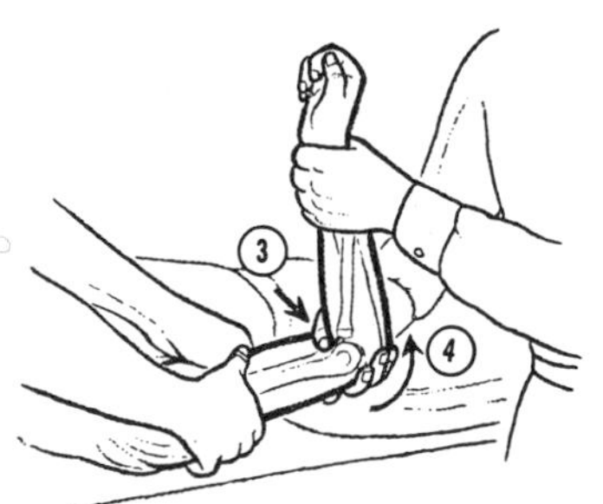

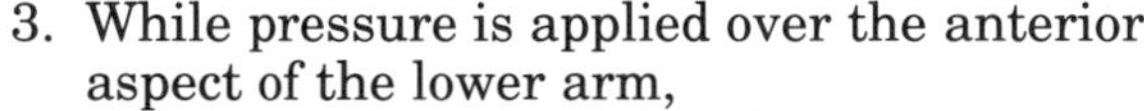

3. While pressure is applied over the anterior aspect of the lower arm,
4. The forearm is flexed acutely.

EVALUATION OF STABILITY

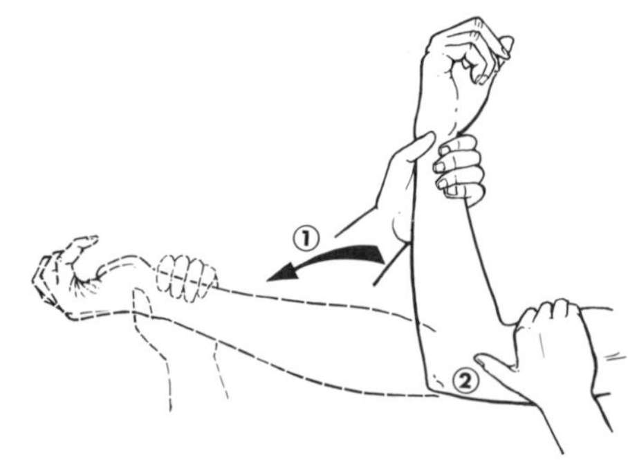

Following reduction,

1. Gently move the elbow through its normal range to check stability in extension.
2. If the elbow is unstable in extension, it must be immobilized for 2–3 weeks to allow for healing of the anterior disruption. Ordinarily, a fracture of the coronoid process does not affect postreduction stability or require prolonged immobilization.

Note: For further discussion of coronoid process fractures see page 1275.

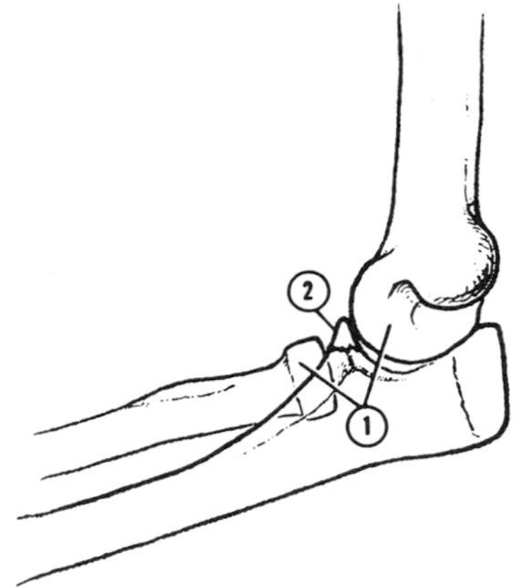

Postreduction X-Ray (Stable Elbow)

1. The radius and ulna are in their normal anatomic positions in relation to the distal end of the humerus.
2. The fragments of the coronoid are in apposition.

Note: Even if the coronoid fragment remains displaced, it usually may be ignored.

Postreduction Management

Observe the patient carefully for the first 24–36 hours for signs of circulatory impairment. If the elbow was stable immediately after reduction, allow gentle active exercises as soon as swelling subsides, usually in 3–5 days. If the elbow was unstable after reduction, treat for soft tissue disruption and immobilize the elbow in flexion for 2–3 weeks.

Emphasize the patient's need for active exercises after immobilization is discontinued. Avoid passive stretching of the elbow, which has been implicated as a cause of myositis ossificans in the brachialis muscle.

Dislocation of the Elbow With Fracture of the Radial Head

REMARKS

An associated fracture of the radial head is relatively common in elbow dislocations in the adult. In contrast to a capitellar fracture, which displaces superiorly into the radial fossa, a radial head fracture displaces distally when associated with an elbow dislocation (also see the section on fractures of the capitellum).

Aspirate the elbow at the time local anesthetic is instilled, and evaluate the ranges of elbow motion and forearm rotation after reduction. If the elbow is stable when range of motion is tested after reduction, it may be treated as a dislocation without a fracture; that is, after 3–5 days range of motion may be started and the sling may be gradually discarded.

If the elbow proves unstable due to the radial head fracture, operative treatment is indicated. The radial head fracture is best repaired and fixed internally to permit stabilization of the unstable elbow. An alternative to internal fixation, if the radial head is extremely comminuted, is replacement of the radial head with interpositional arthroplasty (Swanson or other type).

Prereduction X-Ray

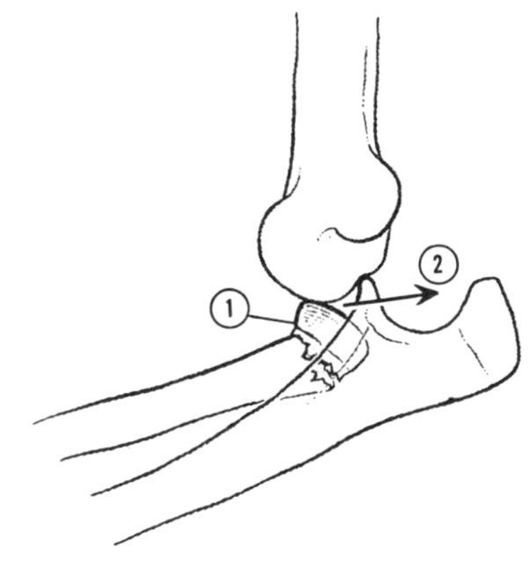

1. Posterior dislocation of the elbow.
2. Fracture of the radial head with displacement of the fragments.

Management

Manipulative Reduction

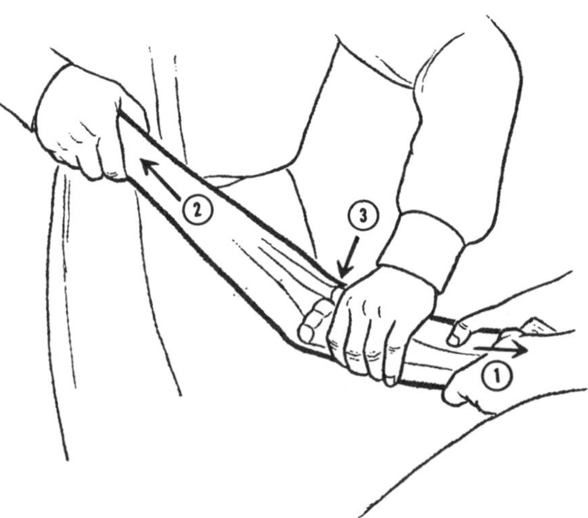

Note: Aspiration of the elbow will relieve pain from hemarthrosis and allow instillation of local anesthetic.

1. While an assistant holds the arm and makes steady countertraction,
2. Grasp the wrist with one hand and make steady traction on the forearm in the position in which it lies.
3. While traction is maintained, apply direct pressure to the radial head fracture.

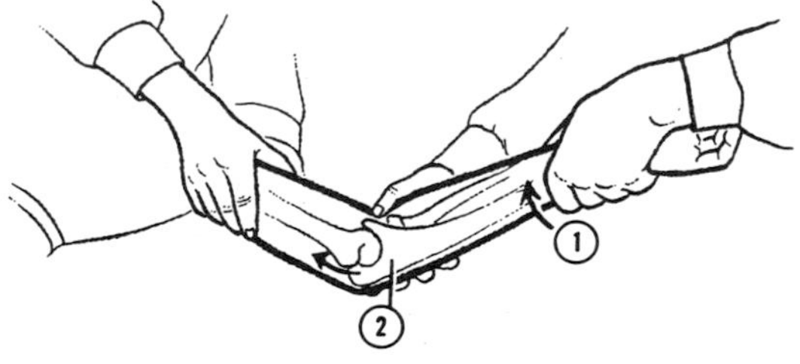

1. Supinate the forearm with direct pressure over the radial head.
2. Push the ulna upward around the end of the humerus.

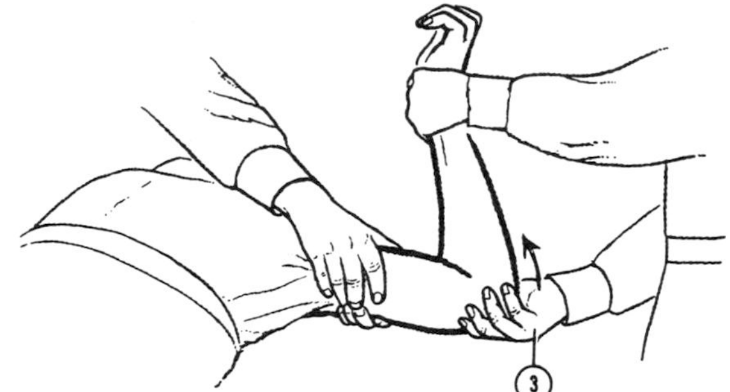

3. Flex the elbow after reduction of the dislocation to the point permitted by soft tissue swelling.

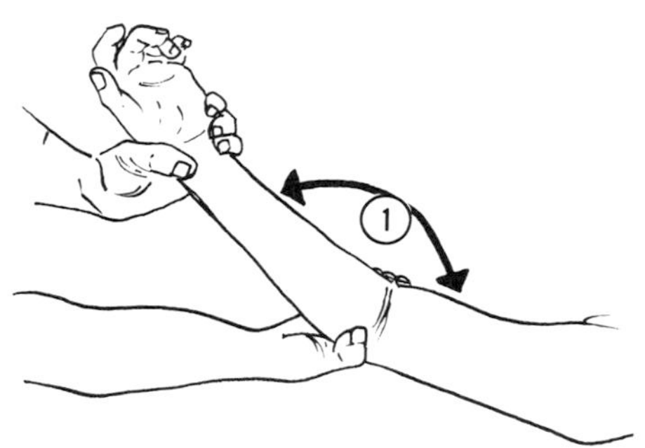

Evaluation of Stability Following Reduction

1. Gently move the elbow through normal range of motion in flexion and extension and

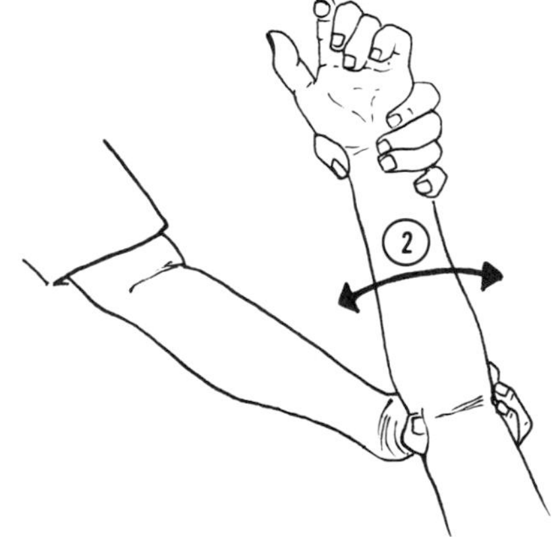

2. Medial and lateral stressing. If the elbow is unstable several diagnoses are possible: (a) in a child, entrapment of the medial epicondyle; (b) in an adult, an unstable fracture of the radial head or olecranon; or (c) medial and lateral disruption of the capsule.

Postreduction X-Ray (Stable Elbow)

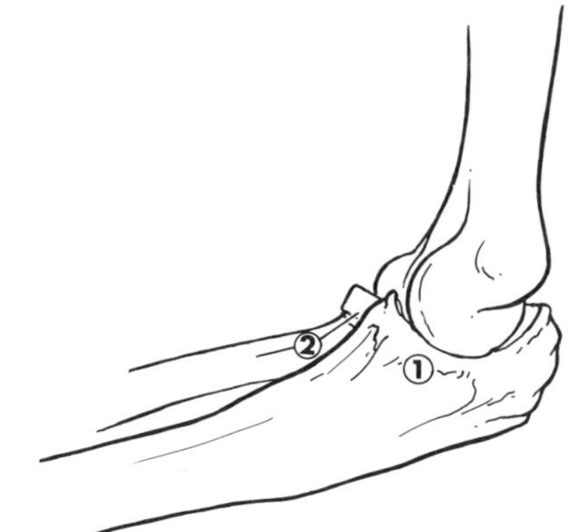

1. The elbow dislocation has been reduced.
2. The radial head fracture remains angulated slightly but does not cause the elbow to be unstable.

Note: This stable type of injury may be treated by early mobilization (5–7 days) of the elbow as soon as the swelling subsides and the patient's symptoms allow. Careful follow-up, however, is necessary to be sure that the dislocation does not recur in the first several weeks as elbow motion begins.

Immobilization

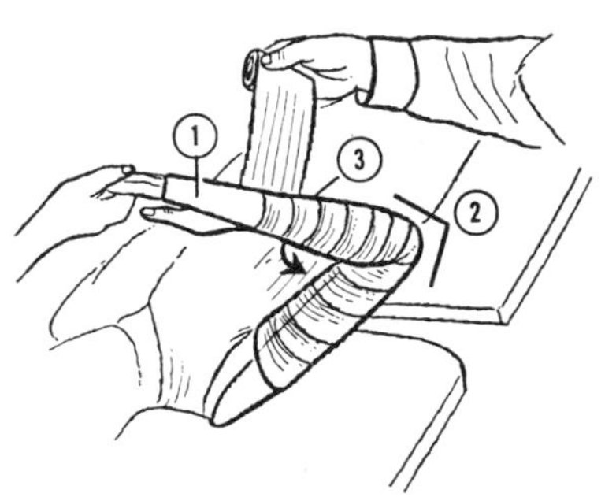

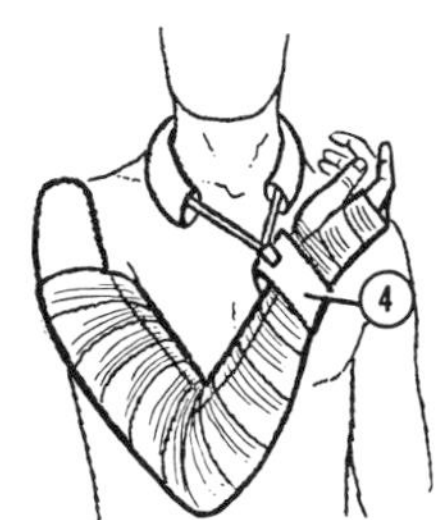

1. Apply a posterior plaster slab from the axilla to the base of the fingers.
2. The forearm is in flexion.
3. The forearm is fully supinated.
4. Suspend the arm with a collar-and-cuff sling.

Note: Avoid the use of a circular cast, which would add considerably to the risk of ischemic muscle injury. Always check carefully before and after reduction for alteration in distal CMS (circulation, motor, sensory) function.

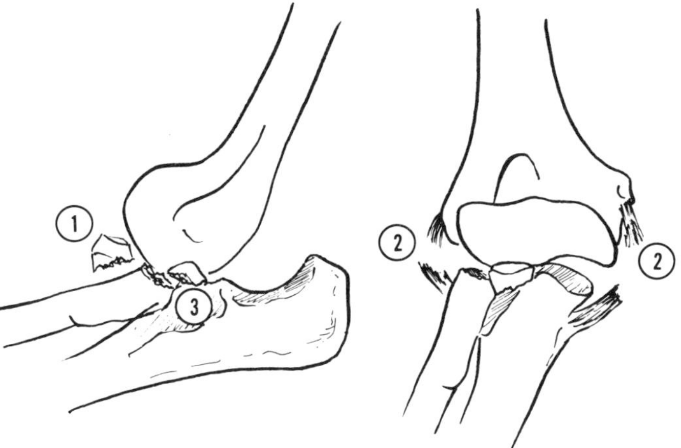

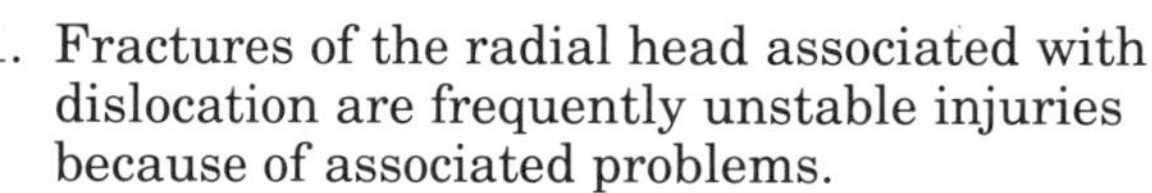

1. Fractures of the radial head associated with dislocation are frequently unstable injuries because of associated problems.
2. Frequently the collateral ligaments or
3. The anterior aspect of the olecranon may also be injured.

Caution: Particularly avoid excising the radial head if there is any evidence of injury to the coronoid process or medial capsular structure. Excision of the radial head in this situation only leads to further instability.

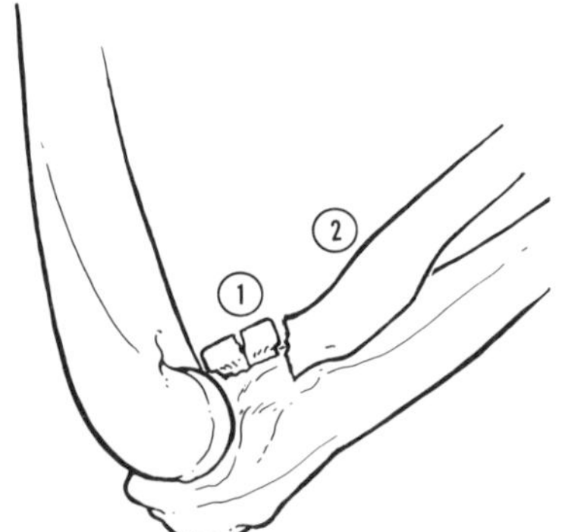

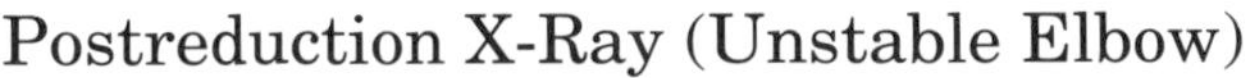

Postreduction X-Ray (Unstable Elbow)

1. The radial head fracture has displaced.
2. This causes subluxation of the elbow with a flexion or medial-lateral stressing.

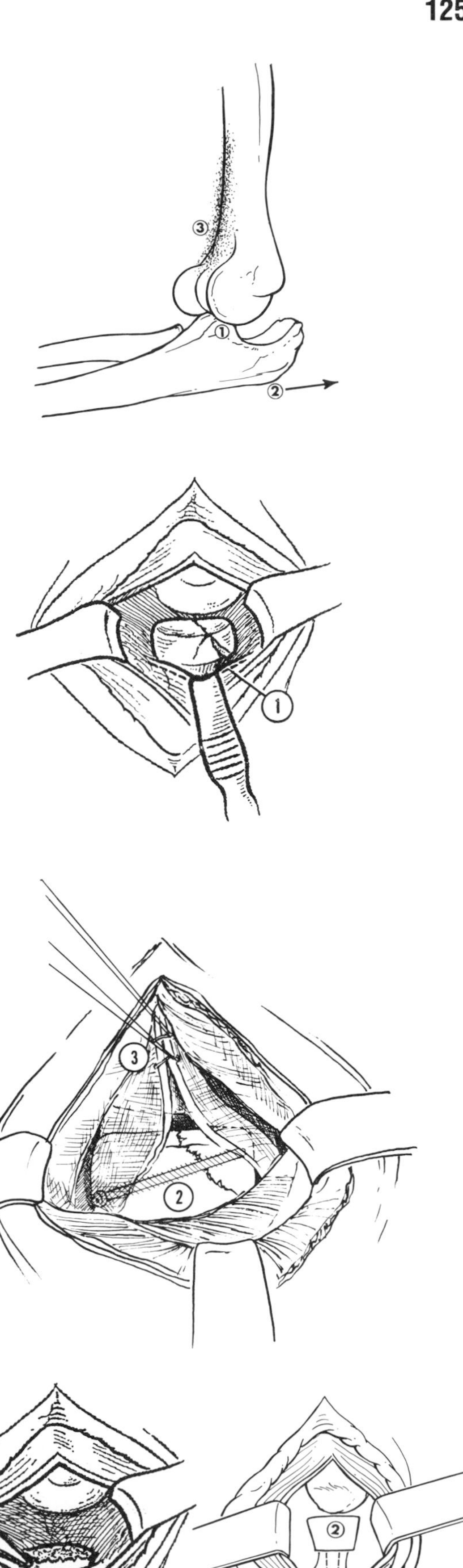

Pitfalls of Excising Radial Head Fracture Associated With Dislocation

1. Excising the radial head fragments without restoring stability can lead to
2. Posterior subluxation and
3. Problems with myositis ossificans in the anterior aspect of the elbow. The result is not only instability but considerable stiffening and loss of elbow function under these circumstances.

Operative Repair of the Radial Head Fracture Causing Instability

1. The radial head fracture is opened and the fracture fragments are reduced as anatomically as possible.
2. Fragments are then fixed with a small cancellous screw.
3. The surrounding posterolateral capsular ligaments are repaired to add further to stability.

Alternative Method for Comminuted Radial Head Fracture with Dislocation

1. The fracture fragments are surgically excised.
2. The radial head is replaced with interpositional arthroplasty to add stability to the elbow.

Note: The surrounding posterolateral capsule ligaments are also repaired to aid in elbow stability.

Forward Dislocation of the Elbow With Fracture of the Olecranon

REMARKS

Generally there is anterior subluxation or dislocation of both bones of the forearm. Usually the radius retains its relationship with the ulna because of the orbicular ligament attachment and moves forward with the ulna. Occasionally the ligamentous support will be completely disrupted and the radius will dislocate separately from the ulna.

The radial nerve as well as the ulnar nerve may be injured. Always check for nerve as well as circulatory deficit. The injury is reduced readily by applying traction to the extended forearm. Maintenance of reduction requires internal fixation of the fracture in adults. In children, closed treatment usually permits stable reduction. (see also the discussion of Monteggia's fracture in Chapters 2 and 15)

Prereduction X-Ray

1. Comminuted fracture of the olecranon.
2. The radius and ulna have moved together to an anterior position.

Operative Management

Reduction

1. The fracture and dislocation are reduced by traction on the extended forearm.
2. The fragments are held in apposition by towel clips.

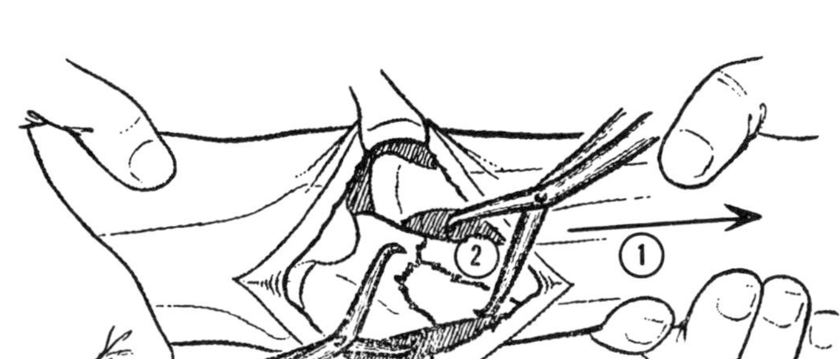

Tension-Band Wiring

1. Steinmann pins are drilled down to the medullary canal to stabilize the fracture and a tension-band wire is inserted transversely into the ulnar cortex distal to the fracture.

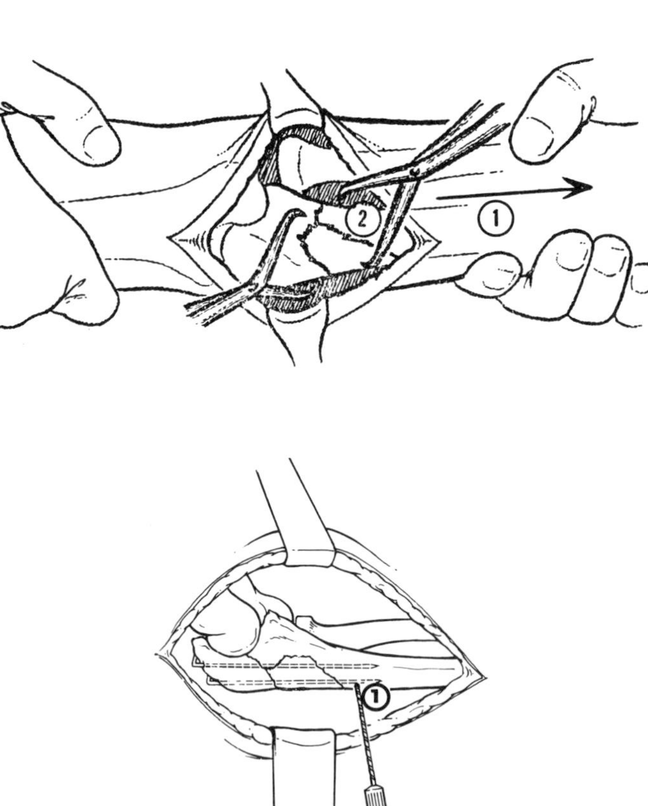

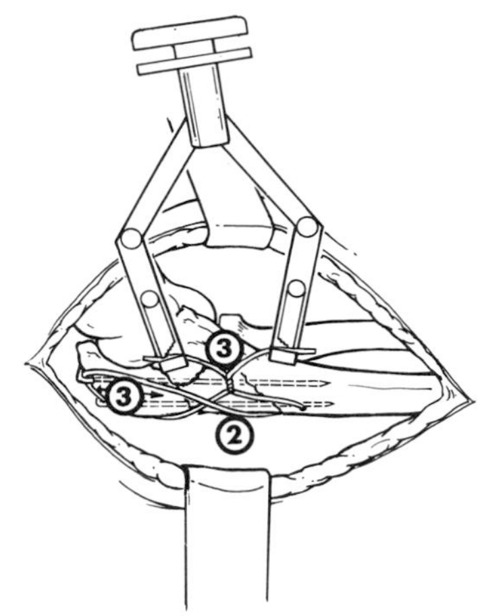

2. A 20-gauge wire is passed through the hole in the distal ulna and tightened to further stabilize the fracture. This is called a *tension wire* to neutralize the pull on the triceps and to close the fracture through the articular surface.
3. The wire may be tightened with a wire tightener or a Kirschner wire bow.

Note: The stability of the fractured ulna usually is sufficient to reduce the dislocated elbow. However, the stability of the fixation needs to be evaluated by flexing and extending the joint.

Intraoperative X-Ray

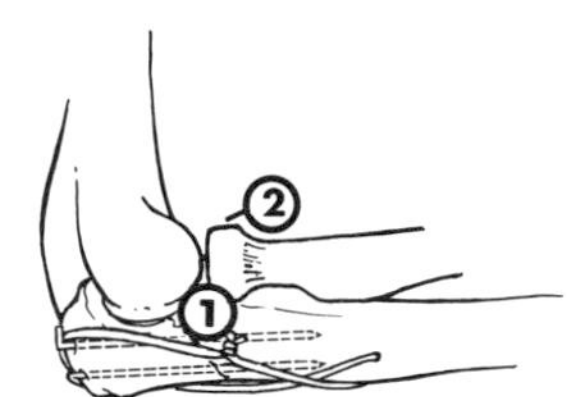

1. The fragments of the olecranon are in normal anatomic alignment.
2. The ulna and radius are in normal positions in relation to the articular surface of the humerus.

Postoperative Immobilization

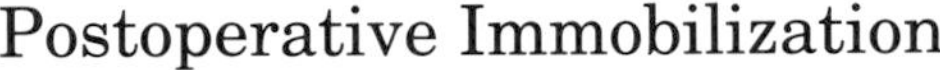

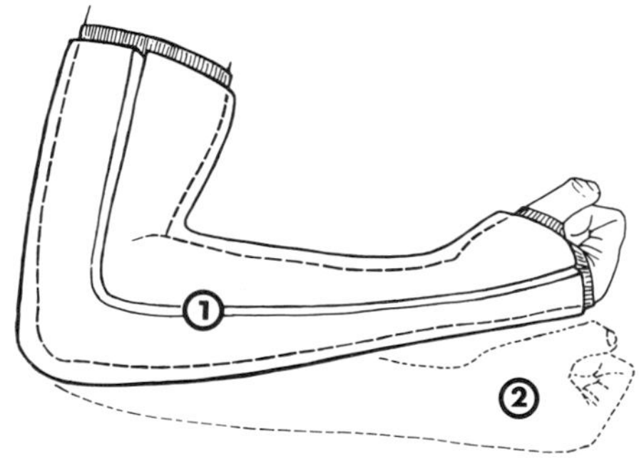

1. A bivalved cast or splint is applied.
2. Active range of motion is begun out of the plaster as soon as the swelling subsides around the elbow. This should concentrate particularly on regaining elbow flexion.

Anterior Displacement of the Radius and Ulna (Side-Swipe Fracture) With Multiple Fractures

REMARKS

Generally the lesion comprises:

- Fracture of the shaft of the humerus.
- Fracture of the olecranon.
- Fracture of the shaft of the ulna.
- Anterior displacement of the radius and ulna.

Note: Occasionally the shaft of the radius is fractured or the radial head may be fractured or dislocated.

The prime concern is reduction of the dislocation and maintenance of the position. Lag-screw fixation of the olecranon and tension-band plating of the ulna shaft fracture generally give effective stability. Closed treatment is usually possible for the humeral fracture if elbow motion is allowed.

Prereduction X-Ray

1. Fracture of the olecranon.
2. Fracture of the shaft of the ulna.
3. Fracture of the shaft of the humerus.
4. Forward displacement of the radius and ulna.

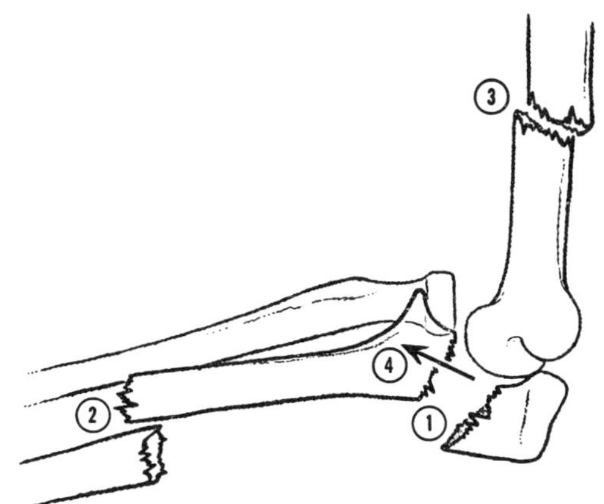

Management

Operative Reduction

1. The olecranon fracture and radial head dislocation are reduced and held with a tenaculum.
2. Several lag screws are inserted across the olecranon fracture or

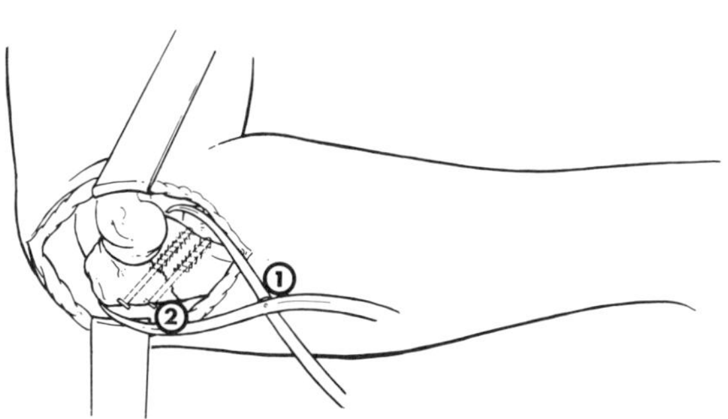

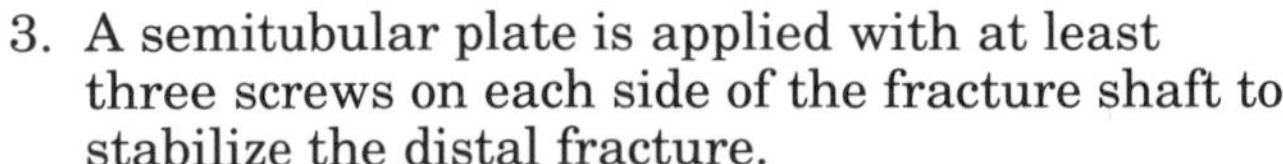

3. A semitubular plate is applied with at least three screws on each side of the fracture shaft to stabilize the distal fracture.

Note: When there is significant comminution of the fracture, a cancellous bone graft should also be utilized.

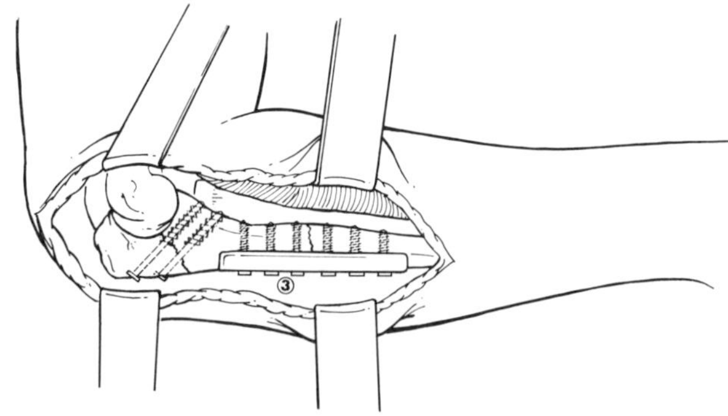

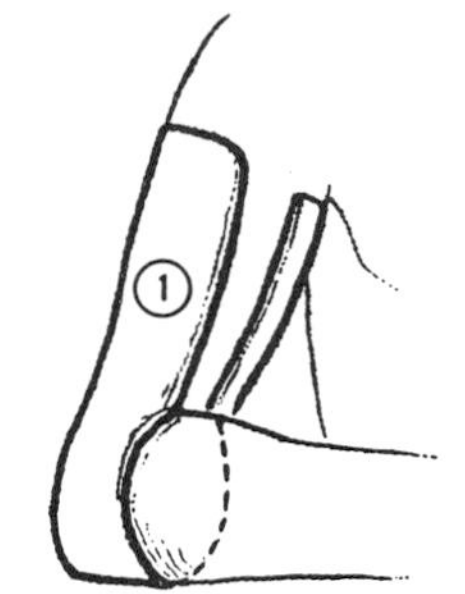

1. Apply a long plaster slab extending from the axilla along the posterior aspect of the arm, around the elbow (flexed 90°) and up on the anterior aspect of the arm.

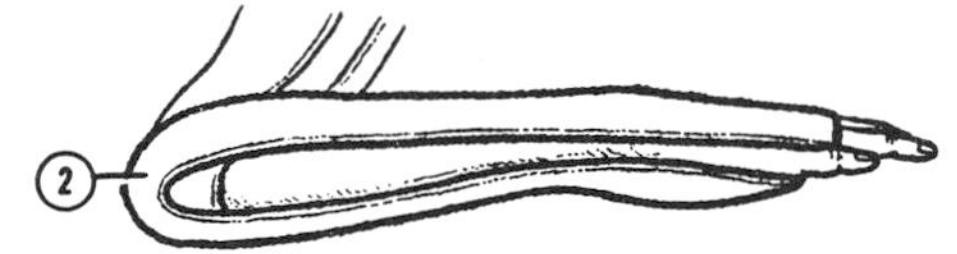

2. Apply a second plaster slab to the forearm in the form of a sugar tong extending around the elbow to the base of the fingers. Fix the slabs with cotton elastic bandages.

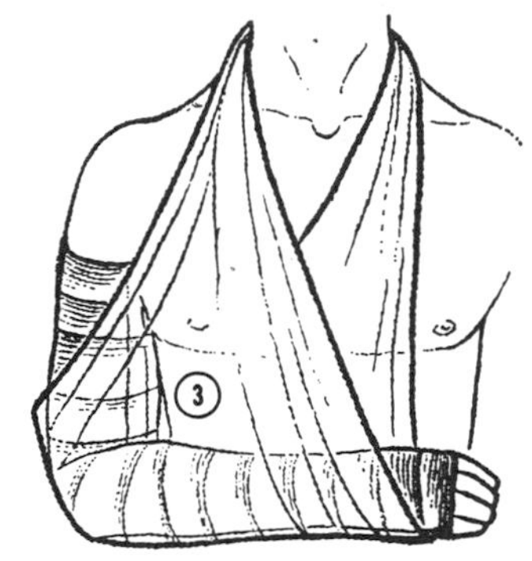

3. Support the arm in a triangular sling.

Postimmobilization Management

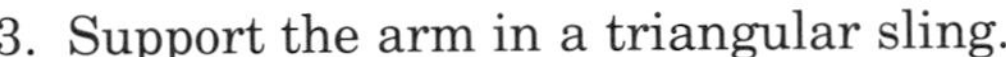

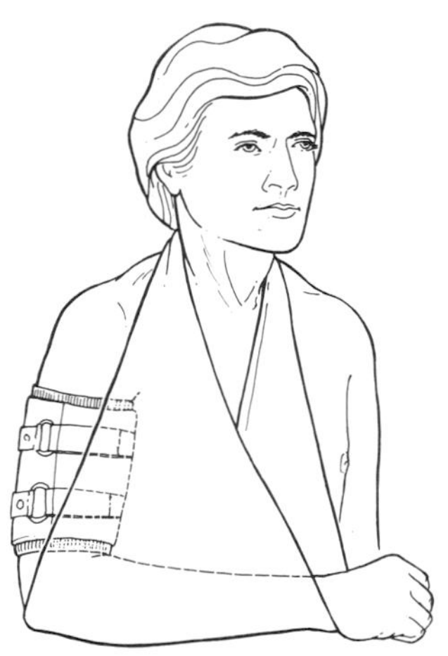

Maintain the plaster support for 3–5 days until the postoperative swelling subsides. Next, place the arm in a humeral brace and the forearm in a sling and allow active range-of-motion exercises.

Discard the sling by 4–6 weeks if reduction remains stable. Avoid passive stretching of the elbow. The humeral brace may be discarded generally by 8–10 weeks when the humeral fracture has consolidated.

Fracture-Dislocation With Forward Displacement of the Forearm Bones and Rupture of the Orbicular Ligament of the Radius

REMARKS

This lesion is best managed by

- Immediate reduction of the forward dislocation of the forearm bones.
- Reduction and stabilization of the olecranon fracture by tension-band wiring.
- Primary repair of the orbicular ligament; if this is not possible, the ligament should be reconstructed.

Note: This injury is frequently associated with motor paralysis of the radial nerve. Evaluate the motor nerve function carefully, particularly wrist and finger extension, before operation. This injury is usually a neurapraxia and can be corrected by prompt reduction of the fracture-dislocation.

Prereduction X-Ray

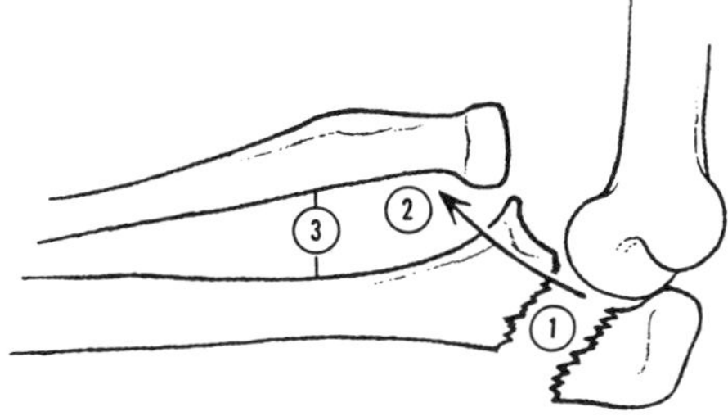

1. Fracture of the olecranon.
2. Forward displacement of the ulna and radius.
3. Displacement of the radius from the ulna indicative of a torn orbicular ligament.

Management

Reduction

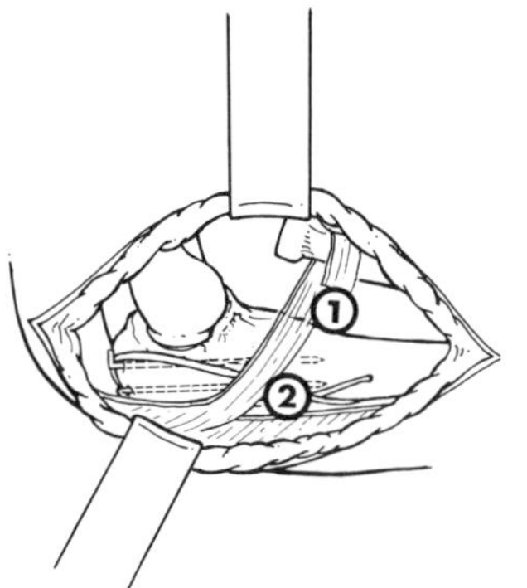

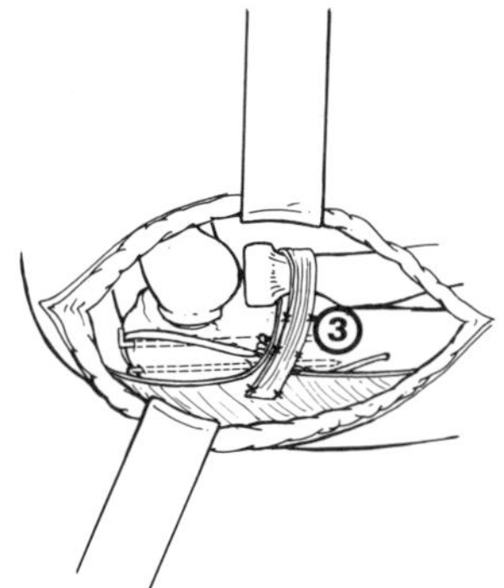

1. Dislocation of the radial head and torn orbicular ligament is repaired using a strip of fascia wrapped around the neck of the radius and taken from the posterior aspect of the olecranon.
2. The olecranon fracture is reduced and stabilized with a Steinmann pin and tension-band wiring.
3. Once the radial head is reduced, the obicular ligament is tightened and sutured to itself around the neck of the radius.

Postreduction X-Ray

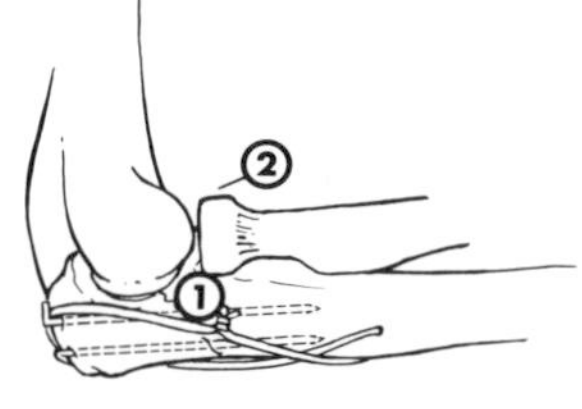

1. The fragments of the olecranon are accurately aligned by the Steinmann pins and tension-band wiring.
2. The radial head is accurately opposed to the capitellum and to the ulna.

Immobilization

1. Apply a bivalved long-arm cast and maintain immobilization for 4 weeks.
2. After 4 weeks begin active gentle exercises on an hourly basis. Between exercises protect the limb in a posterior splint.

Note: Return of elbow function comes slowly after this serious injury. Internal fixation need not be removed unless it causes irritation of overlying soft tissues.

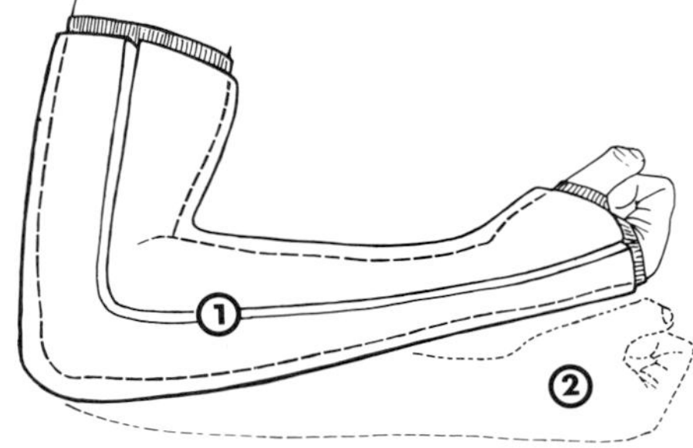

Transcondylar Fracture-Dislocation of the Elbow

REMARKS

This serious injury results from a flexion-type mechanism or a direct posterior blow to the flexed elbow that causes an intracapsular, transcondylar fracture. Both distal humeral condyles are displaced as a single unit. The radius and ulna are dislocated from the fractured condyles. This frequently is an open injury and commonly causes significant vascular and nerve impingement. Temporary longitudinal traction on the forearm with the elbow in extension will usually restore the radial pulse. Open reduction and internal fixation should be done promptly to reduce this unstable fracture dislocation and restore satisfactory function to the elbow.

Preoperative X-Ray

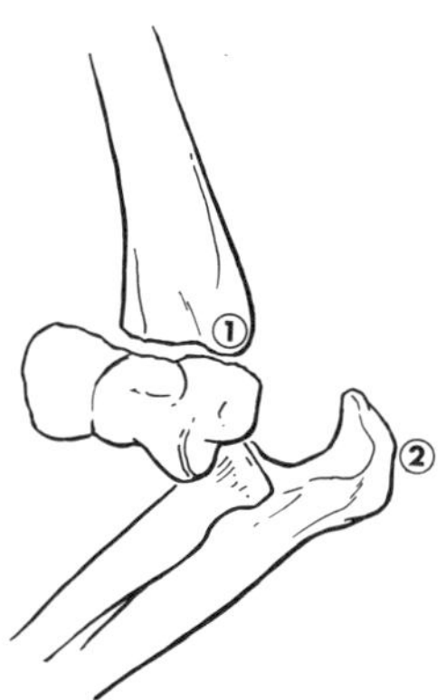

1. Intracapsular, transverse fracture above the capitellum and trochlea with anteromedial rotation.
2. The radius and ulna dislocate medially in relation to the condylar fractures.

Note: Severe displacement compromises the brachial artery. The elbow should be temporarily extended to relieve any circulatory embarrassment.

Management

Reduction Technique

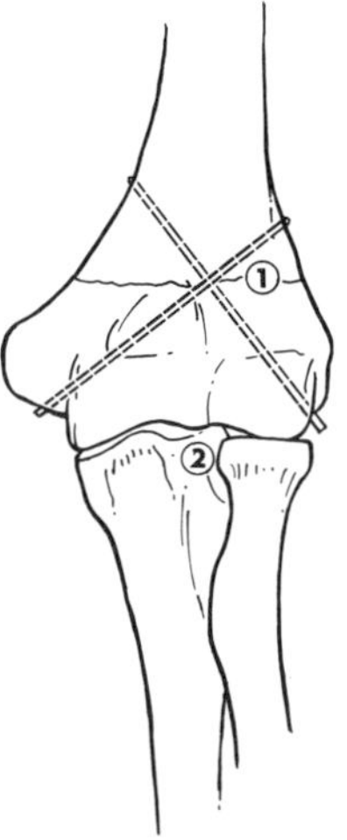

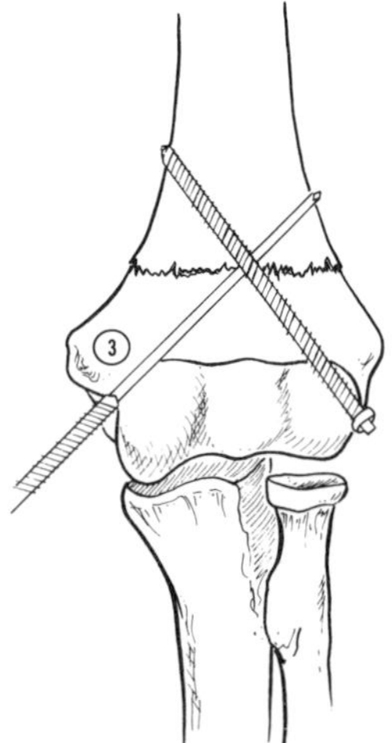

1. The transcondylar fracture must be reduced with an open reduction technique. It is fixed temporarily with guide pins introduced from the medial and lateral cortices.
2. When the condyles are stabilized, the dislocation of the radius and ulna is reduced.

Note: Care should be taken to identify and free the brachial artery and any nerve that may be involved at the fracture site.

3. Cannulated screws are then passed over the guide pins to further achieve stability of the unstable fracture.

Postoperative Immobilization

The elbow is immobilized at 45° of flexion by means of a posterior splint. The radial pulse and circulation are monitored closely for the first 2 days after injury.

Remove the sutures and posterior splint when swelling has subsided, usually by 10 days. If the elbow fracture-dislocation was stable, the patient may begin active exercises by 10 days. If the reduction was unstable, immobilization must be continued for 6–8 weeks, but a stiff elbow is likely to result.

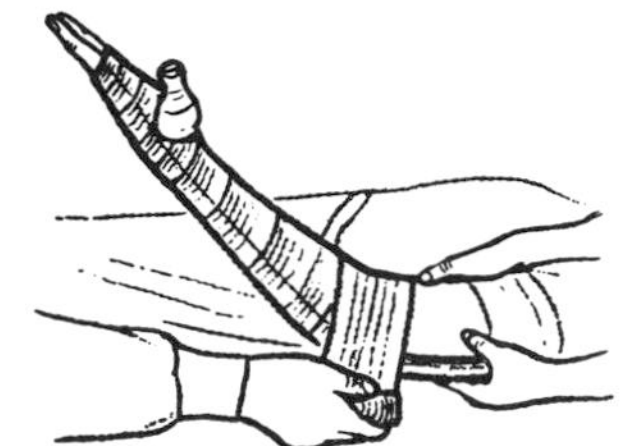

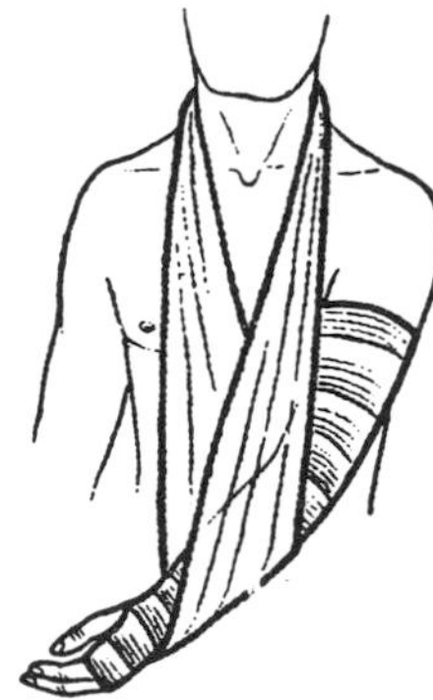

Recurrent Dislocation of the Elbow Joint

REMARKS

Recurrent dislocation is a surprisingly infrequent sequela (1–2 per cent of injuries) from elbow luxation. It should be distinguished from chronic and congenital dislocation. Recurrent dislocation is most likely to follow injury to the child's lax elbow and may be associated with displaced fragments after medial epicondylar or other fractures.

The second most common cause of instability is laxity of the posterolateral capsule. This capsule with its ligament structure ordinarily stabilizes the elbow in full extension but is susceptible to avulsion from its superior attachment at the time of dislocation. Careful testing of stability after initial reduction of the elbow and radiographic assessment of fracture fragments, especially in a child's medial epicondylar fracture, will demonstrate the occasional dislocation that is likely to recur.

Not all elbow instability requires surgical treatment. Subluxation of the radial head may be easily reduced by the patient and may cause only occasional problems of "locking," which may be mistaken for osteochondritis dissecans. In the typical case of recurrent dislocation in a child or adolescent, recurrence is infrequent and may cease as normal growth tightens the capsule and ligament structure.

Surgical repair is indicated for dislocations recurring frequently with trivial injury in the older adolescent and adult. The simplest, most direct way of improving stability is by repairing the lateral ligamentous and capsular laxity (Osborne and Cotterill).

Pathology of Recurrent Dislocation

1. Most dislocations disrupt the lateral and posterior aspects of the capsule.
2. The secondary structure to fail is the anterior lateral capsule.
3. The last structure to fail is the medial capsule.

Note: The commonest source of recurrent dislocation is a lax lateral capsule.

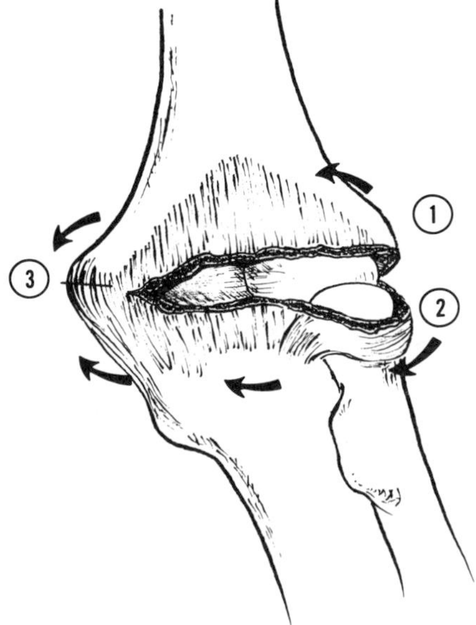

Management

Surgical Repair (After Osborne and Cotterill)

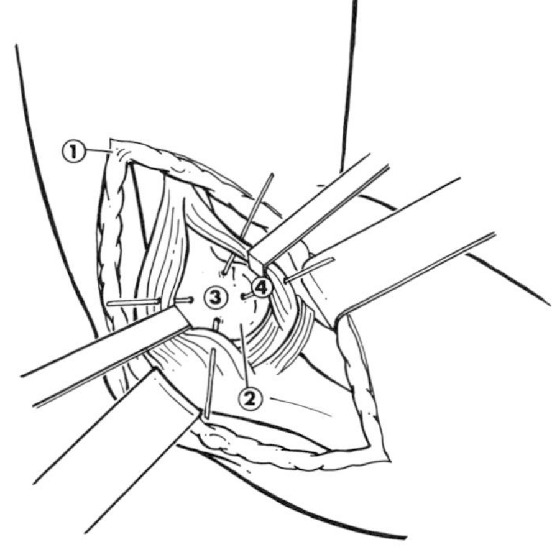

INCISION AND EXPOSURE

1. An incision is made on the lateral side of the elbow from the lateral epicondyle distal to the annular ligament.
2. The elbow is opened behind the lateral ligament, and any fragments of bone are removed.
3. The bone of the lateral condyle is cleared of soft tissue and is scarified.
4. Two transverse drill holes are made in the lateral condyle, and heavy nylon sutures are passed through these holes.

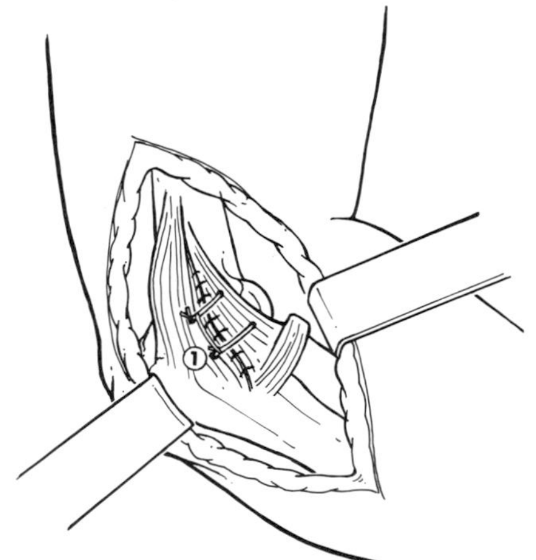

REPAIR

1. The posterolateral capsule is tied down tightly into the scarified site by the suture.

Note: A similar repair may occasionally be necessary for an unstable medial ligament.

Elbow Instability in the Athlete

REMARKS

The post-traumatic recurrent dislocation of the elbow joint should be distinguished from the chronic problem sometimes seen in athletes who throw in the overhead position. These individuals are at risk of developing a variety of elbow problems. Among the problems seen commonly in the high-performance professional athlete is instability due to chronic repetitive stress on the medial collateral ligament of the elbow rather than the lateral capsular structure.

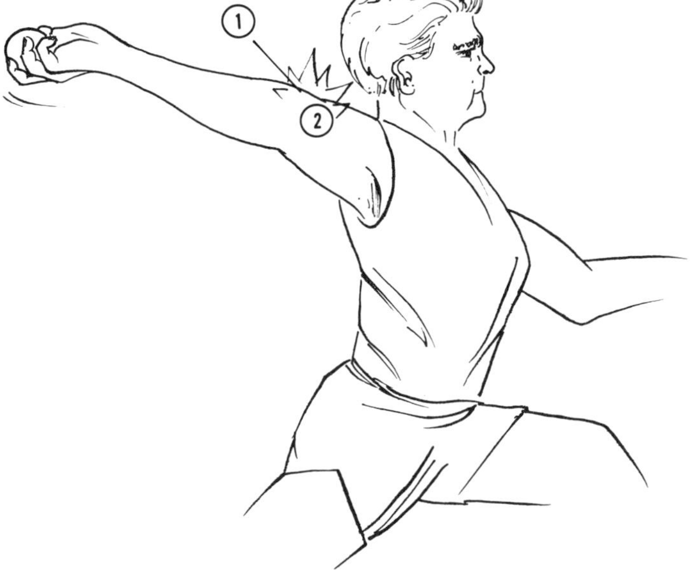

1. The valgus hyperextension strain on the elbow during overhead throwing causes disruption of the medial capsular structures.
2. The individual with poor mechanics, conditioning, or flexibility tends to overload the ulnar collateral ligament of the elbow with resultant instability.

Note: With repetitive stress, dissociation of the ligament occurs and progressive calcification may be evident. The ligament can occasionally be avulsed or rupture in its midsubstance.

Management

The chronic medial instability of the elbow in the throwing athlete is best evaluated by an individual who is expert in the nonoperative rehabilitative as well as the surgical management of the problem.

In most individuals, the problem subsides with avoidance of the overhead throwing. In the professional athlete, reconstructive procedures are available to alleviate the medial instability.

■ Old Unreduced Dislocations of the Elbow Joint

REMARKS

This is a serious and difficult lesion to manage. It usually occurs in individuals who have neglected to obtain medical care because of alcoholism, psychosis, or geographic distance. Chronic traumatic dislocation may rarely be seen in children, but congenital dislocation is more common and is usually bilateral.

If it can be reliably determined that the dislocation is less than 4 weeks old, closed reduction using skeletal traction can be attempted. If the injury is more than 4 weeks old, open reduction is necessary, and the result is likely to be a permanently stiff elbow. Open reduction should be reserved for children and adults with significant preoperative pain who are likely to benefit from the extensive operation to achieve reduction.

Elbow arthroplasty, either resectional or replacement, should be considered as an alternative to open reduction in the older adult with chronic symptomatic dislocation. Total elbow arthroplasty must be reserved for the patient likely to cooperate with long-term postoperative care, which frequently rules out a number of patients presenting with chronic dislocation. The management of this problem requires astute judgment of the patient's needs and personality as well as careful operative technique.

Management

Closed Reduction of Unreduced Dislocation

This method can be used for dislocations less than 4 weeks old. Carefully evaluate neurovascular function before and after any manipulation, because these structures are at higher than usual risk of injury with chronic dislocation.

Reduction in Traction

1. The olecranon pin is inserted, and
2. Traction is begun with the elbow in extension.

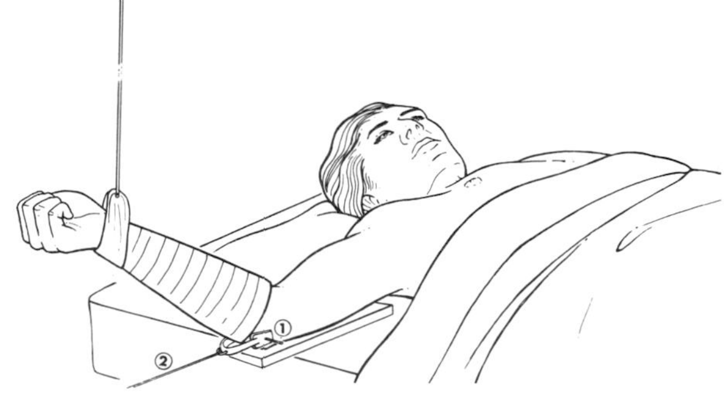

Carefully evaluate neurovascular function.

3. When the radius and ulna have been pulled to the level of the humerus, the position in traction is slowly changed and elbow flexion is accomplished.

Note: General anesthesia is necessary to achieve the flexion-reduction. If reduction in traction fails, open reduction may be carried out.

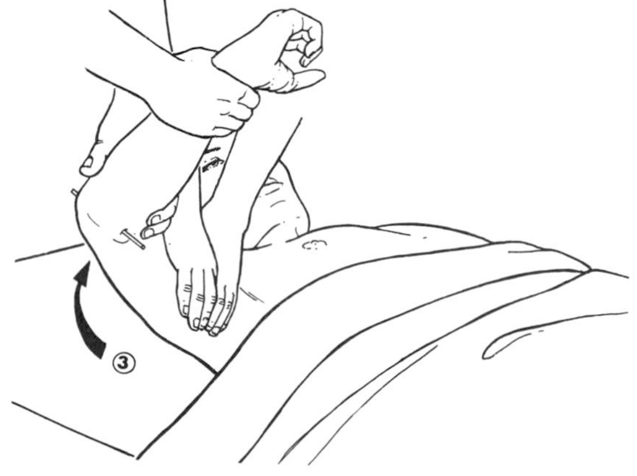

Immobilization After Reduction in Traction

Remove the traction pin and

1. Apply a posterior plaster slab from the axilla to the base of the fingers.
2. The forearm is in acute flexion.
3. The forearm is supinated.
4. Suspend the arm with a collar-and-cuff sling.

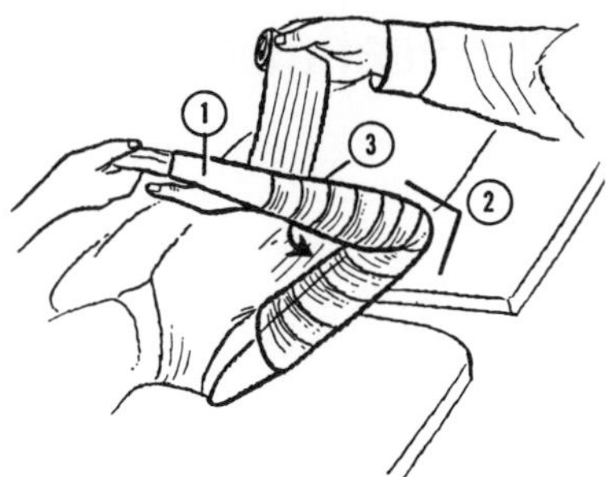

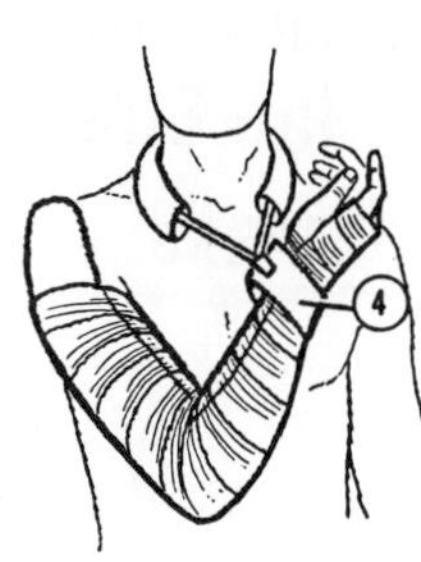

Postreduction Management

Maintain fixation by plaster for 2–3 weeks. Then place the arm in a triangular sling that holds the arm at 90° flexion. Discard the sling after 7–10 days. Institute active exercises for the elbow. Avoid passive stretching of the elbow.

Open Reduction of Unreduced Dislocation

REMARKS

This method may occasionally be useful in cases in which reduction by traction has failed. It is especially applicable to children with old, symptomatic, unreduced dislocations. In general, the results are not as good in adults as they are in children.

The procedure should not be carried out when there is evidence of myositis ossificans. In this instance, the patient should be allowed to regain whatever motion he or she can with active exercises for several months. If the result is still unsatisfactory because of pain and severe limitation of motion, an arthroplasty may be considered.

Technique of Open Reduction

1. Extensive dissection is necessary to expose the dislocated elbow through a triceps reflecting approach.
2. Incision should extend well up into the triceps tendon.
3. All soft tissue scarring and subperiosteal fibrosis must be released to free up the distal end of the humerus anteriorly and posteriorly.
4. Capsular ligamentous structures of the elbow must also be released.
5. Excess callus and fibrosis in the olecranon fossa also blocks reduction and should be removed.
6. Dissection is continued laterally to expose the capitellum and the head of the radius.

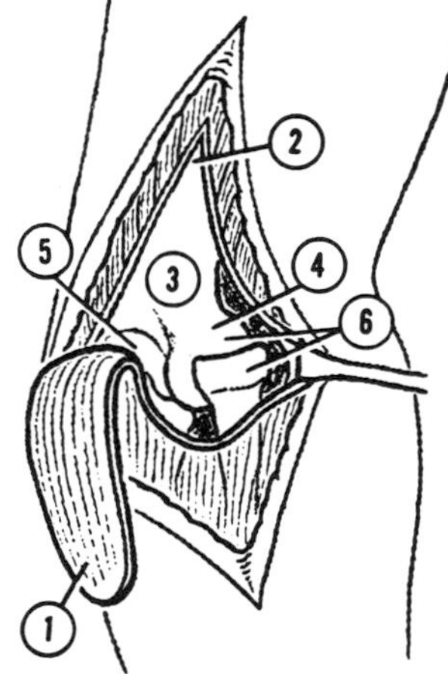

Note: Neural structures also necessitate careful dissection, and occasionally anterior transfer of the ulnar nerve is needed.

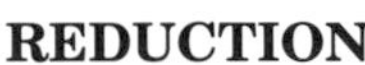

REDUCTION

Reduction is achieved by
1. Rotating the forearm while
2. Downward and backward pressure is applied over the capitellum to engage the radial head on the capitellum.
3. The coronoid process is then slipped forward over the trochlea to complete the reduction.

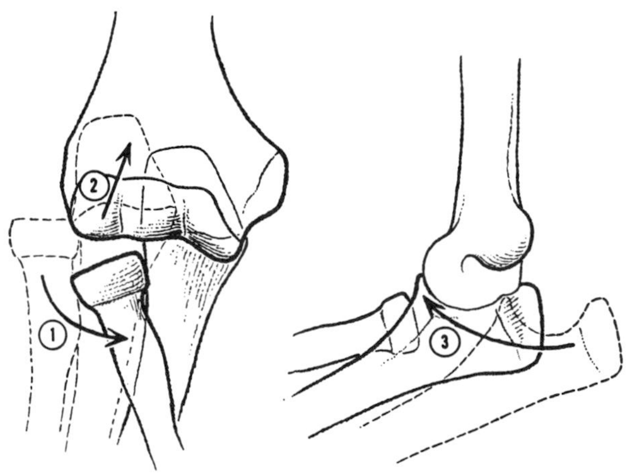

Alternative Method: Resectional Elbow Arthroplasty

REMARKS

Resectional arthroplasty often produces better results for old unreduced dislocations in adults than open reduction. Elbow resectional arthroplasty at present is preferable to artificial joint replacements for symptomatic problems of chronic dislocations. The operation usually affords good relief of pain and a useful increase in both hinge motion and forearm rotation of the elbow. The major complication of resectional arthroplasty is elbow instability, which can be diminished by a period of transarticular pin fixation and cast immobilization following the operative procedure.

1. Extensive bone must be removed from the lower end of the humerus.
2. Bone is also excised from the olecranon, the coronoid process, and the radial head to permit reduction.
3. The reduction must then be maintained by Steinmann pins that cross from the olecranon to the humerus.

Note: After a period of 3–4 weeks in cast immobilization to allow for tightening of soft tissues, the patient may gradually be allowed to begin range-of-motion exercises. The range of motion may slowly improve for many months after the operation; however, instability of the elbow is a fairly common problem after this extensive arthroplasty.

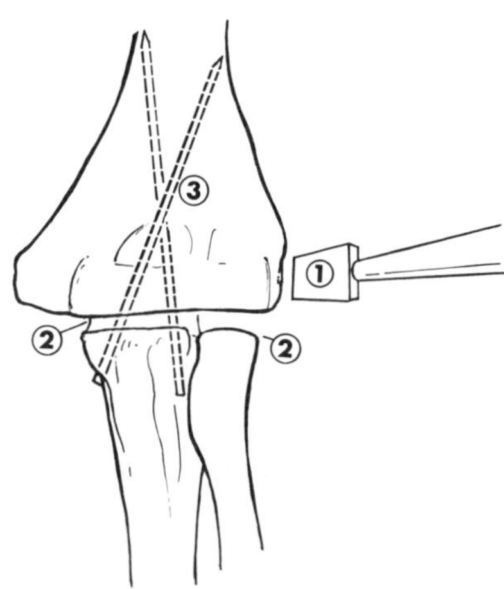

TRAUMATIC MYOSITIS OSSIFICANS

REMARKS

This reactive lesion is apt to follow trauma to the anterior aspect of the elbow as a result of extensive initial injury, overly aggressive surgical intervention, or passive stretching "therapeutic" exercises. Radiographic evidence of this process is evident usually by 3–4 weeks after the injury but may take 4–6 months to completely mature.

Myositis ossificans has become less common after elbow fractures and dislocations than in the past, as the hazards of overvigorous passive stretching have become known. The relationship of the brachialis muscle substance to the anterior capsule makes the muscle area a prime location for reactive calcification. Any insult to this area during the recovery phase is likely to exacerbate the calcification response to trauma.

In elbow dislocation, surgical excision of fragments performed immediately after injury may provoke myositis ossificans. Passive stretching exercises also incite calcification and subsequent blockage of elbow motion. Early (within 3–5 days) active motion within the patient's tolerance is a more physiologic method of regaining elbow function and is less likely to promote reactive calcification.

Myositis ossificans should not be confused with calcification in the medial or lateral capsule, which is seen frequently on x-ray after recovery from elbow dislocation but does not usually affect motion.

Appearance on X-Ray

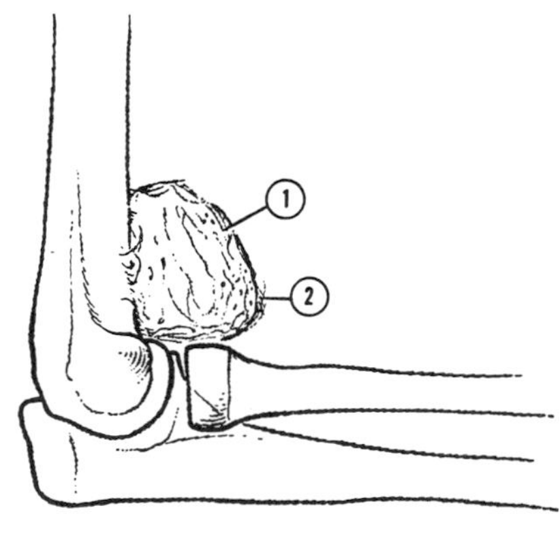

1. Massive calcification in the region of the brachialis muscle following dislocation.
2. This calcification is not sharply demarcated and exhibits no lamellae of ossified bone.

Note: This is usually seen within 3–4 weeks after the injury but takes up to 4–6 months to completely mature.

X-Ray After Active Exercise

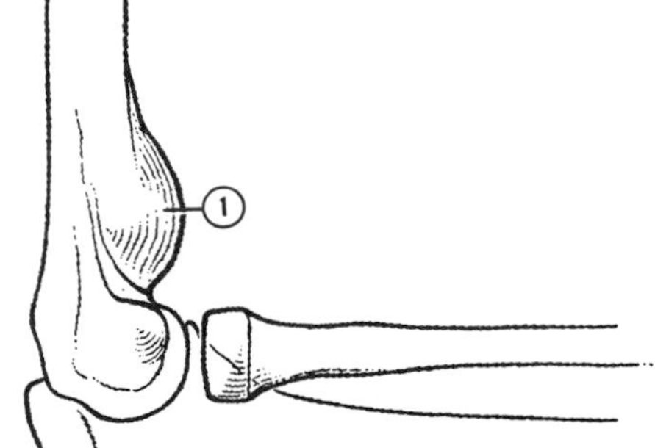

1. After active exercise the bony mass is reduced considerably in size.

X-Ray After Passive Stretching or After Combination Head Injury and Elbow Injury

1. Extensive calcification can occur in the head-injured patient or after passive stretching subsequent to a minor elbow injury.
2. This mass is associated with spastic contraction of the brachialis muscle or stretching of the capsule.

Note: This contracture may require surgical excision as the patient recovers from the head injury. However, surgical excision should be delayed until the ossification process subsides and the head injury improves.

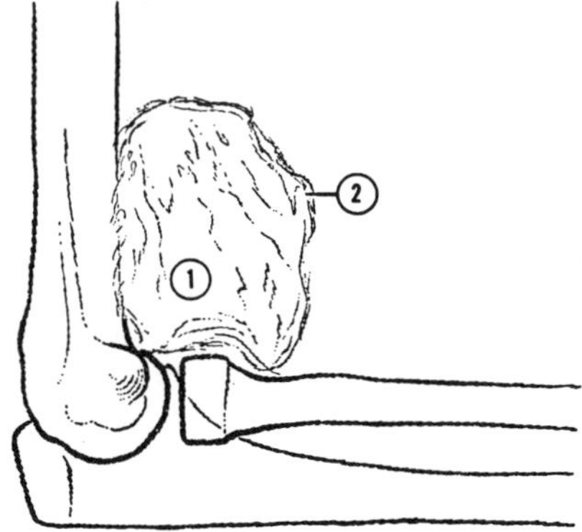

■ Management of Myositis Ossificans

The most desirable method of managing this condition is to prevent its formation initially. To accomplish this goal the arm should be managed with active range-of-motion exercises as soon as possible after the elbow is stabilized. Passive stretching of the injury should be avoided.

Recent evidence has shown that nonsteroidal anti-inflammatory drugs may be useful prophylactically in injuries in which early myositis ossificans becomes evident. These nonsteroidals tend to inhibit soft tissue ossification. If the patient remains symptomatic from the calcification and ossification, surgical excision should be recommended at around 4–6 months.

Operative Management

Indications

Operative intervention is justified only after the bone is mature and only if the lesion acts as a mechanical block to normal function of the elbow. Wait at least 6 months before advising operative excision.

A bone scan is helpful in determining the activity of the soft tissue calcification. It is best to delay until the bone scan is "relatively cool" before recommending surgical excision of the lesion.

Preoperative X-Ray

1. The bone on the anterior aspect of the elbow is smooth and regular, and it exhibits mature bony lamellae.

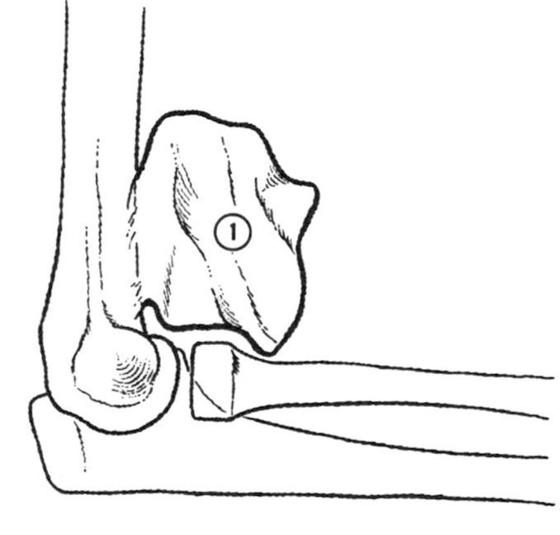

Postoperative X-Ray

1. The bony mass has been completely removed. Mechanical blocking of the joint has been eliminated.

Note: Recurrences of bone formation are not likely to occur if the operation is delayed until the new bone has become mature; on the other hand, violent reformation of new bone may take place if surgical interference occurs during the immature phase of the myositis ossificans process.

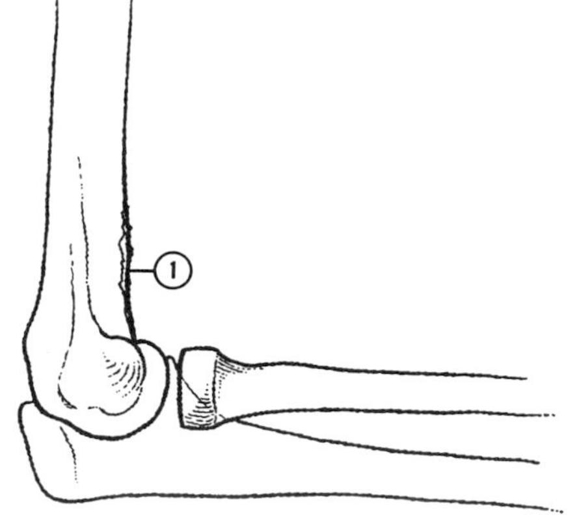

OTHER FRACTURES, DISLOCATIONS, AND INJURIES ABOUT THE ELBOW

Fractures of the Olecranon and Separation of the Olecranon Epiphysis

REMARKS

Reduction of fractures of the olecranon is important for good function and triceps strength. In this respect a fractured olecranon affects elbow function much like a fractured patella affects knee function.

Operative reduction is indicated in any fracture in which the fragments separate when the forearm is brought to 90° of flexion. This applies even if the fragments are in apposition when the arm is extended. Operative excision is feasible for comminuted fractures, but most can be reduced and held with internal fixation.

Separation of the olecranon epiphysis encountered in a patient between the ages of 10 and 16 years is comparable to fracture of the olecranon and is treated in a like manner.

Fractures of the Olecranon Without Displacement

Appearance on X-Ray

1. Complete oblique fracture of the olecranon with no displacement of the fragments.
2. Comminuted fracture of the olecranon with no displacement of the fragments.

Note: An x-ray taken with elbow flexed 90° shows no displacement and indicates that the triceps aponeurosis is intact and prolonged immobilization is unnecessary.

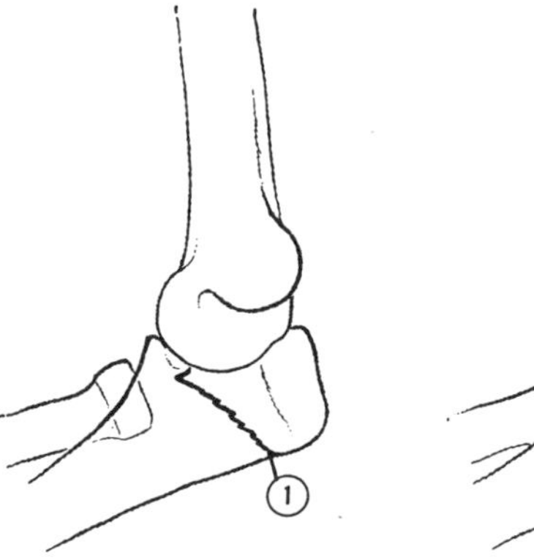

Management

Immobilization

Apply a posterior splint with the elbow in slight (30°) flexion to relax the triceps.

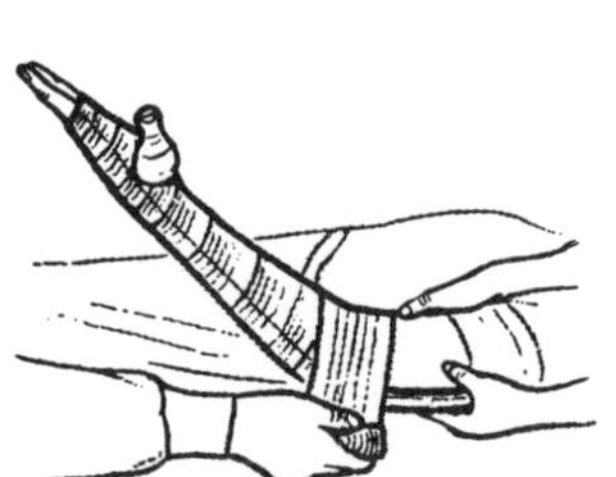

Subsequent Management

The splint may be removed from the elbow when the swelling subsides, usually by 3–5 days. Active exercise may be allowed after the first week to regain elbow motion. The stable fracture should not displace with elbow flexion unless the triceps aponeurosis has been torn. However, the fracture should be re-x-rayed within the first week or two to ascertain its continued stability.

Most of these fractures are clinically healed by 4–6 weeks and radiographically healed by 8–10 weeks. Keep in mind that it is the patient who should be treated rather than the x-ray. Therefore, when the fracture is healed clinically, the patient may be allowed to do light lifting and other functional activities with the elbow.

Fractures of the Olecranon With Displacement

Appearance on X-Ray

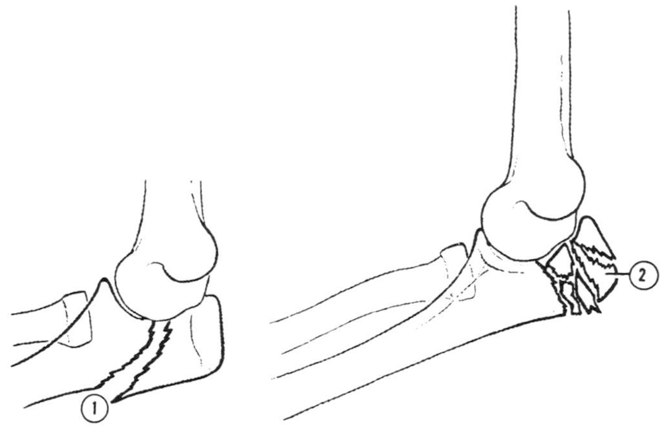

1. Complete oblique fracture with separation of the fragments.
2. Comminuted fracture with separation of fragments. As much as 60 per cent of the comminuted olecranon may be excised without disturbing stability, but internal fixation is usually preferable to operative excision.

Management

Operative Fixation

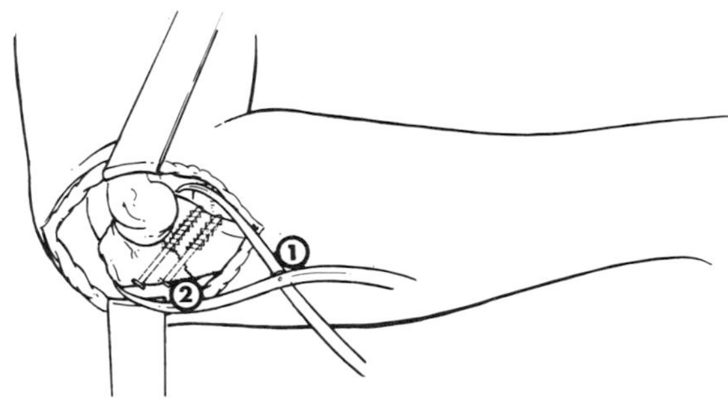

1. The fragments are held in apposition by a tenaculum.
2. The fracture is fixed with two lag screws or two Steinmann pins and

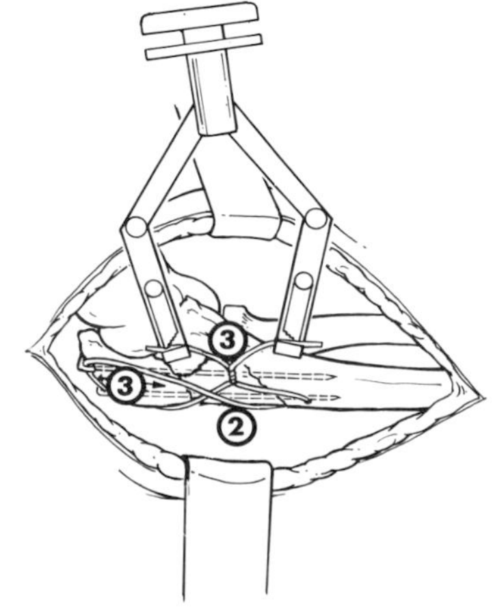

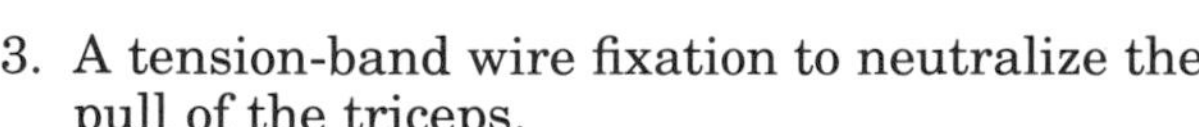

3. A tension-band wire fixation to neutralize the pull of the triceps.

Note: Stability is tested by flexing and extending the elbow. Obtain intraoperative x-ray to determine the completeness of reduction.

Intraoperative X-Ray

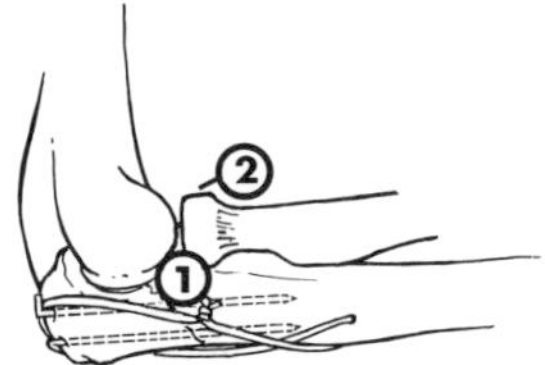

1. The fragments of the olecranon are in normal anatomic alignment.
2. The ulna and the radius are in normal position in relation to the articular surface of the humerus.

Postoperative Management

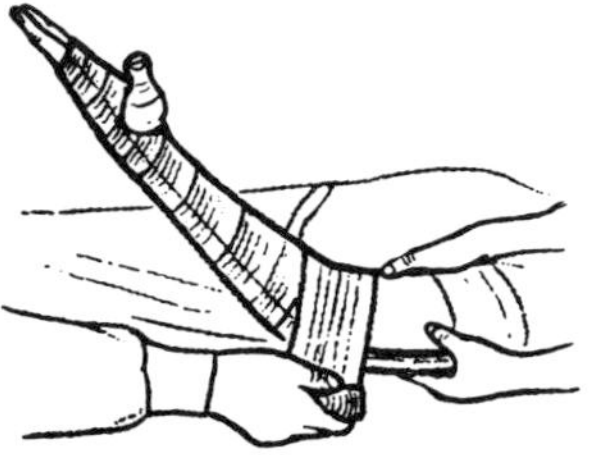

A posterior splint is applied with the elbow near full extension. The limb is elevated for 2–3 days until the swelling subsides. Subsequently the patient may begin guarded active exercises by 5–7 days.

The protective splint device is usually worn for approximately 3 weeks when the patient is not exercising the elbow.

After 3–5 weeks the splint may be discarded. The patient should avoid heavy lifting or pushing with the arm for approximately 3 months.

Alternative Method: Excision of the Olecranon

REMARKS

Isolated comminuted fractures without injury to ulnar or radial head may be treated by excision of the olecranon and secure reattachment of the triceps tendon. This method is useful when internal fixation has failed because of comminution. As much as 60–70 per cent of the olecranon may be excised if the remaining portion of the articulation is undamaged.

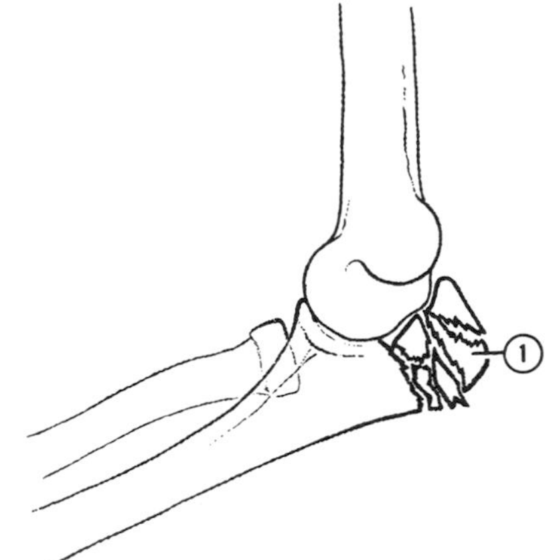

Appearance on X-Ray

1. Severe comminution of the proximal half of the olecranon.

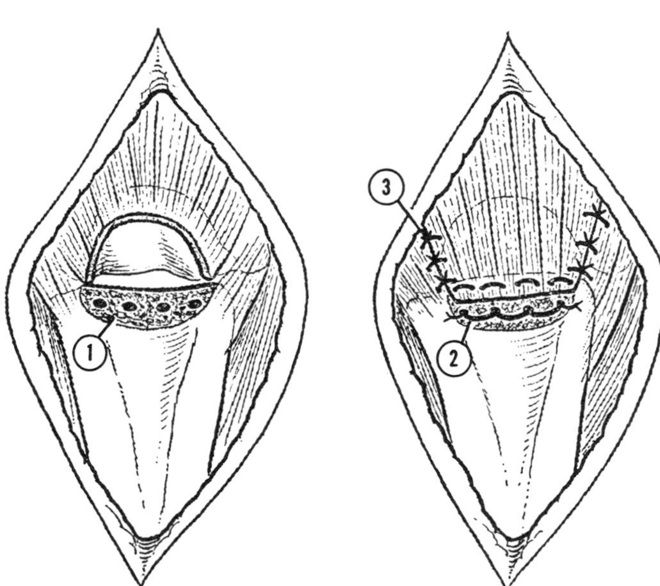

Management

1. The comminuted fracture is approached posteriorly, and the multiple fragments are excised to expose the triceps tendon.
2. The triceps tendon is then reattached to the main surface of the ulna using nonabsorbable sutures placed in holes drilled in the bones.
3. The remaining lacerated portion of the triceps is repaired to the adjacent soft tissue.

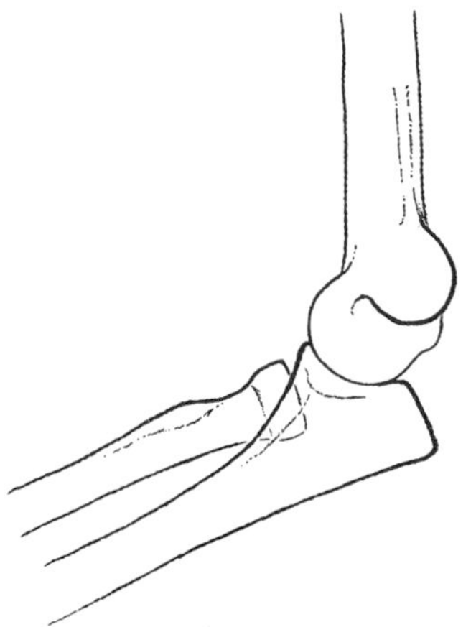

Postexcision X-Ray

All bony fragments have been removed; the end of the ulna is smooth.

Postoperative Management

A posterior splint is applied with the elbow near full extension. The limb is elevated for 2–3 days until the swelling subsides. Subsequently the patient may begin guarded active exercises by 5–7 days.

The protective splint device is usually worn for approximately 3 weeks when the patient is not exercising the elbow. After 3–5 weeks the splint may be discarded. The patient should avoid heavy lifting or pushing with the arm for approximately 3 months.

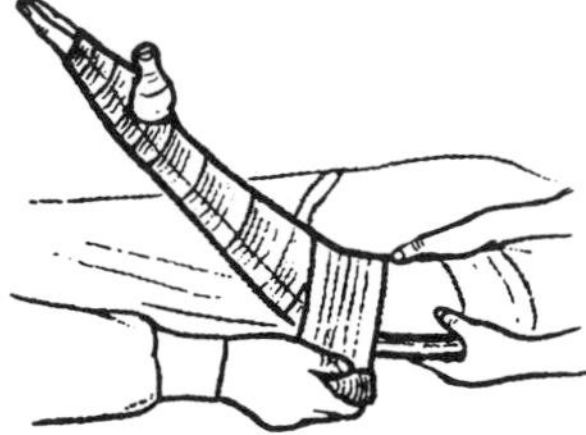

Fractures of the Coronoid Process

REMARKS

Isolated fracture from avulsion of the coronoid process by the brachialis muscle may occur. Most often the fracture is associated with a posterior dislocation of the elbow. The coronoid process fracture may vary in size from a small chip to a large segment.

The small-chip fractures are of little or no significance. It is important not to attack these fragments surgically because an anterior approach to the elbow frequently leads to the loss of elbow motion.

The larger segmental fractures of the coronoid process are usually associated with fracture of the entire ulna as well as dislocation of the elbow. These are considerably more important for elbow stability or instability, and require adequate internal stabilization.

Chip Fracture and Fracture With Minimal Displacement

Appearance on X-Ray

CHIP FRACTURE

1. A small chip of the coronoid process is avulsed and displaced slightly anteriorly.

LARGER FRAGMENT

2. A triangular fragment of bone is detached from the coronoid process; the displacement is minimal.

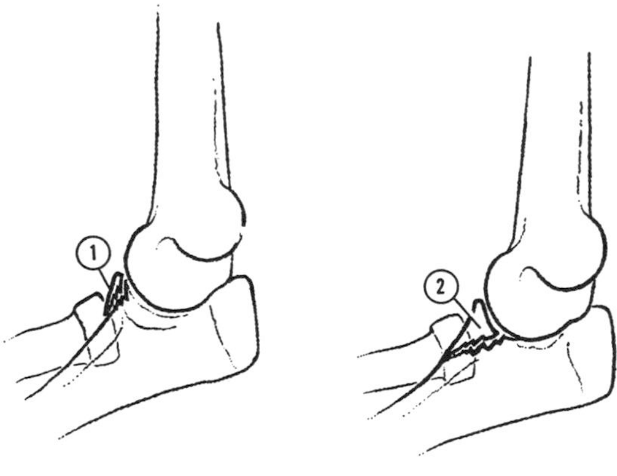

Management

Immobilization

No reduction is necessary.

1. Apply a posterior plaster slab from the axilla to the base of the fingers.
2. The forearm is in acute flexion.
3. The forearm is in full supination.

Suspend the arm with a collar-and-cuff sling.

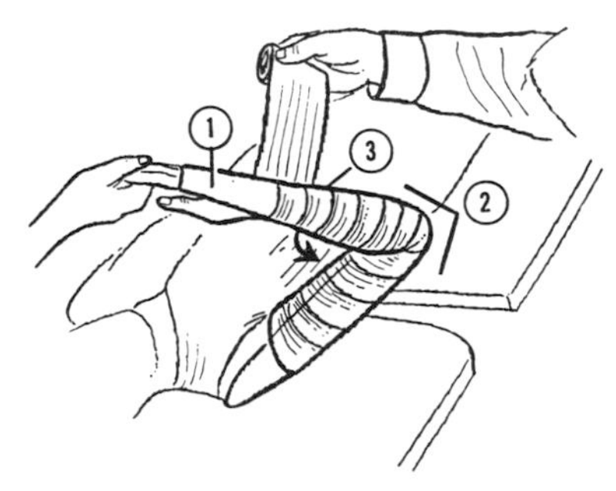

Postimmobilization Management

Maintain the plaster fixation for 7–10 days. Now place the arm in a triangular sling holding the arm at 90° flexion. Discard the sling after 7–10 days. Institute active exercises for the elbow. Avoid passive stretching of the elbow.

Fractures of the Coronoid With Displacements of Fragments

REMARKS

Large fragments from the coronoid process are more difficult to manage than the usual chip fractures. Care should be taken that the injury is not really a posterior Monteggia fracture dislocation. This is usually associated with a triangular or quadrangular fracture at the level of the coronoid process.

Closed treatment of these injuries tends to be unstable. The treatment of choice is open reduction with a plate fixation of the ulna and screw fixation of the coronoid process.

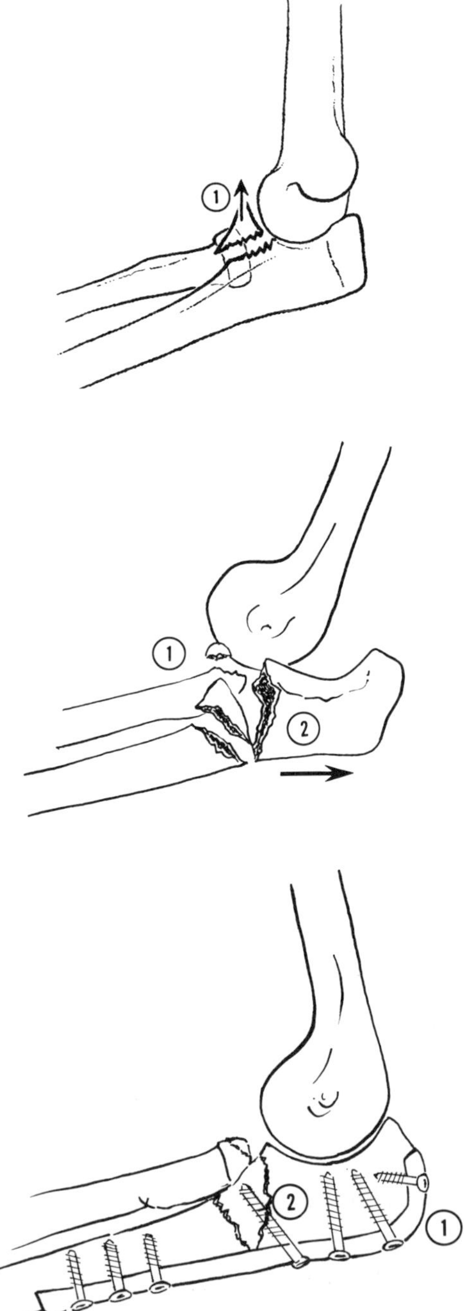

Prereduction X-Ray

1. The large triangular fragment is displaced anteriorly. This my be associated with posterior subluxation of the radius and ulna.

Posterior Monteggia Fracture Dislocation

1. A triangular fracture of the ulna involves the coronoid process.
2. Closed treatment of this injury, which is really a Monteggia fracture dislocation, can result in posterior dislocation, even in a cast.

Management

Operative Fixation

1. The treatment of choice for unstable fractures of the ulna with coronoid involvement is plate fixation.
2. The coronoid process should be fixed with interfragmentary screws that secure the anterior cortical fragment.

Fractures of the Head and Neck of the Radius (in Adults)

REMARKS

Force transmitted through the radius impacts the radial head against the capitellum. The result is radial head or radial neck fractures.

In adults, the radial articular surface is usually involved. In children, the weakened radial physis or growth plate fails without involving the articular surface (see Chapter 2).

Frequently these are very subtle articular fractures that require several views on x-ray to detect. A patient with a fall or direct impact on the elbow with pain localized to the radial head should be suspected of having a fracture, even if the x-ray is inconclusive.

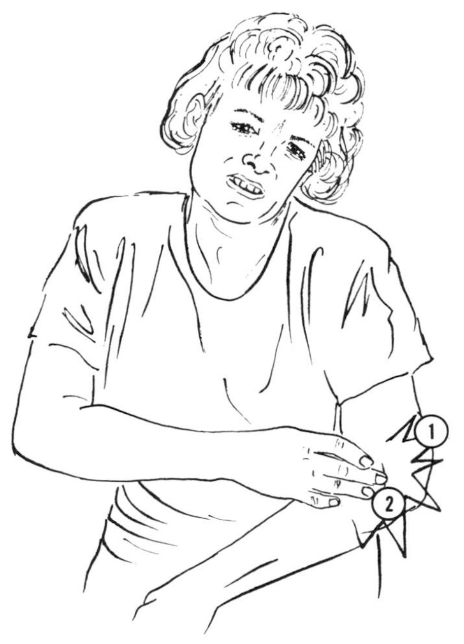

Clinical Diagnosis

1. The patient has painful swollen elbow after a fall on the outstretched hand.
2. The pain is fairly well localized to the lateral aspect in the region of the radial head or capitellum.

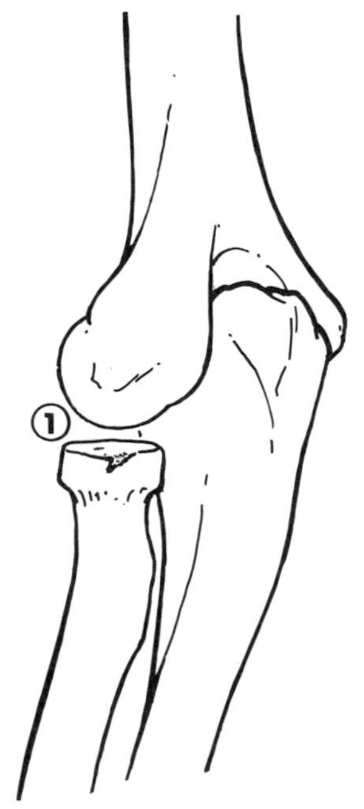

X-Ray Diagnosis of Radial Head Fractures

These are common fractures and frequently are not recognized on cursory x-ray examination. Any adult who falls and complains of pain in the elbow should be considered to have a radial head fracture until proved otherwise.

1. Most often these are linear cracks that may be seen only with an oblique view of the proximal radial head.

Note: Fragments that displace superiorly are produced by fractures of the capitellum and not by radial head fractures (see page 1225).

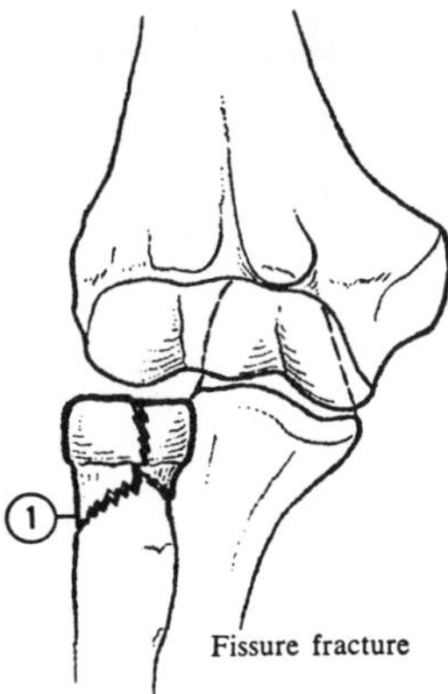

1. Fissure fracture of the head of the radius and fracture of the neck without displacement of fragments.

Management

REMARKS

The most common fracture, the undisplaced type, is best treated by aspiration of the hemarthrosis and temporary sling support. Prompt resumption of active exercises should begin as soon as the acute pain starts to subside.

The displaced fracture in an adult may be treated by an early trial of motion. If motion seems to be blocked by displacement of the fragments, operative excision or internal fixation can be employed.

Internal fixation of some of the fractured radial head fragments may be indicated, but most of those treated operatively are best treated by operative excision of the fragments. However, operative excision of bone fragments should be avoided in a young patient or child in whom subsequent valgus deformity or shortening of the radius may occur.

In the fracture of the radial head combined with symptomatic disruption of the distal radioulnar joint, operative salvage of the radial head, either by internal fixation or silastic prosthetic replacement, is indicated. Stabilization by prosthetic replacement of the radial head fracture is also indicated, as described previously, for fracture-dislocations of the elbow to avoid an unstable recurrent dislocation.

Types of Fractures Treated by a Trial of Motion (After Adler and Shaftan)

1. Marginal fracture of the lateral portion of the radial head with some outward displacement of the fragment.
2. Fracture of the neck of the radius without displacement of the radial head.

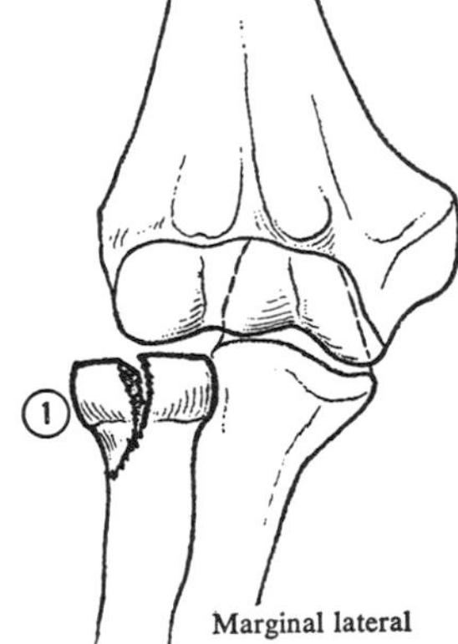

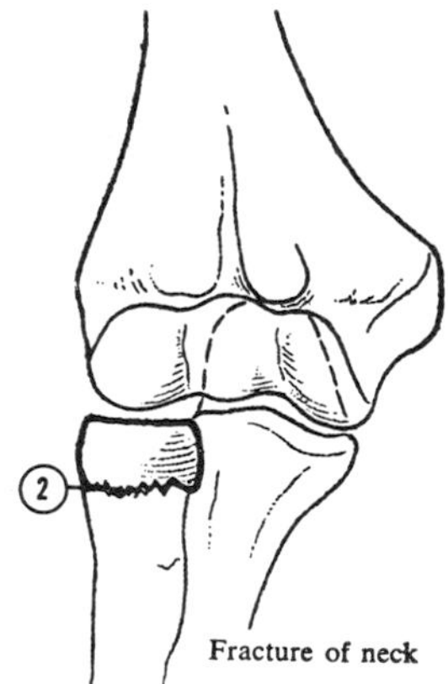

1. Fracture of the neck of the radius with tilting of the radial head.
2. Marginal fracture of the medial portion of the radial head with inward displacement. The radioulnar joint is involved.

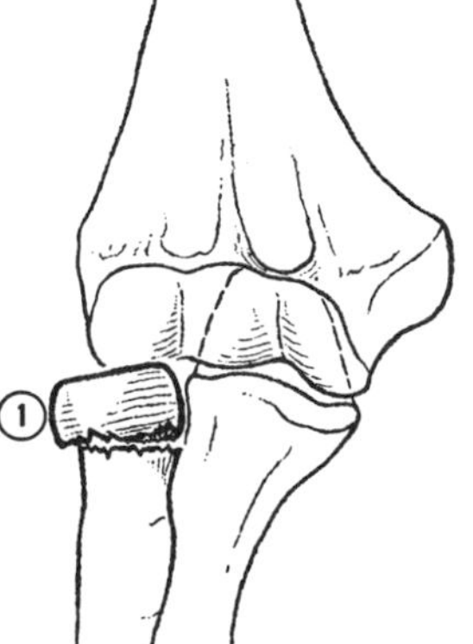

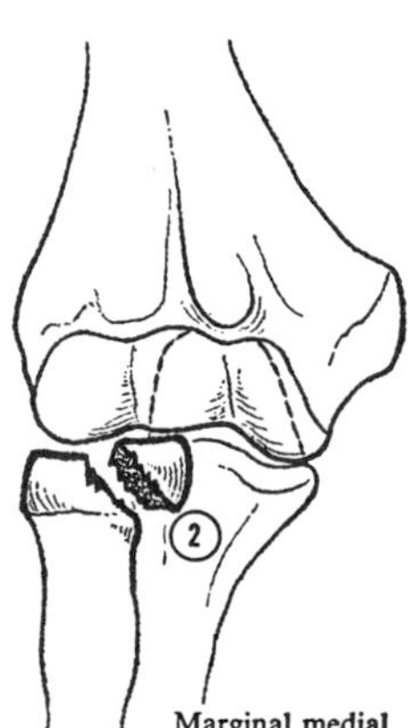

Management

Immediate Management

Aspirate the elbow to relieve pain from hemarthrosis as well as to evaluate motion.

1. An 18-gauge needle is introduced superior to the radial head.
2. Blood is withdrawn.

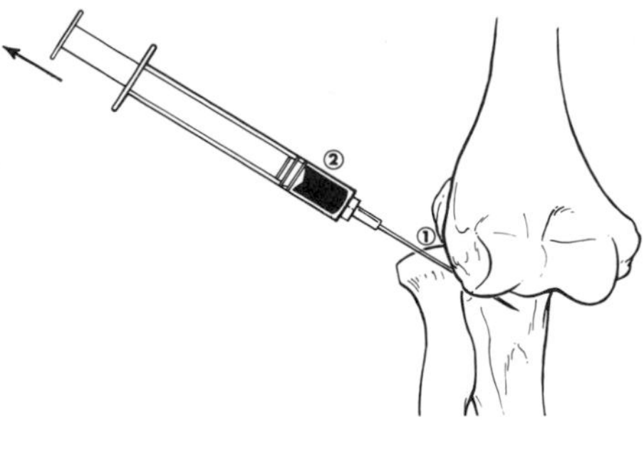

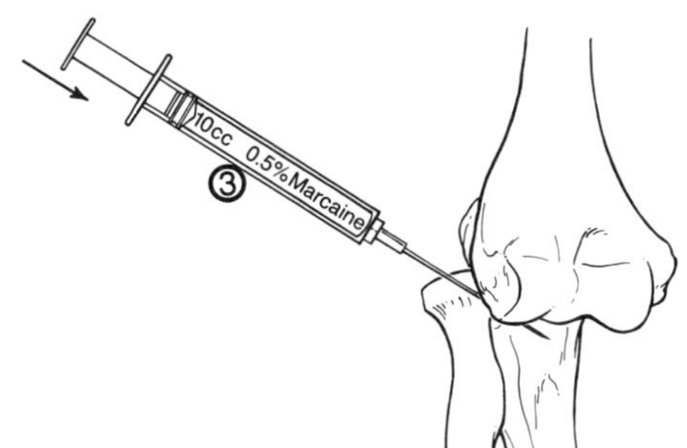

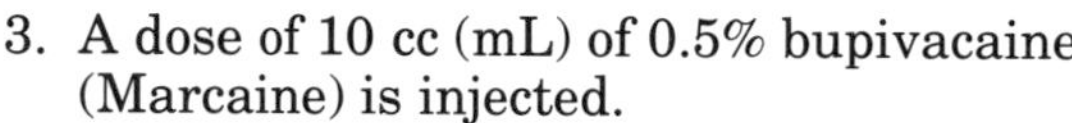
3. A dose of 10 cc (mL) of 0.5% bupivacaine (Marcaine) is injected.

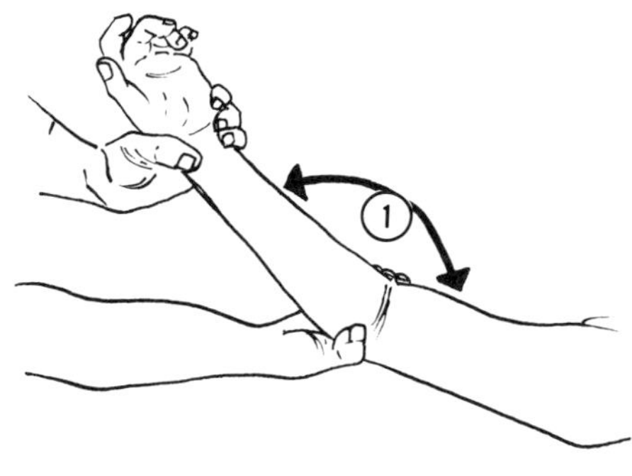

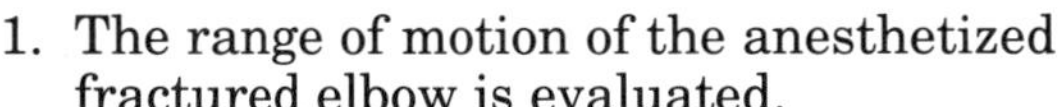
1. The range of motion of the anesthetized fractured elbow is evaluated.

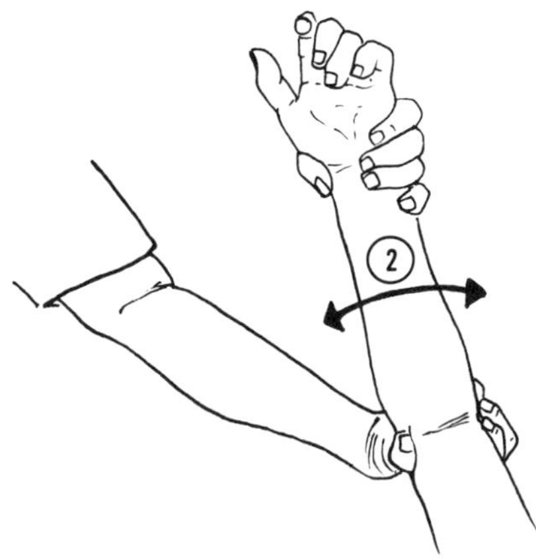

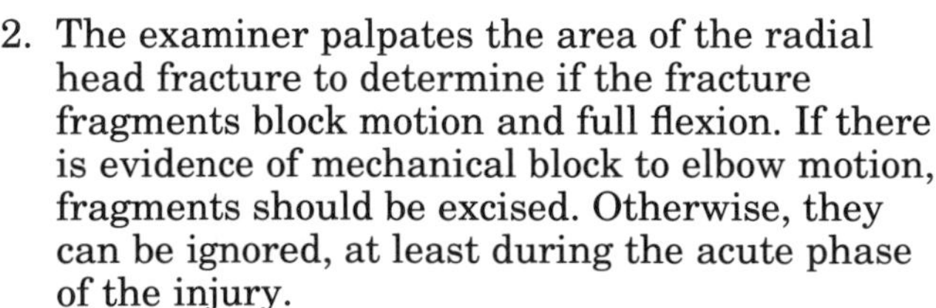
2. The examiner palpates the area of the radial head fracture to determine if the fracture fragments block motion and full flexion. If there is evidence of mechanical block to elbow motion, fragments should be excised. Otherwise, they can be ignored, at least during the acute phase of the injury.

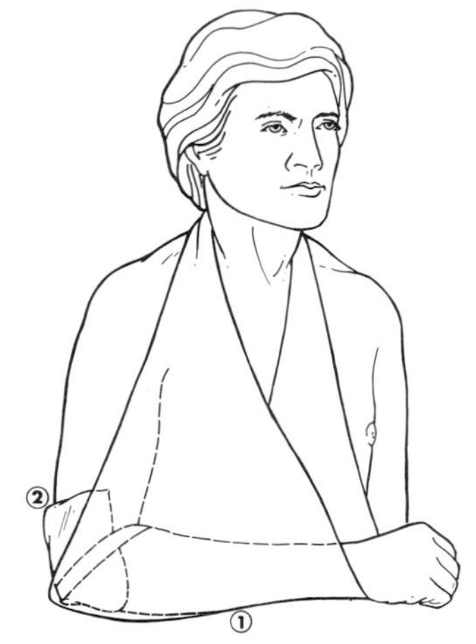

Immediate Immobilization

1. Support the elbow in a sling.
2. For the first 48 hours, apply ice to the radial region to relieve pain.

Trial by Motion

When the pain subsides, the patient may begin forearm rotation exercises with the arm in a sling. By 5–7 days, the pain will have subsided sufficiently to allow active flexion and extension exercises. If extension is slow to return, the patient should use a night splint with the elbow in maximum extension.

Surgical Excision of the Radial Head

Indications

Objective clinical evidence of limitation of flexion from fracture fragments during the acute assessment under local anesthetic or after 8 weeks of trial by motion is the major indication for excision of the radial head. Rarely, the patient will desire excision of radial head fragments because of elbow crepitance, which is usually painless.

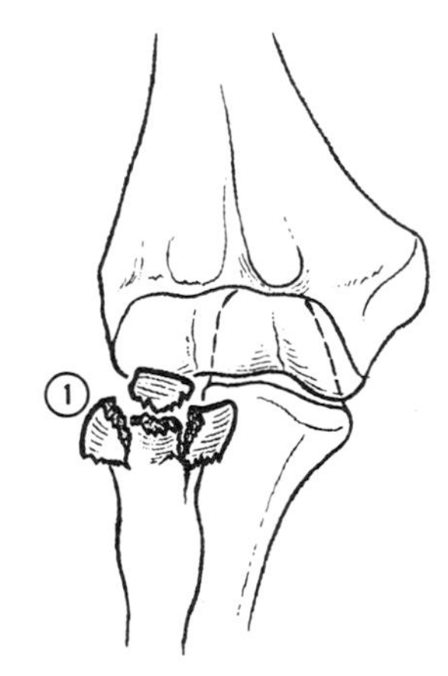

Indications for Surgical Excision

1. Severe comminution of the radial head with displacement of the fragments.

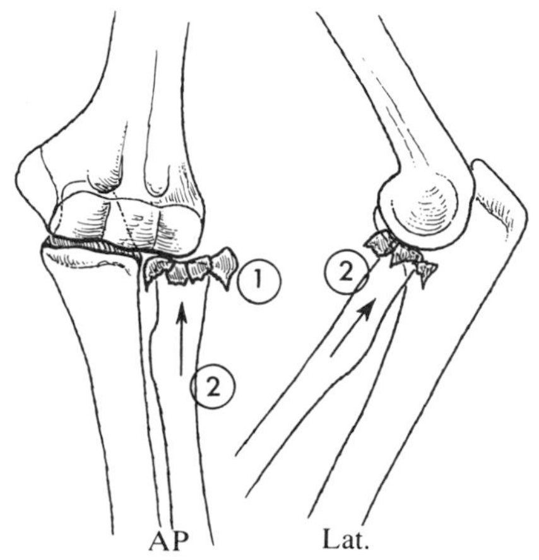

Appearance on X-Ray

1. There is severe comminution and mushrooming of the radial head.
2. The radial shaft is displaced upward against the capitellum.

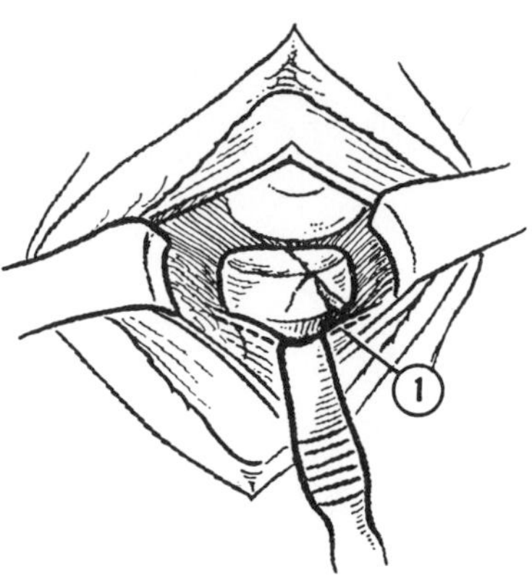

Surgical Technique

1. The fractured radial head is approached through a posterolateral incision. The soft tissue attachments are gently retracted to expose the fracture site.

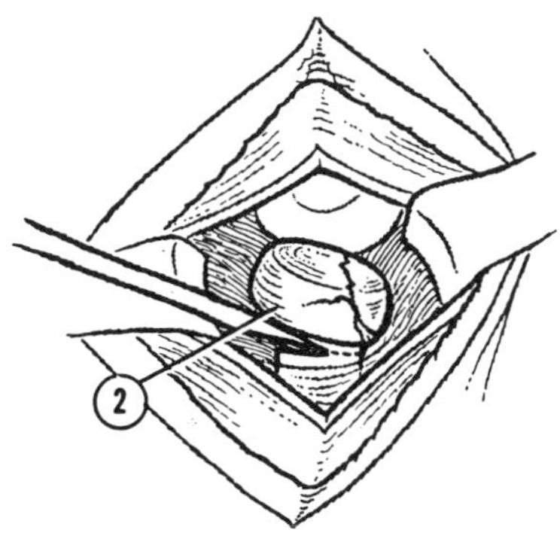

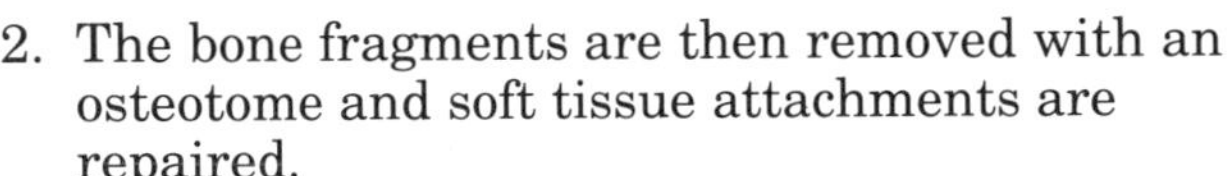

2. The bone fragments are then removed with an osteotome and soft tissue attachments are repaired.

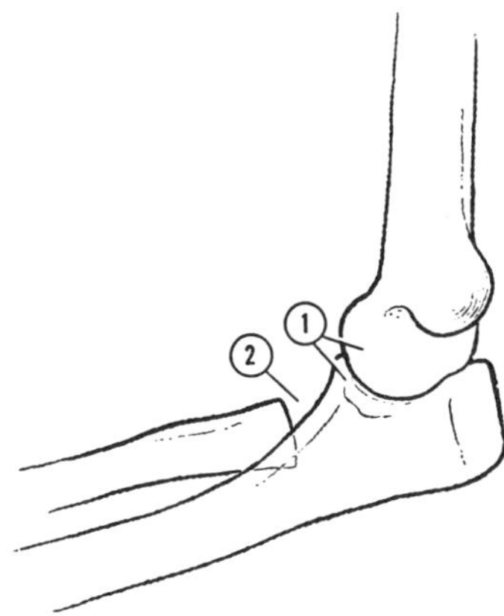

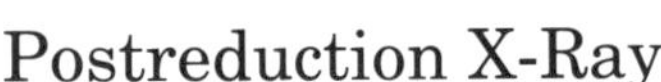

Postreduction X-Ray

1. The articular surfaces of the distal end of the humerus and the ulna are in normal anatomic position.
2. The radial head has been resected.

Comminuted Fracture of the Radial Head With Dislocation of the Distal Radioulnar Joint

REMARKS

This is an infrequent acute lesion. The dislocation at the distal radioulnar joint may be overlooked. It is produced by a severe longitudinal compression force that drives the radius upward. Disruption of the distal joint permits the shaft of the radius to be displaced further upward than is normal with a fracture.

Similarly, symptomatic instability of the distal radial joint may frequently follow excision of the proximal radius. Always suspect this combination when a patient with a fracture of the radial head complains of pain in the wrist. In these patients excision of the radial head will increase the proximal shift of the radius and aggravate the deformity at the wrist. This can be especially disabling in a laborer.

Other problems sometimes seen with proximal migration of the radius include loss of supination and gradual increased valgus angulation at the elbow. If the patient has wrist pain associated with acute injury or is symptomatic from proximal migration of the radius after radial head resection, interpositional arthroplasty may be recommended.

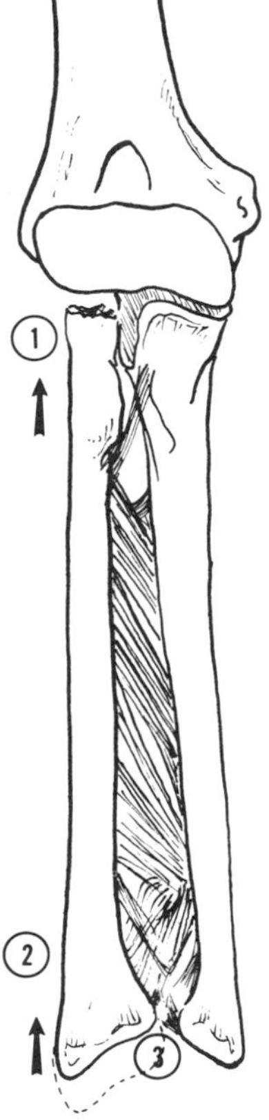

1. Occasionally a comminuted fracture or operative excision of the comminuted fracture will be associated with acute or chronic proximal migration of the radius.
2. This can cause symptomatic wrist discomfort and limitation of supination in some patients.
3. The distal radioulnar ligaments are disrupted and allow proximal displacement of the injured radius.

Appearance on X-Ray of Wrist Showing Disrupted Radioulnar Joint

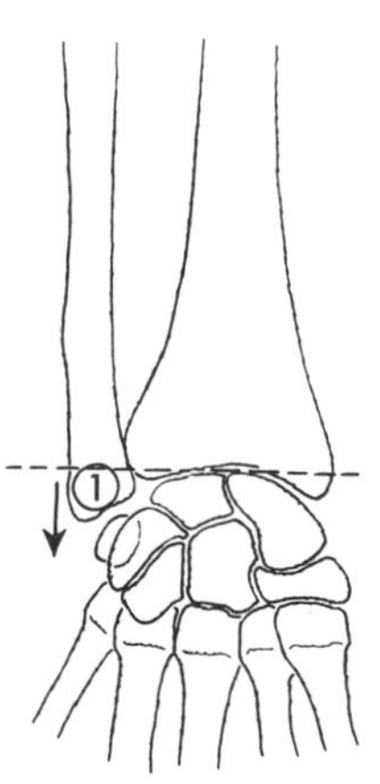

1. The styloid process is at a lower than normal position in relation to the ulna.

Note: Normally the styloid process of the radius extends 1 cm beyond that of the ulna.

Management

Preferred Treatment of Acute or Chronic Proximal Migration of the Radius With Radial Head Fracture

1. The proximal radial fracture site is approached from a posterolateral direction, and the fragments and scar tissue are excised.
2. A radial head prosthesis is inserted into the proximal radius to maintain support and stability against proximal migration. The largest implant accepted by the intramedullary canal is used for stability.

Note: Subsequently the elbow is immobilized until the swelling subsides. Active range-of-motion exercises can usually be started in the first week; however, for unstable fracture-dislocations immobilization for several weeks may be necessary, depending on the stability achieved in surgery.

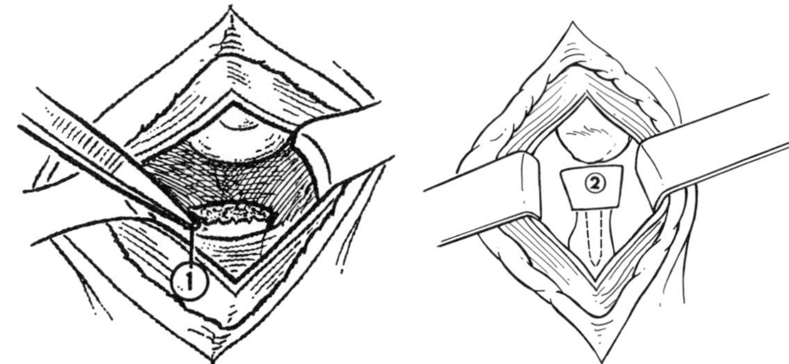

Isolated Anterior Dislocation of the Radial Head

REMARKS

This condition can occur in childhood and may go unrecognized into adulthood. Although there are rare instances of congenital bilateral radial head dislocations, unilateral radial head dislocation is almost consistently the result of a traumatic episode.

A greenstick fracture of the ulna can occur with little force on the child's elbow, and the symptoms and signs of associated radial head dislocation may pass unrecognized unless evaluated carefully by clinical and x-ray examination.

Childhood Injury (Unrecognized)

1. The most frequent cause of a unilateral dislocation of the radial head anteriorly is an unrecognized Monteggia fracture in a child.
2. The callus and angulation of the ulna associated with the radial head dislocation is indicative of a previous Monteggia fracture.

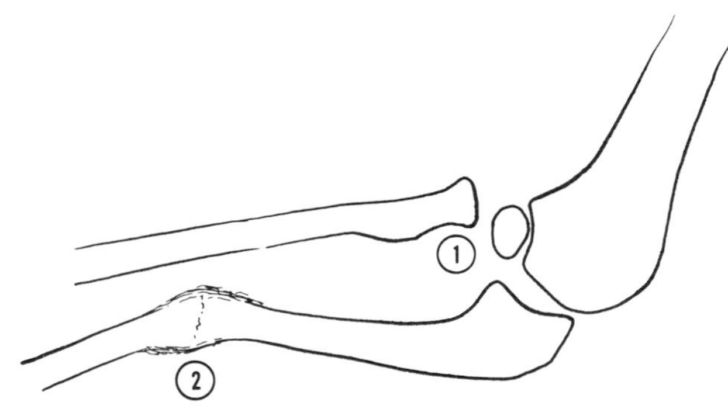

Adult Lesion

1. Failure to recognize a dislocation of the radial head in childhood can lead to persistent dislocation in the adult.
2. Characteristically there is convexity of the proximal radius with resorption of bone.
3. There is flattening of the capitellum.
4. The ulna may angulate in the direction that the radial head is dislocated.

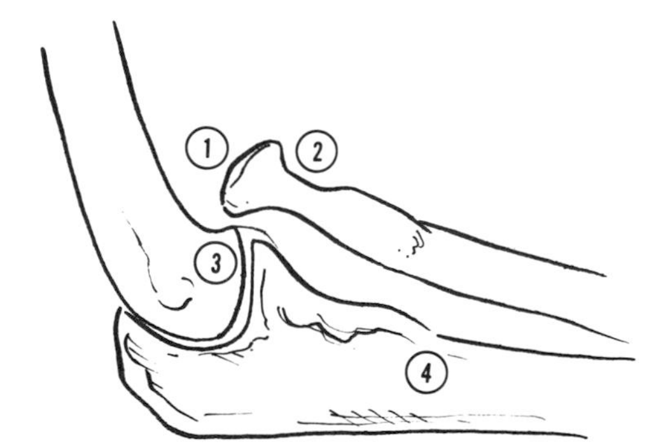

Management

Although in the past it has been recommended that the isolated dislocation of the radial head be managed nonoperatively, Lloyd-Roberts and coworkers have demonstrated that many of these patients lose function and are benefitted by operative repair. This is best carried out as soon as the dislocation is recognized, but the operation may be performed as long as 3 years after this injury.

Posterior Subluxation or Dislocation of the Radial Head

Bell and coworkers discussed problems of posterior subluxation or dislocation of the radial head. Chronic posterior dislocation may occasionally be congenital. However, isolated unilateral dislocations are frequently the result of residual traumatic problems. The subluxation or dislocation is generally one of three types:

1. In type I subluxation the radial head is subluxated and deformed posteriorly but still articulates with the radiohumeral joint.

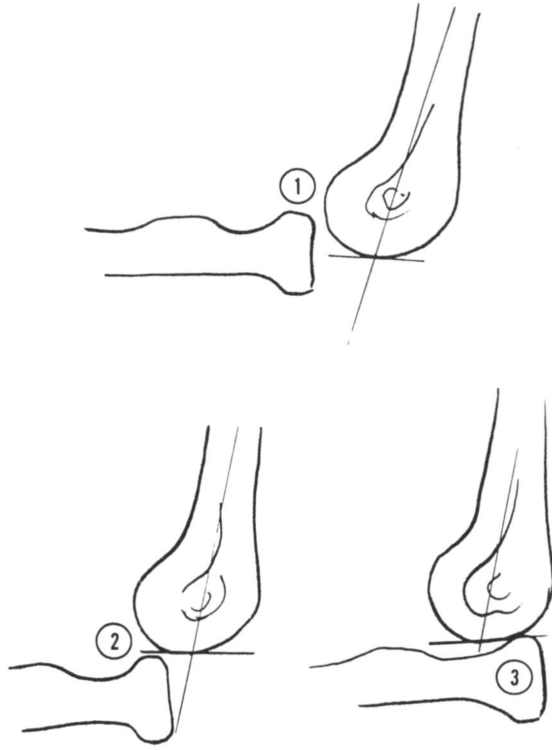

2. A type II radial head dislocation is displaced inferiorly to the capitellum but does not lie posterior to the midline of the humerus.
3. A completely dislocated radial head (type III) lies proximal and posterior to the midline of the humerus.

Management

Pain, limitation of motion, and some cosmetic deformities are the usual complaints associated with chronic posterior dislocation of the radial head. The greatest pain symptoms are associated more with the subluxation type than with dislocation.

Motion, particularly supination, is limited with the completely dislocated radial head. Most patients with posterior subluxation or dislocation of the radial head do not usually have serious impairment of function, except for loss of rotation.

Occasionally the painful symptoms may be sufficiently disabling that radial head resection may be necessary. This, however, is the exception rather than the rule.

BIBLIOGRAPHY

Distal Humeral Fractures

Bledsoe RC, Izenstark JL: Displacement of fat pads in disease and injury of the elbow. A new radiographic sign. Radiology 73:717, 1959.

Bryan RS: Fracture about the elbow in adults. *In* Murray D (ed): American Academy of Orthopaedic Surgeons: Instructional Course Lectures, Vol 30. CV Mosby Co., St. Louis, MO, 1981.

Grantham SA, Teitjen R: Transcondylar fracture-dislocation of the elbow. J Bone Joint Surg Am 58:1030, 1976.

MacAusland WR, Wyman ET: Fractures of the adult elbow. *In* Burke-Evans E (ed): American Academy of Orthopaedic Surgeons: Instructional Course Lectures, Vol 24. CV Mosby Co., St. Louis, MO, 1975.

Morrey BF (ed): The Elbow and Its Disorders. WB Saunders Co., Philadelphia, 1985.

Morrey BF, An K-Y: Functional anatomy of the elbow ligaments. Clin Orthop 201:84, 1985.

Smith FM: Surgery of the Elbow, 2nd ed. WB Saunders Co., Philadelphia, 1972.

Soltanpur A: Anterior supracondylar fracture of the humerus (flexion type). A simple technique for closed reduction and fixation in adults and the aged. J Bone Joint Surg Br 60:383, 1978.

Intercondylar Fracture

Brown RF, Morgan RG: Intercondylar T-shaped fracture of the humerus. J Bone Joint Surg Br 53:425, 1971.

Charnley J: Closed Treatment of Common Fractures, 3rd ed. Williams & Wilkins, Baltimore, MD, 1961.

Evans EM: Supracondylar Y fracture of the humerus. J Bone Joint Surg Br 35:381, 1953.

Gabel GT, Hanson G, Bennett JB, et al.: Intraarticular fractures of the distal humerus in the adult. Clin Orthop 216:99, 1987.

Jupiter JB, Neff R, Holzach P, et al.: Intercondylar fractures of the humerus. J Bone Joint Surg Am 67:226, 1985.

Miller WE: Comminuted fractures of the distal end of the humerus in the adult. AAOS Instructional Course Lectures. J Bone Joint Surg Am 46:644, 1964.

Riseborough FJ, Radin EL: Intracondylar T fractures of the humerus in the adult. J Bone Joint Surg Am 51:130, 1969.

Smith FM: Surgery of the Elbow, 2nd ed. WB Saunders Co., Philadelphia, 1972.

Fractures of the Capitellum

Alvarez E, Patel MR, Nimberg G, et al.: Fracture of the capitellum humeri. J Bone Joint Surg Am 57:1093, 1975.

Christopher F, Bushnell LF: Conservative treatment of fracture of the capitellum. J Bone Joint Surg Am 17:489, 1935.

Collert S: Surgical management of fractures of the capitulum humeri. Acta Orthop Scand 48:603, 1977.

Dushuttle RP, Coyle MP, Zawadsky JP, Bloom H: Fractures of the capitellum. J Trauma 25:317, 1985.

Fowles JV, Kassab MT: Fracture of the capitulum humeri: Treatment by excision. J Bone Joint Surg Am 56:794, 1974.

Morrey BF, Stormont T, An K-N: Force transmission through the radial head. J Bone Joint Surg Am 70:250, 1988.

Richards RR, Khoury GW, Burke FD, et al.: Internal fixation of capitellar fractures using Herbert screws: A report of four cases. Can J Surg 30:188, 1987.

Complications

Ackerman G, Jupiter J: Nonunion of fractures of the distal head of the humerus. J Bone Joint Surg Am 70:75, 1988.

Coventry M: Ectopic ossification about the elbow. *In* Morre BF (ed): The Elbow and Its Disorders. WB Saunders Co., Philadelphia, 1985.

Galbraith KA, McCullough CJ: Acute nerve injury as a complication of closed fractures or dislocations of the elbow. Br J Accident Surg 11:159, 1979.

Hallett J: Entrapment of the median nerve after dislocation of the elbow. J Bone Joint Surg Br 63:408, 1981.

Horne G: Supracondylar fractures of the humerus in adults. J Trauma 20:71, 1980.

Matev I: Radiological sign of entrapment of the median nerve in the elbow joint after posterior dislocation. J Bone Joint Surg Br 58:353, 1976.

Mitsunaga MS, Bryan RS, Linscheid RL: Condylar non-unions of the elbow. J Trauma 22:787, 1982.

Morrey BF, Adams R, Bryan RS: Total elbow replacement for post-traumatic arthritis. J Bone Joint Surg Br 73:400, 1991.

Dislocations

Billett DM: Unreduced posterior dislocation of the elbow. J Trauma 19:186, 1979.

Broberg M, Morrey BF: Treatment of radial head fracture and elbow dislocation. A long-term follow-up study. Clin Orthop 216:109, 1987.

Bruce C, Laing P, Dorgan J, Klenerman L: Unreduced dislocation of the elbow: Case report and review of the literature. J Trauma 35:962, 1993.

Carl A, Prada S, Teixeira K: Proximal radioulnar transposition in an elbow dislocation. J Orthop Trauma 6:106, 1992.

DeLee JC: Transverse divergent dislocation of the elbow in a child. J Bone Joint Surg Am 63:322, 1981.

Dryer R, Buckwalter J, Sprague B: Treatment of the chronic elbow instability. Clin Orthop 100:254, 1974.

Fowles JV, Kassab MT, Douik M: Untreated posterior dislocation of the elbow in children. J Bone Joint Surg Am 66:921, 1984.

Garland DE, O'Hollaren RM: Fractures and dislocations about the elbow in the head-injured adult. Clin Orthop 168:38, 1982.

Grimer RJ, Brooks S: Brachial artery damage accompanying closed posterior dislocation of the elbow. J Bone Joint Surg Br 67:378, 1985.

Hankin FM: Posterior dislocation of the elbow. Clin Orthop 190:254, 1984.

Harrington IJ, Tountas AA: Replacement of the radial head in the treatment of unstable elbow fractures. Injury 12:405, 1981.

Harvey S, Tchelebi H: Proximal radio-ulnar translocation. J Bone Joint Surg Am 61:447, 1979.

Hassmann GC, Brunn F, Neer CS: Recurrent dislocation of the elbow. J Bone Joint Surg Am 57:1080, 1975.

Josepfsson PO, Gentz CF, Johnell O, et al.: Surgical versus nonsurgical treatment of ligamentous injuries following dislocation of the elbow joint. A prospective randomized study. J Bone Joint Surg Am 69:605, 1987.

Jupiter JB, Leibovic SJ, Ribbans W, Wilk RM: The posterior Monteggia lesion. J Orthop Trauma 5:395, 1991.

Linscheid RL, Wheeler DK: Elbow dislocations. JAMA 194:1171, 1965.

Louis DS, Ricciardi JE, Spengler DM: Arterial injury: A complication of posterior elbow dislocation. A clinical and anatomical study. J Bone Joint Surg Am 56:1631, 1974.

Matev I: A radiological sign of entrapment of the median nerve in the elbow joint after posterior dislocation. A report of two cases. J Bone Joint Surg Br 58:353, 1976.

Mehlhoff TL, Noble MS, Bennett JB, et al.: Simple dislocation of the elbow in the adult. J Bone Joint Surg Am 70:244, 1988.

Meyn MA, Quigley TB: Reduction of posterior dislocation of the elbow by traction on the dangling arm. Clin Orthop 103:106, 1974.

Nakano A, Tanaka S, Hirofuji E, et al.: Transverse divergent dislocation of the elbow in a six-year-old boy: Case report. J Trauma 32:118, 1992.

Osborne G, Cotterill P: Recurrent dislocation of the elbow. J Bone Joint Surg Br 48:340, 1966.

Pritchard DJ, Linscheid RL, Svien HJ: Intra-articular median nerve entrapment with dislocation of the elbow. Clin Orthop 90:100, 1973.

Protzmann RR: Dislocation of the elbow joint. J Bone Joint Surg Am 60:539, 1978.

Regan W, Morrey BF: Fractures of the coronoid. J Bone J Surg Am 72:1348, 1989.

Roberts JB, Pankratz D.: The surgical treatment of heterotopic ossification at the elbow following long-term coma. J Bone Joint Surg Am 61:760, 1979.

St. Clair Strange FG: Entrapment of the median nerve after dislocation of the elbow. J Bone Joint Surg Br 64:224, 1982.

Swanson AB, Jaeger SH, LaRochelle D: Comminuted fractures of the radial head. The role of silicone implant replacement arthroplasty. J Bone Joint Surg Am 63:1039, 1981.

Symeonides PP, Paschaloglou C, Stavrou Z, et al.: Recurrent dislocation of the elbow. J Bone Joint Surg Am 57:1084, 1975.

Wheeler DK, Linscheid RL: Fracture-dislocations of the elbow. Clin Orthop 50:95, 1967.

Radial Head Fractures and Dislocations

Adler JB, Shaftan GW: Radial head fractures is excision necessary? J Trauma 4:115, 1964.

Bell SN, Morrey BF, Bianco AJ: Chronic posterior subluxation and dislocation of the radial head. J Bone Joint Surg Am 73:392, 1991.

Broberg M, Morrey BF: Results of delayed excision of the radial head after fracture. J Bone Joint Surg Am 68:669, 1986.

Broberg M, Morrey BF: Treatment of radial head fracture and elbow dislocation. A long term follow-up study. Clin Orthop 216:109, 1987.

Carn RM, Medige J, Curtain D, et al.: Silicone rubber replacement of the severely fractured radial head. Clin Orthop 209:259, 1986.

Charnley J: Closed Treatment of Common Fractures, 3rd ed. Williams and Wilkins, Baltimore, MD, 1961.

Coleman DA, Blair WF, Scherr D: Resection of the radial head for fracture: Long-term follow-up of 17 cases J Bone Joint Surg Am 69:388, 1987.

Geel CW, Palmer AK: Radial head fractures and their effect on the distal radioulnar joint. Clin Orthop 275:79, 1992.

Goldberg I, Peylon J, Yosipovitch Z: Late results of excision of the radial head for isolated closed fractures. J Bone Joint Surg Am 68:675, 1986.

Holdsworth BJ, Clement DA, Rothwell PNR: Fractures of the radial head—the benefit of aspiration: A prospective controlled trial. Injury 18:44, 1987.

Khalfaya EE, Randall WC, Alexander H: Mason type II radial head fractures: Operative versus nonoperative treatment. J Orthop Trauma 6:283, 1992.

Knight D, Rymaszewski L, Amis A, Miller J: Primary replacement of the fractured radial head with a metal prosthesis. J Bone Joint Surg Br 75:572, 1993.

Levin PD: Fracture of the radial head with dislocation of the distal radioulnar joint: Case report. Treatment by prosthetic replacement of the radial ulnar head. J Bone Joint Surg Am 55:837, 1973.

Lloyd-Roberts GC, Bucknill TM: Anterior dislocation of the radial head in children. J Bone Joint Surg 59:402, 1977.

Mackay I, Fitzgerald B, Miller HJ: Silastic replacement of the head of the radius in trauma. J Bone Joint Surg Br 61:494, 1979.

McDougall A, White J: Subluxation of the inferior radioulnar joint complicating fracture of the radial head. J Bone Joint Surg Br 39:278, 1957.

Morrey BF, Chao EY, Hui FC: Biomechanical study of the elbow following excision of the radial head. J Bone Joint Surg Am 61:63, 1979.

Oldenheimer K, Harvey JP, Jr: Internal fixation of fracture of the head of the radius. J Bone Joint Surg Am 61:785, 1979.

Postacchini F, Morace G: Radial head fractures treated by resection: Long-term results. Ital J Orthop Trauma 8:323, 1992.

Radin EL, Riseborough EJ: Fractures of the radial head. J Bone Joint Surg Am 48:1055, 1966.

Shmueli G, Herold HZ: Compression screwing of displaced fractures of the head of the radius. J Bone Joint Surg Br 63:535, 1981.

Swanson AB, Jaeger SH, LaRochelle D: Comminuted fractures of the radial head. The role of silicone-implant replacement arthroplasty. J Bone Joint Surg Am 63:1039, 1981.

Taylor TKF, O'Connor BT: The effect upon the inferior radio-ulnar joint of excision of the head of the radius in adults. J Bone Joint Surg Br 46:83, 1964.

Trousdale RT, Amadio PC, Cooney WP, Morrey BF: Radio-ulnar dissociation. J Bone Joint Surg Am 74:1486, 1992.

Weseley MS, Barenfeld PA, Eisenstein AL: Closed treatment of isolated radial head fractures. J Trauma 23:36, 1983.

Olecranon Fractures

Adler S, Fay GD, MacAusland WR: Olecranon fractures. J Bone Joint Surg Am 41:1540, 1959.

Adler S, Fay GD, MacAusland WR: Treatment of olecranon fractures. Indication for excision of the olecranon fragment and repair of the triceps tendon. J Trauma 2:597, 1962.

Fyfe IS, Mossad MN, Holdsworth BJ: Methods of fixation of olecranon fractures: An experimental mechanical study. J Bone Joint Surg Br 67:367, 1985.

Gartsman GM, Sculco TP, Otis JC: Operative treatment of olecranon fractures. J Bone Joint Surg Am 63:718, 1981.

Jupiter JB, Leibovic SJ, Ribbans W, Wilk RM: The posterior Monteggia lesion. J Orthop Trauma 5:395, 1991.

Murphy DF, Greene WB, Dameron TB: Displaced olecranon fractures in adults: Clinical evaluation. Clin Orthop 224:215, 1987.

15 Fractures of the Shafts of the Bones of the Forearm

EPIDEMIOLOGY OF FRACTURES OF THE FOREARM IN ADULTS (PATIENTS OVER 17 YEARS OF AGE)

REMARKS

Although statistics vary from series to series, the following list represents the usual distribution of forearm fractures in adults:

- Most of the fractures are produced by direct trauma.
- 15 per cent are open fractures.
- 85 per cent occur in men.
- 50 per cent occur in persons under the age of 40.
- 85 per cent occur in persons under the age of 60.
- 40 per cent are fractures of both bones.
- 50 per cent show some comminution.
- 60 per cent involve the middle third of the bones.

Mechanism of Fracture

Direct Injury

The most common mechanism of injury to the forearm is the direct blow, such as frequently causes an isolated fracture of the ulna (nightstick fracture). Greater direct violence may be sustained from motor vehicle accidents, falls, or gunshot wounds, which produce two-bone fracture or, least frequently, solitary fracture of the radius. Direct injury may be sufficient to produce an open fracture, but the majority of forearm fractures do not communicate with the external environment.

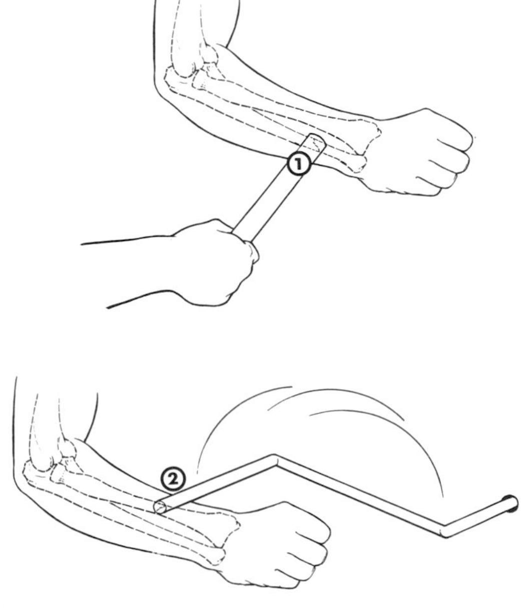

1. Solitary fracture of the ulna from a direct blow (nightstick fracture).

2. Solitary fracture of the distal radius. The distal radioulnar joint is undisturbed, provided that the radius does not shorten.

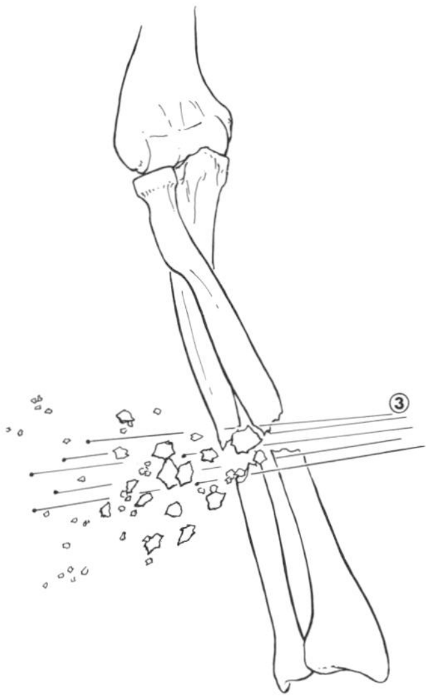

3. Gunshot fracture, both bones.

Indirect Injury

The most common indirect mechanism of forearm fracture is a fall on the outstretched hand. The vertical loading is associated with a rotatory force when the body's weight twists about the axis of the fixed radius, causing either hyperpronation or hypersupination of the forearm. Hyperpronation tends to angulate the fracture dorsally, whereas hypersupination causes the fracture to angulate in a volar direction.

Usually the radius angulates more than the ulna. The most common fracture sustained through the indirect mechanism is the incomplete or greenstick fracture in a child. This quite frequently can be reduced by reversing the rotational force that produced it.

When the adult falls on the outstretched arm with the radius locked and the elbow in extension, the ulna and humerus rotate around the distal radioulnar joint. The extreme torque of this injury disrupts the distal radioulnar joint and fractures the distal radius (Galeazzi's fracture). With the elbow slightly flexed during the fall on the outstretched hand, the torque tends to be absorbed more proximally about the elbow, producing a fracture of the ulna with dislocation of the radial head (Monteggia's fracture-dislocation).

Indirect Torsional Injury from Forceful Pronation

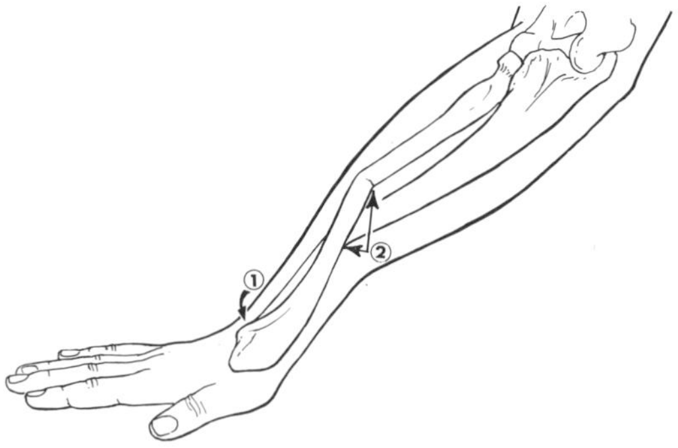

1. Forceful pronation causes
2. The radius to angulate dorsally as it rotates over the ulna.

Indirect Torsional Injury from Forceful Supination

1. Force vectors from supination injury produce
2. Volar angulation of the radius to a greater degree than
3. Angulation of the ulna.

Note: This is the most common type of greenstick deformity. The greater angulation of the radius indicates that the injury occurred while the radius was rotating around the ulna.

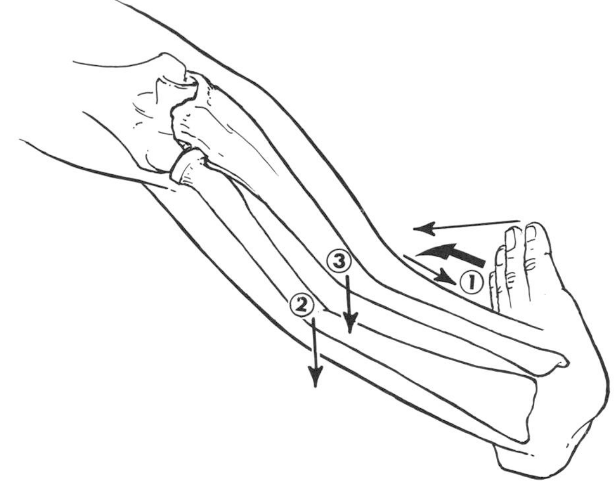

Rotational Injury Producing Galeazzi's Fracture

1. With the elbow extended and the wrist hyperextended,
2. The entire length of the humerus and ulna rotates around the fixed distal radius.
3. The distal radioulnar joint fails.
4. The radius fractures from bending or torque loading.

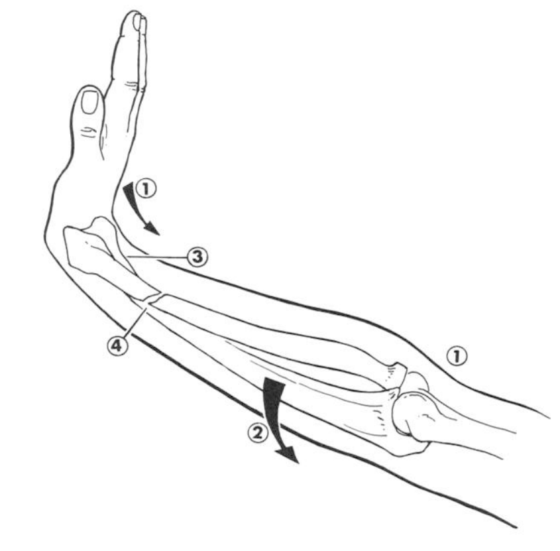

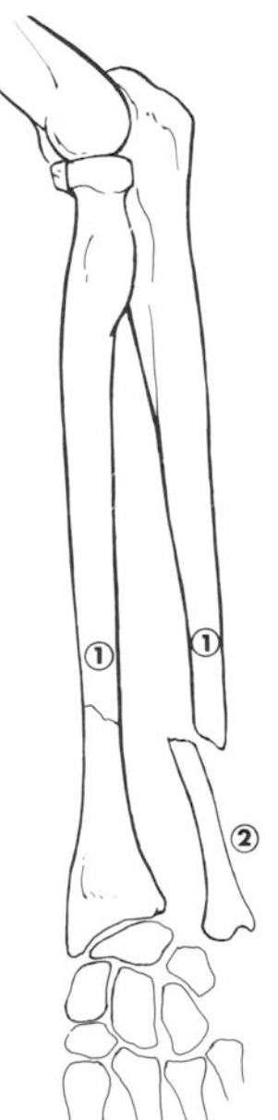

Occasionally,
1. Both the radius and the ulna fail.
2. The distal radioulnar joint also dislocates.

Anterior Monteggia Lesion from Elbow Hyperextension

1. A fall backward forces the forearm into supination.
2. The elbow is hyperextended.
3. Reflex contraction of the elbow flexors dislocates the radial head anteriorly.
4. The force of the injury displaces the ulna through the flexor carpi ulnaris and may displace it through the skin.

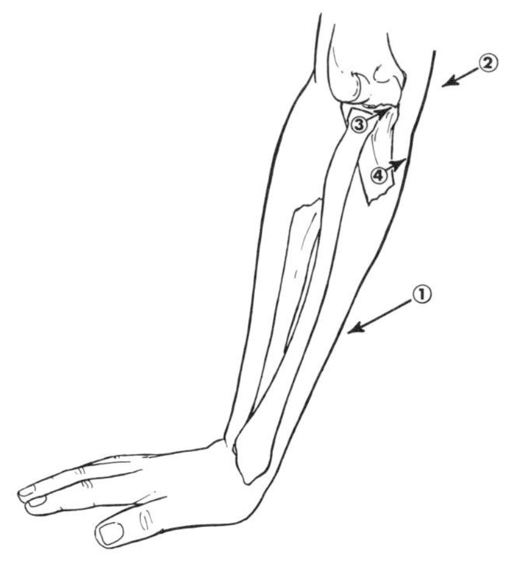

Torsional Injury Producing Anterior Monteggia Fracture-Dislocation

1. With the hand fixed to the ground,
2. The momentum of the fall causes the trunk and arm to rotate externally while
3. The ulna rotates internally around the fixed radius.
4. Fracture of the ulna results.

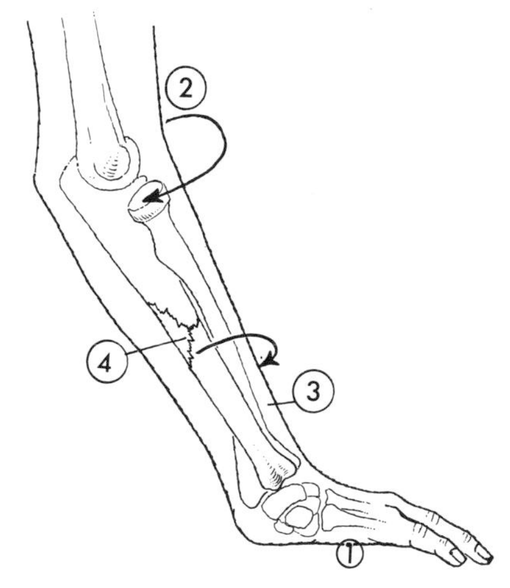

As the force continues,
1. The radius and the proximal fragment of ulna come into contact, and
2. The radial head is levered anteriorly out of the proximal radioulnar joint.
3. Alternatively, a fracture of the radius occurs in the proximal third of its shaft.

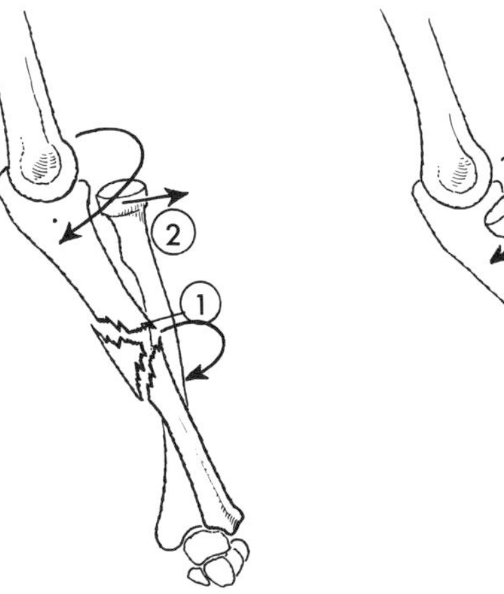

ANATOMIC CONSIDERATIONS

Biomechanics of Forearm Rotation and Forearm Fractures

REMARKS

The function that is significantly most impaired with forearm fractures is the unique rotatory motion necessary for positioning of the hand. This requires rotation of the radius and not of the ulna. Fortunately, loss of forearm rotation can be compensated by shoulder motion, particularly if the loss is in the direction of pronation.

Rotation of 120°–140° is ordinarily possible in the forearm. Maintenance of the normal lateral bow of the radius permits it to clear soft tissues of the forearm and rotate around the ulna. Maintenance of normal interosseous width is also important to permit rotation of the radius.

The interosseous space is widest in neutral rotation and narrowest in full pronation. Maintenance of extreme pronation during fracture treatment may cause permanent contracture and stiffening of the muscles and ligaments, thereby limiting supination. It is thus important to immobilize forearm fractures in either supination or neutral rotation.

Biomechanics of Normal Forearm Rotation

1. The normal 9° bow of the radius permits rotation without soft tissue impingement.

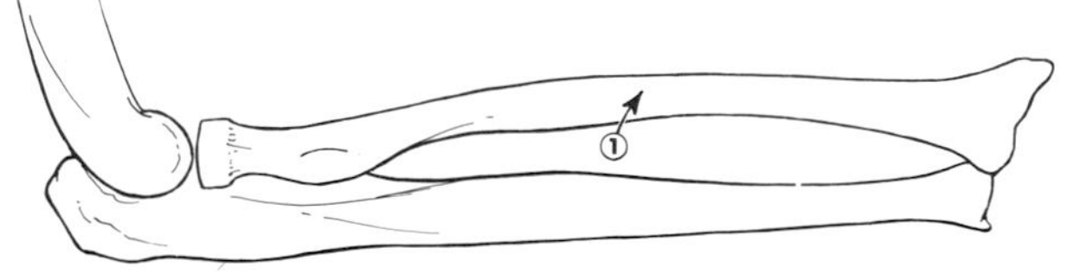

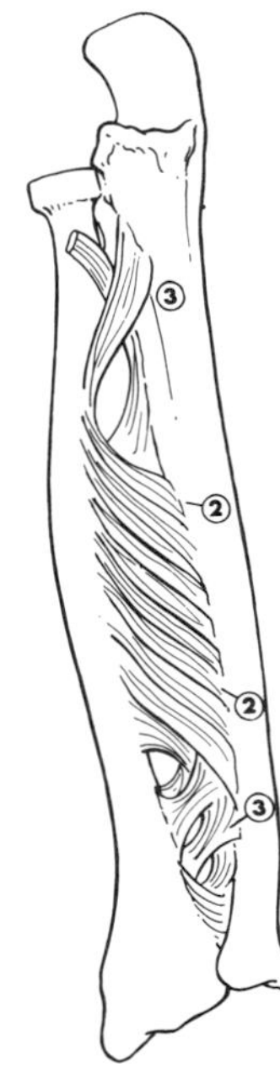

2. The interosseous membrane, which extends from the distal ulna to the proximal radius, prevents upward displacement of the radius and acts as the radioulnar hinge.
3. Superior and inferior oblique cords of the interosseous membrane resist downward pull on the radius.

Note: The major limitation of forearm rotation is due to muscle impingement rather than to the interosseous membrane.

PRONATION AND SUPINATION

1. The pronation and supination range is 120°–140°.

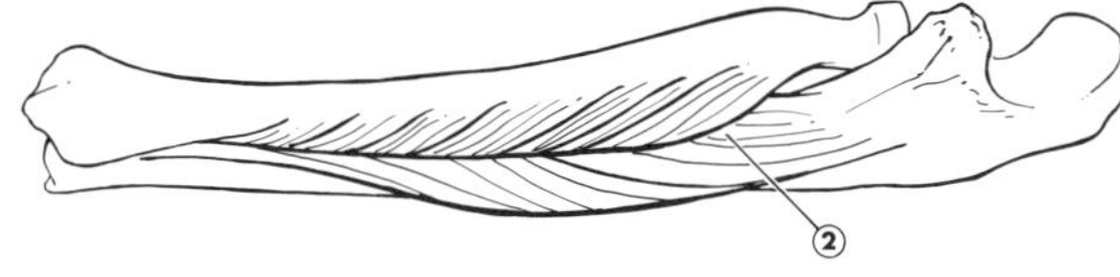

2. The principal impediments to forearm rotation are tight muscles and impingement, particularly of the flexor pollicis longus on the flexor digitorum profundus.

INTEROSSEOUS SPACE

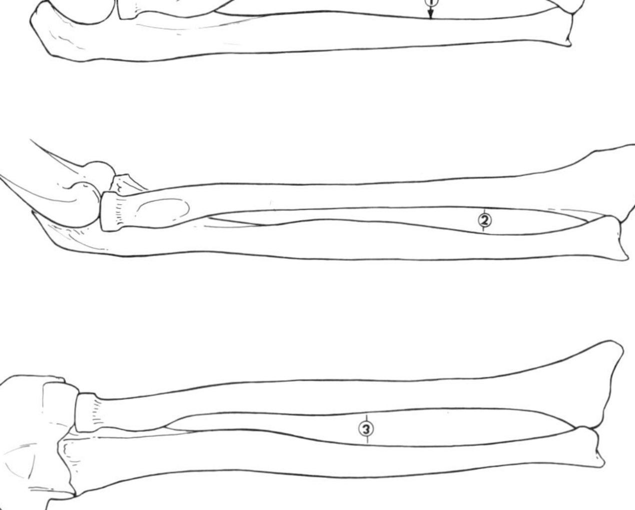

1. The interosseous space is widest in neutral rotation.

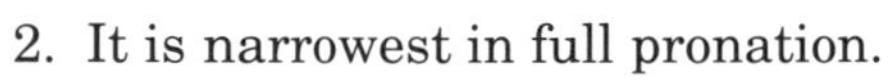

2. It is narrowest in full pronation.

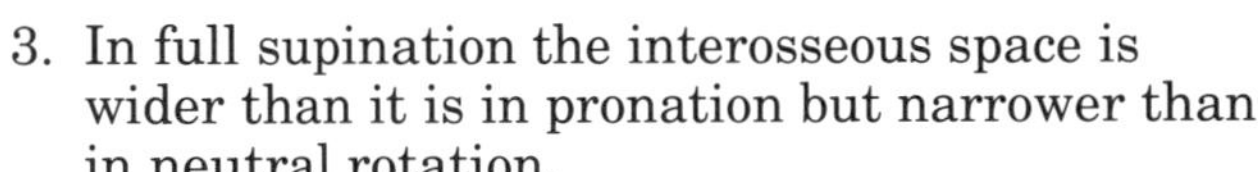

3. In full supination the interosseous space is wider than it is in pronation but narrower than in neutral rotation.

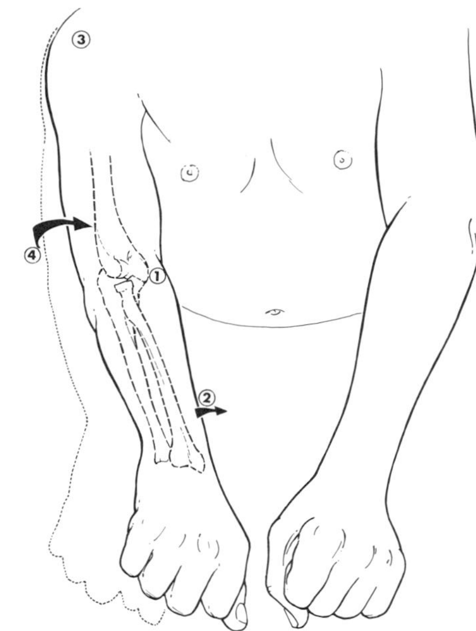

Compensatory Shoulder Motion

LOSS OF FOREARM PRONATION

1. With the elbow extended, the axis of rotation passes through the shoulder.
2. Loss of forearm pronation is accommodated by
3. Shoulder abduction and
4. Shoulder internal rotation.

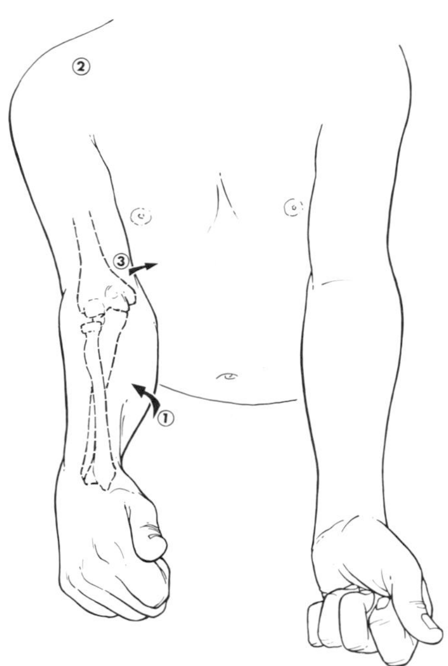

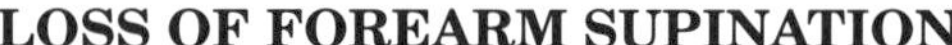

LOSS OF FOREARM SUPINATION

1. Accommodation for loss of forearm supination requires
2. Shoulder external rotation
3. With the arm adducted; adduction is limited by the trunk.

Note: Because shoulder motion can compensate for loss of pronation but not loss of supination, it is preferable to immobilize forearm fractures in supination whenever possible. Then if rotation is lost it is more likely to be lost in pronation, which can be replaced by shoulder motion.

Alterations in Skeletal Anatomy That Can Affect Forearm Function

REMARKS

The forearm can accommodate a great deal of structural alteration and shortening. Shortening of the upper extremity in general is tolerated more and is less functionally impairing than shortening in the lower limb. However, if the radius shortens more than 5–7 mm, it is likely to be associated with disruption of the distal radial-ulnar articulation. In addition, although some angulation of the forearm can be tolerated without impairing rotation, angulation greater than 10°–15° is usually likely to limit rotation and also to be cosmetically unacceptable.

Deformities Resulting from Forearm Fractures

1. Typically there is rotational angulation and displacement of the radius and ulna, with the distal fragment usually pronating relative to the proximal fragments.
2. Shortening and overriding of the radius and ulna occur.
3. The interosseous space is narrowed and the normal radial bow is lost.

Note: The objective of reduction should be to restore the radial bow and rotational alignment as well as to correct shortening of the radius and ulna.

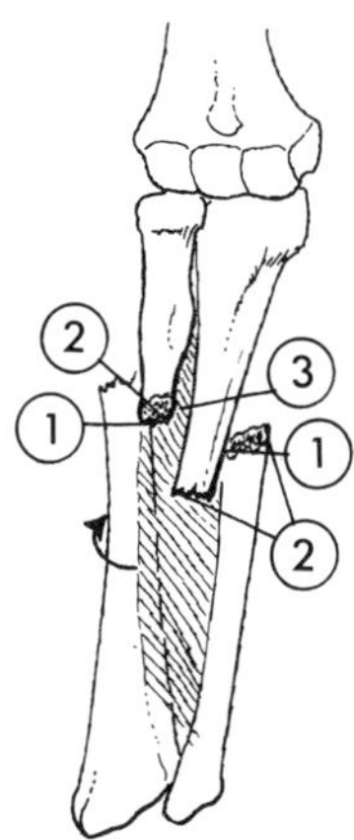

1. Shortening of the radius can be accepted in some fractures, provided it is no greater than 5 mm.
2. If greater shortening occurs, the distal radioulnar joint is likely to be impaired or disrupted.

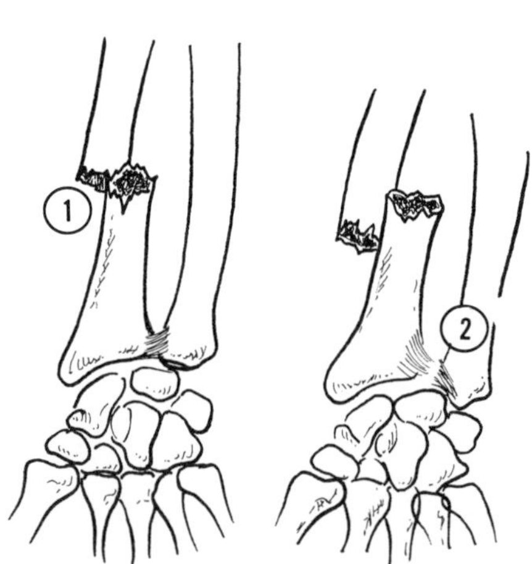

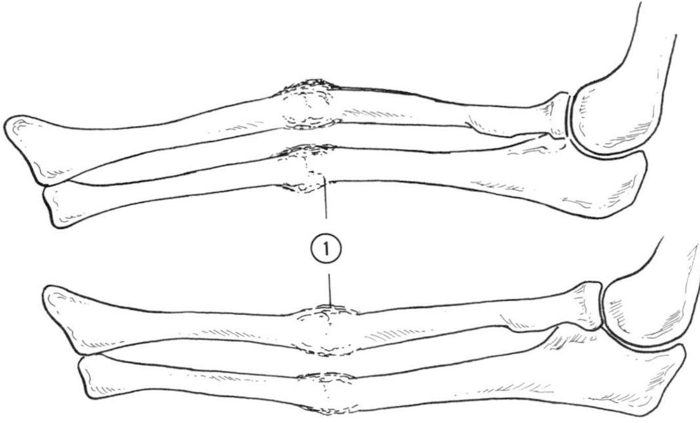

1. Angulation of less than 10° in any plane does not usually significantly impair the forearm rotation.

2. Angulation of 10°–20°, however, is likely to cause visual deformity as well as functional impairment.

GENERAL CONSIDERATIONS IN TREATMENT

REMARKS

Both closed and open treatment of forearm fractures require skill, patience, and a critical appreciation of the indications and limitations of both the technique and the surgeon. Single-bone fractures without associated proximal or distal radioulnar dislocation and two-bone fractures without comminution do well with closed methods.

In the adult, fracture of the radius or ulna associated with dislocation of the adjacent proximal or distal radioulnar joint requires internal fracture fixation to permit reduction of the dislocation. Comminuted fractures with bone loss requiring bone grafting should also be treated by internal fixation.

Except for these categories of fractures in adults, a closed reduction and functional cast or cast-brace treatment may be effective for many forearm fractures. Forearm fractures in children have considerably different physiologic implications and must be considered separately (see Chapter 2).

Closed Reduction and Functional Treatment of Forearm Fractures

REMARKS

Closed reduction is the treatment of choice for fractures of the forearm in children, except for the occasional Monteggia fracture-dislocation, as discussed elsewhere. Closed reduction has also been standard for thousands of years in managing adult forearm fractures. Shang and other investigators in China have shown that the traditional methods of reducing forearm fractures in adults can be quite safe and effective.

Sarmiento and coworkers have shown that closed reduction can be attempted for most adult forearm fractures with the understanding that an unstable fracture may eventually require open reduction and internal fixation. In this situation there is no need to continue persistently with closed management if by 10 days to 2 weeks it becomes evident that desirable reduction cannot be maintained. It is preferable to achieve anatomic reduction, but angulation of 10° or less does not contribute to functional impairment.

The end result from successful closed treatment is frequently equal to or superior to that of operative fixation, particularly for isolated fractures of the radius and ulna without proximal or distal dislocation. In addition, numerous complications of operative fixation can thereby be avoided. Patients who object to forearm scars from surgery are particularly good candidates for attempted closed treatment.

Single Bone Fractures: Indications for Closed Treatment

Isolated Fracture of the Ulna

REMARKS

This is the most common of forearm fractures and is usually isolated and relatively undisplaced. If there is displacement evident, carefully evaluate the proximal and distal radioulnar joints for dislocation.

The isolated ulna fracture has been the forearm fracture most likely to develop nonunion when treated by conventional open or closed techniques. Functional bracing of this difficult fracture, as developed by Sarmiento and coworkers, has given surprisingly better healing and functional results than has standard nonoperative or even operative technique. The reasons for better results with the Sarmiento brace treatment of the ulna fractures are uncertain, except for the possibility that improved blood supply and external callus results from emphasis on function of the wrist and elbow.

In evaluating the progress of the patient, most achieve clinical union several weeks or months before radiographic union. All fractures that reach clinical union eventually heal radiographically. Prolonged immobilization, preventing the patient from returning to work until radiographic union, is unnecessary in most reliable patients.

Fracture angulation of the ulna of 10°–20° does not affect clinical results. However, fractures of the distal ulna and oblique fractures are most prone to angulation, which may be anticipated and corrected initially.

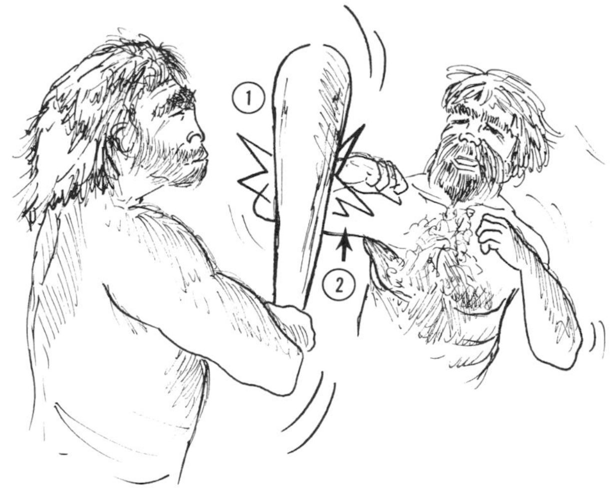

Mechanism of the Isolated Ulna Fracture

1. The classic mechanism of the isolated ulnar fracture through history has been from a direct blow to the forearm.
2. This is characteristically related to some type of assault or accident in which the forearm is raised to protect the head.

Indirect Mechanism

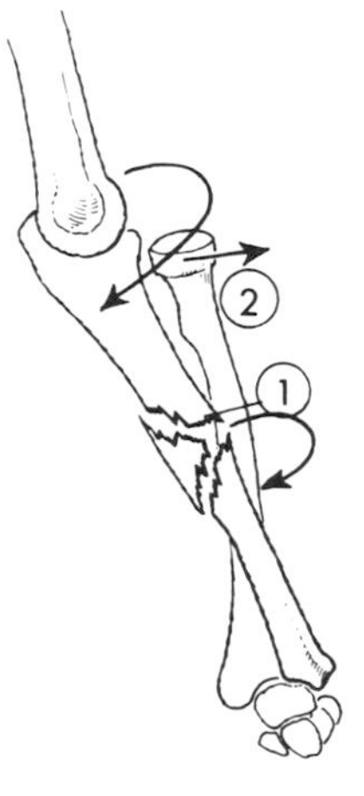

1. An indirect twisting mechanism from a fall on the outstretched forearm may also result in ulnar fracture.
2. This is also associated with a dislocation of the proximal radial head (Monteggia fracture-dislocation). This is an unstable injury, as previously described, and generally requires operative fixation, in contrast to the usual ulnar fracture produced by a direct injury.

Note: A similar rationale applies to the management of the isolated radial fracture. Thus the isolated fracture produced by direct injury can usually be treated closed, whereas the isolated radial fracture resulting from indirect loading usually causes radioulnar instability and necessitates internal fixation. (See section on isolated radial fractures.)

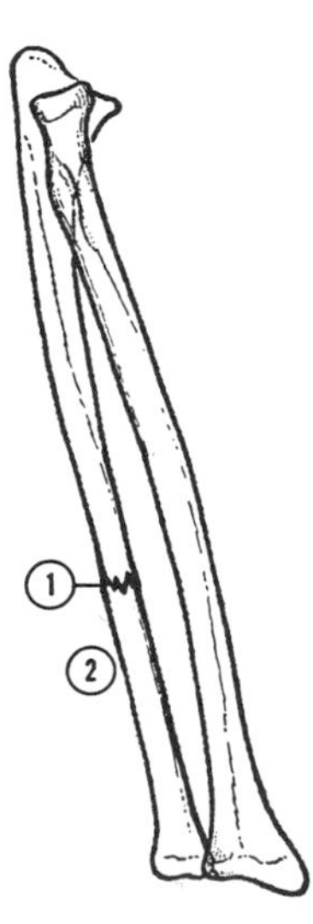

Appearance on X-Ray—Undisplaced Ulnar Fractures

1. Transverse fracture at the junction of the lower and middle thirds.
2. No angulation is evident. If angulation occurs, check carefully for dislocation of the distal or proximal radioulnar joint.

Note: Most isolated ulnar fractures are relatively undisplaced.

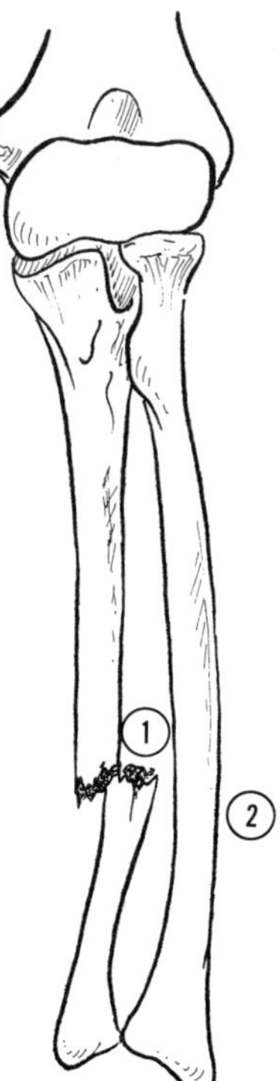

Appearance on X-Ray: Displaced Fracture

1. Fracture of the distal ulna with angulation toward the radius may heal with callus and slight narrowing of the interosseous space.
2. This should affect range of motion and rotation of the forearm minimally, if at all, and is usually an acceptable result.

Management of the Isolated Fracture of the Ulna

REMARKS

This type of fracture is often better treated by closed than by open methods. The fracture initially can be immobilized with a splint or a long arm cast for the first 3–5 days until acute swelling and discomfort subside.

Subsequently a Sarmiento fracture sleeve is applied using plaster or prefabricated brace material. The results with this early fracture brace method is prompt healing with clinical union, usually by 6–8 weeks, and radiographic union by 10–12 weeks.

Functional Sleeve Application

Functional sleeve application is applied when the swelling and pain subside (7–10 days).

1. A plaster sleeve is molded firmly into the interosseous space.
2. The elbow and
3. The wrist are free.

Note: Alternatively, an Orthoplast sleeve, with Velcro straps that permit tightening of the sleeve and allow its removal for personal hygiene, may be used.

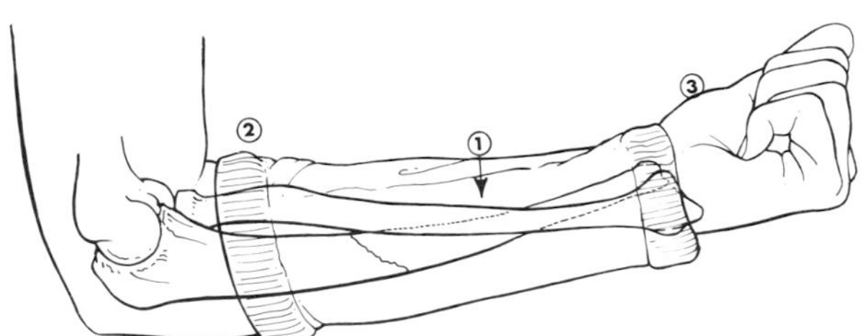

After Fracture-Brace Application

1. The ulnar fracture shows callus with this functional treatment method, usually by 4–6 weeks.
2. It may take an additional 6 weeks for the fracture line to be completely obliterated on x-ray; however, clinically the patient is usually able to function for most activities by 6–8 weeks. Prolonging immobilization until radiographic healing is apparent is usually unnecessary.

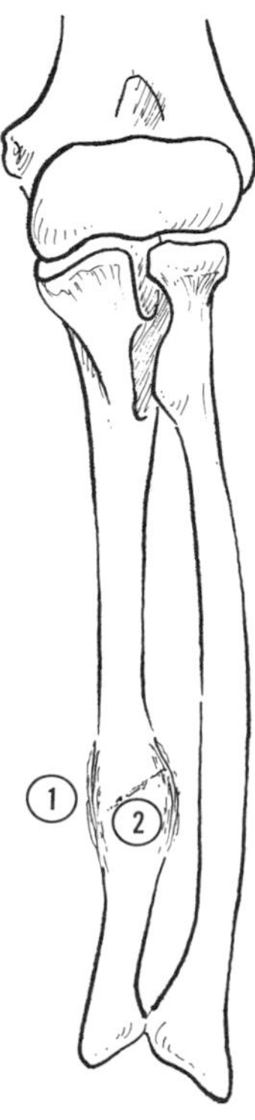

Subsequent Management

Encourage the patient to actively use the wrist and elbow on the fractured side. The ulnar fracture-brace or cast has proved to be the most reliable method of treating the isolated ulnar fracture. The motion in the wrist and elbow, and active muscle exercise of the forearm, maximize healing by external callus.

The ulnar fracture heals clinically, as evidenced by the patient's freedom from pain and absence of motion at the fracture site, usually by 6–8 weeks. Slight displacement of the ulna toward the radius may occur but should not limit forearm rotation.

Use of the ulnar sleeve has proved to be the treatment of choice for isolated ulnar fractures. It has virtually eliminated the need for internal fixation of such injuries.

Fracture of the Ulna With Dislocation of the Radial Head (Monteggia Fracture)

REMARKS

About 7 per cent of forearm fractures are a combination of fracture of the ulna at any level and dislocation of the radial head (Monteggia fracture). Results from this injury in the past have been notoriously bad, because either the dislocation goes unrecognized or nonunion occurs. Awareness of this likely combination and use of adequate operative fixation techniques for Monteggia fractures in the adult have improved results significantly.

In contrast to Galeazzi's fracture (fracture of the distal radius and dislocation of the radioulnar joint), which rarely occurs in children, approximately 25 per cent of Monteggia fracture-dislocations are sustained by patients less than 15 years of age.

The angulation of the ulnar fracture consistently points in the direction of the radial head dislocation. Most commonly (70–85 per cent of cases) the angulation and dislocation are anterior. Less often (10–15 per cent of cases) they are posterior. Lateral angulation of the fracture with lateral dislocation of the radial head is the least common (5–10 per cent of cases); this lesion has been reported only in children, and generally the ulnar fracture is a greenstick type instead of a true fracture.

Occasionally, additional fracture of the radius or a dislocation of the distal radioulnar joint occurs in association with a Monteggia injury. Keep all these possible combinations in mind when evaluating any ulnar fracture at any level in a patient of any age.

Mechanisms of Injury Producing Monteggia Fracture-Dislocation

REMARKS

The Monteggia fracture in adults is usually the result of direct trauma to the proximal posterior aspect of the forearm and elbow. This produces the typical anterior angulation of the ulnar fracture and anterior dislocation of the radius.

Direct trauma produces Monteggia fractures more often in adults. In children an indirect mechanism is the common cause of this fracture-dislocation. The usual indirect mechanism includes a bending and hyperextension of the elbow with forced hyperpronation of the proximal forearm as the individual falls on the extended elbow.

Direct Mechanism of Anterior Monteggia Lesion

1. A blow to the posterior ulnar aspect causes an ulnar fracture with anterior angulation and
2. Anterior dislocation of the radial head.

Note: Direct mechanisms are more common in adult fractures than in the childhood fracture.

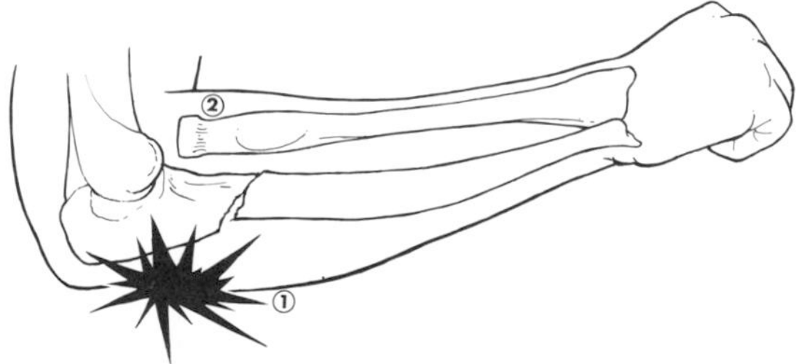

Indirect Mechanisms

ANTERIOR MONTEGGIA LESION FROM TORSIONAL INJURY

1. The hand is fixed to the ground.
2. The momentum of the body forces the humerus and elbow to rotate externally.
3. Floor reaction and muscle response cause the forearm to rotate internally while the humerus and elbow rotate externally.
4. Fracture of the ulna results.

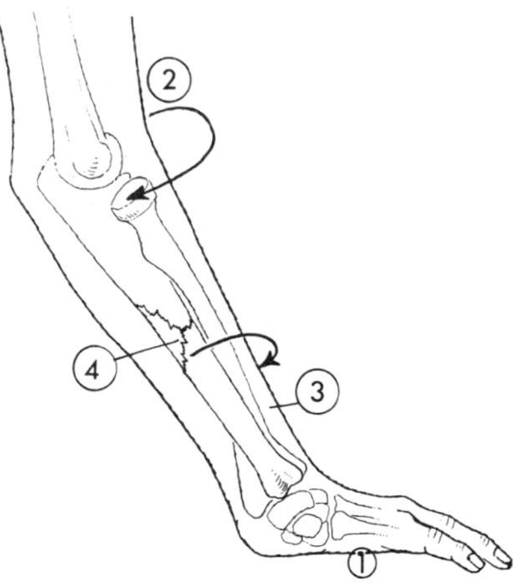

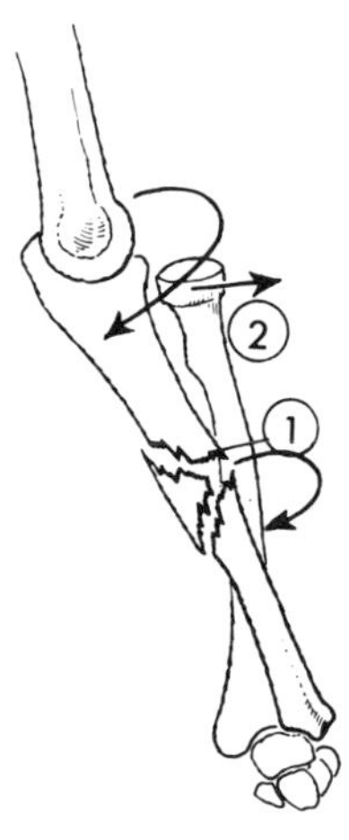

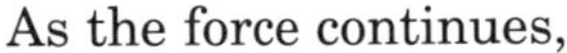

As the force continues,

1. The radius and the proximal fragment of the ulna come into contact.
2. The radial head is levered anteriorly out of the proximal radioulnar joint.

POSTERIOR MONTEGGIA LESION WITH ELBOW FLEXION

The hand strikes the ground with

1. The forearm in supination and
2. The elbow flexed 45°.
3. The axial force up the radius tends to dislocate the radius.

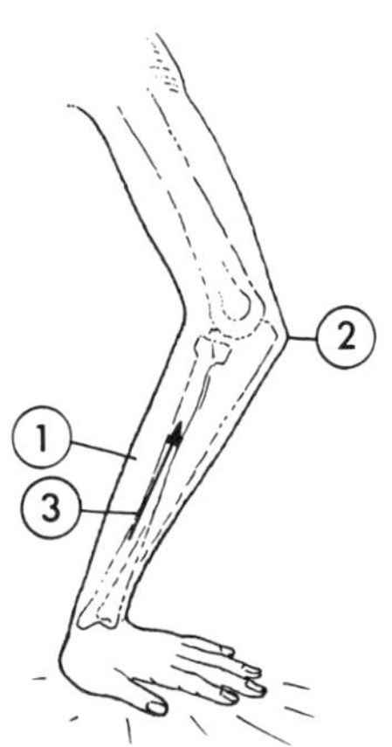

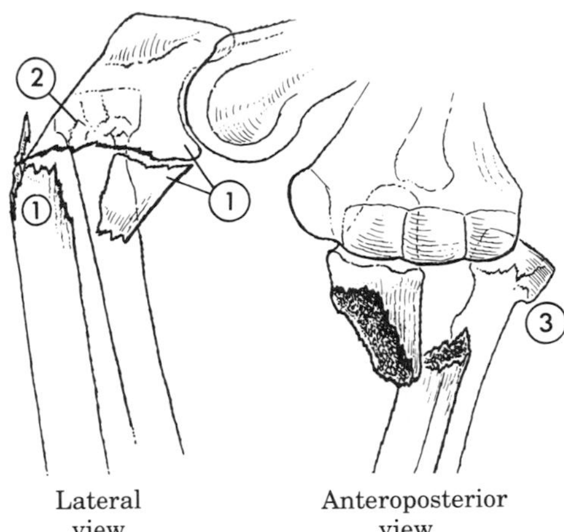

Simultaneously there occurs

1. A comminuted fracture of the upper end of the ulna with posterior angulation and
2. Posterior fracture-dislocation of the head of the radius.
3. The dislocation may be posterior or posterolateral.

Management—Closed Reduction and Splint Immobilization (Limited to Children and Stable Fractures in Adults)

REMARKS

Closed reduction of Monteggia fracture–dislocations in adults in the past has most often led to poor results. Consequently, the treatment of choice for the adult fracture, in contrast to the Monteggia fracture in the child, is usually open reduction.

Occasionally, for stable uncomminuted fractures an attempt can be made initially to achieve reduction by hyperflexing the elbow. This should be done cautiously because the elbow is usually quite swollen and the position of hyperflexion may be enough to occlude distal flow and lead to a compartment syndrome. Shang and others, using traditional Chinese methods, have shown that if care is taken to slowly hyperflex the elbow and reduce the dislocated radial head, reduction of the Monteggia fracture-dislocation can be quite satisfactory, even in adults.

Prereduction X-Ray

1. A classic Monteggia fracture of the proximal ulna has occurred with anterior angulation. The ulna, however, is not comminuted.
2. The radial head is dislocated anteriorly.

Note: Because there is no comminution of the ulna, it is possible to try to correct anterior angulation and reduce the radial head by flexing the elbow, provided the elbow is not extremely swollen.

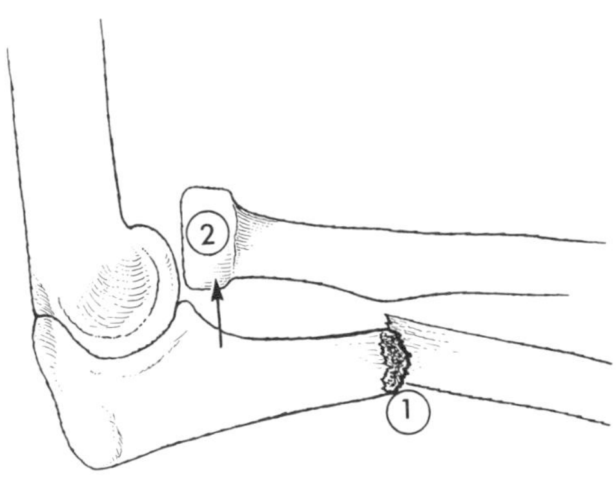

Technique of Reduction

1. The elbow is flexed to approximately 120° to correct the anterior angulation of the ulna.
2. The radial head is manipulated by direct pressure to reduce the dislocation.

Note: The elbow and forearm are immobilized with a well-padded, loosely wrapped posterior splint to maintain the position of 120° of elbow flexion. The forearm is held in supination to maintain the reduction of the radial head.

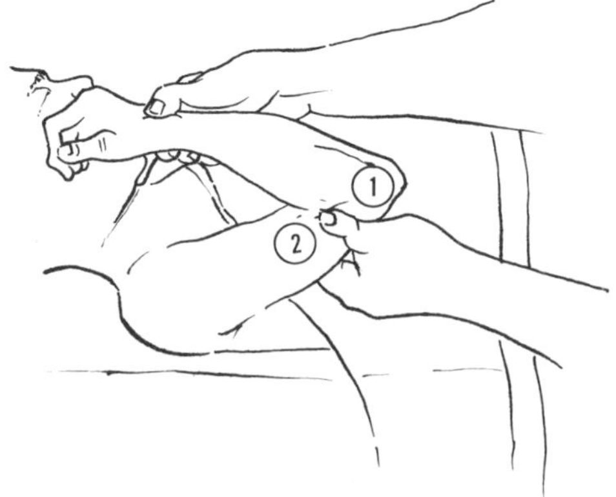

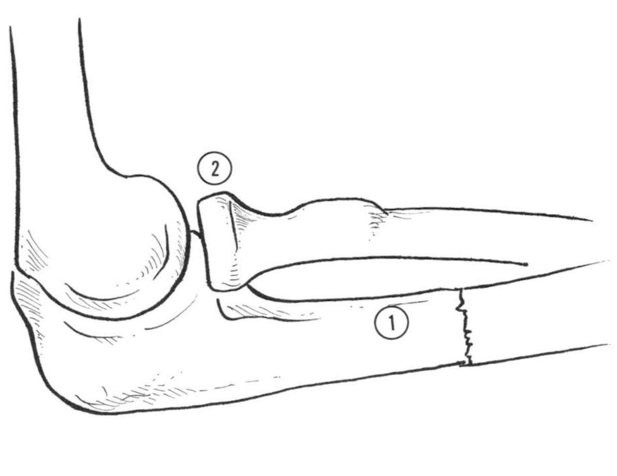

Postoperative X-Ray After Reduction

1. The anterior angulation of the ulna is corrected.
2. The radial head is reduced as shown by its articulation with the capitellum.

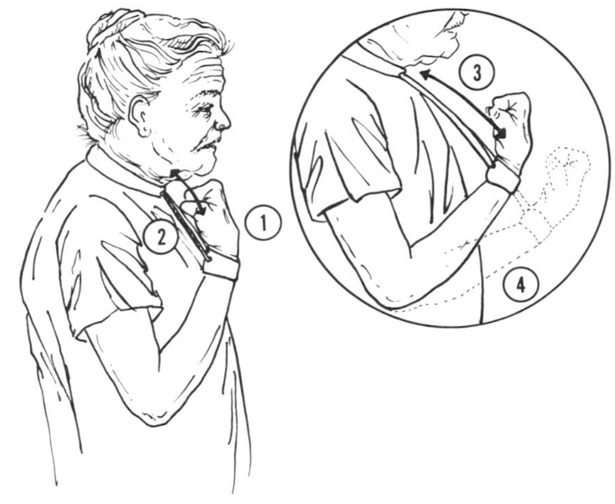

1. As the swelling subsides, usually by 3–5 days, the splint immobilizing the radius is changed to a collar and cuff, maintaining the elbow in maximum flexion.
2. The elbow is also held in supination to maintain the radial head reduced with the capitellum.
3. As the ulna fracture consolidates, elbow motion and extension may be slowly increased. Emphasis should be on flexion rather than extension.
4. By 6–8 weeks the elbow may be slowly extended, provided there is stability of the ulnar fracture.

Note: If the ulna does not reduce by this closed method, open reduction with internal fixation is necessary.

Management of Monteggia Fracture in Adults: Open Reduction and Fixation

REMARKS

Open reduction and rigid internal fixation of the ulnar fracture is the treatment of choice for the usual Monteggia injury in adults. Stabilization of the ulna permits reduction of the radial head. Occasionally, partial disruption of the annular ligament must also be repaired.

In rare instances, the stabilizing annular ligament is so disrupted that a reconstructive procedure is necessary.

Fixation

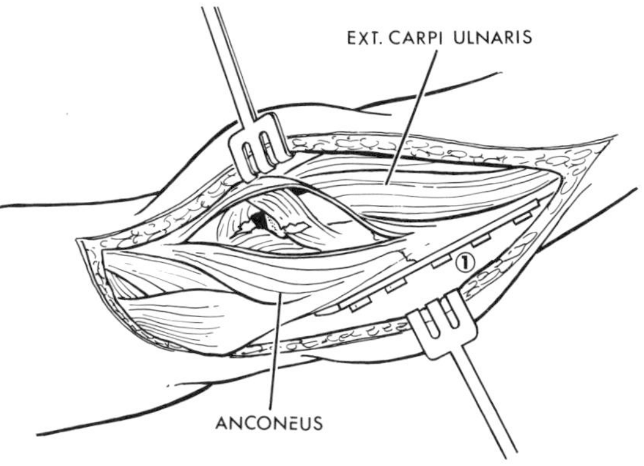

1. After the fracture of the ulna is exposed from a lateral approach, it can be best stabilized with a semitubular plate. Stabilization of the ulna usually reduces the radius if the annular ligament is intact.

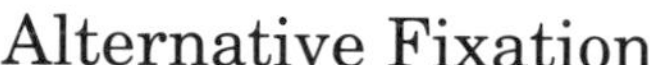

Alternative Fixation

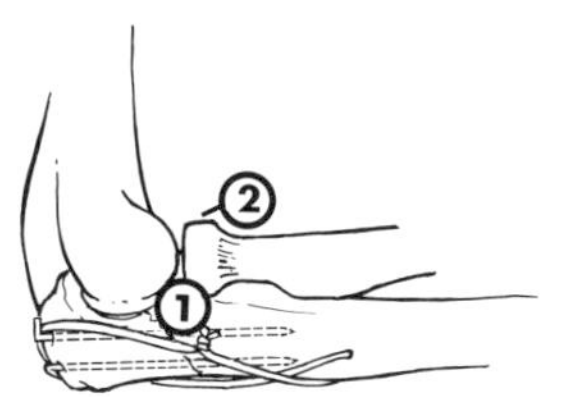

1. The ulna in the proximal area may be best stabilized by tension band wiring.
2. This also should be stable enough to reduce the radial head.

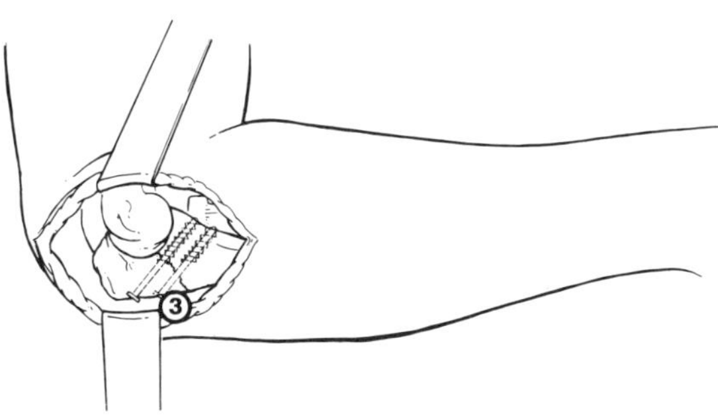

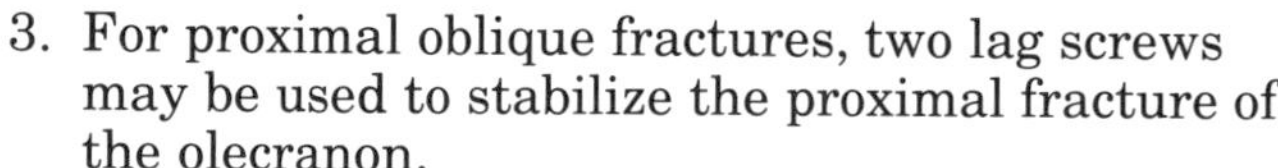

3. For proximal oblique fractures, two lag screws may be used to stabilize the proximal fracture of the olecranon.

Importance of Annular Ligament

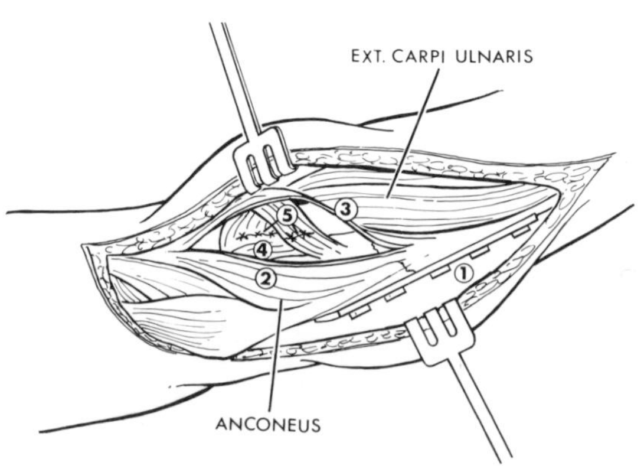

1. After the ulnar fracture is stabilized, the stability of the radial head should be evaluated.
2. This can be best seen by approaching through the anconeus and
3. The extensor carpi ulnaris.
4. The radial head is then visualized.
5. The annular ligament is seen to be intact.

Note: If the annular ligament is torn, it should be repaired or reconstructed.

Subsequent Management

1. The elbow is immobilized after fixation of the ulna and reduction of the radial head using a long arm cast.
2. The forearm is held in a neutral rotation or supination, depending on the position that best stabilizes the radial head.

Note: Subsequently the cast may be removed at 2–3 weeks when the soft tissue swelling has subsided, and active range of motion to the elbow and forearm can be encouraged. For the more unstable fractures of the ulna, particularly if there is comminution, immobilization may be necessary for 6–8 weeks until there are signs of healing radiographically and clinically. The patient should be advised that there is commonly some loss of elbow and forearm motion with these injuries but good function should usually be possible.

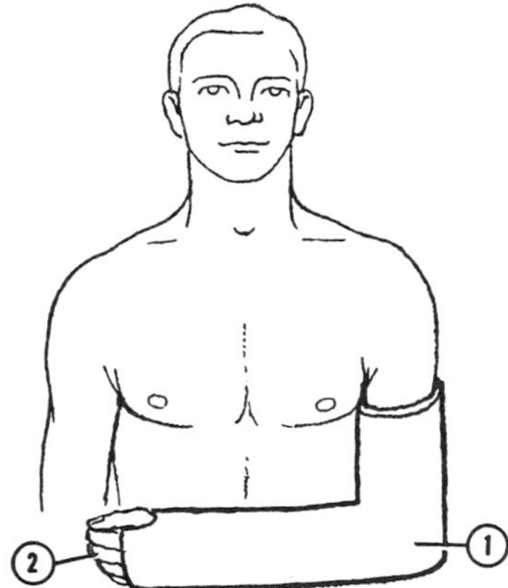

Prevention and Management of Complications of Monteggia Fracture

REMARKS

In the past, Monteggia fracture has been associated with more problems, difficulties, and general failure of treatment than almost any other skeletal injury. The most common complication has been persistent loss of elbow motion and forearm rotation.

Failure to recognize the radial head dislocation associated with ulnar fracture is a common hazard and a common cause of functional loss. Radial head dislocation is especially likely to go unrecognized in a child. Because of this, the alignment of the proximal radius should be carefully assessed by using the Reckling–Cordell method with any fracture of the ulna.

Nonunion is a frequent sequela of this injury, especially if the fracture is comminuted. Rigid dynamic compression fixation, supplemented by autogenous bone graft for comminution, gives the best chance for successful fracture union in the adult. If compression cannot be achieved successfully, the internal fixation should be protected by external immobilization for at least 6 weeks after injury.

Closed reduction is usually successful in children, but the radial head must be completely reduced. If the radial head does not line up anatomically with the capitellum, there may be an interposed capsule, which should be removed in conjunction with annular ligament repair. Radial nerve injury occurs both before and after reduction of the Monteggia fracture-dislocation. Check frequently for both sensory and motor disturbances.

Evaluation of Radial Head Dislocation

In order to detect a dislocation of the radial head with any ulnar fracture, adequate x-rays of the relationship of the radial head to the distal humerus are essential. Reckling and Cordell demonstrated that these are best obtained on the lateral view with the forearm supinated and the elbow flexed to 90°.

X-Ray Determination of Radial Head Reduction

1. On the lateral view with the forearm supinated, a line is drawn tangential to the bicipital tuberosity.
2. A second line is drawn along the opposite radial border.
3. These two lines should encompass the capitellum if there is a normal relationship between the radius and capitellum.
4. Failure of these lines to encompass the capitellum indicates a persistent subluxation or dislocation of the radial head.

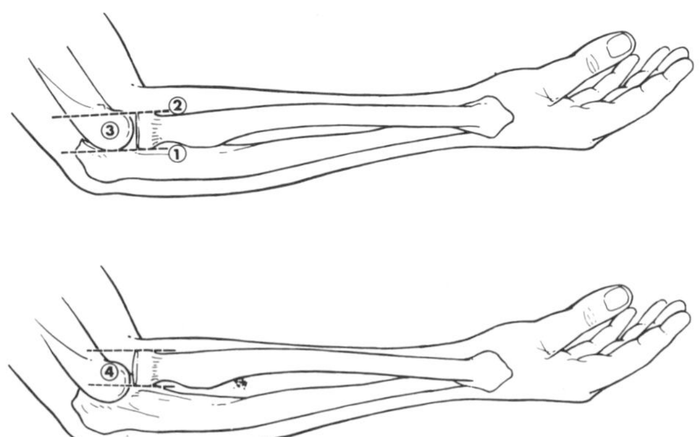

Injury of the Radial Nerve Associated With Monteggia Fracture

Fifteen to 20 per cent of Monteggia fractures injure the radial nerve, either as a result of direct stretch or secondary to entrapment. Most often the neural injury is transitory and due to neurapraxia. This should clear and nerve function should return within 10 weeks.

If the radial nerve is entrapped at the elbow, permanent loss of function is possible. The usual site of entrapment involves the motor branch (posterior interosseous nerve) and occurs at the arcade of Frohse, a fibrous arch through which the nerve enters the supinator muscle.

To differentiate neurapraxia stretch injury from entrapment of the radial nerve, if the neurologic deficit combines sensory and motor loss, it is more likely to have occurred above the branching of the posterior interosseous nerve. Such combined sensory and motor paralysis, therefore, indicates a stretch injury from the displaced radial head.

An isolated motor paralysis most likely indicates compression of the dorsal interosseous nerve in the arcade of Frohse. Such a pure motor lesion usually requires operative exploration to relieve the site of entrapment at the level of the arcade.

1. Posterior interosseous nerve may be scarred down by
2. The arcade of Frohse on the
3. Superior border of the supinator muscle.

Note: Because the nerve entering the arcade of Frohse is purely motor, persistence of a pure motor nerve lesion would indicate the need for surgical decompression of the nerve at this level.

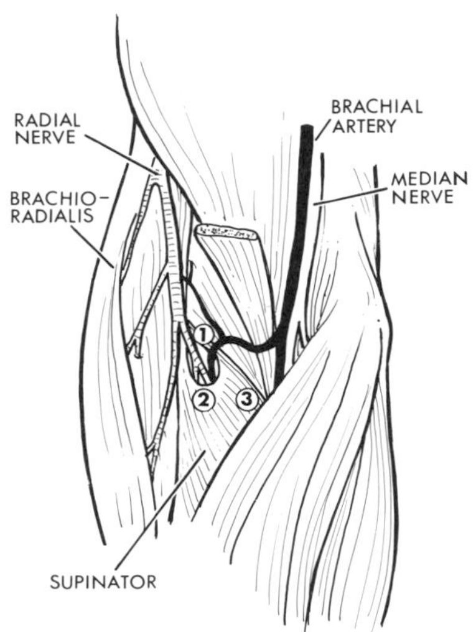

Isolated Fracture of the Radius Without Dislocation of the Radioulnar Joint

REMARKS

Stable single-bone fracture of the radius can be treated effectively by nonoperative methods. Care must be taken to determine that the proximal or distal radioulnar joint has not been damaged. For the undisplaced radial fracture, a short period of long-arm cast immobilization followed by the functional fracture-brace method can achieve satisfactory results without the need for operative fixation.

Closed Treatment of Proximal Radial Fractures

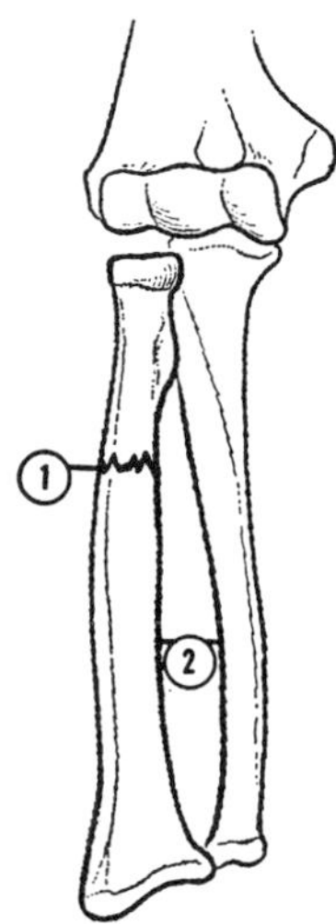

1. The ideal fracture for closed treatment is a moderately displaced or undisplaced fracture of the proximal radius sustained from a direct blow.
2. The interosseous space is preserved, and the distal and proximal radial and ulnar joints are not disrupted.

Initial Immobilization

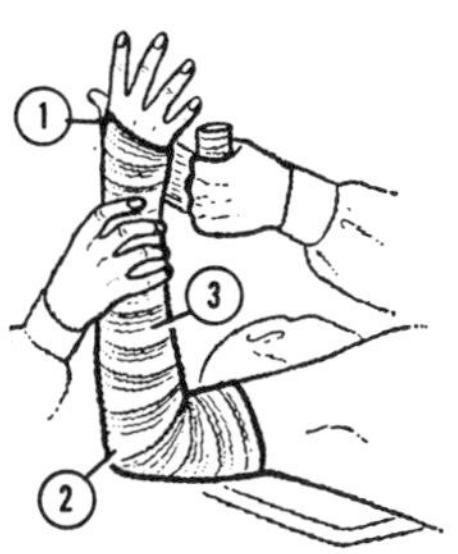

1. A long-arm cast is applied from the axilla to the base of the fingers.
2. The elbow is maintained in 90° flexion.
3. The forearm is supinated to align the distal fragment with the proximal fragment, and the cast is continued for 2–3 weeks until swelling subsides and a fracture-brace can be applied. If a fracture-brace is not available, the cast may be changed to an unpadded long-arm cast.

Functional Cast-Brace Treatment

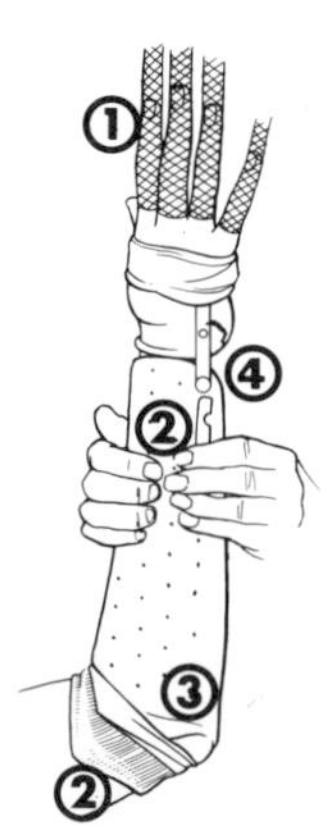

When swelling and initial pain subside (usually by 5–7 days), apply a functional brace.

1. The forearm is suspended in a finger trap.
2. Plaster or orthoplastic material is firmly molded to compress tissues of the interosseous space and to maintain the radial curvature.
3. Supracondylar elbow extension permits flexion and extension but limits pronation and supination.
4. The wrist hinge and hand component permit palmar flexion and dorsiflexion of the wrist.

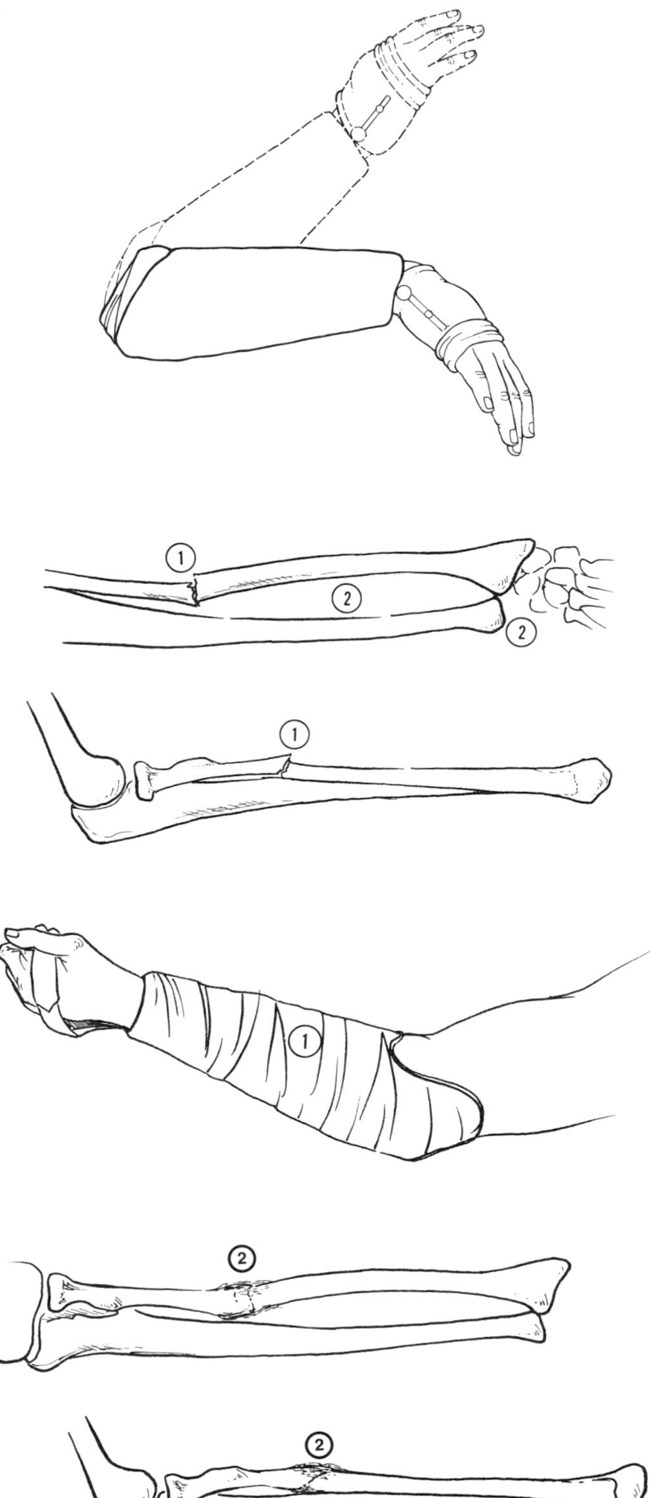

Subsequent Management

Allow the patient to actively exercise shoulder, elbow, wrist, and hand. The cast-brace may usually be discarded by 6–8 weeks if fracture union is evident on x-ray.

Displaced Radial Fracture Before Fracture-Brace Treatment

1. There is slight bayonet apposition and anterior angulation, which can be accepted with the isolated radial fracture provided the proximal and distal radioulnar joints are not injured.
2. The radial bow is not decreased and the interosseous space is widened. There is also no evidence of instability of the radioulnar joint.

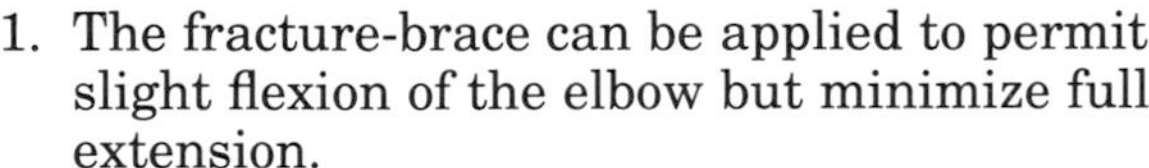

1. The fracture-brace can be applied to permit slight flexion of the elbow but minimize full extension.

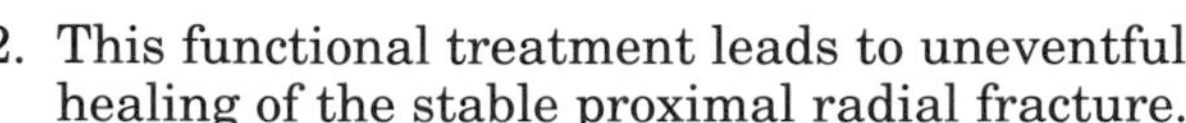

2. This functional treatment leads to uneventful healing of the stable proximal radial fracture.

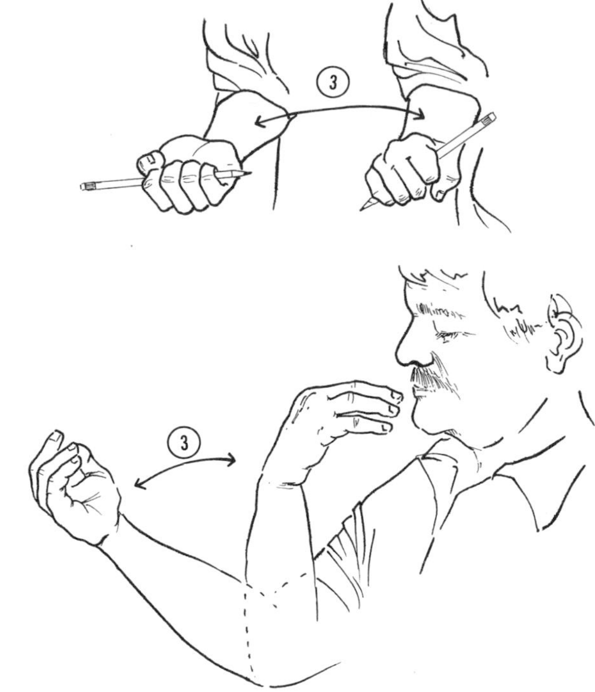

3. The residual impairment of rotation of the forearm, as well as flexion and extension of the elbow, is minimal.

Closed Treatment of Distal Radial Fractures

Mechanisms of Distal Radial Fractures

1. The fracture of the distal radius may result from a direct blow to the bone. This does not significantly displace or angulate the radius.
2. The interosseous membrane and distal radioulnar ligaments remain intact.
3. The distal end of the ulna is not shortened and the fracture is stable.

Note: This type of fracture can be treated quite adequately by closed casting and functional bracing, similar to that for isolated fracture of the proximal radius.

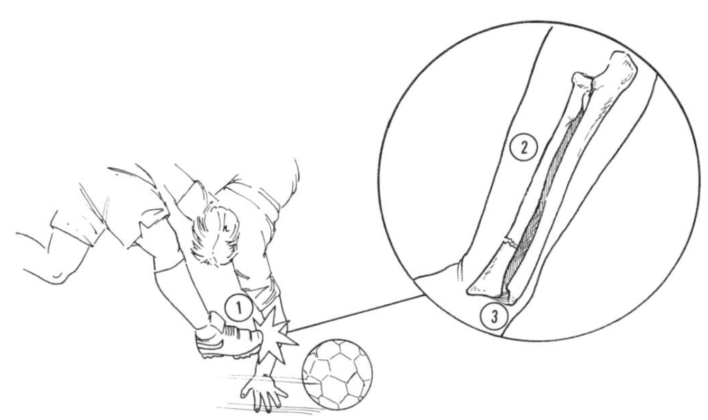

Indirect Injury

1. An isolated fracture of the radius can result from a fall on the outstretched hand. This combines axial loading with
2. Rotational injury.
3. The result is displacement of the radial fracture. Shortening and displacement of more than 5 mm are strong evidence that the interosseous membrane has been disrupted and
4. The distal radioulnar joint is dislocated.

Note: This type of isolated radial fracture with shortening of the fragments and disruption of the distal radioulnar joint necessitates internal stabilization of the radius. This is in contrast to the fracture produced by a direct injury to the radius, which requires operative stabilization.

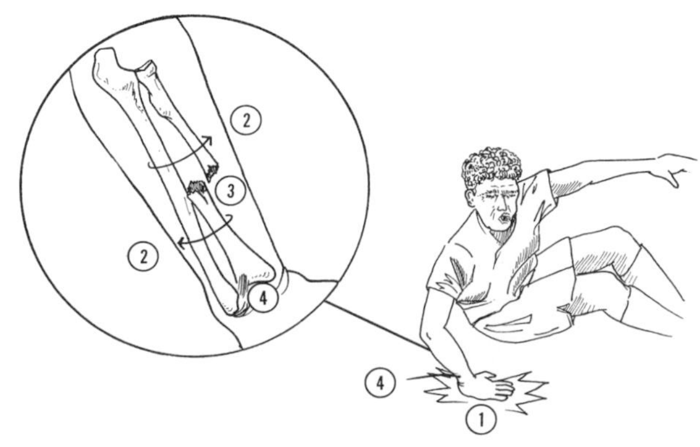

Management of Stable Distal Radial Fracture From Direct Injury

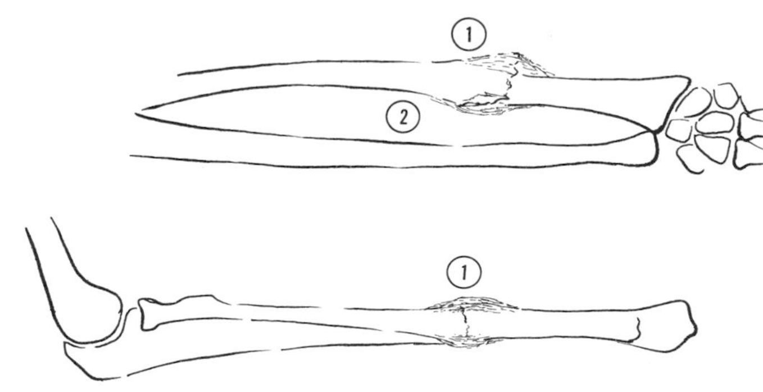

1. The fracture of the distal radius is held in the fracture-brace until it heals, usually by 10–12 weeks.
2. There may be slight bayonet apposition, but the interosseous space is maintained. The functional result allows minimal limitation of pronation and supination.

1. Range of motion of pronation and

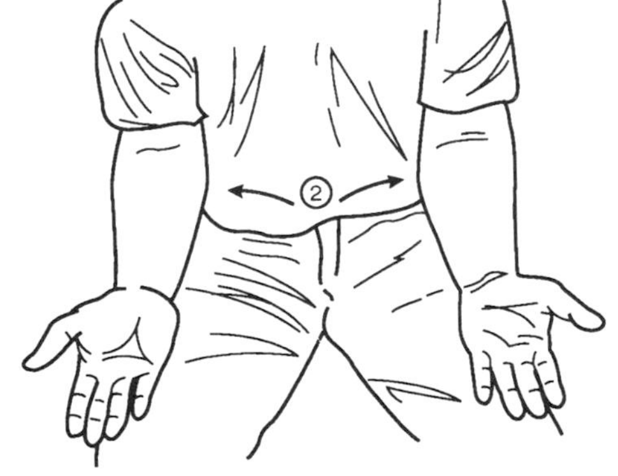

2. Supination is usually quite good as the fracture heals, emphasizing functional treatment and the use of the muscles of the forearm during the healing process.

■ Fractures of Both Radius and Ulna

Indications and Techniques For Closed Reduction of Two-Bone Forearm Fractures

REMARKS

Because the technique of closed reduction is quite demanding, most orthopaedic surgeons prefer open reduction and internal fixation for two-bone fractures of the forearm. However, closed methods can avoid complications, including infections, painful scars, and the need to remove plates, with the uncertainty about the possibility of refracture.

Patients with relatively thin forearms and patients who do not desire a scar on the forearm can be given a trial of closed reduction of the two-bone forearm fracture with the understanding that if the reduction is lost or angulation is unacceptable, a delayed open reduction can be performed without seriously affecting the good result from operative treatment.

The treatment of two-bone forearm fractures has traditionally been by closed methods ranging from ancient Chinese techniques, as described by Shang and coworkers, to fracture bracing techniques, as initially advocated by Sarmiento.

The method of closed reduction consists of a period (5–10 minutes) of sustained steady traction to restore length and apposition of the fractured radius and ulnar fragments.

The next objective is to restore the fracture fragments by correct rotational realignment.

The third maneuver is to maintain the reduced position by molding firmly on the interosseous space to stretch the interosseous ligament maximally. The interosseous ligament is a key stabilizer and is maintained at maximal tension by firmly molding in the interosseous space while plaster is applied. In addition, maximal tension on the interosseous ligament is achieved by separating the radius and ulna in the neutral or supinated position.

The final objective is to maximize healing of the fracture fragments while minimizing scarring and contracture of the muscles of the forearm between the bones. This requires emphasis on early functional restoration of tendon and muscle function in the fingers and wrists.

Both the traditional and the modern methods emphasize early restoration of hand and wrist function as an important component of treatment.

Objectives of Treating Two-Bone Fractures

1. The length of the fractured radius should be restored to normal, although slight bayonet apposition and shortening of less than 5 mm is usually acceptable.
2. The radial bow should be restored to allow maximal return of forearm rotation.
3. The ulnar fracture is usually reduced end to end, although slight bayonet apposition is acceptable. Angulation of either the ulna or the radius should be minimal, although up to 10° of dorsal or volar angulation has not been found to affect functional outcome. Angulation of more than 10° tends to be cosmetically unacceptable.
4. The interosseous space should be kept at its maximal width by maintaining the forearm in supination or neutral rotation. The muscles within the interosseous space should be exercised and utilized functionally in the early period of healing to avoid scarring in the deep compartments of the forearm.

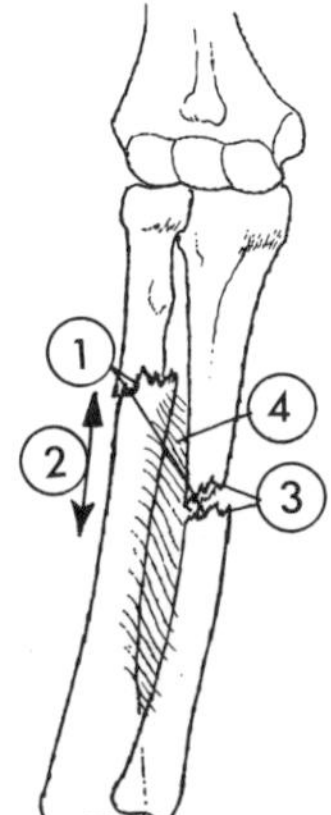

Displaced or Undisplaced Two-Bone Fractures in the Upper Half of the Forearm (In Adults)

REMARKS

Reduction of these fractures should be carried out with attention to rotational alignment so as to avoid fracture displacement during treatment. Varying degrees of supination are necessary to align the distal fragment with the proximal one. However, avoid extreme supination, which closes the interosseous space. The amount of fracture rotation is determined by radiographic study of the bicipital tuberosity compared with the opposite, intact radius.

Prereduction X-Ray

MINIMALLY DISPLACED FRACTURE

1. Fragments of both bones are slightly angulated but firmly engaged and not displaced.
2. The interosseous space at the level of the fractures is reduced in width.

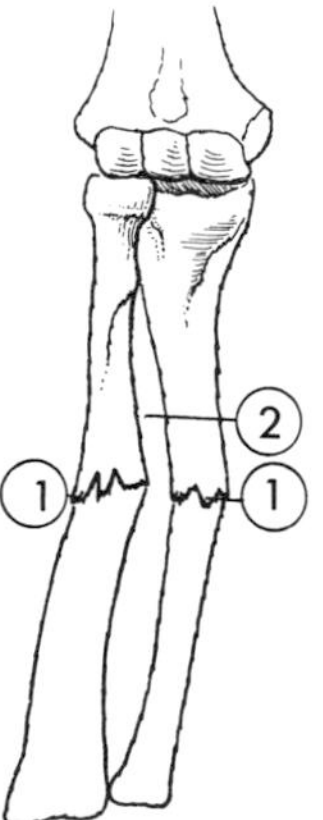

DISPLACED FRACTURE

1. Shortening has occurred.
2. The interosseous space is narrowed.
3. The proximal radial fragment is supinated.

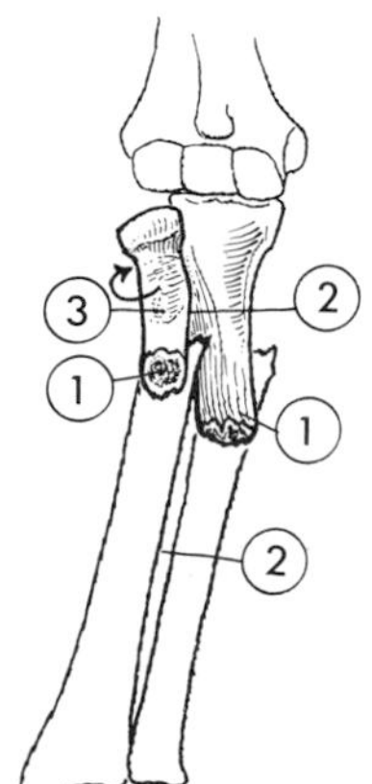

Manipulative Reduction

Reduction is performed with the patient under general or regional intravenous anesthesia.

PREFERRED METHOD OF ACHIEVING ANESTHESIA: INTRAVENOUS REGIONAL ANESTHETIC

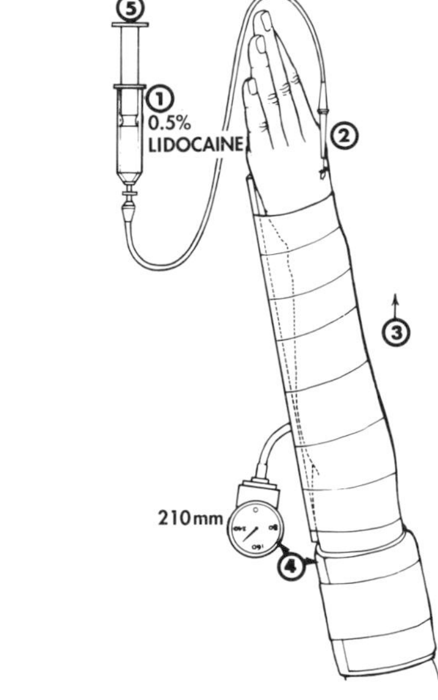

1. Use 0.5% preservative-free lidocaine solution. The dose should be 0.5 mL of this solution per kilogram of body weight.
2. Insert a small butterfly needle into the hand on the fractured side, which is immobilized in a splint.
3. Elevate the limb at least 3 minutes to diminish edema.
4. Using a pretested and securely taped blood pressure cuff, stop circulation by rapid inflation to at least 210 mm Hg.

Note: A specially designed double tourniquet may also be used.

5. Lower the arm and inject an appropriate dose of the lidocaine solution.

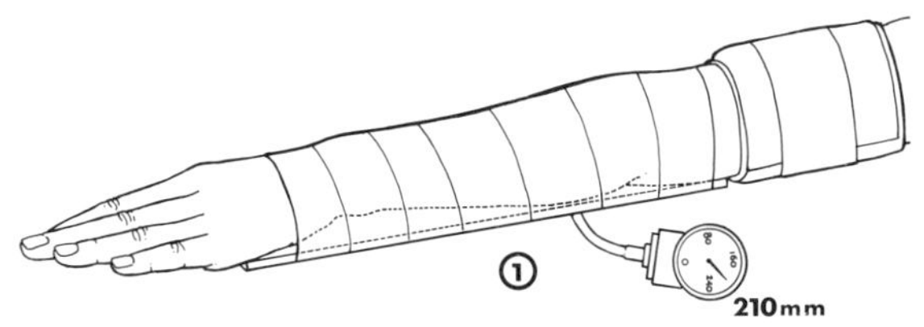

1. The needle is removed, and after a 10-minute interval, the fracture is reduced. Always keep the cuff inflated for at least 15 minutes.

Note: When reduction is satisfactory, deflate the tourniquet for intravenous anesthetic to 80 mm Hg, and after 10 seconds reinflate it to 210 mm Hg. Monitor vital signs and mental status; if these are unchanged, remove the tourniquet completely. Continue monitoring the patient's vital signs and mental status for 10 minutes after release of the tourniquet. The entire procedure requires two assistants, one to monitor the pressure of the cuff during the block and the other to assist in reduction. Minimal tourniquet time should always be in excess of 15 minutes. Resuscitation equipment should be immediately available when anesthetic of any type is administered.

Reduction Technique (Under Local or General Anesthetic)

1. The patient assumes the supine position on the fracture table.
2. The fingers are engaged by a finger traction apparatus.
3. Countertraction is made on the arm in a plane parallel to the forearm by a sling of muslin bandage anchored to a crossbar at the bottom of the table.
4. The elbow is flexed 90°.
5. The forearm is supinated to the degree determined by comparison of the tuberosity views.

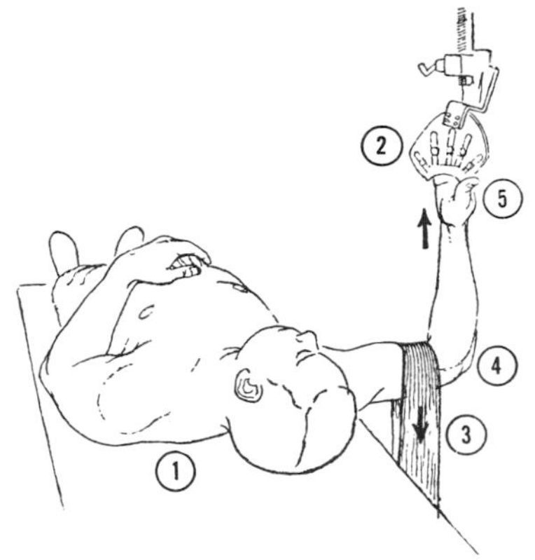

1. Strong traction is applied to the forearm through the finger-traction apparatus until length is restored and angular deformity is corrected. This requires at least 10 minutes of traction.
2. After length is restored, the surgeon squeezes the volar muscle mass between the radius and the ulna, forcing the two bones apart.

Note: If on palpation the radius remains overlapped, it can be corrected by angulating the forearm while maintaining traction.

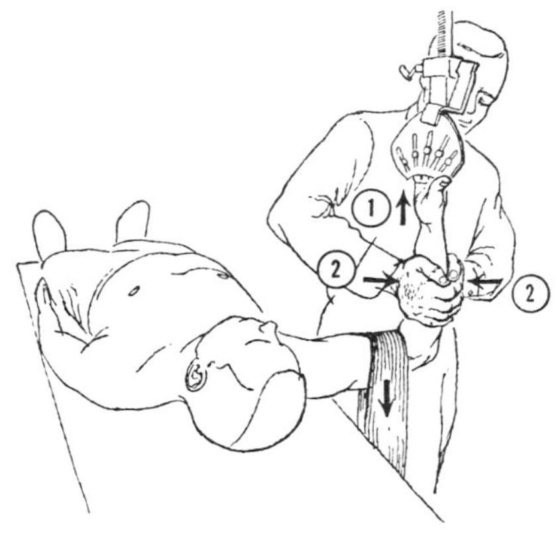

Technique of Achieving Rotational Alignment by Using Bicipital Tuberosity Position

REMARKS

It is important to restore correct rotation of the distal and proximal fragments. Evans pointed out that this can be achieved by rotating the distal fragment to the proximal fragment, using the position of the bicipital tuberosity as a guide. The bicipital tuberosity indicates how much the proximal fragment is supinated and therefore how much the distal fragment must be supinated to line up with the proximal fragment.

1. In full supination, the bicipital tuberosity is directed toward the ulna.
2. In 40° supination, the tuberosity moves posteriorly.
3. In neutral, tuberosity is almost directly posterior.

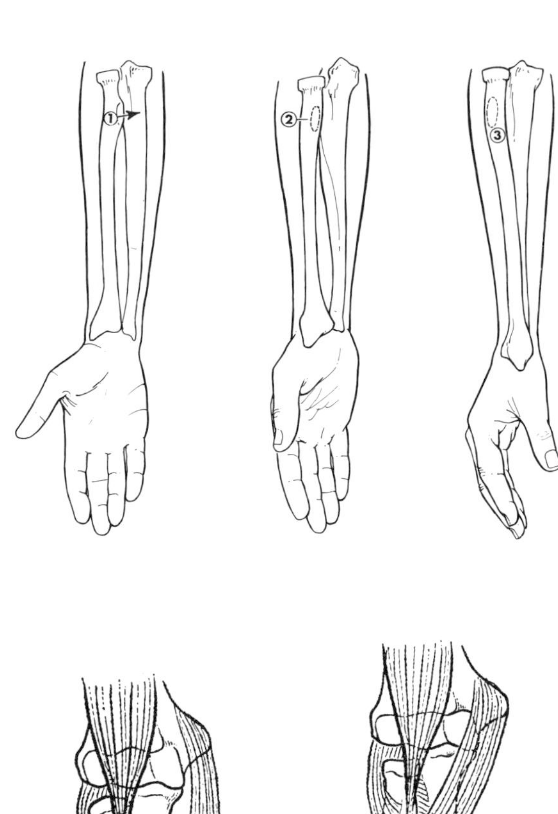

Examples of Fractures Reduced by Supination to Restore Rotational Alignment

1. The proximal fragment is supinated and flexed.
2. The distal fragment is pronated and drawn inward toward the ulna.
3. Because the position of the bicipital tuberosity indicates that the proximal fragment is supinated, the fracture is reduced by supinating the distal fragment.

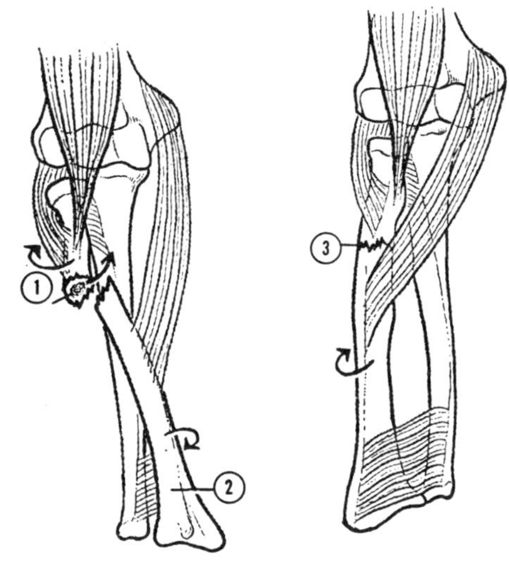

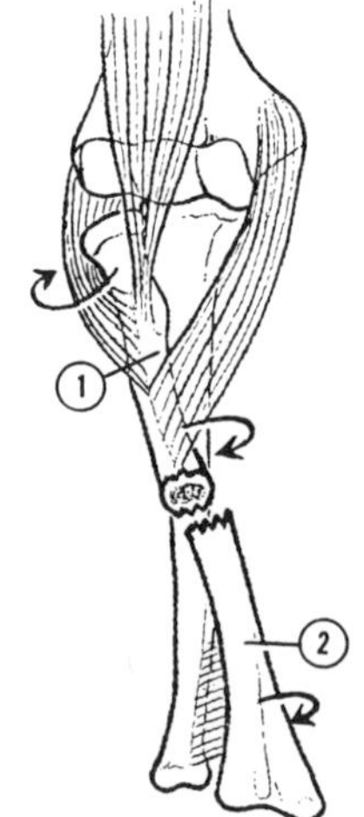

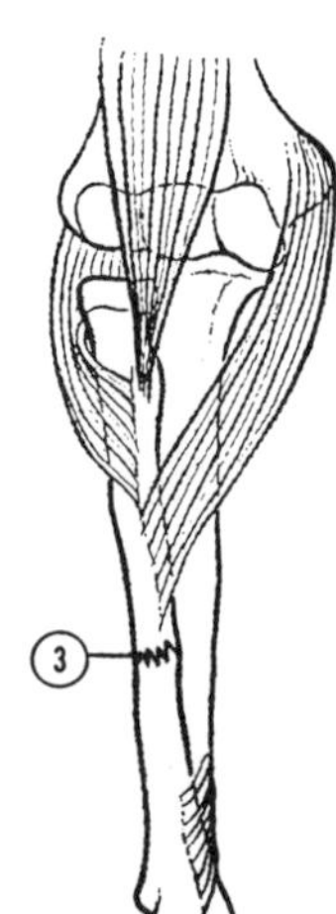

1. The proximal fragment is flexed and is supinated approximately 45° as determined by the position of the bicipital tuberosity.
2. The distal fragment is pronated in relation to the proximal fragment.
3. The fracture is reduced by supinating the distal fragment approximately 45°.

Cast Application

1. Once the fracture is reduced by traction and rotational realignment, a long-arm cast can be applied.
2. A short-arm cast is applied first, molding carefully around the fracture site.
3. The interosseous space is maintained by firm pressure at the fracture site to compress the interosseous space.
4. When the below-elbow portion of the cast is hardened, the counterweight traction may be released and the cast extended above the elbow.

Note: Subsequently, the reduction is carefully monitored by x-ray.

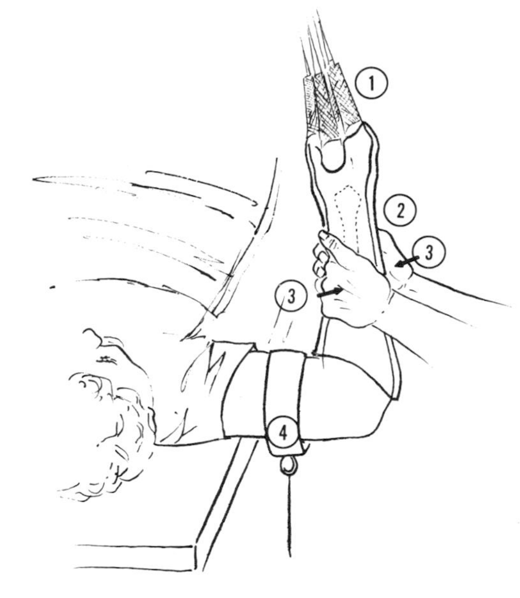

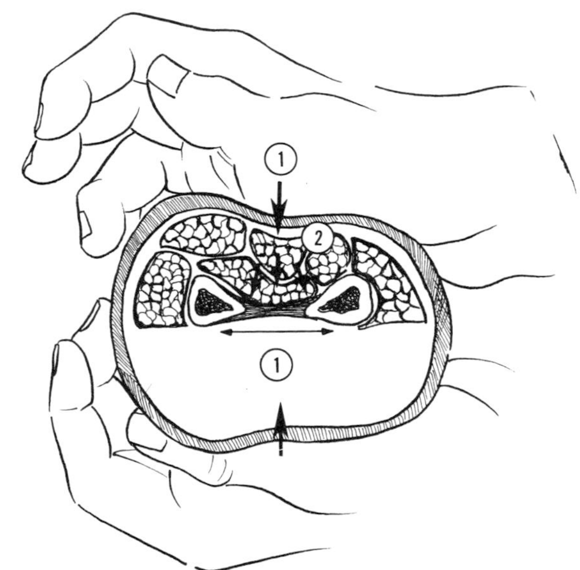

1. The key to maintaining reduction is to mold in the interosseous space between the radius and ulna with the forearm in neutral rotation. This maintains the interosseous space and ligament at maximal width and tension.
2. As the fracture heals, functional use of the hand and wrist is important to prevent scarring of the muscles and soft tissues in the interosseous space, which can subsequently impede forearm rotation or grip strength.

Postreduction X-Rays

MINIMALLY DISPLACED FRACTURE

Note: Ideally, reduction is evaluated by image-intensified fluoroscopy.

1. The angular deformities of both bones are corrected. The radial curve is normal.
2. The interosseous space is restored to normal width.

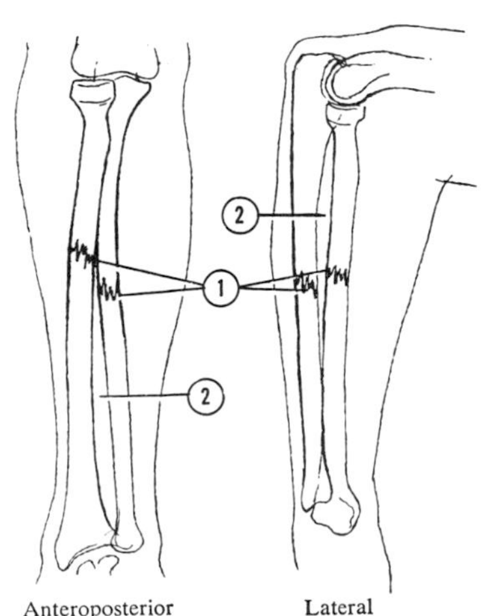

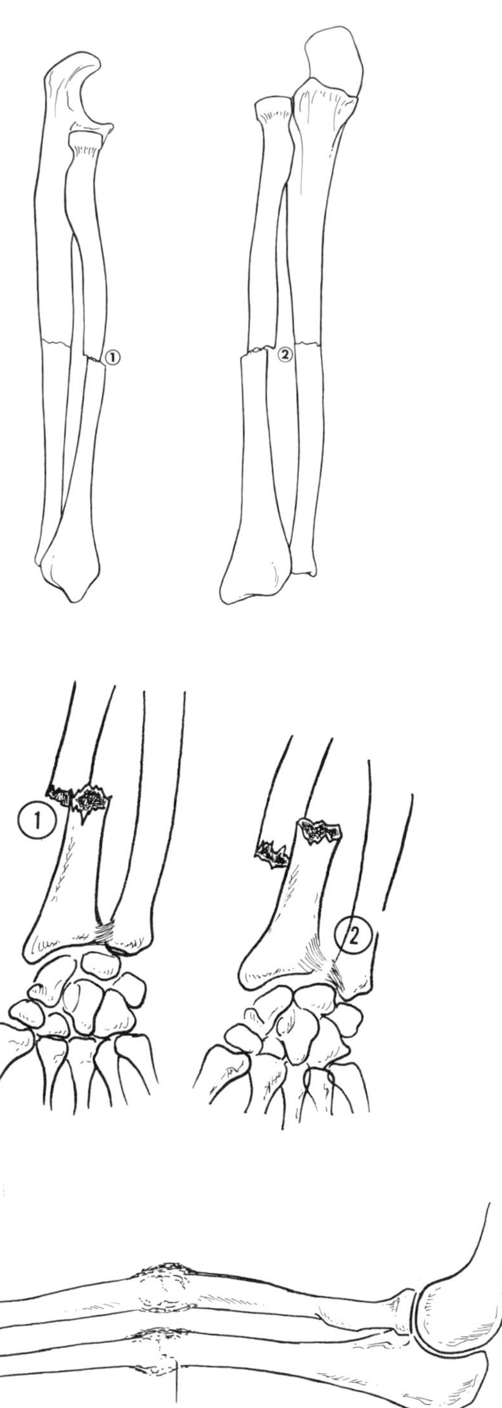

DISPLACED FRACTURE

1. Angulatory deformity has been decreased to less than 10°, although reduction is not anatomic.
2. The interosseous space is restored to close to normal width and the radial bow has been approximated with the radial fracture in slight bayonet apposition.

Note: End-to-end apposition of the ulna and bayonet apposition of the radius is usually acceptable alignment for these fractures.

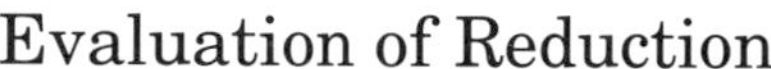

Evaluation of Reduction

1. Shortening of the radius can be accepted in some fractures provided it is no greater than 5 mm.
2. If greater shortening occurs, the distal radioulnar joint is likely to be impaired or disrupted.

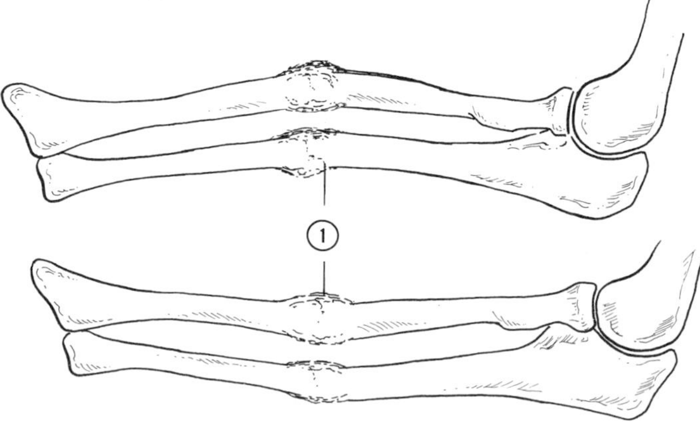

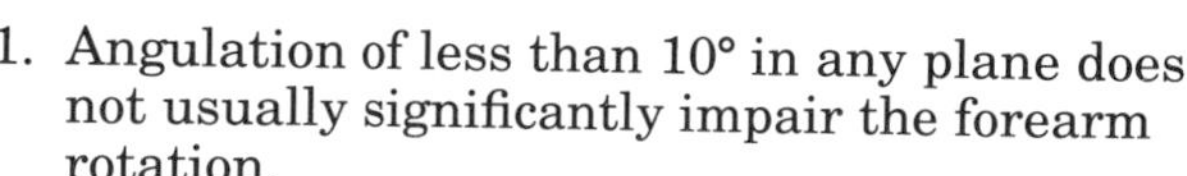

1. Angulation of less than 10° in any plane does not usually significantly impair the forearm rotation.

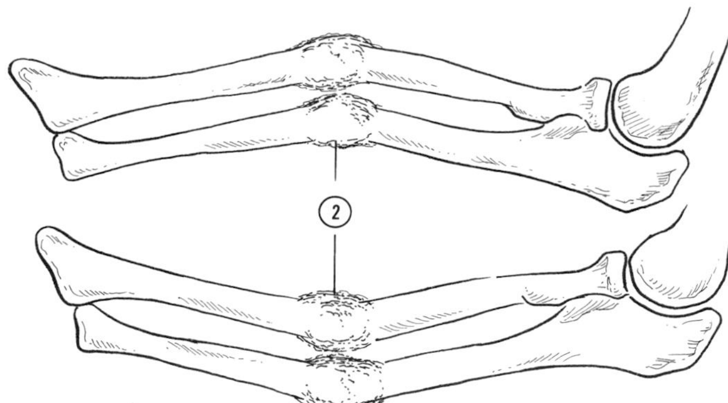

2. Angulation of 10–20°, however, is likely to cause cosmetic deformity as well as functional impairment.

Subsequent Management

REMARKS

As the swelling subsides, the long-arm cast tends to become loose and may be changed to another cast or, preferably, to some type of functional brace treatment. The largest experience ever reported with closed treatment of forearm fractures is that of Shang and coworkers with traditional Chinese methods. These authors had excellent results and minimal complications with the use of closed-reduction techniques and careful monitoring of patient function.

Other functional methods were advocated by Sarmiento and coworkers and have also demonstrated excellent results from forearm fractures treated in this manner. However, the technique is demanding, and careful follow-up is essential. Both methods emphasize maintenance of the forearm in a supinated or neutral rotation and restoration of early functional use of the hand and fingers.

Traditional Chinese Closed Reduction Method (Shang and Coworkers)

1. Over the centuries the traditional method of bone setting in China has proved to be quite effective for forearm fractures. Shang and coworkers showed it can be applied to modern-day fractures by emphasizing the restoration of function and the use of flexible willow wood splints.
2. These are supported by straps that are tightened repeatedly as the swelling subsides.
3. Pads are inserted into the interosseous space at the level of the fracture site to maintain tension on the interosseous ligament and to use the ligament to support and stabilize the fracture.

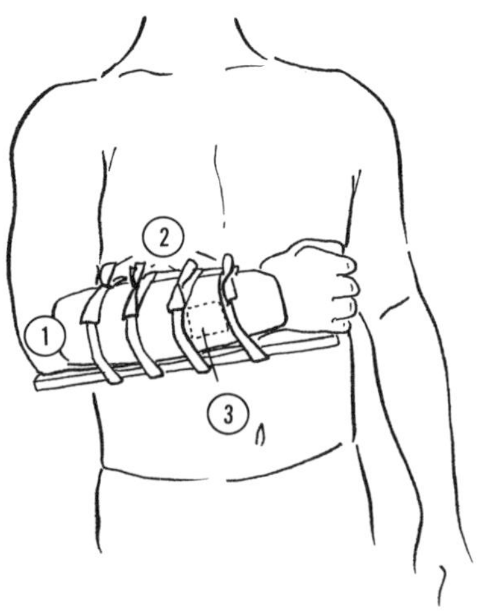

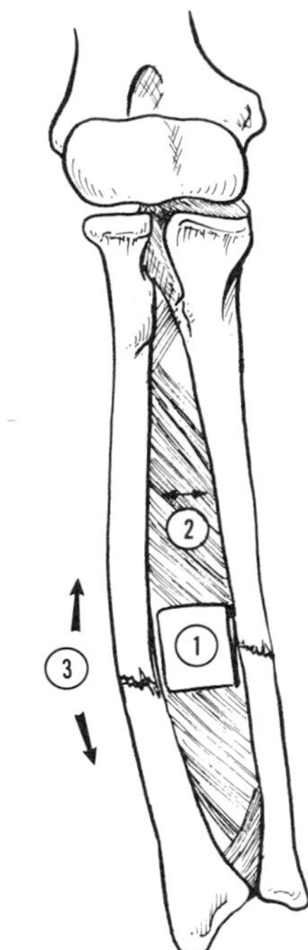

1. The key to reducing the forearm fracture is to compress the interosseous space.
2. This applies tension on the interosseous ligament and uses the ligament to stabilize the fracture.
3. The method of compressing the interosseous space may be done by paper pads, as described by Shang, or by molding of the cast, as described by Sarmiento and others. The objective is to restore radial bowing as much as possible.

Functional Exercises: Shang Method

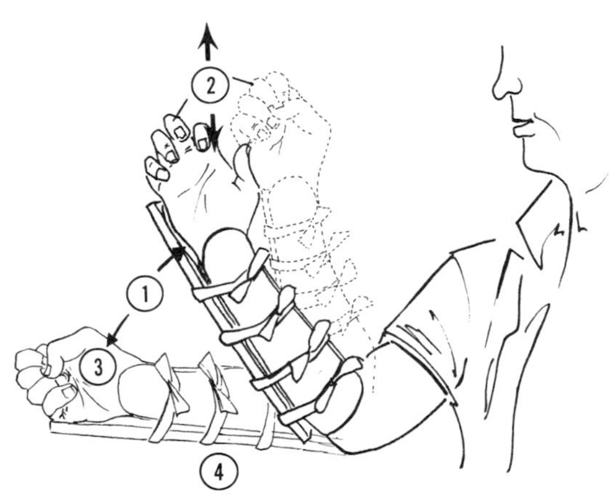

Shang and coworkers emphasized the need for restoration of function to the fractured limb as the fracture is healing. This maintains strength in the forearm muscles and stimulates fracture repair, and also minimizes scarring in the interosseous region that might block rotation of the forearm as the fracture heals.

1. The Chinese exercises include a series of flexion and extension exercises to the elbow and
2. The wrist with
3. The forearm maintained in neutral rotation and
4. The splints progressively tightened as the swelling subsides.

Functional Cast-Brace Application (Sarmiento)

Sarmiento and coworkers have designed a functional cast-brace that can be applied after the initial swelling subsides, usually by 2–3 weeks. This method relies on careful rotational realignment of the fracture and molding the interosseous space to maintain tension on the ligament and radial bow.

The cast-brace can be made of plaster of Paris or orthoplastic material to carefully support the fracture site.

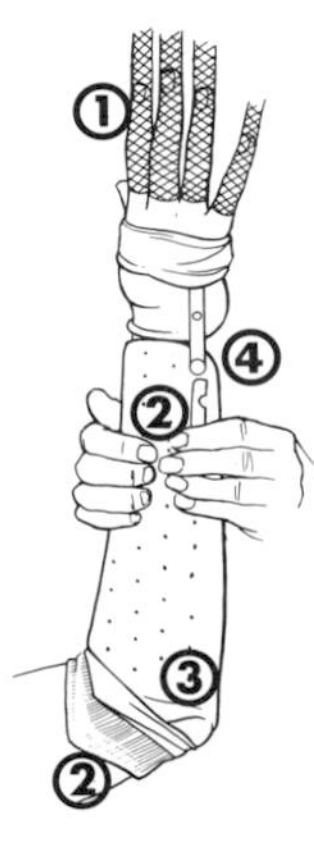

1. To apply the fracture-brace the forearm is suspended in a fingertrap and the patient is lightly sedated.
2. Plaster or orthoplastic material is wrapped and carefully molded to compress the soft tissue and interosseous space and to maintain the radial bow.
3. The material is wrapped over the supracondylar region to limit rotation but permit some flexion and extension.
4. A wrist hinge is applied to the material to allow flexion and extension of the wrist and to encourage finger and hand function.

Postreduction Management

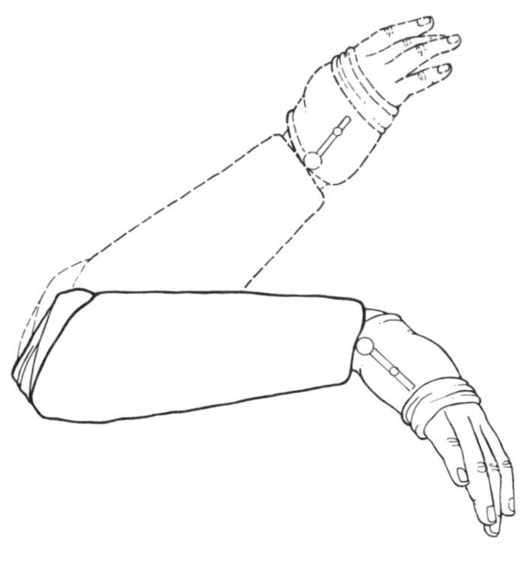

Encourage functional exercises of elbow, wrist, shoulder, and forearm muscles during the period of immobilization.

As pain subsides and confidence returns, the patient will use the fractured limb with greater vigor.

Evaluate the fracture position periodically by x-ray during the first 2–3 weeks after functional cast-bracing.

Most functional braces will last for the period of time required for fracture union and will not require replacement.

Evaluation of Reduction

Reduction is inadequate if the interosseous space becomes narrowed significantly or angulation exceeds 10°. Complete overriding of the fragments is also unacceptable, although end-to-side apposition may be accepted. If the reduction is lost, remanipulate the fracture or perform open reduction and internal fixation.

Follow-Up X-Ray After Cast-Brace Removal

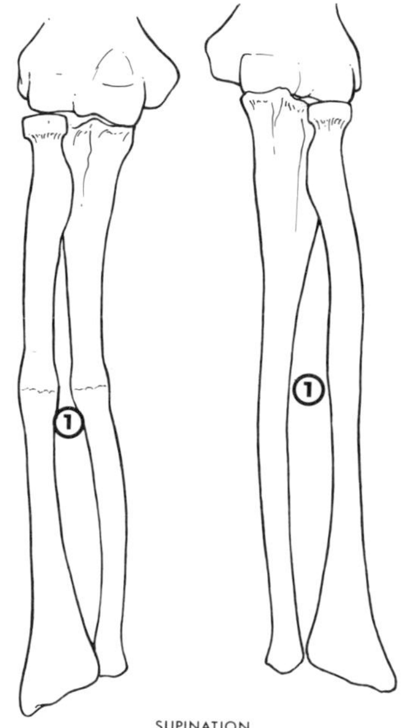

SUPINATION

Slight bayonet or end-to-side apposition permits healing with satisfactory function that is not limited in

1. Supination or
2. Pronation when compared with the opposite intact forearm.

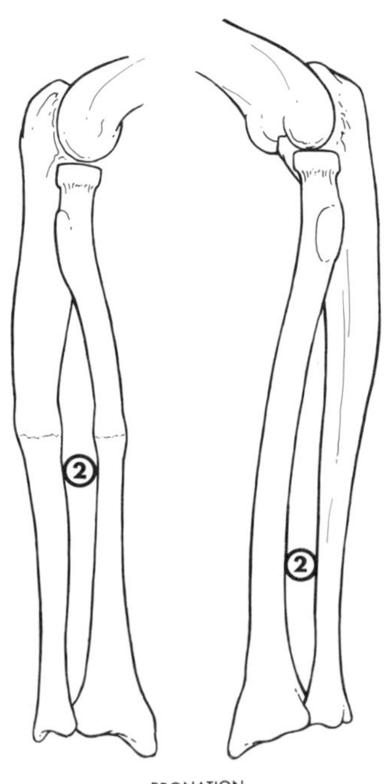

PRONATION

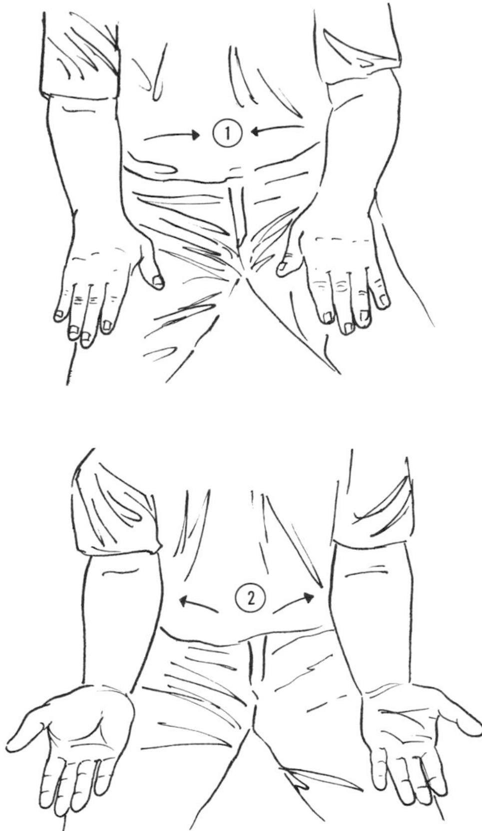

1. Pronation and

2. Supination are also restored clinically to close to normal range.

Note: The key to restoring rotation and grip in the forearm is to maintain the interosseous membrane at maximal tension and to restore the radial bow close to the normal angle. It may be possible to do this, even with bayonet apposition of the radius.

Caution: If adequate reduction cannot be maintained during the early stages of treatment, prompt surgical intervention can be employed, and the limb may then be protected postoperatively with the functional cast-brace technique. The average time for healing of displaced two-bone fractures is 15 weeks. Clinical union, with freedom from pain and absence of motion at the fracture site, always occurs before radiographic healing, but protective splints should be continued until the fracture has consolidated on x-ray. Functional activity during the healing minimizes soft tissue interosseous scarring and muscle contraction, and resultant disability when the immobilization is discontinued.

Displaced or Undisplaced Two-Bone Fractures in the Lower Half of the Forearm (In Adults)

REMARKS

These fractures are managed in the same manner as fractures in the upper half of the forearm, except that the rotation should be closer to a neutral position than to supination. After initial reduction, a long-arm cast is applied until pain and swelling subside (7–10 days). Subsequently, a functional cast or cast-brace is applied, and elbow and wrist motion are encouraged.

Prereduction X-Ray

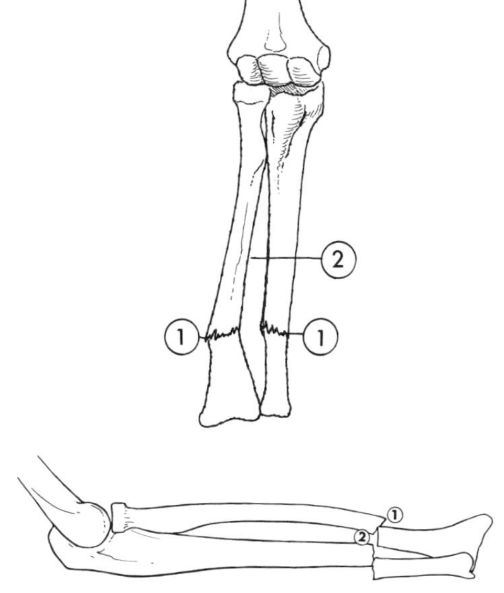

UNDISPLACED FRACTURE

1. Fragments of both bones are angulated but not displaced.
2. The interosseous space between the proximal fragments is decreased in width.

DISPLACED FRACTURE

1. Both the radius and the ulna have shortened and angulated.
2. The interosseous space is extremely narrowed.

Manipulative Reduction

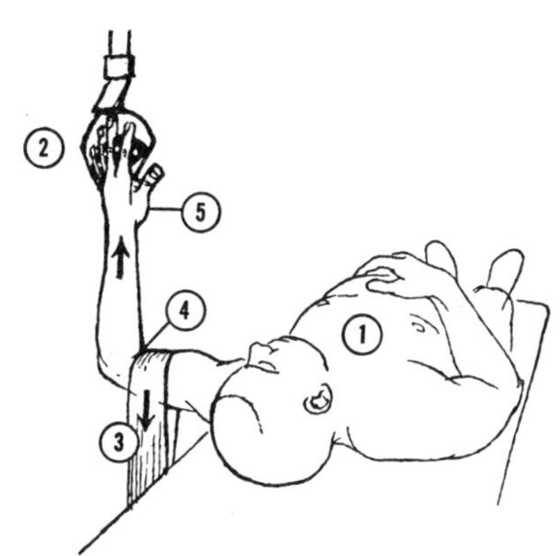

Reduction is performed under general or regional intravenous anesthesia.

1. The patient assumes the supine position on the fracture table.
2. The fingers are engaged by the finger-traction apparatus.
3. Countertraction is made on the arm in a plane parallel to the forearm by a sling of muslin bandage anchored to the crossbar at the bottom of the table.
4. The elbow is flexed 90°.
5. The forearm is in neutral rotation.

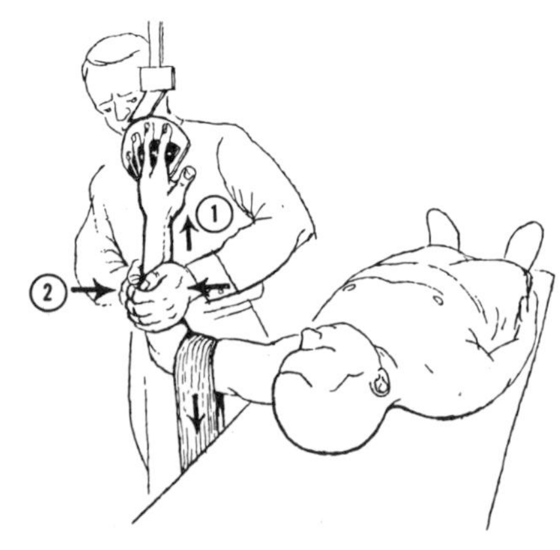

1. Apply strong traction through the finger-traction apparatus until length is restored and angulation is corrected. This requires at least 10 minutes of traction.
2. After length is restored, squeeze the volar muscle mass between the radius and the ulna, forcing the two bones apart.

Postreduction X-Ray

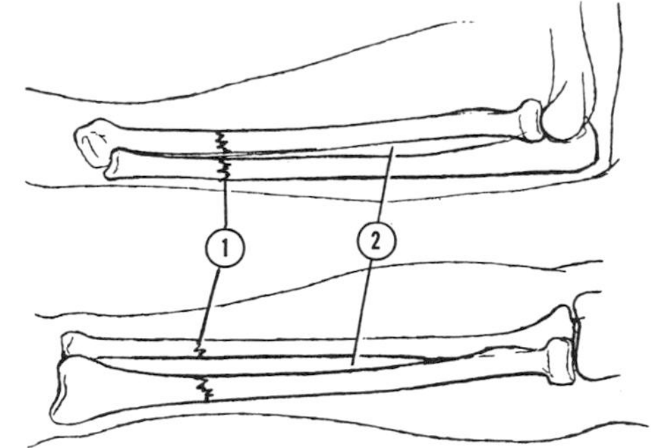

UNDISPLACED FRACTURE

1. Angular deformity of both bones is corrected.
2. The interosseous space is restored to its normal width.

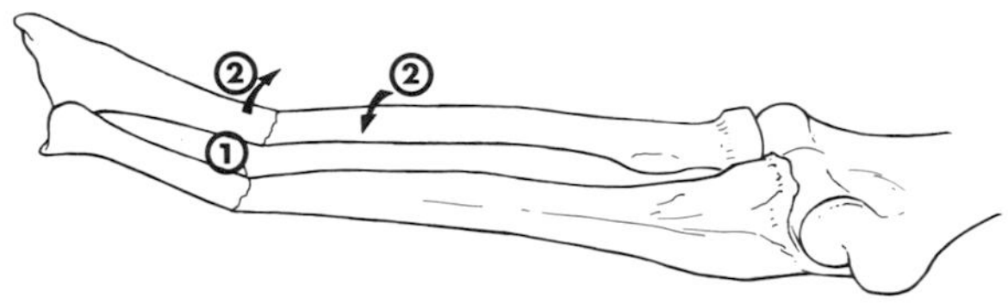

DISPLACED FRACTURE

1. The fractures are aligned but
2. Angulation should not be accepted.

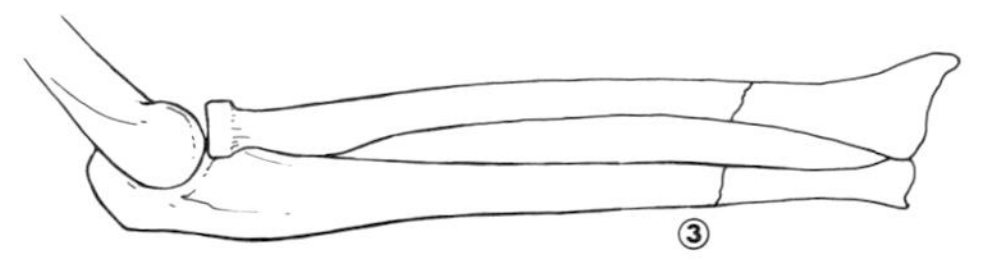

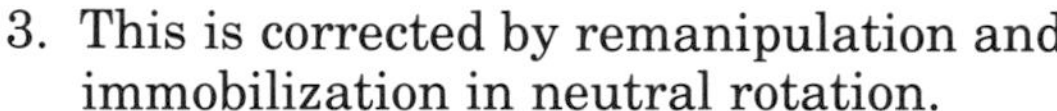

3. This is corrected by remanipulation and immobilization in neutral rotation.

Cast Application

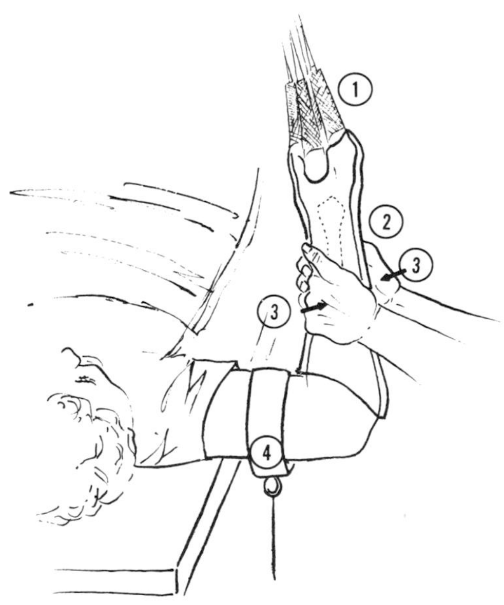

1. When the fracture is reduced by traction and rotational realignment, a long-arm cast can be applied.
2. A short-arm cast is applied first, molded carefully around the fracture site.
3. The interosseous space is maintained by firm pressure at the fracture site to compress the interosseous space.
4. When the below-elbow portion of the cast is hardened, the counterweight traction may be released and the cast extended above the elbow. Subsequently, the reduction is carefully monitored by x-ray.

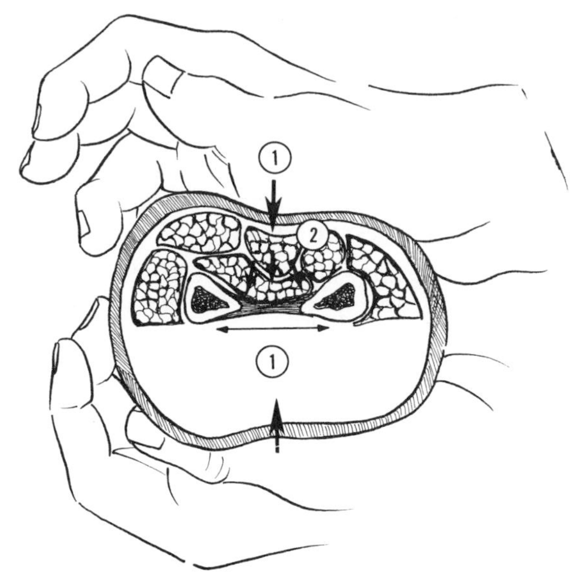

1. The key to maintaining reduction is to mold in the interosseous space between the radius and ulna with the forearm in neutral rotation. This maintains the interosseous space and ligament at maximal width and tension.
2. As the fracture heals, functional use of the hand and wrist is important to prevent scarring of the muscles and soft tissues in the interosseous space, which can subsequently impede forearm rotation or grip strength.

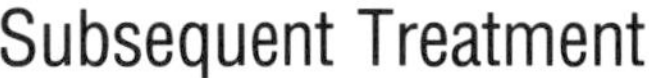

Subsequent Treatment

Check the arm constantly for evidence of circulatory embarrassment; if any signs are noted, bivalve the cast immediately. The cast should allow free motion at the shoulder and at the fingers. When pain and swelling subside, a functional cast-brace can be applied.

Functional Cast-Brace Treatment

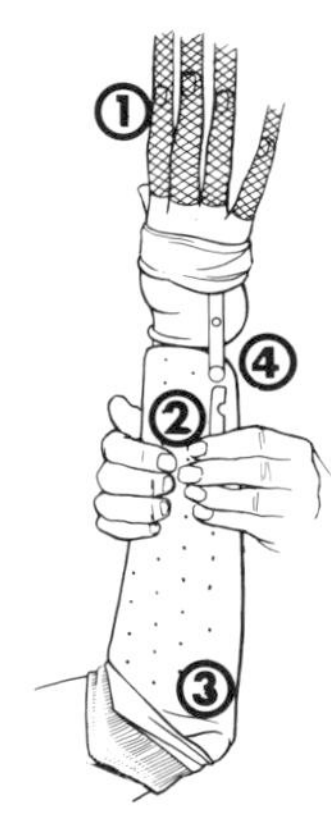

1. The forearm is suspended in fingertraps.
2. The plaster or orthoplast material is firmly molded to compress the tissue in the interosseous space and to maintain radial curve.
3. A supracondylar elbow extensor permits flexion and extension but limits pronation and supination.
4. Wrist hinge and hand component permit palmar flexion and dorsiflexion.

Subsequent Management

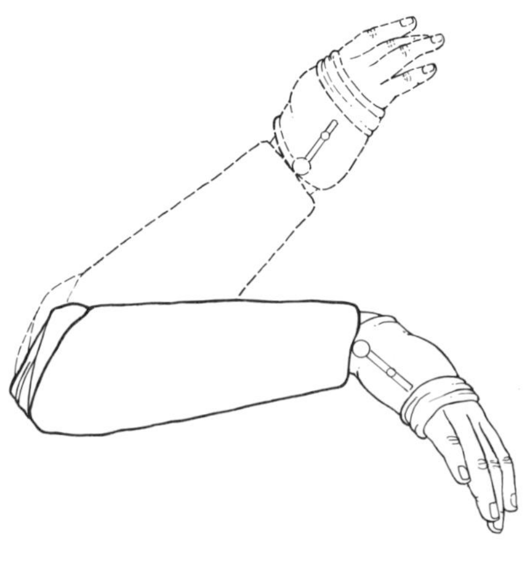

Encourage functional exercises of elbow, wrist, shoulder, and forearm muscles during the period of immobilization. As pain subsides and confidence returns, the patient will use the fractured limb with greater vigor.

Evaluate fracture position periodically by x-ray during the first 2–3 weeks after cast-brace application. Most functional cast-braces last for the period of time required for union and do not require replacement.

The average healing time for two-bone fractures is 15 weeks, but occasionally the process may take as long as 6 months. Functional activity allowed during this slower healing minimizes scarring and muscle contracture, which are present when the plaster is discarded.

X-Ray of Two-Bone Distal Fracture after Functional Treatment

Excellent union is evident at 15 weeks, on the average, despite lack of immobilization of the wrist and elbow. Compression of the soft tissues and interosseous membrane by this snug cast or brace technique maintains fracture stability during the healing.

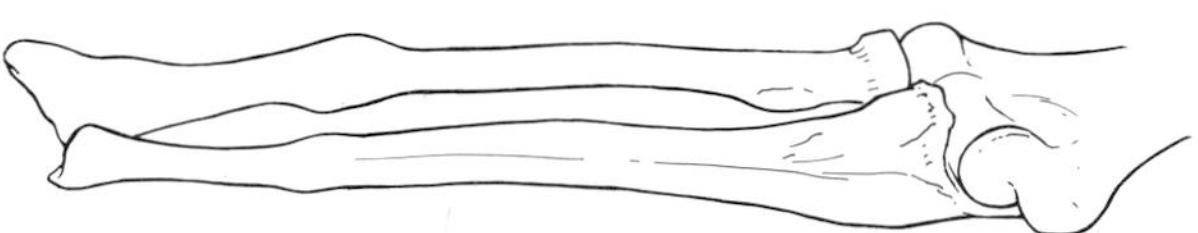

Fracture Deformities to be Avoided With Closed Management and Fracture-Brace Treatment of Forearm Fractures

REMARKS

The major problem with closed reduction of two-bone fracture of the forearm is loss of reduction, even after several weeks in the cast following initial adequate reduction. The decision regarding adequacy of reduction should depend on the fact that less than 10° of angulation has not been shown to impair forearm function and may be quite acceptable in preference to operative treatment. Greater than 10° of angulation should be corrected, especially if it is in a plane likely to produce a cosmetic deformity.

Rotational malalignment of the fracture fragments should also be avoided. The method of Evans by assessing the position of the bicipital tuberosity is helpful to determine reduction. However, rotational alignment can also be assessed by comparing the cortices of the proximal fragment with the distal fragment cortices.

A major concern in dealing with isolated single-bone fractures of the forearm is that the radioulnar joint is not dislocated either proximally or distally. Care must be taken to obtain a full view of the forearm with any isolated forearm fracture in the child or the adult in order to carefully assess the radioulnar relationships (see also section on single-bone fractures).

Effect of Fracture Reduction on Forearm Rotation

1. End-to-end reduction of the ulna and
2. Side-to-side apposition of the radius can be accepted. This alignment maintains the radial bow of the forearm and does not impair forearm rotation if the fracture heals in this position.

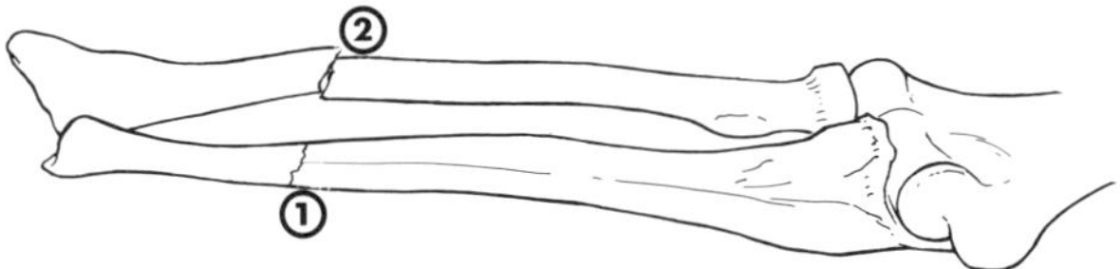

1. Fracture angulation of more than 10° is likely to be unacceptable because it is usually cosmetically unsatisfactory and potentially likely to impair forearm rotation and grip strength.

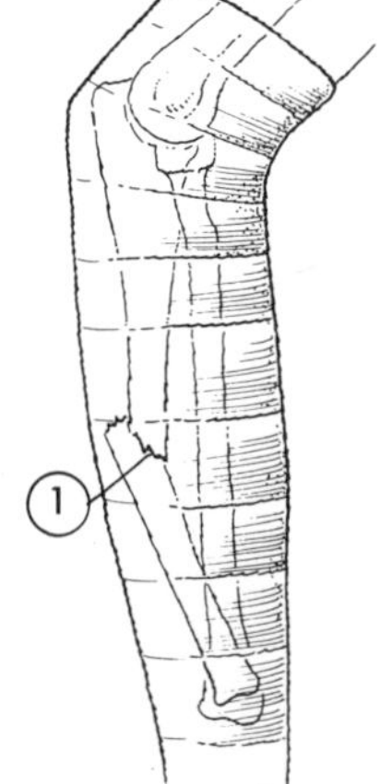

1. Rotational malalignment is frequently associated with angulation of more than 10°.
2. If the distal fragment is pronated while the proximal fragment is supinated, rotational malalignment may be present. This can be assessed by carefully evaluating the width of the cortices of the proximal and distal fragments, which should be equal.

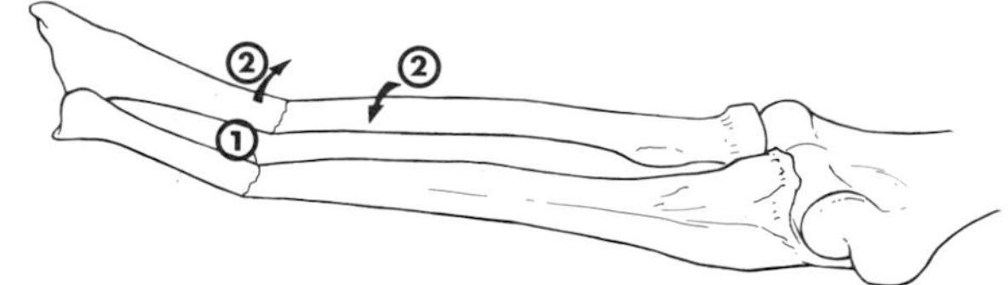

Other Factors Affecting Alignment

WEIGHT OF HAND

Immobilization of forearm fractures in full pronation should be avoided even for fractures in the distal third.

1. Full pronation.
2. Weight of the hand displaces distal fragment downward.

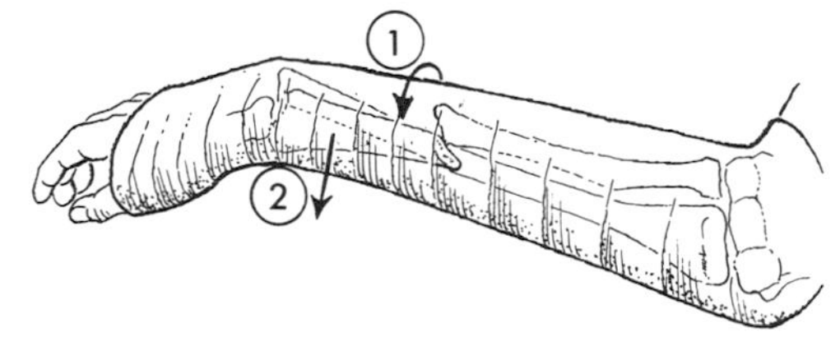

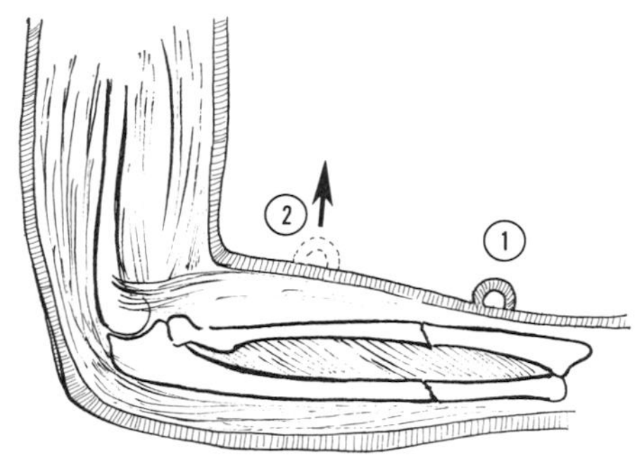

Fracture Angulation in Cast

1. If a loop is attached to the cast to support a sling, the weight of the arm may also cause angulation, even in the cast.
2. To support the cast for the first few days, use a sling or attach the cast loop to the cast in the region of the proximal fragment above the fracture site to avoid deformation caused by the pull of gravity.

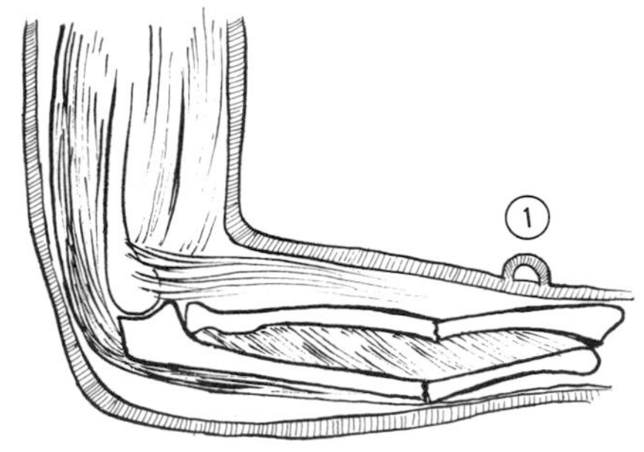

Operative Indications for Forearm Fractures

REMARKS

With skillful management based on the principles of Shang and Sarmiento, many forearm fractures can be treated by closed methods. Nevertheless, the majority of forearm fractures today are treated with open reduction and plate fixation.

The dynamic compression plate (DCP), first described by Bagby and refined by the Swiss Association for the Study of Internal Fixation (ASIF) group, has proven to be an excellent internal fixation method for forearm fractures. The operative technique does carry its own risk of potential complications, including infection, nerve injury, and a painful and unsightly scar, which in some series resulted in a complication rate of 20–25 per cent. In addition, the need to reoperate in order to remove the plate has created problems of refracture and difficulty in determining when the fracture is healed.

In spite of the numerous potential and actual complications, open reduction and internal fixation have significantly improved the management of forearm fractures over the past three decades. Operative fixation is particularly indicated for fractures in which angulation cannot be reduced by closed methods to less than 10°. Open reduction and internal fixation is also the treatment of choice for forearm fractures in patients who sustain multiple injuries. However, the main indication for operative intervention appears to be a reluctance on the part of us surgeons to attempt closed reduction owing to the difficulties of the method and the need for close follow-up to avoid complications and loss of reduction.

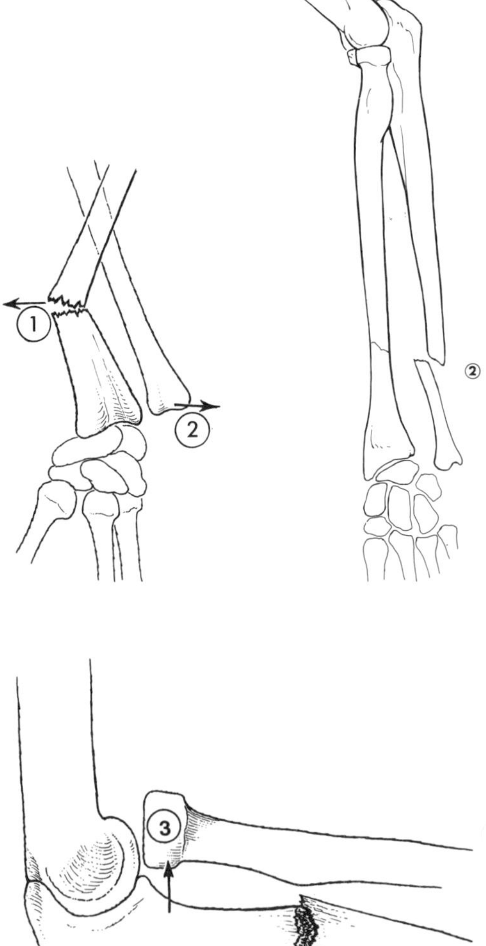

Specific candidates for early internal fixation are

1. Fracture of the radius with ulnar dislocation (Galeazzi's fracture).
2. Two-bone fracture with ulnar dislocation.
3. Fracture of the ulna with radial head dislocation (Monteggia's fracture).

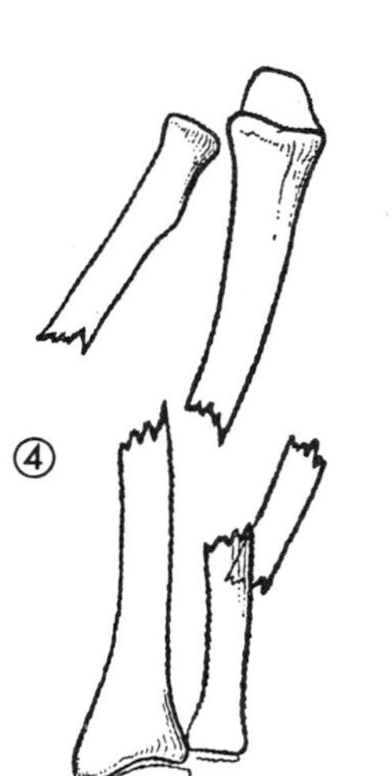

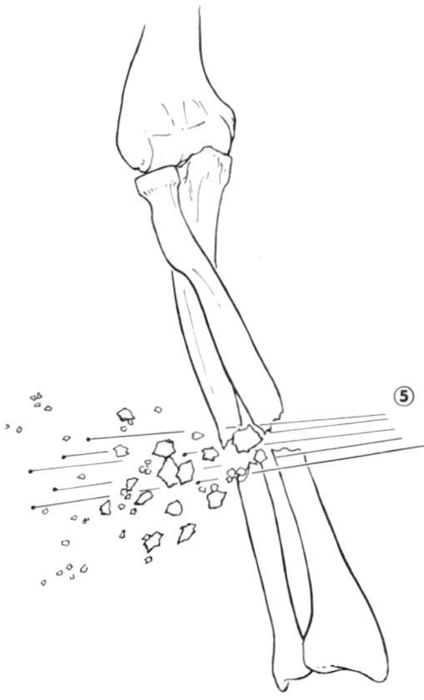

4. Segmental fracture.
5. Comminuted or gunshot fracture with bone loss, necessitating bone grafting.

Fractures of the Proximal Half of the Radius Requiring Internal Fixation

REMARKS

These may not be isolated injuries. Always check the proximal and distal radioulnar joint because dislocation is quite possible. Closed reduction may be attempted and frequently is quite successful. Angulation of more than 10° toward the ulna, however, is unacceptable because this is likely to limit rotation of the radius about the ulna.

If open reduction is chosen, the surgical approach is usually posterior in order to visualize the radial nerve and to allow a dorsal application of the plate. This is less likely to block rotation.

Preoperative X-Ray

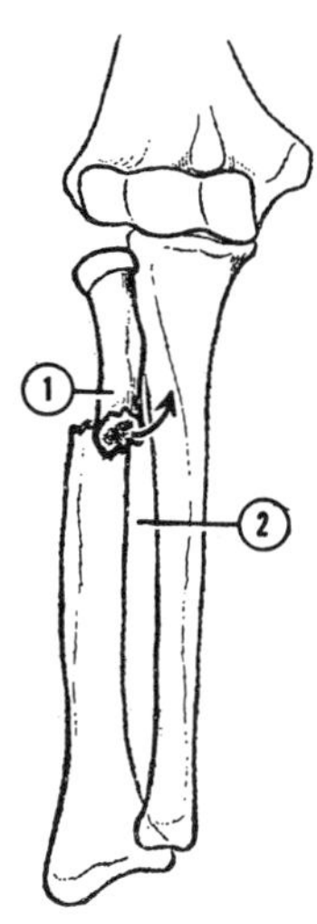

Fracture of the proximal third of the radius.

1. The proximal fragment is supinated and displaced forward.
2. The distal fragment is pronated and drawn toward the ulna.

Note: If angulation cannot be improved by closed reduction, it should not be accepted because it would seriously limit forearm rotation. Dislocation of the distal radioulnar joint should be suspected with radial instability of this severity.

Reduction Technique

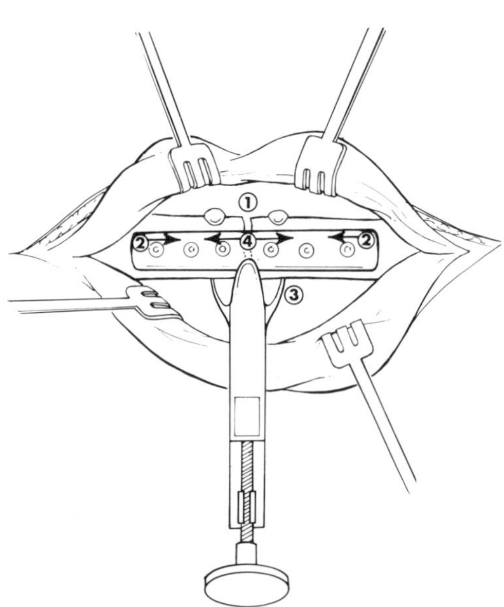

1. After the fracture is exposed, the fragments are reduced and realigned, taking care to be sure that rotation is correct.
2. A five- or six-hole plate is usually necessary to adequately stabilize the fracture.
3. A clamp is applied to maintain the fracture in correct position while the plate is fixed.
4. The alignment of the plate relative to the fracture is carefully evaluated so that screw holes are separated at least 5–10 mm from the fracture site.

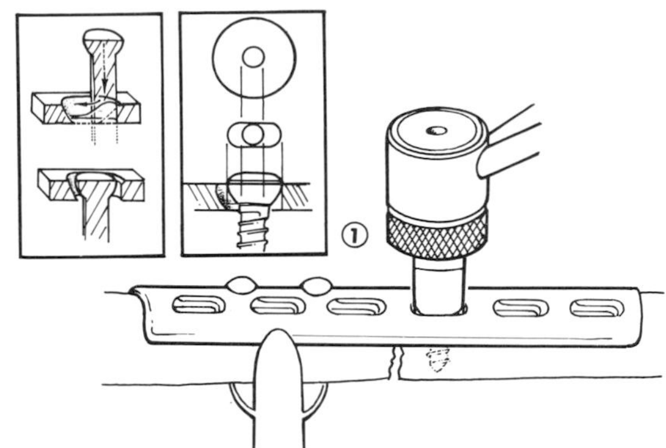

PLATE FIXATION

The ASIF technique of fixation is followed closely.

1. A neutral drill guide is used for the initial fixation of the plate to the bone. This guide is not marked by an arrow, and it centers the chamfered screw at the bottom of the obliquely inclined screw hole. The screw hole is drilled and tapped, and the first screw is inserted at least 1 cm from the fracture.

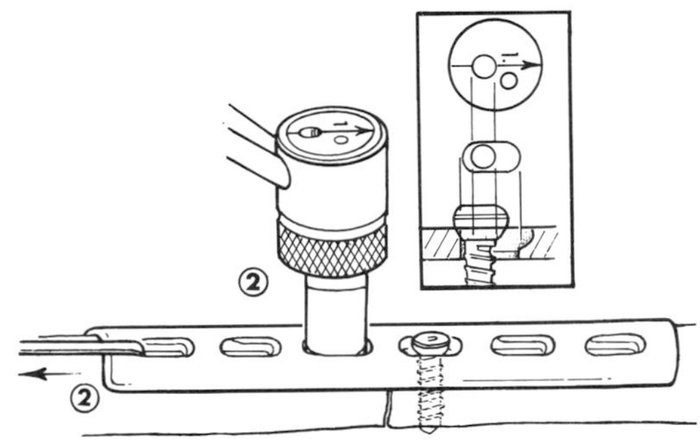

2. With the fracture anatomically reduced, the plate is pulled toward the upper fragment and a second hole is drilled with the load drill guide. This guide locates the hole 1.0 mm eccentrically from the geometric center of the hole. The arrow of this eccentrically designed load drill guide must always point toward the fracture.

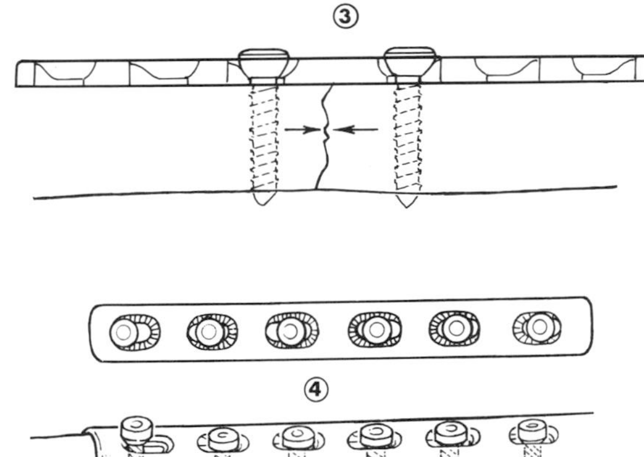

3. As the screw is inserted eccentrically, it glides along the obliquely inclined edge of the screw hole toward the center, at the same time pushing or compressing the fracture.

4. The plate should be of adequate length to permit screw fixation of at least five cortices proximal and five cortices distal to the fracture. These remaining screw holes are drilled using the neutral drill guide.

Postoperative Management

On average, the fracture line will fill in by 8–12 weeks and all external support can be discarded. The patient should be cautioned to avoid heavy lifting as the forearm regains strength. In active individuals, a protective brace is useful during the third and fourth postoperative months.

Routine removal of the plate is usually not necessary unless the patient experiences irritation from a subcutaneous position of the plate. In any event, plate removal should be delayed for at least 2 years until the fracture has healed completely and remodeled to resist bending and secondary refracture.

Fractures of the Distal Half of the Radius With or Without Dislocation of the Distal Radioulnar Joint

REMARKS

In the early part of this century, the eponym for solitary fracture of the distal radius was the "chauffeur's fracture," because the most common mechanism was a violent, direct blow to the radius incurred while a person turned the crank on a motor car. Isolated, undisplaced fractures may still occur from direct blows.

Another mechanism of injury is a forceful rotation, either in a pronation or supination direction, that disrupts the distal radioulnar joint and also fractures the radius. Forceful pronation causes dorsal angulation, whereas supination causes volar angulation as discussed previously under mechanisms.

Single-bone fracture of the distal radius or displaced radial fracture at any level should be carefully evaluated for associated dislocation of the distal radioulnar joint. Dislocation may not be evident on the initial x-ray and may show up only on subsequent studies or even after cast application (Galeazzi's fracture).

Fractures of the distal half of the radius sustained from direct blows to the radius can frequently be treated by closed methods. This type of fracture was discussed earlier in the chapter.

The usual fracture in this location is the result of a combination of axial and torsional loading, which causes a displaced fracture of the distal radius with injury of the distal radioulnar joint. This is a prime indication for early operative stabilization of the distal radius.

Mechanisms of Distal Radial Fractures

Direct Injury

1. Fracture of the distal radius may occur from a direct blow to the bone. This does not significantly displace or angulate the radius.
2. The interosseous membrane and distal radioulnar ligaments remain intact.
3. The distal end of the ulna is not shortened and the fracture is stable.

Note: This type of fracture can be treated quite adequately by closed casting and functional bracing.

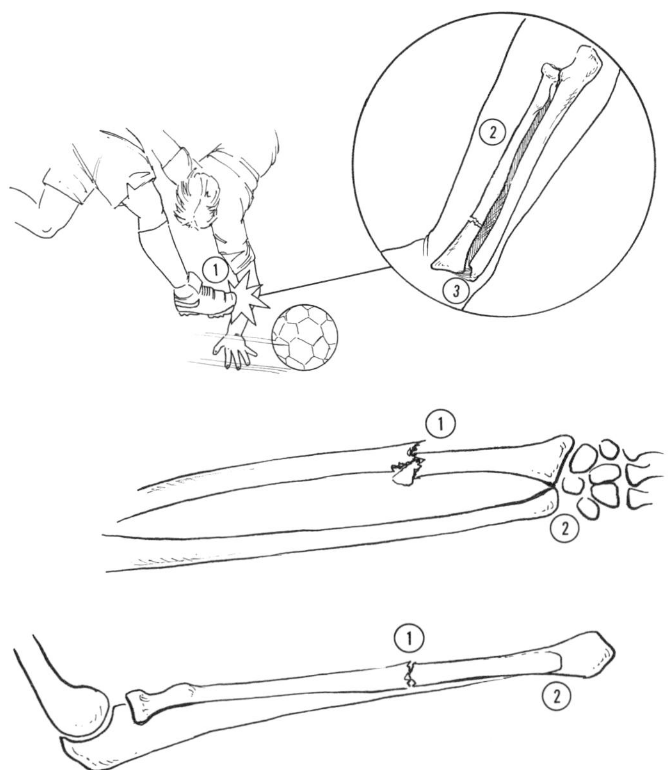

Closed Management for Fractures Sustained by Direct Injuries

1. The isolated fracture of the radius has been sustained by direct injury to the distal radius. The fracture is usually stable.
2. The distal radioulnar joint is intact, and soft tissues are not disrupted.

Note: This can be readily managed by a brief period of long-arm cast followed by fracture-brace to regain wrist and hand function because the fracture is stable.

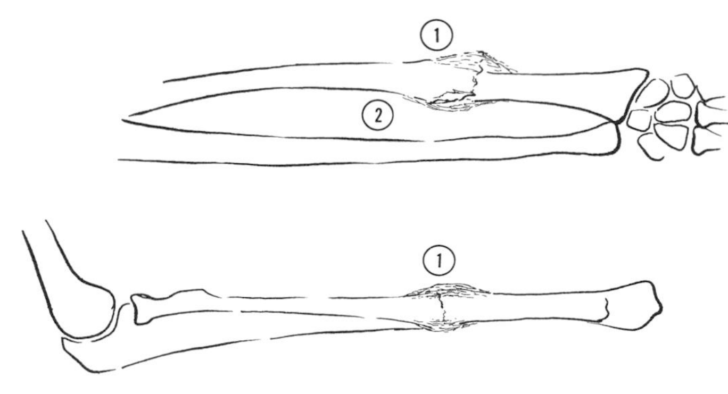

1. As described previously (page 1313), the fracture of the distal radius is held in the fracture-brace with forearm supinated until it heals, usually by 10–12 weeks.
2. There may be slight bayonet apposition, but the interosseous space is maintained. The functional result allows minimal limitation of pronation and supination.

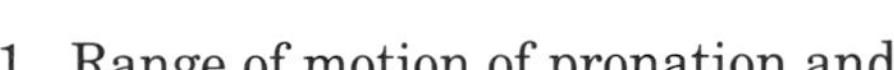

1. Range of motion of pronation and

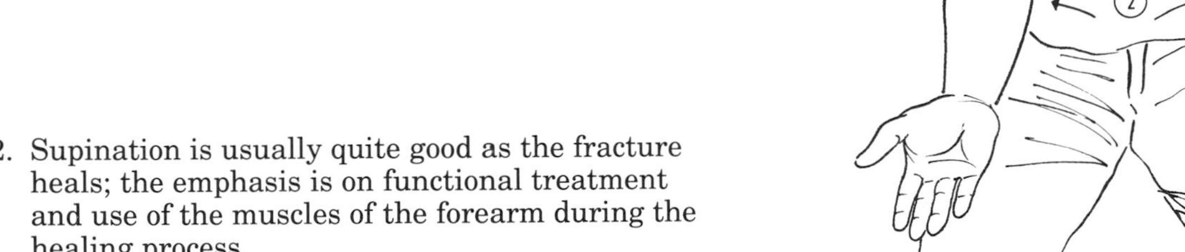

2. Supination is usually quite good as the fracture heals; the emphasis is on functional treatment and use of the muscles of the forearm during the healing process.

Indications for Internal Fixation

Indirect Injury Causing Unstable Fracture

1. An isolated fracture of the radius can occur from a fall on the outstretched hand. This combines axial loading with
2. Rotational injury.
3. The result is displacement of the radial fracture. Shortening and displacement of more than 5 mm are strong evidence that the interosseous membrane has been disrupted and
4. The distal radioulnar joint is dislocated.

Note: This type of isolated radial fracture with shortening of the fragments and disruption of the distal radioulnar joint necessitates internal stabilization of the radius. This is in contrast to the fracture produced by a direct injury to the radius.

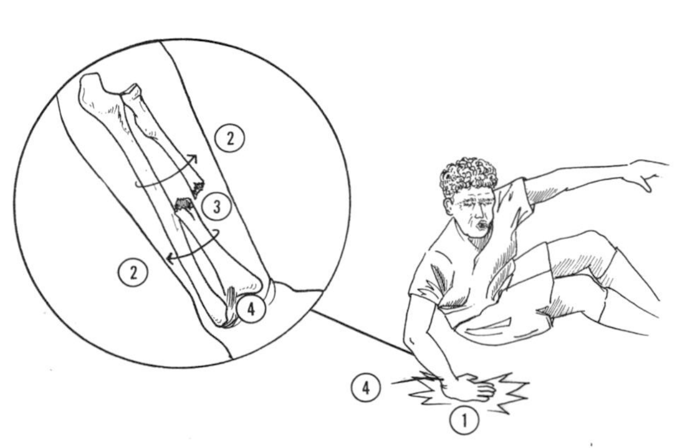

Operative Management of Isolated Radial Fractures From Indirect Loading

REMARKS

An isolated radial fracture resulting from a fall on the outstretched hand is almost inevitably associated with major damage to the support ligaments of the distal radioulnar joint. This is particularly true if there is any angulation or displacement of the fracture site. Failure to correct the disruption of the distal radioulnar joint can result in limitation of forearm rotation and often painful radioulnar joint symptoms.

Because of these potential problems, fractures produced by indirect loading should be anatomically reduced and the reduction should be maintained with internal fixation. Nevertheless, even anatomic reduction in some of these fractures does not guarantee that symptoms of discomfort in the distal joint will not persist.

Preoperative X-Ray

SUPINATION INJURY

1. Fracture of the shaft of the radius proximal to (8 cm from) the radiocarpal joint.
2. The fragments angulate toward the ulna and
3. In a volar direction, indicating that the mechanism was a supination injury.
4. The head of the ulna is dislocated (Galeazzi's fracture).

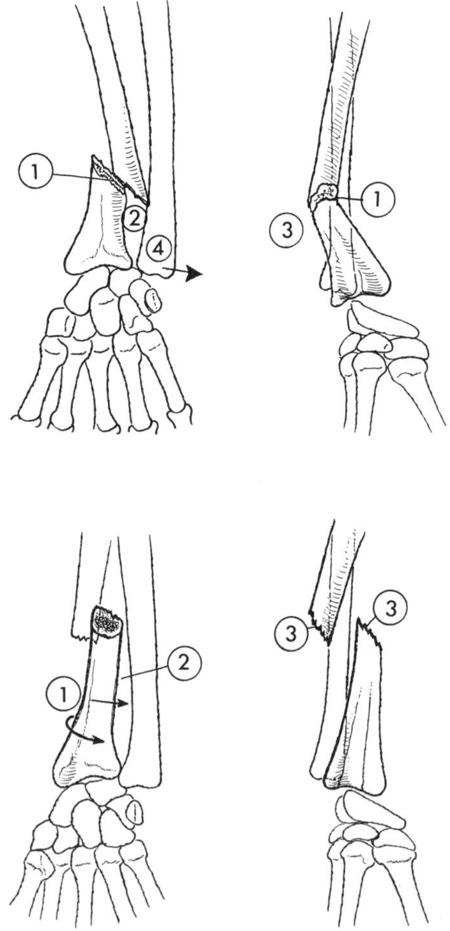

PRONATION INJURY

1. The distal fragment is pronated and displaced toward the ulna, volarly and proximally.
2. The interosseous space is markedly reduced.
3. The fracture is oblique and angulates dorsally, indicating a pronation mechanism.

Note: Fractures with this much displacement and angulation are always associated with disruption of the distal radioulnar joint.

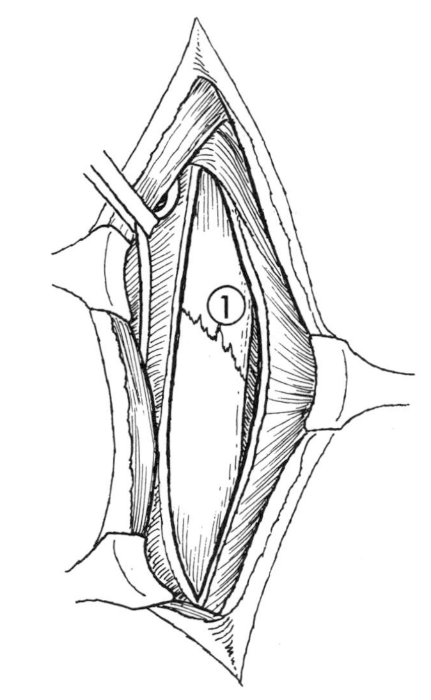

Preferred Management of Displaced Distal Radial Fractures

1. The fracture site should be opened, with care taken to protect the sensory branch of the radial nerve, which is usually directly over the fracture.

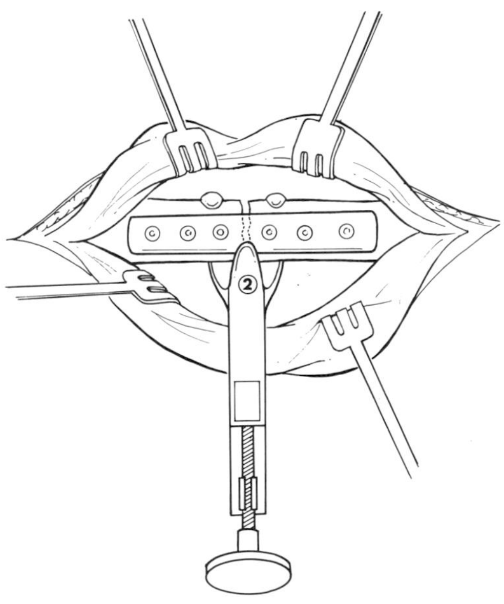

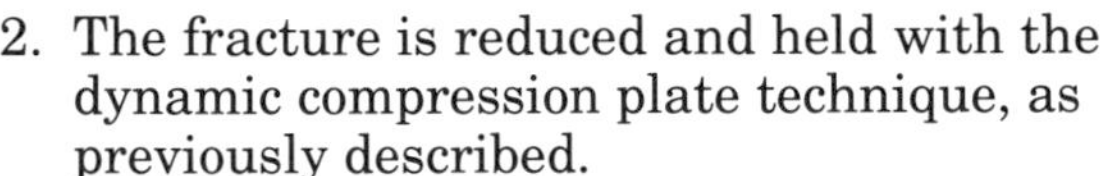

2. The fracture is reduced and held with the dynamic compression plate technique, as previously described.

Postoperative X-Ray After Plate Fixation

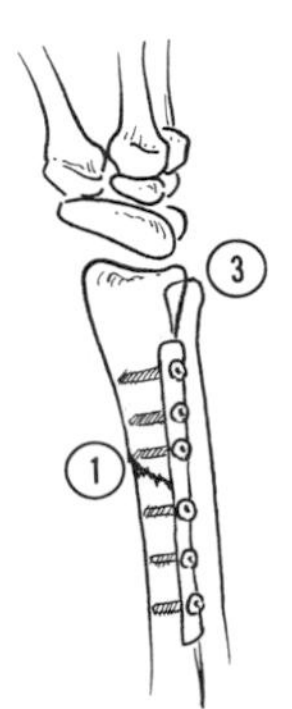

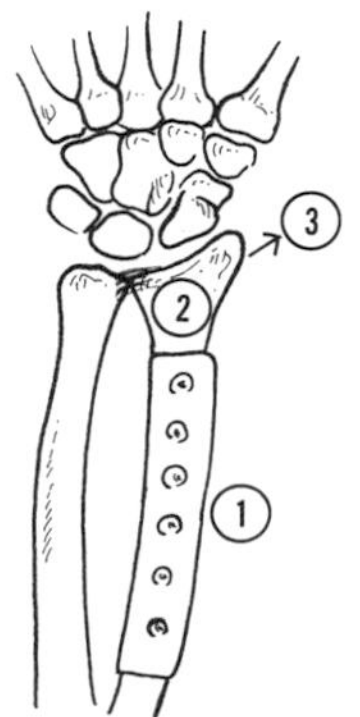

1. The displaced distal radial fracture has been reduced and stabilized with a plate.
2. The distal radioulnar joint has been reduced by reduction of the radius.
3. The forearm is usually held in supination to maintain reduction of the usual dorsal dislocation of the distal ulna.

Note: If the ulna has dislocated in a volar direction, the forearm and wrist can be immobilized in pronation.

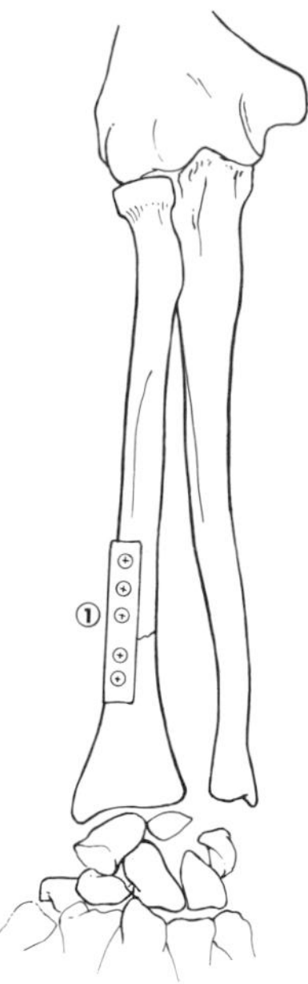

Postreduction X-Ray With Persistent Dislocation of the Distal Radioulnar Joint

1. The reduction of the distal radius rarely may not reduce in a chronic lesion. This may require direct repair of the radioulnar ligaments. Alternatively, the radioulnar joint may be stabilized by percutaneous pin fixation.

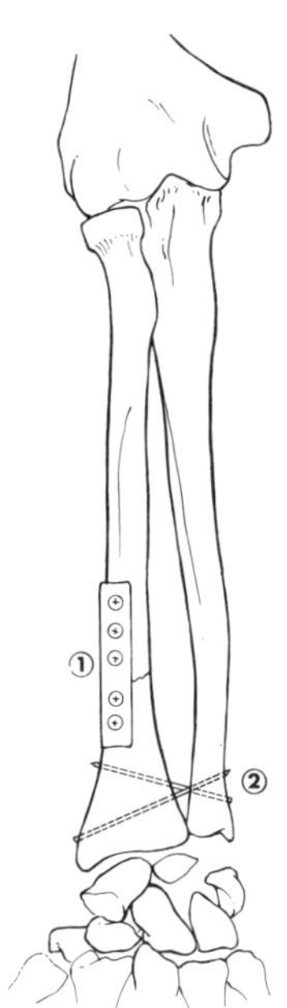

Postoperative X-Ray After Reduction and Stabilization of the Distal Radioulnar Joint

1. The compression plate has reduced the radial fracture.
2. Percutaneous pin fixation may be rarely necessary to reduce an unstable chronic radioulnar dislocation.

Note: Even with repair of this type of injury, chronic pain in the distal radioulnar joint may necessitate later surgical excision of the distal ulna.

Subsequent Management

Immobilization should be individualized according to the type of fracture, the adequacy of the fixation, and the patient's ability to cooperate.

After initial postoperative swelling has subsided, external support may sometimes be discarded, although it is usually safer to employ a functional cast-brace.

If the fracture was unstable and pins were required to immobilize the distal radioulnar joint, postoperative immobilization should be continued for a month, or until the pins are removed. During postoperative immobilization, the patient should actively exercise the shoulder, elbow, and fingers of the injured limb. Remove the pins at 1 month and begin active range-of-motion exercises.

Follow-Up Management

On average, the fracture line will fill in by 8 weeks and the external cast support can be discarded. For active individuals, a protective splint should be continued for an additional 2–3 months. Routine removal of the plate is not necessary, except in athletic individuals who participate in contact sports or in patients in whom the subcutaneous presence of the plate irritates overlying soft tissues.

Segmental Fractures of the Forearm Bones

REMARKS

These fractures are usually the result of considerable violence and may be extensively comminuted. There is frequently soft tissue damage and other multiple injuries.

Open reduction and plate fixation, frequently supplemented by autogenous bone grafting, are the most effective treatment methods for the usual segmental fracture. However, if the segmental fracture involves only one bone, such as the ulna or the radius, closed reduction and functional fracture-brace treatment may be indicated initially. This is particularly true for the occasional segmental fracture of the ulna, which can be treated with the fracture-brace method.

Closed Treatment of a Segmental Fracture of the Radius

1. A gunshot injury has produced an open comminuted fracture of the proximal third of the radius.
2. The ulna is intact and therefore stabilizes the radial fracture.
3. The interosseous ligament is also intact and can be used as an aid to stabilize the segmental radial fracture.

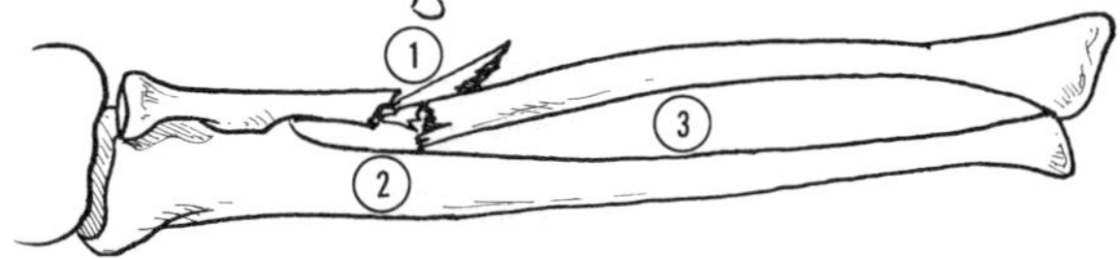

Initial Treatment With a Long Arm Cast

1. A functional fracture-brace can be applied at 2–3 weeks after the initial injury.

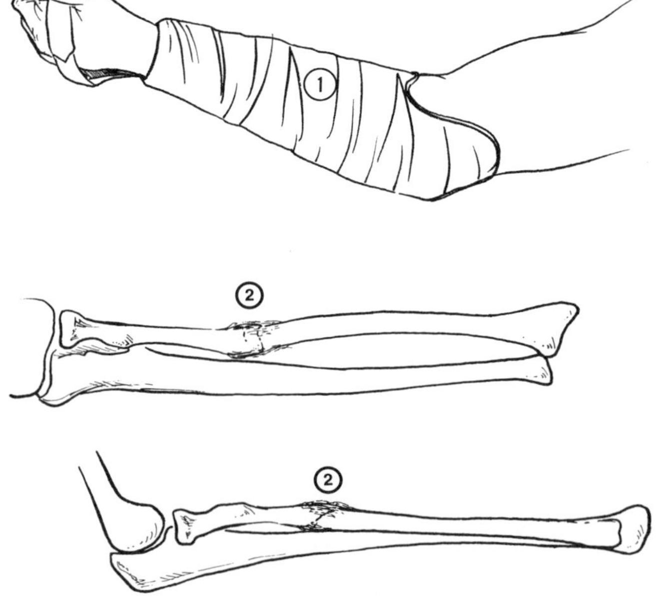

2. This leads to uneventful healing of the comminuted segmental radial fracture.

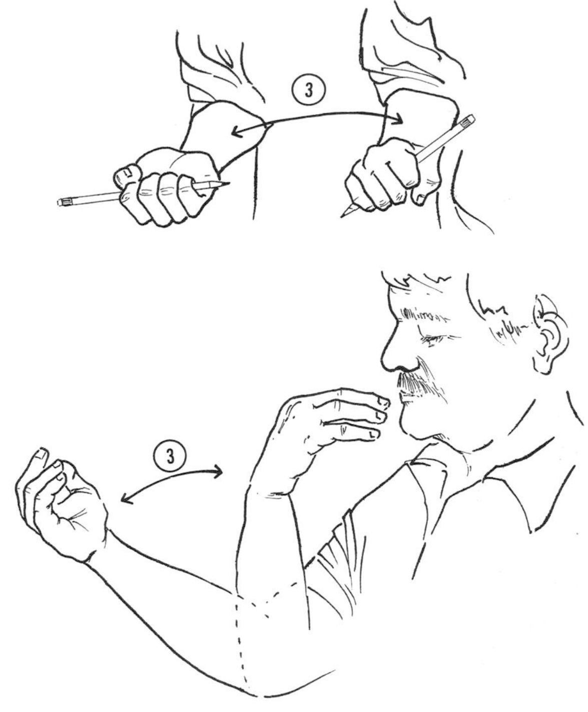

3. The residual impairment of function is barely measurable.

Note: If the comminution produced measurable shortening of the radius, open reduction and internal fixation would be preferable to the closed functional treatment approach.

Segmental Fracture of the Ulna Treated by the Functional Fracture-Brace Method

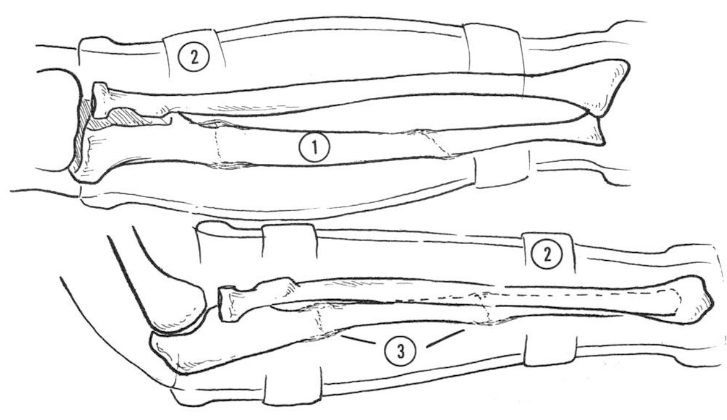

1. A segmental fracture has occurred in the ulna as a result of several blows to the forearm.
2. The fracture sleeve can be applied at 2–3 weeks as the swelling subsides. Prior to this time keep the forearm immobilized in a long-arm cast.
3. The undisplaced segmental fracture should heal as rapidly as the other ulnar fractures treated by this method. Slight loss of rotation may occur as a result of the severity of this injury to the soft tissues.

Segmental Fracture Necessitating Open Reduction and Internal Stabilization

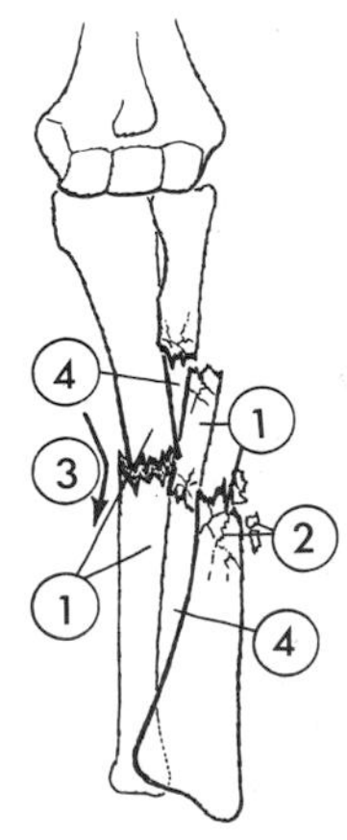

1. A segmental fracture of the radius has resulted from severe direct trauma. This frequently is associated with an open wound over the fracture site.
2. The radial fracture fragments tend to be comminuted.
3. Gross displacement and angulation have occurred.
4. The interosseous ligament has also been damaged, causing distortion of the interosseous space.

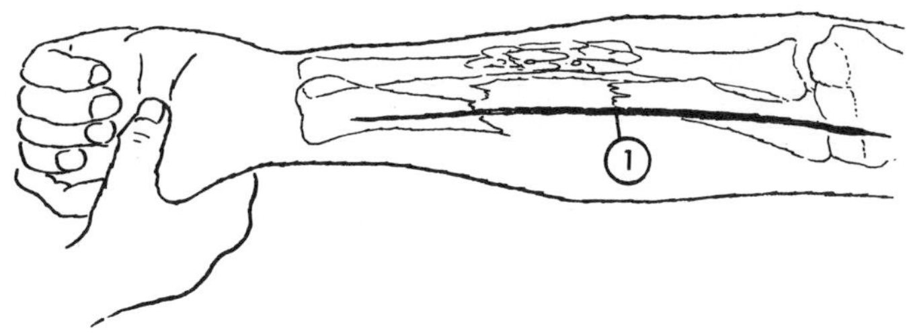

1. The segmental radial fracture must be exposed by an extensile approach through either the anterior or posterior aspect of the forearm.

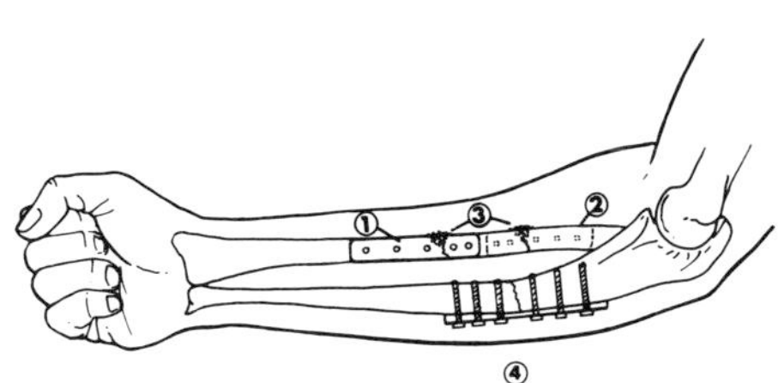

2. A separate incision is made to expose the ulnar fracture.

1. The distal radial fracture is fixed with a dynamic compression plate applied to the volar surface.
2. The proximal radial fracture may require a dynamic compression plate applied on the dorsal surface.
3. Supplemental bone graft is added for any comminution involving more than one third of the cortex.
4. The ulnar fracture is stabilized before stabilization of the radius, to avoid excessive shortening of the radius.

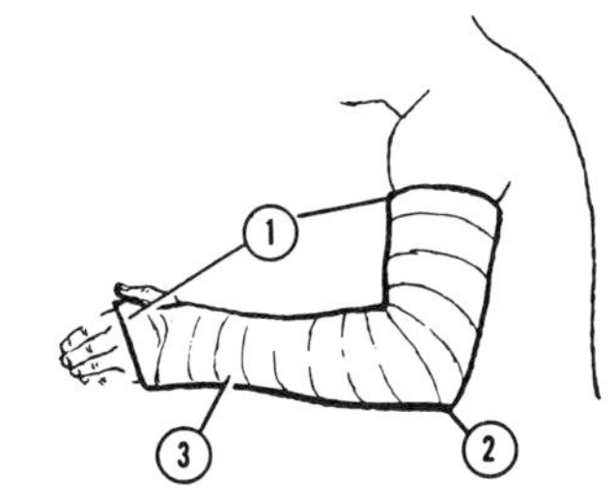

Postoperative Management

1. A circular long-arm cast is applied.
2. The elbow is flexed approximately 90°.
3. The forearm is in neutral rotation.

Subsequent Management

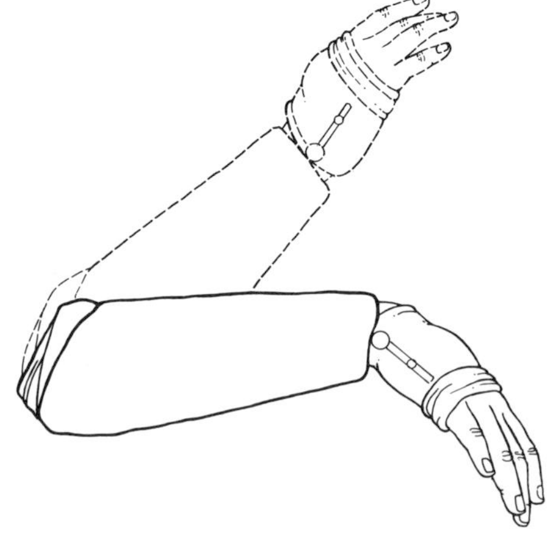

A fracture-brace may be applied as the initial swelling subsides, usually by the second or third postoperative week. The protective brace should be maintained for approximately 8–12 weeks until there is clinical and radiographic evidence of healing of all fractures of the forearm.

The patient should be advised that some limitation of forearm rotation and grip strength is highly likely with this severely comminuted type of fracture.

Management of Open Fractures of the Bones of the Forearm

REMARKS

Approximately 15 per cent of forearm fractures are open injuries that mandate complete wound debridement. The smallest wounds often prove to be the most treacherous, because fracture fragments may have been driven out through the wound to be contaminated by dirt, barnyard manure, or a variety of pathogens and then have returned under the skin.

Avoid the inclination to cleanse only the superficial wound for fear of damaging underlying tendons or nerves. Too often this leaves the patient with a significant deep abscess at the fracture site and a strong chance for amputation or death. All open forearm fractures, even with slight and seemingly insignificant puncture wounds, mandate complete operative cleansing of the bone ends (see Chapter 1), as well as tetanus prophylaxis. If the wound is explored surgically within 6 hours, before bacteria become firmly established in the traumatized tissues, and if the bone ends are found to be clean, the wound may be closed primarily.

All other wounds, especially wounds of an uncertain nature, should be left open to be reexplored and reirrigated within 3 days. Secondary closure may be performed at this time of reexploration, but the edematous wound should never be closed under tension. If there is any doubt, the wound should be allowed to heal spontaneously by intussusception of the wound edges.

Undisplaced open fractures heal well when treated by functional cast-bracing. Comminuted or segmental open fractures that are unstable can be stabilized with plates and screws if the wound is not grossly contaminated at the time of initial debridement. The wound is left open over the fracture site, and repeated debridements are then carried out to achieve wound closure. If the open wound is badly contaminated, secondary stabilization of the fracture may be carried out at the time of the second or third debridement.

Open fractures of the forearm are often associated with injuries to the neurovascular structures and adjacent tendons. Nerve injuries require adequate repair, as do tendon injuries. Vascular injury to a single vessel does not necessitate repair if the distal pulse is adequate. However, a compartment syndrome associated with an open fracture is an indication for prompt fasciotomy. Special problems of the open forearm fracture necessitate adaptable approaches to the functional needs of the patient.

Types of Open Fractures

MOST DANGEROUS WOUNDS

1. Beware of small puncture wounds, which do not always reflect the degree of contamination.
2. Fragments may have been driven through the skin and into the ground or dirt, and then returned beneath the skin.

Note: All open forearm fractures mandate complete wound debridement. (See also forearm fractures in children.)

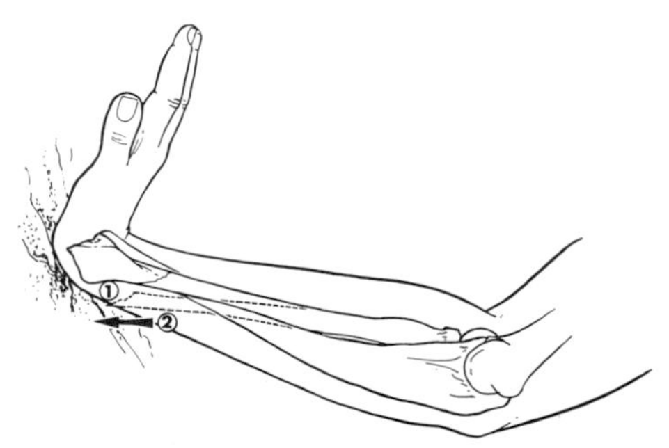

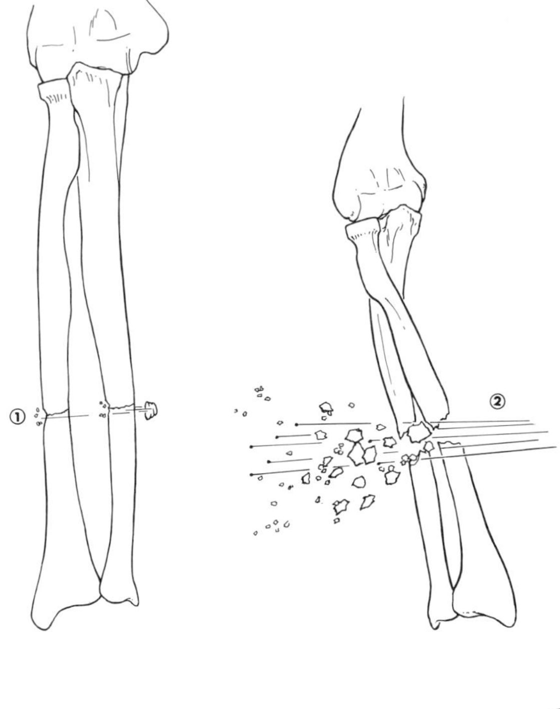

GUNSHOT FRACTURE

1. The undisplaced gunshot fracture may be treated by the functional cast-brace. A low-velocity gunshot wound does not necessitate fracture exploration.
2. Comminuted gunshot fracture necessitates thorough debridement and primary or secondary internal fixation with bone graft.

Note: Comminuted open fractures frequently damage adjacent tendons and nerves, which must also be repaired.

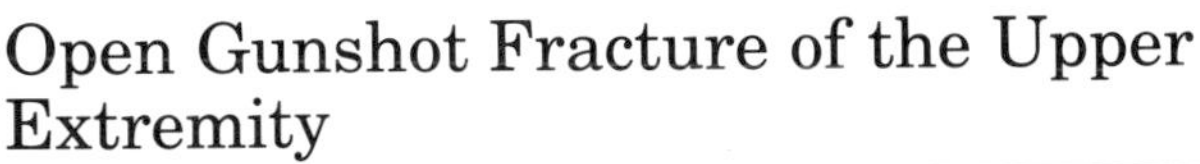

Open Gunshot Fracture of the Upper Extremity

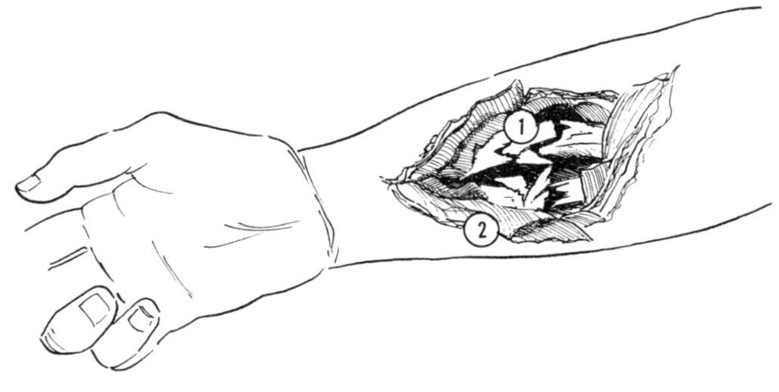

1. There is a comminuted fracture of the radius and ulna as the result of a shotgun injury to the forearm.
2. Soft tissue damage has also occurred as the result of the violent injury.

Primary Treatment

1. The soft tissue wounds are stripped of necrotic muscle and any foreign material.
2. If the soft tissue wounds undergo adequate debridement, the fracture site can be stabilized primarily.
3. Fasciotomies of the anterior and posterior compartments may be necessary if there is excessive swelling.
4. Neurovascular injury as well as tendon injuries can be repaired at the time of internal fixation. Repair of vascular injury depends on the status of the distal circulation.

Caution: If the wound is heavily contaminated, internal fixation should be avoided until the time of secondary debridement.

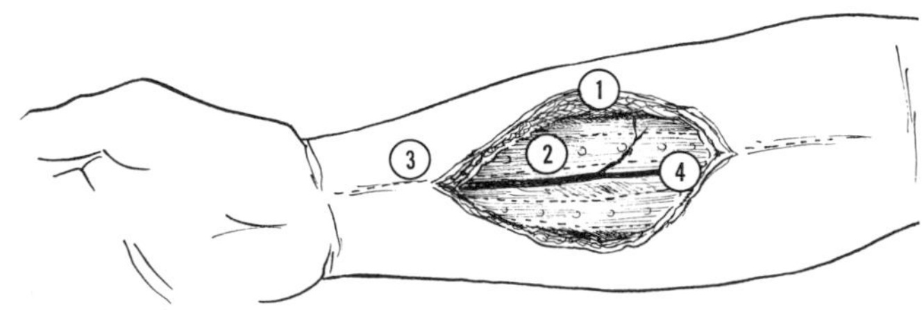

Subsequent Management

The open wound of entrance is left open and allowed to gradually close, either secondarily or by repeat debridement and skin grafting. The surgical wound over the fracture site can be closed primarily.

Antibiotic treatment (not prophylaxis) is continued for 5–7 days, depending on the status of the wound and the bacteria that are cultured from the wound. As the soft tissue wounds heal, functional rehabilitation should emphasize restoration of forearm motion and grip strength of the hand. This postoperative regimen has to be modified in accordance with any associated neurologic or tendon injuries.

Compression Plating Technique After Soft Tissue Healing Occurs

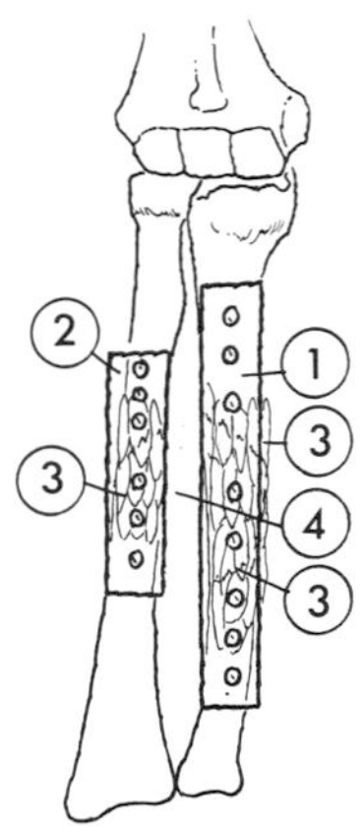

1. The ulnar fracture is fixed with a dynamic compression plate technique using a sufficiently long plate to stabilize a segmental fracture.
2. The radial fracture is fixed with a shorter compression plate because it is not segmental.
3. Cancellous bone graft has been added to the fracture site because of comminution.
4. The interosseous space should be restored to near normal width.

Alternative Method of Managing Open Forearm Fractures: Pins in Plaster or External Fixation

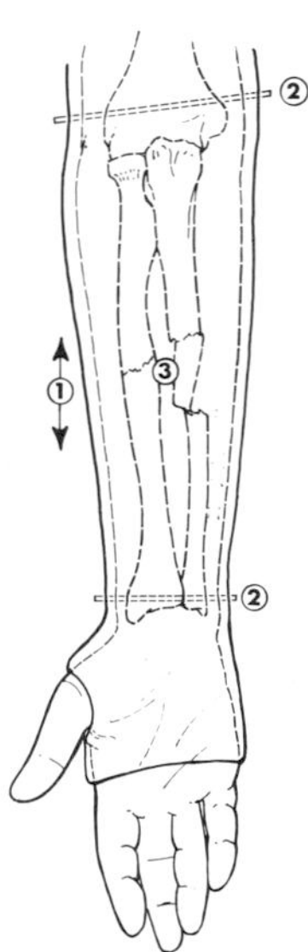

1. For an extensive open soft tissue wound with fracture comminution, primary internal fixation can be avoided until soft tissue healing is evident. During this time length can be maintained with the pins-in-plaster technique.
2. Proximal and distal pins are incorporated in plaster to maintain alignment until the soft tissues heal.
3. The interosseous space may not be restored to normal width by this method; therefore, early compression plate fixation with bone grafting is usually necessary to restore normal anatomy and to permit functional restoration.

Special Problems

Traumatic Bowing of the Forearm

REMARKS

Bowing fractures result from low-velocity injuries that plastically deform the bone without fracturing it. Microfractures often occur at the concavity of the bone, but these may not be evident on x-ray. Plastic deformation of bone is more common in children and is discussed in Chapter 2. In adults, however, it may result from direct, severe compression injury to the forearm, such as when the arm is compressed in machinery.

Typical Bowing Fracture of the Forearm

1. A severe compression injury has occurred as a result of the patient's forearm being caught in heavy machinery. There are multiple excoriations and contusions on the forearm.
2. X-ray shows bowing of the fracture of more than 20°, which is likely to impede forearm function.

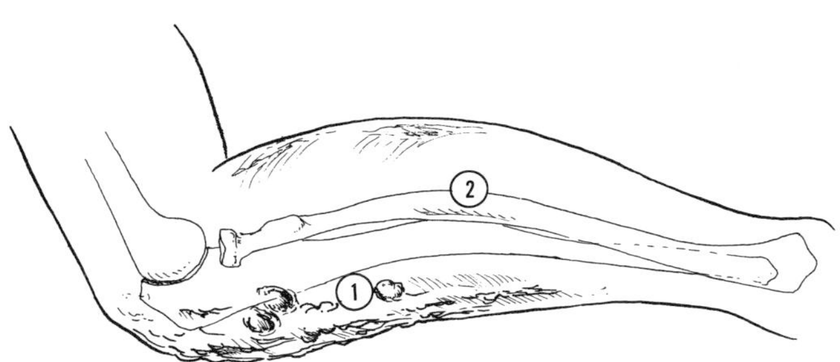

Management (After Van Den Wildenberg and Greve)

1. After the initial swelling subsides within 3–4 days, the patient's forearm can be subjected to manipulation with gradual force over a padded fulcrum.
2. When the plastic deformation is corrected, internal stabilization is obtained with intramedullary rods inserted in the radius and the ulna.

Note: The intramedullary rod is preferable to plate fixation because of the soft tissue injury and the extent of the plastic deformation in a large portion of the shaft.

If fracture occurs during manipulation of the plastically deformed bone, the forearm may be treated by closed functional cast methods; however, intramedullary fixation is useful to maintain the straight position and to avoid recurrence of the plastic bowing.

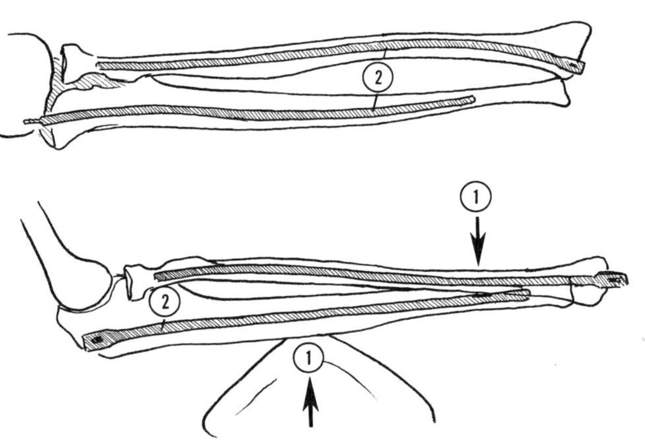

Subsequent Management

If stabilization is satisfactory, the patient can be treated with soft tissue support and compression dressing until the swelling subsides. Gradual rehabilitation is then begun by the second or third week as the swelling subsides. By 3 months the fracture usually heals without malalignment and without restriction of function.

Bone Loss Associated With Ulnar Fractures

REMARKS

Bone loss produced by fractures of the radius necessitates bone grafting and internal fixation. Severe bone loss associated with isolated fractures of the ulna may be amenable to treatment by producing a pseudoarthrosis, resulting in a "three-bone forearm."

The ulna is analogous to the fibula in that a sizable defect may not cause pain symptoms or instability, whereas an undisplaced unhealed fracture may well cause pain. A good portion of the ulna may be expendable, especially from the distal half toward the wrist. This should be kept in mind before carrying out any extensive bone grafting procedures to heal an un-united ulnar fracture with large defects. Operative grafting of an ulnar defect may actually decrease forearm rotation because of the associated scarring and prolonged immobilization required to achieve healing of the defect.

The Three-Bone Forearm

Appearance Immediately After Injury

1. Gunshot fracture to the ulna has produced a large defect.
2. The ulnar nerve is also damaged.
3. The radius is intact.

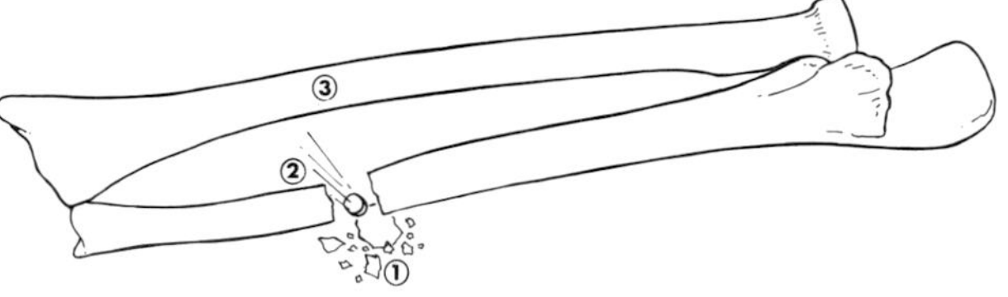

Range of Motion After Healing of Soft Tissue and Ulnar Nerve

1. Forearm rotation is minimally limited despite ulnar defect. This is essentially a "three-bone" forearm.
2. Occasionally with this instability, the proximal or distal end of the defect will become prominent and can be treated by surgical excision.

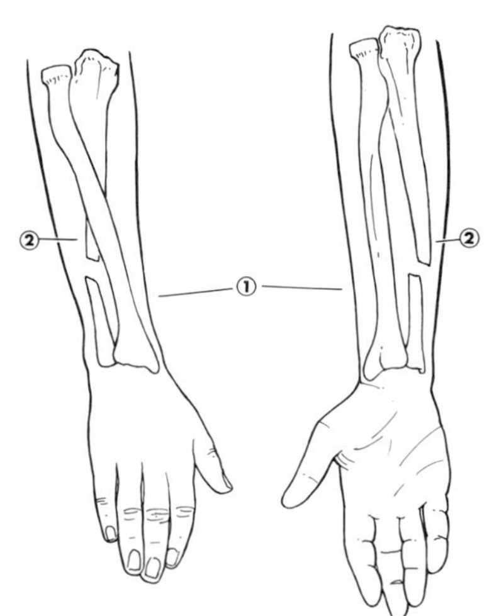

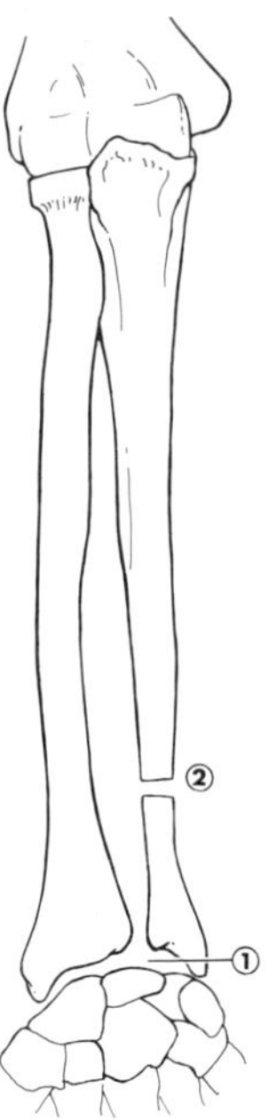

CONTRAINDICATION FOR CREATION OF THREE-BONE FOREARM

1. The stability of the distal radioulnar joint is essential to allow function of the three-bone forearm; if the distal radioulnar ligament is disrupted, as illustrated here, the distal ulna may displace laterally.
2. The defect of the ulna in this situation may be best treated by internal stabilization with bone grafting or, if the defect is distal enough, resection of the distal ulna should be considered (Darrach procedure) or stabilization of the distal ulna to the radius should be considered (see also Chapter 16, on wrist injuries).

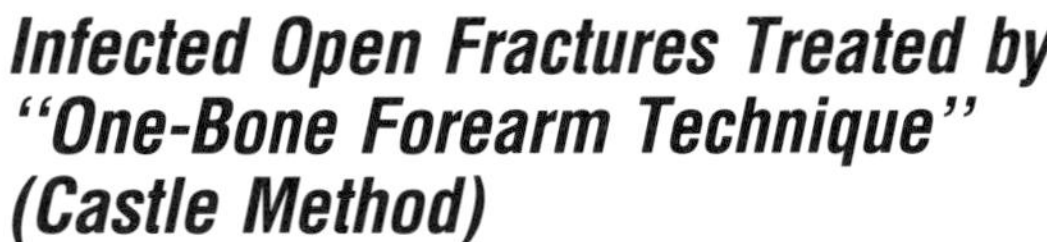

Infected Open Fractures Treated by "One-Bone Forearm Technique" (Castle Method)

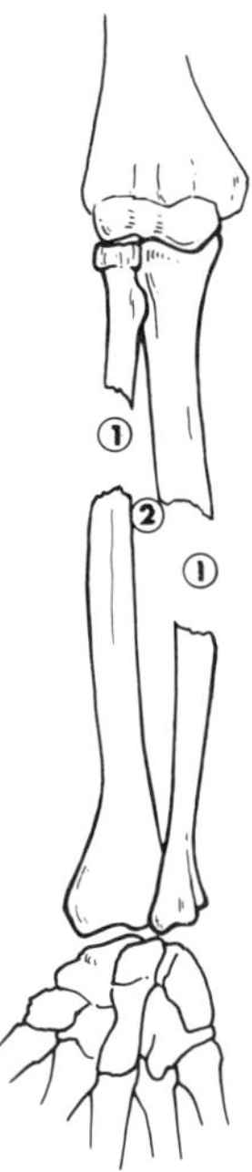

If extensive bone loss or infection makes loss of forearm rotation inevitable, functional recovery of the patient can be expedited by creating a one-bone forearm in which the distal radial segment is fixed to the proximal ulnar fragment.

Preoperative X-Ray

1. Infection has left nonunions with 5-cm gaps in both the radius and the ulna.
2. The proximal ulna fragment is adjacent to the distal radius.

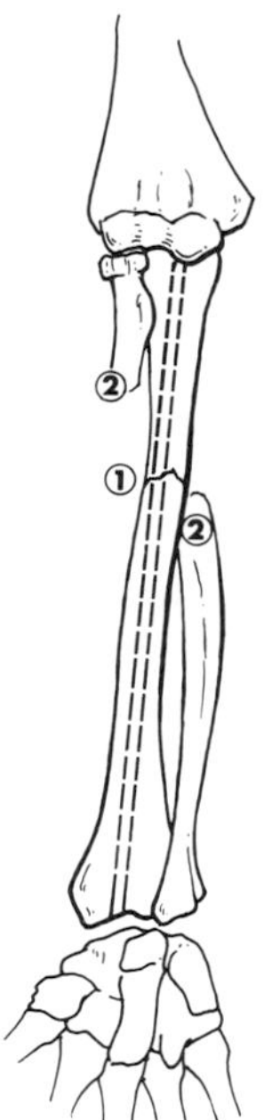

Postoperative X-Ray

Rather than attempting bone graft of both defects with resultant radial-ulnar ankylosis,

1. The proximal ulna is aligned with the distal radius and both are fixed with intramedullary pins.
2. The remaining radial and ulnar fragments are left free to permit forearm rotation.

Other Complications

Cross-Union of the Radius and Ulna Following Fracture of the Forearm

REMARKS

Cross-union between the radius and ulna may occasionally occur as a result of severe local trauma. Bone fragments in the interosseous space may be a source of excessive callus, producing bridging between the radius and ulna. The result may be a complete loss of forearm pronation and supination.

Although severe trauma or complications of the fracture are usually implicated, cross-union can occur after a stab or puncture wound without a fracture or after almost any kind of injury to the forearm. Overall, the incidence of this complication is approximately 1–2 per cent of forearm fractures. Cross-union, however, is often higher after Monteggia fracture-dislocations or other injuries with severe trauma.

Other conditions accompanied by high incidence of cross-union include head injuries or multiple trauma. Under these circumstances, surrounding undifferentiated connective tissue cells apparently can be stimulated to develop into osteoblastic (bone-forming) cells and produce heterotopic ossification.

Operative fixation with primary bone grafting is associated with a higher-than-normal incidence of cross-union. Any method of treatment should emphasize maintenance of the maximal width of the interosseous space and early restoration of forearm function to avoid the complication of cross-union.

Types of Fractures Associated With Cross-Union

1. The typical fracture resulting in cross-union is a comminuted two-bone fracture treated by operative reduction and internal fixation.
2. There is early evidence of bone in the interosseous space and callus forming in the interosseous region.

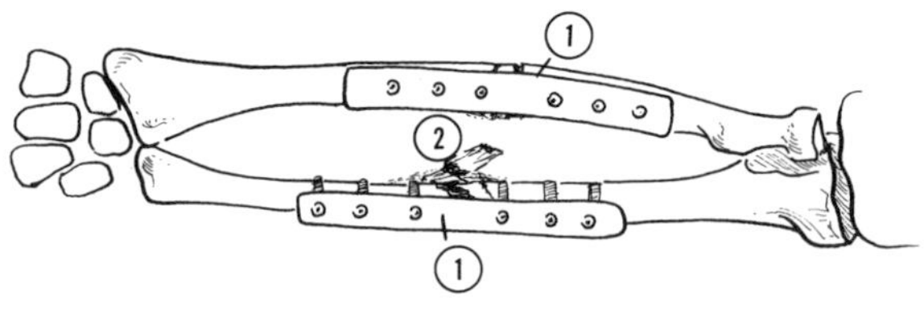

1. Cross-union is evident as the fracture heals and is sufficient to eliminate all forearm rotation.

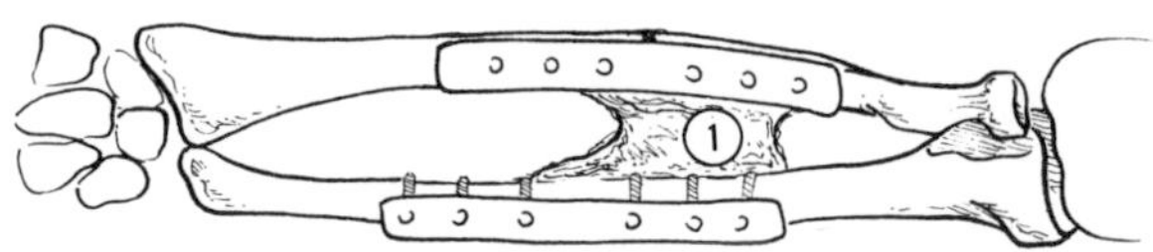

Management

Vince and Miller reported fairly satisfactory results in managing cross-unions in the common location of the middle forearm. These are amenable to resection, which is best done 1–2 years after the fracture. Formation of the callus should be quiescent. A bone scan may be indicated in order to demonstrate decreased activity before surgical resection of the cross-union.

Resection of a cross-union in the proximal forearm is prone to considerable complication because of the proximity of the posterior interosseous nerve and the likelihood of nerve damage. The removal of the bony bridge or cross-union can be supplemented by interposition of a Silastic sheet between the forearm bones in order to avoid recurrence of the problem.

Postoperative X-Ray After Plate Removal and Bone Bridge Resection

1. Resection has been carried out, and a Silastic sheet has been interposed between the radius and ulna. This results in a satisfactory arc of rotation of approximately 80°, allowing functional range of motion.

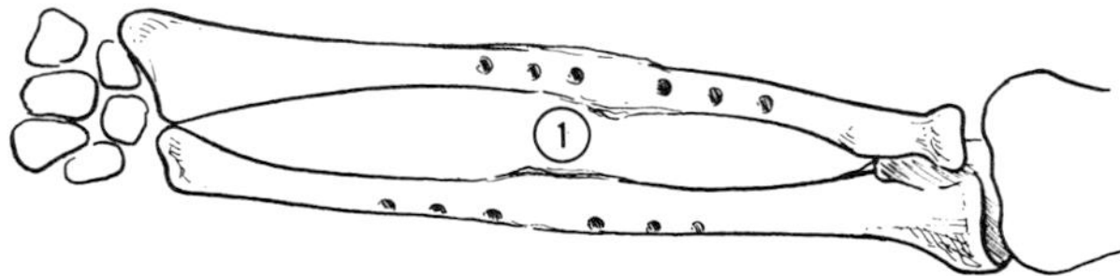

Note: Plate removal should be carried out only if the fracture is solidly united. The patient should be cautioned to avoid any strenuous lifting or activity with the forearm because it may be subject to refracture for many months after plate removal; this in turn is because complete remodeling of both the fracture site and the screw hole defects takes many months.

BIBLIOGRAPHY

Monteggia Fracture Dislocations

Austin R: Tardy palsy of radial nerve from a Monteggia fracture. Injury 7:202, 1976.

Boyd HB, Boals JC: The Monteggia lesion. Clin Orthop 66:94, 1969.

Bruce HE, Harvey JP, Wilson JC: Monteggia fractures. J Bone Joint Surg Am 56:1563, 1974.

Engber WD, Keene JS: Anterior interosseous nerve palsy associated with a Monteggia fracture. Clin Orthop 174:133, 1983.

Fowles JV, Sliman N, Kassab MT: The Monteggia lesion in children. J Bone Joint Surg Am 65:1276, 1983.

Jessing P: Monteggia lesions and their complicating nerve damage. Acta Orthop Scand 46:601, 1975.

Lichter RL, Jacobsen T: Tardy palsy of the posterior interosseous nerve with a Monteggia fracture. J Bone Joint Surg Am 57:124, 1975.

Mueller ME, Allgoewer M, Schneider R, Willenegger H: *Manual of Internal Fixation*, 2nd ed. Springer-Verlag, Berlin, 1979.

Pavel A, Pitman JM, Lance EM, Wade PA: The posterior Monteggia fracture. A clinical study. J Trauma 5:185, 1965.

Reckling FW: Unstable fracture-dislocation of the forearm (Monteggia and Galeazzi lesions). J Bone Joint Surg Am 64:857–863, 1982.

Stein F, Grabia SL, Deiffer PA: Nerve injuries complicating Monteggia lesions. J Bone Joint Surg Am 53:1432, 1971.

Closed Treatment Of Forearm Fracture

Charnley J: *The Closed Treatment of Fractures*, 3rd ed. Churchill Livingstone, New York, 1961.

Connolly JF: Torsional fractures and the third dimension of fracture management. South Med J 73:884, 1980.

Du Toit FP, Grabe RP: Isolated fractures of the shaft of the ulna. South Med J 56:21, 1979.

Evans EM: Fractures of the radius and ulna. J Bone Joint Surg Br 33:548, 1951.

Hoffer M, Schobert W: The failure of casual treatment of nondisplaced ulna shaft fractures. J Trauma 24:771, 1984.

Knight RA, Purvis GD: Fractures of both bones of the forearm in adults. J Bone Joint Surg Am 31:755–764, 1949.

Matthew LS, Kaufer H, Garver DF, et al.: The effect of supination-pronation of angular malalignment of fractures of both bones of the forearm. J Bone Joint Surg Am 64:14, 1982.

Sarmiento A, Cooper JS, Sinclair WF: Forearm fractures. J Bone Joint Surg Am 57:297, 1975.

Sarmiento A, Kinman P, Murphy RB, et al.: Treatment of ulnar fractures by functional bracing. J Bone Joint Surg Am 58:1104, 1976.

Sarmiento A, Latta LL: *Closed Functional Treatment of Fractures*. Springer-Verlag, New York, 1981.

Schiller MG: Intravenous regional anesthesia for closed treatment of fractures and dislocations of the upper extremities. Clin Orthop 118:25, 1976.

Shang T, Gu Y, Dong F: Treatment of forearm bone fractures by an integrated method of traditional Chinese and Western medicine. Clin Orthop 215:56, 1987.

Stewart TD: Nonunion of fractures in antiquity, with descriptions of five cases from the New World involving the forearm. Bull NY Acad Med 50:875, 1974.

Operative Treatment of Forearm Fractures

Anderson LD, Sisk TD, Tooms RE, Park WI III: Compression-plate fixation in acute diaphyseal fractures of the radius and ulna. J Bone Joint Surg Am 57:287, 1975.

Bagby GW: Compression bone-plating: Historical considerations. J Bone Joint Surg Am 59:625, 1977.

Chapman MW, Gordon JE, Zissimos AG: Compression plate fixation of acute fractures of the diaphysis of the radius and ulna. J Bone Joint Surg Am 71:159, 1989.

Deluca PA, Lindsey RW, Rowe PA: Refracture of bones of the forearm after the removal of compression plates. J Bone Joint Surg Am 70:1372, 1988.

Fisher WD, Hamblen DL: Problems and pitfalls of compression fixation of long bone fractures: A review of results and complications. Injury 10:99, 1978.

Grace TG, Eversmann WW Jr: Forearm fractures: Treatment by rigid fixation with early motion. J Bone Joint Surg Am 62:433, 1980.

Hidaka S, Gustilo RB: Refracture of bones of the forearm after plate removal. J Bone Joint Surg Am 66:1241, 1984.

Langkamer VG, Ackroyd CE: Internal fixation of forearm fractures in the 1980s: Lessons to be learnt. Injury 22:97, 1991.

Moed BR, Kellam JF, Foster JR, et al.: Immediate internal fixation of open fractures of the diaphysis of the forearm. J Bone Joint Surg Am 68:1008, 1986.

Mueller ME, Allgoewer M, Schneider R, Willenegger H: *Manual of Internal Fixation*, 2nd ed. Springer-Verlag, Berlin, 1979.

Stern PJ, Drury WJ: Complications of plate fixation of forearm fractures. Clin Orthop 175:25, 1983.

Tile M, Petrie D: Fractures of the radius and ulna. J Bone Joint Surg Br 51:193, 1969.

Galeazzi Fracture Dislocations

Galeazzi R: Ueber ein besonderes Syndrom bei Verletzungen im Bereich der Unterarmknochken. Arch Orthop Unfallchir 35:557, 1934.

Hughston JC: Fracture of the distal radius shaft. Mistakes in management. J Bone Joint Surg Am 39:249, 1957.

Kraus B, Horne G: Galeazzi fractures. J Trauma 25:1093, 1985.

Mikic ZD: Galeazzi fracture-dislocations. J Bone Joint Surg Am 57:1071, 1975.

Moore TM, Klein JP, Patzakis MJ, Havey JP Jr: Results of compression plating of closed Galeazzi fractures. J Bone Joint Surg Am 67:1015, 1985.

Moore TM, Lester DK, Sarmiento A: The stabilizing effect of soft tissue constraints in artificial Galeazzi fractures. Clin Orthop 194:189, 1985.

Reckling FW: Unstable fracture-dislocation of the forearm (Monteggia and Galeazzi lesions). J Bone Joint Surg Am 64:857, 1982.

Sarmiento A, Latta LL: Closed functional treatment of fractures. Springer-Verlag, New York, 1981.

Shang T, Gu Y, Dong F: Treatment of forearm bone fractures by an integrated method of traditional Chinese and Western medicine. Clin Orthop 215:56, 1987.

Open Fractures And Other Problems

Breit R: Post-traumatic radioulnar synostosis. Clin Orthop 174:149, 1983.

Castle ME: One-bone forearm. J Bone Joint Surg Am 56:1223, 1974.

Chapman MW, Gordon JE, Zissimos AG: Compression plate fixation of acute fractures of the diaphysis of the radius and ulna. J Bone Joint Surg Am 71:159, 1989.

Elstram JA, Pankovich AM, Eqwele R: Extra-articular low velocity gunshot fracture of the radius and ulna. J Bone Joint Surg Am 60:335, 1978.

Fee NF, Dobranski A, Bisla RS: Gas gangrene complicating open forearm fractures. J Bone Joint Surg Am 59:135, 1977.

Garland DE, Dowling V: Forearm fractures in the head injured adult. Clin Orthop 176:190, 1983.

Greene WB: Traumatic bowing of the forearm in an adult. Clin Orthop 168:31, 1982.

Hart GB, Lamb RC, Strauss MB: Gas gangrene: I. A collective review. J Trauma 23:991, 1983.

Kersley JB, Scott BW: Restoration of forearm rotation following malunited fractures: Baldwin's operation. J Hand Surg 15:421, 1990.

Langkamer VG, Ackroyd CE: Internal fixation of forearm fractures in the 1980s: Lessons to be learnt. Injury 22:97, 1991.

Langkamer VG, Ackroyd CE: Removal of forearm plates. J Bone Joint Surg Br 72:530, 1990.

Moed BR, Kellam JF, Foster JR, et al.: Immediate internal fixation of open fractures of the diaphysis of the forearm. J Bone Joint Surg Am 68:1008, 1986.

Nimityongskul P, Anderson LD, Sri P: Plastic deformation of the forearm: A review and case reports. J Trauma 31:1678, 1991.

Vince KG, Miller JE: Cross-union complicating fractures of the forearm. Part I–Adults. J Bone Joint Surg Am 69:640, 1987.

Yong-Hing K, Tchang SPK: Traumatic radioulnar synostosis treated by excision and a free fat transplant. A report of two cases. J Bone Joint Surg Br 65:433, 1983.

16 Fractures and Dislocations in the Region of the Wrist

FRACTURES OF THE LOWER END OF THE RADIUS: COLLES', SMITH'S, AND BARTON'S FRACTURES

REMARKS

Like most fractures of the upper limb, these eponymic fractures result from a fall on the outstretched hand. Varying force vectors produced by the fall, the position of the wrist, and the differing structural properties of bones account for the differences in fracture types. Forceful hyperextension with the forearm and wrist pronated drives the carpals into the distal radius and produces a bending and compressive failure of the cancellous subchondral bone (Colles' fracture).

Colles' fracture is a typical fracture of weakened osteoporotic bone; 60–70 per cent of these fractures occur in postmenopausal women. The same hyperextension mechanism in the young adult male is more likely to produce a fracture of the scaphoid. The hyperextension injury to the child's wrist usually results in failure through the physis or produces a distal greenstick fracture.

Occasionally, the force vector of the injury drives the carpal bones in a volar direction. This results in a fracture that angulates volarly instead of dorsally, that is, Smith's fracture. The same force vectors with a volar direction in a young adult male shear off the articular surface of the distal radius and produce a Barton's fracture with volar dislocation of the carpus.

Each of these fracture types carries different implications regarding stability of reduction and prognosis; however, each is managed with the same ultimate objective—restoration of painless function.

■ Colles' Fracture

REMARKS

Colles' fracture with the dinner-fork deformity in the older female patient is the commonest fracture seen in emergency rooms. Like fractures of the hip and the proximal humerus, this is a typical fracture in an older patient with osteoporotic bone.

Ten to 15 per cent of Colles' fractures occur in younger patients due to more violent injuries, such as a fall from a height directly onto the outstretched hand. These fractures can be considerably more unstable and more complex to manage.

The usual Colles' fracture presents with a characteristic fork deformity of the wrist. This consists of three components: radial shortening, dorsal tilt, and radial deviation of the distal fragment.

Although these are usually isolated injuries, it is important to evaluate the patient for occasional associated fractures, such as a fracture of the scaphoid or the elbow area. In addition, 5–10 per cent of these injuries are associated with an injury to the median nerve, which can complicate the problem and lead to long-term and persistent symptoms.

Colles' Fracture Without Comminution

Dinner-Fork Deformity

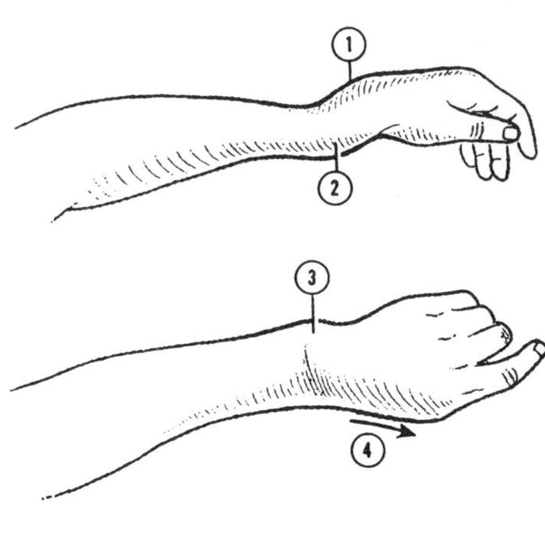

1. Abrupt dorsal prominence.
2. Gently rounded volar prominence.

3. The wrist is broadened.
4. The hand is deviated radially.

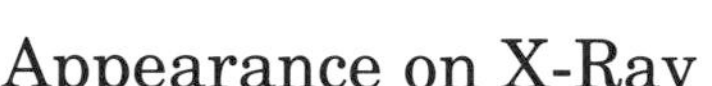

Appearance on X-Ray

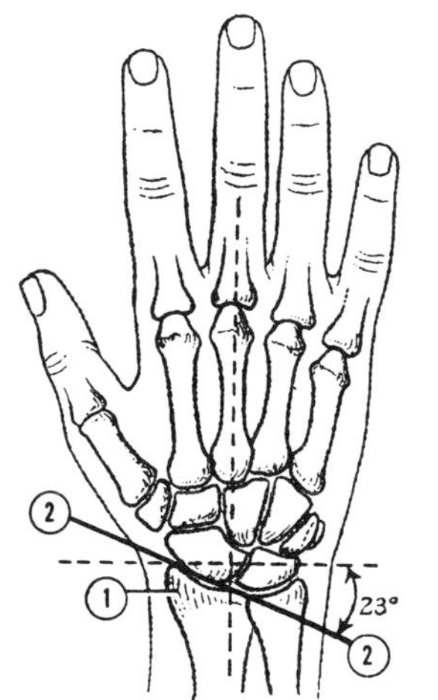

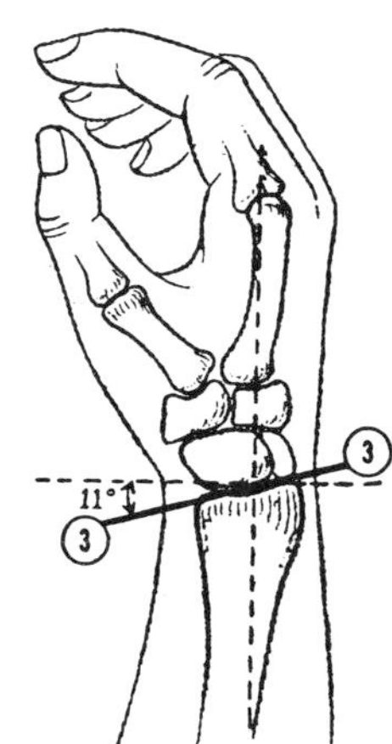

NORMAL WRIST

1. The styloid process of the radius extends 1 cm beyond that of the ulna.
2. The articular surface of the radius projects toward the ulna 15°–30° (average 23°).
3. The plane of the radial articular surface slopes downward and forward 1°–23° (average 11°).

Note: Compare these anatomic features with those seen in Colles' fracture.

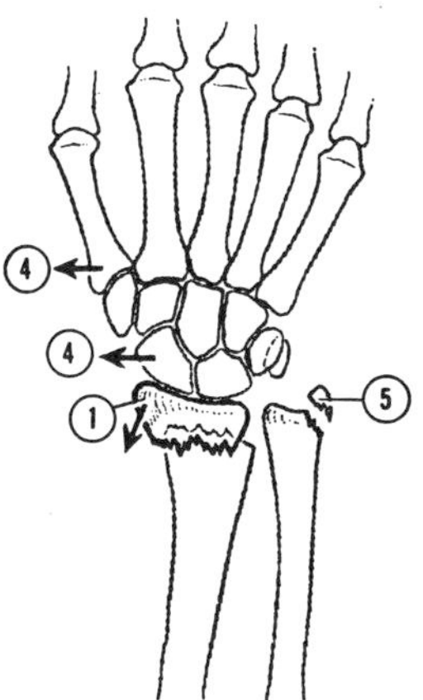

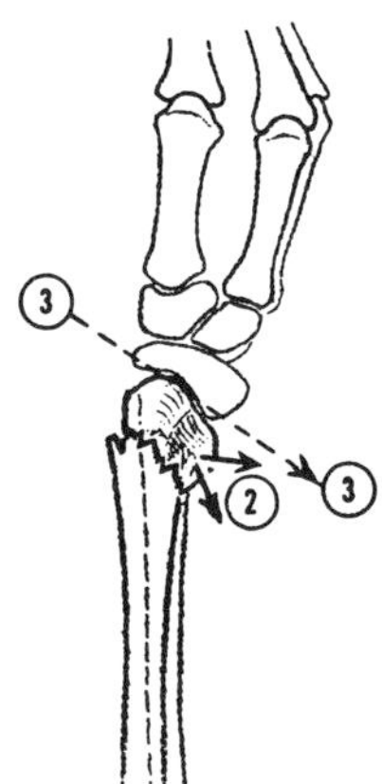

COLLES' FRACTURE

1. The distal radial fragment is displaced proximally. (The radial styloid may be on the same plane as the ulnar styloid or proximal to it.)
2. The distal radial fragment displaces dorsally and proximally.
3. The plane of the articular surface of the radial fragment tilts dorsally. (This angle varies greatly in different patients.)
4. The carpus and hand deviate toward the radius.
5. The ulnar styloid may or may not be fractured.

Management

REMARKS

Correcting the dinner-fork deformity of Colles' fracture is accomplished by initial steady traction to pull the radius out to length. Secondly, the normal volar orientation of the surface is restored, and finally the radial tilt of the distal end of the fracture is corrected.

The reduction must be maintained until the weak subchondral bone heals sufficiently to prevent redisplacement. This is the difficult aspect. A large percentage (20–30 per cent) of these deformities recur in spite of initially adequate reduction. Shortening of the radius is particularly common because of the egg-shell structural properties of the fractured bone in this region. In most elderly patients with Colles' fracture, overtreatment should be avoided. Some swelling and settling is acceptable, although maintenance of a good reduction is also consistent with good functional outcome and a satisfied patient.

If the fracture is judged to be unstable or if significant redisplacement occurs despite initial reduction, other methods of fixation should be considered. This is particularly necessary for the 10–15 per cent of cases of Colles' fractures in younger individuals with more unstable injuries. The choices besides cast or splint immobilization include pin fixation through the distal radius and external fixation to maintain alignment.

Whatever method of reduction and fixation is chosen, it is important to use adequate anesthesia for adequate reduction. For the minimally displaced Colles' fracture, injection of local anesthetic into the hematoma usually provides adequate anesthesia. However, most of these injuries require either intravenous block or a general anesthetic.

In most elderly patients with Colles' fracture, open treatment should be avoided. Some swelling and settling of the fracture is acceptable, but redisplacement, and particularly recurrence, of radial deviation should be avoided.

Immobilization of the swollen wrist in an awkwardly flexed position or tight cast should be avoided. The commonest problem associated with Colles' fracture develops from tight cast application, which causes pain, discomfort, and sometimes even compartment syndrome of the forearm or wrist.

Because of this common problem with swelling after Colles' fracture, it is preferable and highly recommended to use sugar-tong splints rather than a circular cast in immobilizing the initially injured wrist. As the swelling subsides, the splints may be changed to a short-arm cast, which allows the patient elbow and finger motion on either side.

Preferred Method of Anesthesia: Regional Intravenous Anesthetic

1. Use 0.5% preservative-free solution of lidocaine. The dosage should be 0.5 mL of this solution per kilogram of body weight.
2. Insert a small butterfly needle into the hand on the fractured side, which is immobilized in a splint.
3. Elevate the limb for at least 3 minutes to diminish edema.
4. Using a pretested and securely taped blood pressure cuff, stop circulation by rapid inflation to at least 250 mm Hg.

Note: Specially designed double tourniquets may also be used. An assistant should carefully monitor the patient.

Then lower the arm and inject the lidocaine solution in the appropriate dose.

1. The needle is removed, and after 10 minutes the fracture is reduced. Always keep the cuff inflated for at least 15 minutes, and monitor the patient carefully after the tourniquet is released.

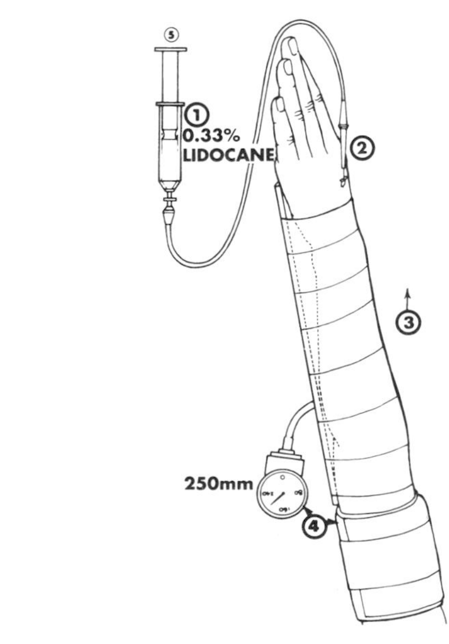

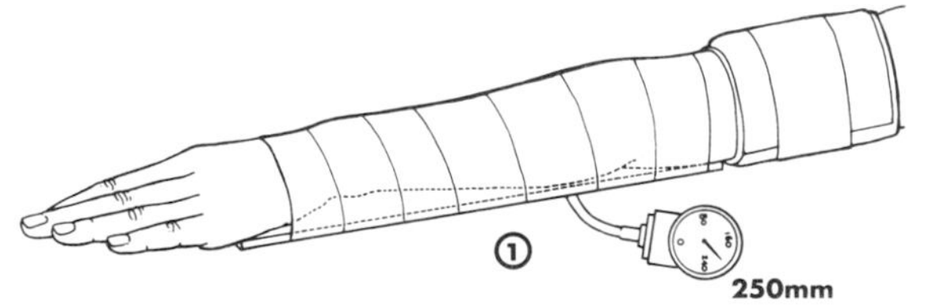

Closed Reduction Method

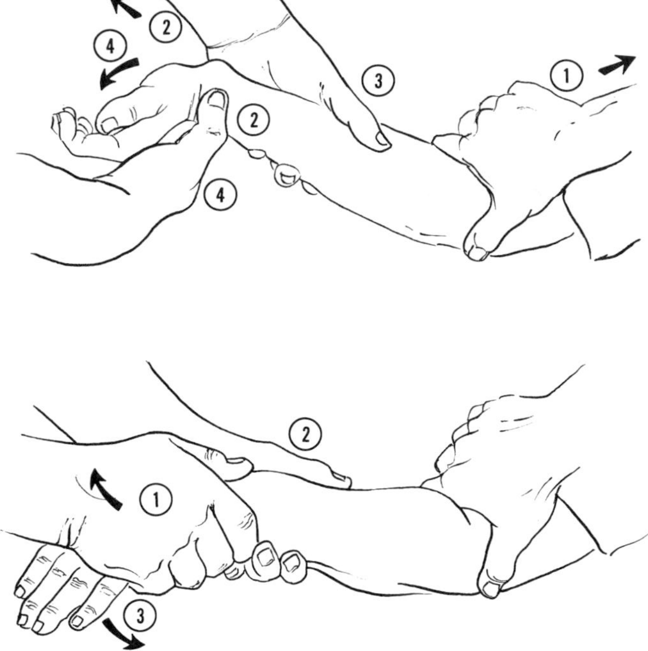

1. An assistant holds the elbow and offers countertraction.
2. The surgeon applies traction with the right hand and thumb applied to the distal fragment.
3. The forearm is supinated and held with the surgeon's opposite hand.
4. The fracture is then disimpacted by allowing dorsal angulation while maintaining the supinated position.

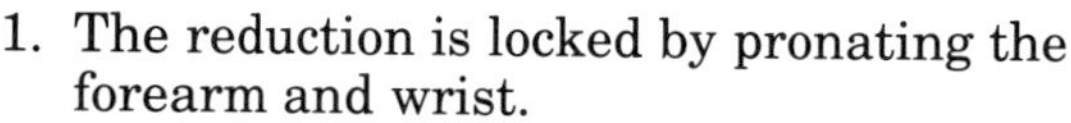

1. The reduction is locked by pronating the forearm and wrist.
2. The left hand remains stationary while the pronation is done entirely by the reducing hand.
3. The wrist is directed into ulnar deviation by this maneuver to correct a radial and dorsal angulation of the distal fragment.

Application of Sugar-Tong Splint (Miller-Gilmer Method)

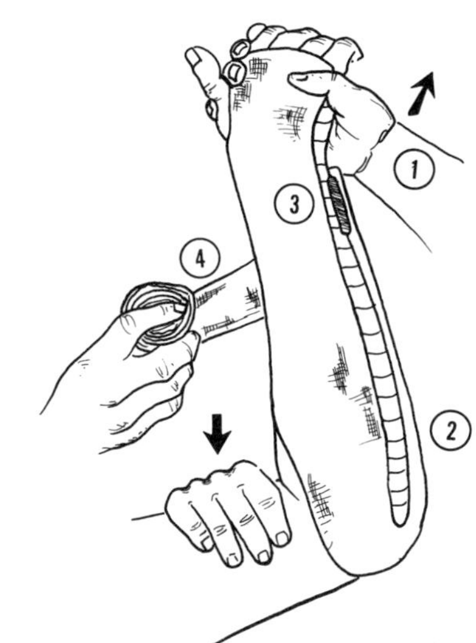

Avoid applying a cast to a swollen wrist after Colles' fracture. This can lead to increased swelling and discomfort, and even the compartment syndrome. The most reliable and safe method is a sugar-tong splint, as described by Miller and Gilmer.

1. The position of the wrist and forearm is held by an assistant, who maintains steady traction on the elbow and hand.
2. Cast padding is applied from the metacarpal heads to above the elbow.
3. A felt pad is applied to the volar surface of the proximal fragment.
4. A 10-cm sugar-tong plaster splint of 12 thicknesses is wrapped around the forearm and held using circumferential gauze bandage. This avoids having to apply a cast to the swollen wrist after Colles' fracture.

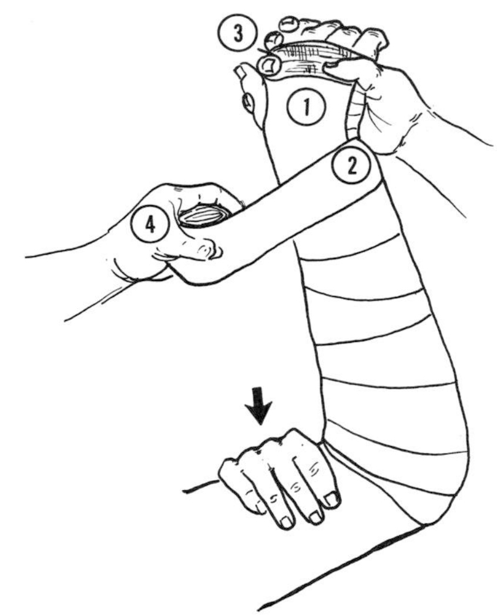

1. The dorsal half of the splint ends at the metacarpal heads and is molded over the distal fragment.
2. The volar half ends 1–2 cm proximal to the fracture.
3. To maintain the wrist in ulnar deviation, a strip of plaster is wrapped around the distal end of the splint and metacarpal heads to prevent radial deviation. This strip should not extend beyond the distal palmar crease.
4. The entire sugar-tong splint is then wrapped with a circumferential bandage or elastic bandage wrap to maintain the position of the forearm and wrist.

Subsequent Management

If the reduction is satisfactory, deflate the tourniquet used for the intravenous anesthetic to 80 mm Hg. After 10 seconds reinflate it to 250 mm Hg. Monitor vital signs and mental status during this time. If they are unchanged, the tourniquet may be completely removed. Continue monitoring vital signs and mental status for 10 minutes following release of the tourniquet.

This entire procedure requires at least two assistants, one to monitor the pressure of the cuff during the block and the other to assist in reduction. The minimum tourniquet time should always exceed 15 minutes. Resuscitation equipment should be immediately available when administering anesthetic of this type.

While the patient is being monitored after anesthetic, the postreduction x-rays can be evaluated. If reduction is acceptable, the patient can be followed on an outpatient basis in a few days. Avoid immobilizing the fractured arm entirely in a sling because prolonged use of a sling can lead to stiffness of the hand and shoulder.

Alternative Method: Reduction by Traction and Manipulation

The patient assumes the supine position on the fracture table.

1. Finger traction is applied.
2. The elbow is flexed to a right angle.
3. The forearm is in neutral rotation.
4. Countertraction is applied using a muslin sling with a water bucket for traction.
5. Traction is maintained for approximately 5 minutes to pull the radial styloid distal to the ulnar styloid.

Note: The tourniquet for intravenous anesthesia is maintained during reduction.

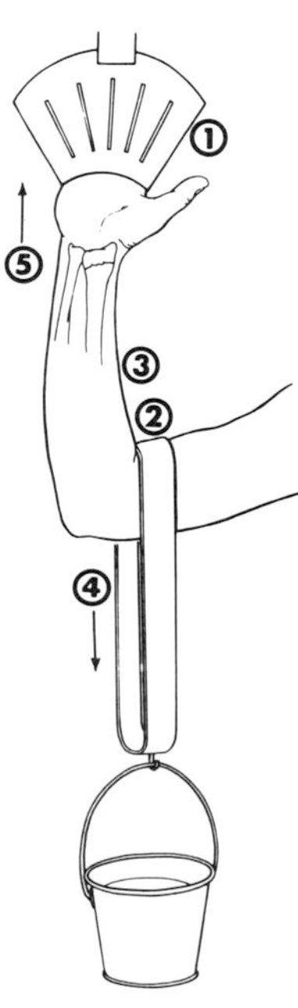

Correction of Dorsal and Radial Angulation

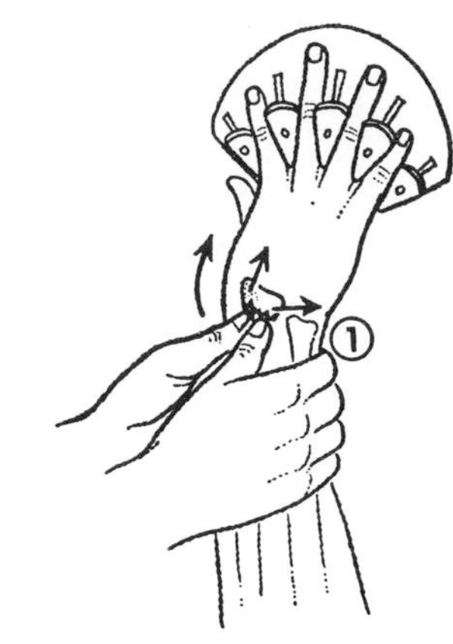

1. The fingers of both hands support the proximal fragment on the volar side. The thumbs then push the dorsally angulated distal fragment volarly and in an ulnar direction to correct both the dorsal and radial angulation.

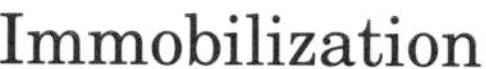

Immobilization

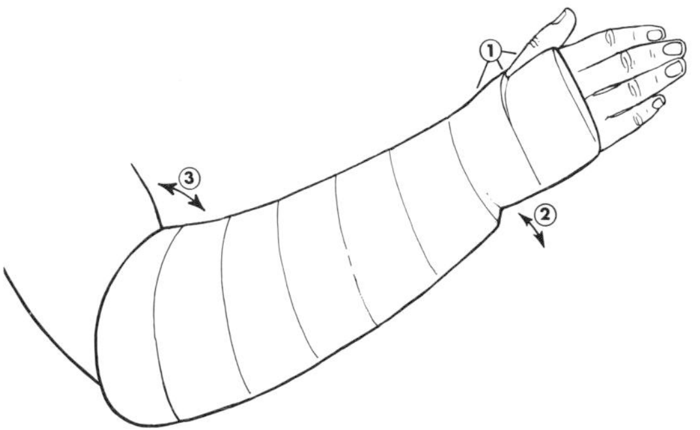

1. A sugar-tong splint is applied to allow room for swelling after reduction.
2. Limited wrist flexion permits volar angulation of the distal fragment.
3. Limited elbow flexion is possible without forearm rotation.

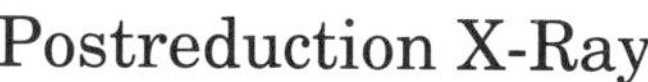

Postreduction X-Ray

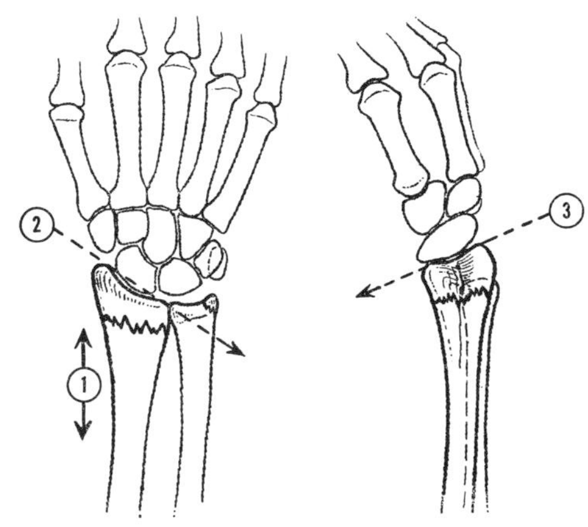

1. The normal length of the radius has been restored. The radial styloid is distal to the ulnar styloid.
2. The articular plane of the radius is now directed toward the ulna.
3. The articular surface of the radius is directed downward, forward, and inward.

Postreduction Management

Once the sugar-tong splint is applied, x-rays are obtained to determine the adequacy of reduction. If the reduction is not satisfactory a second manipulation may be needed, but repeated manipulation should be avoided.

The splint allows room for swelling, which might compromise circulation. If there is any evidence of circulatory embarrassment, the splint should be loosened or the padding removed down to the skin.

The patient should be advised to keep the arm elevated and to apply ice to the wrist because swelling with these injuries is very common. Follow-up evaluation of the patient should be carried out in 1–2 days to ensure that the patient is comfortable and that the splint has not become excessively tight.

By 5–7 days the fracture can be re-x-rayed and a short-arm cast applied. At 4–6 weeks clinical healing is usually present, although the fracture may still be evident on x-ray. A wrist support or cast may be continued for 2–3 weeks until the pain and tenderness subside at the fracture site.

At all times during the recovery period, it is important that the patient actively exercise the fingers and shoulder on the injured side because these are very frequently subject to stiffening and cause problems in regaining function long after Colles' fracture heals. Prolonged use of a sling for more than a few days after Colles' fracture tends to lead to a stiff shoulder, particularly in elderly patients, who tend to develop joint stiffness. The sling is only necessary for a few days until the acute pain and swelling subside. After this time, encourage the patient to begin active exercise of the shoulder and fingers.

Unstable Colles' Fractures

REMARKS

Twenty to thirty per cent of Colles' fractures are unstable and tend to lose reduction after adequate initial reduction and splint application. Cooney and coworkers have identified several characteristics of the unstable Colles' fracture. These include severe comminution with intra-articular components and more than 20° of dorsal angulation or 10 mm of radial shortening.

An additional problem of distal radial or Colles' fractures is the "die-punch" fracture, which causes a step-off between the scaphoid and lunate fossa of the distal radius. These are more often seen in younger patients and require adequate reduction and stabilization of the displaced lunate fossa or ulnar aspect of the radius to maximize the chances of adequate functional recovery of the wrist.

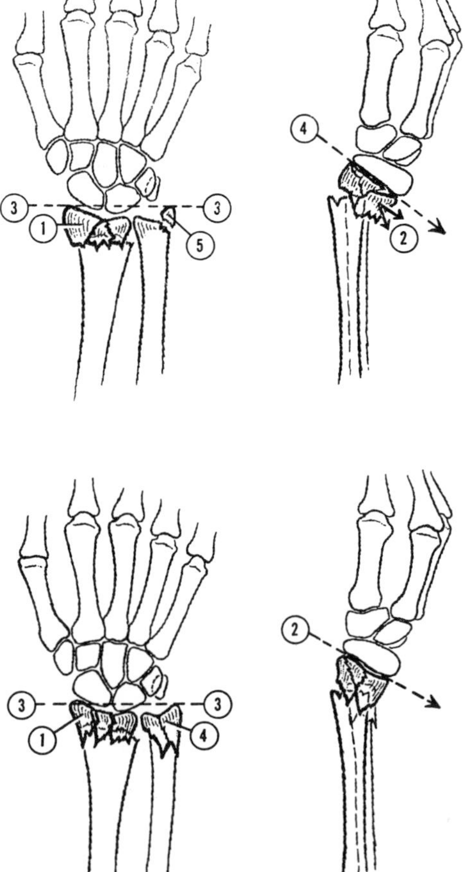

Types of Fractures Likely to be Unstable

1. There is comminution of the distal radial articular surface.
2. The distal fragment is dorsally angulated more than 20°.
3. The radius has shortened more than 10 mm so that the radial styloid is at the level of the ulna.
4. The articular surface of the radial fragment is oriented dorsally and radially.
5. The ulnar styloid is usually fractured, although this is not by itself a sign of instability.

Other Indication of Instability—Recurrence of Deformity After Reduction

1. There is a persistent comminution of the articular surface of the distal radius.
2. Dorsal angulation may be diminished but not corrected, and this angulation is likely to worsen.
3. The radial shortening has not corrected, and so the radius remains at the level of the ulna.
4. There is comminution of the distal end of the ulna and involvement of the radioulnar joint.

Management of Unstable Colles' Fractures

REMARKS

If the articular surface comminution, dorsal or radial angulation or shortening, or recurrence of the deformity after reduction indicates instability, the options are several. Remanipulation and cast treatment may be indicated for Colles' fracture in the young individual that is not comminuted. A preferable method of managing an unstable fracture with one or two articular fragments is with percutaneous pin fixation. For a more severely comminuted and unstable fracture, external fixation is preferable.

Percutaneous Pin Fixation

Reduction by traction, manipulation, and transfixion pin is accomplished under either general or regional intravenous anesthetic.

The patient assumes a supine position on the fracture table. Ideally, image-intensified fluoroscopy should be used if available.

TRACTION

1. The fingers are supported with a finger-traction apparatus.
2. The elbow is flexed 90°.
3. The forearm is in neutral rotation to relax the brachioradialis.
4. Countertraction is applied using the weight of a water bucket.
5. Traction is continued until the radial styloid is pulled distal to the ulnar styloid.

Note: A tourniquet is maintained for intravenous anesthetic during traction maneuvers as previously described.

MANIPULATION

1. Place the fingers of both hands on the volar side of the forearm and
2. Use the thumbs on the dorsal aspect of the wrist to push the distal fragment volarly and distally.

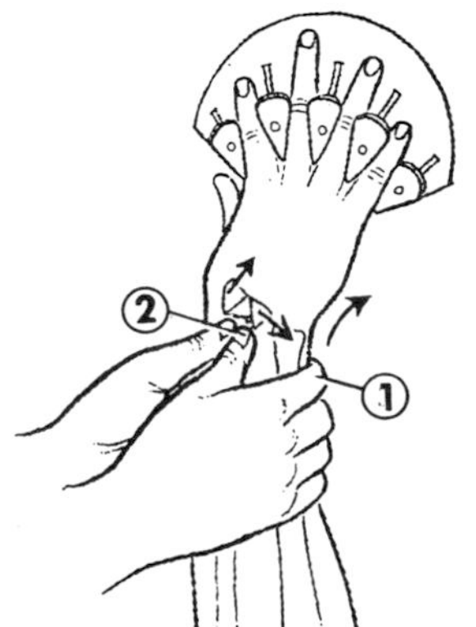

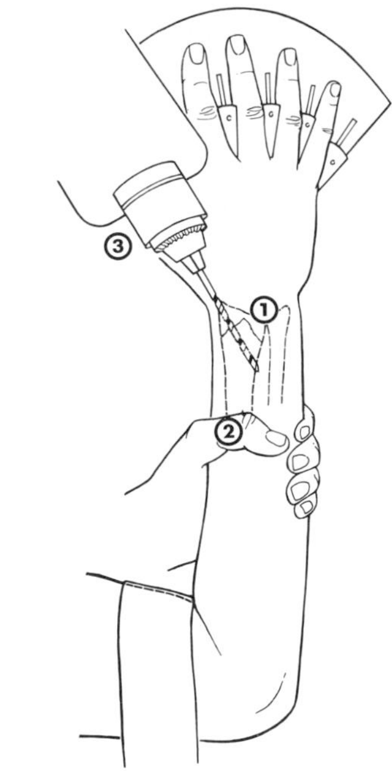

INSERTION OF TRANSFIXION PIN

1. Confirm the reduction by fluoroscopy and then prepare the distal forearm for surgery.
2. While traction and the position of the wrist are maintained by an assistant,
3. Pass a threaded Steinmann pin, 2.0 mm in diameter, from the radial styloid across the fracture and into the opposite radial cortex. The pin is directed from the radial styloid at approximately a 45° angle. Confirm the position of the pin by fluoroscopy.

Note: The pin should be heavy enough that it does not break and should be threaded so that it does not loosen.

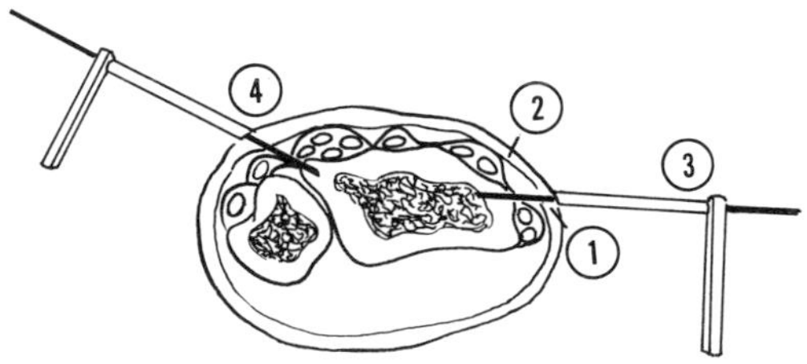

Site for Insertion

1. The insertion site should be on the volar aspect of the radial styloid.
2. It should avoid the extensor tendons in the first and second compartments, as well as the sensory branch of the radial nerve in the snuff box.
3. A pin guide is used to protect the nerve and tendons in this area from injury by the pin.
4. A second pin may be inserted from the ulnar side of the radius if there is a dye-punch fracture that causes disruption of the distal radius.

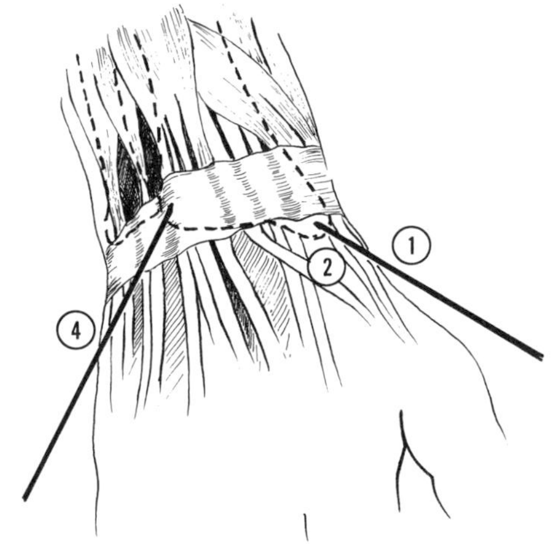

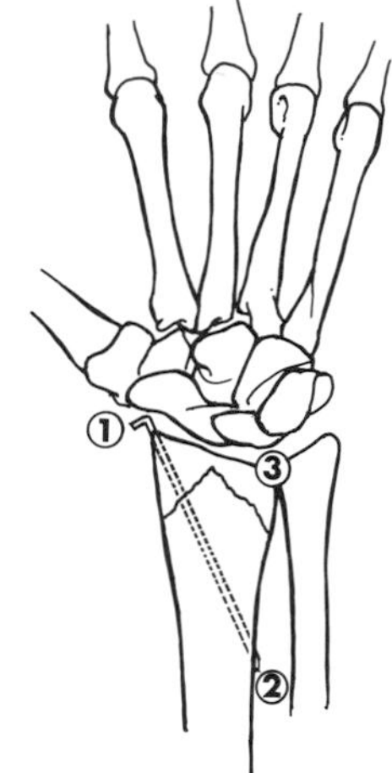

Postreduction X-Ray

1. The pin from the radial styloid crosses the fracture site and reduces the radial aspect of Colles' fracture.
2. The pin should be long enough to penetrate through the opposite cortex but not into the surrounding soft tissues.
3. The radial shortening and radioulnar joint relationships should be restored.

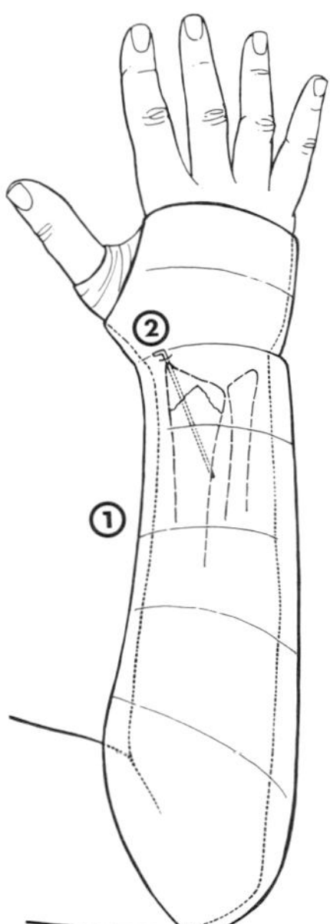

Application of Sugar-Tong Splint

1. Apply a sugar-tong splint.
2. The pin is cut off outside the skin but is not incorporated in the plaster.

Alternative Method—External Fixation of Unstable Fractures

REMARKS

External fixation techniques have recently become more popular for Colles' fractures. They have a number of advantages, including the fact that the fracture can be reduced and held closer to the anatomic position. In addition, the tendency to secondary displacement is diminished by these external fixators.

The wrist joint can be held in a neutral position and excessive wrist flexion can be avoided, thereby diminishing the chance of median nerve injuries. In addition, the fixator should allow motion of the radioulnar joint, which can improve the pronation and supination function of the wrist and forearm.

However, complications do occur from these devices at a fairly high frequency, and therefore they should be used only with the fracture that shows signs of instability or articular surface comminution, particularly in the younger patient.

Technique of External Fixation

1. After adequate anesthesia is administered, traction is applied to the hand for 10 minutes to distract the fracture fragments and allow gentle reduction.
2. The objective is to restore alignment of the volar cortex as anatomically as possible.
3. In addition, length should be restored. This is evident when the radial styloid has been pulled at least 10–13 mm beyond the distal ulna.

Note: Reduction may be aided by supinating rather than pronating the forearm and wrist to achieve a stable position.

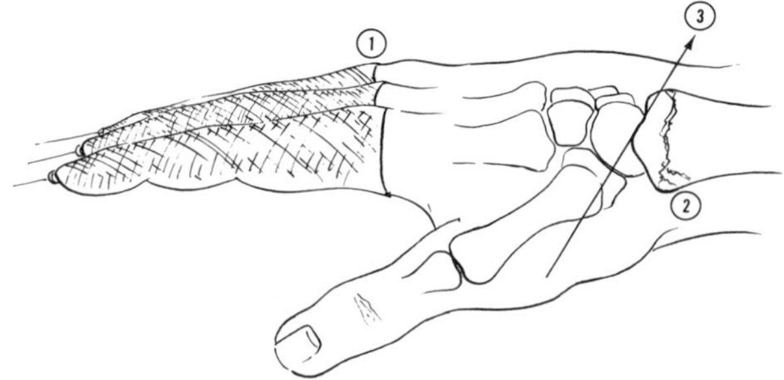

Application of External Fixation System

A number of wrist fixators are available. A commonly used type is that produced by the Association for the Study of Internal Fixation (ASIF) group, which is summarized as follows:

1. A 2.5-mm Kirschner wire is inserted into the dorsal-radial aspect of the index metacarpal. After blunt dissection of soft tissue, a guide sleeve is used to direct the Kirschner wire at a 45° angle into the distal end of the metacarpal. The Kirschner wire must engage both cortices of the bone.
2. With the forearm pronated, a 2.5-mm pin is drilled into the radius, while being careful to avoid the sensory branch of the radial nerve and tendons. The Kirschner wire must engage both cortices.

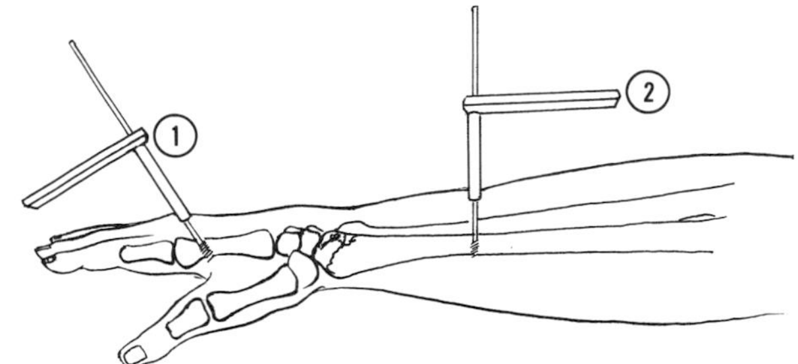

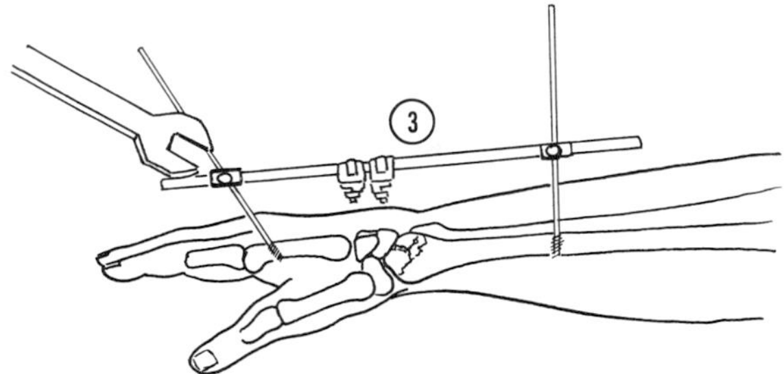

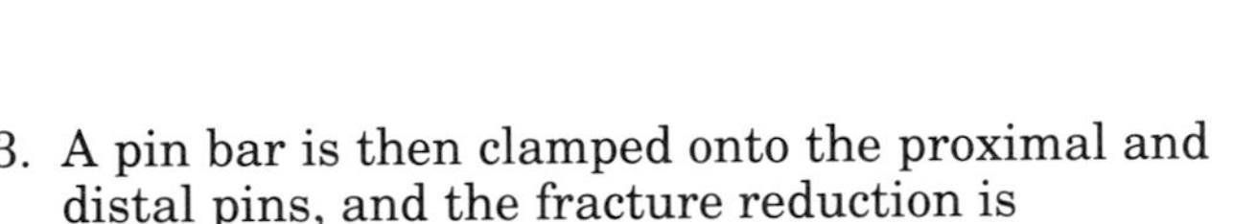

3. A pin bar is then clamped onto the proximal and distal pins, and the fracture reduction is checked again under x-ray.

1. A second metacarpal pin is inserted into the same plane as the first metacarpal pin with a 40°–60° convergence.
2. The second radial pin is inserted through a skin incision, while being careful to avoid the sensory nerve and tendons.
3. The clamp on the bar is used as a guide for insertion of these Kirschner wires into the same plane as the previously inserted Kirschner wires.
4. After final reduction is evaluated on x-ray, the fixator nuts are tightened.

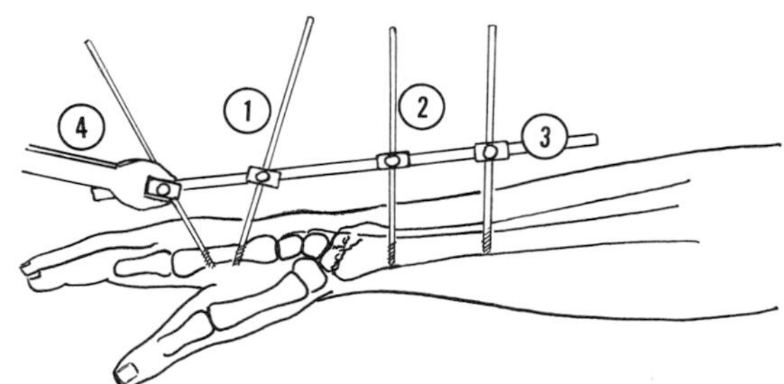

1. To increase the fixator rigidity, a second bar can be applied to the pins.
2. The nuts are tightened with a wrench, and each pin is cut above the clamps and protected with a protective cap.

Note: For fractures that require flexion or ulnar deviation, two short bars may be used with interlocking spring-loaded nuts.

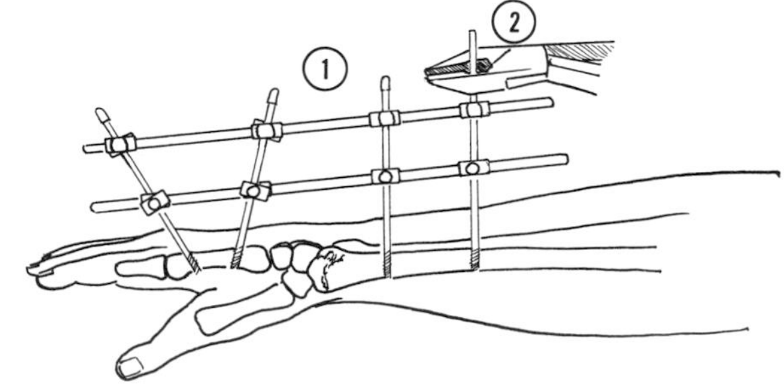

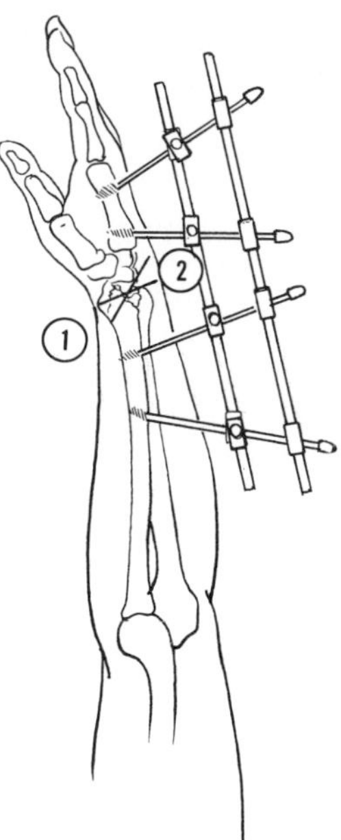

Percutaneous Fixation Combined With External Fixation

1. For comminuted fractures, particularly in young adults without osteoporotic bone, percutaneous fixation may be combined with external fixation.
2. After the reduction is achieved with the external fixator, percutaneous pins are inserted through the radial and ulnar side of the fracture, as previously described.

Note: Once the position of the percutaneous pins are satisfactory, cannulated screws can be inserted if the bone is not osteoporotic.

Subsequent Management

The external fixator is maintained for at least 6–8 weeks, but sometimes as long as 10 weeks is necessary for the more comminuted fracture. It should be emphasized that early motion of the fingers, elbow, and shoulder is necessary to avoid contractures of these joints and should be started in the first 1–2 days after injury. After the pins are removed at 8–10 weeks, a temporary wrist splint should be applied, and the patient should be started on exercises to regain full range of wrist motion.

Other Fractures Likely to Cause Problems of Instability—Die-Punch Fractures

These intra-articular fractures of the distal radius occur most often in young adults due to high-energy impact. The carpus is driven into the distal end of the radius, which results in an asymmetric step-off. The lunate fossa tends to displace more than the scaphoid fossa, so there is inherent instability of the articular surface.

These are difficult to reduce anatomically without some type of pin fixation or external fixation device. Occasionally open reduction is necessary to realign the joint surface.

1. An impaction fracture of the carpus against the distal radius characteristically produces a die-punch fracture.
2. There is step-off between the lunate and scaphoid fossa, which results in instability of the distal radius.

Note: This frequently requires pin fixation or even open reduction to restore the normal support of the distal radius to the carpus.

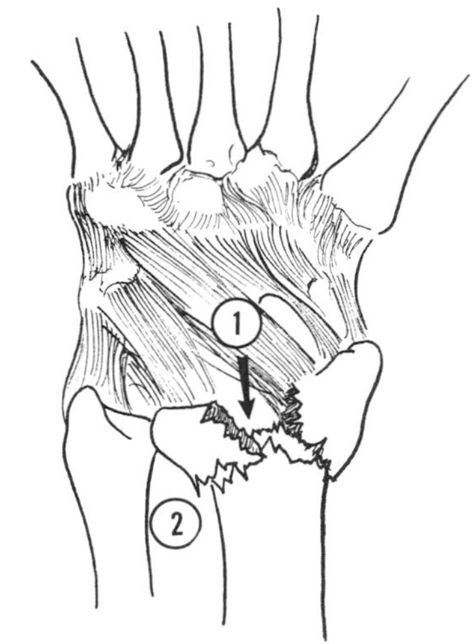

1. Application of an external fixation device to apply ligamentotaxis to a die-punch fracture may not reduce the ulnar fragment. This is due to minimal ligamentous attachment to this fragment.
2. Occasionally transverse pin fixation between the articular fragments may be necessary to realign the joint surface. This can be done in conjunction with the external fixation, and the fracture may then be treated like a standard fracture with external fixation.

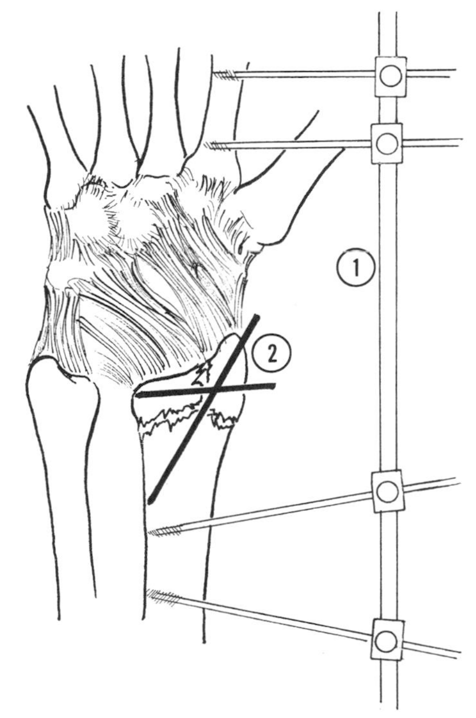

Complications of Colles' Fracture: Joint Pain and Stiffening

REMARKS

The most common complications of Colles' fractures include loss of finger and wrist motion, diminished grip strength, and loss of shoulder motion. These complications can be temporary but occasionally may be the source of permanent impairment.

The painful joint stiffening is most often associated with malposition of the fracture as well as failure of the patient to work vigorously at regaining hand and shoulder function while the fracture is healing.

Shoulder stiffness can be a frequent problem, particularly if the patient holds the injured arm continuously in a sling and fails to move the shoulder. For this reason, the arm sling should be avoided or discarded early, and the patient should be encouraged to move the shoulder to the overhead position at least hourly.

Preventive Treatment

Although painful stiffening is common, it can be combatted with preventive active therapy that includes the following:

1. Avoid tight casts and use sugar-tong splints for immobilizing the fracture.
2. Emphasize active range of motion to the fingers on the injured side during the early phases of fracture healing.
3. Avoid the use of a sling and prescribe active range of motion to raise the arm to the overhead position hourly.

Caution: Failure of the patient to follow this regimen can result in a syndrome of persistent pain and tenderness, which has been termed *reflex sympathetic dystrophy, Sudeck's atrophy,* or *algodystrophy*. It progresses from vasomotor instability and loss of joint mobility to painful skin and subcutaneous tissues with joint contractures. Because of the difficulties in managing the chronic painful stiff hand and wrist, it is important to emphasize this program of preventive treatment.

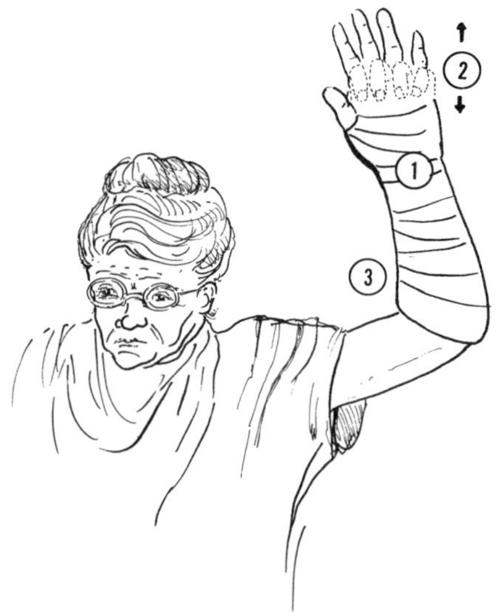

Other Complications: Compartment Syndrome From Cast Application

REMARKS

A tight constrictive cast applied to the swollen wrist may produce a compartment syndrome of the hand or forearm. If the patient complains of severe pain after application of the cast, it should quickly be bivalved and loosened down to the skin. The acute fracture is best managed by sugar-tong splinting (see Miller-Gilmer technique).

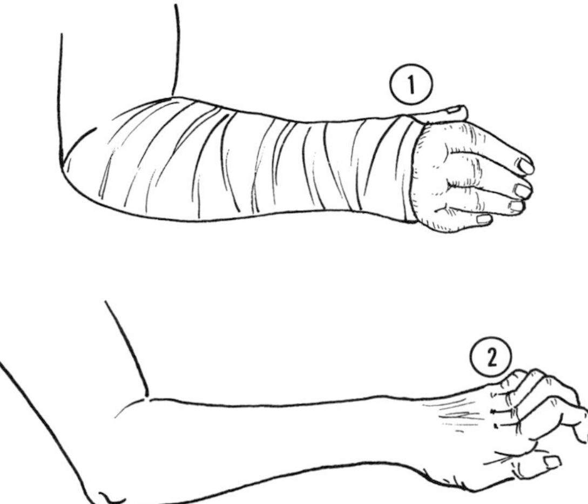

1. A patient can develop a compartment syndrome of the hand after application of a cast that becomes tight due to a swollen wrist.
2. This may lead to persistent clawing of the fingers, which significantly impairs function of the hand.

Note: It is important to relieve any pressure on the swollen wrist in patients who are being treated acutely for Colles' fracture because treatment of the swelling of the wrist and hand is more significant initially than is maintenance of fracture reduction under these circumstances.

Management to Prevent Compartment Syndrome and Other Complications From Extensive Swelling With Colles' Fracture

REMARKS

The acute management of a swollen wrist should emphasize elimination of swelling, even before reduction of the fracture. In the severely swollen wrist this may require a specific boxing-glove-type of dressing and elevation for 24–48 hours before reducing the fracture. This is essential to keep in mind, because occasionally there may be a tendency to focus on the fracture rather than on the more serious acute problem and the potentially dangerous wrist and hand swelling.

Application of a Boxing-Glove Dressing to Combat Extensive Swelling of the Wrist and Hand

This dressing applies compression to the hand and wrist to diminish swelling before attempted reduction of the fracture.

1. The wrist is slightly extended. The metacarpophalangeal joints are flexed, and the interphalangeal joints are extended.
2. The thumb is in apposition with the fingers.
3. Soft tissue fluffs are applied liberally in the palm and between the fingers.

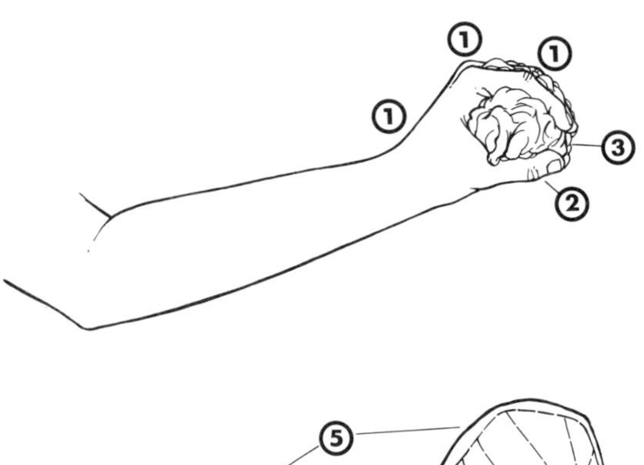

4. Rolled gauze is wrapped around the soft tissue fluffs from the elbow to the fingertips.
5. Plaster is applied over the rolled gauze.

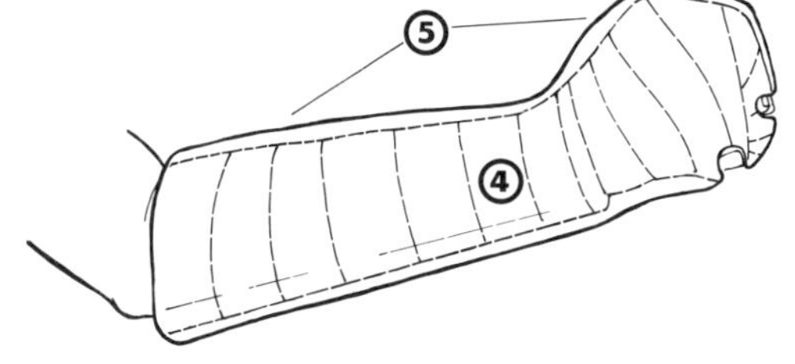

6. The limb is elevated for 24–48 hours before reducing the fracture. When the swelling has subsided by 24–48 hours, the boxing-glove dressing may be removed and the fracture then reduced without risk of worsening the swelling or producing a compartment syndrome of the hand.

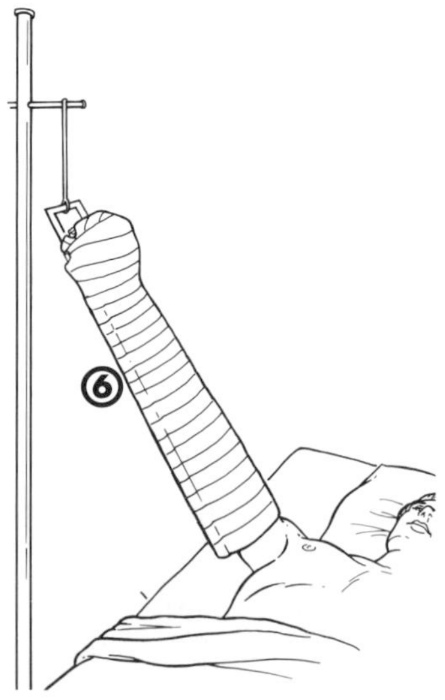

Other Complications: Tendon Rupture

1. The commonest tendon injury associated with Colles' fracture is rupture of the extensor pollicis longus tendon.
2. This is commonly associated with irregularity around Lister's tubercle, which leads to attrition. This frequently may not occur acutely, but rather weeks or months after the fracture.

Note: The ruptured extensor pollicis tendon is best replaced by transfer of the extensor indicis proprius to the thumb rather than attempting to repair a tendon that has become worn and frayed at the fracture site.

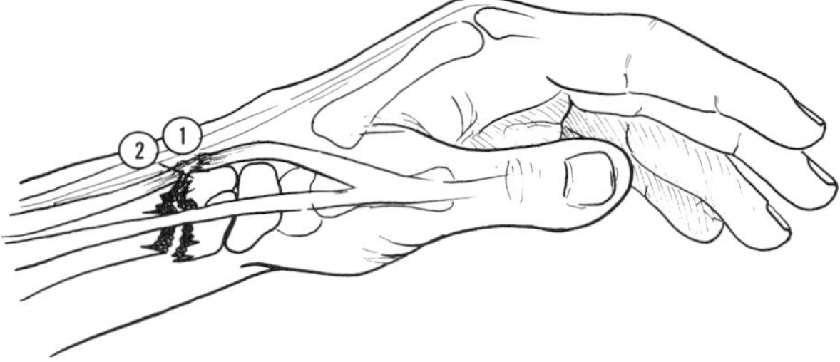

Other Complications: Median Nerve Injury

REMARKS

Approximately 3–5 per cent of Colles' fractures injure the median nerve. Median neuropathy is usually transient if the wrist is not forced into a hyperflexed position during the reduction maneuver.

Rarely the median nerve may be compressed by bone spicules or callus that form on the anterior aspect of the fracture site. This indicates the need for prompt surgical decompression.

Persistent median nerve symptoms, which include sensory loss in the median nerve distribution and dysesthesias in the fingers, can be a persistent source of functional impairment and are best prevented by early decompression of the carpal tunnel. Median nerve symptoms that persist after reduction of Colles' fracture may lead to reflex sympathetic dystrophy. Consequently, it is preferable to proceed with early decompression of the median nerve if reduction of the fracture does not relieve the painful symptoms.

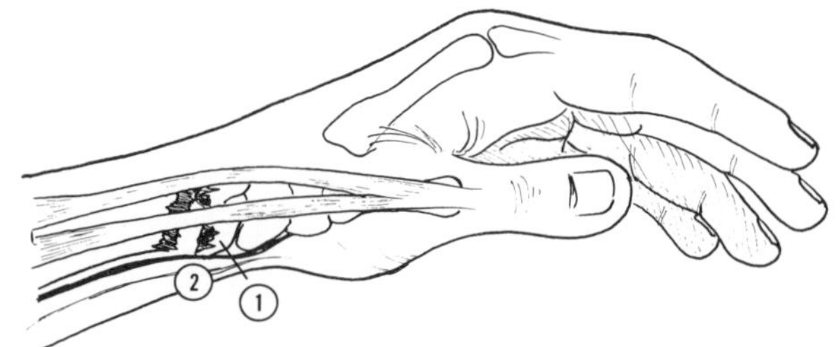

1. A typical fracture associated with median nerve injury is Colles' fracture with a displaced fragment on the volar side of the wrist.
2. This impinges on the median nerve in the carpal tunnel and requires surgical decompression.

Other Complications: Associated Scaphoid Fractures

REMARKS

Approximately 3–5 per cent of Colles' fractures are complicated by a fracture of the scaphoid or the carpal bones. This is especially likely in younger patients without osteoporotic bone.

The initial and subsequent x-rays should be carefully evaluated to look for evidence of scaphoid fractures or disruption of the carpal bones. These are usually undisplaced but still require appropriate treatment.

Colles' Fracture Complicated by Fracture of the Carpal Scaphoid

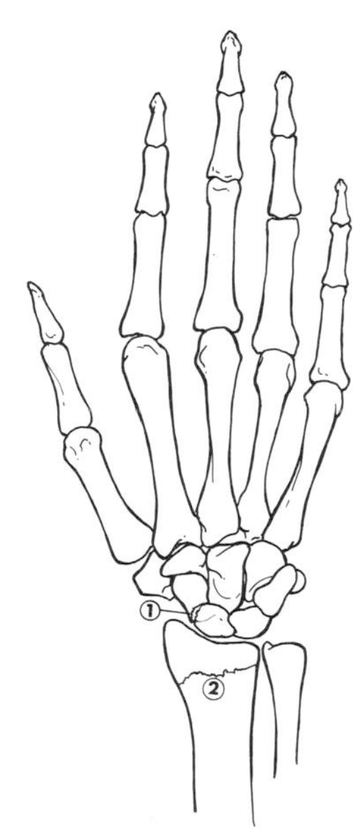

Appearance on X-Ray

1. Fractured carpal scaphoid.
2. Comminuted Colles' fracture.

Immobilization

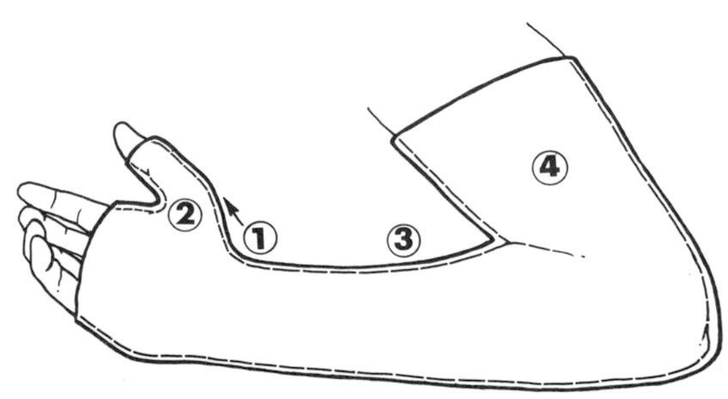

1. The wrist is held in 25° of extension and 20° of radial deviation.
2. The cast includes the thumb, with the first metacarpal aligned along the long axis of the radius.
3. The forearm is in neutral rotation.
4. The cast extends above the elbow to immobilize both the distal radial and scaphoid fractures.

Note: If Colles' fracture is unstable, insert a pin across the fracture from the radial styloid as described previously.

Other Complications: Disruption of the Radioulnar Joint From Shortening in Adults or Growth Arrest in Children

REMARKS

Disruption of the distal radioulnar joint can be a source of persistent pain and limitation of forearm rotation after Colles' fracture. It is most commonly the result of shortening of the radial fracture. Occasionally it may follow a growth arrest or acute injury to the distal physis in the child.

If pain and deformity from radioulnar disruption are persistently symptomatic, they can be best managed by resection of the distal 1–2 cm of the ulna. If there is significant ulnar slant of the radius, an osteotomy of the ulna with fusion of the distal radioulnar joint may be preferable to avoid increasing instability of the wrist.

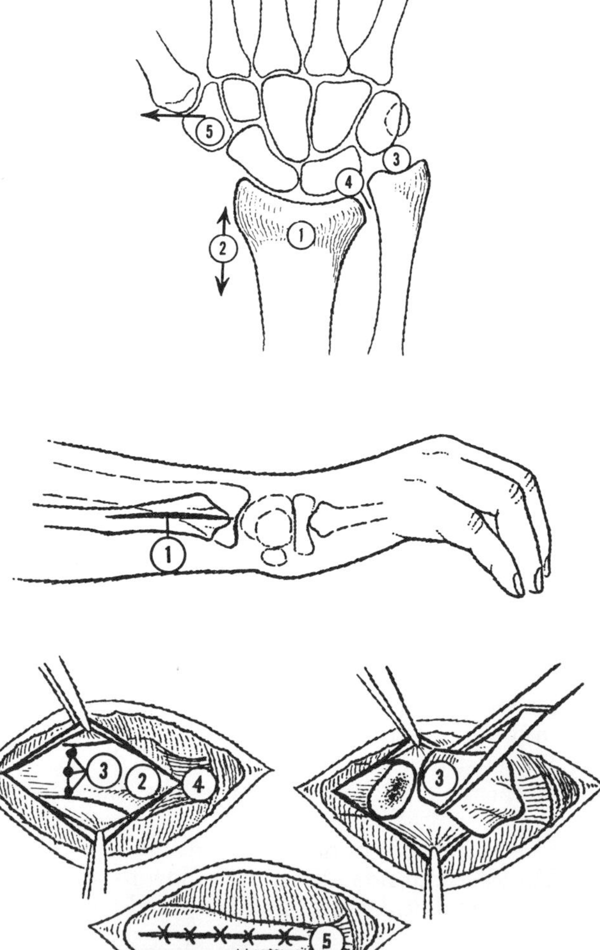

Preoperative X-Ray

1. The radius has impacted on itself due to fracture or physeal growth arrest.
2. Radial shortening is significant because it causes
3. The ulna to extend distally and
4. The radioulnar joint to dislocate.
5. The hand is pushed into radial deviation.

Resection of the Ulna in the Older Adult

Resection of the Distal Ulna

1. An incision is made over the prominence of the distal ulna.
2. The flap is made dorsally and volarly to expose the bony prominence.
3. A 1- to 2-cm segment of bone is removed from the distal ulna down to the styloid.
4. The flaps are repaired to stabilize the remaining ulna.
5. The extensor carpi ulnaris is rerouted to pass directly over the resected segment.

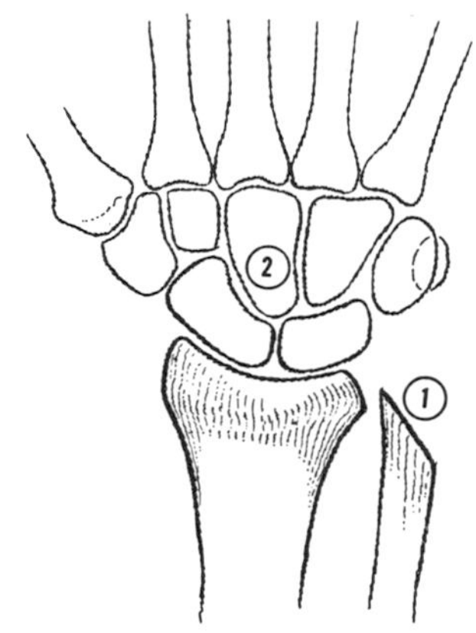

Postoperative X-Ray

1. The distal end of the ulna has been resected.
2. The hand is now in neutral position.

Alternative Method—Distal Ulnar Pseudoarthrosis With Arthrodesis of the Radioulnar Joint

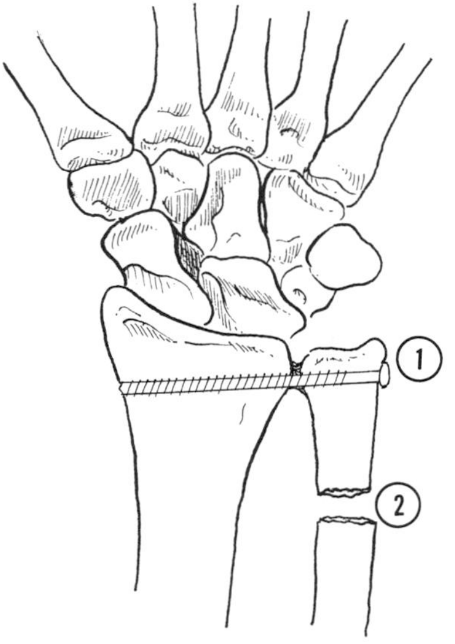

If the wrist shows a tendency for the carpus to slide in the ulnar direction, it is best stabilized by arthrodesis of the distal radioulnar joint.

1. A screw fixation with bone grafting of the distal ulna to the radius is usually effective in achieving arthrodesis of the joint.
2. The ulna is resected from 1 to 2 cm proximal to the arthrodesis to allow forearm rotation.

Note: This stabilizes the distal radial and ulnar joint, and maintains necessary support for the carpus, and is preferred by some authors to resection of the ulna. However, the distal ulnar resection remains the treatment of choice for most of these deformities produced by excessive shortening after Colles' fracture in the elderly.

Other Complications Producing Severe Infection and Gas Gangrene

REMARKS

Fractures of the distal radius are infrequently open injuries. However, when they are associated with penetration through the skin, the risk of serious complications is always present.

One of the commonest sources of gas gangrene leading to amputation of the limb is the "minor puncture wound" over a distal radial fracture that is incompletely debrided in the emergency room and develops life-threatening gangrene and infection.

Severe infections are particularly to be feared in the elderly diabetic patient, who may develop gas gangrene. The other problem fracture is a distal radial fracture in the child that is contaminated by dirt on the bone fragments and may lead to life-threatening infections.

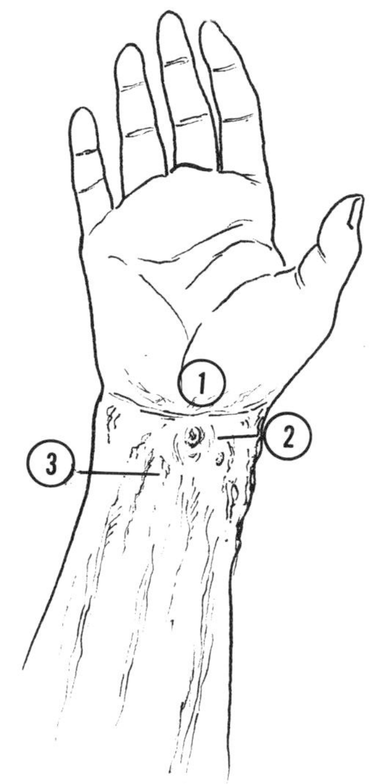

1. A small penetrating wound on the volar aspect of the wrist was associated with
2. A displaced Colles' fracture.
3. Incomplete debridement of this "puncture wound" or "poke hole" in the emergency room led to life-threatening gas gangrene infection. The result was an above-elbow amputation. There is no such thing as a "minor" open distal radial fracture. All open fractures in this area require complete cleansing and debridement under operating room conditions.

Management of Open Wrist Fractures

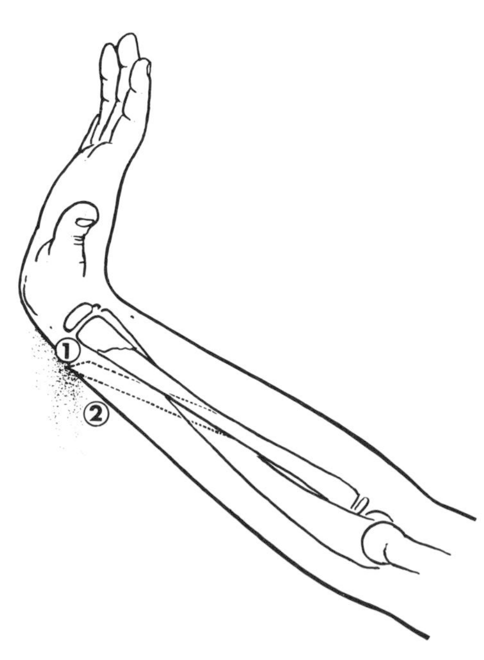

1. Small puncture wounds may not reflect the degree of contamination of fractures of the distal forearm in children or adults.
2. The fragments are frequently driven through the skin and are contaminated by dirt and then returned beneath the skin. The relatively small puncture wound associated with these injuries may be deceiving and lead to incomplete "wound cleansing" in the emergency room. The result can be rapid, life-threatening infections.

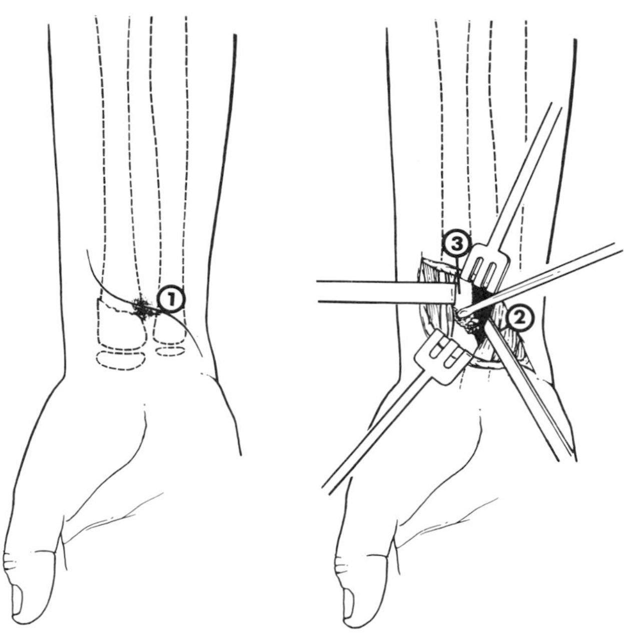

Operative Management

1. The fracture should be exposed by an S-shaped incision that includes and excises the puncture wound.
2. The flexor tendons and median nerves are identified and protected.
3. The fracture fragments are visualized and curetted, as well as washed thoroughly.

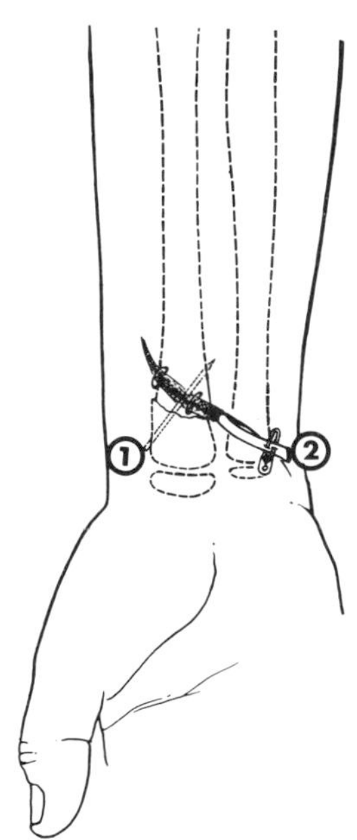

1. These fractures are generally unstable and should be supported by transcutaneous Steinmann pin fixation for 3 weeks while the soft tissues heal.
2. The wound is drained with a Penrose drain and is not closed primarily. Use loose wire sutures.

Note: Antibiotic treatment for presumed *Staphylococcus* infection of these wounds should be started in the emergency room after cultures have been taken. Continue broad-spectrum antibiotics for 5–7 days, depending on the healing of the wound and the absence of pathogens on reculturing. Reinspect and redebride the fracture site in the operating room within 3–5 days.

Subsequent Management

The transcutaneous Steinmann pins are removed after 3 weeks, when soft tissue healing is adequate and swelling has subsided. The fracture may then be immobilized in a long-arm cast with the forearm in pronation. Cast immobilization is continued for at least 8 weeks, because these open fractures tend to be slower to heal than a usual fracture.

Other Complications: Malunion of the Distal Radius After Colles' Fracture

REMARKS

Numerous gradations of malunited Colles' fracture are encountered. Many cases with only minor deformity give rise to no dysfunction. Such a deformity can be accepted and requires no surgical intervention, particularly in the typical older patient.

If there is significant radial deviation or radial displacement along with radial shortening, corrective osteotomy of the fractured radius should be considered. Avoid recommending corrective osteotomy, however, until the patient has regained function in the hand and wrist, and has been allowed to evaluate function for herself or himself. Particularly avoid operating on patients with disuse atrophy or Sudeck's atrophy, because surgical intervention may aggravate the clinical problem.

Clinical Appearance Commonly Seen After Colles' Fracture

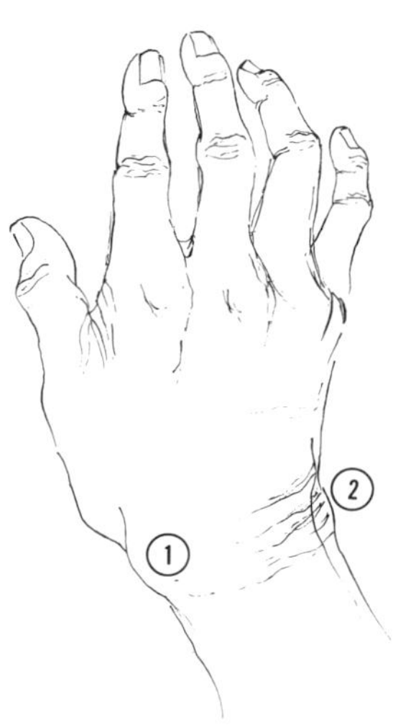

1. Commonly Colles' fracture produces chronic swelling and shortening of the radius resulting in
2. Prominence of the distal ulna.

Note: This common physical appearance after healed Colles' fracture is not functionally impairing, and the vast majority of cases do not require any further treatment.

Clinical Appearance of Malunion

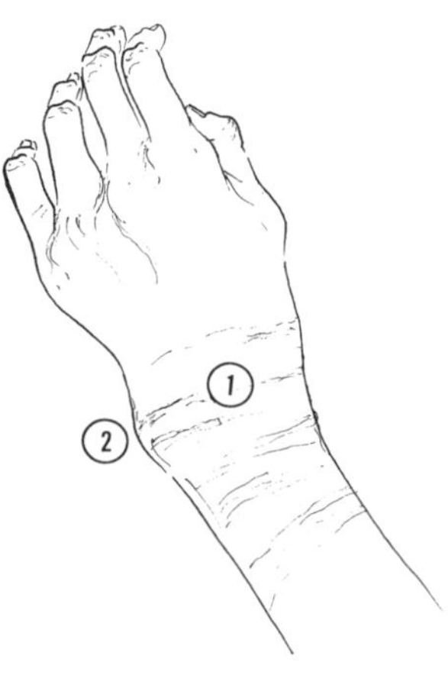

1. Excessive shortening to
2. Radial deviation causes symptomatic radioulnar pain and impairment of function.

Note: This occasionally is persistently symptomatic and does require corrective osteotomy.

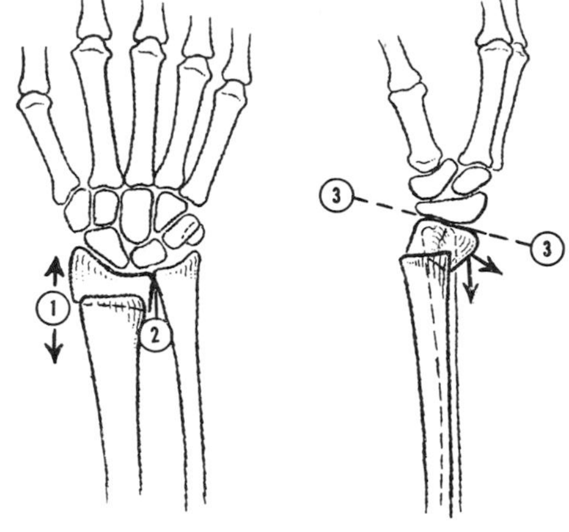

Radiographic Appearance: Malunion of Colles' Fracture

1. The radius is shortened
2. Relations of the radioulnar joint are disturbed.
3. The articular surface of the radius is directed upward and backward.

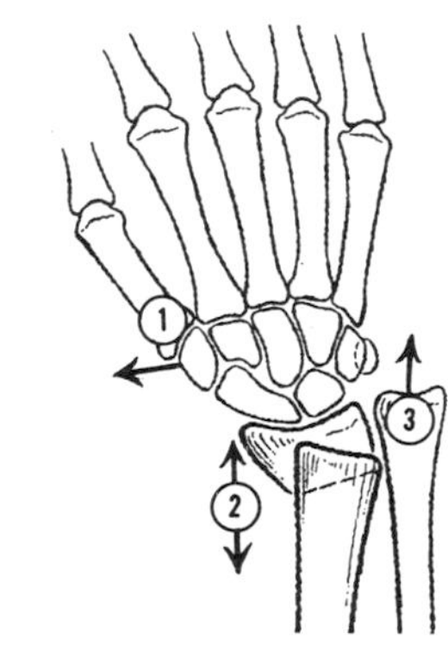

Malunion of Colles' Fracture

1. Radial deviation of the wrist and hand.
2. The radius is shortened.
3. The distal end of the ulna extends beyond the styloid of the radius.

Corrective Osteotomy

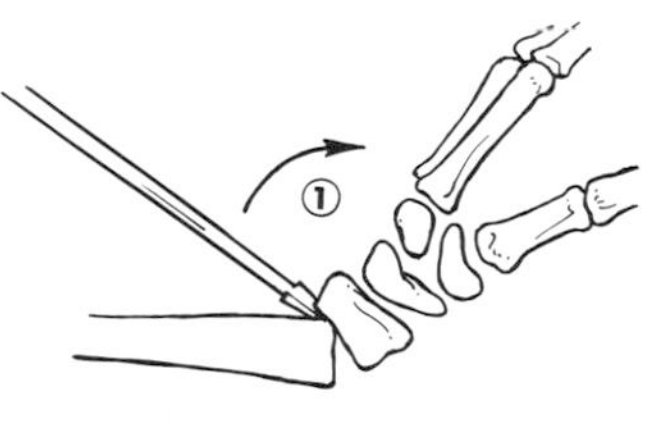

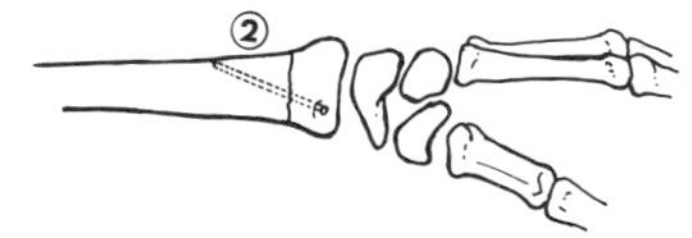

Caution: This should be carried out only after the patient has been allowed to regain function in the hand and wrist, and swelling and signs of painful stiffness have subsided.

1. An open reduction of the deformity is carried out with an osteotomy, preferably through the old fracture site.
2. The osteotomy is fixed in a corrected position with a pin, screw, or plate.

Note: A buttress plate may also be used to stabilize the distal fragment.

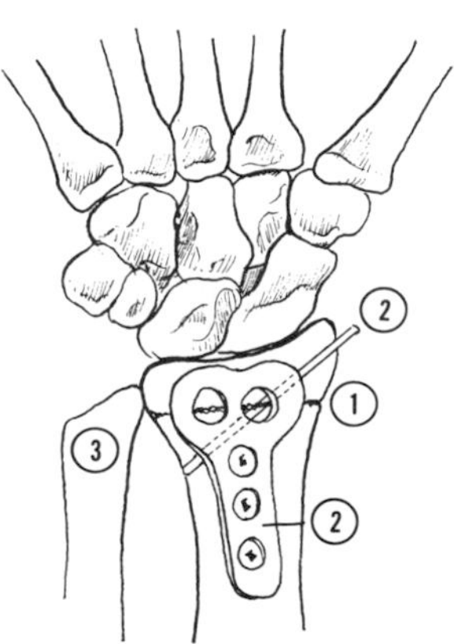

Postoperative X-Ray

1. The malunion has been corrected by osteotomy through the old fracture site.
2. Fixation with a buttress plate or Steinmann pin stabilizes the distal radius in the corrected position.
3. The distal end of the ulna may be resected minimally to correct any displacement of the radioulnar joint.

■ Smith's Fracture

REMARKS

Robert Smith, like Abraham Colles, was an 18th-century Dublin surgeon who described the clinical manifestations of distal radial fractures. In contrast to the dorsally displaced Colles' fracture, the less common Smith's fracture displaces volarly. Smith's fracture occurs about one tenth as often as Colles' fracture. It frequently is extremely unstable and may cause significant disability if mistaken for and treated as Colles' fracture.

The usually described mechanism that produces Smith's fracture is a direct blow to the dorsum of the wrist. Motorcyclists are especially susceptible to Smith's fracture during accidents, when the wrists are hyperextended as the motorcyclist is being thrown over his or her grip on the handlebars.

The force vectors from this injury displace the carpus and the distal radius in a volar rather than a dorsal direction. Extension of the wrist accentuates the displacement, and wrist function may be seriously impaired by recurrence of the deformity.

Usually this unstable fracture can be reduced by supinating the wrist to tighten the pronator quadratus muscle and the volar capsule of the wrist. For an unstable Smith's fracture, the distal radius can be fixed by pins.

Smith's fracture, which occurs 1–2 cm above the articular surface of the metaphyseal bone, must be distinguished from Barton's fracture-dislocation, which occurs through the volar articular surface. Smith's fracture can usually be managed by closed methods. Open reduction and buttress plate fixation are necessary for the unstable Barton's fracture-dislocation.

Mechanism of Injury

1. A fairly common mechanism producing Smith's fracture is hyperextension-pronation overload to the distal radius in a motorcyclist thrown over the handlebars of a motorcycle.
2. The result is an oblique fracture in the metaphyseal region with volar displacement of the distal fragment.

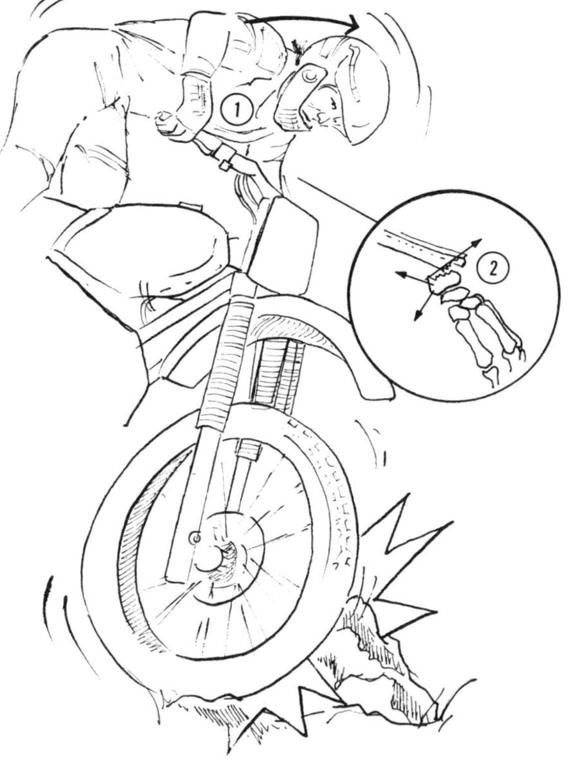

Garden-Spade Deformity

1. Dorsal prominence of the distal end of the proximal fragment.
2. Fullness of the wrist on the volar side due to the displaced distal fragment.
3. Deviation of the hand toward the radial side.

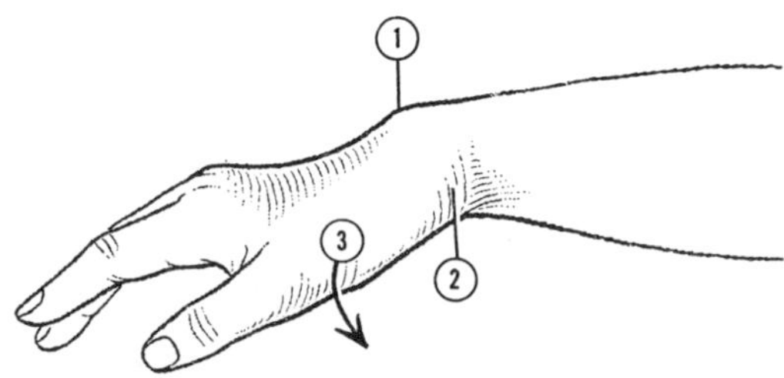

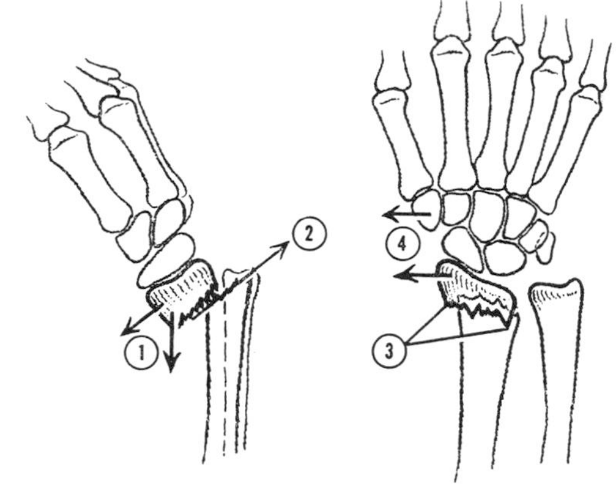

Prereduction X-Ray

1. The distal fragment displaces volarly and proximally.
2. The fracture line runs obliquely through the metaphyseal bone approximately 1–2 cm proximal to the articular surface.
3. The fracture runs through the full width of the metaphysis.
4. The hand and distal fragment displace radially.

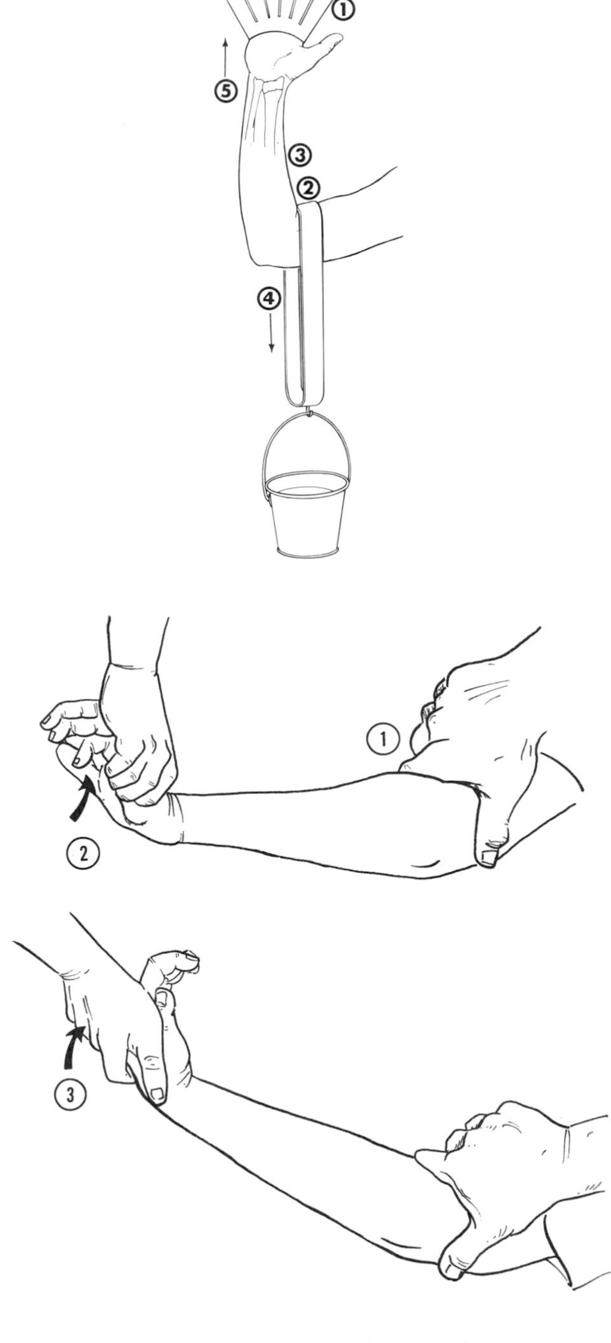

Reduction by Traction and Manipulation

The patient is under regional intravenous anesthesia as described previously (see page 1361).

TRACTION

1. Apply the finger-traction apparatus.
2. Flex the elbow at a right angle.
3. Supinate the forearm.
4. Apply countertraction with a muslin bandage and a water bucket for weight.
5. Maintain traction for at least 5 minutes, until the radial styloid is distal to the ulnar styloid.

Note: Keep the tourniquet inflated during manipulation to maintain intravenous anesthesia.

Reduction by Supination

1. After the fracture is pulled out to length, the hand is taken from the finger-trap device while traction is maintained proximally and distally.
2. The forearm is at first pronated and the wrist is extended to disimpact any of the fracture fragments that are still locked.
3. The forearm is supinated and the wrist is slightly flexed and held in ulnar deviation.

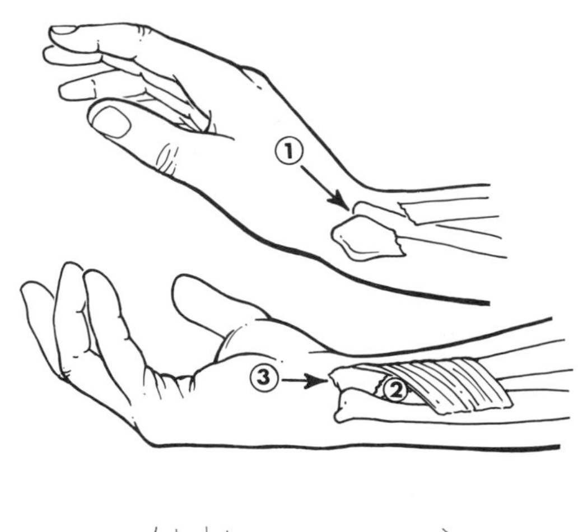

Mechanics of Reduction

1. Wrist extension usually reproduces the force vectors of injury and displaces the fracture volarly.
2. Supination tightens the pronator quadratus as a buttress against volar displacement.
3. A neutral or slightly flexed position of the wrist eliminates shear across the fracture.

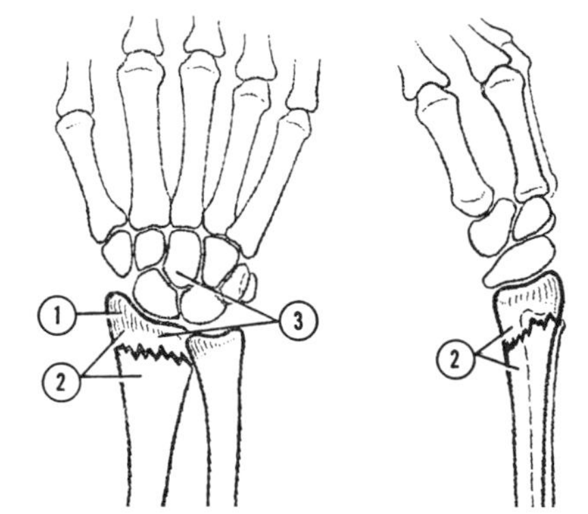

Postreduction X-Ray

1. The radial styloid is distal to the ulnar styloid.
2. The distal fragment is restored to its normal relationship with the proximal fragment. The wrist is slightly flexed to impact the fracture.
3. Radial deviation of the lower fragment and hand has been corrected.

Note: If reduction is satisfactory, deflate the tourniquet for intravenous anesthetic to 80 mm Hg, and after 10 seconds reinflate it to 210 mm Hg. Monitor vital signs and mental status; if these are unchanged, remove the tourniquet completely. Continue monitoring vital signs and mental status for 10 minutes following release of the tourniquet. The entire procedure requires two assistants, one to monitor the pressure of the cuff during the block and the other to assist in reduction. The minimum tourniquet time should always exceed 15 minutes.

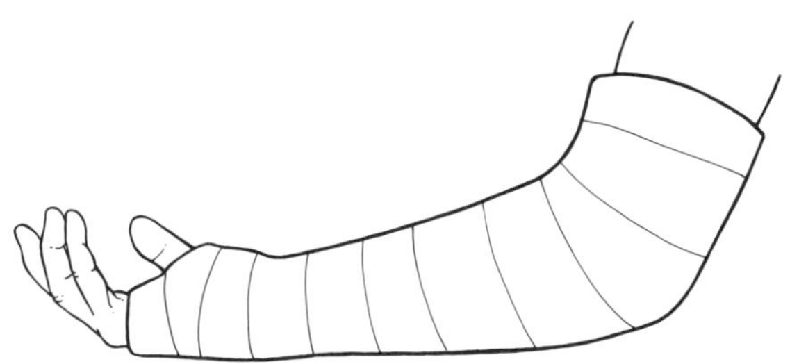

The cast should be applied firmly so as to prevent loss of position but not so tightly as to cause circulatory embarrassment. Elevate the arm with the fingers pointed toward the ceiling for the first 24 hours and apply ice bags.

Postreduction Management

Evaluate reduction by means of image-intensified fluoroscopy or standard x-rays. If reduction is unsatisfactory, repeat manipulation to achieve accurate alignment of the fracture. If the fracture remains unstable, employ pin-fixation technique through the radial styloid, as described for unstable Colles' fractures. If the patient complains that the cast is too tight, bivalve the cast down through the padding. After 24–48 hours encourage active exercises of the fingers and shoulder.

Take x-rays again within 5–10 days to evaluate the position. After 2–3 weeks a new cast that allows some elbow flexion but prevents wrist extension and forearm rotation may be applied. During the healing period, supervise active finger and shoulder motion exercises. Avoid the use of a support sling, which discourages shoulder and finger exercises. Remove the plaster cast after 6 weeks and allow the patient to begin active wrist exercises.

Unstable Smith's Fracture of the Lower End of the Radius With Comminution

REMARKS

In a number of Smith's fractures, because of fracture obliquity or comminution, redisplacement frequently occurs. Volar displacement of Smith's fracture causes significantly more functional disability than does dorsal displacement of Colles' fracture. The fracture deformity and instability can be prevented by distal-radial pin fixation or open reduction and plate fixation.

Prereduction X-Ray

1. The distal radial fragment is comminuted.
2. Displacement has recurred volarly.
3. The distal fragments have also redisplaced into a radial deviated position.
4. The styloid process of the ulna is avulsed, which indicates potential instability.

Note: This unstable Smith fracture is best stabilized internally with either percutaneous-pin or plate fixation.

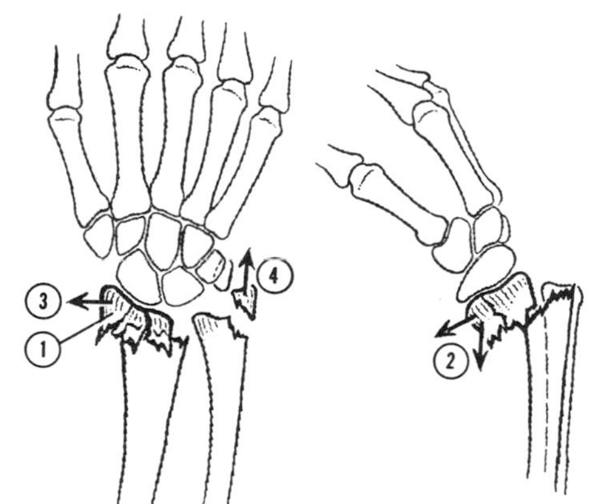

Reduction by Traction, Manipulation, and Transfixion Pin

The patient is under general or regional intravenous anesthesia.

TRACTION

1. Apply a finger-traction apparatus.
2. The elbow is flexed 90°.
3. The forearm is supinated fully.
4. Apply countertraction using a muslin bandage and water bucket for weight.
5. While maintaining forearm supination, continue traction until the radial styloid is distal to the ulnar styloid.

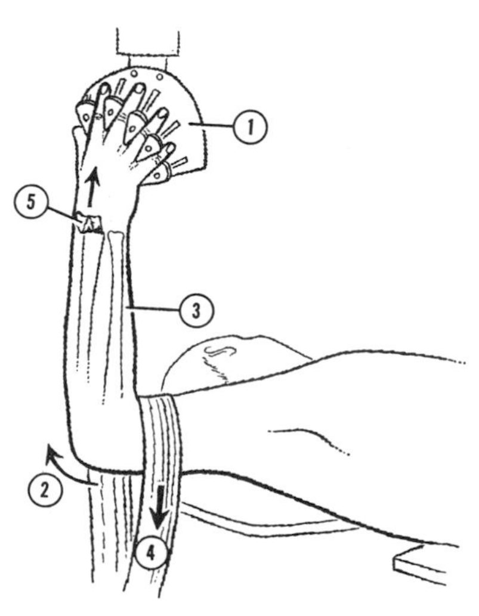

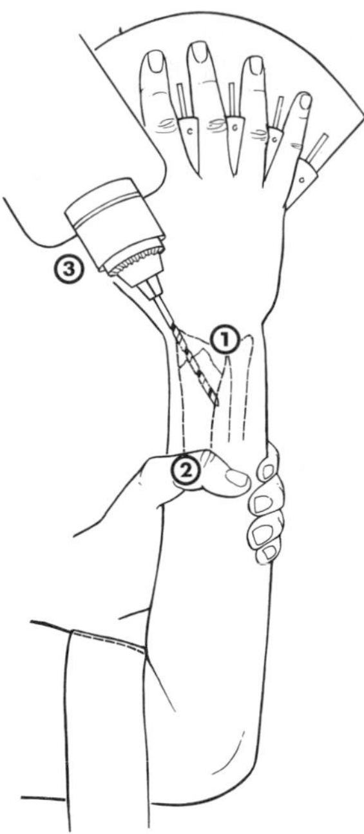

Insertion of Transfixion Pin

1. Confirm the reduction by fluoroscopy and then prepare the distal forearm for surgery.
2. While traction and the position of the wrist are maintained by an assistant,
3. Pass a threaded Steinmann pin, 2.0 mm in diameter, from the radial styloid across the fracture and into the opposite radial cortex. The pin is directed from the radial styloid at approximately a 45° angle. Confirm the position of the pin by fluoroscopy.

Note: The pin should be heavy enough so that it does not break and should be threaded so that it does not loosen.

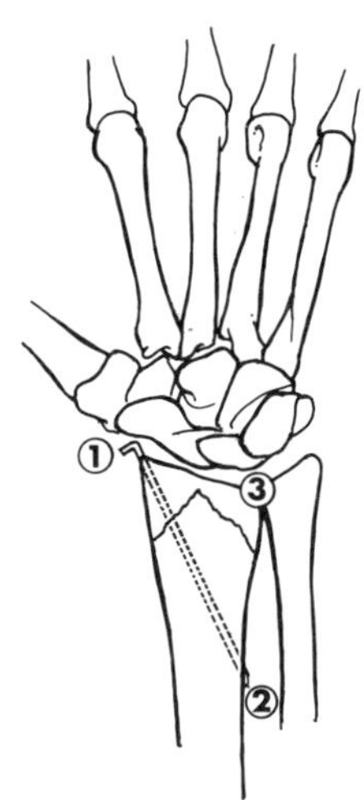

Percutaneous Pin Through a Radial Styloid

1. A pin is inserted from the radial styloid across the fracture site to the opposite radial cortex.
2. Transfixion to the opposite radial cortex adds stability to the reduction.
3. Reduction of the radioulnar joint should also be achieved. If necessary, a second pin may be inserted through the ulnar fragment of the fracture.

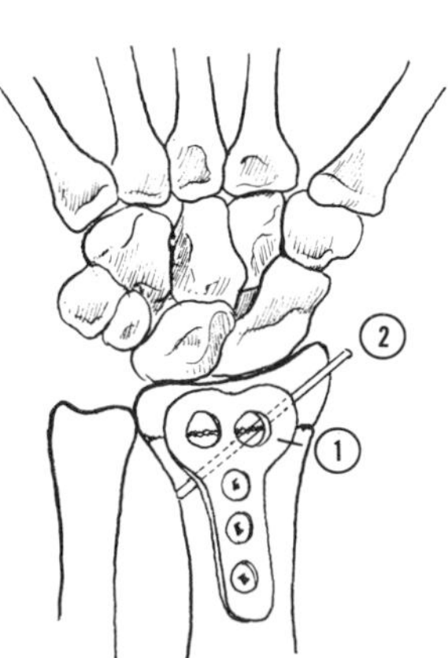

Alternative Method for Fixing Unstable Smith's Fractures: Plate Fixation

1. A buttress plate applied to the volar aspect of the wrist is also an effective way of stabilizing comminuted unstable Smith's fractures.
2. The distal fragment may be fixed with screws or simply supported with a buttress plate, depending on the amount of comminution.

Note: This technique is further discussed in the section on Barton's fracture.

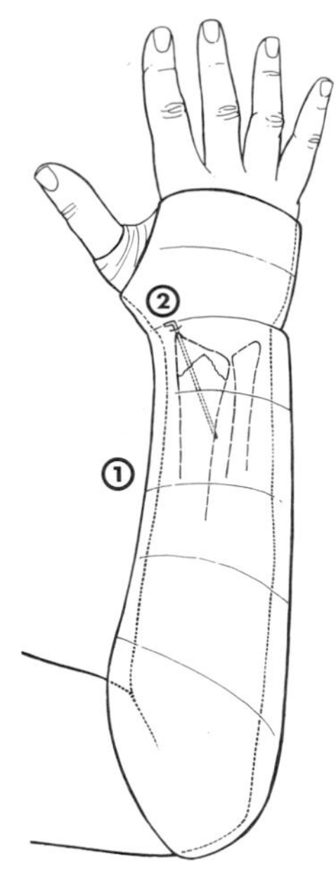

Application of Sugar-Tong Splint

1. A sugar-tong splint is also applied to stabilize the fracture.
2. The pin is cut off outside the skin but is not incorporated in the plaster.

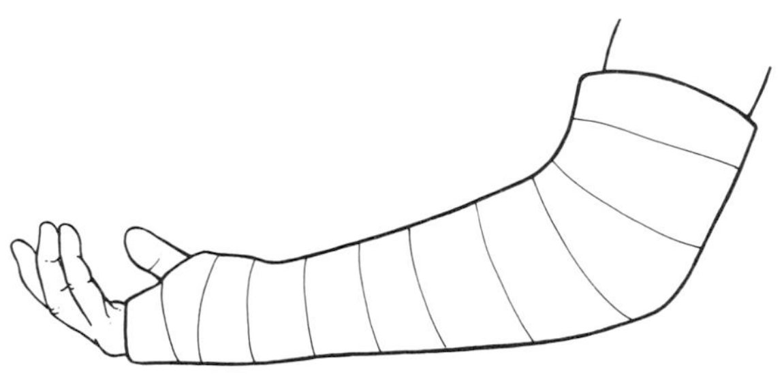

The splint should not be applied so tightly as to cause circulatory embarrassment. If at any time the patient complains that the splint is too tight or the hand is swollen, loosen the splint and padding. Elevate the arm with fingers pointing toward the ceiling for the first 24 hours and apply ice bags.

Avoid the use of a sling and insist on active finger and shoulder exercise from the start. By 2–3 weeks the cast may become loose and may have to be changed. Keep the forearm in the supinated position for at least 6–8 weeks.

Remove the cast at the end of 6–8 weeks, depending on the status of the healing, and, under local anesthetic, remove the pin fixation. Continue active range-of-motion exercises to the wrist after the cast and pin are removed.

Barton's Fracture

John Rhea Barton in 1838 described posterior and anterior marginal fractures of the distal radial articular surface. Barton's posterior marginal fracture is best classified as Colles' fracture.

The term *Barton's fracture* should be confined to describing an anterior fracture-dislocation in which a wedge-shaped articular fragment shears off the volar surface of the radius and displaces with the carpus forward and proximally.

In contrast to Colles' fracture, Barton's fracture is produced by a violent direct injury to the carpus and wrist. Seventy per cent of Barton's fractures occur in young male laborers or motorcyclists.

Usually the dislocated fragment includes all of the anterior portion of the lower metaphysis. The radial styloid may occasionally be separated as well.

Because of the extreme instability of this injury, it is best managed by prompt open reduction and buttress plate fixation. Screws are usually not inserted into the distal fragment, in order to avoid comminuting it further. If the radial styloid is fractured and separated, it is held with a Kirschner wire or screw fixation.

Prereduction X-rays

SIMPLE BARTON'S FRACTURE-DISLOCATION

1. A large fragment of the anterior articular surface of the radius is displaced anteriorly and proximally.
2. The carpus follows the radial fragment.
3. Some comminution of the radial fragment exists.

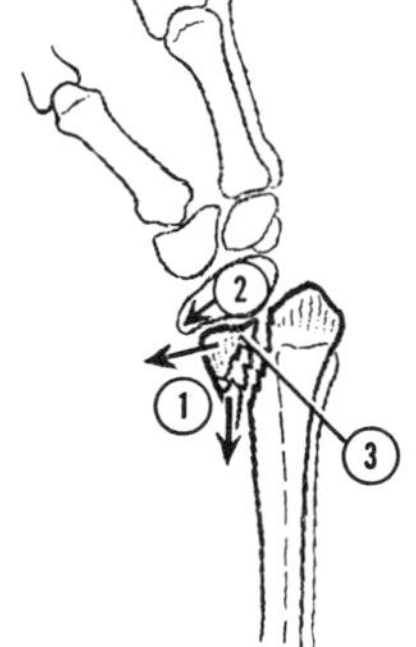

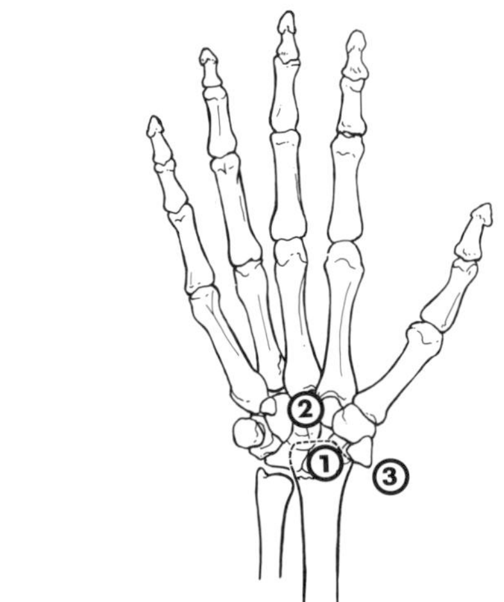

COMMINUTED BARTON'S FRACTURE-DISLOCATION

1. The comminuted fracture of the volar articular surface is associated with
2. Volar dislocation of the carpus.
3. Occasionally, the radial styloid process is also fractured.

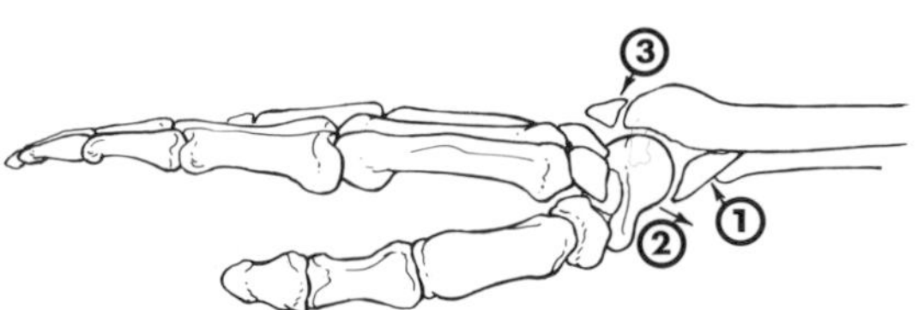

Open Reduction and Buttress Plate Fixation

1. A volar approach is made along the radial aspect of the fracture site.

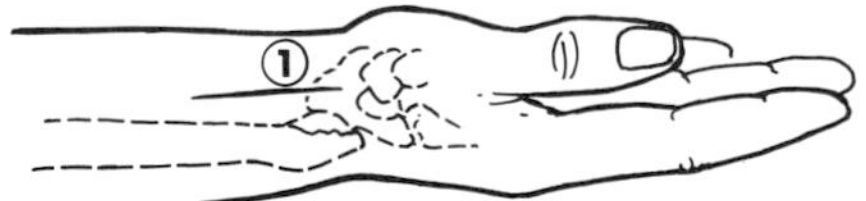

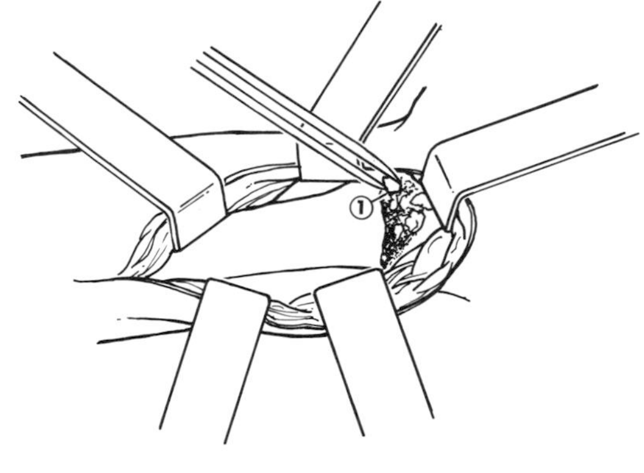

1. The fracture fragments that are loose are removed from the joint. The major articular fragments, however, are left in place.

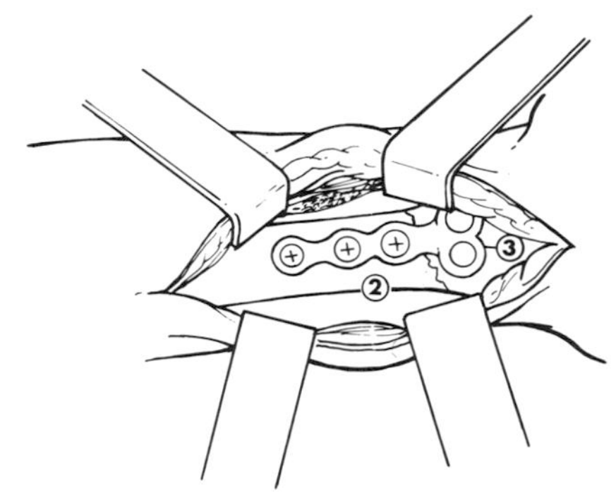

2. A small, angled plate is fixed to the intact shaft with screws.
3. The pressure of the lower end of the plate over the distal fragment reduces and holds the articular surfaces.

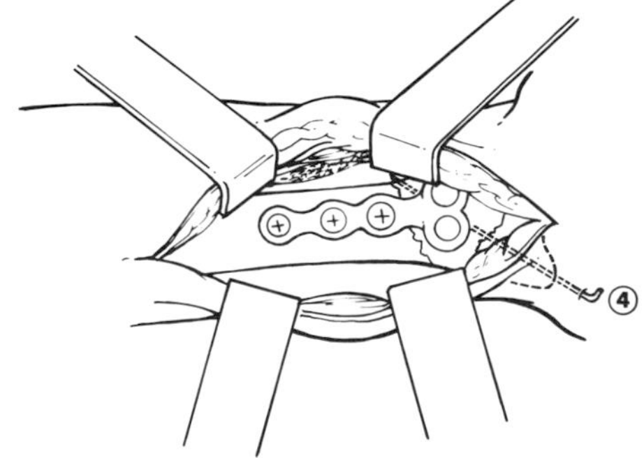

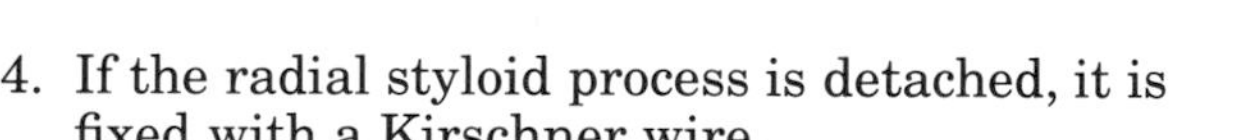

4. If the radial styloid process is detached, it is fixed with a Kirschner wire.

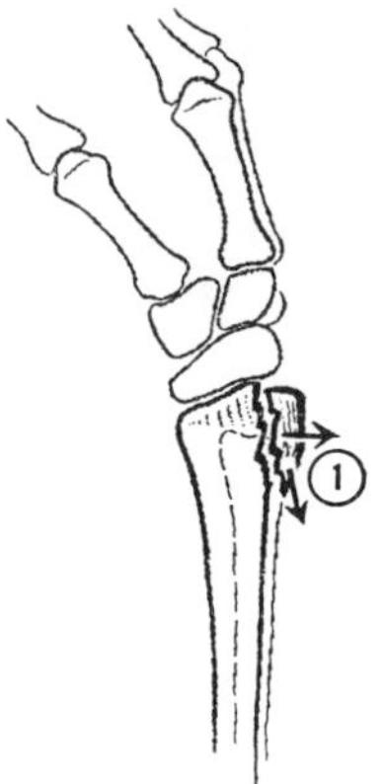

Reverse Barton's Fracture

1. Occasionally the displaced articular fragment may come from the dorsal surface.

The reverse Barton's fracture, or a fracture of the dorsal articular surface, is best classified as Colles' fracture. It must, however, be treated with the wrist in extension rather than in flexion, which is the normal position for immobilization of Colles' fracture.

1. Dorsiflexion of the wrist often reduces the dorsal radial fracture and aligns the lunate against the volar surface of the radius.
2. The articular surface of the radius shows no incongruity.

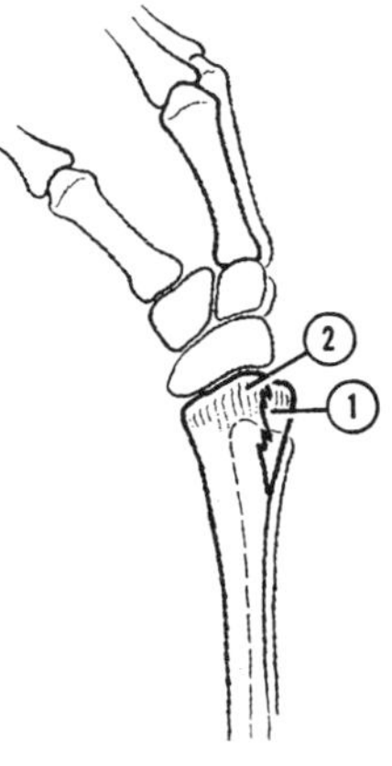

Note: If reduction of the articular fragment is not accurate, open reduction and internal fixation should be carried out as with Barton's fracture and volar dislocation.

FRACTURES OF THE RADIAL STYLOID PROCESS

REMARKS

This lesion is important because it implicates the articular surface of the radius. In most instances there is no displacement of the radial fragment; hence, simple immobilization in a plaster cast for 4–6 weeks is all that is required.

If there is displacement and reduction fails to restore perfect anatomic congruity of the articular surface, percutaneous pin or screw fixation is indicated. Occasionally a styloid fracture may be associated with a significant carpal injury, such as a perilunate dislocation. Always evaluate thoroughly for any associated injuries.

Undisplaced Fracture

1. The radial fragment is maintained in its anatomic position.
2. The articular surface of the radius is congruous.
3. The radial length and alignment are maintained.

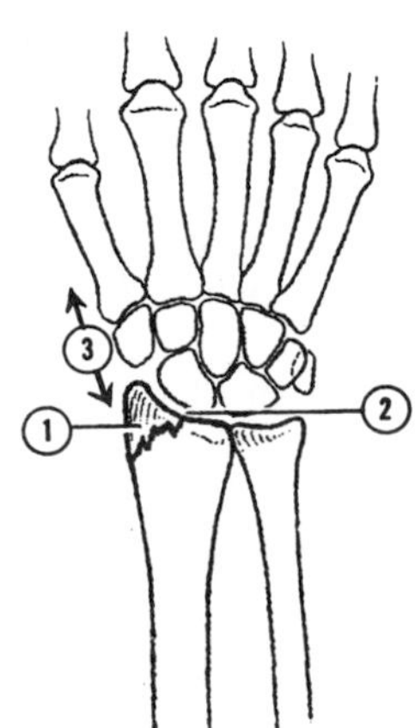

Cast Management

Immobilization is adequate in a short-arm cast. The undisplaced fracture usually heals by 6 weeks, when the cast can be removed. The patient may have some residual aching in this prominent radial styloid region for several weeks or months after the injury. However, function should return rapidly to a normal range of motion.

Management of Displaced Fractures

Prereduction X-Ray

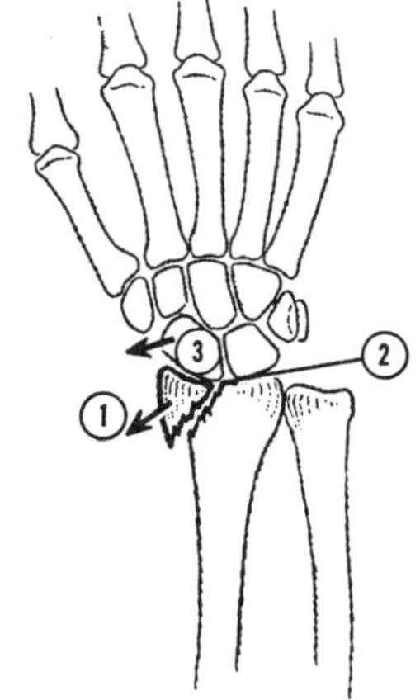

1. The fracture line is directed upward and outward.
2. The articular surface of the radius is involved.
3. The carpus is shifted slightly to the radial side along with the radial fragment.

Reduction Technique for Styloid Fracture

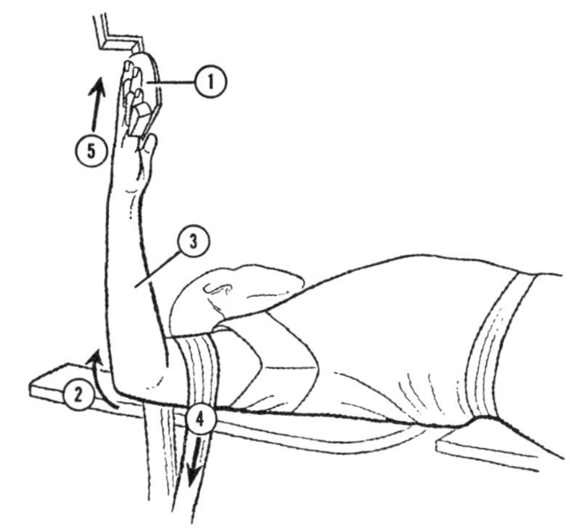

The procedure is performed with the patient under general or regional intravenous anesthesia.

TRACTION

1. Apply finger-traction apparatus.
2. The elbow is flexed 90°.
3. The forearm is in neutral rotation.
4. Make countertraction by using a muslin sling and a water bucket for weight.
5. Continue the strong traction upward until the radial styloid is pulled out to length.

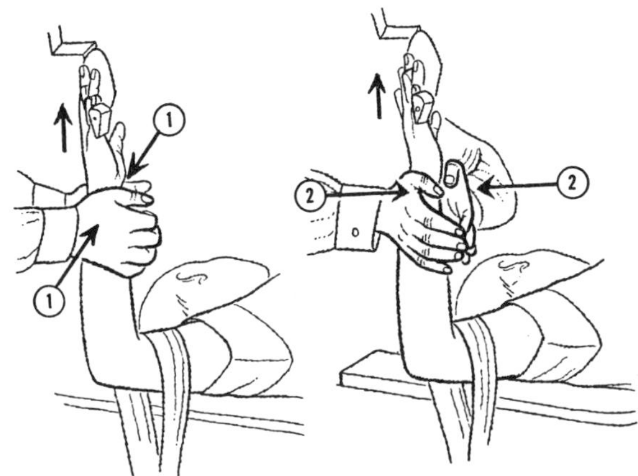

MANIPULATION

While traction is maintained,

1. Compress the fragment firmly with the heels of both hands; first compress the fragment laterally, and then
2. Compress the volar and dorsal surfaces.

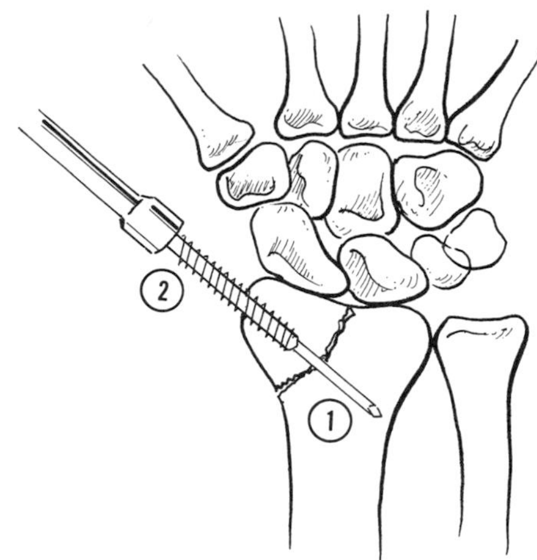

1. A guide pin is inserted percutaneously through the radial styloid region, while being careful to avoid the sensory branch of the radial nerve as well as the tendons in the snuff box.
2. When the position of the guide pin is confirmed on anteroposterior and lateral image-intensified fluoroscopy, a cannulated screw is inserted over the guide pin to stabilize the fracture.

Postreduction Management

The forearm is immobilized in a long-arm cast with supination and ulnar deviation of the wrist. The cast is kept in place for 4–6 weeks, depending on the radiographic and clinical progress of the fracture. Most of these fractures heal by 6 weeks, and after this, active range of motion of the wrist, forearm, and elbow can be instituted.

TRAUMATIC DISLOCATION AND SUBLUXATION OF THE DISTAL END OF THE ULNA (WITH AND WITHOUT FRACTURE)

REMARKS

Dislocation of the distal ulna must be recognized promptly when it is associated with a fracture of either the radius or ulna. Dislocation or subluxation of the joint can occur as an acute injury without fracture. The most serious problem associated with this type of injury is making the correct diagnosis. In about half of these isolated injuries, the diagnosis is overlooked clinically and radiographically. In some instances the deformity may be strikingly obvious, with narrowing of the transverse diameter of the wrist, dorsal or volar prominence of the distal ulna, and inability to pronate or supinate the wrist.

If the wrist has become swollen after injury, the clinical deformity may not be apparent, and the diagnosis depends on radiographic interpretation. The wide variation of possible radioulnar relationships on x-ray causes both the surgeon and the radiologist to ignore inconsistencies in this region. To visualize the distal radioulnar joint adequately, the x-ray beam must be centered over the wrist rather than the forearm, and the elbow must be flexed so as to prevent compensatory shoulder rotation. The diagnosis of an ulnar subluxation depends on a characteristic x-ray showing a lateral shift of the ulnar styloid with forearm pronation.

Forceful pronation of the wrist can also produce subluxation rather than complete dislocation of the ulna. This is a unique condition in that there is pain without clinical deformity. Ulnar subluxation can also result from forceful pronation imposed on the wrist as treatment for a distal radial fracture. Changing the position of the forearm from pronation to supination corrects this condition.

Pathomechanics of Injury (Snook and Coworkers)

The three structures that support the distal radioulnar joint are as follows:

1. Dorsal radioulnar ligament.
2. Volar radioulnar ligament.
3. Triangular fibrocartilage ligament.

Note: Disruption of either the dorsal or the volar ligament must occur along with partial disruption of the triangular fibrocartilage in order for the joint to be dislocated.

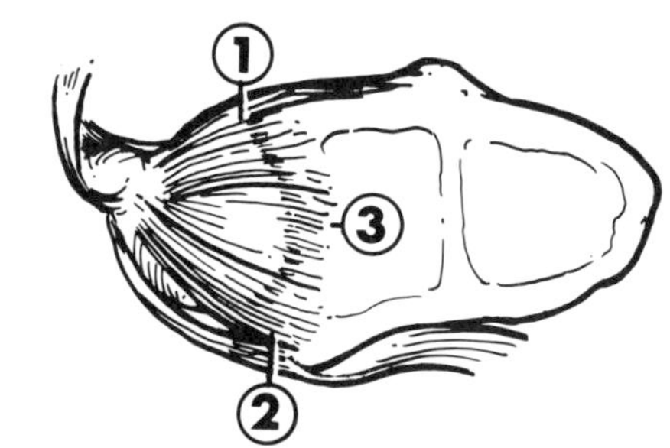

Relationship of Distal Ulna and Radius

1. The ulnar head is round for the usual 140° of rotation. Beyond this range it is irregular.
2. Forceful supination displaces the ulna volarly if the dorsal radioulnar ligament is torn.
3. Pronation displaces the ulna dorsally if the volar radioulnar ligament is torn.
4. If the ligaments remain intact, the radius locks on the incongruent surface of the ulna, causing the ulna to remain subluxed.

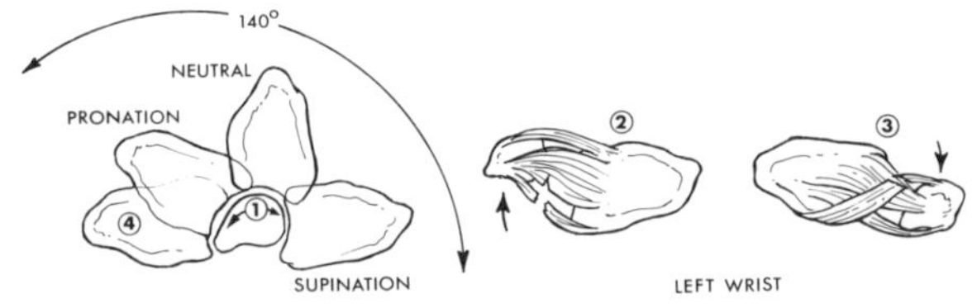

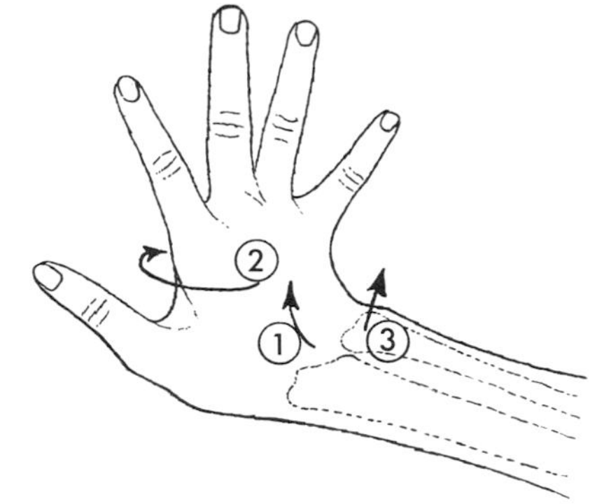

Mechanism of Dorsal Dislocation

1. The wrist and hand are forcefully extended and
2. Pronated.
3. Dorsal dislocation results if the ligament supports are ruptured.

Clinical Features of Dorsal Dislocation

Marked prominence of the head of the ulna on the dorsum of the wrist. The hand is locked in pronation. The transverse diameter of the wrist appears to be narrower than normal. Any attempt to supinate the hand elicits severe pain.

Note: In half the cases, extreme swelling after injury obscures the position of the ulna.

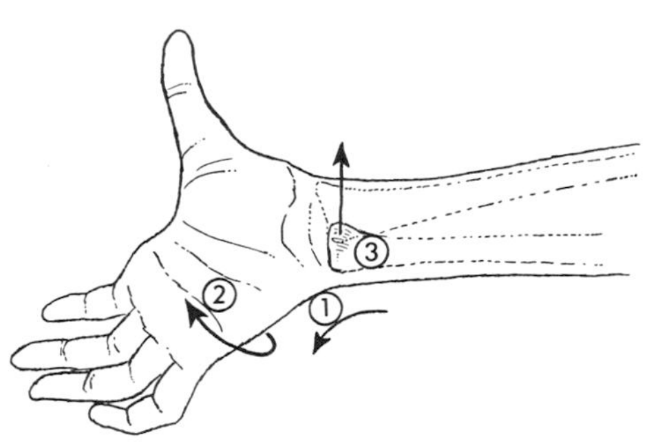

Mechanism of Volar Dislocation

1. The wrist and hand are forcefully extended and
2. Supinated.
3. Volar dislocation results if the ligament supports are ruptured.

Clinical Features of Volar Dislocation

The normal prominence of the head of the ulna on the dorsum of the wrist is absent. The hand is locked in supination. The prominence of the head of the ulna is on the volar aspect of the wrist. The transverse diameter of the wrist is narrower than normal. Any attempt to pronate the hand is painful.

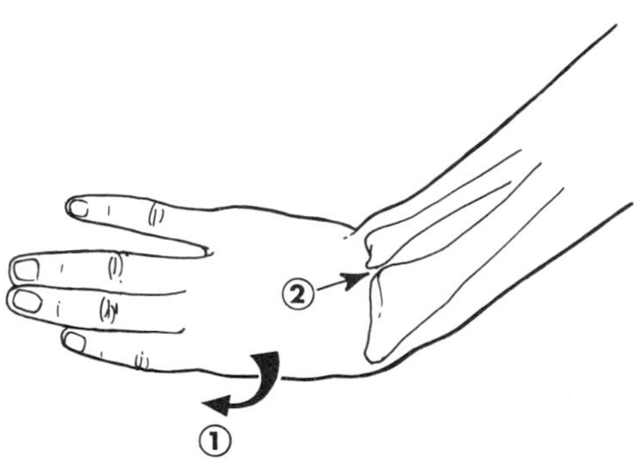

Mechanism of Subluxation

1. Hyperpronation applied to the wrist is insufficient to rupture the ligaments.
2. The radius locks on the incongruent surface of the ulna.

Clinical Features of Subluxation

If there is no fracture of the radius, ulnar subluxation has no presenting deformity. Symptoms include extreme pain and tenderness with marked reluctance to move the wrist out of the pronated position.

■ Radiographic Appearance of Dislocations

Note: Radiographic interpretation may be erroneous if it is made on the basis of anteroposterior and oblique views that are not properly centered on the wrist.

Volar Dislocation

On the anteroposterior view,
1. The head of the ulna has shifted radially.
2. A true lateral view centered on the wrist will demonstrate the dislocation and volar displacement of the ulna, particularly when compared with the opposite wrist.

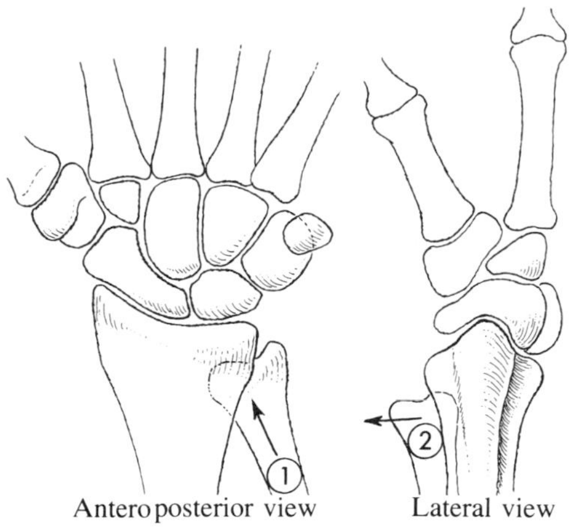

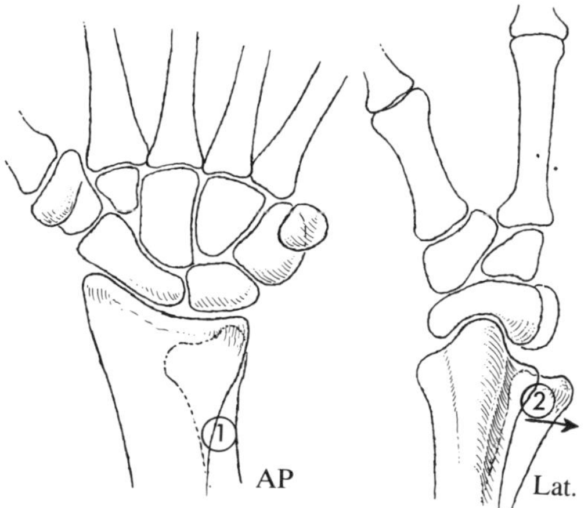

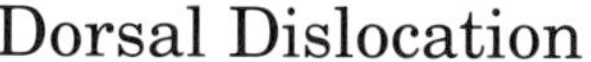

Dorsal Dislocation

1. The anteroposterior view shows some lateral shift of the ulna.
2. A true lateral view demonstrates dorsal displacement of the ulna, particularly when compared with the opposite wrist.

Subluxation From Hyperpronation

The diagnosis of a subluxated ulna is entirely dependent on anteroposterior and oblique views of the pronated wrist taken with the elbow flexed so as to prevent compensatory motion of the shoulder.
1. A pronated view of the normal wrist shows the ulnar styloid positioned on the lateral aspect of the ulna.
2. In the pronated view of a subluxated wrist, the ulnar styloid is displaced to the center of the bone or sometimes to the radial side.

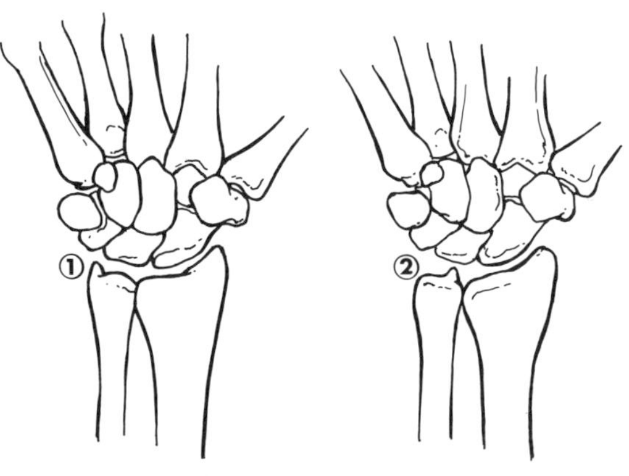

Ulnar Subluxation With Radial Fracture

1. Hyperpronated immobilization of a distal radial fracture can be associated with
2. Subluxation of the ulna, as indicated by displacement of the ulnar styloid.

Note: This should be corrected by changing the position of the wrist to supination.

Subluxation in Children

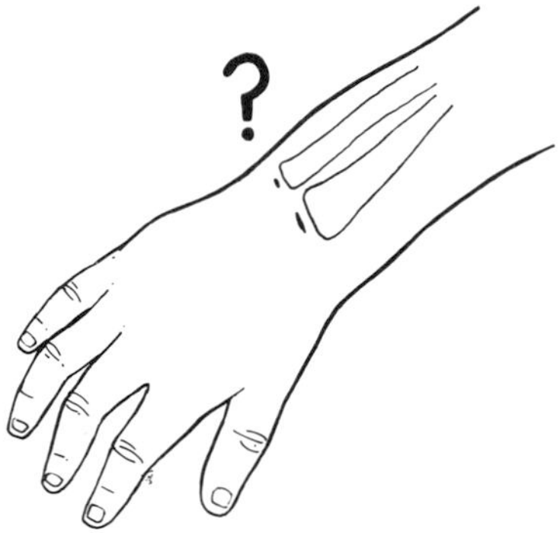

In children subluxation from forceful pronation cannot be diagnosed by x-ray if the distal ulna epiphysis has not ossified.

This injury is analogous to a pulled elbow and should be treated, on the basis of clinical findings, by firm supination.

Manipulative Reduction

The patient is given general or regional intravenous anesthetic.

Volar Dislocation of Right Wrist

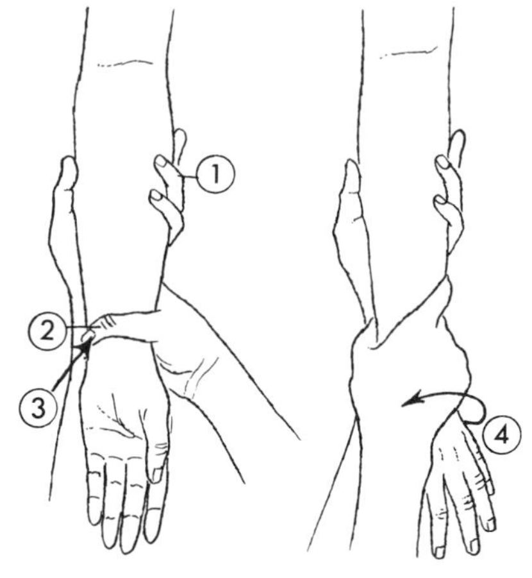

1. Grasp and steady the patient's supinated forearm with your left hand.
2. With the right hand, grasp the patient's hand and place your thumb over the prominence of the head of the ulna.
3. While making firm backward pressure on the head of the ulna,
4. Forcefully pronate the hand and wrist.

Note: Reduction is accompanied by a definite snap.

Dorsal Dislocation or Subluxation of Right Wrist

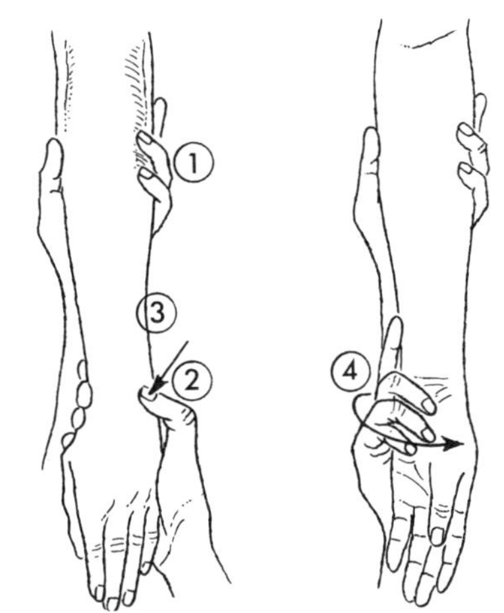

1. Grasp and steady the patient's pronated forearm with your left hand.
2. With your right hand grasp the patient's hand and place your thumb over the prominence of the head of the ulna.
3. While making steady and firm forward pressure on the head of the ulna,
4. Forcefully supinate the hand and wrist.

Note: Reduction is accompanied by a definite snap.

Immobilization

VOLAR DISLOCATION

Apply a plaster cast from the middle of the arm to just proximal to the metacarpal joints.

1. The elbow is flexed 90°.
2. The forearm is fully pronated.

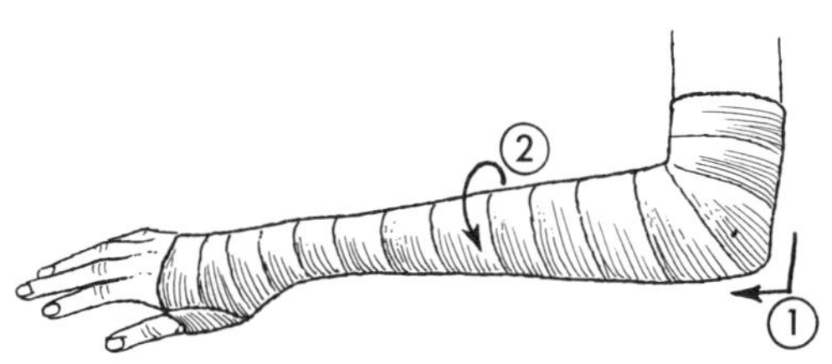

DORSAL DISLOCATION OR SUBLUXATION

1. The elbow is flexed 90°.
2. The forearm is fully supinated.

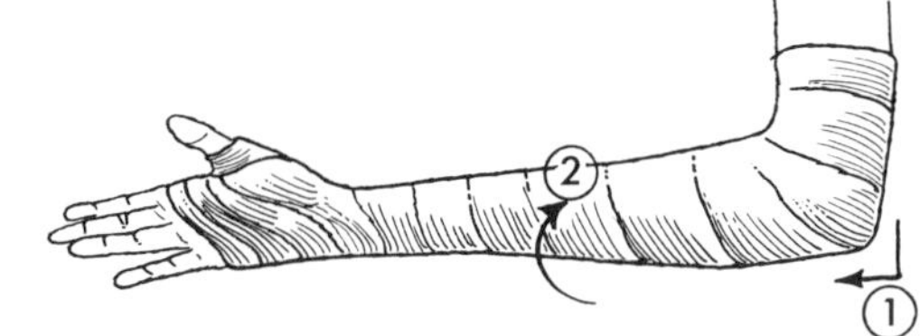

Postreduction Management

The cast is maintained for 4 weeks. After removal of the cast allow free use of the limb within the patient's tolerance. Avoid any forceful rotation of the hand and wrist, especially against resistance.

Habitual or Recurrent Subluxation of the Distal Radioulnar Joint

REMARKS

Occasionally a subluxation or dislocation of the distal radioulnar joint may pass unrecognized or untreated after an acute injury to the wrist. The result may be recurrent subluxation or clicking of the radioulnar joint, which impairs rotation of the forearm and wrist.

If the condition is present for only 4–6 weeks the subluxation or dislocation may be reduced, as described in the preceding section. However, the joint requires stabilization with percutaneous Kirschner wires in addition to cast immobilization.

Alternatively, an excision of the distal ulna (Darrach procedure) may be used to eliminate painful subluxation and dislocation of the joint. This is generally preferable to more extensive soft tissue stabilization procedures with this structure.

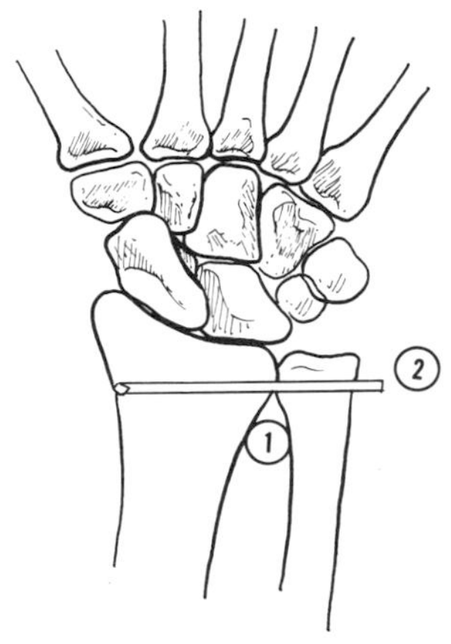

1. An unrecognized chronic subluxation or an unrecognized dislocation of the distal radioulnar joint seen at 4 weeks or more after injury may be reducible by closed manipulation, as previously illustrated.
2. This unstable joint usually requires percutaneous transosseous pin fixation for stability and soft tissue healing.

Subsequent Management

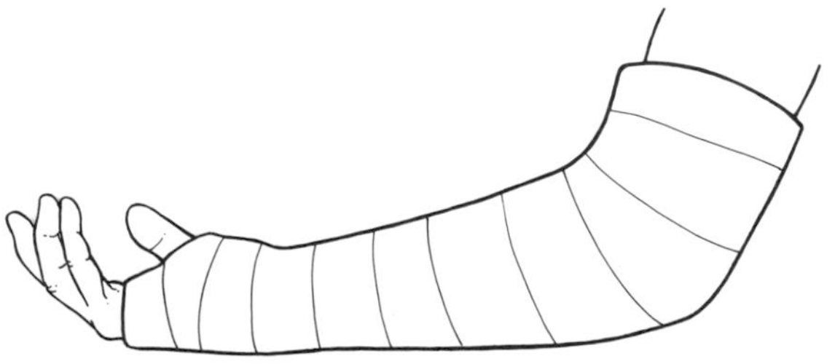

The injury is immobilized in supination for the dorsally dislocated ulna and in pronation for the volar dislocation, as previously illustrated.

After 4 weeks the cast and pin are removed and gentle range of motion in the wrist and forearm is allowed. If the joint remains symptomatic or unstable, resection of the distal ulna may be considered.

FRACTURES AND DISLOCATIONS OF THE CARPAL BONES: GENERAL PRINCIPLES

Injuries to the wrist implicating the carpal bones are common lesions in all age groups, particularly in young adults. Knowledge of the mechanics of the wrist is important to understand the mechanisms of injury and the rationale of treatment.

Anatomic Considerations

The Mechanics of Wrist Motion

REMARKS

Rotation does not occur through the radiocarpal and carpal joints. Only flexion-extension and abduction-adduction are possible. The absence of rotation is compensated for by pronation and supination movements of the forearm. Although the exact measurement of wrist motion varies depending on the subject and observer, approximately 40 per cent of wrist palmar flexion takes place in the radiocarpal joint and 60 per cent in the carpal joint.

The proximal and distal rows move simultaneously but in opposite directions. When the wrist is extended, the proximal row glides volarly and the distal row rotates dorsally. When the wrist is flexed, the proximal row of carpal bones glides dorsally and abuts against the dorsal lip of the distal articular surface of the radius; the distal row shifts volarly.

When the hand is deviated toward the radius, the proximal row shifts toward the ulna, while the distal row and the metacarpal bones move toward the radius. Conversely, when the hand deviates toward the ulna, the proximal row moves toward the radius, while the distal row and metacarpals move toward the ulna. Radial deviation of the wrist is slight, usually not more than 15°, whereas ulnar deviation may reach up to 40°.

Due to its connecting and supporting function for the synchronous motion between the proximal and distal carpal rows, the scaphoid is subjected to the greatest shear forces and the highest incidence of injury of all the carpal bones.

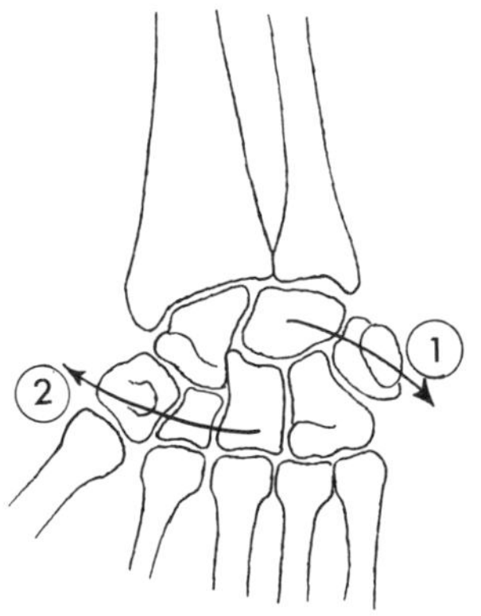

Radial Deviation of the Wrist

1. The proximal row glides toward the ulna.
2. The distal row with the metacarpals moves toward the radius.

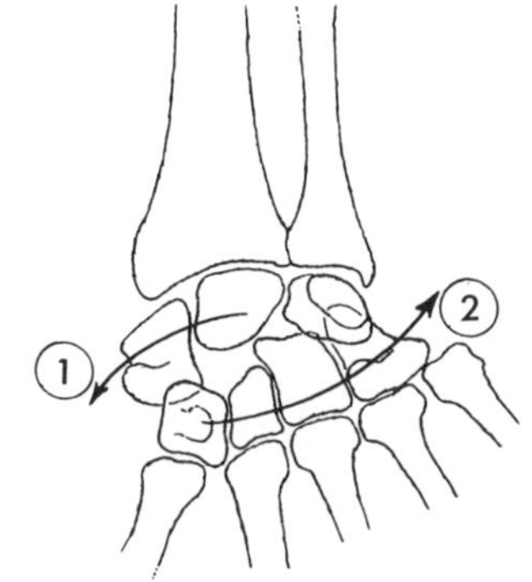

Ulnar Deviation of the Wrist

1. The proximal row glides toward the radius.
2. The distal row and the metacarpals move toward the ulna.

Flexion of the Wrist

1. The proximal row moves dorsally. The slope of the distal radius limits motion in the radiocarpal joint.
2. The distal row moves anteriorly.

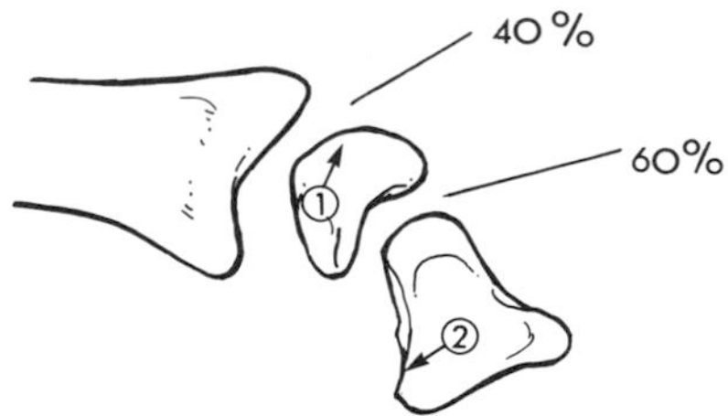

Extension of the Wrist

1. The proximal row moves volarly. The slope of the distal radius allows greater motion in the radiocarpal joint.
2. The distal row moves dorsally.

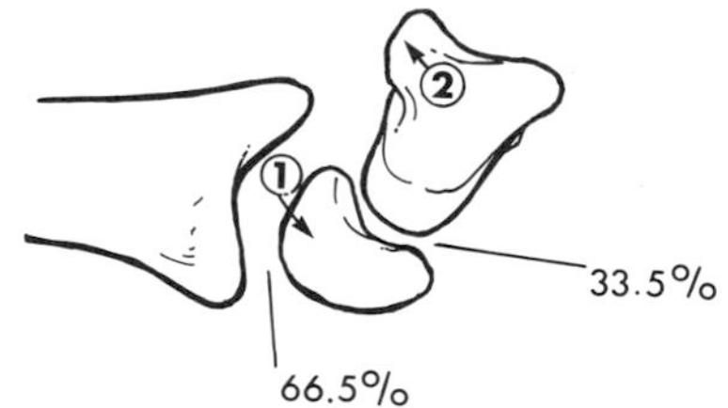

Carpal Ligaments

The strength of the wrist depends on the numerous strong bands that encircle it and also on a tough intricate complex of ligaments, of which the volar component is the strongest. The strong ligaments anchor the bones in place and to each other, to the radius, and to the metacarpal bones; this is especially true on the volar surface of the bones. The pisiform bone actually lies within the tendon of the flexor carpi ulnaris, which in turn continues onto the carpus and metacarpals and hamate through strong ligaments extending from the pisiform to these bones.

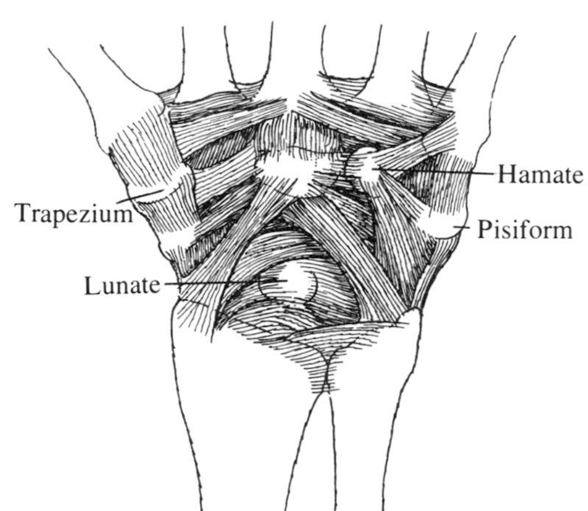

Carpal Stability

1. The scaphoid acts as a mechanical shaft that stabilizes the intercarpal area by its oblique position between the proximal and distal rows.
2. The strong scapholunate and scaphocapitate ligaments permit synchronous carpal motion in flexion, extension, and radial and ulnar deviation.

Note: Carpal instability may result from either a displaced fracture of the scaphoid or disruption of the scaphocarpal ligaments.

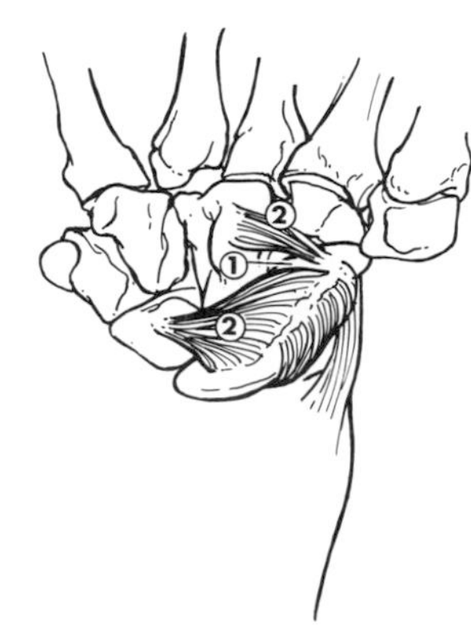

Radiographic Diagnosis of Fractures and Dislocations of Carpal Bones

REMARKS

Adequate x-ray technique is critical for prompt diagnosis and proper treatment of these common injuries. Injuries to the carpal bones are among the most likely to be missed or to be subject to delayed diagnosis.

Occasionally the fracture may be so subtle that it becomes radiographically apparent only after 2–4 weeks of vascular response and osteoclastic resorption. Complete dislocation may not be recognized if an incomplete radiographic study is relied on.

Radiographic evaluation of the injured wrist should often include anteroposterior views with the wrist in neutral, maximal ulnar deviation, and maximal radial deviation. In addition, a true lateral view and lateral views with the wrist in flexion and extension should also be obtained, particularly if the diagnosis is uncertain.

If pain symptoms are located on the volar aspect, a carpal tunnel view is necessary to rule out such injuries as fracture of the hook of the hamate. Occasionally if careful radiographic study with plain films fails to find the injury, more elaborate and expensive studies, including bone scan, computed tomography, or magnetic resonance imaging, may rarely be indicated. However, most injuries can be diagnosed by careful analysis of standard plain radiographic studies.

Standard X-Ray Views of the Injured Wrist

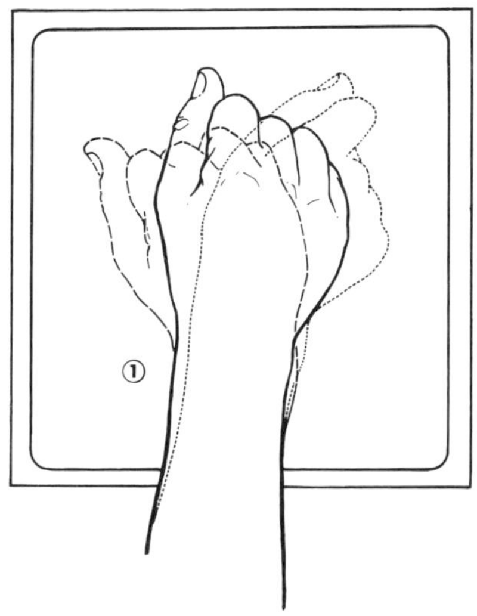

1. Anteroposterior views with the wrist in neutral, ulnar deviation, and radial deviation.

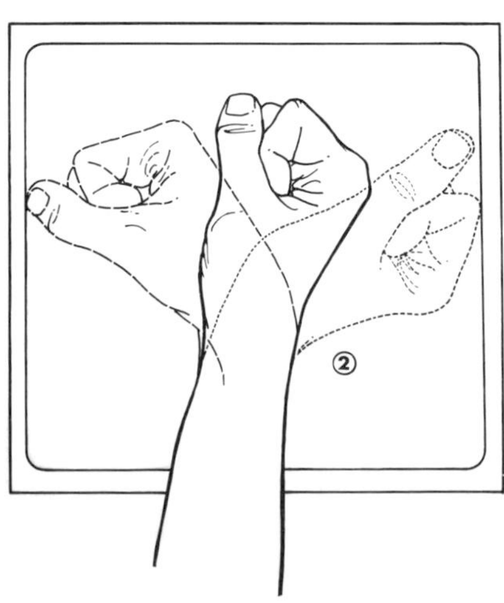

2. True lateral views with the wrist in neutral, flexion, and extension.

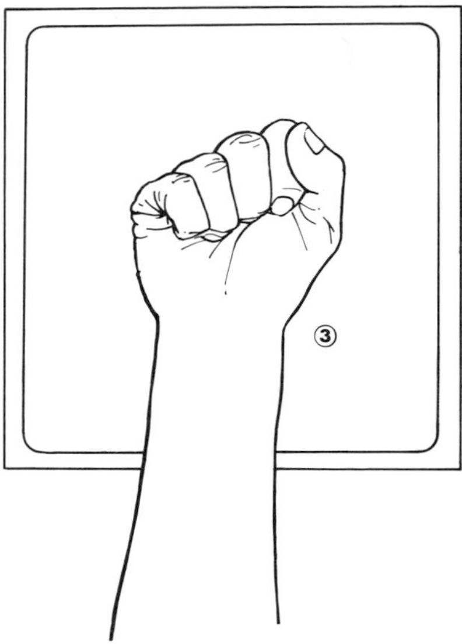

3. A view of the supinated wrist is often necessary if carpal dislocation or subluxation is suspected.

Note: Even if standard x-rays are normal, treat the patient with acute wrist pain after injury by protective immobilization. Undisplaced fractures or subluxations of the carpal bones may not become evident radiographically for several weeks after injury.

FRACTURES OF THE SCAPHOID

REMARKS

Of all the carpal bones, the scaphoid is the most frequently fractured. Its relationship to the radius and its linkage to both proximal and distal carpal rows render it vulnerable to injury. During dorsiflexion the scaphoid is sheared, as its proximal half is locked against the distal radius and its distal half is forced into further dorsiflexion because of its linkage with the distal carpal row. This results most frequently in a fracture through the midscaphoid. With sufficient violence, the scaphoid may fracture and dislocate with the distal carpal row.

The rapidity of scaphoid fracture healing depends on the degree of circulatory damage as well as the displacement and instability of the fracture. The scaphoid circulation enters the bone, for the most part, through the distal half, on both the dorsal and volar surfaces. Fractures through the proximal third tend to disrupt blood flow proximally and are slower to heal.

Fracture lines that run transversely or slightly obliquely across the long axis of the scaphoid tend to be compressed by finger-muscle forces and to heal quickly. The vertical, oblique fracture, which is uncommon, is sheared by finger-muscle forces and heals more slowly.

Fractures in which a longer than normal healing period can be anticipated include fractures in the proximal third with poor blood supply, oblique fractures that are unstable, and fractures that are displaced initially in either an axial or a transverse direction, particularly if associated with dislocation of the carpus.

Mechanisms of Scaphoid Fracture

1. The mechanism of the scaphoid fracture is a fall on the outstretched hand with the force absorbed by the thenar eminence.
2. The forceful extension of the wrist wedges the scaphoid against the dorsal rim of the radius.
3. This produces a typical transverse fracture in the middle third of the scaphoid, which begins on the palmar surface and propagates dorsally.

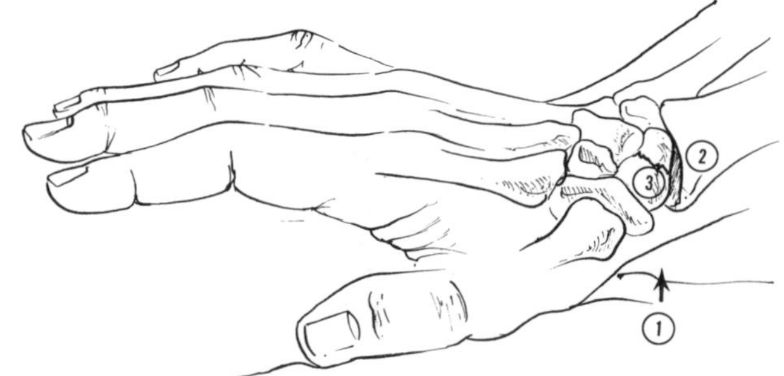

Epidemiology

The fracture occurs in all age groups, but the highest incidence is in young adult males. Approximately 50 per cent occur in patients less than 30 years of age. It also occurs in children more generally than appreciated. Approximately 85 per cent of scaphoid fractures occur in men.

The right hand is involved more frequently than the left (70 per cent). Bilateral involvement occurs in 2–3 per cent of cases. Approximately 85 per cent of all fractures of the scaphoid occur through the middle third, 5 per cent through the proximal third, and 5–7 per cent through the distal third. Most scaphoid fractures (85 per cent) are isolated injuries; however, there may also be injuries to adjacent structures, such as

- transscaphoid perilunate dislocation.
- fractured scaphoid with a scapholunate dissociation.
- a scaphoid fracture with Colles' fracture.

Mechanism of Unstable Scaphoid Fracture-Dislocation

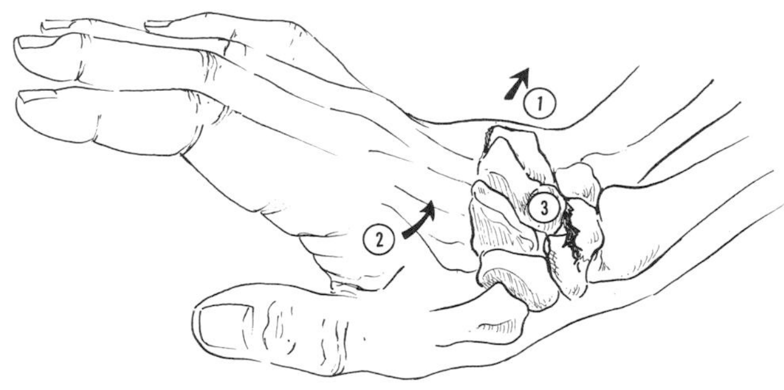

1. If ulnar deviation and forceful supination are combined with
2. Forceful hyperextension,
3. A transscaphoid perilunate dislocation or perilunate dislocation occurs.

Note: This unstable mechanism should be suspected if there are abrasions on the thenar side of the palm or excessive swelling about the wrist.

Types of Fractures

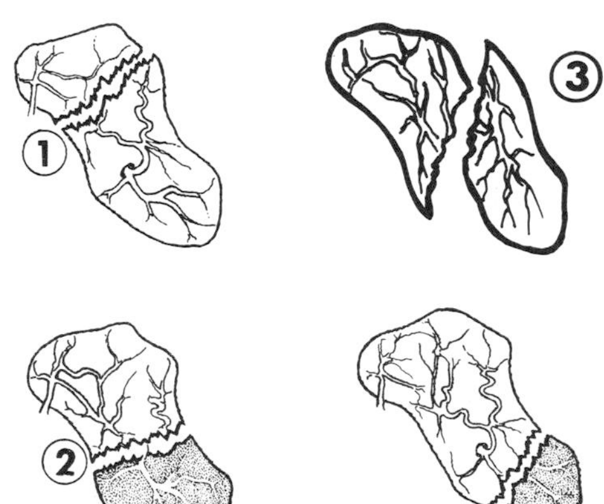

The type of fracture sustained depends on the position of the wrist at the time of impact and in general can be categorized into one of four groups:

1. Fracture of the distal third or fracture of the tuberosity.
2. Transverse fracture of the middle third; this is the usual stable fracture.
3. Vertical oblique fracture; this is an unstable fracture.
4. Fracture of the proximal third; this is slow to heal because of impaired blood supply.

Intraosseous Blood Supply

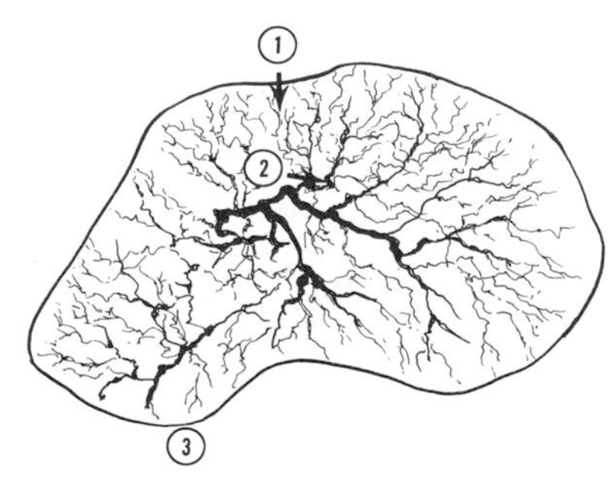

1. Most of the intraosseous blood supply flows in a retrograde fashion from the dorsal vessels entering at the waist of the scaphoid.
2. The vessels entering through the dorsal area flow retrogradely toward the proximal pole.
3. The tuberosity is supplied by a separate palmar scaphoid branch distally.

Note: Because of this retrograde vascular flow, the proximal third of the scaphoid is subject to avascular necrosis with displaced fractures.

■ Clinical Diagnosis

REMARKS

Fractures of the carpal scaphoid are among the most frequent injuries that are not detected on initial evaluation. Any patient with wrist pain, particularly localized to the snuff box, should be suspected of having sustained this injury. The "O" sign is a typical physical sign of a carpal scaphoid fracture.

1. The pain is usually localized to the snuff box region.
2. The patient localizes the pain by encircling the snuff box with the opposite index finger and thumb so as to form an "O."

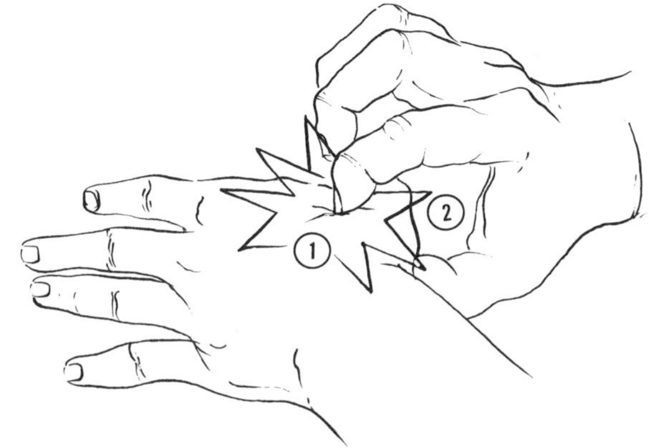

Radiographic Diagnosis

REMARKS

Most scaphoid fractures can be diagnosed from standard x-ray studies of the wrist, as described previously. An anteroposterior view of the wrist in ulnar deviation is particularly useful because this position demonstrates the full length of the scaphoid.

Occasionally initial adequate x-rays do not demonstrate a fracture. In this case the symptomatic wrist can be protected with a cast or brace for 1–2 weeks. After this time if the scaphoid or snuff box pain is still present despite the period of immobilization, x-rays should be repeated.

If the x-ray remains negative but the symptoms persist, further studies with either computed tomography or bone scan are indicated. If the bone scan is negative, a scaphoid fracture has been ruled out. If the bone scan is positive, conditions such as an osteoid osteoma or other inflammatory processes may be the source of the pain, although the most likely diagnosis is an undisplaced scaphoid fracture.

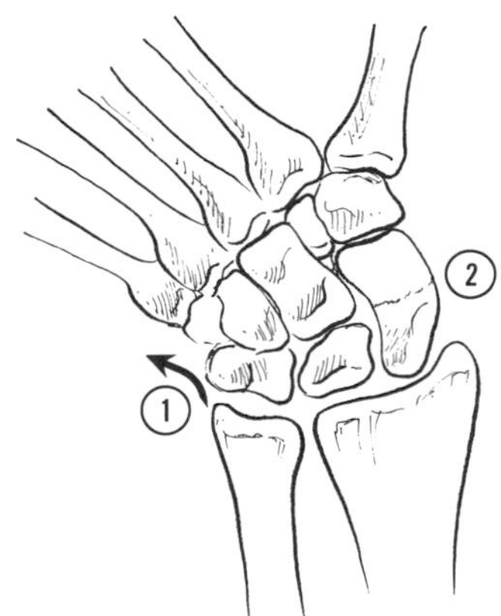

1. The most useful x-ray technique is a posterioanterior view with the wrist in ulnar deviation.
2. This shows the elongated scaphoid and is most useful in demonstrating the typical fracture of the waist of the scaphoid.

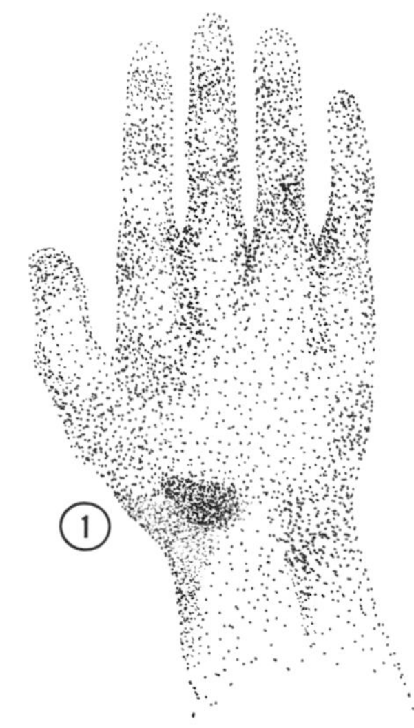

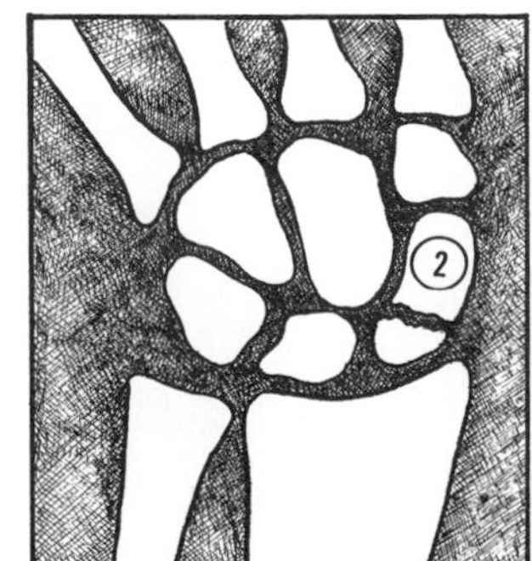

1. Radioactive bone scanning or
2. Computed tomography may be necessary to diagnose the occasional undisplaced fracture carpal injury not evident from careful standard radiographic evaluation.

Note: These nonstandard techniques are also useful for evaluating healing of nonunions and delayed union of carpal bone injuries.

■ Prognosis

Ninety-five per cent of acute fractures of the scaphoid, including those not treated for 3–4 weeks after injury, heal with plaster immobilization for 6–10 weeks. In fact, 70–75 per cent of fractures in which diagnosis is delayed and treatment is not instituted for several months will heal with adequate immobilization.

Fractures that require longer than normal immobilization include those in the proximal third, those with an oblique fracture line that is unstable, and those with initial axial or transverse displacement. In general, treatment should be based on the patient's freedom from pain and ability to grip without discomfort. Clinical evidence of union frequently precedes radiographic evidence by several months.

■ Management of Scaphoid Fractures That Heal Rapidly

Most scaphoid fractures are undisplaced and should heal within 8 weeks. These include the following.

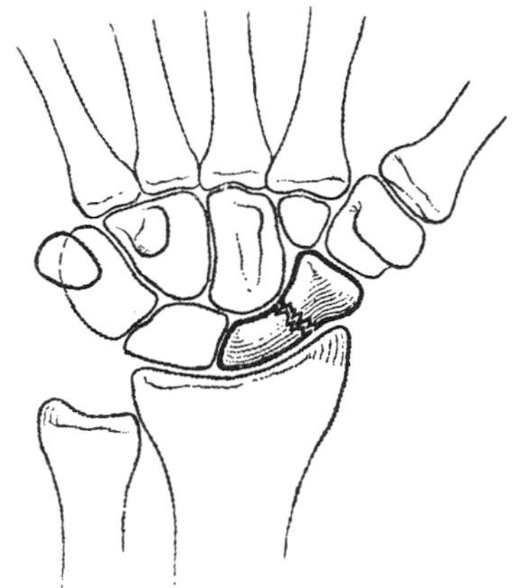

Prereduction X-Rays

Fracture through the mid-third.

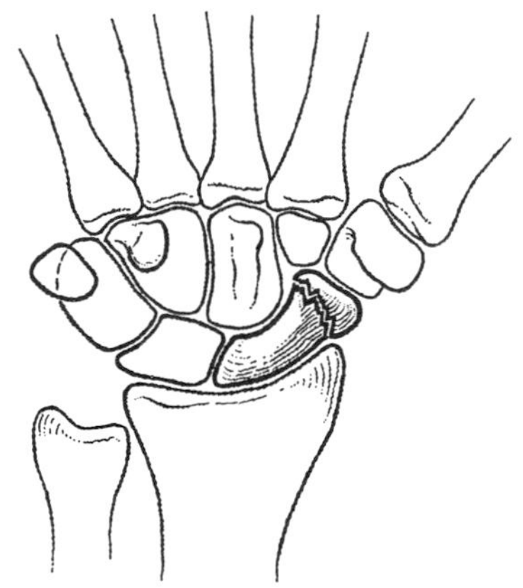

Fracture through the distal third.

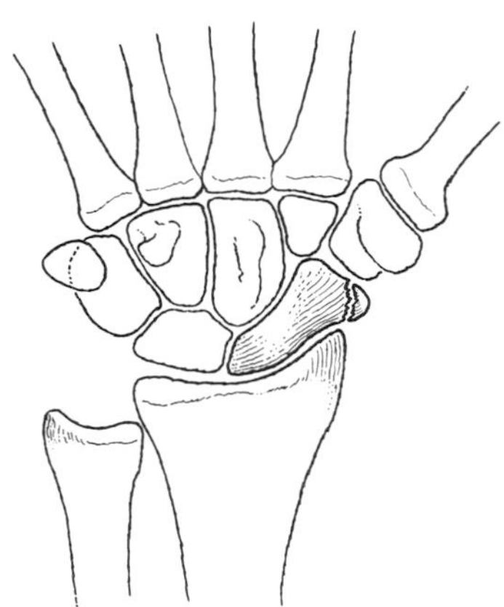

Fracture through the tubercle.

Initial Immobilization

If the patient is seen immediately after injury and has considerable swelling, apply an anterior and posterior splint.

1. The splint extends from below the elbow to the metacarpophalangeal joints.
2. The thumb is in a grasp position and is included in the plaster beyond the interphalangeal joint.
3. The wrist is in slight extension and slight radial deviation.

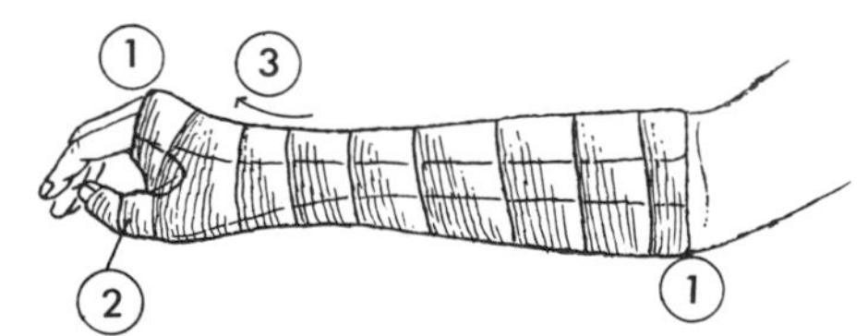

Subsequent Immobilization After Swelling Subsides

Swelling usually subsides within 5–7 days. At this time a circular cast over a lightly padded stockinette can be applied.

1. The cast extends from just below the elbow to the metacarpophalangeal joints.
2. The wrist is in slight dorsiflexion and radial deviation.
3. The thumb is in the grasp position and
4. The cast extends across the interphalangeal joint of the thumb.
5. The cast is molded carefully to support the proximal carpal row and is contoured between the hypothenar eminences.
6. The cast extends to the distal palmar crease.

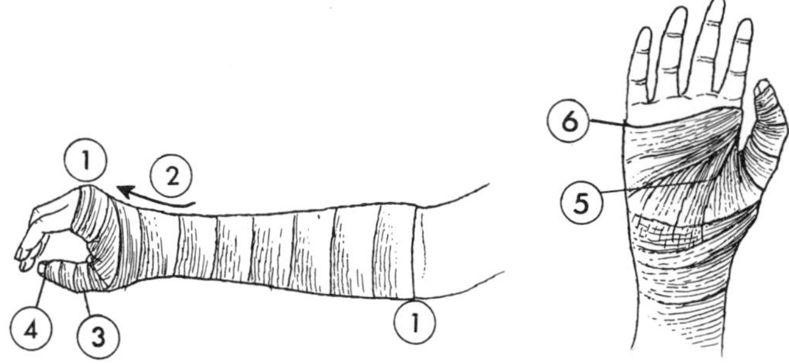

Symptomatic Follow-Up and Management

Ninety to ninety-five per cent of scaphoid fractures heal in 8–12 weeks with adequate immobilization. These fractures heal clinically much earlier than they do radiographically. Treatment, therefore, is based primarily on clinical symptoms rather than radiographic changes, which are difficult to interpret.

An initial period of cast immobilization is planned for 6–8 weeks. During this time immobilization should be complete with a short-arm cast. However, if the patient has persistent symptoms after the cast is applied, consider extending the cast above the elbow or occasionally operative fixation may be necessary. The cast is inspected every 2 weeks, and if it becomes loose a new, snugly fitting cast is applied.

At the end of 8 weeks the cast is removed and the patient is carefully examined. If the patient has a pain-free wrist, a reasonable range of motion, and is able to grip with little or no localized tenderness, the plaster may be discarded. However, the wrist should be protected with a splint and contact sports should be avoided until complete union is evident on x-ray.

If the patient has persistent discomfort, weakness, pain, or tenderness in the wrist snuff box, the cast is reapplied for 4–6 more weeks. Cast immobilization is continued for no longer than 3 months. If at the end of this time the fracture is still clinically symptomatic, operative treatment with internal fixation and bone grafting should be considered. The fracture may still be visible after the plaster is discarded; however, it is usually obliterated in the subsequent 6- to 12-month follow-up x-rays.

This protocol is applicable to the usual stable scaphoid fracture. For the unstable scaphoid fracture in 5–10 per cent of cases, early operative internal stabilization is generally indicated. Signs of instability include displacement of the fracture initially by more than 2 mm, an oblique fracture rather than the usual transverse fracture, and a comminuted fracture, particularly in the proximal third of the scaphoid.

Management of Unstable, Displaced, or Slowly Healing Fractures

Types

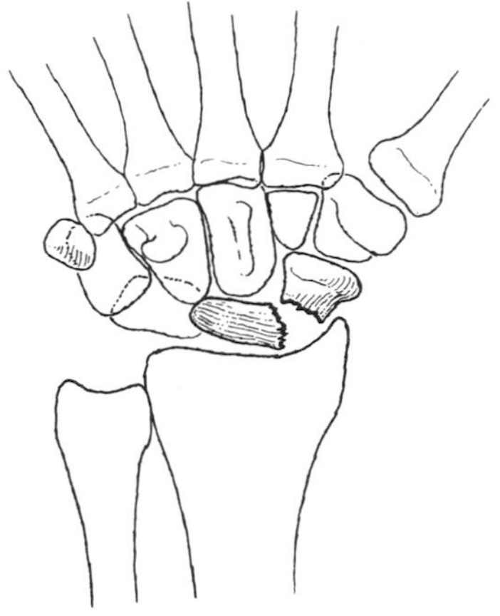

A fracture with horizontal displacement and a fracture gap, which takes longer to fill in.

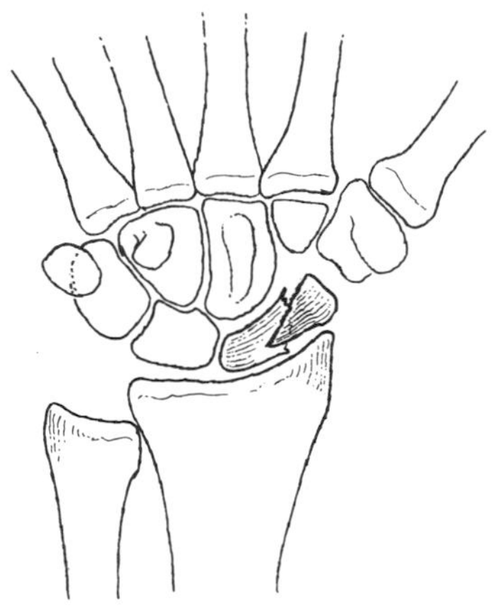

An oblique fracture, which is displaced by intrinsic and extrinsic muscle pull.

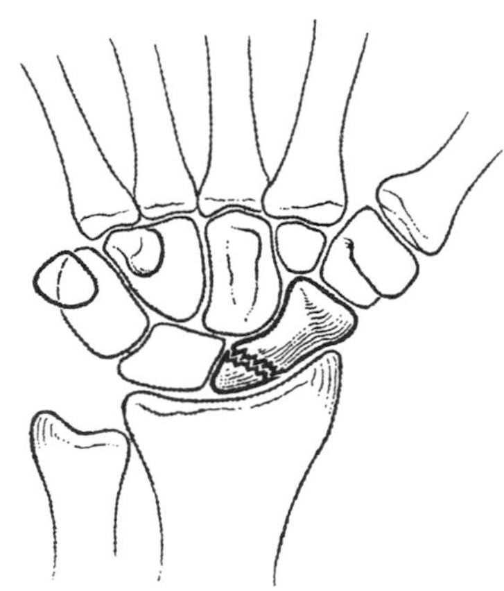

A fracture of the proximal third. This heals more slowly due to deprivation of blood supply, which must enter from the distal fragment.

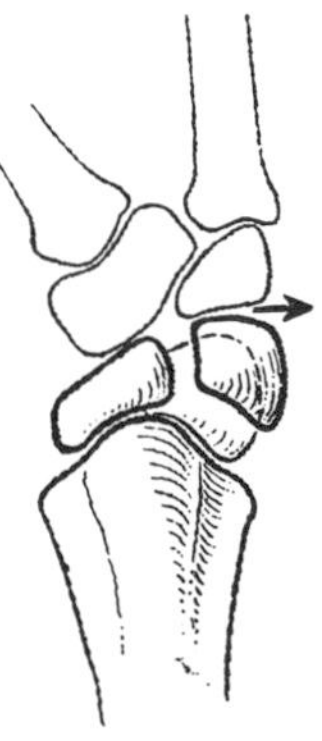

A scaphoid fracture associated with a perilunate dislocation. Unless anatomic reduction is achieved by closed manipulation of this unstable injury, it should be opened and the scaphoid should be fixed and stabilized internally.

Effect of Instability of the Scaphoid on Carpal Stability

1. A stable transverse scaphoid fracture maintains normal orientation and support for the proximal and distal rows of the carpus.
2. An unstable displaced scaphoid fracture angulates dorsally and produces a "humpback deformity."
3. The volar displacement of the distal fragment leads to loss of support between the proximal and distal carpal rows.

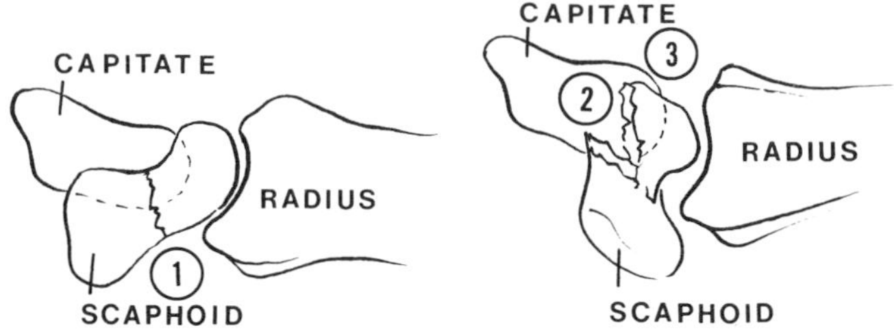

Closed Management of a Fracture With Displacement of the Fragments

Prereduction X-Ray

1. Fracture of the mid-third of the scaphoid.
2. The normal relationship of the fragments to the surrounding carpal bones is disturbed.
3. The fragments are angulated.

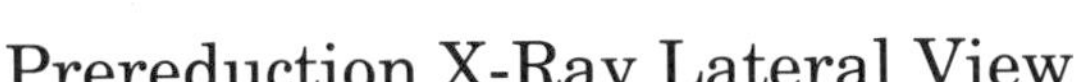

Prereduction X-Ray Lateral View

1. The displaced fracture has developed a "humpback" deformity.
2. This causes malalignment of the scaphoid with the proximal and distal carpal rows and is likely to lead to carpal intercalary dorsal collapse.

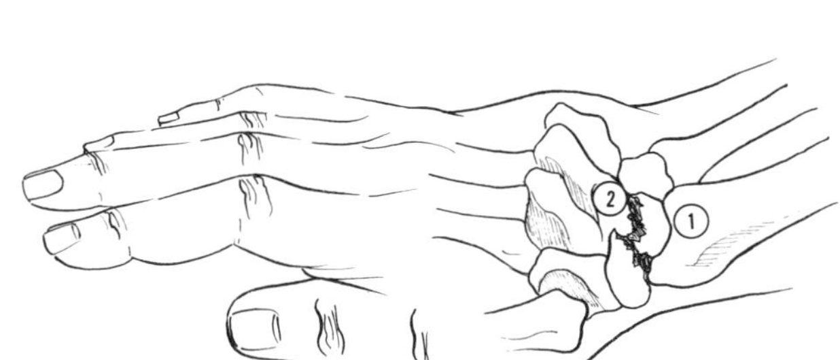

Reduction

Fluoroscopic study revealed that a position of moderate radial deviation of the hand realigned the fragments.
1. The hand is deviated toward the radius.
2. The fragments are in normal alignment.

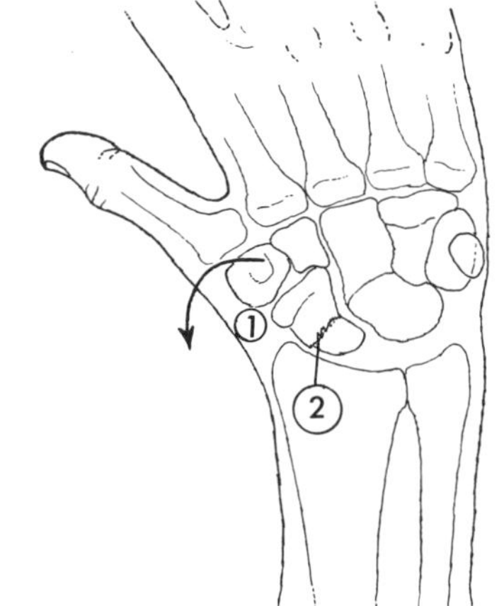

1. A fracture that is stable on fluoroscopy in both the anteroposterior and lateral views may be immobilized simply with a cast that includes the index and long fingers as well as the thumb.
2. The wrist is in slight extension and radial deviation to maintain reduction of the scaphoid.

Note: If the fracture is likely to be unstable in the cast, percutaneous Kirschner wires or intraosseous screw fixation is indicated.

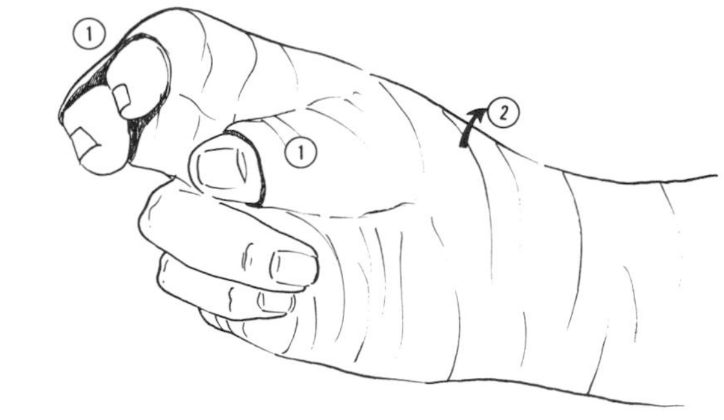

Postreduction

LATERAL VIEW

1. The scapholunate angle is close to normal on the lateral view of the carpus.
2. The volar angulation or "humpback" deformity of the scaphoid has been corrected so that the scaphoid is again properly aligned with the proximal and distal carpal rows.

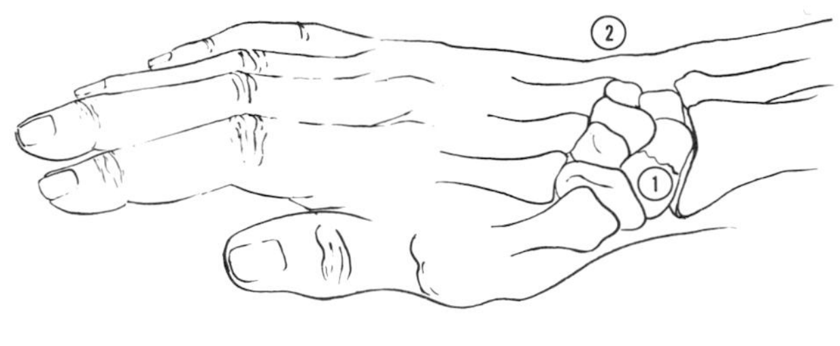

KIRSCHNER WIRE FIXATION

1. A percutaneous Kirschner wire is passed through the scaphoid and
2. Into the capitate and lunate to temporarily support the reduction.

Note: These pins are cut and buried beneath the skin. They may be removed in an outpatient procedure at 4–6 weeks.

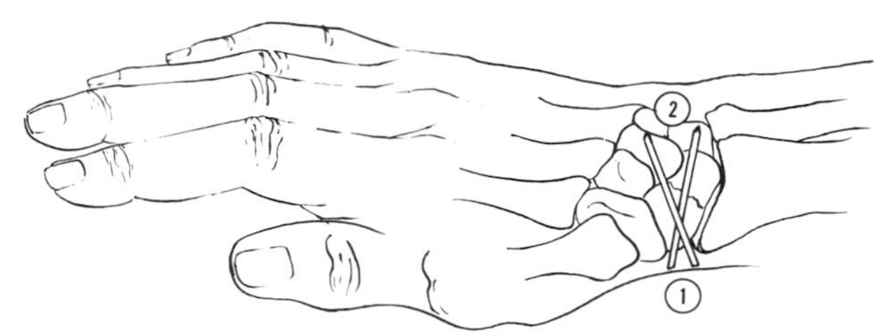

Cast Immobilization

- the fracture is immobilized in a three-finger cast after pin fixation.
- the cast is removed at 4–6 weeks to permit removal of the pins.
- additional cast immobilization is necessary for 12–16 weeks with these unstable scaphoid fractures.
- if adequate reduction of the fracture is not achieved initially or if the humpback deformity is not corrected, open reduction and internal fixation should be carried out.

Choices for Managing Unstable Displaced Fractures by Open Reduction

REMARKS

In managing the potential or the truly unstable scaphoid fracture, the physician should select methods that effectively add to the stability. Occasionally a cast that includes three fingers including the thumb may increase stability. This can be supplemented by subcutaneous pin fixation of the scaphoid if the fracture can be adequately reduced.

In attempting a closed reduction of these fractures, it is important to determine that the scapholunate angle has been restored so that the chances for subsequent collapse of the carpal alignment are mitigated by correcting the "humpback position." If this cannot be accomplished by closed methods, operative open reduction and internal fixation are indicated.

Open Reduction and Screw Fixation

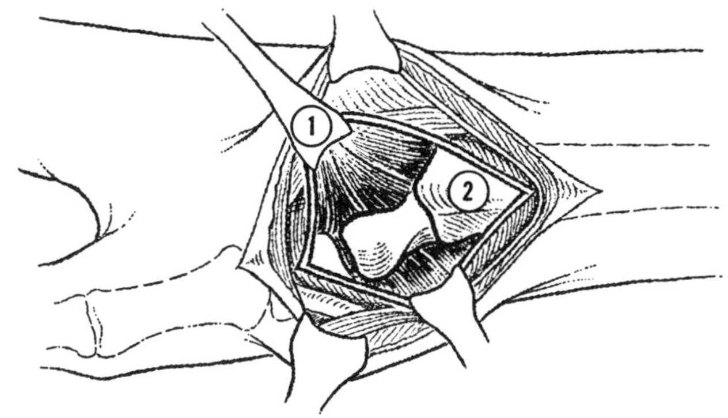

1. The unstable or displaced scaphoid fracture that cannot be adequately reduced by these methods is best opened and transfixed with a Herbert screw.
2. This is inserted from a palmar radial approach, which does not disrupt the blood supply.

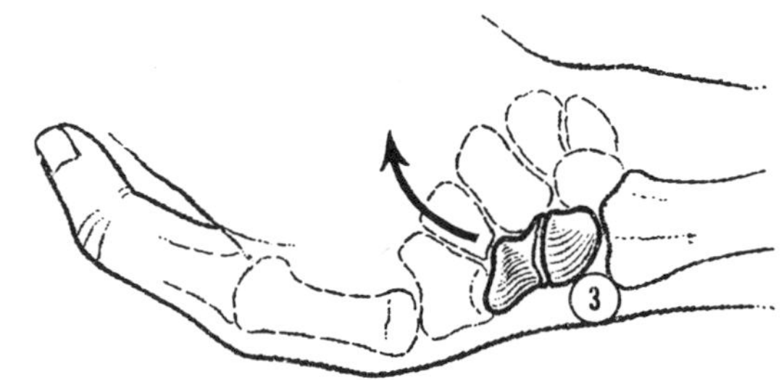

3. The fracture site is carefully identified with the wrist in ulnar deviation.

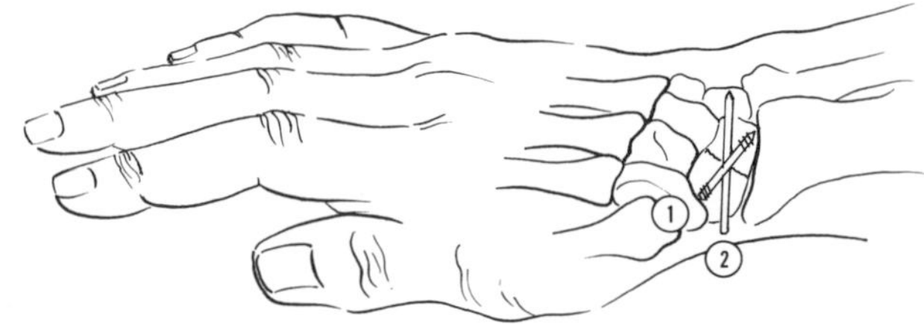

1. The screw is inserted from the distal to the proximal poles and provides adequate stability for most displaced scaphoid fractures.
2. If there are additional injuries to the carpal ligaments or a transscaphoid perilunate dislocation, these ligaments should also be stabilized.

Alternative Method of Kirschner Wire Fixation With Bone Graft

1. A bone graft may be necessary to fill in defects with a comminuted fracture.
2. The fracture may be stabilized with a transarticular Kirschner wire passed from the greater multangulum into the scaphoid.

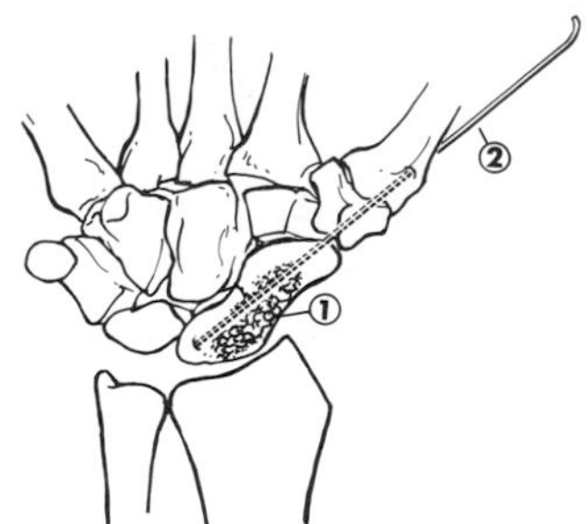

■ Subacute Fractures of the Scaphoid (Diagnosed Three or More Months After Injury)

REMARKS

Many of these fractures are initially unrecognized or are treated as wrist sprains or not treated at all. By the time the diagnosis is made after 3 or more months, bone resorption has occurred and cysts are frequently evident in the fracture fragments. There may also be some evidence of bony sclerosis of the proximal fragment, which may indicate some avascular necrosis.

Cysts or bone sclerosis do not preclude bony union with closed treatment. Fifty to 75 per cent of these initially unrecognized fractures can heal with closed reduction and cast immobilization. Conversely, approximately half of them do require operative stabilization.

If there is no evidence of arthritis or carpal collapse, a trial period of cast treatment may be warranted for the patient with a scaphoid fracture of 3 months or more, or of uncertain, duration.

If there is evidence of carpal collapse from a humpback deformity, operative correction is indicated.

Nonunion of the Scaphoid

REMARKS

Most un-united scaphoid fractures require treatment. This statement would seem unnecessary except for the fairly common problem of the asymptomatic nonunion found incidentally on x-ray of the wrist. In the past many of these scaphoid nonunions were considered as congenital bipartite scaphoids. However, careful review by Louis and others has shown that they are traumatic, not congenital, in origin.

Asymptomatic nonunions can cause progressive instability and eventual osteoarthritic changes. There is a strong correlation between the severity of degenerative changes in the wrist and the duration of scaphoid nonunion. Degenerative arthritis is most commonly seen 10–20 years after the nonunion develops. Based on the high probability that degenerative changes will occur, it is recommended that a scaphoid nonunion that demonstrates displacement or carpal instability (scapholunate dissociation) be reduced, fixed internally, and grafted, preferably before arthritic changes occur.

Occasionally a patient with an asymptomatic scaphoid nonunion reinjures the wrist and becomes symptomatic. It is at this time of reinjury that the old nonunion is detected. Under these circumstances, a period of symptomatic cast immobilization and nonsteroidal anti-inflammatory medications may be indicated, particularly in the older patient with a previously asymptomatic nonunion.

Management of the nonunion must be based partially on the patient's age and functional demands. The usual candidate for operative correction is a young adult, less than 30 years old, who has symptomatic or unstable nonunion that has not responded to a trial of cast immobilization for 2–3 months.

Chronic Scaphoid Nonunion of Fifteen Years' Duration

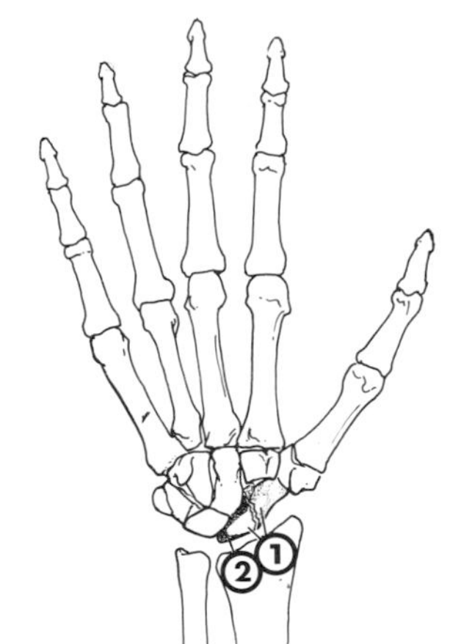

1. There are cystic changes and evidence of rotational deformity of the scaphoid found on x-ray of a previously "asymptomatic" patient approximately 15 years after the first injury.
2. There is spurring and evidence of early degenerative changes secondary to the chronic nonunion and moderate instability of the wrist.

Note: This patient with a chronic nonunion who was previously asymptomatic can be treated with a period of cast immobilization to alleviate the acute symptoms. The patient should be advised that the possibility of subsequent progressive degenerative changes is present but the period of cast support may relieve most of the present symptoms.

Nonoperative Management

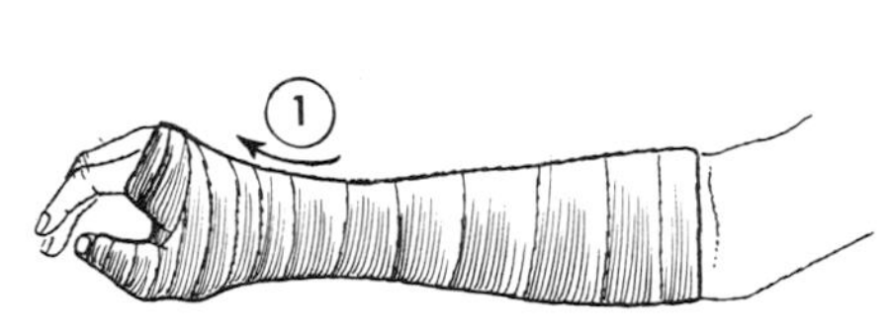

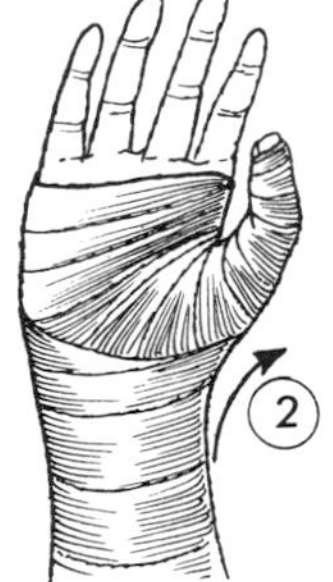

Apply a circular cast over a stockinette without padding.

1. Hold the wrist slightly dorsiflexed and
2. In moderate radial deviation. (Evaluate the ideal position for fracture reduction under image-intensified fluoroscopy.)

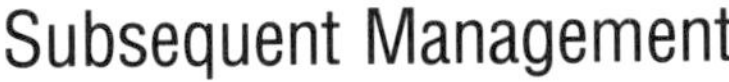

Subsequent Management

The cast is applied for 4–6 weeks. Nonsteroidal anti-inflammatory medication may be helpful to alleviate symptoms associated with acute injury of a chronic nonunion.

If the wrist symptoms have not been alleviated by this temporary trial of immobilization, operative stabilization and treatment of the chronic wrist problem should be recommended. However, results of stabilization of the scaphoid nonunion of this duration are likely to be much less satisfactory than they are for the acute scaphoid fracture or a nonunion of recent duration.

Surgical Management of Delayed Union and Nonunion

REMARKS

The usual candidate for operative treatment is a young working adult less than 30 years of age with pain, loss of grip strength, and limitation of wrist motion. A trial of nonoperative treatment is worth employing before deciding on operative treatment to relieve the symptoms.

An asymptomatic patient who is found to have an undisplaced nonunion and no evidence of wrist instability should be advised of the possibility of late degenerative changes. However, this advice should be tempered by the patient's age and functional demands.

The surgical procedure most often employed for scaphoid nonunion is open reduction with bone grafting and internal fixation using a Herbert screw. For patients who do heavy work and have signs of carpal collapse, a wrist arthrodesis may be necessary to alleviate symptoms.

Appearance on X-Ray

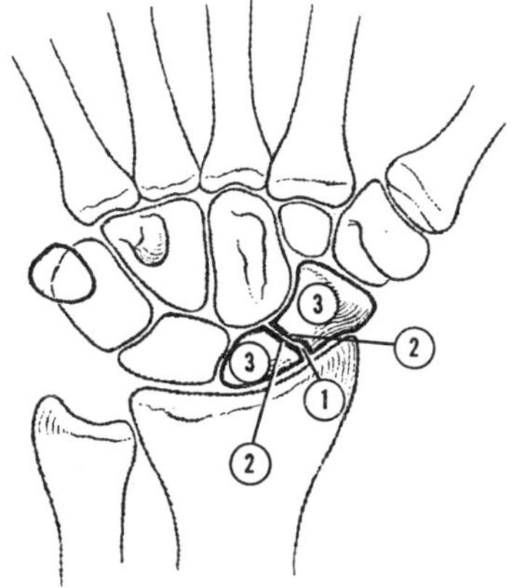

1. Old un-united fracture through the body.
2. Fractured surfaces are smooth and sclerotic.
3. Sclerosis of fragments does not alter the prognosis for healing.

Note: There is slight evidence of arthritis in the radiocarpal joint adjacent to the fracture.

Preoperative X-Rays

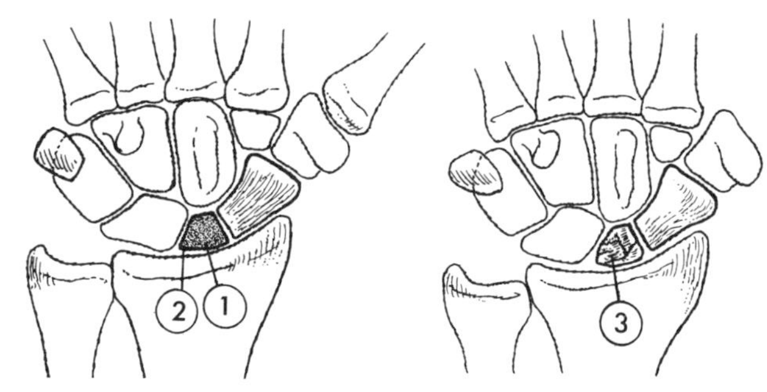

1. The proximal fragment is a third of the scaphoid.
2. The fragment is dense and
3. Comminuted.

Symptomatic Nonunion

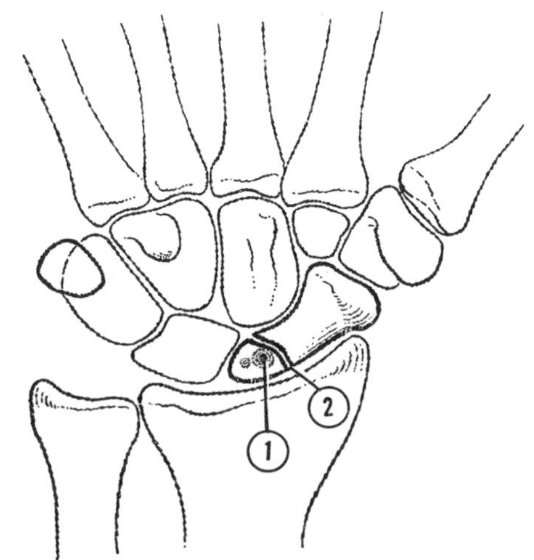

1. Cystic fragmentation persists despite previous attempt at bone grafting.
2. There is slight radiocarpal arthritis but not generalized involvement.

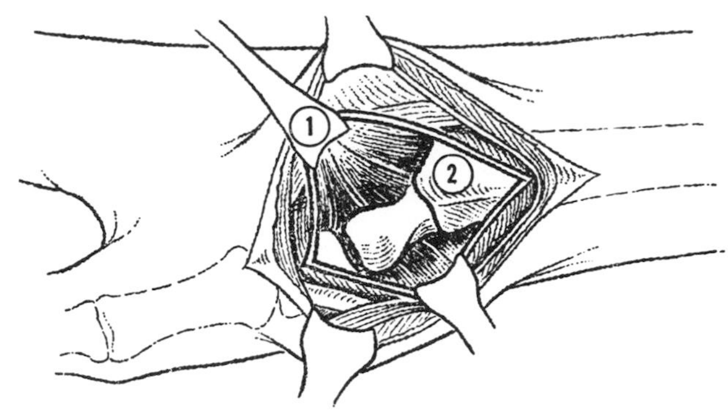

Surgical Alternative

1. A volar approach is used to expose the scaphoid and to minimize damage to the circulation.
2. Occasionally the radial styloid may be removed to allow better visualization and better decompression of the scaphoid nonunion.

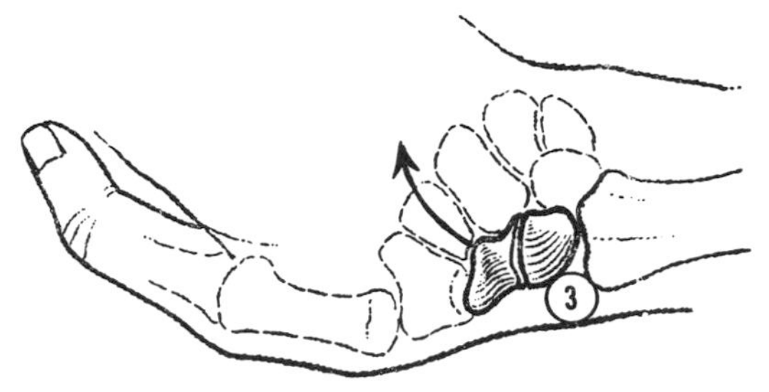

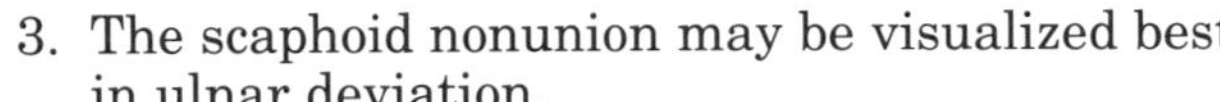

3. The scaphoid nonunion may be visualized best in ulnar deviation.

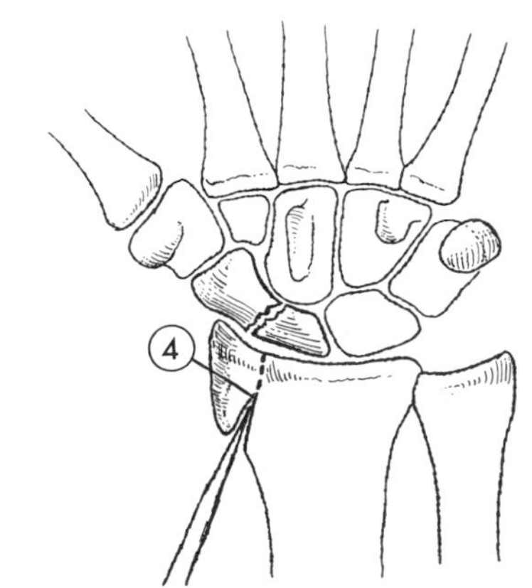

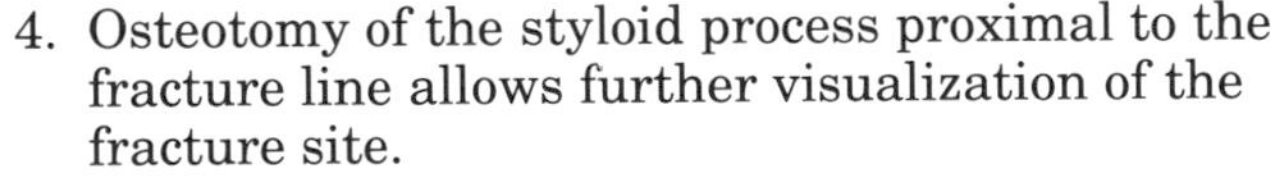

4. Osteotomy of the styloid process proximal to the fracture line allows further visualization of the fracture site.

Note: An intraoperative x-ray is important to be sure of the location of the nonunion.

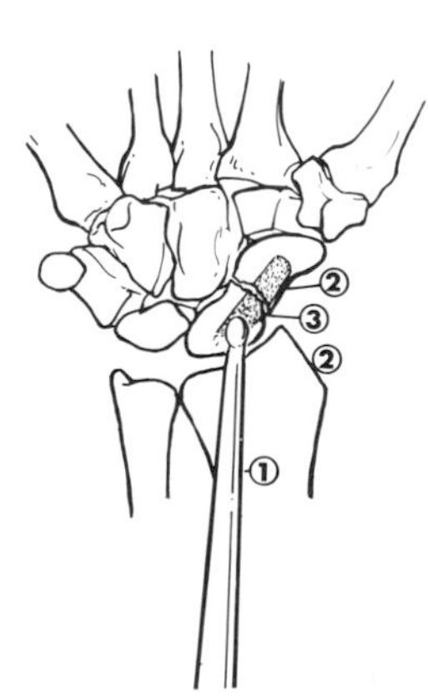

1. A gauge is used to remove a trough across the nonunion site.
2. This is filled with autologous graft taken from the radial styloid.
3. Additional chips are packed around any cystic changes in the scaphoid.

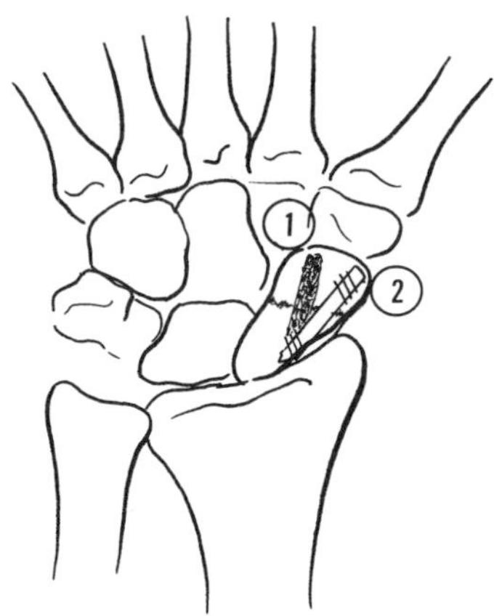

1. After bone grafting is accomplished, the fracture site usually requires stabilization.
2. This is best accomplished with a Herbert screw or a similar device to stabilize the scaphoid proximally and distally or with Kirschner wires.

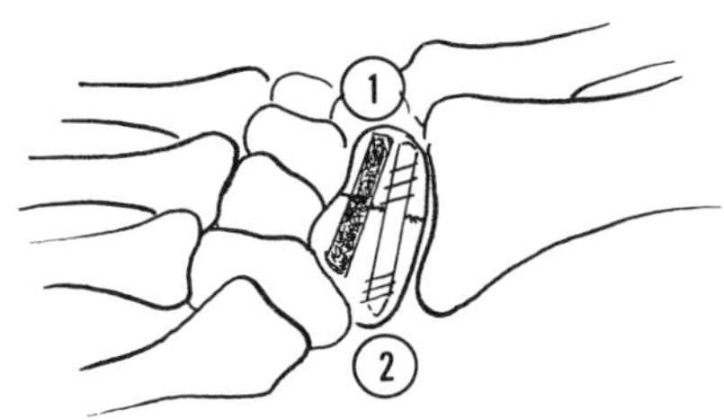

1. The reduction of the scaphoid on the lateral view should demonstrate correction of any "humpback" deformity.
2. The relationship of the scaphoid to the proximal and distal carpal row should be restored with the use of Kirschner wires if necessary.

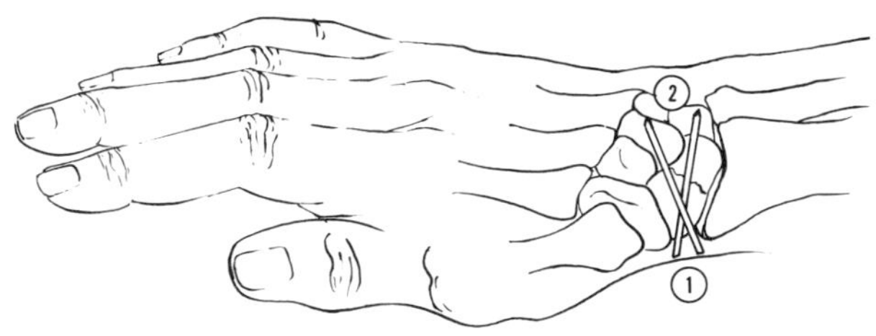

1. If the nonunion of the scaphoid is associated with a humpback deformity and secondary carpal collapse, the fracture can be stabilized with a Kirschner wire through the scaphoid into the proximal and
2. Into the distal carpal row.

Follow-Up Management

External cast immobilization is continued and changed as necessary every 2 weeks as the cast becomes loose. If a transarticular Kirschner wire is used, it may be removed in 4–6 weeks. Immobilization is continued until the fracture is clinically and radiographically healed. This may take as long as 3–5 months.

If radiographic union is not complete by the end of 4–6 months and the patient is asymptomatic, the cast may be removed and the patient allowed free use of the limb. Subsequently radiographic obliteration of the fracture site may occur in 4–6 months after clinical healing. Some residual wrist stiffness should be anticipated, but pain relief and fracture union occur in the majority of nonunions treated by this method.

Management of Chronic Post-Traumatic Arthritis—Arthroplasty or Arthrodesis

REMARKS

Occasionally, nonunion of the scaphoid fracture will produce severe symptomatic arthritis years later. This is especially likely if carpal instability and dorsiflexion collapse have resulted from the loss of scaphoid stability. Most patients with generalized carpal arthritis are older.

Frequently the symptoms are intermittent and are the result of overuse. Local intra-articular cortisone injection, splint immobilization, and systemic anti-inflammatory agents will relieve periodic symptoms for many years.

If the wrist pain and functional loss cause permanent and significant disability despite these nonoperative measures, a limited or complete arthrodesis of the wrist is the preferred method of treatment. Wrist arthroplasty may be considered in the sedentary individual, but these have not proved as satisfactory as arthrodeses for most patients with this type of chronic traumatic arthritis.

Appearance on X-Ray I

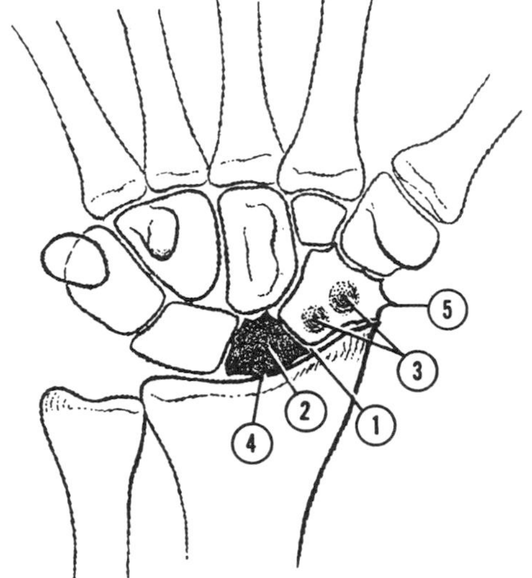

1. Nonunion of the fracture of the scaphoid.
2. The ulnar fragment is dense and sclerotic.
3. The radial fragment shows cystic changes.
4. The joint space is narrowed, indicative of degeneration of articular cartilage.
5. Bony spurs are consistent with osteoarthritis.

Appearance on X-Ray II

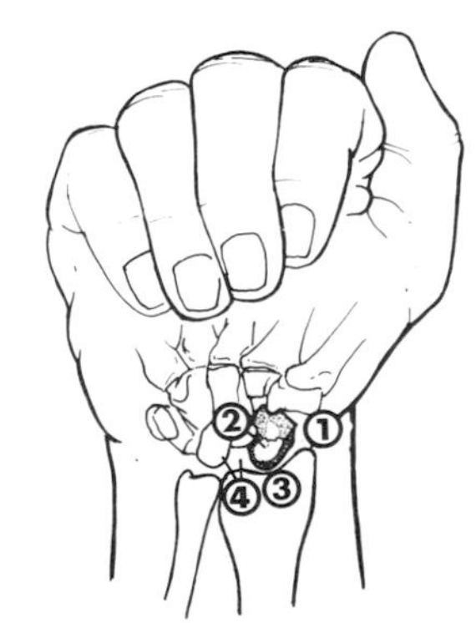

ANTEROPOSTERIOR VIEW

1. Persistent nonunion of the scaphoid.
2. The scaphoid is cystic and irregular with osteophytes.
3. The radiocarpal joint space is narrowed.
4. The palmar horn of the lunate has shifted distally on the neck of the capitate, and the scapholunate space is widened.

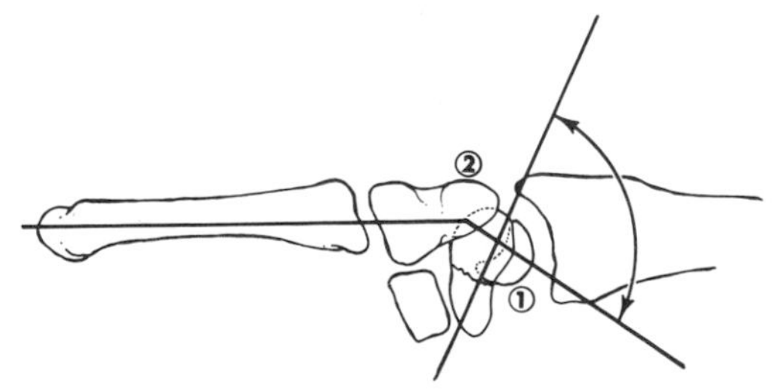

LATERAL VIEW

1. The lunate has dorsiflexed as the result of loss of scaphoid stability.
2. The capitate has shifted proximally and dorsally.

Wrist Arthrodesis

1. A bone graft is removed from the radius and carpus, and its position is reversed.
2. The graft is fixed to the radius and the carpus with small fragment screws.

Note: An alternative method if the radiocarpal joint is not damaged is a limited arthrodesis of the scaphoid to the greater and lesser multangulum. In most instances chronic long-standing nonunion of the scaphoid produces radiocarpal arthritis and requires radiocarpal fusion.

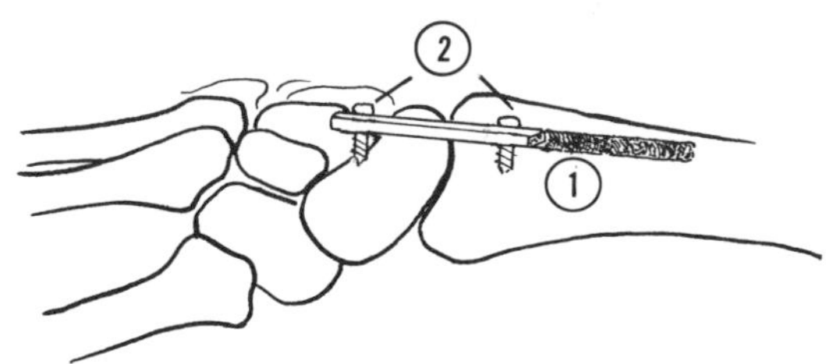

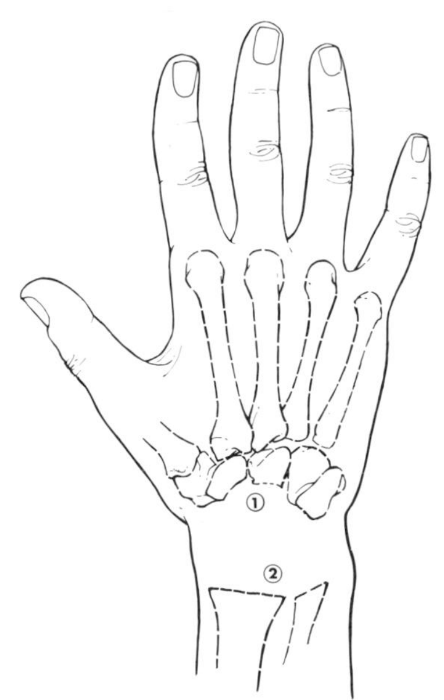

Alternative Method—Resectional Arthroplasty

1. Occasionally motion of the wrist may be salvaged by removing the proximal carpal rows. This is indicated only if there is reasonable articular surface on the capitate.
2. The resection of the proximal row leaves a large gap, which is stabilized with the surrounding capsule. The results of this procedure are less predictable than arthrodesis.

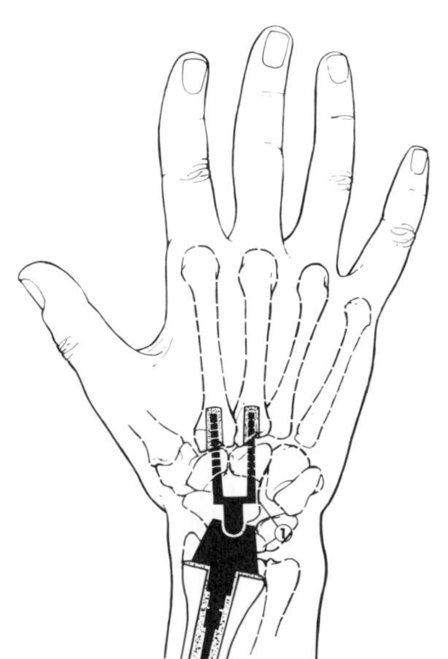

Alternative Method—Arthroplasty

1. Arthroplasty of the wrist may be considered in the individual who is relatively sedentary and will place less demand on the arthritic wrist. This has the advantage of maintaining wrist motion but gives less stability and is subject to failure in the individual who makes heavy demands on the wrist.

LUNATE AND PERILUNATE DISLOCATIONS AND SUBLUXATIONS

Perilunate and Lunate Dislocations: Post-Traumatic Carpal Dissociation

REMARKS

Most hyperextension forces on the wrist that fracture the scaphoid may also disrupt the scapholunate and perilunate ligaments to some extent. Such dissociation is particularly likely when hyperextension forces combine with a rotatory or supination overload on the wrist.

This sequence of injury includes first fracture of the scaphoid then disruption of the carpal ligaments, which produces a perilunate dislocation of the carpus on the lunate. The other outcome of a hyperextension-supination injury may be a complete dislocation of the lunate out of its articulation with the radius.

These fairly common injuries cause severe disruptions of carpal stability. Surprisingly, they may not be appreciated at times if the emergency room x-rays do not adequately visualize the relationships of the carpal bones and are not carefully analyzed for signs of instability.

Impairment from chronic scapholunate or perilunate instability may, like the un-united scaphoid fracture, range from minimal limitation of motion to an extremely painful traumatic arthritis of the wrist. Any swollen wrist should be carefully evaluated to determine if there are signs of lunate or perilunate instability. This analysis should be based on an understanding of the normal carpal relationships, as well as the abnormal, as seen on adequate radiographic studies.

Mechanism of Dorsal Perilunate Dislocation

1. The patient falls on the outstretched hand with the wrist in slight extension. The force acts directly on the palm of the hand.
2. A second force is applied to the wrist to produce a supination mechanism.
3. The capitate-lunate articulation is disrupted.
4. The carpal bones are driven dorsally behind the lunate.
5. The result is a dislocation of the carpus from the lunate (perilunate dislocation).
6. The radiolunate articulation is preserved.

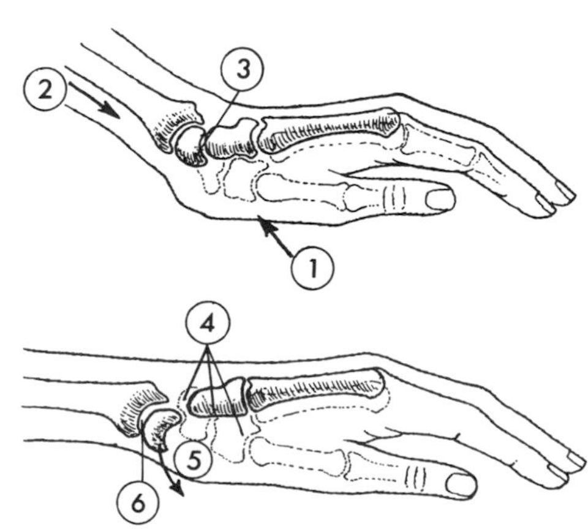

Mechanism of Lunate Dislocation

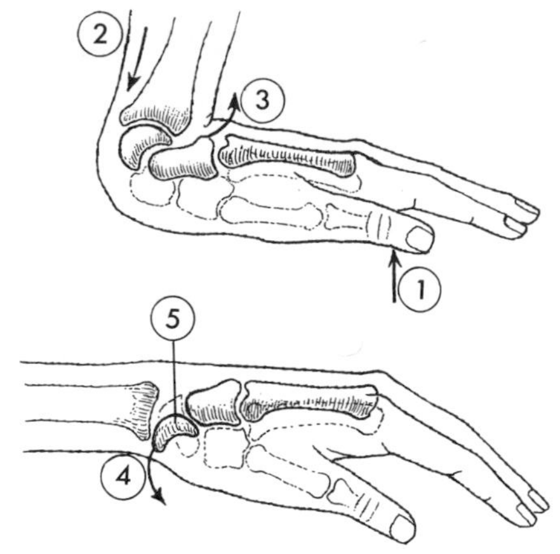

The hand and carpus are severely hyperextended by

1. The force acting upward on the fingers and metacarpal heads and
2. The force acting downward in the line of the radius.
3. The capitate rotates dorsally on the lunate.
4. The lunate is squeezed out of the wrist joint.
5. The rotated lunate lies anterior to the wrist joint.

Transscaphoid Perilunate Dislocations

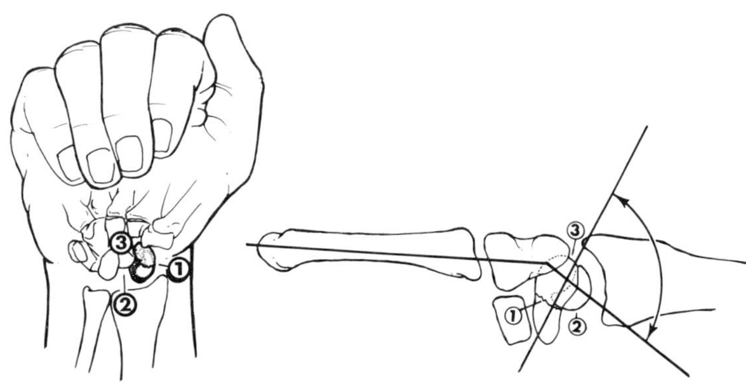

1. One of the commonest causes of carpal or perilunate dislocations is a fracture through the scaphoid. The fracture to the scaphoid eliminates the support to the proximal distal carpal rows.
2. The space between the lunate and scaphoid is widened as the scapholunate ligaments are torn.
3. The scaphoid rotates in a volar direction and the carpus dislocates dorsally. Usually the lunate remains articulating with the radius.

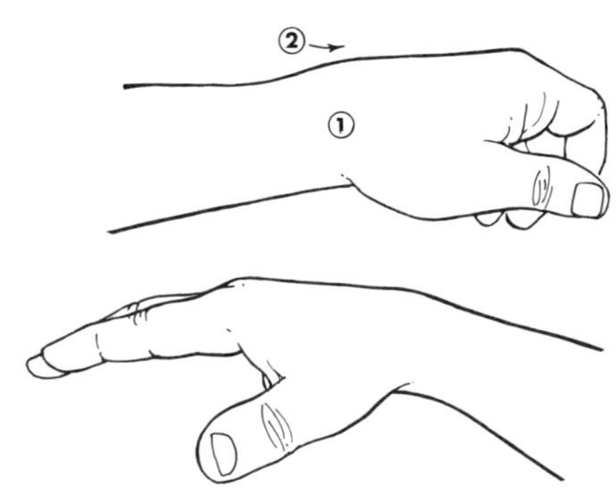

Clinical Deformity

1. The injured wrist is always swollen after these injuries.
2. There is a distal dinner-fork deformity as a result of the dorsal displacement of the distal carpal row.

Assessment

1. Suspect carpal disruption and instability with any grossly swollen wrist after an injury in spite of initial inconclusive x-ray assessment.
2. Fractures of the radial styloid are often associated with carpal instability and should be carefully evaluated.

Note: Signs of chronic instability include repeated clicking or pain in the wrist on radial and ulnar deviation associated with scaphoid subluxation over the dorsal rim of the radius. Keep in mind that there is such a thing as a sprained wrist, that is, a disruption of the ligamentous attachments to the carpal bones. Such injuries are best recognized and treated acutely because reconstruction of the problem is frequently quite difficult.

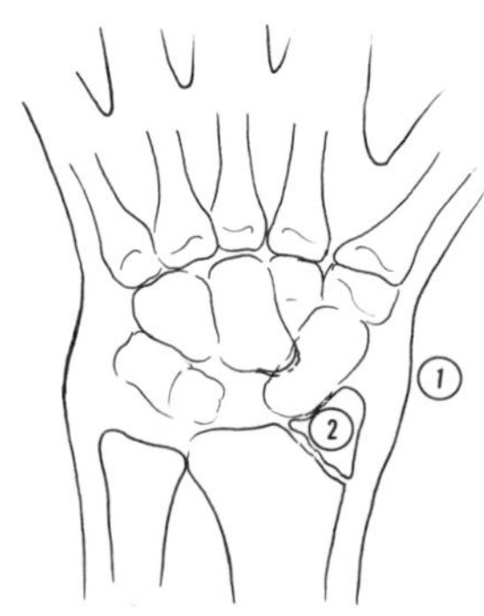

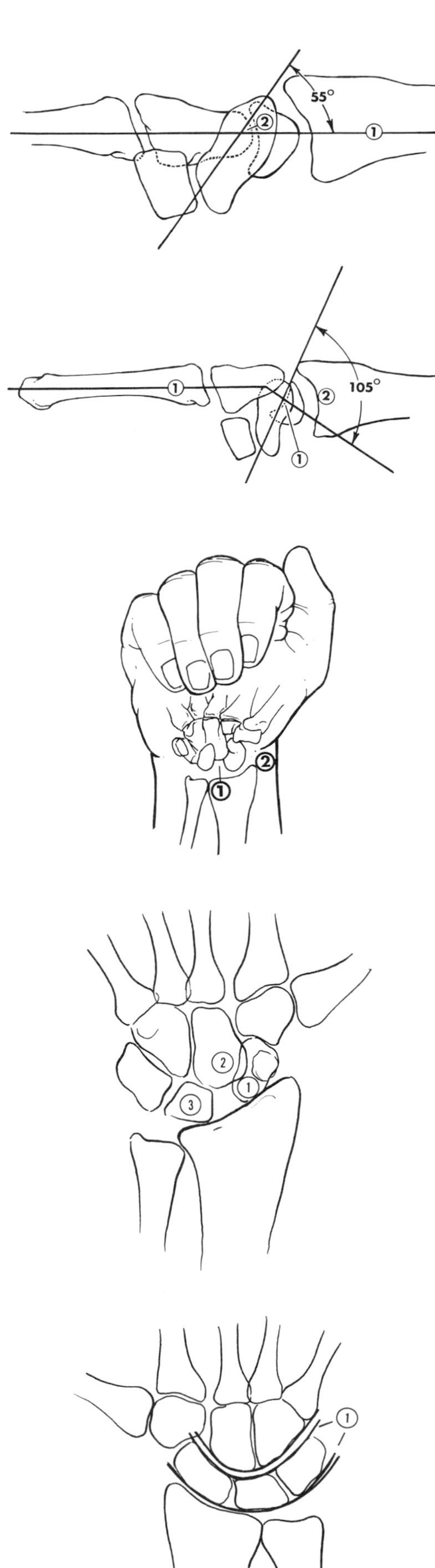

Normal Carpal Relationships

On a true lateral view,
1. The axes of the radius, lunate, and capitate form a straight line.
2. The axis of the scaphoid intersects the radial-lunate-capitate axis at an angle of 30°–60°.

Perilunate Instability

LATERAL X-RAY

1. The lunate is dorsiflexed and the radial-lunate-capitate axis is no longer a straight line.
2. The scapholunate angle exceeds 70°.

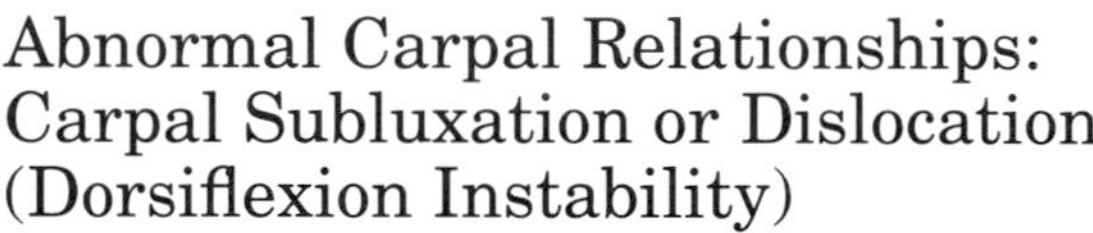

Abnormal Carpal Relationships: Carpal Subluxation or Dislocation (Dorsiflexion Instability)

This is best seen on a posteroanterior view taken with the wrist supinated and the fist clenched.
1. The space between the scaphoid and lunate exceeds 2 mm.
2. The length of the scaphoid is decreased.

Additional X-Ray Findings of Carpal Dissociation or Dislocation Seen on Anteroposterior View

1. A foreshortened scaphoid with a cortical ring sign due to overlapping of the distal scaphoid on the proximal scaphoid.
2. Overlapping of the scaphoid on the capitate.
3. A change in the shape of the lunate from trapezoid to wedge shape.

1. These findings contrast with the normal smooth arc and anatomy seen on the anterior posterior view of the wrist. If there is any break in these three lines, malalignment should be suspected.

Uncomplicated Dorsal Perilunate Dislocations

REMARKS

This lesion is relatively common. The lunate is the focal point around which the dislocation of the remaining carpus occurs. The lunate maintains its normal anatomic position in relation to the radius; the rest of the carpus is displaced upward, backward, and outward. This injury can usually be reduced by closed methods. However, because of the disruption of the carpal ligaments and risk of carpal collapse, internal stabilization is frequently needed.

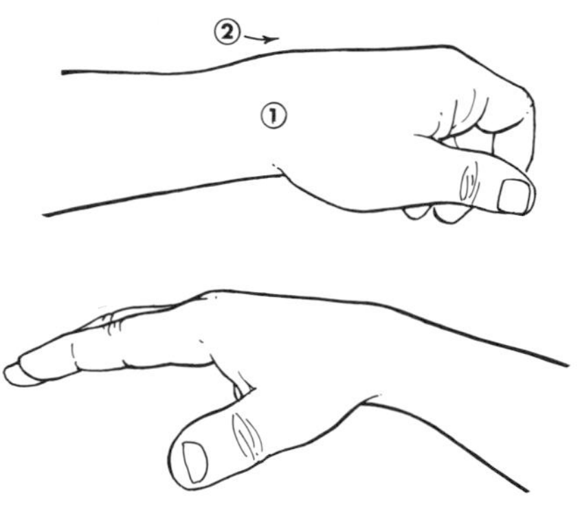

Clinical Deformity

1. The injured wrist is always swollen after these injuries.
2. There is a distal dinner-fork deformity as a result of the dorsal displacement of the distal carpal row.

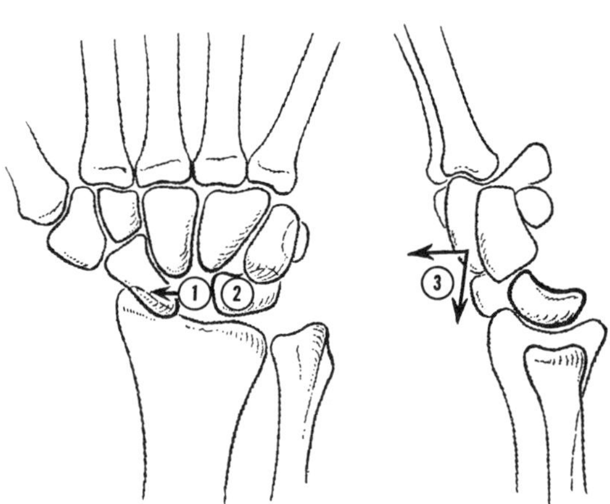

Prereduction X-Ray

1. The normal relationship of the lunate to the remaining carpal bones is lost; the carpus is displaced to the radial side.
2. The lunate is in normal relation to the radius.
3. The remaining carpus is displaced upward and backward.

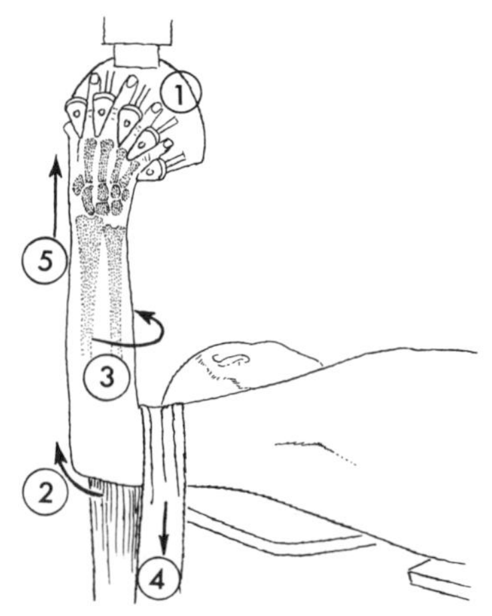

Reduction by Traction and Manipulation

TRACTION

1. Apply finger traction.
2. The elbow is flexed at a right angle.
3. The forearm is fully supinated.
4. Countertraction is accomplished by a muslin bandage attached to a water bucket.
5. Traction is maintained for at least 5–10 minutes to overcome carpal shortening.

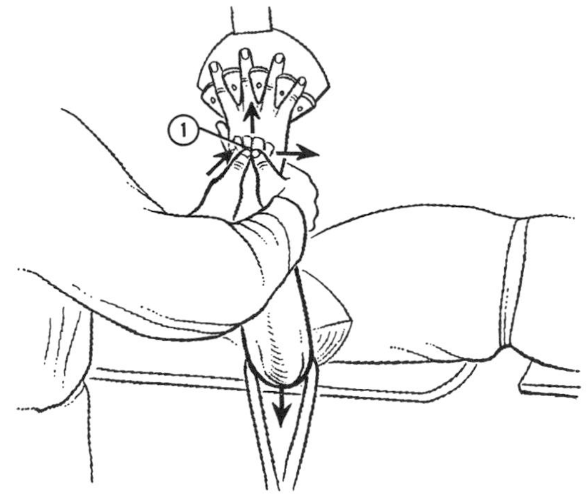

MANIPULATION

While traction is maintained,

1. Place both thumbs against the posterior aspect of the carpus and apply strong pressure forward and outward, and at the same time flex the wrist.

Note: Check the position of the carpus by x-ray before applying the plaster cast.

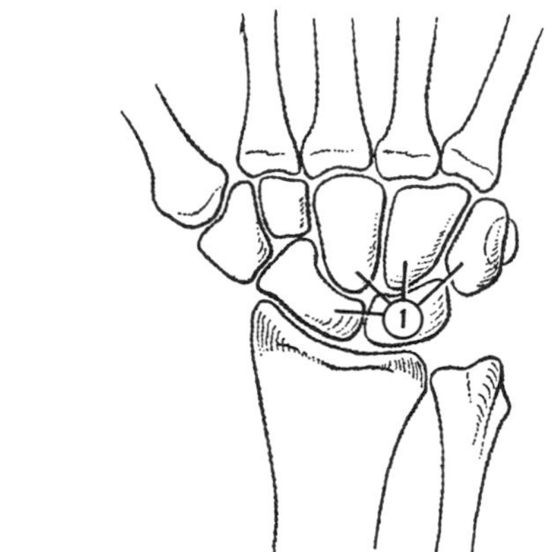

Postreduction X-Ray

1. The carpus is in normal anatomic alignment, and the scapholunate space is less than 2 mm.

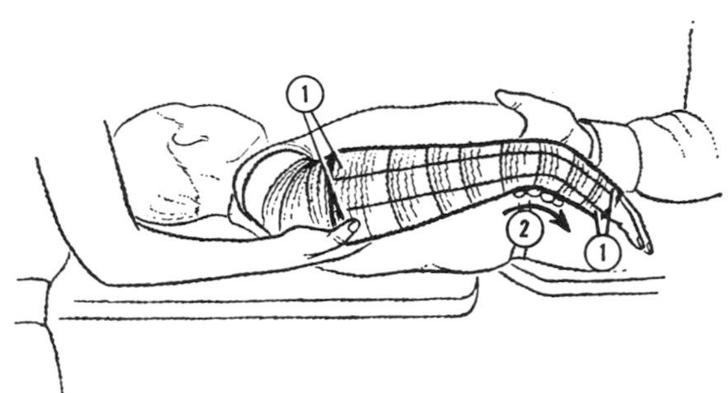

Immobilization

1. Apply anterior and posterior plaster slabs from just below the elbow to just proximal to the metacarpophalangeal joints.
2. The wrist is flexed 45°.

Note: If the reduction proves unstable, the carpus may be fixed with percutaneous pins.

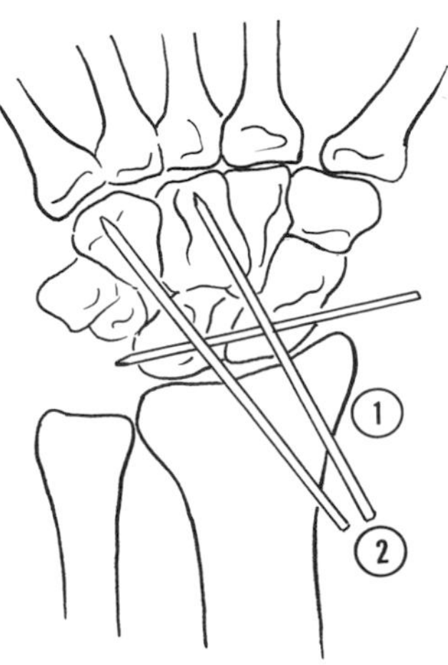

Alternative Method of Immobilization for Unstable Reduction

1. Multiple Kirschner wires are inserted percutaneously to stabilize the scaphoid to the lunate and
2. To the capitate.

Note: These wires are bent and maintain reduction for 4–6 weeks prior to removal.

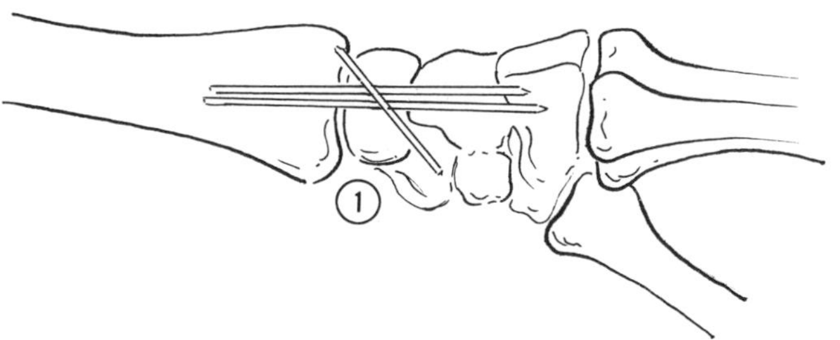

1. Reduction should restore the normal scapholunate angle and the relationship of the scaphoid to the proximal and distal carpal row, as seen on the lateral view.

Postreduction Management

The plaster splints are changed to a cast after the swelling subsides, usually by 5–7 days. Immobilization is continued for 2–3 weeks. During immobilization encourage active exercise of the fingers.

The plaster cast and/or percutaneous pins are removed by 3–4 weeks, after which time an active exercise program is started. The prognosis for recovery of function is usually good for injuries recognized acutely. However, if the diagnosis is not made in the first week or two, operative reduction is necessary, and the wrist is likely to be unstable.

Dorsal Perilunate Dislocation Complicated by Fracture or Dislocation of Other Carpal Bones

Dorsal perilunate dislocation is frequently complicated by lesions of the other carpal bones; the scaphoid is most frequently involved.

Dorsal Perilunate Dislocation With Fracture of the Scaphoid With Displacement of the Fragments

REMARKS

The proximal fragment remains with the lunate and the distal fragment is displaced dorsally with the rest of the carpus. This is the usual occurrence with these fracture-dislocations.

Mechanism

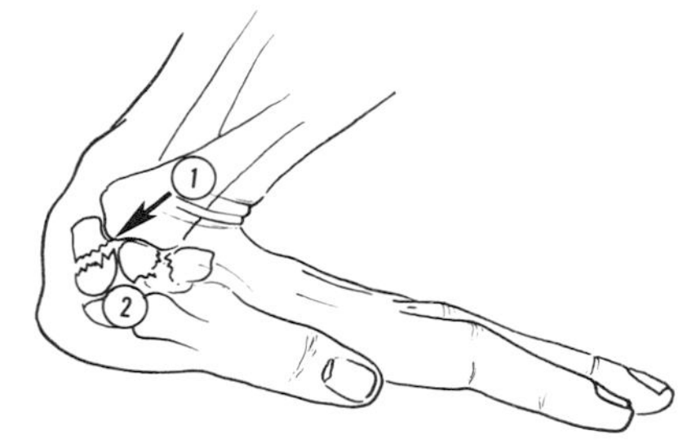

1. A hyperdorsiflexion injury to the wrist places an extreme load against the scaphoid as well as the capitate.
2. This can fracture both the scaphoid and the capitate, or produce a perilunate dislocation.

Appearance on X-Ray

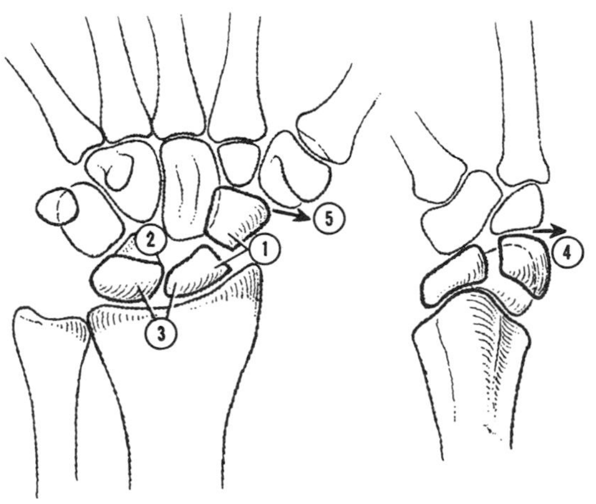

1. Fracture through the waist of the scaphoid.
2. The normal relationship of the carpal bones is disturbed; note the wide gap between the lunate and the capitate.
3. The lunate and the proximal half of the scaphoid are in normal relationship to the radius.
4. The carpus and the distal half of the scaphoid are displaced backward.
5. The carpus distal to the lunate and the proximal half of the scaphoid are displaced radially.

Note: A scaphoid fracture with this much displacement and instability of the carpus is best managed by primary internal fixation.

Management

The perilunate dislocation is reduced by traction and direct manipulation as described previously. The scaphoid fracture is then exposed and fixed internally with either a Kirschner wire or a Herbert screw or both.

Dorsal Perilunate Dislocation With Fracture of the Capitate and Scaphocapitate Syndrome

REMARKS

Hyperdorsiflexion of the wrist can fracture through the waist of the scaphoid and the neck of the capitate, as well as produce a perilunate dislocation. Frequently the head of the capitate and the proximal fragment of the scaphoid rotate together so that the capitate fragment remains completely displaced. Closed reduction usually fails. Reduction and internal fixation are usually necessary to stabilize this unstable injury.

Mechanism

1. A hyperdorsiflexion injury to the wrist places an extreme load against the scaphoid as well as the capitate.
2. This can fracture both the scaphoid and the capitate or produce a perilunate dislocation.

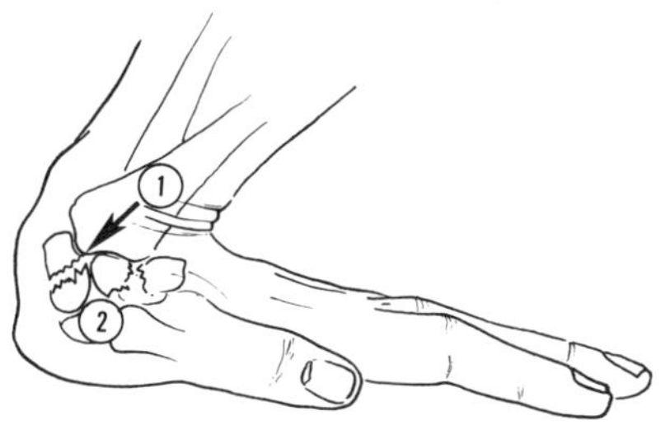

Appearance on X-Ray

1. Fracture of the capitate.
2. Fracture of the scaphoid with displacement.
3. Dorsal displacement of the carpus distal to the lunate.

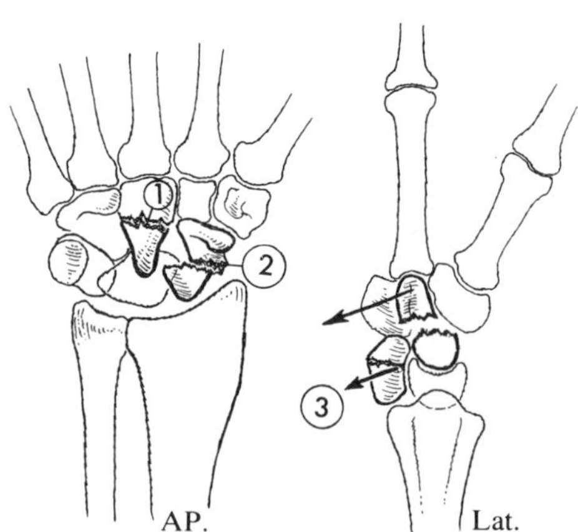

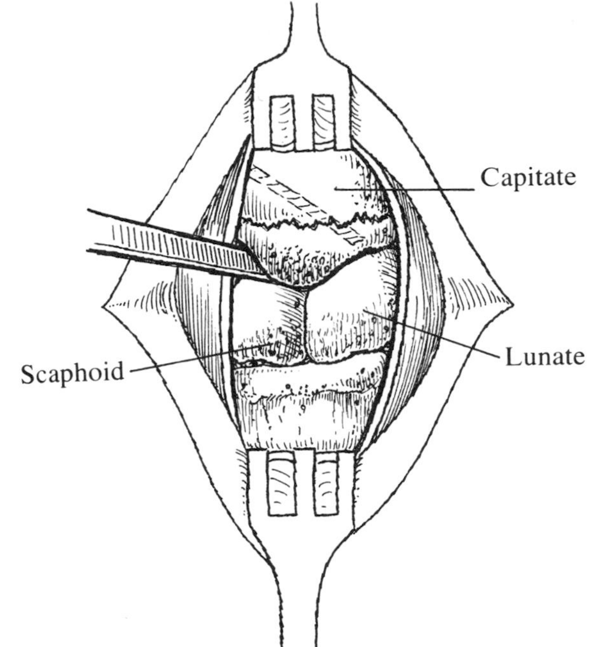

Management

The fracture of the scaphoid and capitate is sufficiently unstable to mandate internal stabilization. The fragments of both the capitate and scaphoid are visualized by a direct surgical approach and are fixed internally with either Kirschner wires or small fragment screws or both.

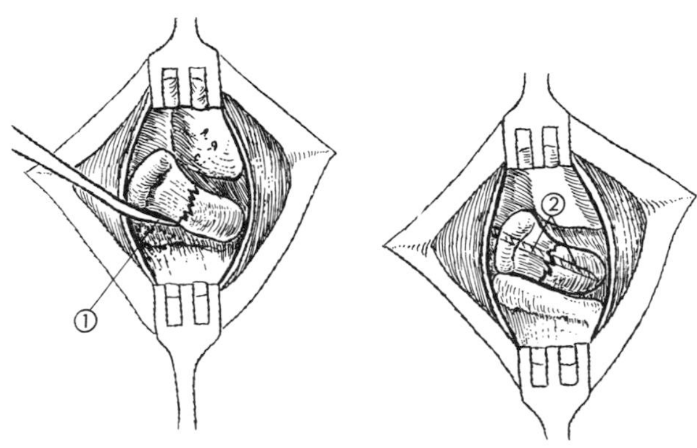

Management of Associated Unstable Fracture of the Scaphoid

1. The associated scaphoid fracture is approached via a separate incision on the volar aspect of the wrist to demonstrate the displaced fracture.
2. The fracture is fixed with either a Kirschner wire or Herbert screw, as described previously.

Volar Dislocation of the Lunate Bone

REMARKS

Replacement of the lunate by closed methods is generally achieved if the reduction is performed early; in rare instances closed methods fail even in fresh lesions, making open reduction necessary.

After 2 weeks, closed methods rarely achieve a reduction; therefore, when the dislocation is more than 2 weeks old, an open reduction through the posterior approach should be performed. Excision of the lunate is not indicated because reduction gives a much more satisfactory result. Avascular necrosis of this bone after dislocation is rare, and poor wrist function often follows excision of the lunate.

Prereduction X-Ray

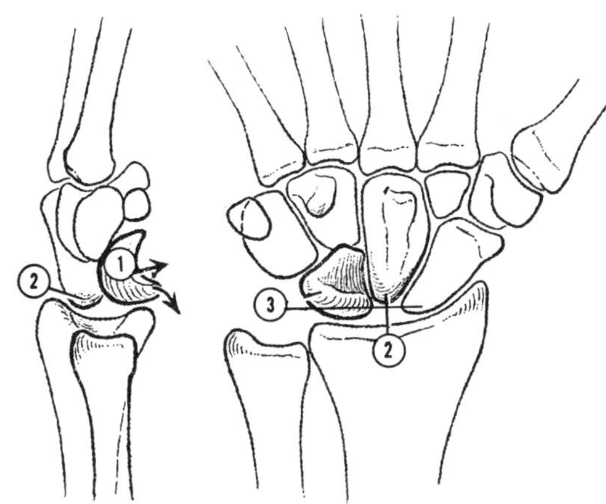

1. The lunate lies in front of the wrist and its articular surface tilts forward.
2. The capitate articulates with the articular surface of the radius.
3. In the anteroposterior view, the lunate appears to be triangular instead of quadrilateral and the scapholunate joint space is widened.

Reduction by Traction and Manipulation

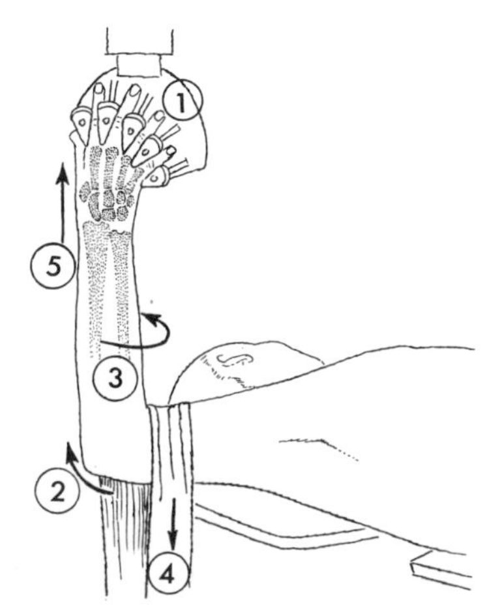

1. Apply finger traction.
2. The elbow is flexed at a right angle.
3. The forearm is supinated.
4. Countertraction is applied with a muslin bandage and a water pail for weight.
5. Traction is maintained for approximately 5 minutes.

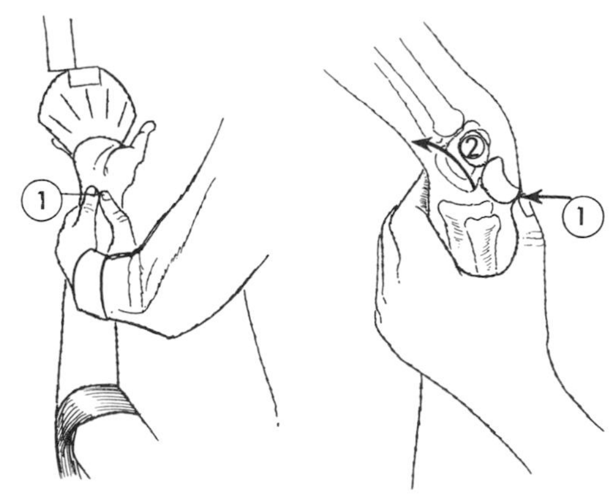

While traction is maintained,
1. Place both thumbs against the front of the lunate and apply strong pressure directly backward while
2. The wrist is dorsiflexed.

Note: Check the position of the lunate by x-ray before applying the plaster slabs.

Postreduction X-Ray

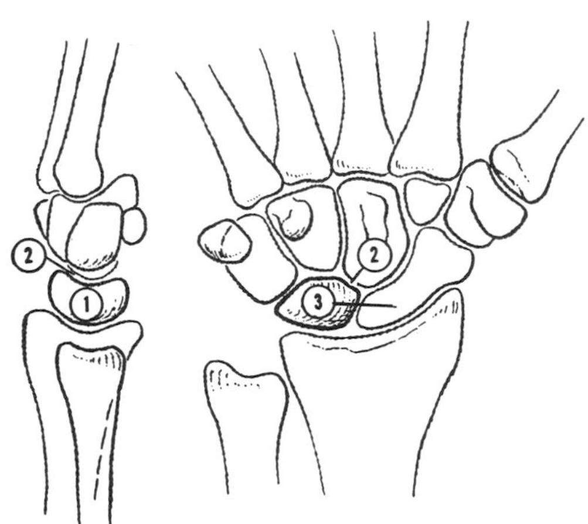

1. The lunate is in its normal anatomic position and articulates with the radius.
2. Its concave articular surface articulates with the capitate.
3. In the anteroposterior view, the profile of the lunate is quadrilateral and the scapholunate joint space has been restored to normal.

Note: Closed reduction is usually feasible if the injury is recognized acutely, but the stability of the carpus must be carefully assessed. If there is any question about carpal instability or dissociation, percutaneous fixation or internal repair of the torn ligaments is warranted. There is often a problem with median nerve compression when the lunate is completely displaced in a volar direction at the carpal tunnel. In this instance anterior exposure is required to decompress the median nerve in the carpal tunnel.

Percutaneous Pin Fixation for Unstable Lunate Dislocation

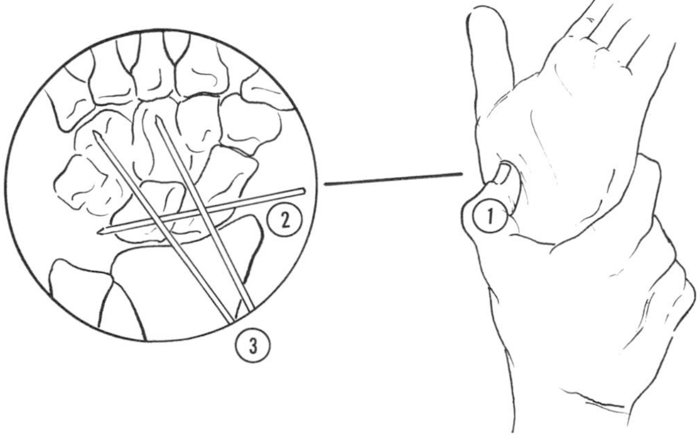

Note: This can be a difficult technique but can be accomplished under careful fluoroscopic control.

1. The forearm and wrist are stabilized by the surgeon holding his or her thumb over the dorsum of the capitate and
2. A second surgeon inserts multiple Kirschner wires to stabilize the proximal and distal carpal row. This is done under careful fluoroscopic guidance.
3. Multiple Kirschner wires are drilled to fix the scaphoid to the lunate and the capitate to the lunate, thereby stabilizing the proximal and distal carpal rows.

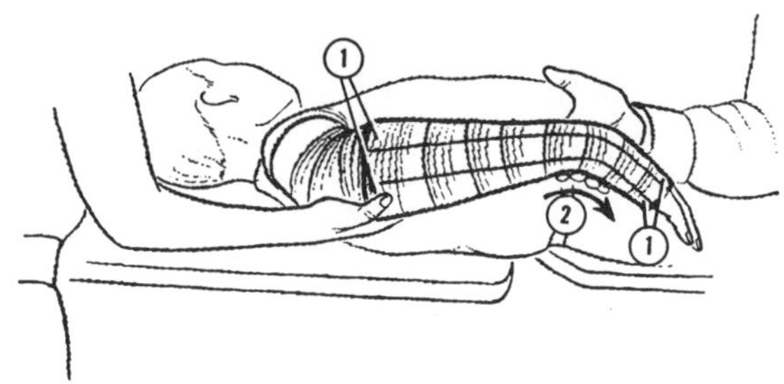

Immobilization

1. Apply anterior and posterior plaster slabs from just below the elbow to just proximal to the metacarpophalangeal joints.
2. The wrist is flexed 45°.

Subsequent Management

Casts are changed every 2–3 weeks as the swelling subsides. The pins may be removed at 4–6 weeks, but continued immobilization is necessary for approximately 8–12 weeks.

If the closed reduction and percutaneous fixation are not successful, open reduction and internal fixation with repair of the torn carpal ligaments are necessary. Because this injury involves complete disruption of most of the ligaments supporting the carpus, if there is any question about the reduction it is preferable to perform open operative exploration and repair.

Open Reduction

REMARKS

Open reduction is indicated if closed reduction fails in a fresh injury or if the dislocation is more than 2 weeks old. A dorsal approach is most applicable. This may have to be combined with a volar approach to decompress the median nerve. The relationship of the scaphoid to the reduced lunate must be carefully evaluated and must be corrected if there is rotational malalignment of the scaphoid (scapholunate subluxation).

A dorsal approach is also applicable to fix a fracture of the scaphoid associated with transscaphoid-perilunate dislocation. In all these instances, carefully evaluate the reduction achieved by means of intraoperative x-rays.

Volar Dislocation of the Lunate With Subluxation of the Scapholunate Joint

REMARKS

After closed or open reduction of the lunate, there may be persistent subluxation or dissociation of the scaphoid and lunate. The subluxation should be corrected and fixed by open reduction. Failure to correct this dissociation may result in dorsal instability and poor function.

Intraoperative X-Ray of Scapholunate Subluxation After Reduction of the Lunate Dislocation

1. The lunate has been restored to normal.
2. The scaphoid is rotated volarly and appears to be beneath the trapezoid and trapezium.
3. The scapholunate space is greater than 2 mm.

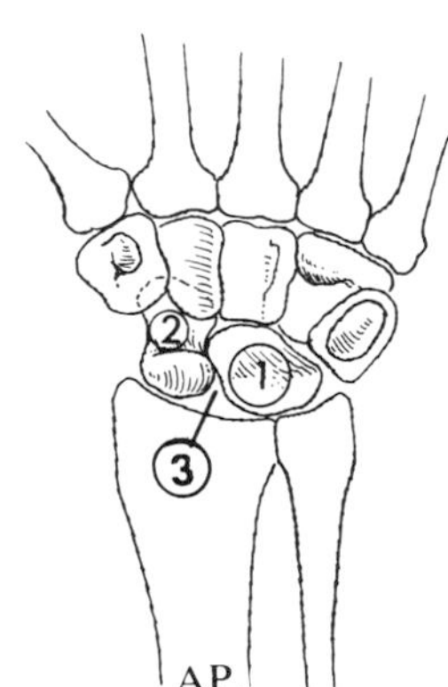

Open Repair Technique

1. With a dorsal approach the scaphoid is visualized and reduced to its normal anatomic position with a blunt dissector or periosteal elevator.
2. The scapholunate space and articulation is closed down and fixed with a 2-mm Kirschner wire. The wire is bent and cut below the level of the skin. In addition, the scapholunate ligament and any other dorsal ligaments that are torn are repaired.

Note: Stabilization of the distal scaphoid to the distal carpal row may also be necessary, as with a fractured scaphoid.

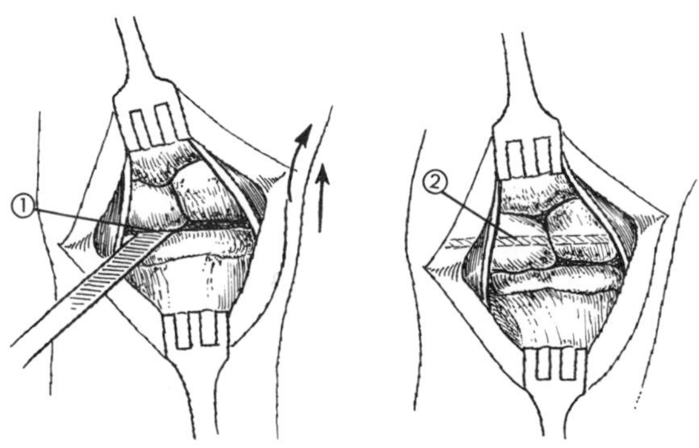

■ Scaphoid Fracture With Lunate Dislocation

Stabilization of Displaced Fragments of the Fractured Scaphoid

After closed or open reduction of the lunate, displacement of the fragments from associated fracture of the scaphoid generally persists. Internal fixation is necessary to hold this unstable injury. Use either a lag screw (Herbert screw) or a threaded Kirschner wire.

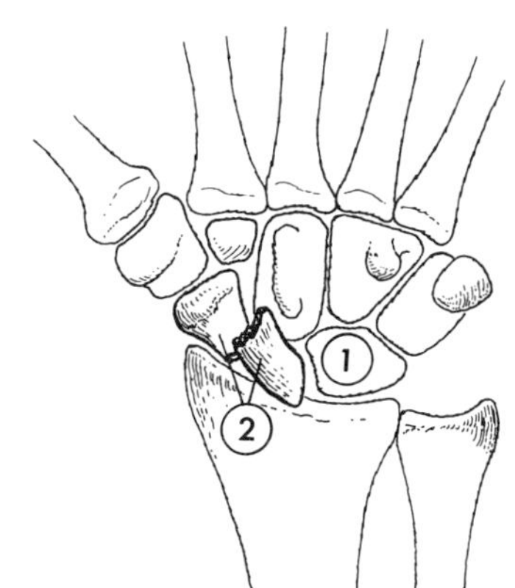

Appearance on X-Ray After Closed Reduction of Lunate Dislocation

1. The lunate is in normal alignment with the capitate and radius.
2. Displaced fragments of the scaphoid.

Operative Procedure

1. The scaphoid fragment is realigned and is fixed temporarily by a Kirschner wire drilled through a double-barreled guide.
2. After the second barrel of the guide is drilled through, a lag screw is inserted while fracture fixation is maintained with a Kirschner wire. Following lag screw fixation, the wire is removed.

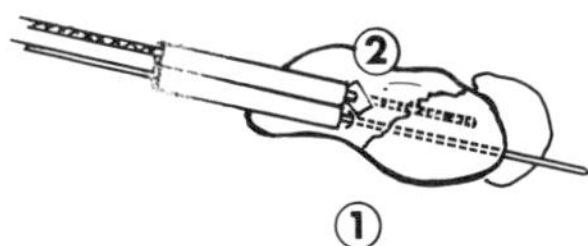

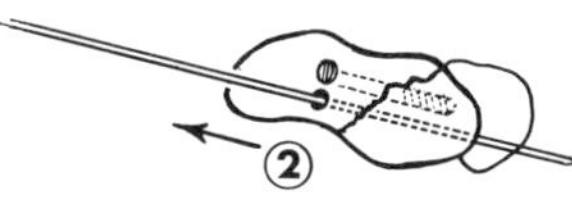

Note: Occasionally the fragment will be too small for lag screw fixation, and transcarpal Kirschner wire fixation can be used.

1. After the scaphoid fracture is stabilized with the screw,
2. The scapholunate and scaphocapitate may be stabilized with percutaneous Kirschner wires.

Subsequent Management

The hand is immobilized initially postoperatively in anterior and posterior splints. A thumb spica is then applied as the swelling subsides. The transcarpal pins can be removed by 6 weeks. The cast is kept in place until the scaphoid fracture shows clinical and radiographic signs of healing, which may require 12–16 weeks of continued immobilization.

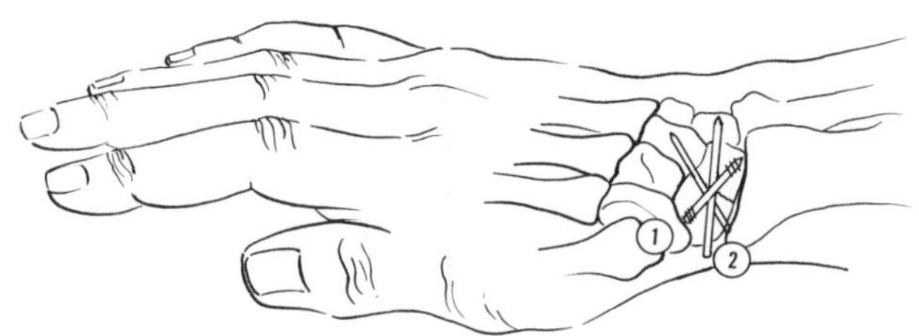

■ Chronic Lunate Dislocation With Avascular Necrosis

REMARKS

Open reduction through the posterior approach, as previously described, should be performed for chronic dislocation of the lunate, provided that the bone is not destroyed. If avascular necrosis develops, either before or after reduction of the lunate, excision with Silastic replacement arthroplasty is a useful reconstructive procedure. Excision of the lunate without replacement arthroplasty generally does not permit satisfactory wrist function.

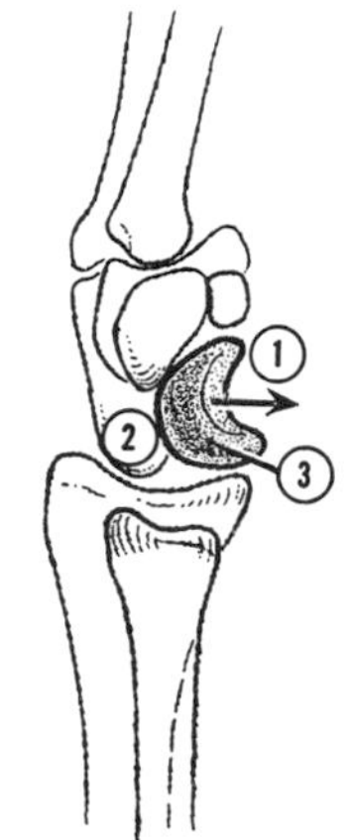

Preoperative X-Ray

Dislocation of the lunate is 8 months old.

1. The lunate is in front of the wrist.
2. The capitate is in line with the radius.
3. The lunate is dense and sclerotic, indicative of aseptic necrosis.

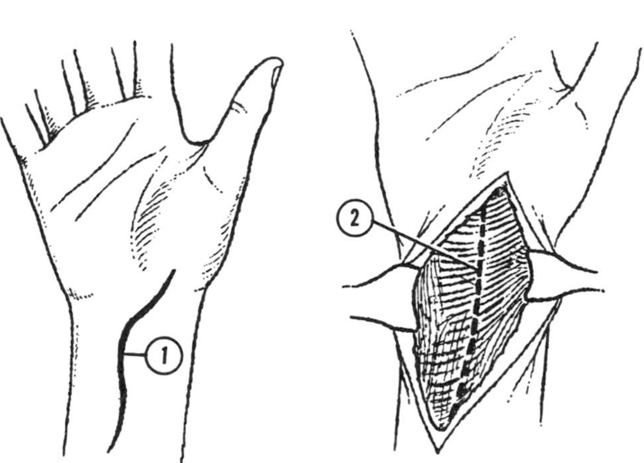

Preferred Management—Swanson Silastic Arthroplasty

1. The chronically dislocated lunate is approached through a volar incision, which also exposes the median nerve.
2. The fascia and transverse carpal ligament are divided to visualize the underlying structures.

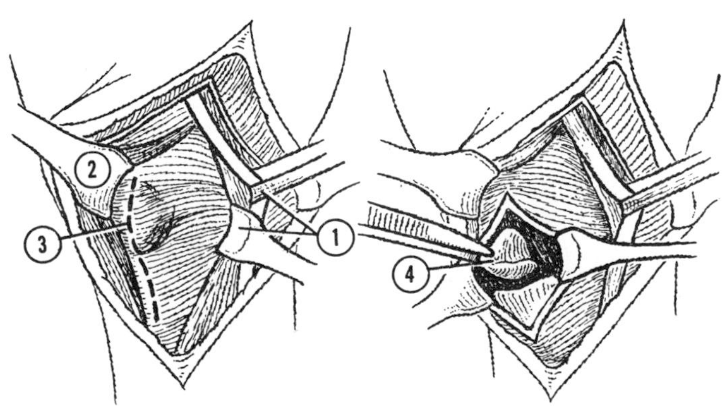

Operative Procedure: Swanson Silastic Arthroplasty

1. The median nerve is decompressed.
2. The flexor tendons of the fingers are protected.
3. The capsule is exposed over the dislocated lunate.
4. The lunate is removed.

The palmar radiocarpal and ulnar carpal ligaments are later repaired to maintain some stability in the wrist.

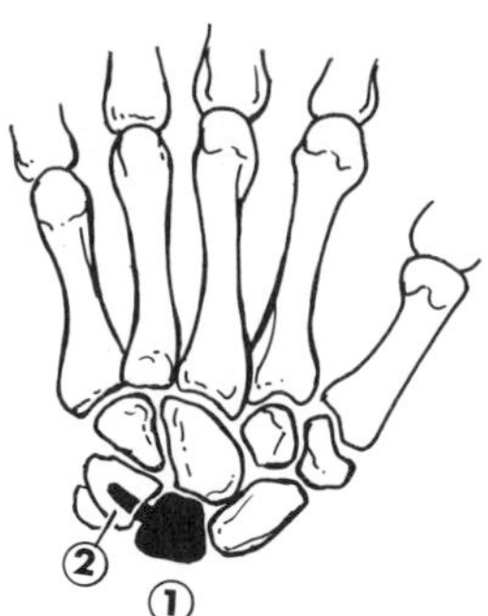

1. A Silastic implant is inserted snugly into the space of the resected lunate.
2. The lunate can be fixed to the triquetrum by the stem fixation device.

Note: An alternative method if the Silastic implant is not available is to fill the space with a rolled-up segment of the palmaris longus tendon (anchovy procedure).

Subsequent Management

A postoperative dressing is applied to the wrist for several days until the swelling subsides. Subsequently a short-arm cast is applied for 4–6 weeks. Full wrist activity is usually possible after 12 weeks.

The silastic replacement arthroplasty has been occasionally associated with breakdown of silastic fragments, but for purposes of a space filler in this area it generally serves quite satisfactorily. If the silastic replacement arthroplasty cannot be successfully accomplished, subsequent wrist fusion or proximal row resection may be a useful alternative procedure.

OTHER DISLOCATIONS AND SUBLUXATIONS OF THE CARPUS

Rotatory Subluxation of the Scaphoid-Scapholunate Dissociation

Rotatory subluxation of the scaphoid with its proximal pole displaced dorsally and its distal pole displaced volarly may persist after incomplete reduction of carpal dislocation. Rotatory subluxation can also occur independent of a carpal dislocation in individuals such as carpenters, who use their wrists frequently in heavy labor.

The diagnosis can be recognized if it is specifically sought. The patient characteristically has

- pain in the radioscaphoid region, particularly on wrist extension.
- a palpable click on extension of the wrist.
- loss of grip strength and decreased wrist motion.

For the gap between the scaphoid and lunate to be produced, the dorsal and palmar radiocarpal ligaments as well as the scapholunate interosseous ligaments must have ruptured. Reconstruction of these ligamentous structures is difficult, and results are generally less satisfactory than with early treatment.

Even when recognized, early treatment of the dissociation can be difficult. Occasionally closed reduction can be successful, but realigning the scaphoid as a link between the proximal and distal carpal rows may require internal fixation. If there is any doubt about the adequacy of closed reduction of the scaphoid, operative reduction with repair of the torn ligaments may be indicated.

Clinical Findings (Watson Test)

The patient with symptomatic scapholunate dissociation may complain of intermittent wrist pain, weakness, and instability.

1. The instability of the scaphoid may be demonstrated by producing a click when moving the proximal pole of the scaphoid over the dorsal rim of the radius.
2. The distal pole of the scaphoid is pressed upward by the examiner, who rocks the patient's wrist back and forth in radial and ulnar deviation, thereby producing the click of the unstable carpus.

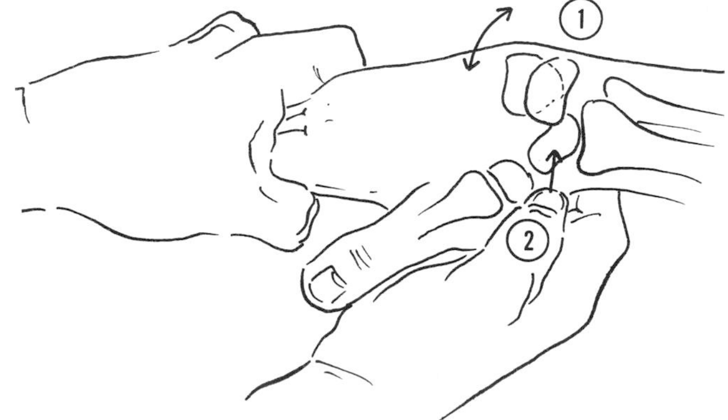

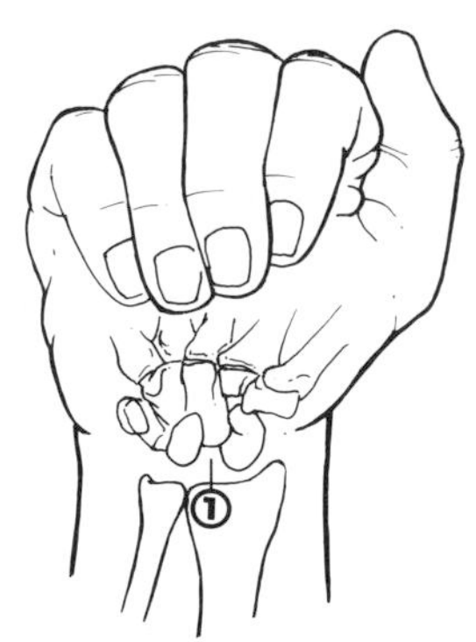

Appearance on X-Ray

On the anteroposterior view of the supinated wrist,

1. The scapholunate space is widened more than 2 mm.

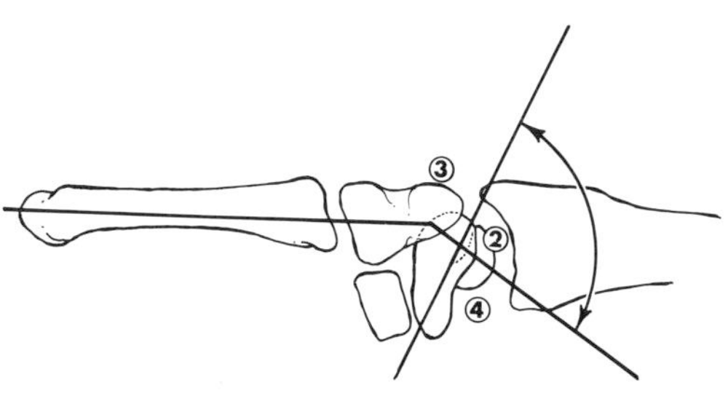

On the lateral view,

2. The scapholunate angle exceeds 70°.
3. The capitate is subluxating proximally through the space between the scaphoid and the lunate.
4. The lunate is dorsiflexed and is not aligned with the long axis of the radius.

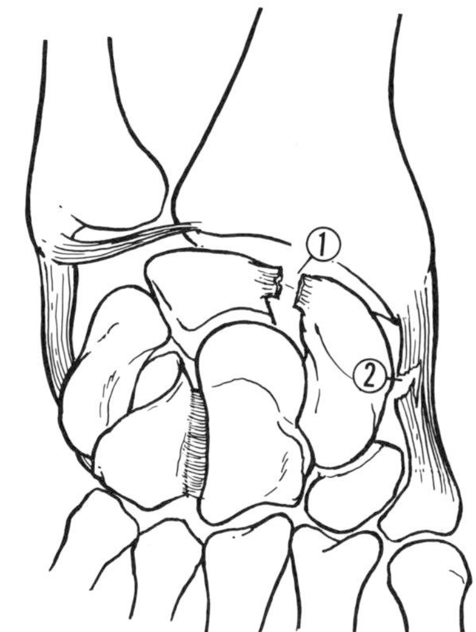

Pathomechanics

1. Disruption of the scapholunate ligaments on the dorsal and volar surface and
2. Rupture of the radioscaphoid ligaments allow rotatory displacement of the scaphoid and dorsiflexion collapse.

Note: Dorsiflexion collapse may also occur with a nonunion of the scaphoid as described previously.

Closed Treatment

Reduction of the unstable scaphoid may be difficult but is not impossible. The reversal of the mechanism by which the injury was sustained helps to achieve alignment. If the injury occurred with the wrist in ulnar deviation, reduce it by radial deviation. Alignment of the capitate with the lunate is best achieved by wrist extension.

Reduction must be confirmed on fluoroscopy. The alignment is then best maintained by two smooth Kirschner wires through the scaphoid into the capitate and the lunate.

Reduction Technique (Under Anesthesia)

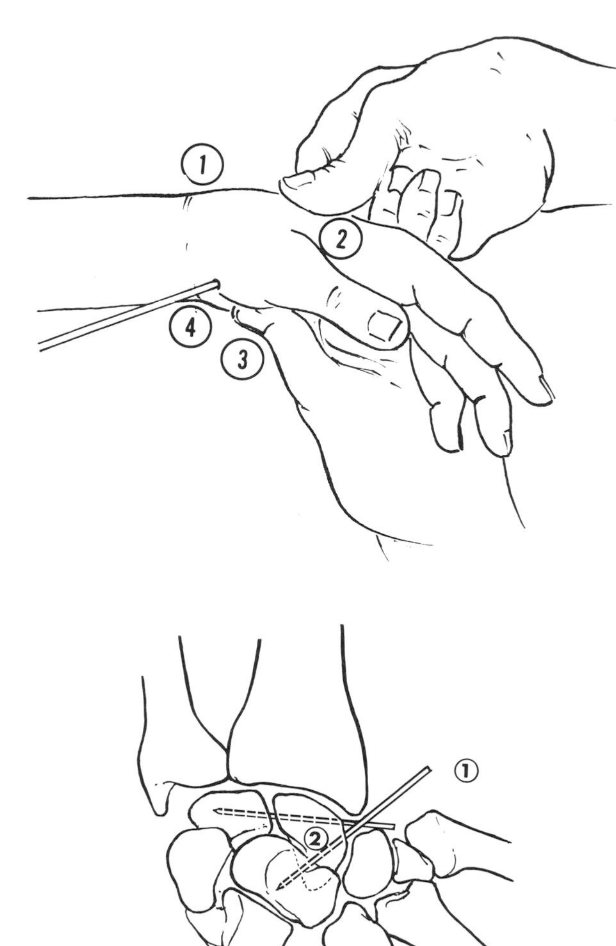

1. To reduce the distal scaphoid the wrist is held in the neutral position.
2. The capitate is stabilized by direct pressure dorsally.
3. The scaphoid is rotated upward by direct pressure on the distal pole.
4. A pin is placed percutaneously between the scaphoid and the capitate.

Note: The position of the capitate and the scaphoid should be carefully evaluated on lateral fluoroscopy. If the scaphoid remains rotated downward, this should be corrected.

1. After the scaphoid is pinned to the capitate, the wrist is extended slightly and placed in radial deviation to close the scapholunate space.
2. A smooth Kirschner wire is inserted percutaneously through the scaphoid into the lunate to maintain the position of the scapholunate articulation.

Note: Again the position must be carefully monitored under fluoroscopy, and the reduction should be carefully monitored in both the anteroposterior and lateral positions.

Subsequent Management

The hand and wrist are supported in a long-arm cast. The pins are bent and allowed to be buried beneath the skin. The cast and pins are removed after 6–8 weeks depending on the stability of the injury. The patient is encouraged to begin active range-of-motion exercise to the wrist.

If the carpal instability persists after closed treatment, operative repair of the ligaments is indicated. However, results from operative repair of these ligaments of the wrist are not as good as they are in other joints of the body. Some stiffness and limitation of function can be expected after this type of injury. The patient should be so informed from the start of treatment. A limited wrist arthrodesis may eventually be needed for persistent symptomatic instability.

■ Dorsal Periscapholunate Dislocation

REMARKS

In this lesion the lunate and scaphoid remain articulated with the radius, while the remaining carpus displaces dorsally. The scaphoid may be forced into a volar position as the carpus is shortened. After reduction always check for any malposition of the scaphoid. Usually realignment is achieved by closed reduction. Percutaneous pin stabilization may be needed after reduction.

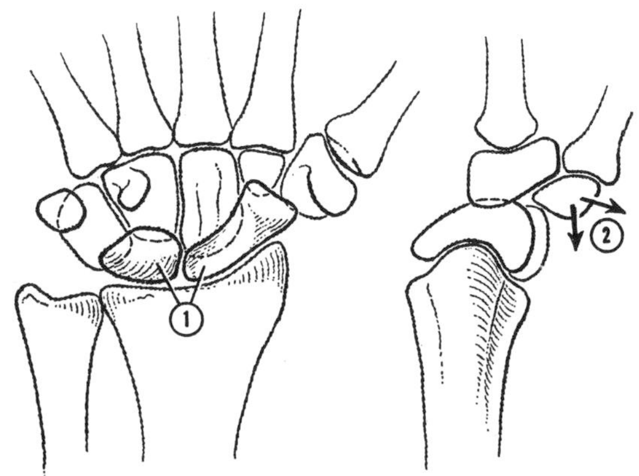

Appearance on X-Ray

1. The scaphoid and lunate articulate with the radius.
2. The remaining carpus is displaced dorsally and proximally.

Management

Reduce the dislocation by traction and manipulation as described for perilunate dislocation.

Dislocation of the Lunate and the Proximal Half of the Scaphoid

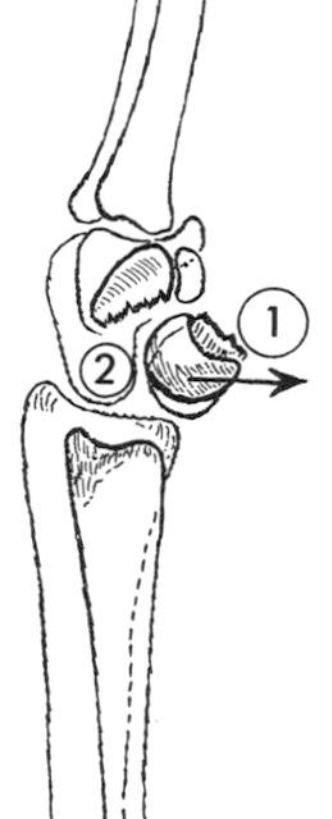

Appearance on X-Ray

1. The lunate and the proximal half of the scaphoid do not articulate with the radius but are in an anterior position.
2. The capitate articulates with the radius.

After reduction the fragments of the scaphoid usually remain displaced. Open reduction and internal fixation are generally needed, as described for transscaphoid perilunate dislocations.

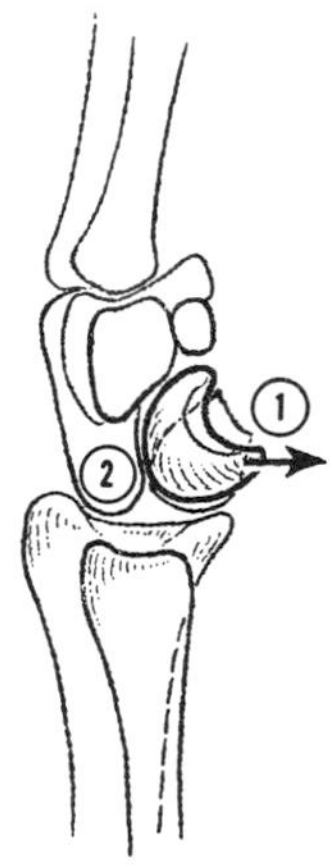

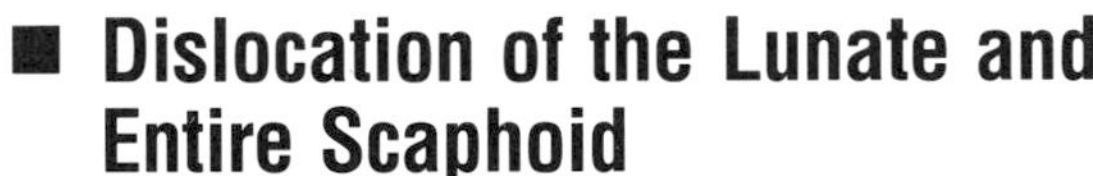

Dislocation of the Lunate and Entire Scaphoid

Appearance on X-Ray

1. The lunate and the entire scaphoid are displaced anteriorly.
2. The capitate articulates with the radius.

Management

Reduce the dislocation by traction and manipulation as described for dislocation of the lunate. Percutaneous pin stabilization of the proximal and distal carpal rows is usually indicated.

Dislocation of the Metacarpal Bones on the Carpus

Appearance on X-Ray

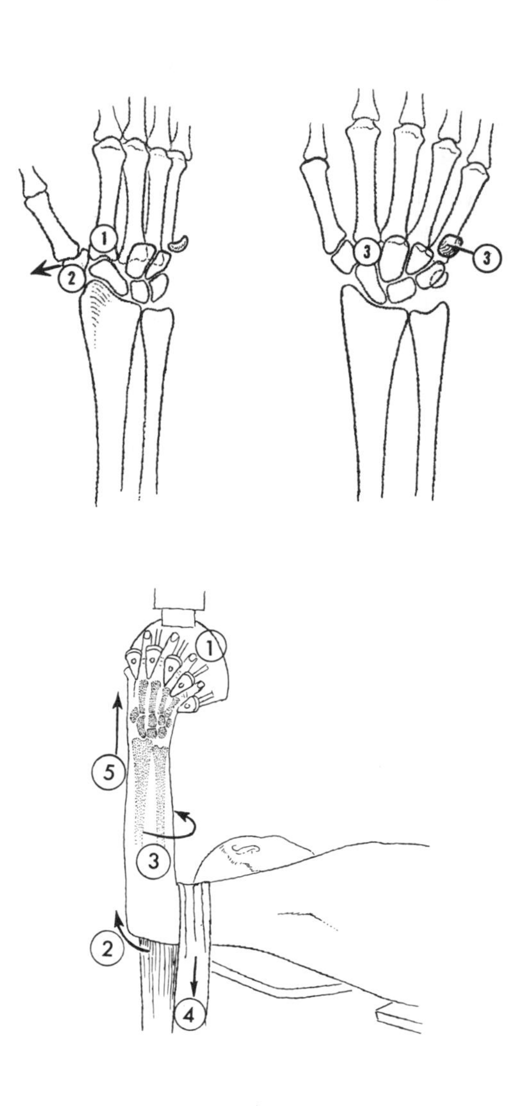

1. The metacarpal bones together with
2. The trapezium are displaced anterior to the remaining carpus.
3. The trapezoid is displaced to the dorsum of the wrist on the ulnar side. (In this instance this bone was excised.)

Note: This degree of disruption is likely to damage the motor branch of the ulnar nerve. Check ulnar nerve function carefully before and after reduction. If the nerve is involved, perform open reduction and pin fixation.

Reduction by Traction and Manipulation

Note: This method applies to most carpal dislocations. The direction of manipulation varies with the direction of displacement.

TRACTION

1. Apply finger traction.
2. The elbow is flexed at a right angle.
3. The forearm is fully supinated.
4. Countertraction is applied by a muslin bandage with a weight attached.
5. Apply strong traction directly upward for at least 5 minutes.

MANIPULATION

While traction is maintained, pressure is applied on the displaced elements.

1. If one or two metacarpal bones are displaced anteriorly, pressure is applied directly backward, and at the same time
2. The wrist is dorsiflexed.
3. If these elements are displaced posteriorly, pressure is applied directly forward and
4. The wrist is flexed in a palmar direction.

Note: If lateral displacement is present, pressure is directed in the opposite direction to correct it.

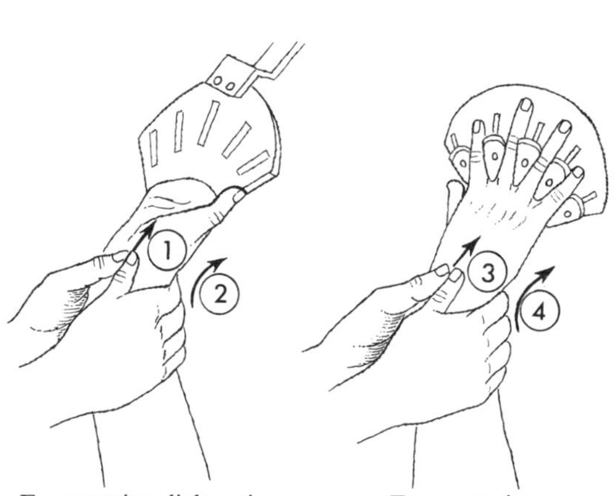

For anterior dislocation

For posterior dislocation

Percutaneous Pin Fixation

1. These dislocations tend to be unstable and are best stabilized by percutaneous pin fixation.
2. The pin is inserted from the ulnar border of the fifth metacarpal under fluoroscopic control through the fifth and fourth metacarpals into the distal carpal row.

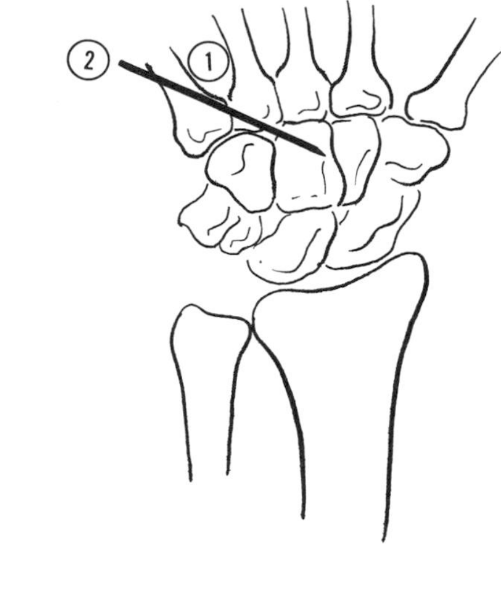

Subsequent Immobilization

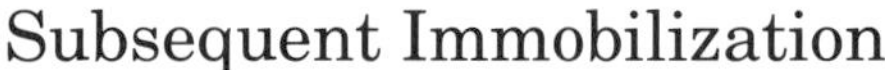

1. An anterior and posterior plaster splint is applied with the wrist flexed for stability. The transcutaneous pins inserted into metacarpals are bent, cut, and buried beneath the skin.

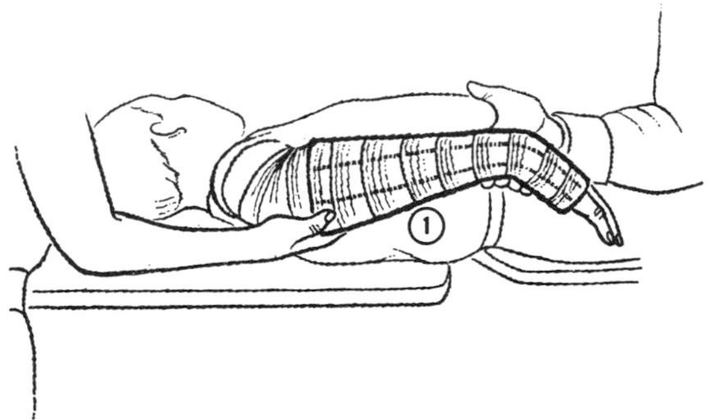

Postreduction Management

Carefully evaluate the postreduction x-ray to ensure that an anatomic reduction has been achieved. If the carpus has not been completely reduced, open reduction is indicated. Following adequate closed reduction, change the plaster splints to a long-arm cast when the swelling subsides, usually by 5–7 days.

For dislocations without fracture, the cast may usually be removed by the end of 4 weeks. Fracture-dislocations require immobilization until bony union of the fractured carpal bone is complete. Pins inserted for stabilization are also removed at 3–4 weeks.

■ Dislocation of the Trapezoid (Lesser Multangular)

REMARKS

This is a rare lesion. It may occur as an isolated injury or with other lesions of the carpal bones. The dislocation is usually dorsal, but in rare instances it is volar. Aseptic necrosis of the bone is a common sequela.

Management

Closed reduction rarely is successful. Excision of the bone is the procedure of choice, whether dislocation has occurred as an isolated lesion or with other carpal injuries.

Disruption of the Proximal Row of the Carpus

REMARKS

Occasionally, as a result of severe violence, the proximal carpal row can be completely disrupted and the scaphoid and lunate can be fractured and dislocated. Because of the multiplicity of injury and the likelihood of persistent traumatic arthritis, particularly from the lunate fracture, excision of the proximal carpal row may be justified rarely as a primary procedure.

This involves excision of the lunate, scaphoid, and triquetrum. Although the result is usually not an excellent one, the patient generally has a painless wrist with varying degrees of restriction of motion. This procedure is preferable to primary arthrodesis of the wrist.

Wrist immobilization should be maintained for 6 weeks to achieve a fibrous ankylosis. Should the patient suffer persistent pain with motion after a proximal row resection, a total wrist arthroplasty or arthrodesis may be employed as a secondary procedure.

Appearance on X-Ray

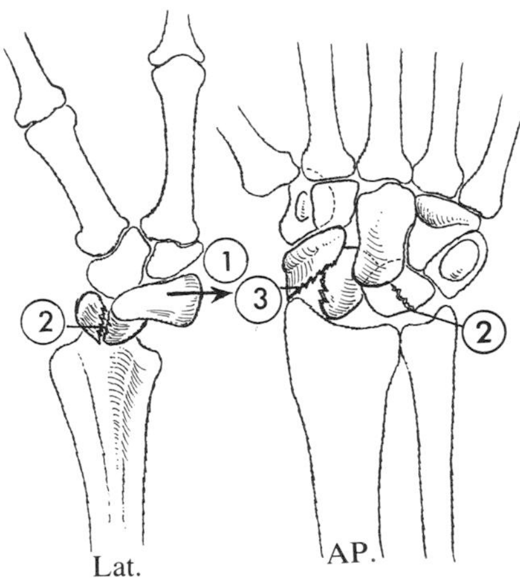

1. Dorsal perilunar dislocation of the carpus.
2. The lunate is fractured.
3. The scaphoid is fractured and its distal fragment is dislocated on the radius.

Postoperative X-Ray

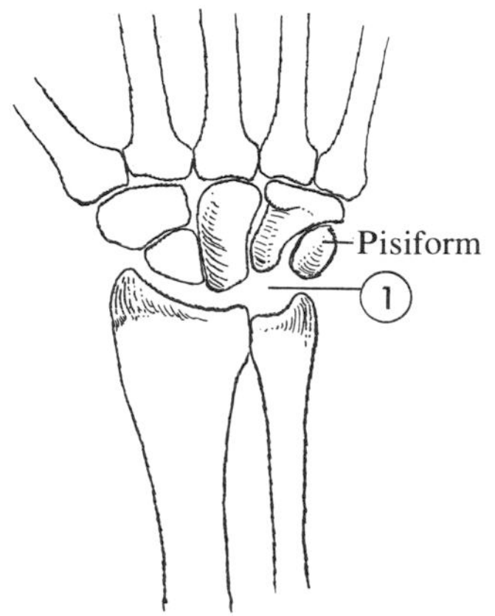

1. The proximal row of carpal bones (except the pisiform) has been excised.

Note: Immobilize the wrist for at least 6 weeks to achieve a fibrous ankylosis. If the patient has persistent pain on wrist motion, a total wrist arthroplasty or arthrodesis may be used as a secondary procedure.

Disruption of the Distal Row of the Carpus (Proximal Carpal Arch)

REMARKS

Crush injuries to the hand can disrupt the stabilizing transverse arch, which includes the distal carpal row. Damage to the bony and ligamentous support that is provided by the capitate and hamate is particularly likely to disrupt the stability of the arch. This is reflected clinically as rotational finger deformities and flattening of the palm, which should be corrected by restoring the continuity between the capitate and hamate. Because the distal carpal row also forms the floor of the carpal tunnel, decompression of the median nerve is often necessary with these injuries.

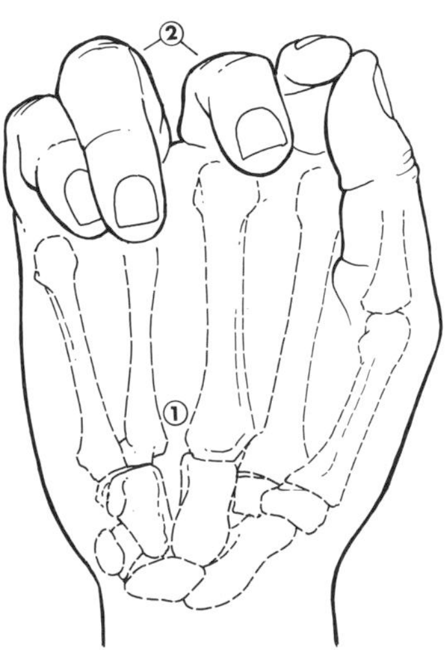

Preoperative X-Ray

1. Crush injury to the hand leaves the patient with a widening of the capitate-hamate articulation.
2. Clinical malrotation of the ring and small fingers may go unexplained if there is no fracture of the metacarpal bones or phalanx.

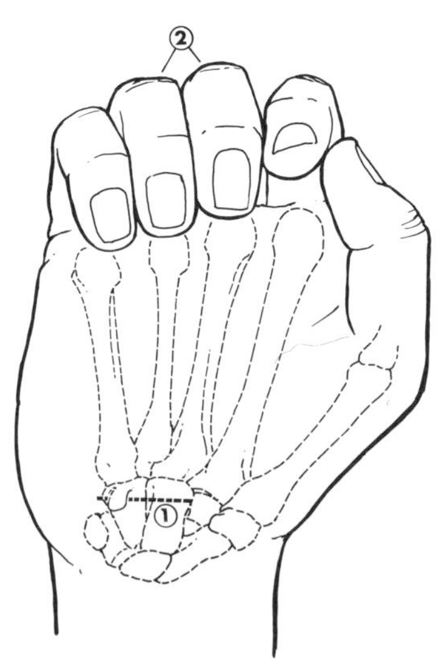

After Open Reduction of the Distal Carpal Row

1. The capitate-hamate articulation has been reduced and fixed with Kirschner wire.
2. There is normal convergence with finger flexion.

Note: Decompression of the median nerve in the carpal tunnel is often necessary.

■ Volar Perilunate Dislocation and Fracture-Dislocation

REMARKS

These are indeed rare lesions. Volar perilunate dislocation may be complicated by fracture or fracture-dislocation of the scaphoid, just as in the dorsal lesion.

Volar Perilunate Dislocation

1. The lunate is in normal relation to the radius.
2. The remaining carpus is displaced anterior to the lunate.

The principles of management are the same as for dorsal dislocation with or without associated fractures of other carpal bones.

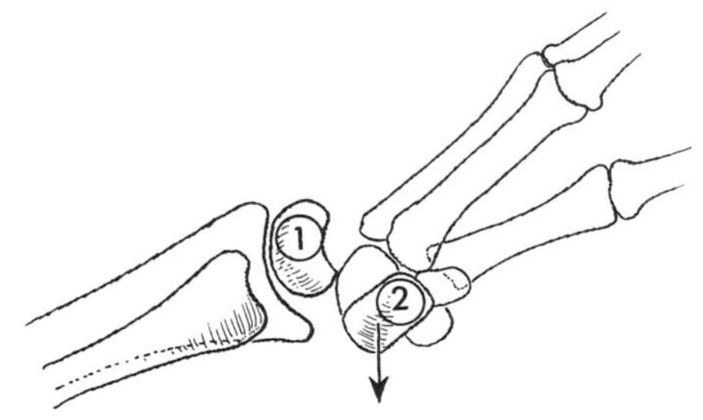

FRACTURES OF THE CARPAL BONES

Fracture of the Capitate

Anatomic Considerations

The size and relationships of the capitate to the other carpal bones make the capitate vulnerable to injury; it is the largest of all the carpal bones and articulates with seven bones: the scaphoid and the lunate proximally, the lesser multangular on the radial side, the hamate on the ulnar side, and the second, third, and fourth metacarpals distally.

The capitate receives its blood supply from vessels penetrating the dorsal surface of the neck and waist of the bone, so that trauma may sever a portion of the bone from an adequate blood supply, thus causing aseptic necrosis of the affected segment.

The capitate is firmly anchored to the bases of the second, third, and fourth metacarpal bones by an intricate system of tough intercarpal ligaments. The capitate is intimately related to the axial motion of the third metacarpal bone.

1. The capitate, the largest bone, occupies a central position in the carpus.
2. Distally it articulates with the second, third, and fourth metacarpals.
3. Proximally it articulates with the scaphoid and lunate.
4. It is related to the axial movements of the third metacarpal.

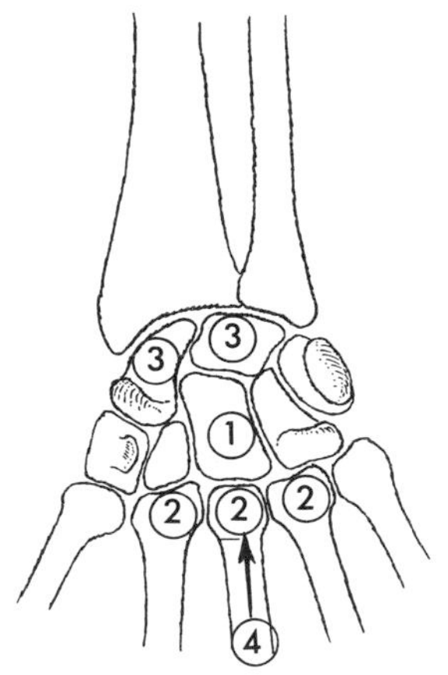

Mechanism of Fracture

Fractures of the capitate are produced either as the result of direct or indirect violence:

- direct violence causes injury to other carpal bones.
- indirect violence due to a fall on the outstretched hand is by far the most common mechanism. The type of lesion produced depends on the direction of the hand and wrist.

  If the hand and wrist are dorsiflexed and are deviated toward the ulna, the lunate is caught between the radius and the capitate, and is squeezed volarly out of the wrist joint. This lesion may be associated with a fracture of the distal tip of the radius or the capitate.

  If the hand and wrist are dorsiflexed and are deviated toward the radius, the styloid process of the radius digs into the waist of the scaphoid, producing a fracture; with continuance of the force, the capitate is also fractured through its waist and the proximal fragments may rotate as much as 180° (see scaphoid-capitate fracture syndrome).

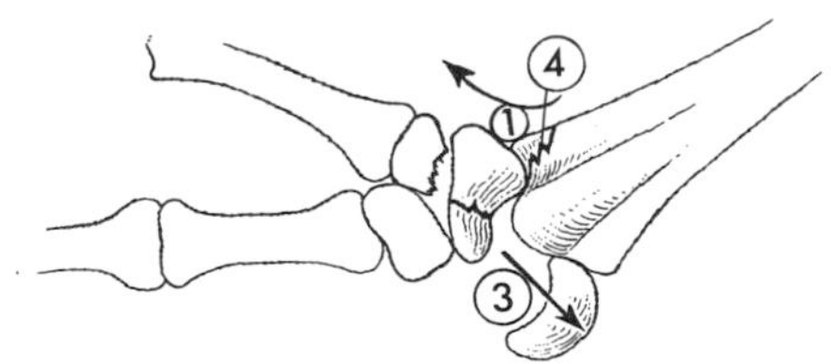

Also, trauma to the radial side of the dorsum of the hand with the wrist flexed in a palmar direction may result in a fracture of the capitate.

1. The wrist is in extreme dorsiflexion.
2. The wrist and the hand are deviated toward the ulna.
3. The lunate is forced volarly out of the wrist joint.
4. The distal tip of the radius may fracture.
5. The capitate may fracture; also, a fracture may occur through the proximal head of the scaphoid.

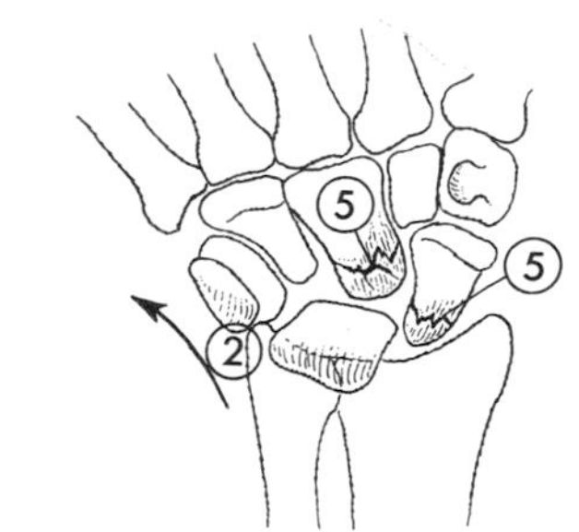

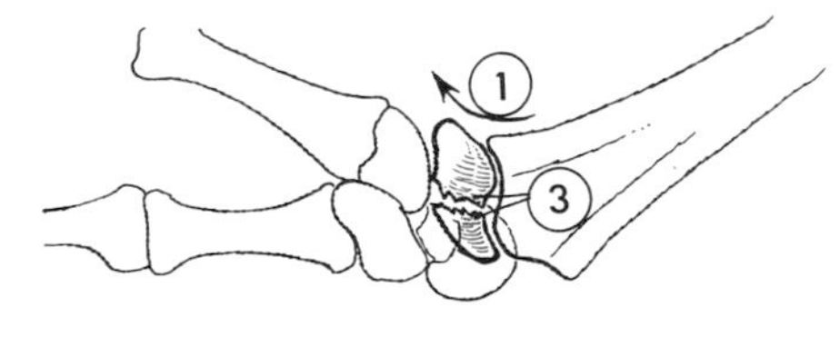

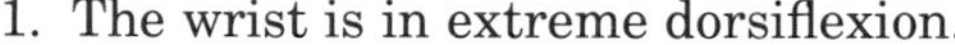

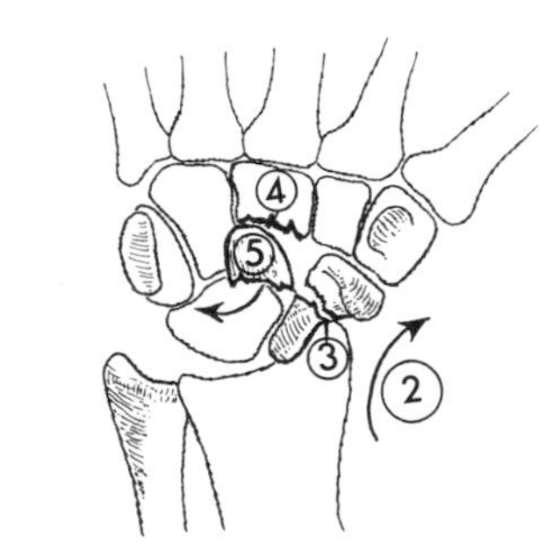

1. The wrist is in extreme dorsiflexion.
2. The wrist and the hand are deviated toward the radius.
3. The styloid process of the radius impacts into the waist of the scaphoid, producing a fracture. With continuance of the force,
4. The capitate fractures through the waist and
5. Its proximal fragment rotates (almost 180°).

Many fractures of the capitate may be difficult to detect; take oblique x-rays and laminograms to establish the diagnosis, especially if symptoms localized to the region of the capitate persist. The fractures may be transverse (the most common), oblique, vertical, and incomplete.

Most of the fractures are isolated lesions, although many are associated with other carpal injuries. When the scaphoid and capitate bones alone are involved, the combination is referred to as the *scaphoid-capitate fracture syndrome.*

Management of Isolated Fracture of the Capitate

REMARKS

Most of these lesions are the result of a fall on the palm of the hand. Most fractures are transverse and show little or no displacement. Simple plaster fixation for 8 weeks is adequate treatment. Bony union is the rule. If fibrous union or avascular necrosis of a fragment occurs and produces painful disability, the fragment can be excised.

Immobilization

1. Apply a plaster cast from below the elbow to the metacarpophalangeal joints.
2. The thumb is in the grasp position and is included in the cast up to the base of the thumbnail.
3. The wrist is only slightly dorsiflexed; otherwise, it is in the neutral position.

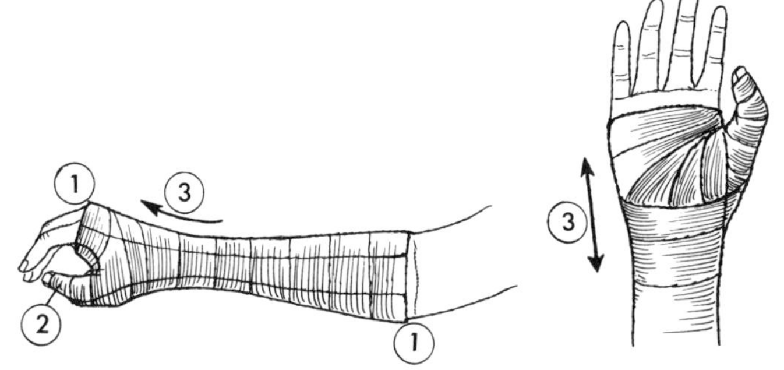

Subsequent Management

Cast immobilization for 4–6 weeks is usually adequate. If the cast becomes loose, it should be changed during this time. After 6 weeks the cast is removed and an exercise program is prescribed to restore finger and wrist motion. If there is evidence of a symptomatic fibrous union or avascular necrosis of the proximal fragment, excision of the fragment can be carried out.

Management of Scaphoid-Capitate Fracture Syndrome

REMARKS

As a rule, the fracture of the capitate is transverse and the proximal fracture is rotated up to 180°. This lesion may have been produced in association with a dorsal perilunate dislocation that reduced spontaneously. In these instances the proximal capitate fragment may remain in a displaced position on the dorsum of the wrist.

In most instances the fracture of the capitate should be fixed internally, but very small displaced fragments may be excised. The incidence of traumatic arthritis when the fragments are unreduced, particularly if the proximal fragment is rotated, is very high. Operative reduction gives the best chance for a satisfactory result as described previously.

Management of Capitate Fracture Associated With Other Carpal Injuries

In general, treatment of these injuries is the same as that described for isolated capitate fracture and the scaphoid-capitate fracture, except that the treatment is also directed to the other associated injuries, which in some instances may be more severe than the fracture of the capitate; for example, a fracture of the distal end of the radius. If the principles of the treatment of capitate fracture just described are adhered to when the fracture is associated with other carpal injuries, a plan of adequate management should readily evolve.

■ Fractures of the Triquetrum

REMARKS

The triquetrum is frequently fractured, but it is rarely displaced because of its strong ligamentous support. These fractures may frequently be difficult to detect on x-ray unless an oblique projection is obtained.

Mechanism of Fracture

- by direct violence to the dorsum of the hand.
- extreme dorsiflexion, as in a fall on the outstretched hand (this is the most common mechanism), or extreme palmar flexion due to a fall on the flexed hand.
- twisting movements against resistance.
- the type of fracture may be a chip fracture, varying in size, of the dorsum of the bone with some separation of the fragments or a fracture of the body, which may also be comminuted.
- separation of fragments is never marked; bony union is the rule; fibrous union occurs rarely. Aseptic necrosis does not occur.
- the lesions may be isolated or associated with other injuries, such as fractures of the scaphoid or of the distal end of the radius.
- untreated cases frequently masquerade as chronic sprains of the wrist.

Appearance on X-Ray

LATERAL VIEW

1. Chip fracture from dorsum of the bone.

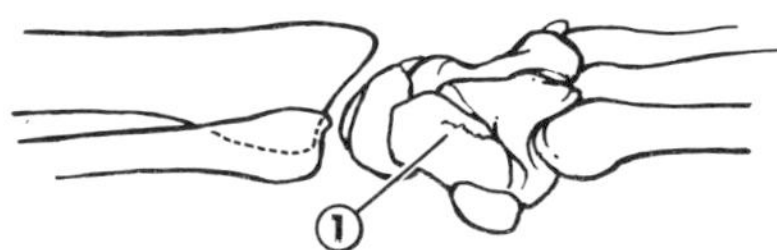

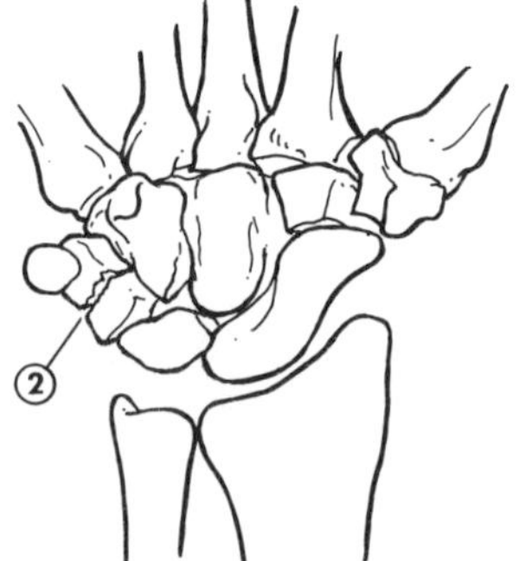

OBLIQUE VIEW

2. Fracture through the body of the bone.

Management of Isolated Fractures

Immobilization

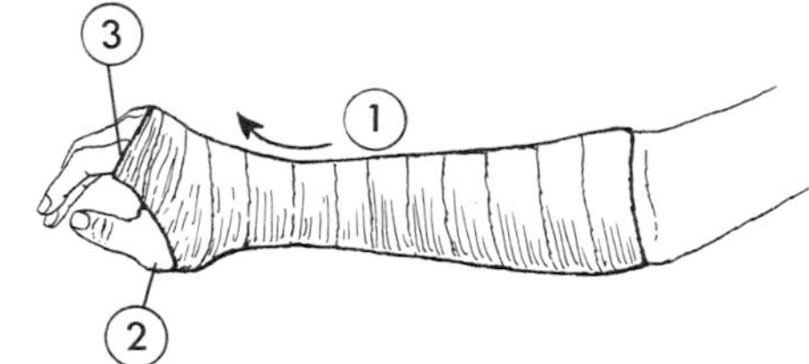

1. Apply a well-molded short-arm cast from below the elbow to the metacarpal joints. The wrist is slightly dorsiflexed.
2. The thumb is free.
3. The fingers are free to flex and extend fully.

Subsequent Management

Remove the cast after 6–8 weeks, regardless of what the status of union may be as interpreted on x-ray. The wearing of a wrist support for several weeks after the cast is removed may be helpful in some instances. Institute a program of physical therapy and exercises to restore normal motion of the fingers and wrist.

Note: Union may be delayed, especially in fractures with separation of the fragments. Bony union may not occur for many weeks after the cast is removed; fibrous union or delayed union does not preclude achievement of good wrist function without pain.

Management of Fractures of the Triquetrum Associated With Other Injuries

When a triquetrum fracture is associated with other injuries, attention should be directed to the treatment of the other injuries, because they are usually more serious. The most common associated fractures are fracture of the scaphoid and fracture of the distal end of the radius.

Fractures of the Pisiform

REMARKS

The anatomic features of this bone render it vulnerable to injury. Its volar surface is attached to the volar ligament and the tendon of the flexor carpi ulnaris, which sends fibrous strands to the hamate and metacarpal bones, forming the pisohamate and pisometacarpal ligaments. The dorsal surface of the pisiform articulates with the triquetrum, forming the pisotriquetrum joint, which is enclosed in a tough fibrous capsule.

Mechanism of Injury

The bone may be fractured by direct trauma (the most common mechanism) or by forceful hyperextension, as in a fall on the outstretched hand, or with forceful dorsiflexion of the wrist against resistance.

The types of fracture produced are as follows:

- avulsion fracture by the action of the flexor carpi ulnaris.
- transverse or linear fracture of the body of the pisiform.
- comminuted fracture.

Because the capsule and ligaments are attached to the bone, separation of the fragments is never marked. The fractures may be isolated lesions or may be associated with other carpal injuries. The diagnosis is often missed; oblique x-ray projections are necessary to show the lesions.

Appearance on X-Ray

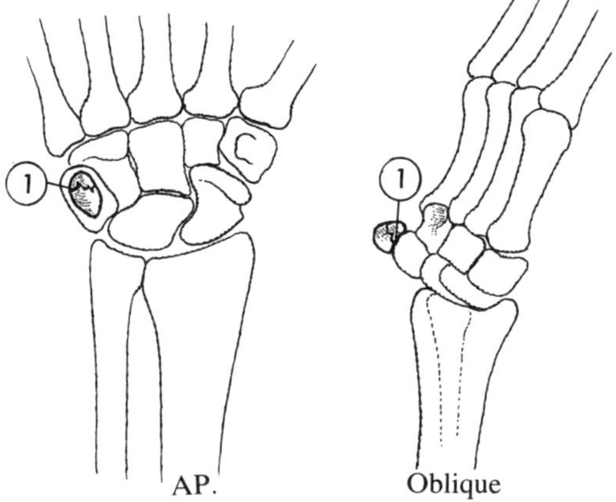

1. Fracture of pisiform involving the articular surface.

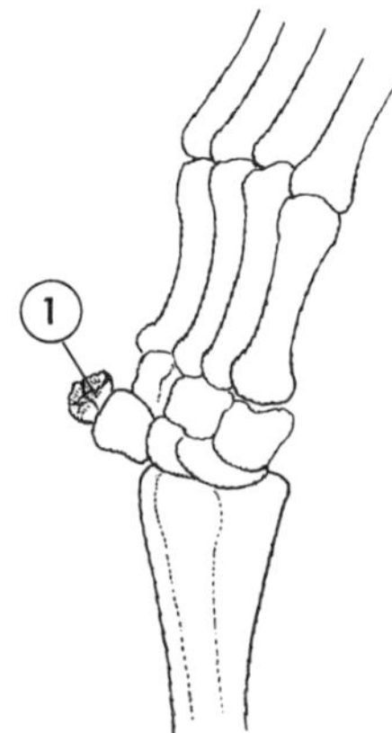

1. Comminuted fracture of the pisiform can be seen on the oblique view.

Nonunion is rare but may occur; bony union is nearly always achieved and recovery is usually complete.

Management of an Isolated Lesion

Immobilization

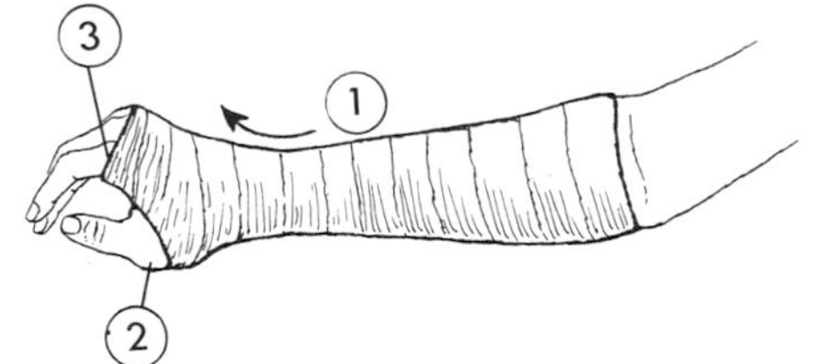

1. Apply a well-molded short-arm cast from below the elbow to the metacarpophalangeal joints.
2. The thumb is free.
3. The fingers are free to flex and extend fully.

This lesion is best treated as a sprain. Occasionally injection of corticosteroid into the area of the pisiform may be effective. Rarely, for persistent symptoms excision of the pisiform bone may be indicated; however, care should be exercised to avoid injury to the ulnar nerve.

Occasionally, calcification may occur around the tendon of the flexor carpi ulnaris and produce this chronic strain syndrome. This lesion can be treated as a calcific deposit for nonsteroidal medication, rest, and occasionally steroid injections.

Subsequent Management

Remove the cast after 4 weeks. Institute a program of physical therapy and exercises to restore normal finger and wrist motion.

Chronic Sprain of the Pisotriquetral Joint

Persistent pain localized over the pisiform and aggravated by radial deviation of the wrist may be caused by a chronic sprain of the pisotriquetral joint, usually seen in women. Pain may be referred to the fourth and fifth fingers.

Management of Fracture of the Pisiform Associated With Other Carpal Injuries

When the pisiform fracture is associated with other injuries, attention should be directed to treatment of the other injuries, because they are usually more serious. The most common associated fractures are fractures of the triquetrum, hamate, and distal end of the radius.

■ Fracture of the Hook of the Hamate

REMARKS

Fracture of the hook of the hamate may be caused by a fall or a crushing injury. It is most often a diagnostic problem in athletes who sustain a direct blow against the hamate by the handle of a tennis racquet, golf club, or bat during an unbalanced swing. The hamate hook is not fractured by indirect forces of attached ligaments or muscle, but these structures interfere with bone healing by exerting intermittent forces on the hamate.

Characteristically, the diagnosis is delayed one or more months because the x-ray views usually taken of the wrist do not demonstrate the lesion. Occasionally, rupture of the finger flexor tendons, secondary either to the fracture or to cortisone injections, may occur.

Typically, the patient has pain localized to the dorsal ulnar aspect of the wrist rather than over the hamate, because the fracture is usually at the base of the hook. Diagnosis depends on a suspicion from the history and the physical examination, and particularly on adequate carpal tunnel x-rays.

Although this fracture may unite if the hand and wrist are immobilized in plaster after the acute injury, in most instances excision of the fracture fragment is necessary.

Mechanism of Injury

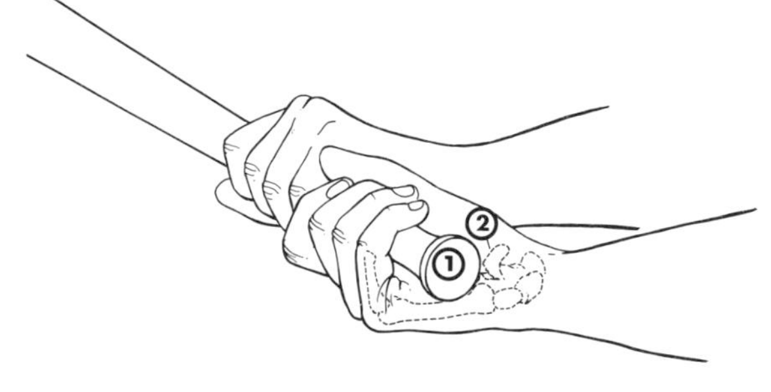

1. The fracture always occurs in the hand that grasps the end of the club, bat, or racquet.
2. The butt end of the club strikes the hook of the hamate when the patient loses control of his or her swing.

Clinical Symptoms

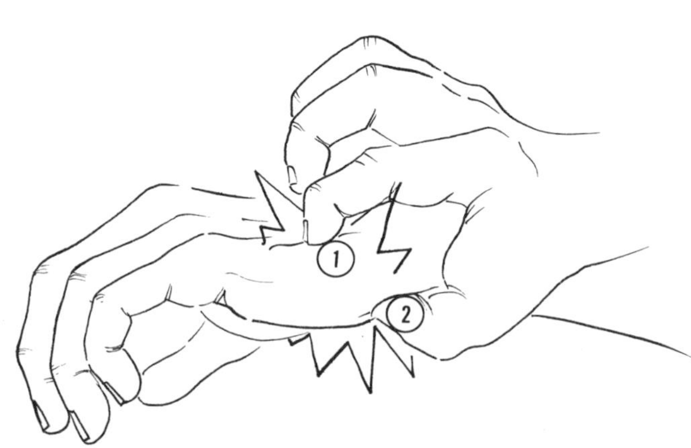

1. The clinical symptoms may be confusing because the pain is usually located at the base of the fifth metacarpal on the dorsal surface of the hand.
2. The swelling of the hypothenar eminence may not be readily visible, and the patient may not localize the pain to the palm of the hand despite the fracture in the hamate.

X-Ray Technique for Carpal Tunnel View

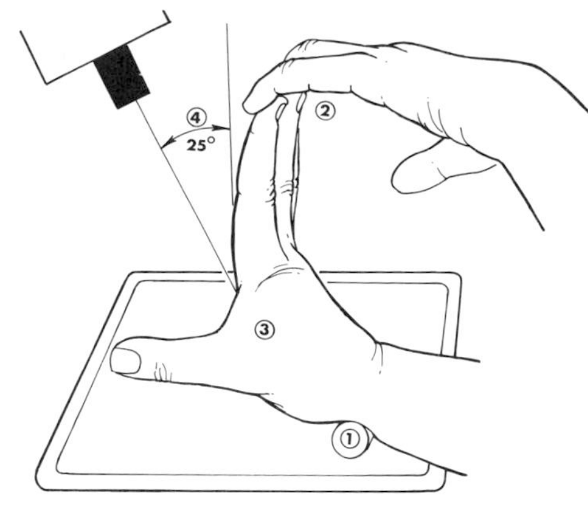

1. Place a radiolucent pad 2 cm thick between the wrist and the cassette.
2. Have the patient hold the wrist in maximum dorsiflexion by pulling the fingers dorsally with the opposite hand.
3. Direct the central ray to a point approximately 2.5 cm distal to the base of the fourth metacarpal.
4. Angle the tube 25° toward the horizontal from the long axis of the hand.

X-Ray Appearance

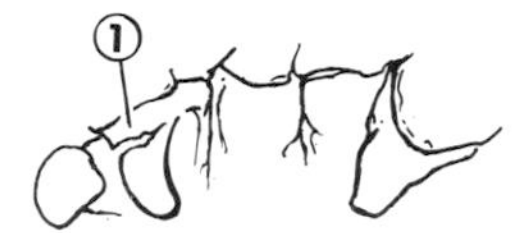

1. The carpal tunnel view shows a 1-month-old fracture of the hook of the left hamate in a baseball player.

Cast Management

A trial cast period of 4–6 weeks is indicated to determine if the localized symptoms from this fracture can be relieved by simple immobilization. A well-padded short-arm cast is applied with the wrist in slight flexion and ulnar deviation, and is changed if it becomes loose.

The fracture heals clinically more rapidly than it does radiographically. The patient may be symptom-free by 6 weeks but may require an additional 3–6 months for the fracture line to be completely obliterated on x-ray. If the patient remains symptomatic after 6–8 weeks of trial cast immobilization, operative excision of the fracture fragment is indicated to relieve pain and improve grip strength.

Operative Treatment for Persistently Symptomatic Fractures of the Hamate

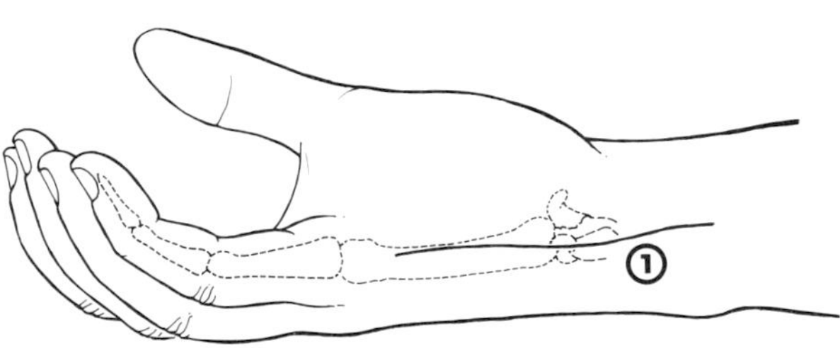

1. The fracture site must be carefully exposed through a medial approach along the ulnar border of the fifth metacarpal.

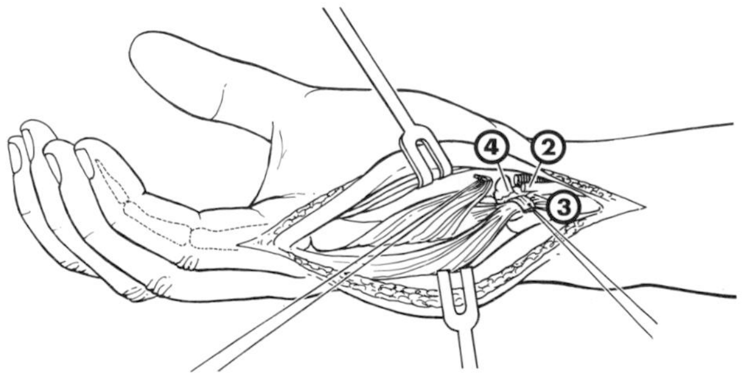

2. The superficial and
3. The deep branches of the ulnar nerve are identified and protected.
4. After the periosteum is stripped, the hamate fragment is removed, the base of the hamate is smoothed, and the wound is closed.

Fracture of the Trapezium (Greater Multangular)

Mechanism of Injury

Fracture of the trapezium is produced by direct trauma to the radiodorsal aspect of the joint or by extreme dorsiflexion of the wrist, as occurs in a fall on the outstretched hand. The bone is caught between the styloid process of the radius and the base of the first metacarpal bone.

The fracture may be an isolated lesion or may be associated with other carpal lesions, the most common being fracture of the first metacarpal and fracture of the distal end of the radius.

Anatomic Features

The trapezium (greater multangular) is trapezoid in shape and articulates with the first and second metacarpals, the scaphoid, and the trapezoid (lesser multangular). The articulation with the first metacarpal is saddle-shaped and is enveloped in a loose capsule, permitting a wide range of motion.

Fractures may be of various types: vertical, comminuted, or avulsion fractures. The vertical type is by far the most common and is invariably associated with dislocation of the first metacarpal bone.

Management

Accurate restoration of the fragments is useful for normal function of the thumb; therefore, open reduction and internal fixation, unless contraindicated, are the treatment of choice. Excision of the fragments may be carried out for extremely comminuted fractures.

Appearance on X-Ray

1. Fracture of the trapezium.
2. The outer fragment is displaced proximally.
3. The articular surface of the first metacarpal is subluxated.

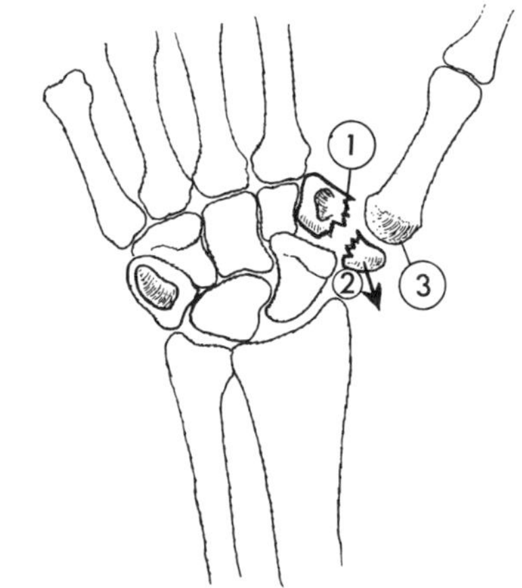

Operative Repair for Large Fragments

1. The fracture is visualized with a direct dorsal surgical incision.
2. Traction is applied to the thumb to bring the fracture fragments into alignment.

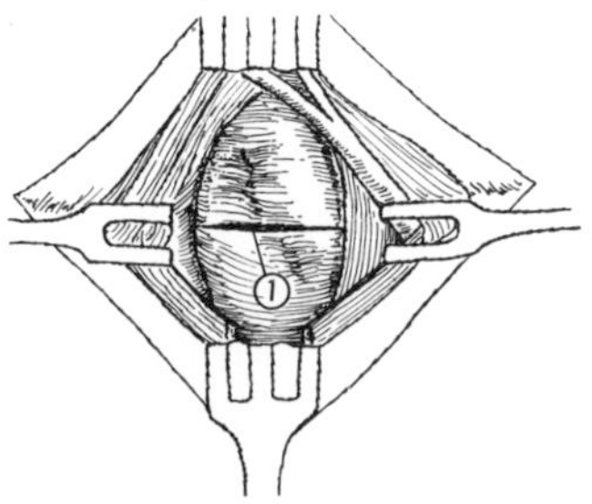

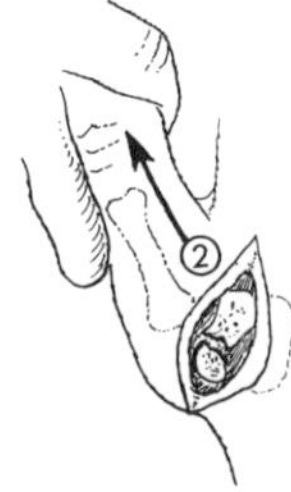

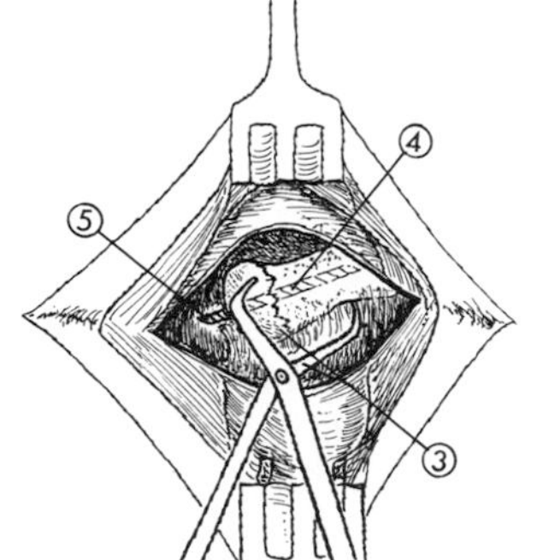

3. The fragments are then approximated with a bone clamp.
4. A 2-mm wire or small fragment screw is used to fix the fragments.
5. The wire or screw is buried beneath the skin.

Management of Severely Comminuted Fractures of the Trapezium

REMARKS

In this instance, excision of the bone fragments is preferable. The thumb is immobilized in the position of function for 6 weeks to allow for soft tissue healing and stability. Subsequent circumduction of the thumb should then be pain-free.

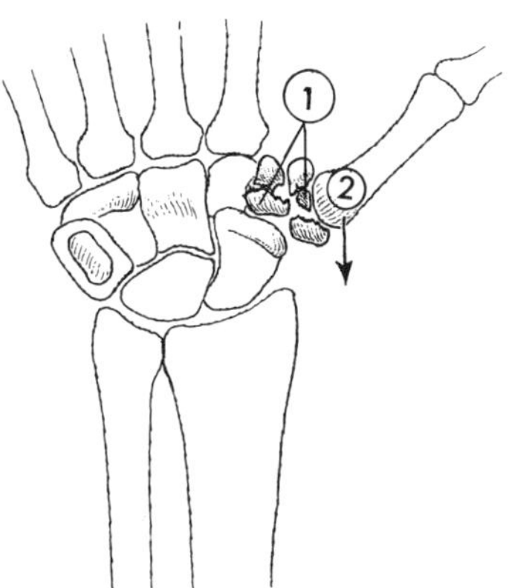

Preoperative X-Ray

1. Severe comminution of the trapezium.
2. Proximal displacement of the first metacarpal.

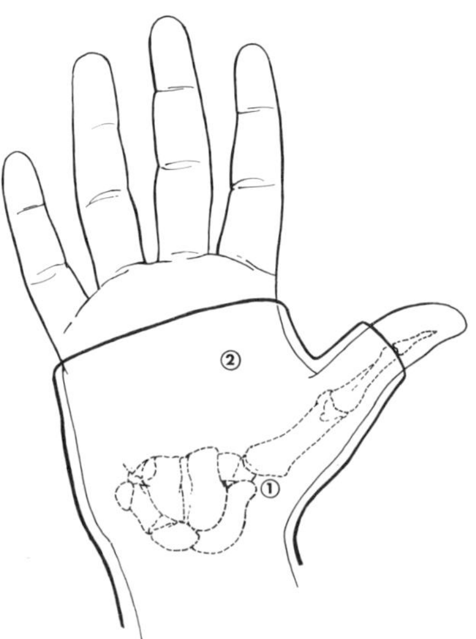

Postoperative X-Ray

1. The comminuted fracture fragments have been surgically excised.
2. The thumb and first metacarpal are stabilized externally in a position of function using a cast for 6 weeks.

NEUROLOGIC COMPLICATIONS OF CARPAL INJURIES

Ulnar Nerve Involvement

REMARKS

In closed fractures of the pisiform, hamate, triquetrum, and fourth and fifth metacarpals, the motor branch of the ulnar nerve, which is the chief motor nerve of the hand, may be injured; the sensory branch is rarely affected. Blunt trauma to the hypothenar eminence of the hand may also contuse the ulnar nerve.

Following fracture or soft tissue injuries, the nerve may be compressed by edema or hemorrhage. Intraneural fibrosis may result, as indicated by delayed or progressive paralysis of the intrinsic muscles of the hand.

Management

If there is a large hematoma, it can be evacuated. Generally, spontaneous recovery occurs; however, if there is no recovery after 6–8 weeks, the ulnar nerve should be explored. If the nerve is being compressed, excise any tight ligament in Guyan's canal. If a neuroma is present, excise it. Decompression and neurolysis of the nerve may be necessary, particularly with injuries to the hamate or to the bases of the fourth and fifth metacarpals.

Median Nerve Involvement

Carpal Tunnel Syndrome

REMARKS

This disorder is characterized by sensory disturbances in the index and middle fingers such as tingling. Pressure over the volar ligament accentuates pain and paresthesia along the course of the median nerve. Late in the disorder the thenar eminence exhibits muscular atrophy.

Implication of the median nerve is the result of compression due to (1) constriction of the osseofibrous tunnel containing the flexor tendons of the fingers and the median nerve or (2) swelling of the structures within the tunnel, as in tenosynovitis of the flexor tendons. Direct trauma to the volar aspect of the wrist may cause swelling of the volar ligament.

The commonest sources of carpal tunnel syndrome are a displaced Colles' fracture or a fracture of one of the proximal carpal bones or perilunate dislocation. The patient who complains of numbness and tingling in the hand in association with a fracture of the wrist should be evaluated carefully before and after fracture reduction.

If the symptoms do not respond to prompt reduction of the fracture and elevation for a day or so, decompression of the median nerve in the carpal tunnel is indicated. In addition, any operative repair of the fracture site generally warrants decompression of the carpal tunnel at the same time.

Persistent compression of the median nerve has been associated with persistent painful dysesthesias and even a Sudeck type of atrophy. Therefore, early decompression of the carpal tunnel is preferable to a prolonged "wait and see" management.

Appearance on X-Ray

RECENT LESION

1. Perilunar dislocation.
2. Fracture of the scaphoid.

This patient had an acute compression of the median nerve.

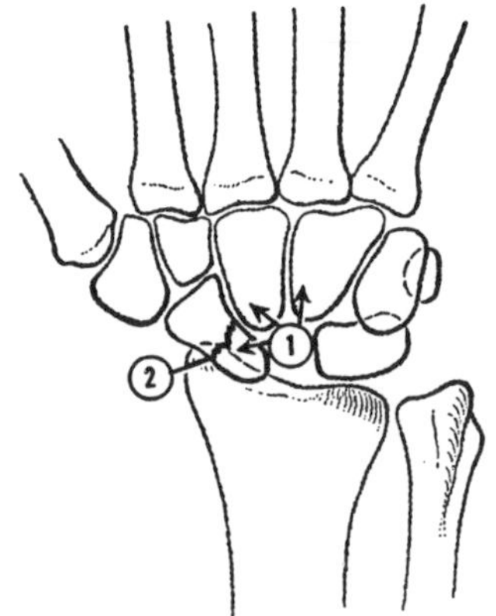

Carpal Tunnel Syndrome With Colles' Fracture

1. A displaced Colles' fracture is the commonest cause of the carpal tunnel syndrome with wrist injury.
2. The distal radial fracture fragment impinges upon the medial nerve and the tight canal.

Note: Progressive swelling or immobilization of Colles' fracture in a hyperflexed position can aggravate the entrapment of the median nerve. Any persistent painful numbness, tingling, or dysesthesias after reduction of Colles' fracture is best treated by early decompression of the nerve to avoid prolonged painful dysesthesia and Sudeck atrophy.

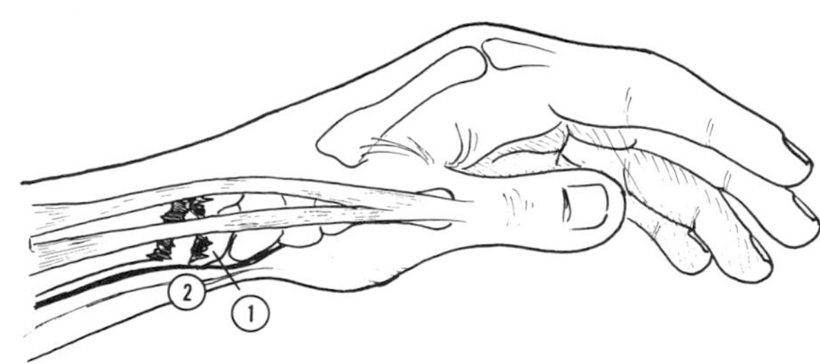

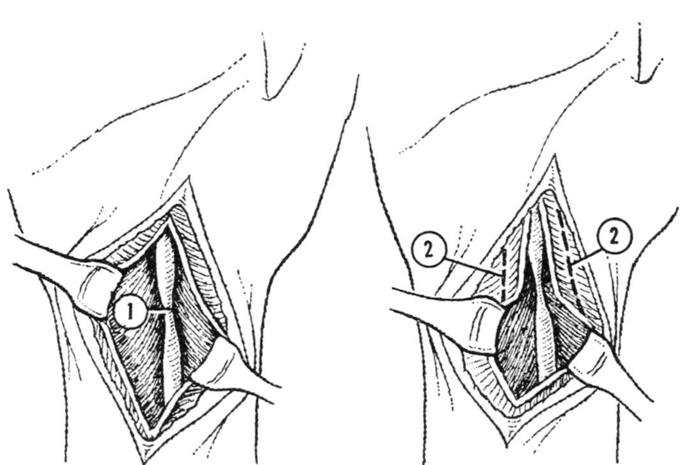

1. The median nerve is exposed through a wrist incision between the flexor carpi radialis and the palmaris longus. This demonstrates the area of compression of the median nerve and usually an area of constriction or narrowing.
2. The carpal tunnel is completely released to decompress the median nerve. In addition, any displaced fracture fragment should be reduced as well.

Immobilization

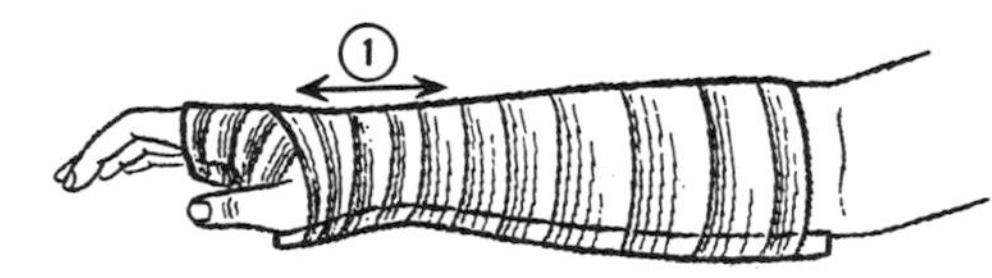

1. Apply an anterior plaster slab, holding the wrist in the neutral position.

Subsequent Management

The fracture is treated with either splints or a cast if not fixed internally. The median nerve symptoms should be relieved promptly with decompression of the carpal tunnel. Subsequently immobilization is continued for the period of time necessary to achieve adequate healing of the fracture.

BIBLIOGRAPHY

Colles' Fractures

Atkins RM, Duckworth J, Kanis JA: Algodystrophy following Colles' fracture. J Hand Surg 14B:161, 1989.

Axelrod T, Paley D, Green J, McMurtry RY: Limited open reduction of the lunate facet in comminuted intraarticular fractures of the distal radius. J Hand Surg 13A:372, 1988.

Bickerstaff DR, Bell MJ: Carpal malalignment in Colles' fractures. J Hand Surg 14B:155, 1989.

Bradway J, Amadio PC, Cooney WP: Open reduction and internal fixation of displaced, comminuted intraarticular fractures of the distal end of the radius. J Bone Joint Surg Am 71:839, 1989.

Chapman DR, Bennett JB, Bryan WJ, Tullos HS: Complications of distal radius fractures: Pins and plaster treatment. J Hand Surg 7:509, 1982.

Clancey GJ: Percutaneous Kirschner-wire fixation of Colles' fractures. J Bone Joint Surg Am 66:1008, 1984.

Clyburn TA: Dynamic external fixation for comminuted intraarticular fractures of the distal end of the radius. J Bone Joint Surg Am 69:248, 1987.

Cooney WP: Management of Colles' fractures. Editorial. J Hand Surg 14B:137, 1989.

Cooney WP, Linscheid RL, Dobyns JH: External pin fixation for unstable Colles' fractures. J Bone Joint Surg Am 61:840, 1979.

Cooney WP, Dobyns JH, Linscheid RL: Complications of Colles' fractures. J Bone Joint Surg Am 62:613, 1980.

De Oliveira JC: Barton's fractures. J Bone Joint Surg Am 55:586, 1973.

DePalma AF: Comminuted fractures of the distal end of radius treated by ulnar pinning. J Bone Joint Surg Am 34:65, 1952.

Dias, JJ, Wray CC, Jones JM, Gregg PJ: The value of early mobilization in the treatment of Colles' fractures. J Bone Joint Surg Br 69:463, 1987.

Ellis J: Smith's and Barton's fractures—a method of treatment. J Bone Joint Surg Br 47:724, 1965.

Field J, Protheroe D, Atkins R: Algodystrophy after Colles' fracture is associated with secondary tightness of casts. J Bone Joint Surg Br 76:901, 1994.

Ford D, Ali M: Acute carpal tunnel syndrome. J Bone Joint Surg Br 68:758, 1986.

Green DP: Pins and plaster treatment of comminuted fractures of the distal end of the radius. J Bone Joint Surg Am 57:30, 1975.

Haberneck H, Weinstabl R, Fialka C, Schmid L: Unstable distal radius fractures treated by modified Kirschner wire pinning: Anatomic considerations, technique, and results. J Trauma 36:83, 1994.

Howard PW, Stewart HD, Hind RE, Burke FD: External fixation or plaster for severely displaced comminute Colles' fractures? J Bone Joint Surg Br 71:68, 1989.

Jupiter J: Fractures of the distal end of the radius. J Bone Joint Surg Am 73:461, 1991.

Knirk JL, Jupiter JB: Intraarticular fractures of the distal end of the radius in young adults. J Bone Joint Surg Am 68:647, 1986.

Lewis MH: Median nerve decompression after Colles' fracture. J Bone Joint Surg Br 60:195, 1978.

McQueen MM, Maclaren A, Chalmers J: The value of remanipulating Colles' fractures. J Bone Joint Surg Br 68:232, 1986.

Melone CP: Open treatment for displaced articular fractures of the distal radius. Clin Orthop 202:103, 1986.

Pattee GA, Thompson GH: Anterior and posterior marginal fracture-dislocations of the distal radius. Clin Orthop 231:183, 1988.

Peltier LF: Fractures of the distal end of the radius. An historical account. Clin Orthop 187:18, 1984.

Sarmiento A, Zagorski JB, Sinclair WF: Functional bracing of Colles' fractures: A prospective study of immobilization in supination vs. pronation. Clin Orthop 146:175, 1980.

Stein AH: The relation of median nerve compression to Sudeck's syndrome. Surg Gynecol Obstet 115:713, 1962.

Taleisnik J, Watson HK: Midcarpal instability caused by malunited fractures of the distal radius. J Hand Surg 9A:350, 1984.

Tountas A, Waddell J: Simultaneous fracture of the distal radius and scaphoid. J Orthop Trauma 4:312, 1988.

Tulipan D, Eaton R, Eberhart B: The Darrach procedure defended. J Hand Surg Am 16:438, 1991.

Weber SC, Szabo RM: Severely comminuted distal radial fracture as an unsolved problem: Complications associated with external fixation and pins and plaster techniques. J Hand Surg 11A:157, 1986.

Werry D, Meek R: Clostridial gas gangrene complicating Colles' fracture. J Trauma 26:280, 1986.

Younge D: Haematoma block for fractures of the wrist: A cause of compartment syndrome. J Hand Surg Br 14:194, 1989.

Carpal Fractures and Dislocations

Bellinghausen H, Gilula LA, Young LV, Weeks PM: Posttraumatic palmar carpal subluxation. J Bone Joint Surg Am 65:998, 1983.

Bora FW Jr, Osterman AL, Woodbury DF, Brighton CT: Treatment of nonunion of the scaphoid by direct current. Orthop Clin North Am 15:107, 1984.

Botte MJ, Gelberman RH: Fractures of the carpus, excluding the scaphoid. Hand Clin North Am 3:149, 1987.

Bunker TD, McNamee PB, Scott TD: The Herbert screw for scaphoid fractures. J Bone Joint Surg Br 69:631, 1987.

Campbell RD Jr, Thompson TC, et al.: Indications for open reduction of lunate and perilunate dislocations of the carpal bones. J Bone Joint Surg Am 47:915, 1965.

Carter PR, Eaton RG, Littler JW: Ununited fracture of the hook of the hamate. J Bone Joint Surg Am 59:583, 1977.

Cooney WP, Dobyns JH, Linscheid RL: Fractures of the scaphoid: A rational approach to management. Clin Orthop 149:90, 1980.

Cordrey LJ, Ferrer-Torells M: Management of fractures of the greater multangular. J Bone Joint Surg Am 42:1111, 1960.

Crabbe WA: Excision of the proximal row of the carpus. J Bone Joint Surg Br 46:708, 1964.

Dehne E, Deffer PA, Feighney RE: Pathomechanics of the fracture of the carpal navicular. J Trauma 4:96, 1964.

Duppe H, Johnell O, Lundborg G, Karlsson M, Redlund-Johnell I: Long-term results of fracture of the scaphoid. J Bone Joint Surg Am 76:249, 1994.

Ebraheim N, Spie M, Saudaine E, et al: Coronal fracture of the body of the hamate. J Trauma 38:169, 1995.

Fisk GR: The wrist. J Bone Joint Surg Br 66:396, 1984.

Garcia-Elias M, Abanco J, Salvador E, Sanchez R: Crush injury of the carpus. J Bone Joint Surg Br 67:286, 1985.

Gelberman RH, Menon J: The vascularity of the scaphoid bone. J Hand Surg 5:508, 1980.

Gelberman RH, Wolock BS, Siegel DB: Fractures and non-unions of the carpal scaphoid. J Bone Joint Surg Am 71:1560, 1989.

Green DP: Proximal row carpectomy. Hand Clin North Am 3:163, 1987.

Green DP, O'Brien ET: Classification and management of carpal dislocations. Clin Orthop 149:55, 1980.

Herbert TJ, Fisher WE: Management of the fractured scaphoid using a new bone screw. J Bone Joint Surg Br 66:114, 1984.

Horii E, Nakamura R, Wanatabe K, Tsunoda K: Scaphoid fracture as a "puncher's fracture." J Orthop Trauma 8:107, 1994.

King RJ, MacKenney RP, Elnur S: Suggested method for closed treatment of fractures of the carpal scaphoid: Hypothesis supported by dissection and clinical practice. J Soc Med 75:860, 1982.

Kleinman WB: Management of chronic rotary subluxation of the scaphoid by scapho-trapezio-trapezoid arthrodesis. Hand Clin North Am 3:113, 1987.

Lawlis J, Gunther S: Carpometacarpal dislocations. J Bone Joint Surg Am 75:56, 1991.

Linscheid RL, Dobyns JH: Athletic injuries of the wrist. Clin Orthop 198:141, 1985.

Linscheid RL, Dobyns JH, Beabout JW, Bryan RS: Traumatic instability of the wrist. J Bone Joint Surg Am 54:1612, 1972.

London PS: The broken scaphoid bone: The case against pessimism. J Bone Joint Surg Br 43:237, 1961.

Mack GR, Bosse MJ, Gelberman RH, Yu E: The natural history of scaphoid nonunion. J Bone Joint Surg Am 66:504, 1984.

Mayfield JK, Johnson RP, Kilcoyne RK: Carpal dislocations: Pathomechanics and progressive perilunar instability. J Hand Surg 5:226, 1980.

Palmer AK, Dobyns JH, Linscheid RL: Management of posttraumatic instability of the wrist secondary to ligament rupture. J Hand Surg 3:507, 1978.

Rand JA, Linscheid RL, Dobyns JH: Capitate fractures. Clin Orthop 165:209, 1982.

Reagan DS, Linscheid RL, Dobyns JH: Lunotriquetral sprains. J Hand Surg 9A:502, 1984.

Ruby LK, Stinson J, Belsky MR: The natural history of scaphoid nonunion: A review of 55 cases. J Bone Joint Surg Am 67:428, 1985.

Sarrafian SK, Melamed JL, Goshgarian GM: Study of wrist motion in flexion and extension. Clin Orthop 126:153, 1977.

Smith D, Cooney W, An KN, et al.: The effects of simulated unstable scaphoid fractures on carpal motion. J Hand Surg 14A:283, 1989.

Stark HH, Jobe FW, Boyes JH, et al.: Fracture of the hook of the hamate in athletes. J Bone Joint Surg Am 59:575, 1977.

Stein F, Siegel MW: Naviculocapitate fracture syndrome: A case report. New thoughts on the mechanism of injury. J Bone Joint Surg Am 51:391, 1969.

Taleisnik J: Post-traumatic carpal instability. Clin Orthop 149:73, 1980.

Taleisnik J: Subtotal arthrodeses of the wrist joint. Clin Orthop 187:81, 1984.

Taleisnik J, Kelly PJ: The extraosseous and intraosseous blood supply of the scaphoid bone. J Bone Joint Surg Am 48:1125, 1966.

Tiel-van Buul M, van Beek E, Broeckhuizen A, et al: Radiography and scintigraphy of suspected scaphoid fracture. J Bone Joint Surg Br 75:61, 1993.

Vance R, Gelberman R: Acute ulnar neuropathy with fractures at the wrist. J Bone Joint Surg Am 60:962, 1978.

Watson HK, Ryu J, Akelman E: Limited triscaphoid intercarpal arthrodesis for rotatory subluxation of the scaphoid. J Bone Joint Surg Am 68:345, 1986.

17 Fractures and Dislocations of the Hand

APPLIED ANATOMY

REMARKS

The great versatility of the hand, which permits actions ranging from precision pinch to power grip, depends on a well-tuned interplay of intrinsic and extrinsic muscle function.

Normal mobility of joint and skeletal support is critical for hand function.

Thorough knowledge of applied anatomy is essential in managing all injuries, major or minor, that disrupt the delicate balance that is hand function.

Longitudinal and Transverse Arches of the Hand

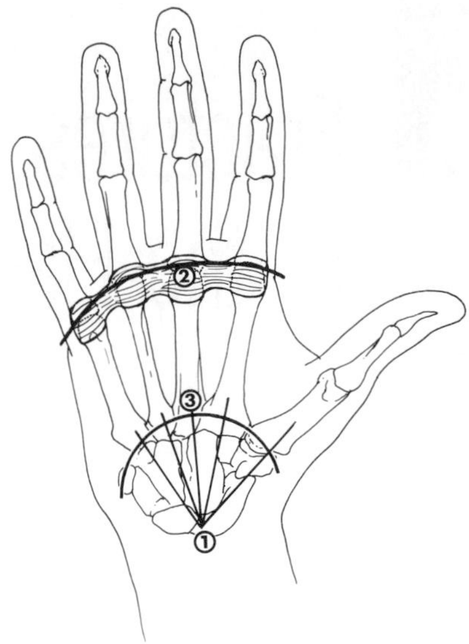

The hand is composed of five longitudinal and two transverse arches. Disruption of these arches frequently produces rotational deformities of the fingers.

1. Longitudinal arches are composed of carpals, metacarpals, and phalanges.
2. Mobile distal transverse arch is composed of the intermetacarpal ligaments (intervolar plate) with the interposed metacarpal heads.
3. Proximal transverse arch is a rigid semicircular structure consisting of the distal row of carpal bones and the intercarpal ligaments with the keystone of the arch at the capitate bone.

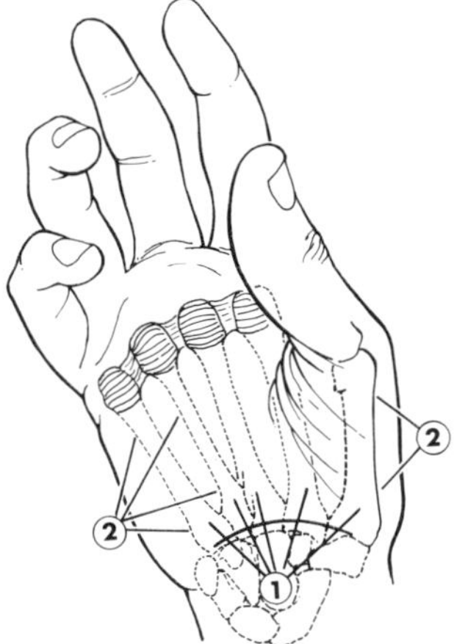

1. Proximal transverse arch combined with the heads of the second and third metacarpals to which it firmly attaches is the fixed unit of the hand.
2. Mobile proximal and distal structures rotate about the rigid unit.

Metacarpophalangeal Joints of the Fingers

REMARKS

Each metacarpophalangeal (MP) joint is so fashioned that, on flexion of the corresponding digit, the distal phalanx points to the tubercle of the scaphoid, and the fingers do not overlap. This is an important anatomic arrangement and must always be borne in mind when fractures of the phalanges of the fingers are treated.

Malunion with rotation of a phalanx produces overlapping of the finger when the hand makes a fist.

The sphericity of the metacarpal head is slightly eccentric, so that the capsular structures tighten with full flexion. This is important for adduction-abduction motion of the joint.

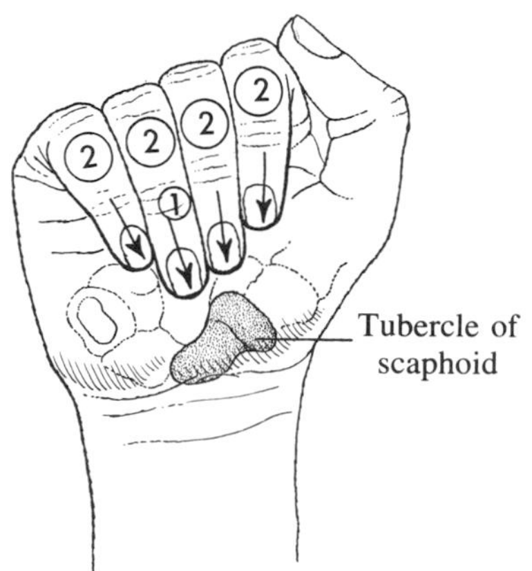

Normal Position of Finger on Flexion

1. Distal phalanges all point to the tubercle of the scaphoid.
2. Fingers do not overlap.

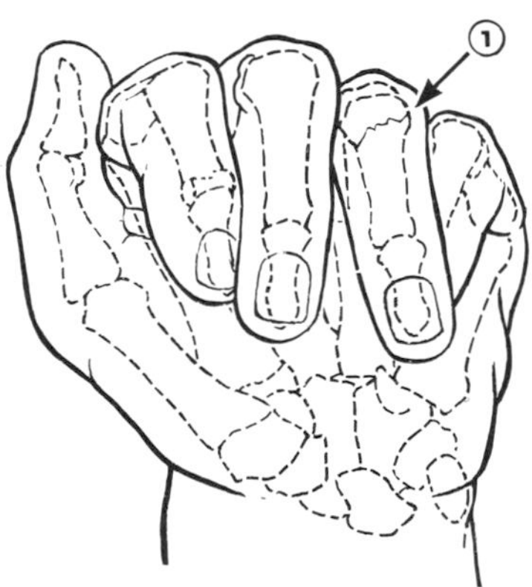

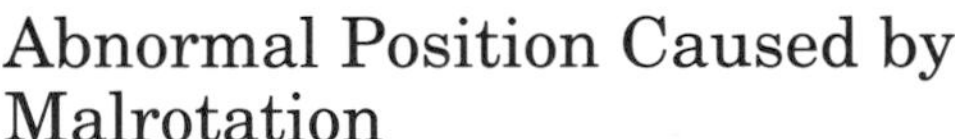

Abnormal Position Caused by Malrotation

1. Fracture of a phalanx or metacarpal.

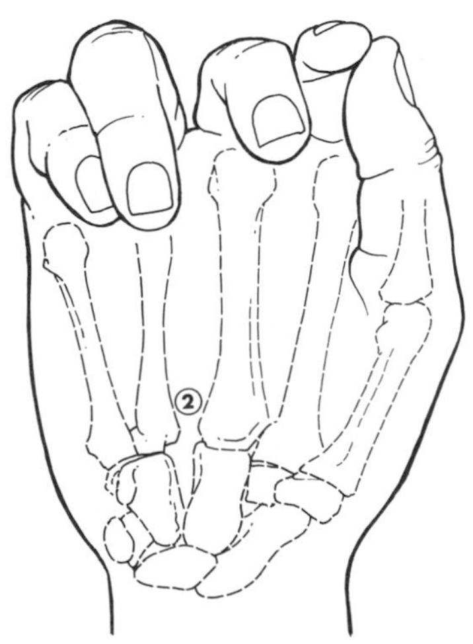

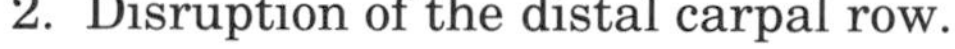

2. Disruption of the distal carpal row.

The MP joint also permits abduction of the finger away from the midline and some circumduction. This motion is greater in the index and little fingers than in the long and ring fingers.

The stability of the MP joint depends largely on its capsular ligaments and collateral structures.

The eccentric shape of the metacarpal head makes these ligaments tight in flexion and loose in extension.

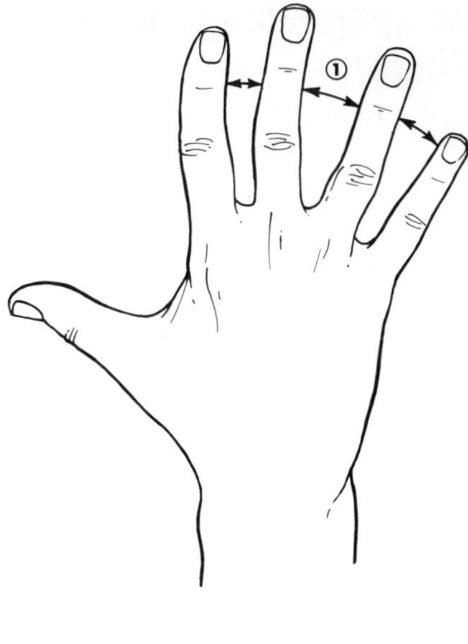

Test the stability in your own fingers.

1. In extension, 40° of lateral (abduction or adduction) motion is present at the MP joint.

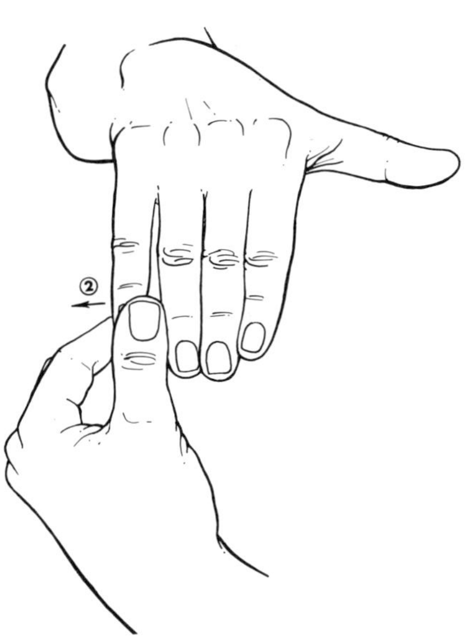

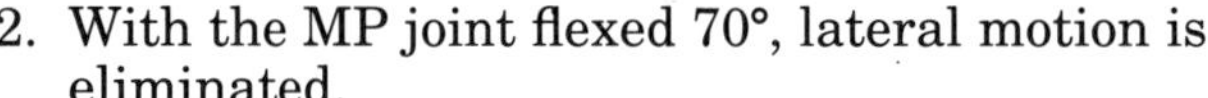

2. With the MP joint flexed 70°, lateral motion is eliminated.

Metacarpophalangeal Joint of the Thumb

REMARKS

The MP joint of the thumb must be stable for the important pinch mechanism. Consequently, the joint has more of the characteristics of a hinge joint and functions like an interphalangeal (IP) joint of the finger.

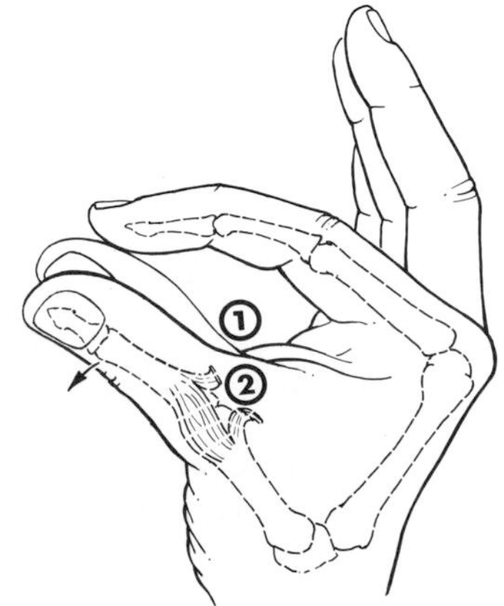

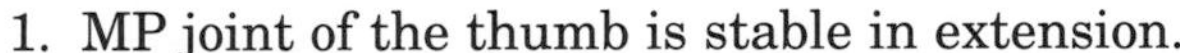

1. MP joint of the thumb is stable in extension.
2. Disruption of the thumb support ligaments causes considerable loss of pinch strength.

Positions for Immobilizing Joints (Position of Function)

REMARKS

The shape of the IP joints permits motion in only one plane, flexion and extension.

The IP joints have the same capsular structure, collateral ligaments, and volar plates as do the MP joints.

Owing to their different shapes, the MP joint support structures are stretched to their fullest, in full flexion, while the IP joint support structures are tightest, in very slight flexion. This is essentially the intrinsic-plus position.

Capsule and Collateral Ligaments of Metacarpophalangeal and Interphalangeal Joints

The shape of the articular surfaces has the following effect on the joint capsule.

1. Collateral ligament of the MP joint is slack in extension but
2. Tight in flexion.

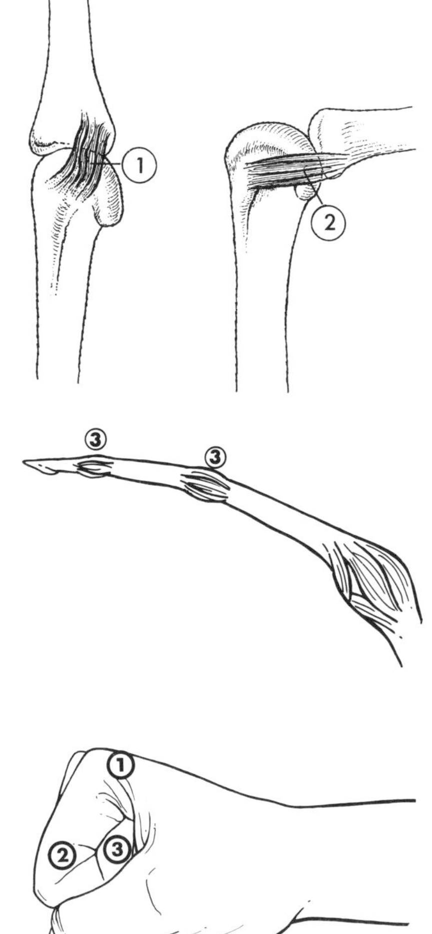

3. Collateral ligament of the IP joint is tight in slight flexion.

Normal Finger Flexion

The synchrony between intrinsic and extrinsic muscle function allows normal finger flexion consisting of

1. 70°–80° of MP flexion.
2. 110°–120° of proximal IP flexion.
3. 90° of distal IP flexion.

Abnormal Finger Flexion: Intrinsic-Minus Position

Absence of intrinsic function, as in median and ulnar nerve palsy, produces grossly inefficient flexion or clawing of the hand.

Intrinsic-minus hand flexion consists of

1. Hyperextension of the MP joint and
2. Inability to flex the fingertips into the palm for grasp.

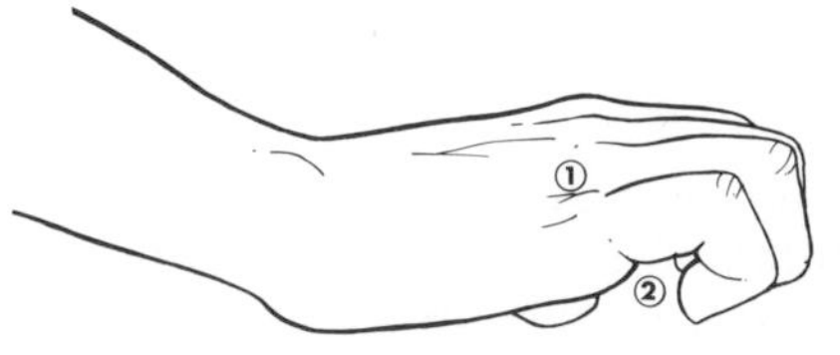

Importance of Immobilizing the Injured Hand in the Position of Function

REMARKS

The position of function is the intrinsic-plus position.

The position of rest, which is the classic grasp or beer glass position, does not take into account the need of the joint support structures to be stretched to their fullest.

The worst position and the one most likely to impair hand function permanently is the position of failure. This is also known as the intrinsic-minus position, which allows hyperextension of the MP joints and flexion of the IP joints, with adduction contracture of the thumb.

Preferred Method—Intrinsic-Plus Position for Immobilization (Position of Function)

To minimize stiffening of joints, the MP joints and IP joints are held in the intrinsic-plus or safe position, which maintains the capsules and ligaments at maximal length. This minimizes chronic stiffening after immobilization.

1. MP joints are flexed as near to 70° as possible.
2. IP joints are in slight (15°) flexion.
3. Thumb is abducted and opposed to the fingers.

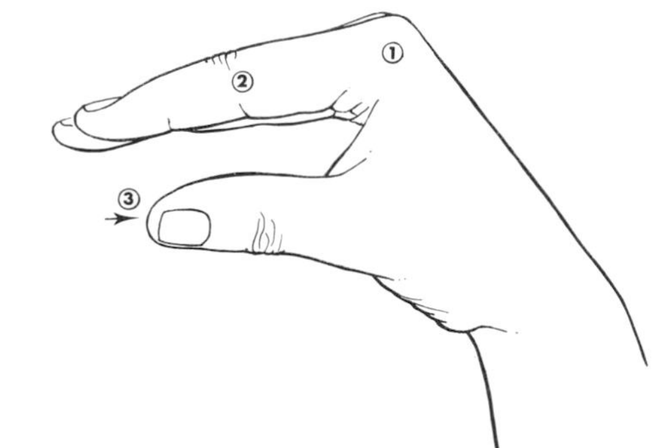

Position of Rest or Beer Glass Position

The position of rest or beer glass position has been recommended for immobilizing the injured hand in the past. However, this does not meet the requirement of maintaining the capsule and joint structures at their maximal lengths and sometimes contributes to stiffening.

1. MP joints are not flexed maximally to keep the capsule and ligament structures lengthened.
2. IP joints are flexed too much, which leads to loss of full extension.

Note: The position of rest should be abandoned in preference to the intrinsic-plus position.

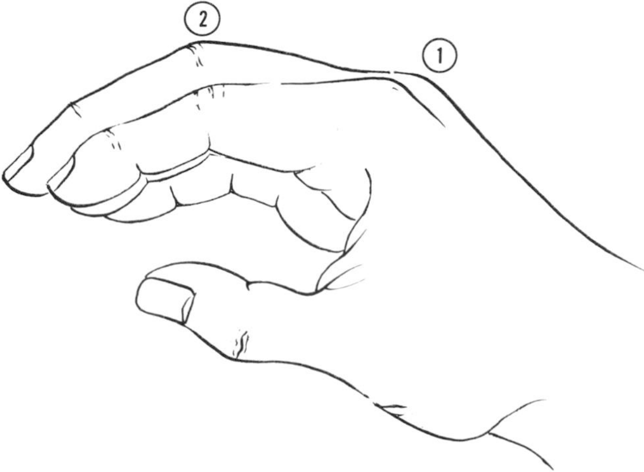

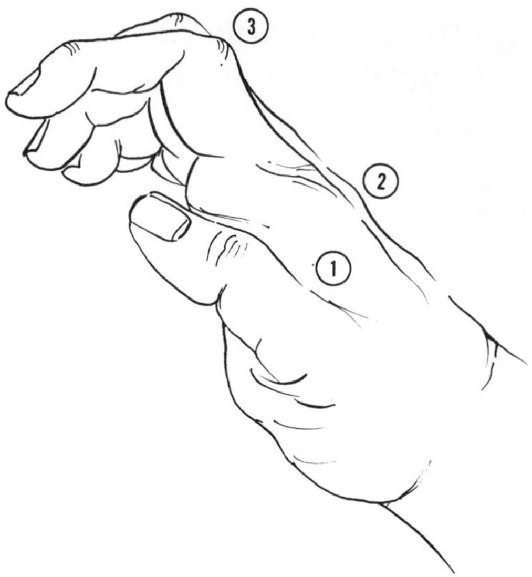

Position of Failure

The hand at all times should be kept out of the position of failure or the intrinsic-minus position.

1. This leads to *ad*duction of the thumb (rather than *ab*duction).
2. Hyperextension of the MP joints.
3. Flexion of the IP joints.

Chronic stiffening of the hand in this position significantly impairs the ability of the hand to grasp or pinch and must be prevented. This is particularly likely to occur with fractures associated with burns or soft tissue injuries, which contribute to scar contracture.

BASIC PRINCIPLES IN MANAGING HAND FRACTURES AND INJURIES

REMARKS

By far, most fractures and dislocations of the hand are best treated by simple closed methods. Exceptions to this general principle include irreducible dislocations, angulated unstable fractures of the proximal or middle phalanx, and multiple fractures in the same hand.

A prime objective in the management of hand fractures and joint injuries is to permit early active motion and thereby allow a "pumping out" of the swollen soft tissues. Early active motion restores the delicate gliding mechanism of tendon and joint systems, which can be severely disrupted by fractures and dislocations.

Prolonged immobilization (more than 3 weeks) should be avoided for most injuries because this leads to permanent stiffness and impaired hand function.

Open injuries are common in the hand and require thorough wound cleansing and meticulous excision of wound edges. Particularly, we should be aware of "minor hand injuries" over joints. Some of the worst infections of the hand develop from human bites over knuckles.

Methods of Fracture Management

Splint for Mallet Finger

1. Distal IP (DIP) joint is in slight hyperextension.
2. Proximal IP (PIP) joint is free.

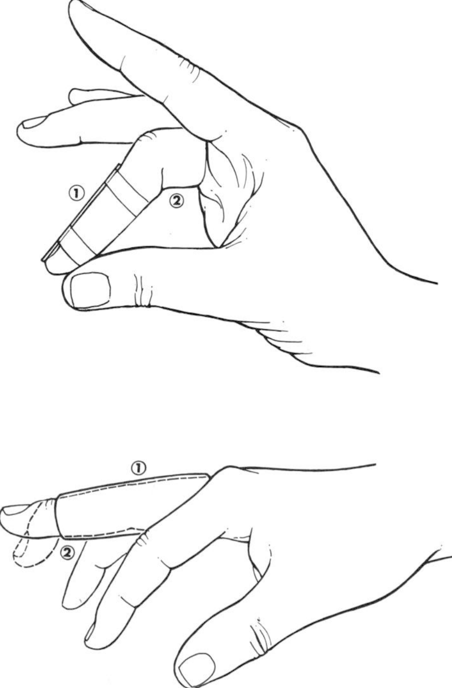

For Boutonnière Deformity

1. PIP joint is extended.
2. DIP joint is free.

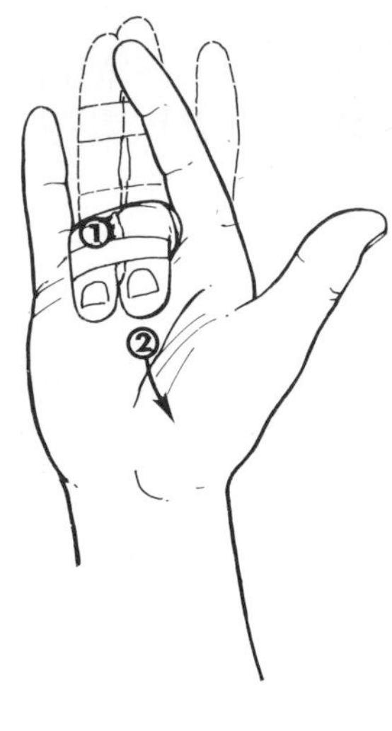

For Stable Phalangeal Fractures

1. Fractured finger is taped to the adjacent finger.
2. Tips of both fingers point to the scaphoid tuberosity in flexion.

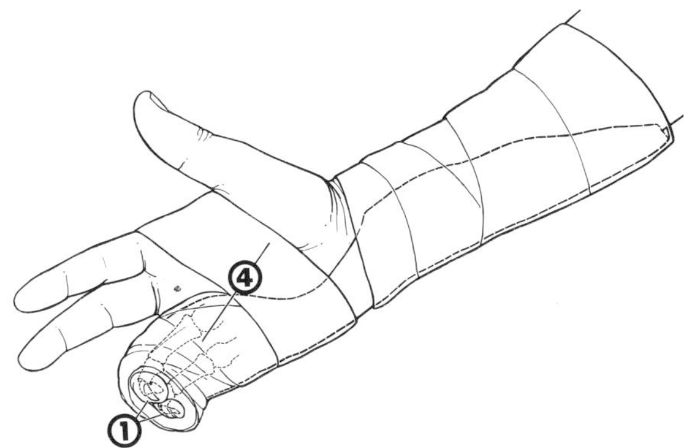

Cast-Splint Immobilization After Reduction of Phalangeal or Metacarpal Fracture

The fractured finger and adjacent finger are immobilized together.

1. Incorporate the fractured and the adjacent unfractured finger.
2. MP joints are flexed 70°.
3. IP joints are in slight flexion.
4. Tips of the fingers are aligned to point toward the scaphoid tuberosity for correct rotational alignment.

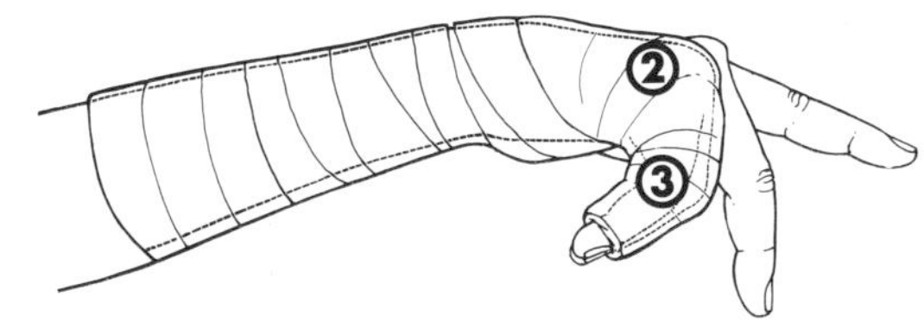

Immobilization of the Swollen Hand by Compressive Dressing

It is important to eliminate swelling and edema from the injured hand as quickly as possible before and after treatment.

This can best be accomplished by using a compressive dressing and elevating the hand.

1. Wrist is slightly extended, and the MP joint and IP joints are immobilized in the intrinsic-plus position.
2. Thumb is in apposition with the fingers.
3. Soft tissue fluffs are applied liberally in the palm between the fingers.

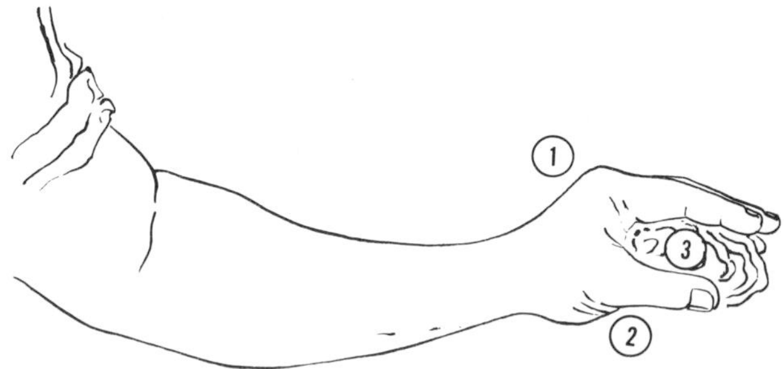

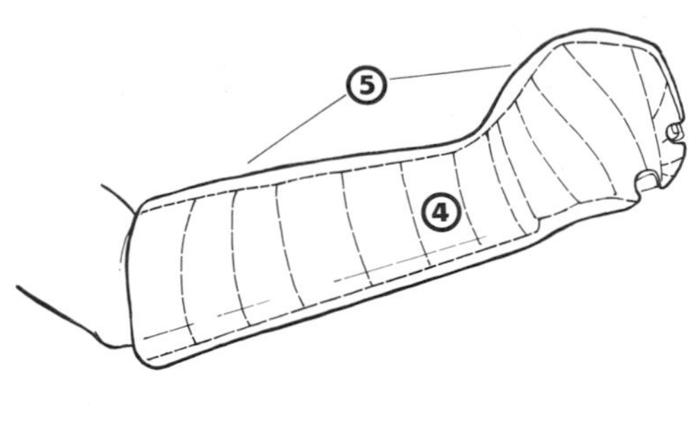

4. Rolled gauze is wrapped around the soft tissue from the elbow to the finger tips.
5. Light plaster is applied with the rolled gauze.

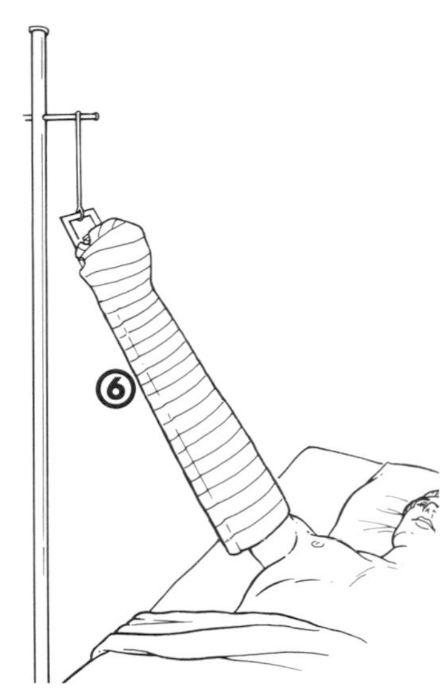

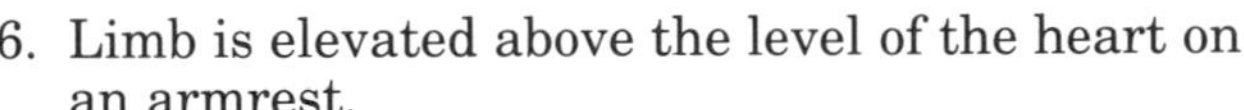

6. Limb is elevated above the level of the heart on an armrest.

When the swelling has subsided, usually by 2–3 days, the compressive dressing can be removed, and a cast or other support can be applied.

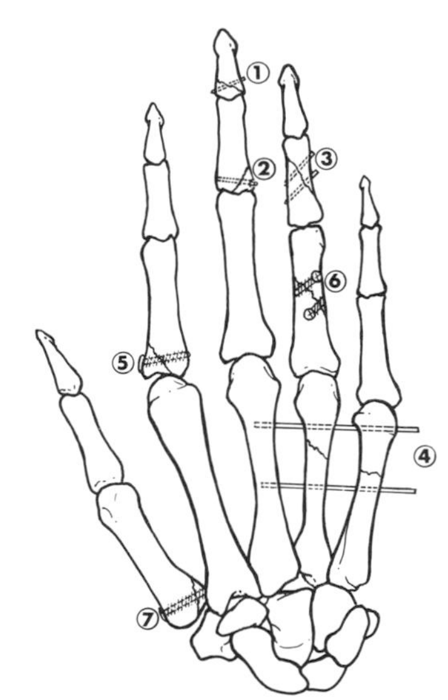

Methods of Internal Fixation

Closed treatment is not always the most "conservative" method. Operative fixation of unstable injuries permits early restoration of hand and finger function.

Kirschner wire fixation is used for

1. Avulsion fracture of the distal phalanx,
2. Fracture-dislocation of the PIP joint, or
3. Shortened oblique fracture of the middle phalanx.
4. Transverse Kirschner wires are used for multiple metacarpal fractures.

Small fragment screw is used for

5. Condylar fractures,
6. Angulated fractures of the proximal phalanx, or
7. Bennett fracture-dislocations.

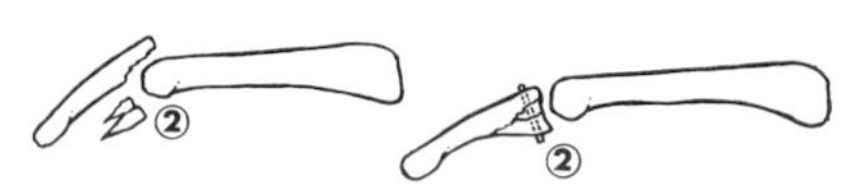

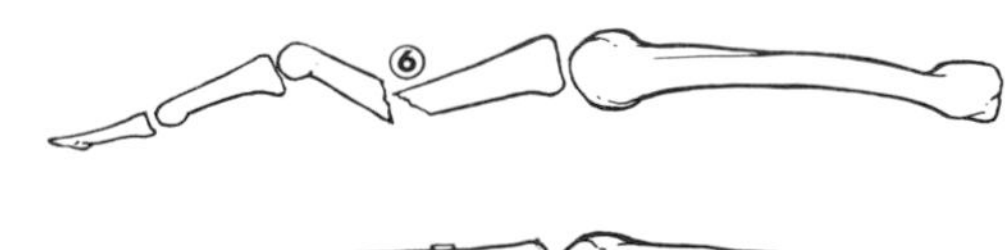

■ Open Wounds of the Hand

All open wounds of the hand require complete wound excision and cleansing. Be particularly wary of the following.

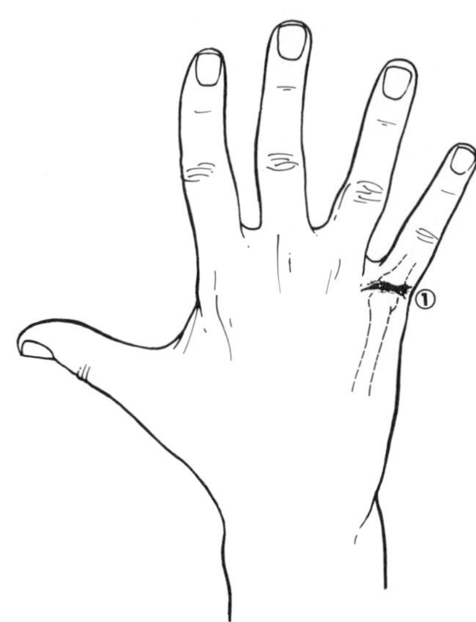

1. Open wounds over MP knuckles sustained from a human bite, which inevitably become infected if closed primarily. These are extremely contaminated and must be thoroughly excised, cleansed, and left open.

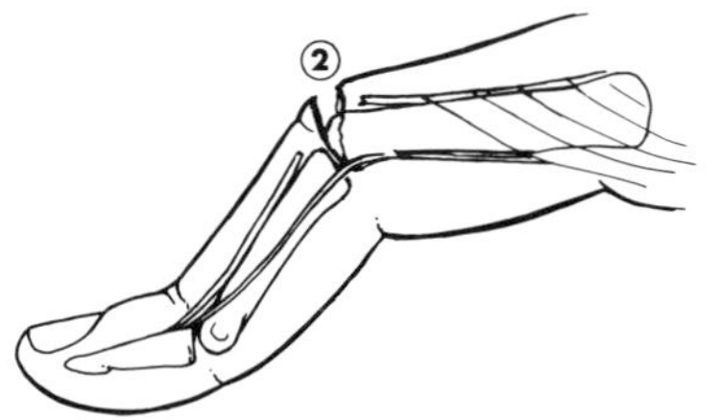

2. Laceration over PIP joint that detaches the extensor central slip insertion and leads to boutonnière deformity.

Management of Crushing, Open Wounds

Open fractures from high-velocity wounds or crushing injuries are best treated by staged wound management. Initial debridement should be thorough and antibiotics should be used. At times, it is necessary also to do the following.

1. Release tight carpal ligaments.
2. Free intermetacarpal fascia compartments by dorsal fasciotomy.

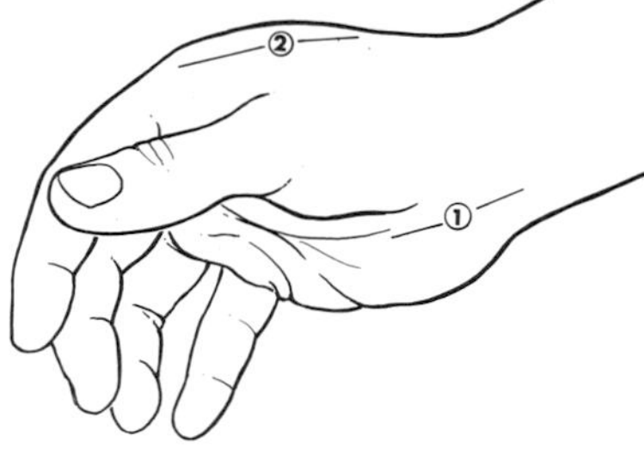

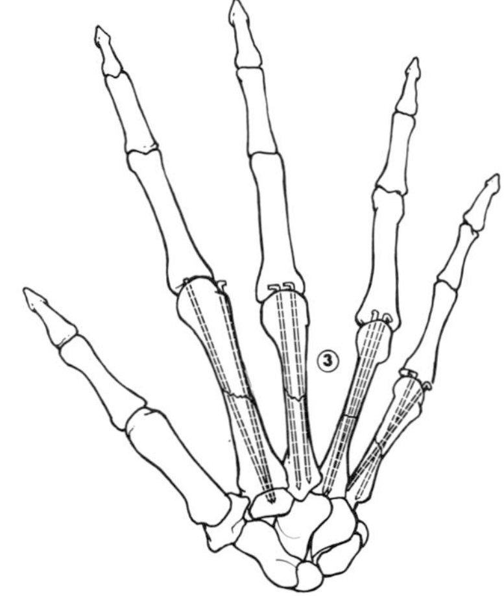

3. Fix multiple fractures with Kirschner wires.

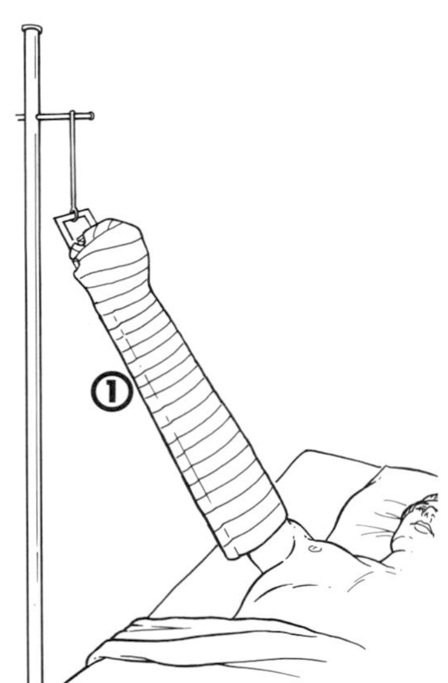

Secondary wound excision and closure is performed in 3–5 days with assurance that the wound is clean. To eliminate edema before closure,

1. Elevate the limb in a hand compression dressing, and maintain it constantly until closure.

■ Anesthetic Techniques for Reduction of Finger and Metacarpal Fractures

REMARKS

Fractures and dislocations of the metacarpals are best anesthetized by the intravenous block technique described previously for distal radial fractures (see Chapter 16).

Fractures and dislocations of the fingers can be adequately anesthetized by local digital blocks.

Technique of Digital Block

1. Preferred location for digital block of the dorsal and volar nerves is in the web space.

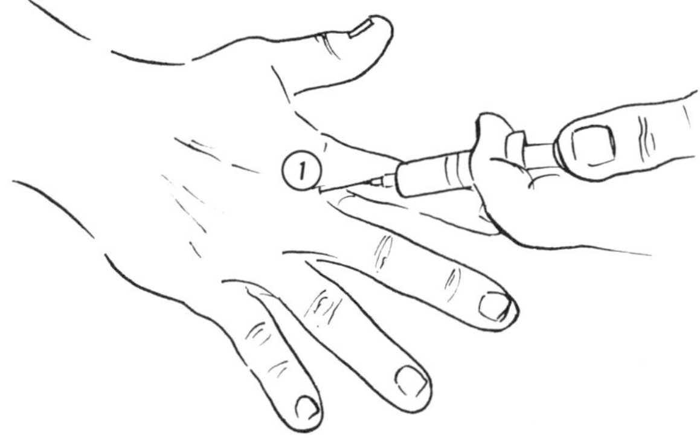

2. Alternative method is to block the digital nerves at the distal palmar crease.

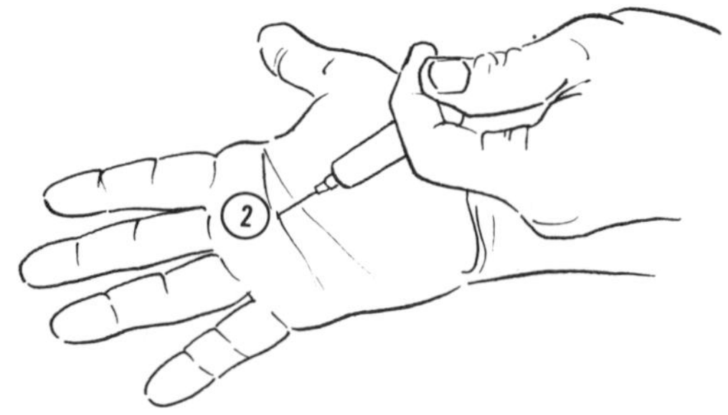

Note: Avoid injecting the anesthetic circumferentially about a finger because this has been associated with vasospasm and gangrene of the digit. Epinephrine or other vasoconstrictive agent should also be avoided when the local anesthetic is injected.

DISLOCATIONS AND FRACTURE-DISLOCATIONS OF THE THUMB

REMARKS

The thumb is the most mobile component of the hand. Through the carpometacarpal (CM) joint, which may be considered the thumb's MP joint, the thumb is capable of almost universal motion. This great range of mobility is necessary for the hand to function effectively in prehension. Complete loss of thumb function is equivalent to the loss of at least 50 per cent of hand function.

The bony architecture of the CM joint provides little stability. The stability of this joint is chiefly derived from its capsule and collateral ligaments.

The very nature of the thumb's position and function renders it vulnerable to injury, varying from sprains to complete disruption of its linkage system.

The most common injuries to the thumb's linkage system include

- Bennett fracture—fracture-dislocation of the CM joint.
- Rolando fracture—fracture comminuted into the CM joint.
- Transverse fracture of the first metacarpal.
- Dislocation of the MP joint.
- Skier's thumb—subluxation of the MP joint from ulnar collateral tear.
- Fracture of the phalanges and dislocation of the IP joint.

Fracture-Dislocation of the Carpometacarpal Joint of the Thumb (Bennett Fracture)

REMARKS

Essentially, the Bennett fracture is an oblique fracture through the base of the first metacarpal with dislocation of the radial portion of its articular surface. The medial portion of the articular surface, which is triangular and smaller than the radial shaft fragment, remains attached by its ligaments to the trapezium.

A Bennett fracture is usually produced by direct violence applied to the end of the metacarpal, driving the shaft proximally and dorsally.

The dislocated portion of the metacarpal disrupts the dorsal capsular structures.

The objective of treatment for this fracture is to maintain the width of grip to allow the hand to grasp glass tumblers and other wide objects. Consequently, the thumb should be immobilized in wide abduction and opposition.

Charnley and others have shown that closed reduction can work for most of these fractures if proper manipulation is used. Operative measures should be reserved for occasions when closed methods have failed.

Prereduction X-Ray

1. Shaft fragment is displaced radially and dorsally.
2. Triangular ulnar fragment maintains its normal relationship to the trapezium.

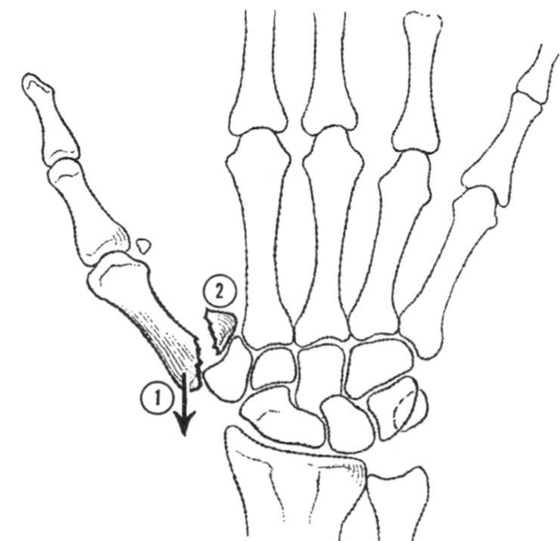

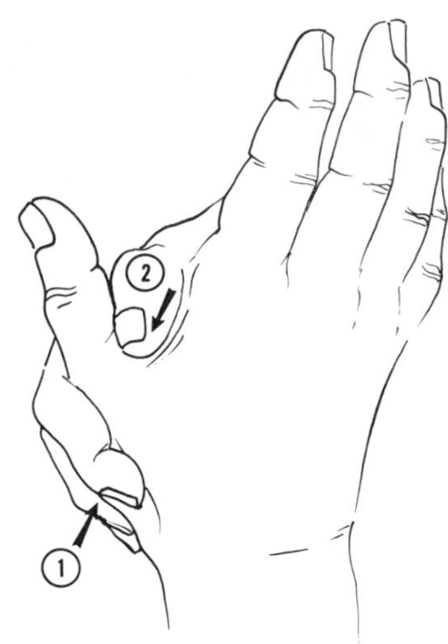

Charnley Method of Manipulation

1. Reduction of this unstable fracture requires direct application of pressure to the base of the first metacarpal to reduce the dislocation.
2. Second force is applied to the distal head of the metacarpal to maintain the thumb in abduction.

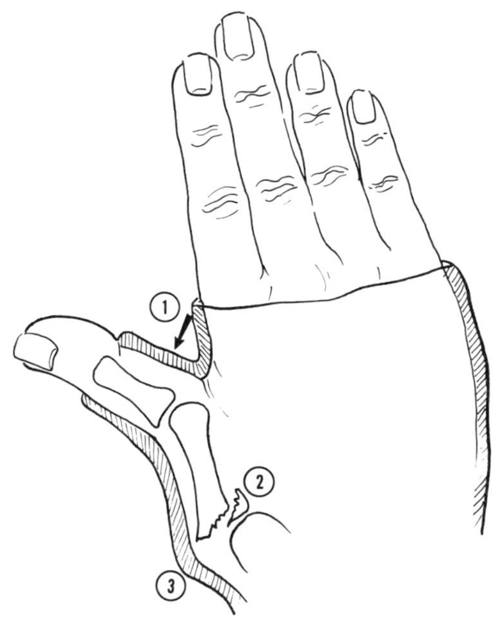

1. Avoid extending the thumb at the MP joint. This does not reduce the metacarpal but only hyperextends the MP joint.

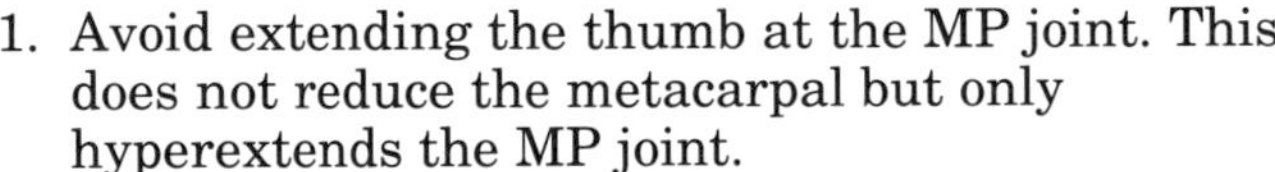

2. The result is the fracture-dislocation at the base of the metacarpal remains unreduced unless the extension position of the metacarpal is maintained.
3. Plaster should be molded on the palmar aspect of the metacarpal and on the dorsal aspect.

Technique of Plaster Application

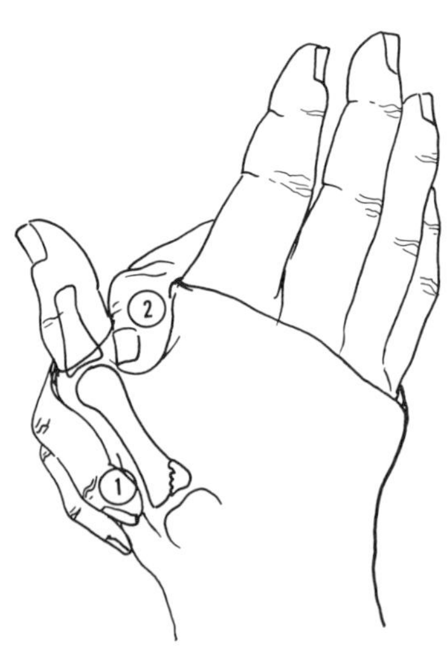

1. Cast padding is applied lightly to the fractured hand and forearm, and padding is particularly applied carefully to the base of the metacarpal of the thumb.
2. As the plaster is applied and setting, the fracture is reduced by dorsal pressure on the base of the thumb metacarpal and distal metacarpal joint.

As the surgeon's pressure is applied against the metacarpal, the bone can be felt to reduce into position.

Note: This gentle pressure is maintained until the plaster has hardened sufficiently. After the plaster has hardened over the metacarpal and hand, the cast is continued to below the elbow.

Closed Reduction and Fixation With Kirschner Wire

This technique is used for the more unstable fracture-dislocations that require internal stabilization.

1. Thumb metacarpal is abducted to align the radial portion of the dislocated fracture with the intra-articular fragment. Reduction is checked by fluoroscopy or standard x-ray.
2. Smooth Kirschner wire is then inserted through the shaft fragment dorsally into the trapezium. The ulnar fracture fragment is not fixed, but a pin is used to restore stability to the joint surface.

Note: Occasionally, if closed reduction and either cast or Kirschner wire fixation does not adequately reduce the fracture, open reduction may be indicated.

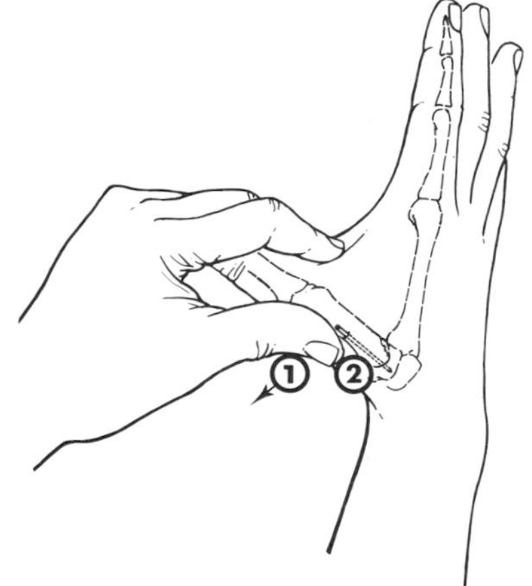

Postreduction X-Ray (After Closed Kirschner Wire Fixation)

1. Relationship between the radial and ulnar fragments and the articular surface is restored.
2. Pin through the metacarpal shaft fragment crosses the articular surface into the trapezium.

Note: If closed reduction and Kirschner wire fixation do not restore the joint surface satisfactorily, open the fracture, and fix the fragments internally.

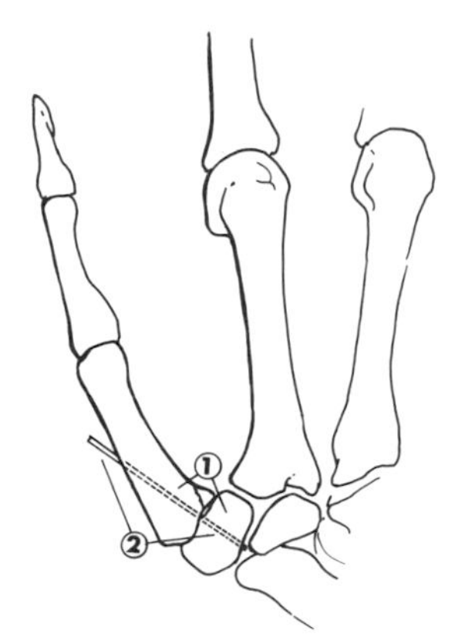

Alternative Method

POSTOPERATIVE X-RAY (AFTER OPEN REDUCTION)

1. Fracture-dislocation is adequately reduced.
2. Small fragment screw stabilizes the fracture in anatomic position.

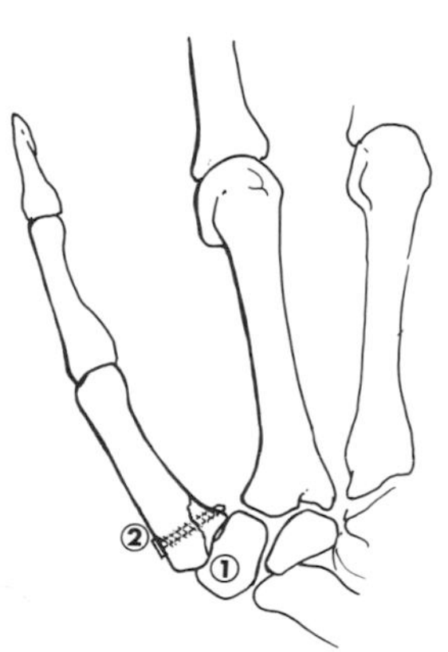

Postoperative Management

If Kirschner wire fixation has been used, remove the wire at 3 weeks and permit the patient to do active exercises. If the fracture is still tender, use a protective splint for 2 more weeks.

If small fragment screw fixation has been used, immobilize for 3 weeks and then remove the plaster. The screw need not be removed unless it causes local tenderness.

Rolando Intra-Articular Fracture

REMARKS

In contrast to a Bennett fracture, a Rolando fracture consists of multiple intra-articular fragments. Anatomic reduction is frequently impossible.

If the metacarpal shaft can be realigned with the trapezium, the comminution of the joint surface may be accepted. Attempted operative reduction of the fragments usually only worsens the joint disruption.

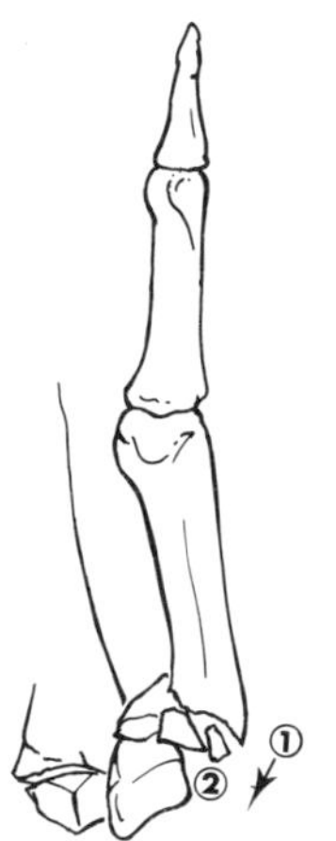

Preoperative X-Ray

1. Metacarpal fragment has displaced radially and dorsally.
2. Base of the metacarpal is shattered.

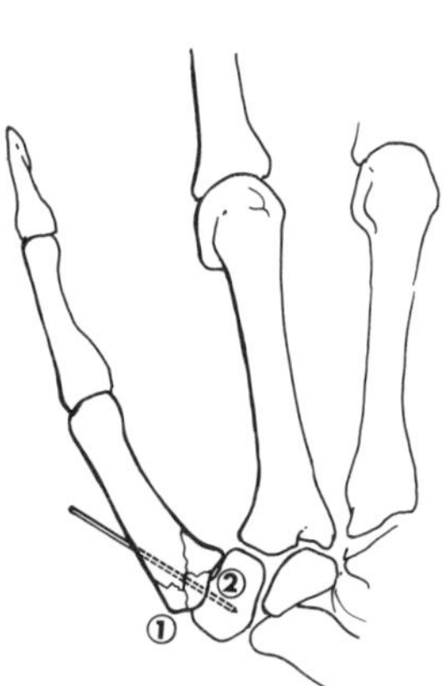

X-Ray After Closed Reduction and Kirschner Wire Fixation

1. Metacarpal shaft fragment is realigned with the trapezium.
2. Comminuted articular surface remains incompletely reduced.

Postoperative Management

Immobilize the hand in a thumb spica cast for 3 weeks and then remove the cast and pin.

Evaluate the degree of healing clinically and radiographically.

If the shaft fragment is stable, begin guarded range-of-motion exercises to regain as much circumduction as possible in the thumb.

Traumatic arthritis of varying degrees is likely to follow this injury.

Subluxation of the Carpometacarpal Joint of the Thumb

Like most highly mobile joints, the CM joint of the thumb is subject to a number of strains and capsular injuries.

This joint is a common site for osteoarthritis in later years because of its susceptibility to "wear and tear."

Acute injuries of the CM joint without fracture-dislocation can be treated by rest with cast immobilization for 2–3 weeks.

Prereduction X-Ray

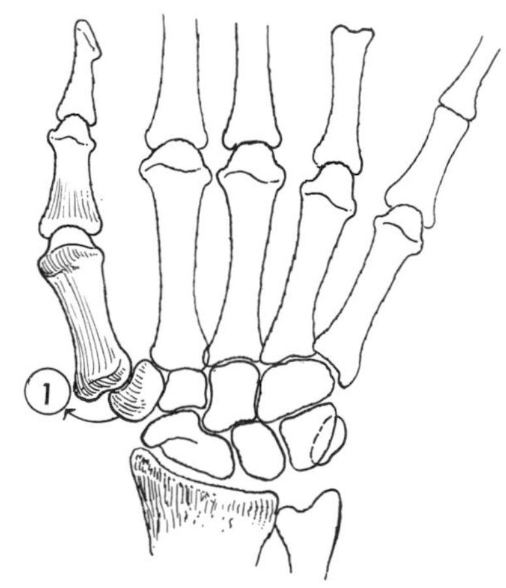

1. Metacarpal has subluxated radially and dorsally.

Closed Treatment

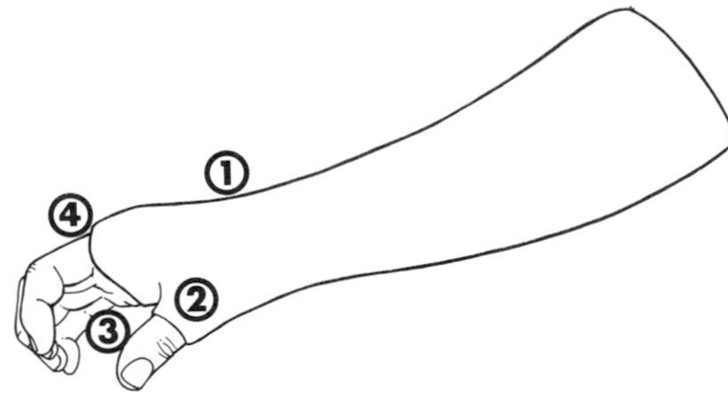

Apply a short-arm cast.

1. Cast extends above the wrist.
2. Thumb is apposed to the fingers, and the cast is molded over the CM joint.
3. IP joint of the thumb is free to move.
4. Unaffected fingers are free to move.

Subsequent Management

Maintain the thumb in the plaster cast for 3 weeks.

Encourage free use of the unaffected fingers.

After 3 weeks, remove the cast, and permit active range of motion.

The patient should avoid heavy usage or contact sports, which are likely to reinjure the thumb, for 3–4 weeks longer.

■ Unstable Subluxations or Dislocations of the Carpometacarpal Joint of the Thumb

REMARKS

If the capsular tissues are severely disrupted, the CM joint is very unstable and may subluxate even in plaster.

It is essential that the tissues heal with the articular surfaces of the joint in the normal anatomic position.

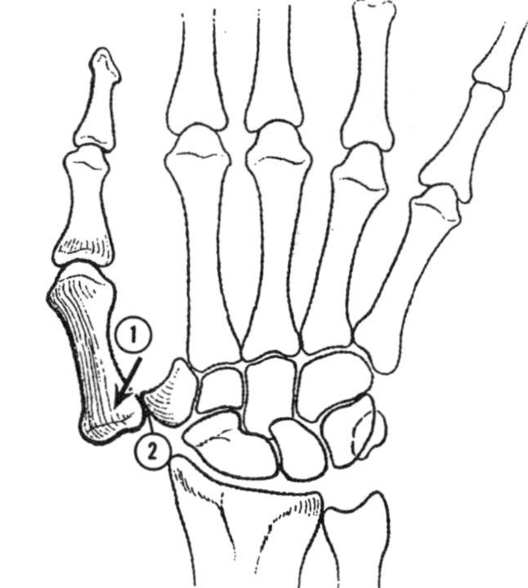

Prereduction X-Ray

1. Metacarpal is displaced upward and backward.
2. Metacarpal rests on the posterior aspect of the trapezium.

Manipulative Reduction

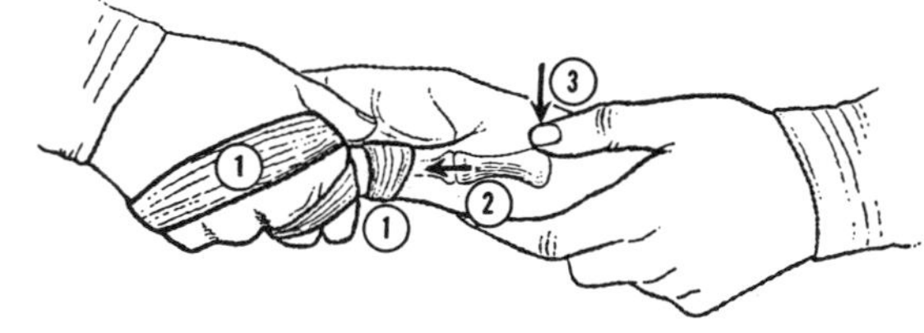

1. Bandage is looped first around the patient's thumb and then around the operator's hand.
2. While traction is applied along the long axis of the thumb, the thumb is gradually abducted, and at the same time,
3. Direct pressure is exerted against the head of the metacarpal bone.

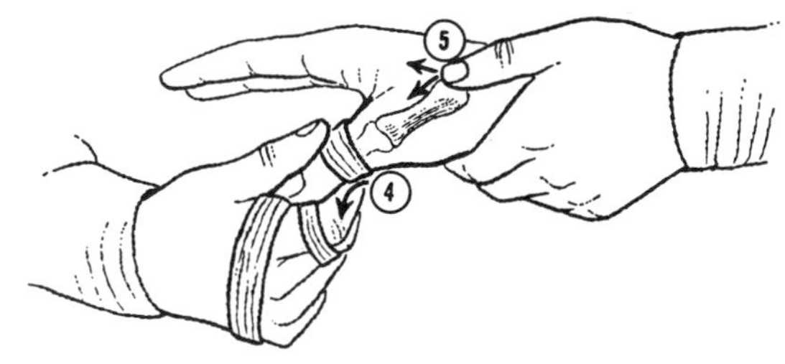

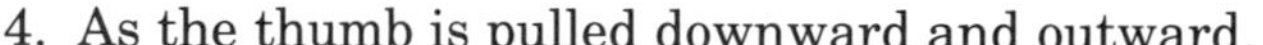

4. As the thumb is pulled downward and outward,
5. The head of the metacarpal is pushed forward and inward.

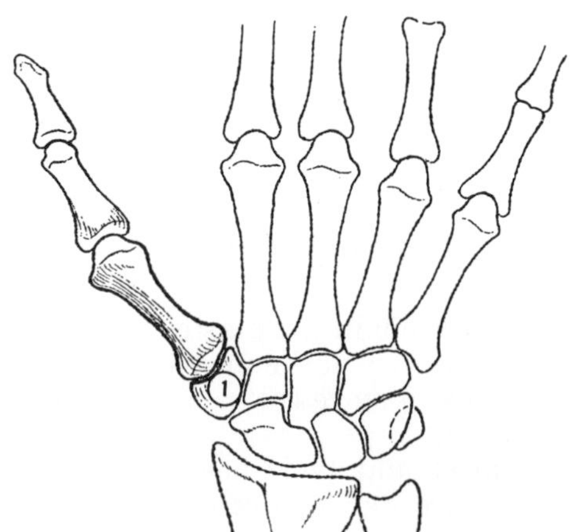

Postreduction X-Ray

1. Head of the metacarpal is in normal relationship to the trapezium.

Note: If the reduction is unstable, use Kirschner wire fixation.

Immobilization

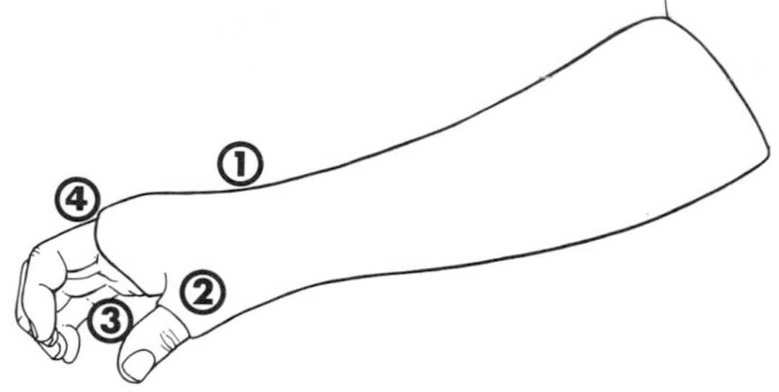

1. Apply a cast from below the elbow.
2. Thumb is abducted and plaster is molded over the CM joint.
3. IP joint of the thumb is free.
4. Unaffected joints are allowed to move freely.

Postreduction Management

Take x-rays on the fifth and tenth days. Check the position of the articular surfaces of the joint.

Encourage active exercises of the unaffected fingers.

Remove the cast at the end of 3 weeks, and have the patient begin active exercise to the joint.

If the dislocation or subluxation recurs in plaster, use Kirschner wire fixation through the joint.

Closed Reduction With Internal Fixation

If the CM joint is unstable or displaces while in plaster, internal fixation becomes necessary.

Persistent subluxation of the joint is likely to result in traumatic arthritis and impairment of thumb function.

Percutaneous Pin Technique

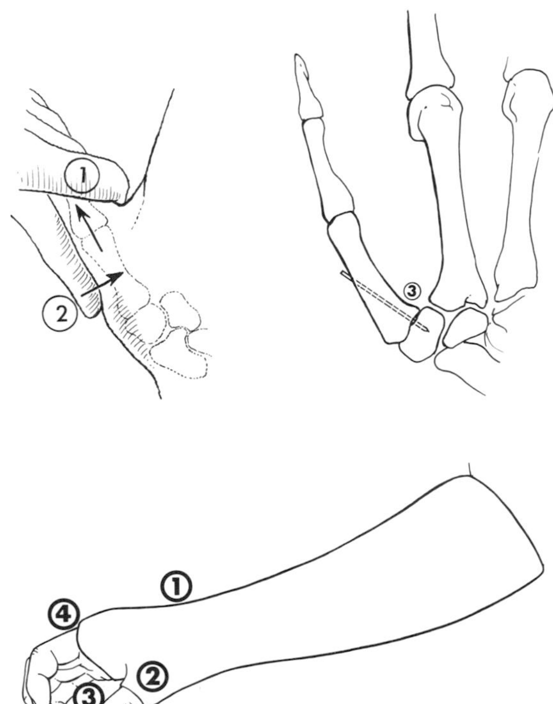

1. Assistant applies traction on the abducted thumb and, at the same time,
2. Applies inward pressure on the metacarpal with his or her thumb.
3. While this position is maintained, pass a smooth Kirschner wire through the base of the metacarpal into the trapezium. Cut the wire off below the level of the skin.

Immobilization

1. Apply a cast from below the elbow.
2. Thumb is abducted, and plaster is molded over the CM joint.
3. IP joint of the thumb is free.
4. Unaffected joints are allowed to move freely.

Subsequent Management

Remove the cast after 3 weeks, and permit active motion of the thumb.

If Kirschner wire fixation was necessary, remove the wire after 3 weeks, and begin protected active motion.

If the patient is going to use the thumb in heavy labor or sports, a protective bandage should be applied for 3 more weeks.

■ Fractures at the Base of the Metacarpal of the Thumb

REMARKS

Fractures at the base of the thumb metacarpal may be transverse, oblique, or comminuted.

Generally, they occur in men. In children, the lesion is essentially an epiphyseal separation with a triangular fragment of the diaphysis displaced with the epiphysis.

Usually, the deformity is posterior with outward bowing.

Most lesions are readily reduced by traction and manipulative maneuvers and are stable; they can be treated by immobilizing the thumb in abduction.

Unstable fractures can be treated by open reduction and fixation with a small fragment screw.

Stable Fractures

PREREDUCTION X-RAY

1. In an adult man, fracture through the base of the metacarpal.
2. Distal fragment is displaced upward and backward.
3. Usual deformity is posterior with outward bowing.

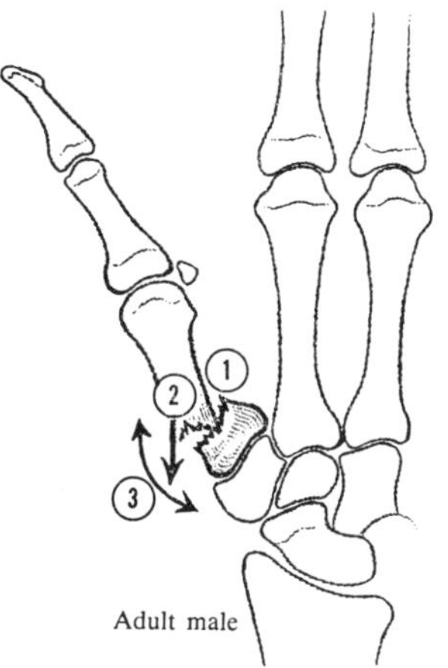

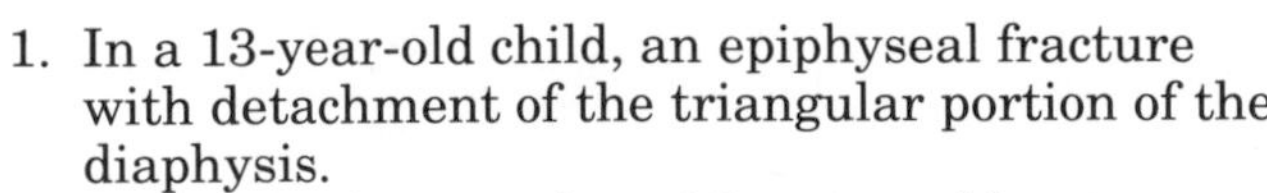
1. In a 13-year-old child, an epiphyseal fracture with detachment of the triangular portion of the diaphysis.
2. Deformity is posterior with outward bowing.

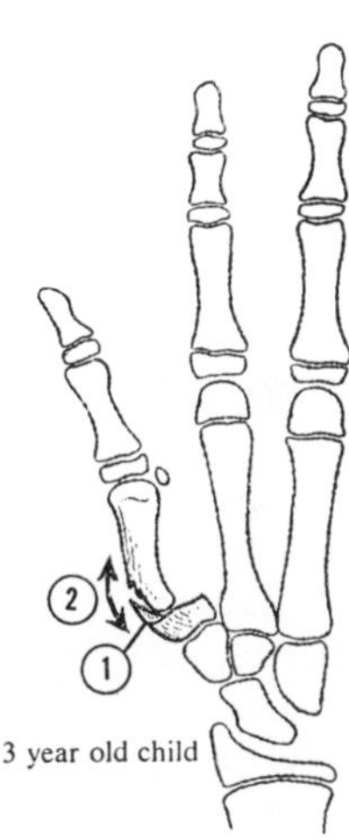

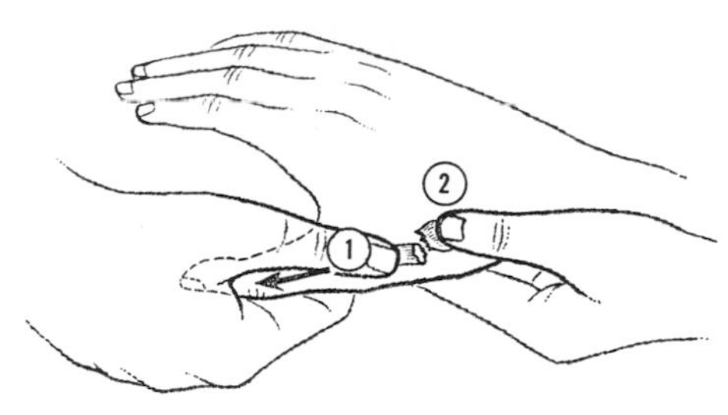

MANIPULATIVE REDUCTION (UNDER LOCAL ANESTHESIA)

1. Apply strong traction to the abducted thumb.
2. Surgeon places the thumb of his or her other hand at the base of the metacarpal.

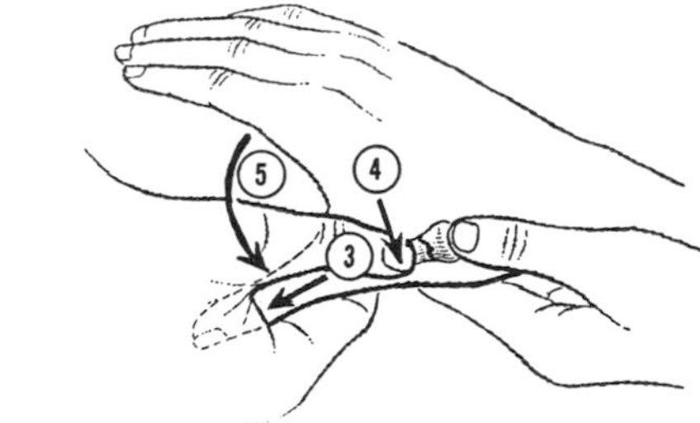

3. While traction is maintained,
4. Firm pressure is applied over the proximal end of the distal fragment.
5. Thumb is hyperabducted.

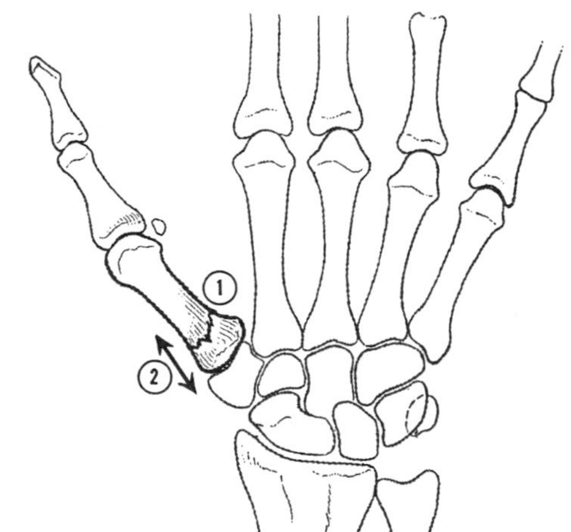

POSTREDUCTION X-RAY

1. Fragments are engaged and in normal alignment.
2. Posterior and outward bowing is corrected.

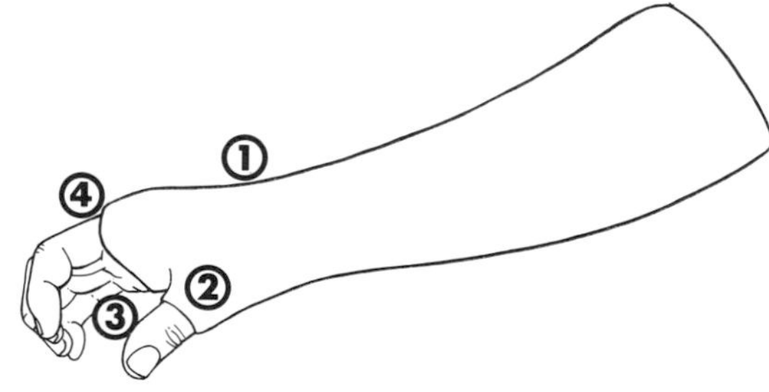

IMMOBILIZATION

1. Apply a cast from below the elbow.
2. Thumb is abducted, and plaster is molded over the MP joint.
3. IP joint of the thumb is free.
4. Unaffected joints are allowed to move freely.

Postreduction Management

Check the position by x-ray within 1 week.

Encourage the patient to use the uninjured fingers of the hand during immobilization.

Reapply a new cast at the end of 10–14 days if the original cast becomes loose.

The patient should actively exercise all the joints of the fingers that are not immobilized on a regular daily basis.

Remove the cast at the end of 3 weeks, and evaluate healing of the fracture clinically and radiographically.

Usually, the fracture is sufficiently stable clinically by 3 weeks so that active, protected motion is possible. If the fracture site is still tender, apply a light finger splint that can be removed for regular exercises of the thumb.

Do not wait for complete radiographic union to permit some active exercises. Clinical union precedes radiographic evidence of healing by several weeks.

Unstable Fractures of the Base of the Metacarpal of the Thumb

PREREDUCTION X-RAY

1. Oblique fracture through the base of the metacarpal.
2. CM joint is not involved. This is in contrast to Bennett or Rolando fracture.

Note: If plaster fixation does not hold this fracture, operative reduction with screw fixation is necessary.

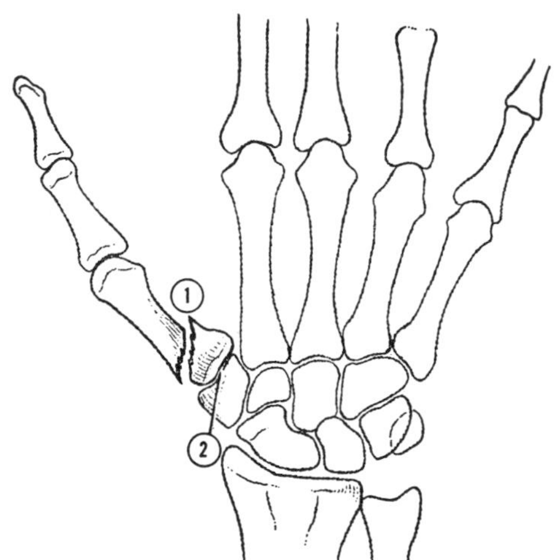

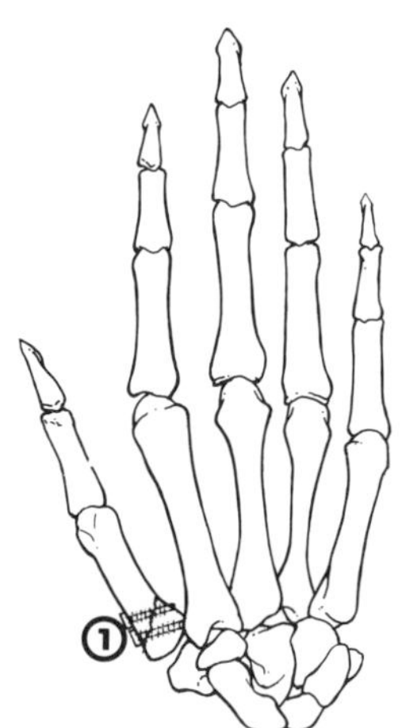

POSTOPERATIVE X-RAY

1. Fracture is reduced and is held by two small fragment screws, which stabilize the fragment sufficiently to permit early exercises of the hand.

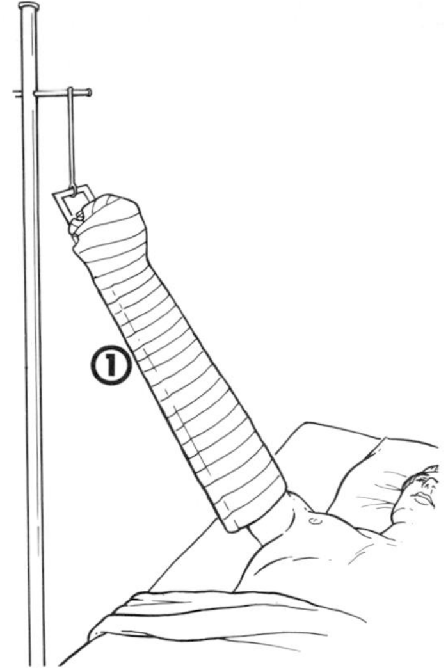

IMMOBILIZATION FOR SWOLLEN FRACTURED HAND

1. If the hand is swollen, a compressive dressing is applied, and the limb is elevated for 24–48 hours to diminish the swelling.

Subsequent Management

By 3–5 days, remove the compression hand dressing, and permit the patient to do guarded active exercises.

When the patient is not exercising the hand, a protective splint is worn.

The fixation must be secure to permit this early exercise program. If there has been any comminution of the fracture, cast immobilization must be continued for at least 3 weeks.

Fractures of the Shaft of the Metacarpal of the Thumb

REMARKS

In general, what has been noted for fractures of the base of the first metacarpal is applicable to the entire metacarpal shaft. The fractures can be grouped into stable and unstable types.

Stable fractures are treated by plaster immobilization with the thumb in abduction.

Unstable fractures may be treated by open reduction with fixation by a small fragment screw or plate.

Stable Fractures of the Shaft of the Metacarpal of the Thumb

Prereduction X-Rays

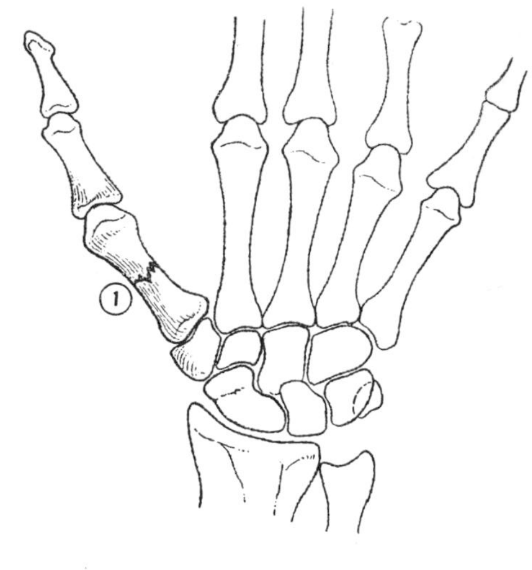

1. Fracture of the shaft of the thumb metacarpal with no displacement.

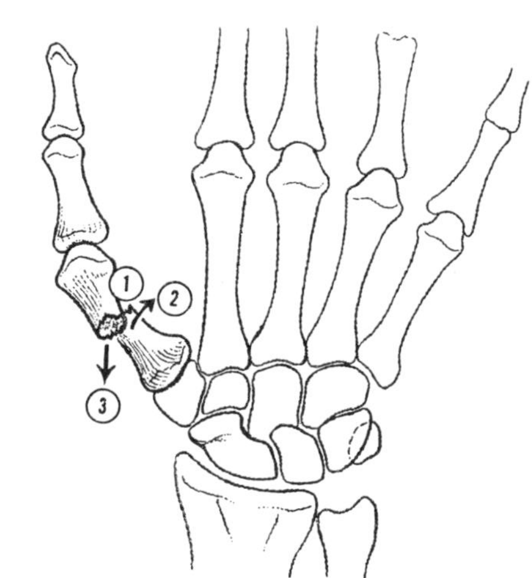

1. Fracture of the shaft of the thumb metacarpal with backward displacement.
2. Proximal fragment is tilted forward.
3. Distal fragment is displaced upward and backward.

MANIPULATIVE REDUCTION FOR DISPLACED FRACTURES (UNDER INTRAVENOUS BLOCK ANESTHESIA)

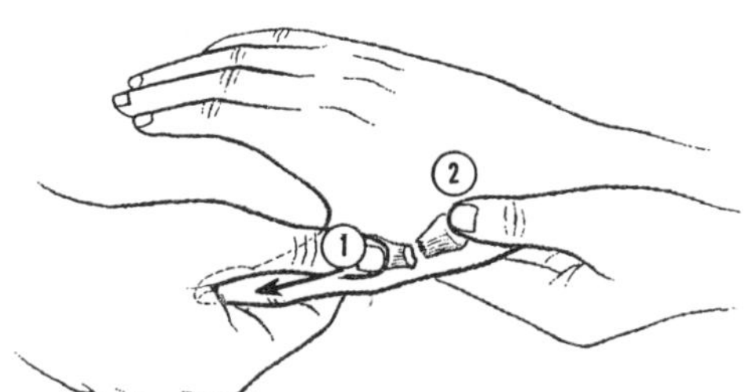

1. Apply strong traction on the abducted thumb.
2. Place the thumb of your other hand over the end of the proximal fragment.

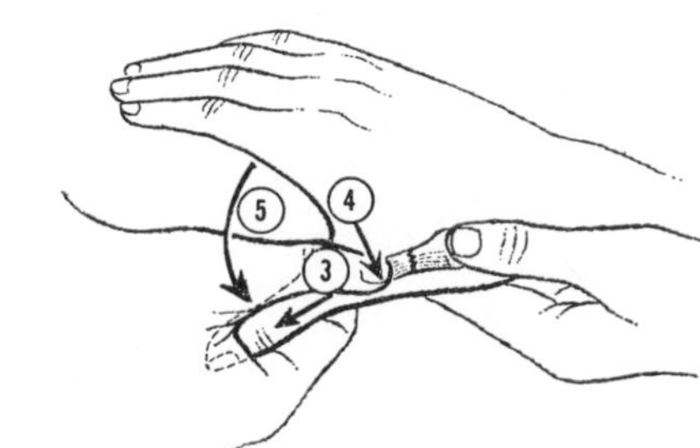

3. While traction is maintained,
4. Apply firm pressure to the proximal end of the distal fragment and
5. Hyperabduct the thumb.

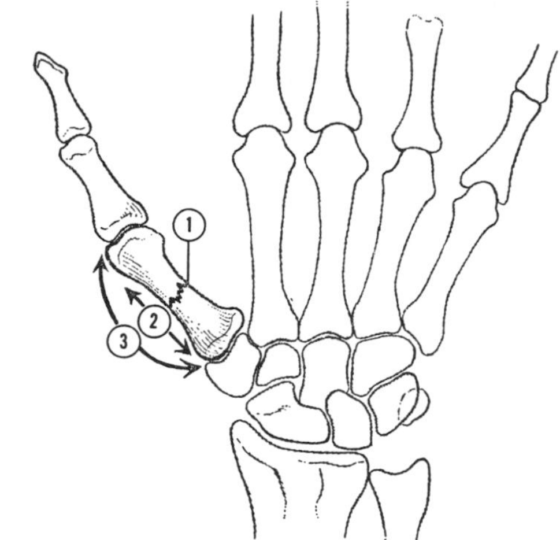

POSTREDUCTION X-RAY

1. Fragments are engaged and in normal alignment.
2. Posterior angulation is corrected.
3. Length of the shaft is restored.

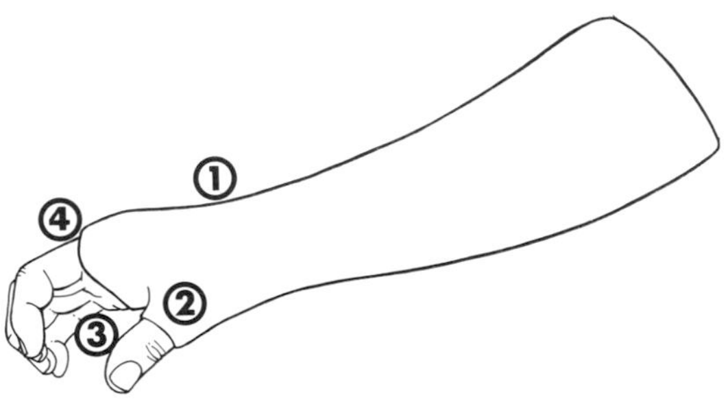

IMMOBILIZATION

1. Apply a cast from below the elbow.
2. Thumb is abducted, and plaster is molded over the CM joint.
3. IP joint of the thumb is free.
4. Uninjured fingers are free to exercise.

Postreduction Management

Check the fracture position by x-ray within 1 week.

Encourage the patient to use the nonimmobilized fingers actively during immobilization.

The cast may be removed at 3 weeks, and fracture healing may be evaluated clinically and radiographically.

If there is still localized tenderness at the fracture site, apply a protective splint; otherwise, encourage the patient to begin active exercises with the plaster removed.

The patient should avoid contact sports or activities that are likely to reinjure the hand for 3 weeks after the cast is removed.

Clinical union usually precedes radiographic union of these metacarpal fractures by several weeks or 1 month. Do not wait for complete radiographic union of the fracture to permit active, protected range-of-motion exercises for the thumb.

Unstable Fractures

Open Reduction and Fixation by Small Fragment Screw

REMARKS

Open reduction with internal fixation and small fragment screw or plate placement is the procedure of choice for the unstable thumb metacarpal fracture.

Most often, a closed reduction is possible, but fixation is necessary to maintain alignment.

If closed reduction is impossible, carry out open reduction with internal fixation as described for fractures of the base of the metacarpal.

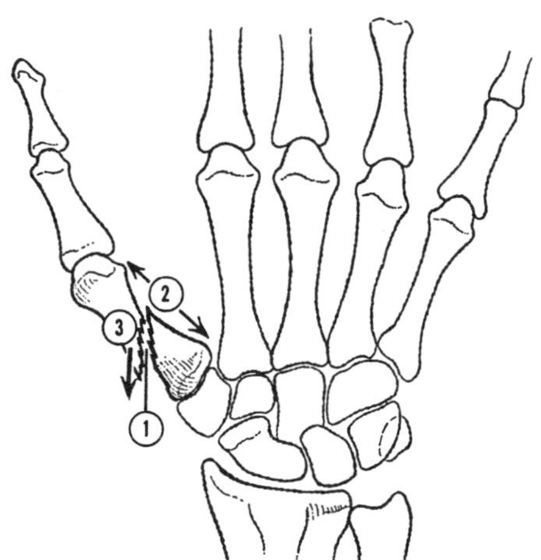

Prereduction X-Ray

1. Oblique fracture of the shaft of the metacarpal.
2. Metacarpal is shortened.
3. Distal fragment is displaced upward and backward.

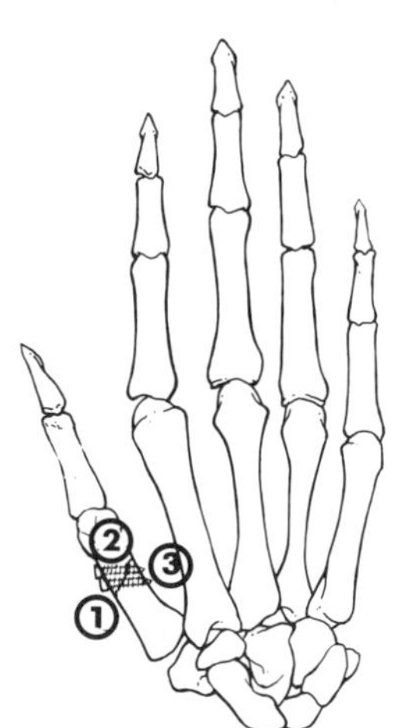

X-Ray After Open Reduction and Screw Fixation

1. Shortening of the metacarpal has been corrected.
2. Displacement and rotational malalignment of the fracture has been reduced.
3. Fracture is held by two small fragment screws applied perpendicular to the oblique fracture.

Postreduction Management

Apply a compression hand dressing and elevate the limb for several days until the edema subsides.

By 3–5 days, remove the compression hand dressing, and permit guarded active exercises.

The fixation must be secure to permit this early, active exercise program. If there has been any comminution of the fracture, cast immobilization should be continued for at least 3 weeks.

The internal fixation need not be removed unless it causes local tenderness.

Dislocations and Subluxations of the Metacarpophalangeal Joint of the Thumb

REMARKS

Dislocations and disruptions occur as frequently in the MP joint of the thumb as in the CM joint.

The mechanism of injury may be either a hyperextension force, which produces an anterior dislocation, or a lateral strain, which disrupts the collateral ligament.

Lateral strain with instability is frequently known as "skier's thumb" because it most often results from a skier jamming the thumb while falling into a bank of hard-packed snow.

Complete anterior dislocation of the MP joint has been classified by McLaughlin as either simple or complex, depending on whether the volar platc is blocking reduction.

Simple MP dislocation may be recognized by the perpendicular relationship of the proximal phalanx to the first metacarpal. Reduction of a simple dislocation can be done by closed means if the surgeon avoids trapping the volar plate in the MP joint by direct traction.

A complex MP dislocation is recognized clinically by the relationship of the proximal phalanx, parallel to the metacarpal. Dimpling of the skin directly over the metacarpal head also indicates that the volar plate has become trapped within the joint. Radiographically, a complex dislocation can be diagnosed by the fact that the sesamoid bone in the volar plate can be seen within the joint.

Normal Joint

1. Normal arrangement of the collateral ligaments and volar plate of the MP joint.

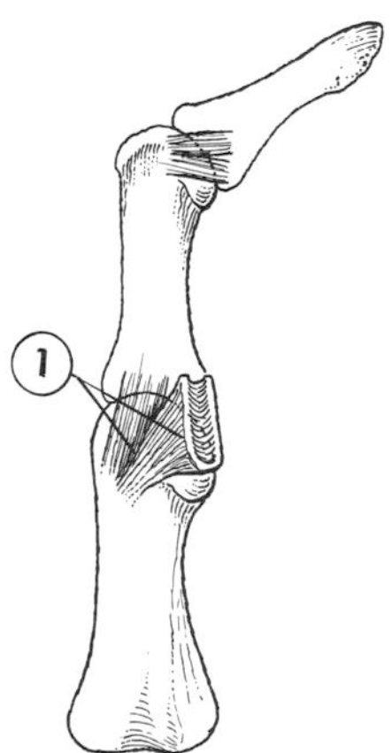

Simple Dislocation

1. Phalanx sits on the back of the metacarpal in a vertical position.
2. Volar plate hangs in front of the metacarpal head but has not become trapped within the joint. Note that the plate is always detached from its weaker metacarpal insertion.

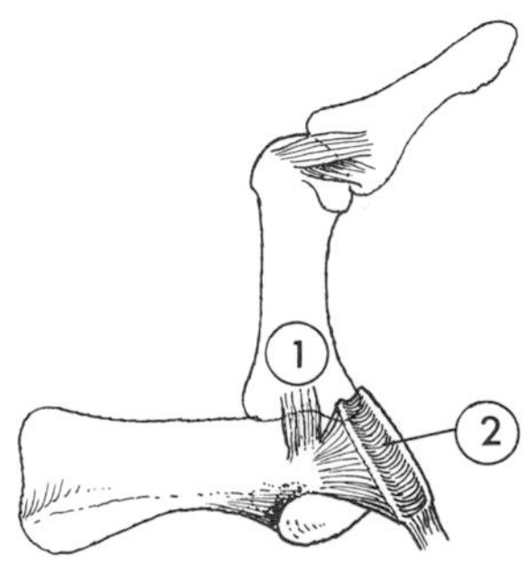

Conversion of a Simple Dislocation to a Complex Dislocation by Traction

If traction is applied directly to a simple dislocation, the volar plate frequently becomes trapped in the joint and produces an irreducible or complex dislocation.

1. Proximal phalanx is now parallel to the metacarpal.
2. Volar plate has become interposed in the joint.

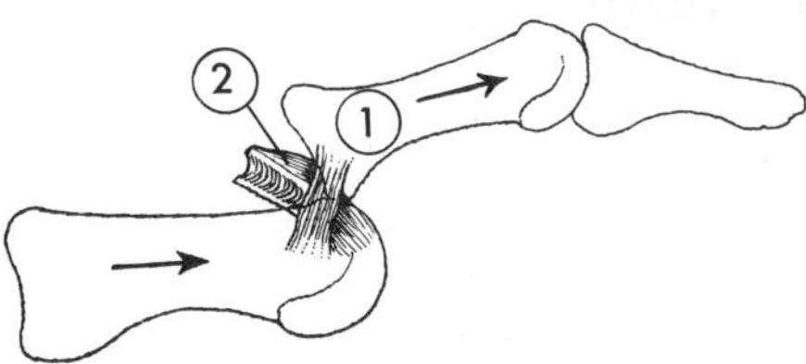

The intrinsic muscles of the thumb may also obstruct reduction.

1. Proximal phalanx.
2. Protruding head of the metacarpal.
3. Intrinsic muscles of the thumb.

A complex MP dislocation requires open reduction through a volar approach to remove the volar plate, which has become trapped within the joint and is preventing reduction.

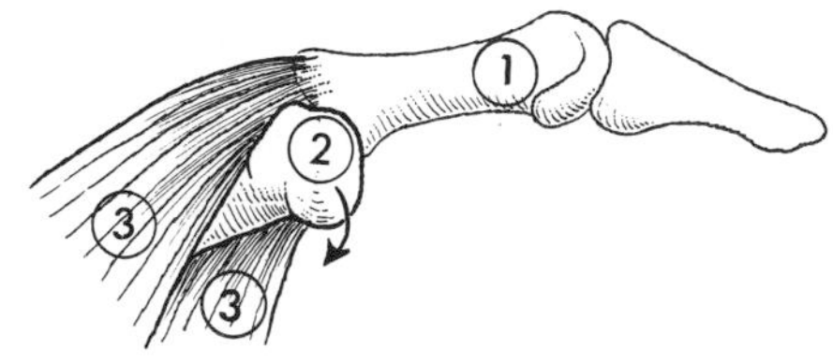

Reduction of a Simple Dislocation of the Metacarpophalangeal Joint of the Thumb

REMARKS

The technique of reduction is to push rather than pull the dislocated phalanx into the MP joint.

If this reduction is not possible after one or two attempts, open reduction is indicated.

Avoid damage to the thumb by repeated and futile attempts at closed reduction when the probability is that the volar plate is interposed in the joint.

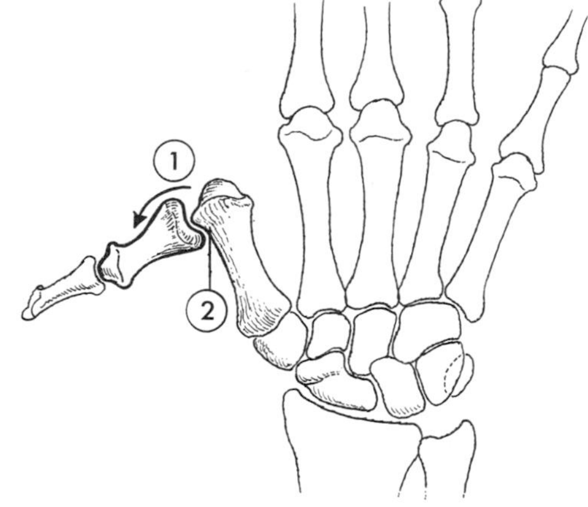

Prereduction X-Ray

1. Phalanx is hyperextended and is displaced upward and backward.
2. Base of the phalanx rests on the head of the metacarpal at a right angle.

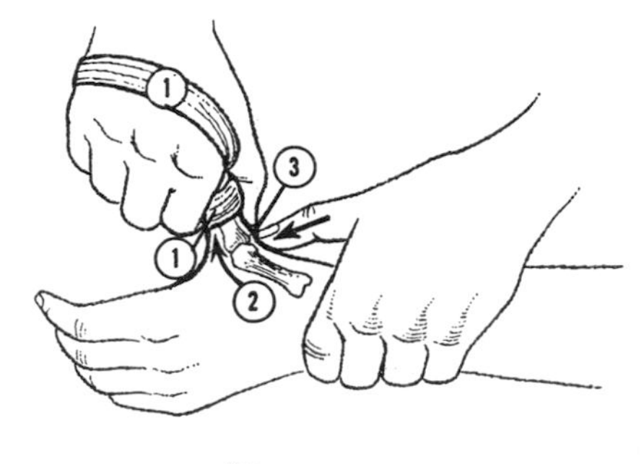

Manipulative Reduction (Under Intravenous or General Anesthesia)

1. Bandage is looped around the patient's thumb and then around the operator's hand.
2. Grasp the patient's thumb, and hyperextend the dislocated phalanx about 90° on the metacarpal.
3. Push the dorsal surface of the dislocated phalanx to reduce the dislocation. Avoid reducing this dislocation by traction alone.
4. While continuing to push against the dorsal surface of the phalanx, flex the thumb, and reduction should be accomplished.

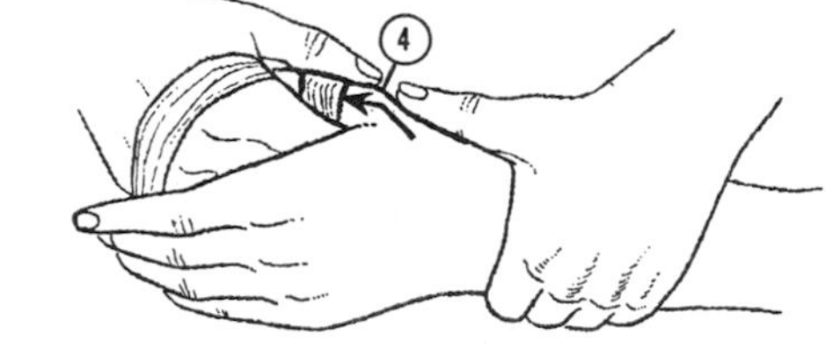

Note: If this simple dislocation is manipulated by traction alone, a complex or irreducible dislocation is likely to result.

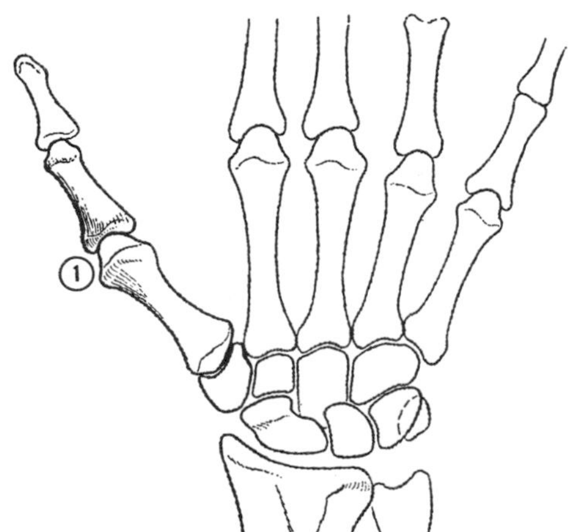

Postreduction X-Ray

1. Base of the phalanx is in a normal relationship to the head of the metacarpal.

Immobilization

Always test stability and motion after reduction. Usually, the joint is stable after closed reduction. A minimum amount of external support is necessary. Avoid immobilizing the injury for longer than 10 days because this is likely to produce a stiff MP joint.

Apply 1-cm strips of adhesive.

1. Strapping encircles the MP joint.
2. IP joint is left free.
3. Basket-weave strapping extends above the wrist.
4. Anchor the strips of adhesive encircling the thumb by strips encircling the wrist.
5. Thumb is strapped in the grasp position for 5–7 days.

Note: Allow the patient to use the hand actively. After 5–7 days, remove the strapping, and permit full active exercises.

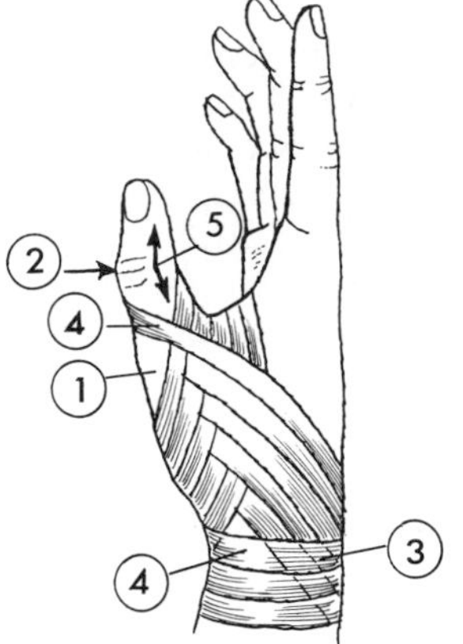

Open Reduction of Complex Dislocation of the Metacarpophalangeal Joint of the Thumb

REMARKS

A trapped volar plate is always the major obstacle to reduction. Occasionally, the flexor pollicis brevis or longus may also block relocation.

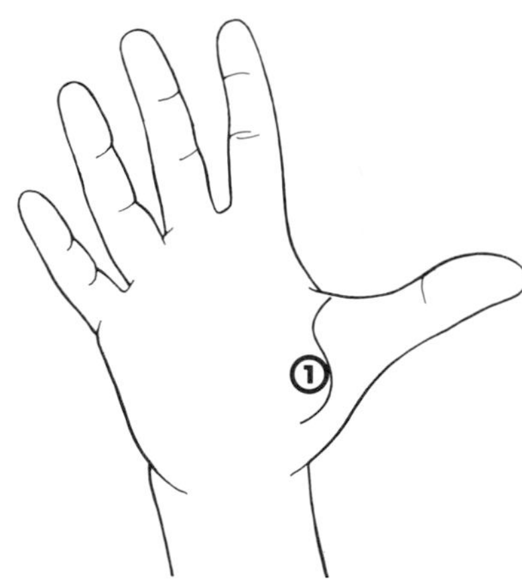

1. Curved volar incision is made to approach the MP joint.

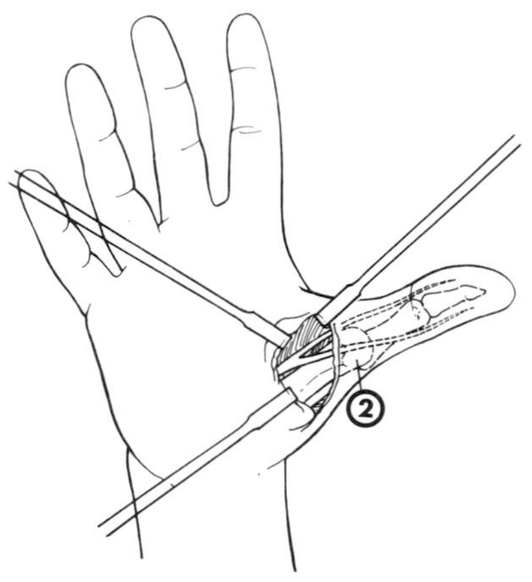

2. Neurovascular structures that are displaced immediately beneath the skin have to be carefully identified and protected.

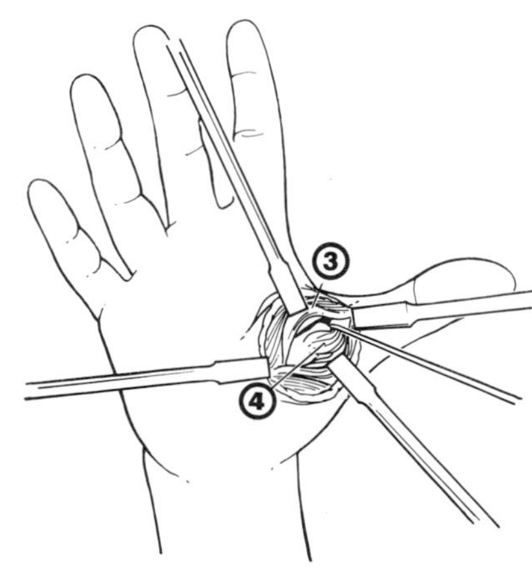

3. Short thenar muscles frequently envelop the metacarpal head and can be released by hyperextending the thumb.

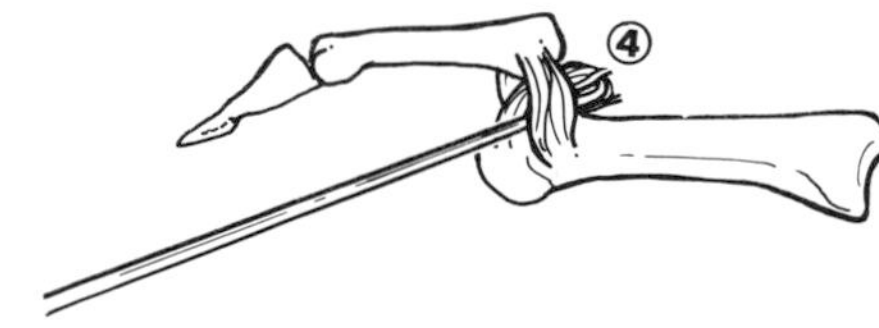

4. Longitudinal incision is used to release the capsular attachment to the volar plate. This is pulled out of the joint with a skin hook.

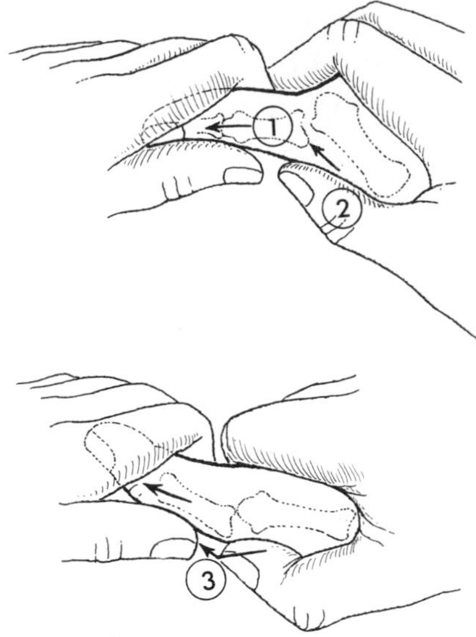

When the volar plate has been released from the joint, the reduction can be accomplished with a maneuver for simple dislocation.

1. Phalanx is hyperextended to approximately 90°.
2. Dislocated phalanx is then pushed forward over the metacarpal head.
3. Reduction is achieved by continuing to push the phalanx and flexing the metacarpophalangeal joint.

The postoperative immobilization is as described for closed treatment.

Volar Dislocation of the Metacarpophalangeal Joint of the Thumb

REMARKS

Volar dislocation of the MP joint is an extremely rare injury of the thumb that occurs from injuries that cause hyperflexion of the MP joint.

Although most case reports recommend open treatment, closed reduction can be satisfactory.

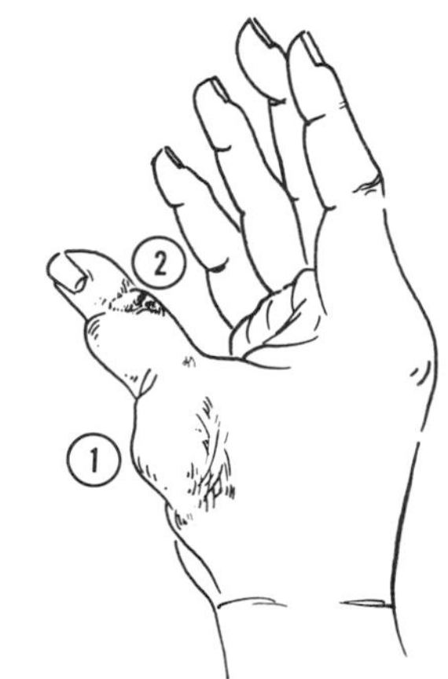

Clinical Appearance

1. MP joint is swollen and locked in a flexed position.
2. There are bruises and lacerations evident on the dorsal aspect of the thumb.

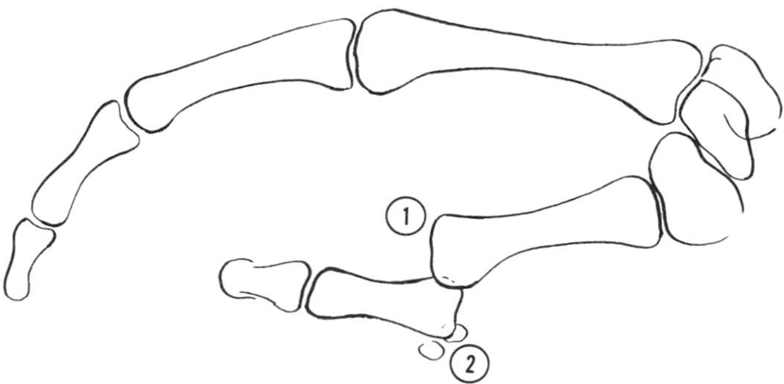

X-Ray

1. X-rays show volar dislocation of the MP joint of the thumb.
2. Sesamoid bones of the thumb are displaced with the proximal phalanx.

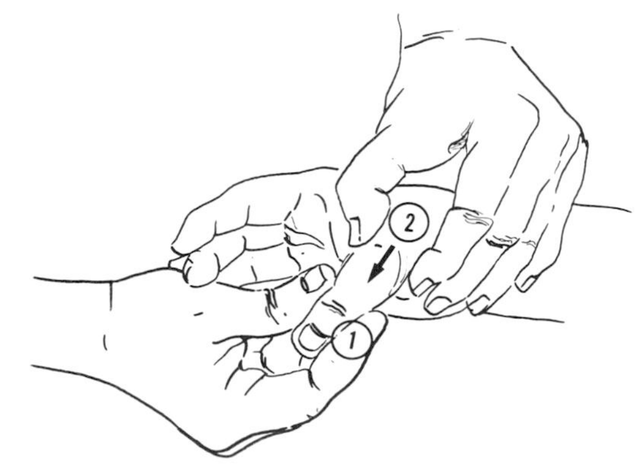

Management

1. Apply longitudinal traction while stabilizing the metacarpal head. The traction is applied initially in the direction of the deformity.
2. As the proximal phalanx is pulled over the metacarpal head, the joint may be reduced by extending the MP joint.

Subsequent Management

The stability of the dislocation is tested, particularly in adduction of the thumb. If the reduction is stable a thumb spica cast is applied for 2–3 weeks. After this time, the patient may begin full range of motion of the joint. If reduction cannot be achieved or, if the joint is grossly unstable, operative repair is indicated.

Skier's Thumb: Collateral Ligament Disruption

REMARKS

Acute abduction injury to the MP joint of the thumb occurs frequently when a skier falls and jams the thumb into hard-packed snow. This may cause either partial or complete rupture of the ulnar collateral ligament.

Occasionally, the radial collateral ligament may be injured instead.

Clinically, the joint is swollen, and the thumb is tender in the region of the ulnar collateral ligament. Injecting local anesthesia into the painful region permits adequate clinical and radiographic evaluation of joint stability with stress testing.

For the most part, these injuries may be treated by immobilization in a thumb spica cast for 4 weeks, which permits healing with adequate stability for pinch. Should the joint be completely unstable on stress x-ray, primary surgical repair is advisable because the disrupted ligament usually folds back on itself and winds up beneath the proximal end of the adductor tendon insertion.

Radiographic evidence of an avulsion fracture at the base of the phalanx is also an indication for operative fixation.

Mechanism of Injury

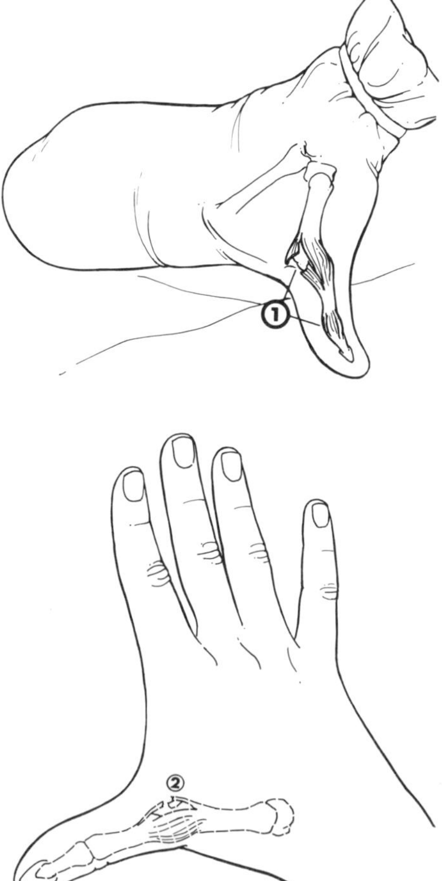

1. Abduction strain to the thumb may cause either partial or complete disruption of the ulnar collateral ligament.

2. Avulsion fracture of the phalanx may also occur.

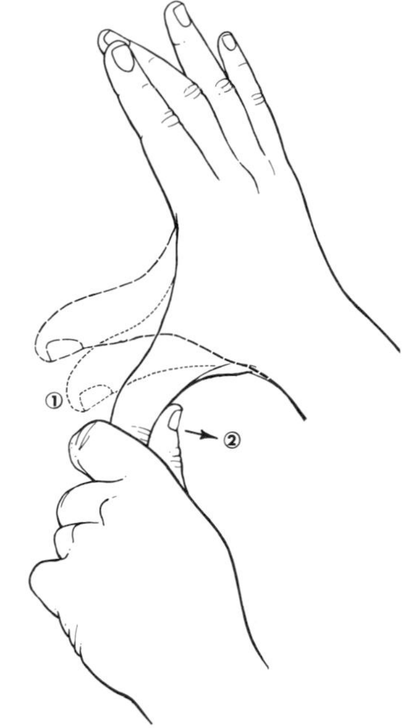

Clinical Appearance

Evaluate stability with stress testing under local anesthesia. The injury may cause

1. Partial instability compared with the uninjured side or
2. Complete disruption.

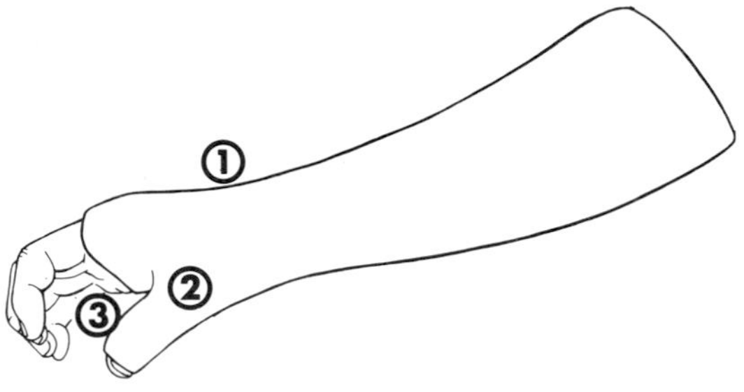

Closed Treatment for Partial Tear

1. Apply a thumb spica cast that includes the wrist and forearm.
2. MP joint of the thumb is in slight flexion to relax the collateral ligament, and the thumb is apposed to the other fingers.
3. IP joint is immobilized in slight flexion.

Subsequent Management

Continue cast immobilization for 3–4 weeks, and then evaluate the stability of the MP joint.

If the joint is still significantly unstable, offer the patient operative repair. Otherwise, allow active exercises with protection against abduction reinjury for 4 more weeks.

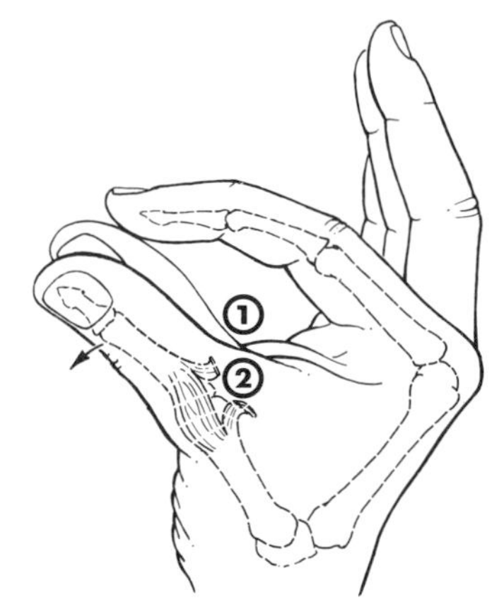

Operative Repair for Complete Disruption or Avulsion Fracture

For treatment of a complete tear or an avulsion fracture,

1. Normal pinch requires stability of the MP joint's ulnar collateral ligament.
2. Complete disruption of the ligament impairs key pinch significantly and should be corrected surgically.

Surgical Procedure for Complete Disruption

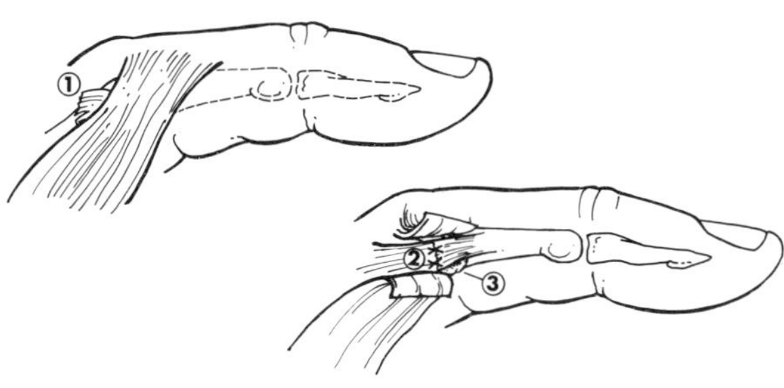

1. Ulnar collateral ligament is usually turned outward and separated from its attachment by the adductor tendon.
2. Repair is accomplished after the adductor tendon is opened transversely.
3. Small, loose avulsion fractures may be removed. Fix larger fragments with a screw.

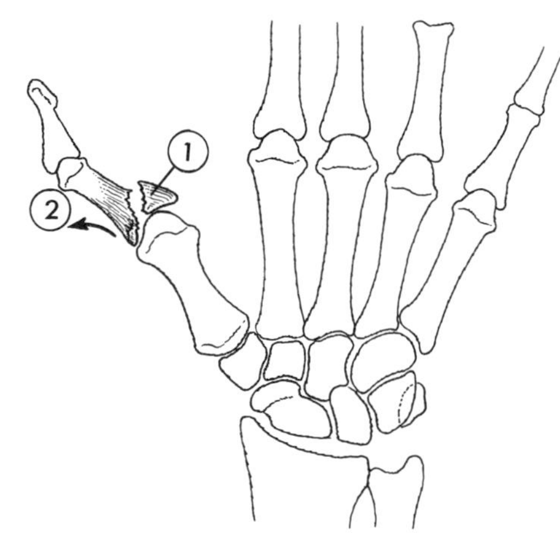

Avulsion Fracture

PREOPERATIVE X-RAY

1. Large triangular fracture avulsed from the proximal phalanx.
2. Radial deviation of the finger.

Note: This is best repaired by open reduction and screw fixation.

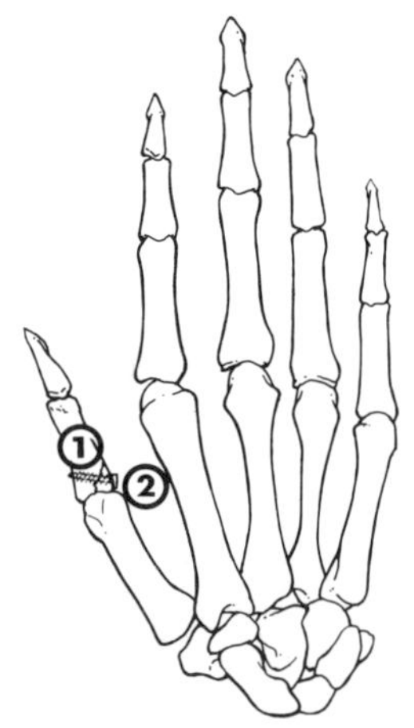

POSTOPERATIVE X-RAY

1. Radial deviation of the finger is corrected.
2. Fragment is fixed by a small fragment screw.

Note: The screw may be removed at the end of 3 weeks under local anesthesia if it is palpable beneath the skin.

Injury to the Radial Collateral Ligament of the Metacarpophalangeal Joint of the Thumb

Injury to the radial collateral ligament of the MP joint is less common than disruption of the ulnar collateral ligament because the other metacarpals protect the thumb against extreme adduction.

As with ulnar collateral ligament injury, indications for closed or open treatment depend on the degree of instability.

Occasionally, an avulsed fragment from the phalanx may require operative fixation.

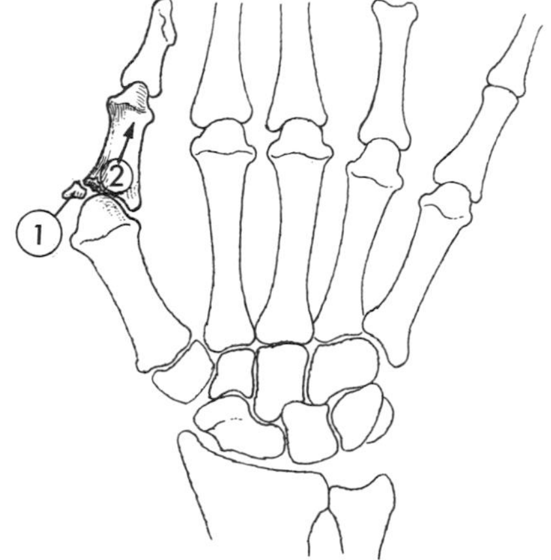

Preoperative X-Ray

1. Small fragment avulsed from the dorsoradial margin of the proximal phalanx.
2. Ulnar deviation of the proximal phalanx.

Note: If this fragment is not in the joint, the injury may be treated closed with thumb spica cast immobilization. If the fragment is in the joint, it should be removed, and the collateral ligament should be repaired.

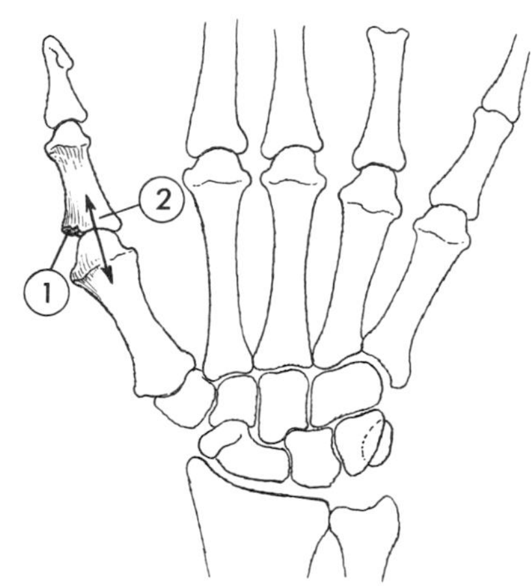

Postoperative X-Ray

1. Defect after removal of the fragment.
2. Phalanx is in normal alignment with the head of the metacarpal. Collateral ligament has been reattached.

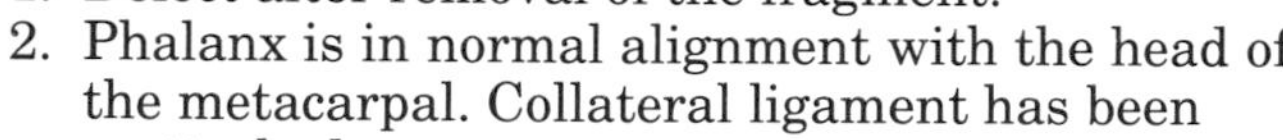

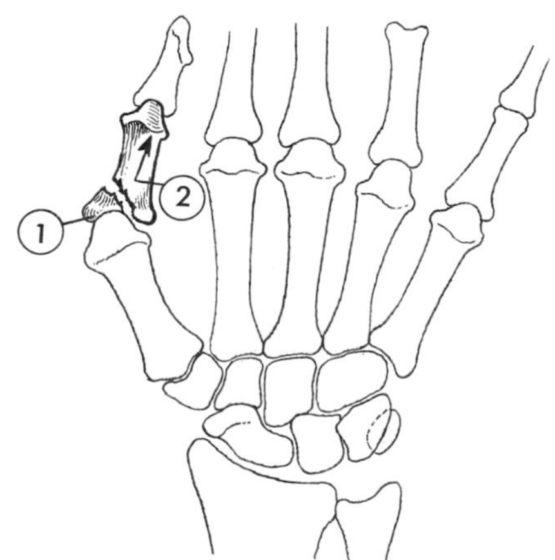

Preoperative X-Ray

1. Large triangular fragment avulsed from the proximal phalanx.
2. Ulnar deviation of the proximal fragment.

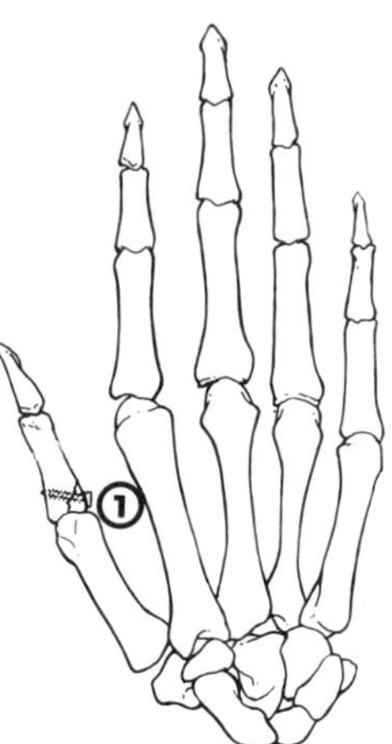

Postoperative X-Ray

1. Fragment has been reduced and fixed with a small fragment screw. The alignment between the proximal phalanx and metacarpal is restored.

■ Injuries to the Interphalangeal Joint of the Thumb

REMARKS

Because of the stability that is provided by the insertions of the flexor and extensor tendons and by the strong collateral ligaments, dislocation of the IP joint is rare.

Occasionally, such a dislocation may be irreducible because of an interposition of the volar plate or the flexor pollicis longus tendon.

A dislocation or subluxation may be unstable because of a fracture of the phalanx.

Indications for closed or open treatment depend on the degree of instability and the reducibility of the injury.

Frequently, these dislocations are open injuries and require thorough wound excision and appropriate fixation.

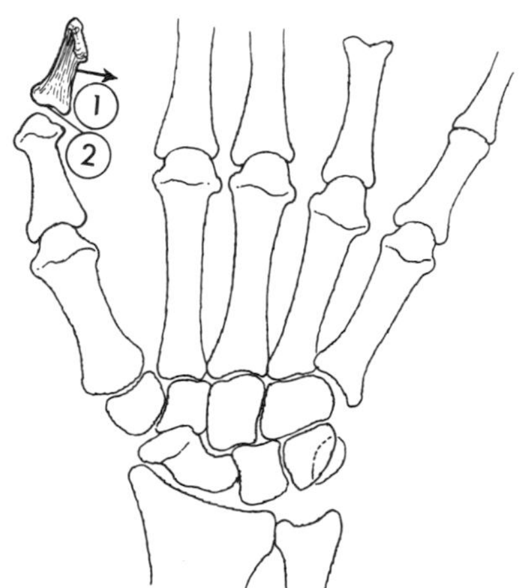

Subluxation of the Interphalangeal Joint of the Thumb

Appearance on X-Ray

RUPTURE OF ONE OF THE COLLATERAL LIGAMENTS

1. Lateral deviation of the distal phalanx.
2. Widening of the IP joint.

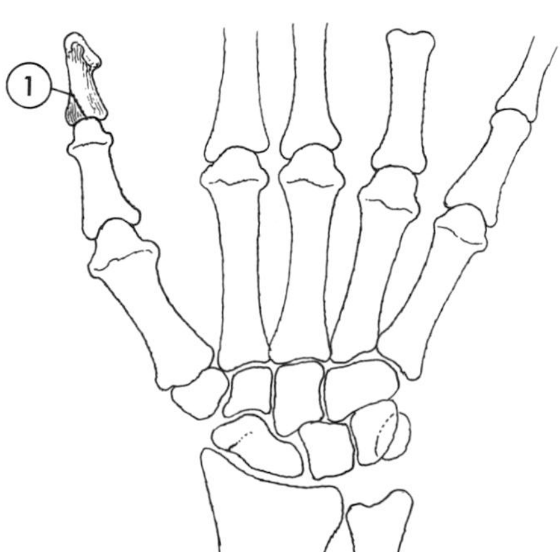

FRACTURE WITHOUT DISPLACEMENT

1. Marginal fracture without displacement.

Immobilization With Thumb Spica

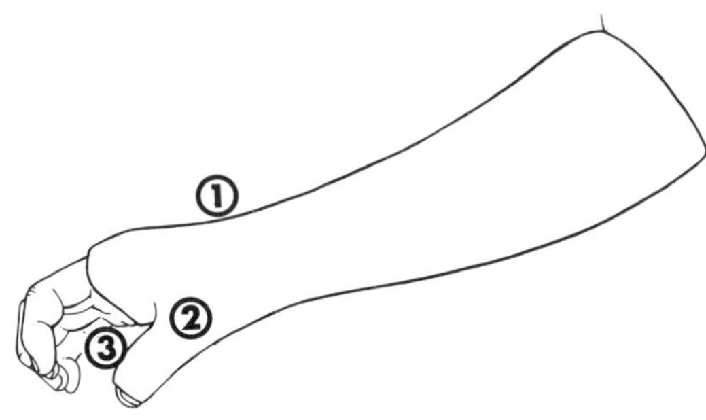

1. Apply a cast from below the elbow.
2. Thumb is abducted, and the plaster is molded over the arches of the hand.
3. IP joint of the thumb is immobilized in slight flexion, and the thumb is apposed to the fingers.

Subsequent Management

Remove the cast at the end of 10 days, and evaluate the joint's stability clinically and radiographically.

If the joint is stable, allow the patient to begin guarded active range-of-motion exercises.

Immobilization for longer than 10 days tends to produce stiffness of these joints and, if at all possible, should be avoided.

Dislocation of the Interphalangeal Joint of the Thumb

Prereduction X-Ray

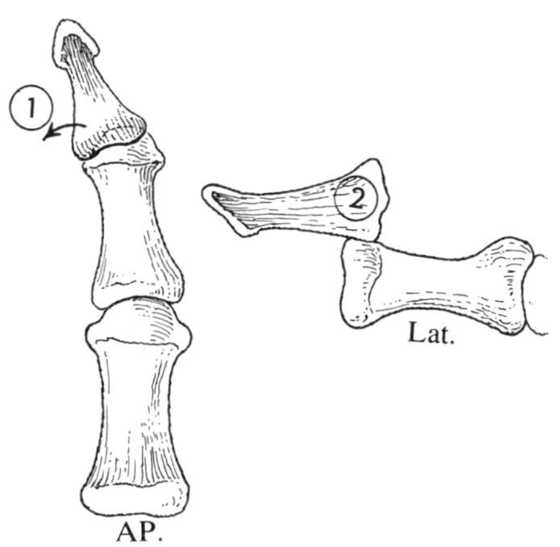

1. On the anteroposterior view, the distal phalanx is displaced laterally.
2. On the lateral view, the distal phalanx sits on the dorsum of the proximal phalanx.

Note: This relationship is analogous to complex dislocation of the MP joint and may indicate volar plate interposition in the joint.

Reduction

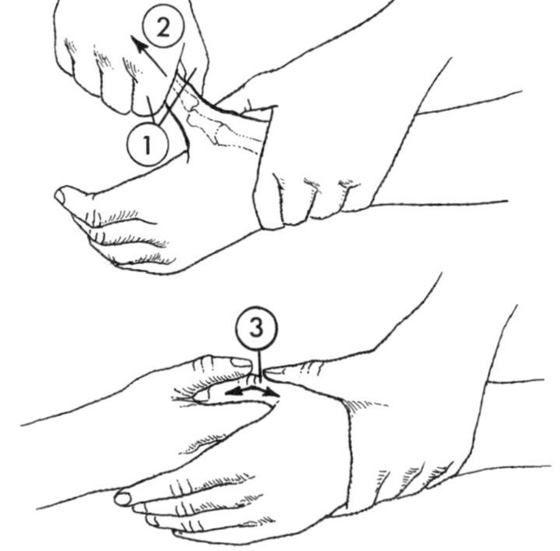

1. Grasp the patient's thumb with your thumb and index finger.
2. Apply steady traction in the line of deformity of the distal phalanx.
3. While traction is maintained, flex the IP joint.

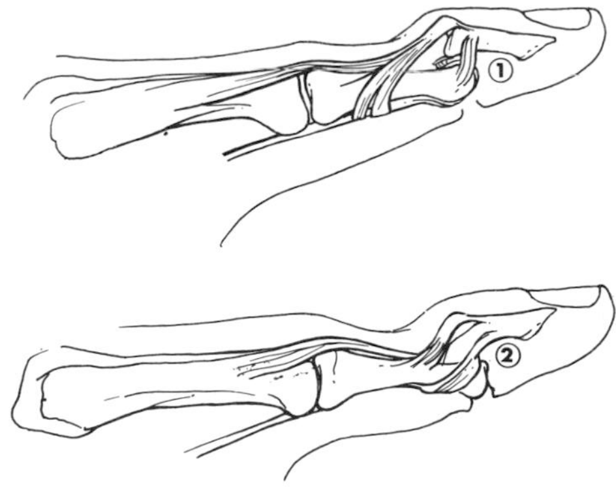

Reduction should be relatively simple. If the joint does not reduce with this maneuver, there is either

1. Entrapment of the volar plate in the joint or
2. Entrapment of the flexor pollicis longus, which is wrapped around the ulnar condyle of the proximal phalanx.

Note: Both of these situations require open reduction to remove the obstacle.

Immobilization

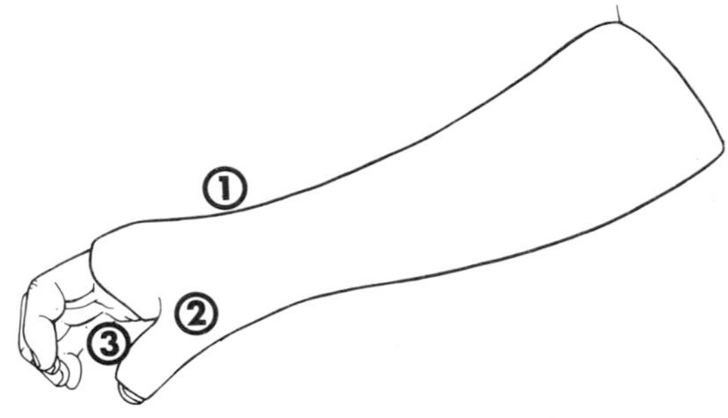

After reduction, the joint is usually stable.

If there is evidence of instability or if there is a small fracture, immobilize the thumb in a spica cast.

1. Apply a cast from below the elbow.
2. Thumb is abducted, and the plaster is molded over the arches of the hand.
3. IP joint of the thumb is immobilized in slight flexion, and the thumb is apposed to the fingers.

Remove the cast after 10 days, and evaluate the joint for instability.

Healing is usually satisfactory by 10 days. Prolonged immobilization of the joint tends to produce joint stiffness and should be avoided if at all possible.

FRACTURES, DISLOCATIONS, AND FRACTURE-DISLOCATIONS OF THE FINGERS

Carpometacarpal Joints

REMARKS

Dislocation of the CM joint is rare because of the strong ligamentous support in this region.

The injury frequently is associated with extensive soft tissue damage, and the dislocation may go unrecognized unless true lateral x-rays visualize the CM relationships.

Severe hyperextension or hyperflexion of the carpus may cause a rupture of the ligaments and may produce either dorsal or volar dislocation. The former is more common than the latter.

Complete dislocation of the metacarpals is rare. Isolated dislocations can occur at either the fourth or the fifth CM joint because these joints are more mobile than the middle two.

Most commonly, dislocation of a single metacarpal is associated with a fracture of its base. Oblique fractures at the base of the metacarpal must be carefully assessed for the possibility of an associated dislocation.

Fracture-dislocations of the fifth metacarpal with volar displacement commonly involve the motor branch of the ulnar nerve, which should be decompressed.

Dislocations of the CM joint usually are unstable and require Kirschner wire fixation to maintain reduction.

The patients who are most likely to experience unsatisfactory results are those with injuries to the normally stable second or third CM joint.

The patient with concomitant ulnar nerve injury is also likely to have permanent grip weakness unless the problem is recognized and corrected early.

Diagnosis of a Carpometacarpal Dislocation

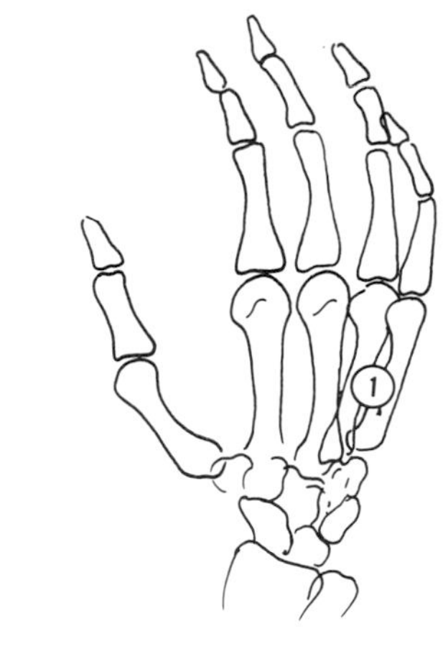

1. Dislocation may not be evident clinically or on x-ray because of the usual extreme swelling of the hand after a severe injury of this type.

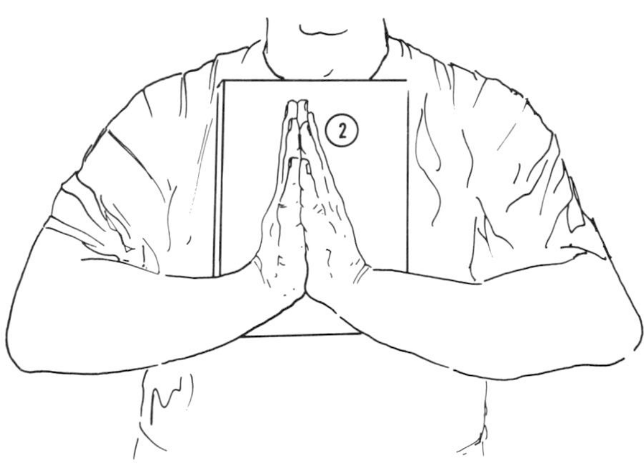

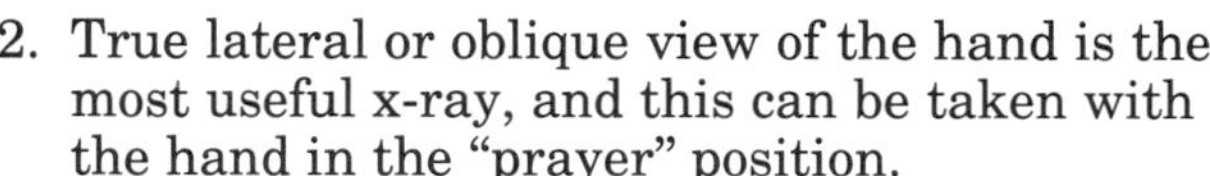

2. True lateral or oblique view of the hand is the most useful x-ray, and this can be taken with the hand in the "prayer" position.

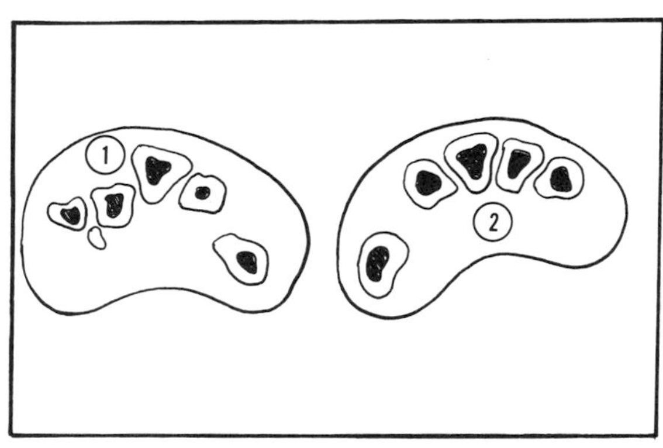

1. If the standard x-rays do not provide adequate visualization of the metacarpal articulation, a computed tomographic (CT) scan is useful. This injury is sometimes difficult to interpret on standard lateral views, but CT shows the dislocation of the fourth and fifth metacarpals.
2. This is evident particularly when compared with the opposite hand.

Dislocations of the Carpometacarpal Joint

Prereduction X-Rays

DORSAL DISLOCATION

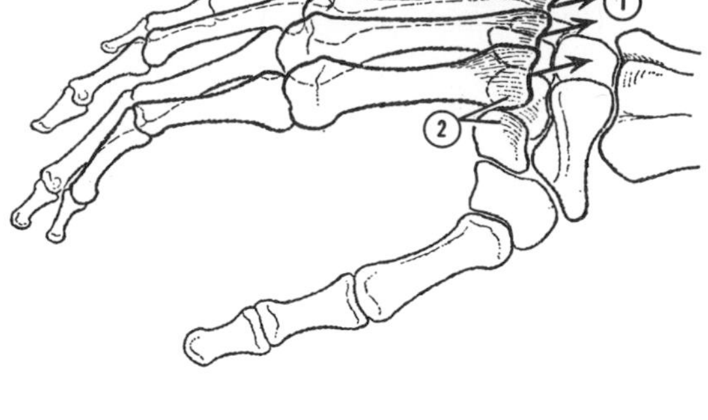

1. Four metacarpals are displaced dorsally en masse.
2. Bases of the metacarpals lie on the dorsum of the distal row of carpal bones.

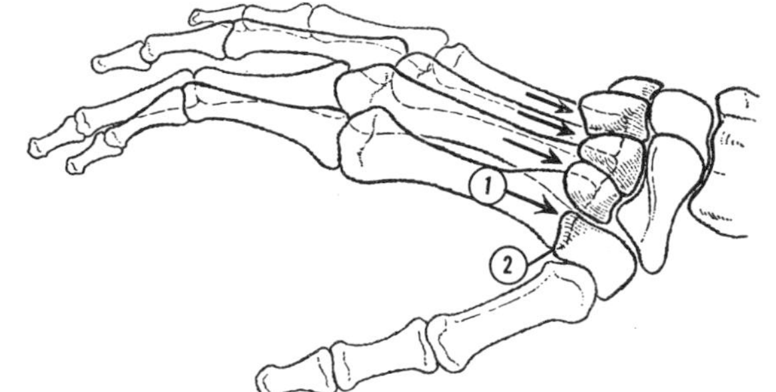

VOLAR DISLOCATION

1. Four metacarpals are displaced volarly.
2. Bases of the metacarpals are in the palm.

Note: Volar dislocations are extremely rare, but when they occur, they are likely to cause significant neurovascular injury. Therefore, prompt reduction is essential.

Reduction by Traction and Manipulation for Dorsal Dislocation

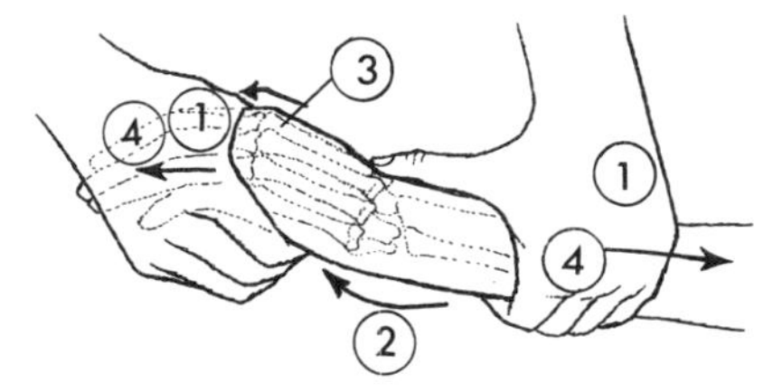

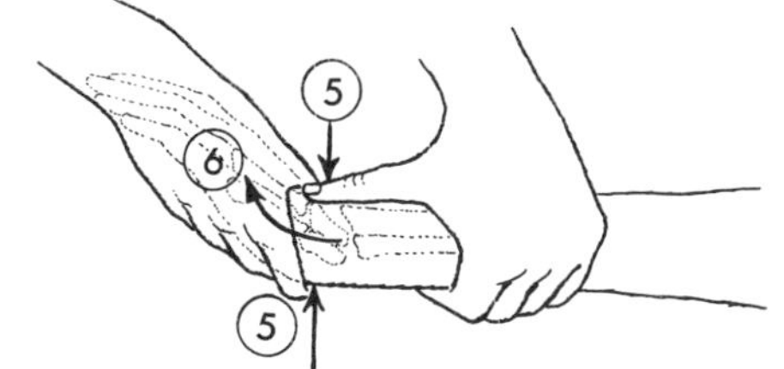

1. One hand of the operator encircles the patient's wrist while the other encircles the patient's hand.
2. Wrist is slightly dorsiflexed.
3. Fingers are flexed.
4. While countertraction is applied to the wrist, apply strong traction on the hand.
5. While the thumb of the proximal hand applies first downward pressure over the bases of the metacarpal bones, the fingers of the distal hand apply upward pressure on the shafts of the metacarpals. At the same time, the
6. Wrist is dorsiflexed further.

Note: For volar dislocation, the manipulative maneuvers are reversed, and the wrist is immobilized in slight flexion.

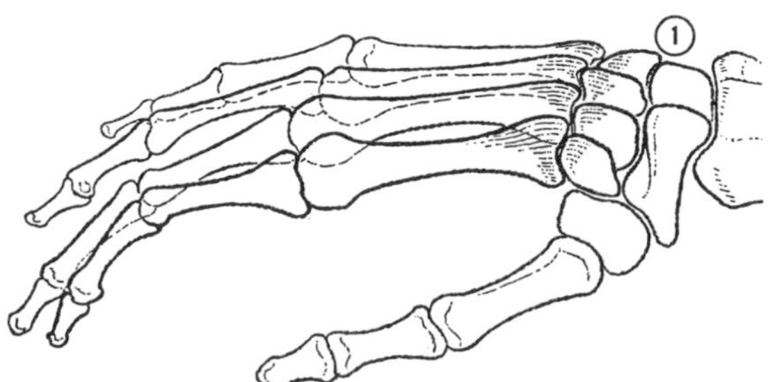

Postreduction X-Ray

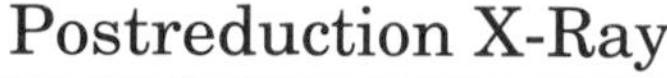

1. Bases of the metacarpals are now in a normal relationship with the distal row of carpal bones.

Stabilization With Kirschner Wires

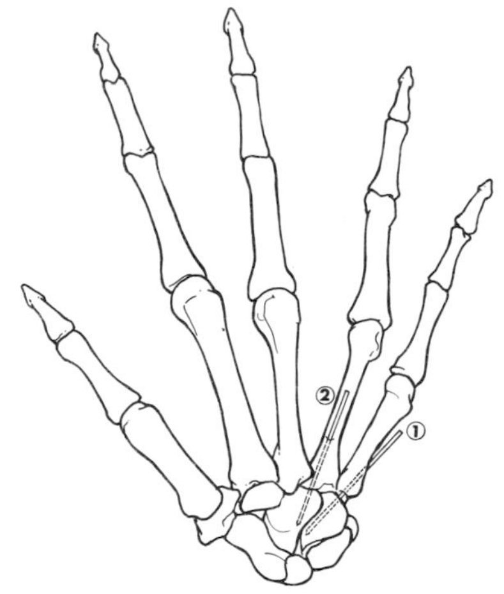

1. Smooth Kirschner wire is inserted from the fifth metacarpal into the carpal bones to prevent redislocation.
2. Occasionally, a second pin through the fourth metacarpal into the carpus is necessary.

Note: For injuries that involve the second and third metacarpal, arthrodesis with screw fixation is usually the treatment of choice because these unstable injuries are likely to cause grip weakness.

Fasciotomy and Carpal Tunnel Release for Swollen Hand

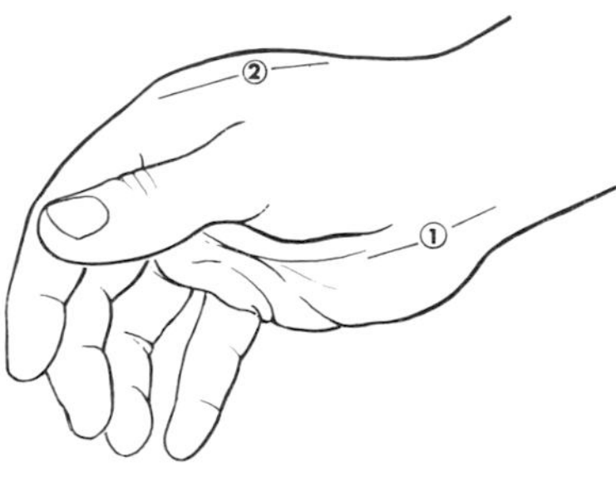

1. If the dislocation of the metacarpal has caused median nerve entrapment, the nerve can be released through a carpal tunnel incision.
2. There may be extreme swelling of the intrinsic muscle compartments of the hand, requiring multiple dorsal fasciotomies.

Note: The need for fasciotomy can be determined by measurements of compartment pressures, as discussed previously.

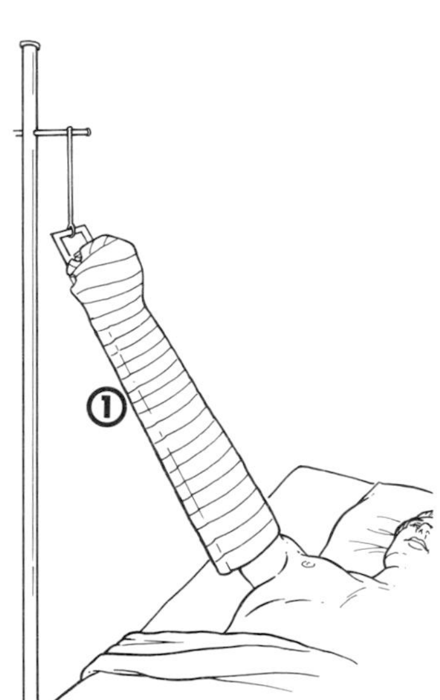

Immobilization

1. Apply a postoperative hand dressing, and elevate the limb for several days to diminish edema. Monitor the circulation to the finger tips closely.

Subsequent Management

After the edema has subsided, apply a short-arm cast with the hand in dorsiflexion.

Remove the pins at the end of 3 weeks, and evaluate stability. If the injured CM joint is stable, allow the patient to begin guarded active range-of-motion exercises. Have the patient avoid hyperextension of the hand for at least 6 weeks.

Fracture-Dislocations of the Carpometacarpal Joints

REMARKS

CM dislocations may be accompanied by a marginal fracture of the base of the metacarpal.

The dislocation may not be recognized unless true lateral views or even CT scan of the hand are scrutinized for the altered metacarpal-carpal relationships.

These are usually unstable injuries and require internal fixation with Kirschner wires.

Fractures with volar displacement of the fourth or fifth metacarpal frequently impinge on the motor branch of the ulnar nerve and cause intrinsic paralysis. Evaluate these fractures carefully for nerve injury and reduce them anatomically.

Fracture-Dislocations of the Third Carpometacarpal Joint

REMARKS

The second and third CM joints are the stable joints of the distal palmar arch. Instability of either one of these joints is likely to weaken grip.

Because of the long-term disability or discomfort from these injuries, primary stabilization or arthrodesis is usually indicated.

Prereduction X-Ray

1. Fracture-dislocation is evident at the base of the third metacarpal.
2. There is dorsal displacement of the shaft of the metacarpal.

Note: Displacement is difficult to detect unless a true lateral x-ray or CT scan is obtained, as previously described.

The dislocation of either the second or third CM joint is best treated by open reduction and internal stabilization of the joint.

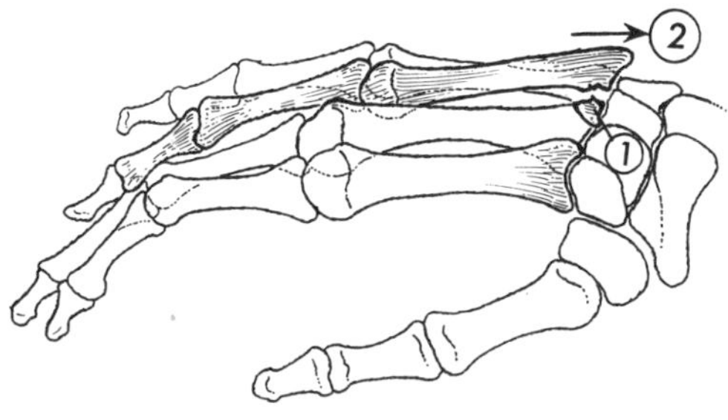

Postreduction X-Ray

1. Base of the third metacarpal has been restored to normal articulation with the carpus.
2. Joint is further stabilized, and arthrodesis is done with Kirschner wires or small fragment screw fixation.

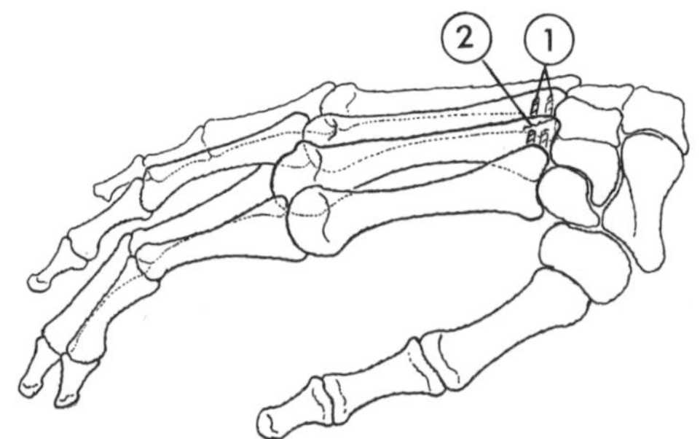

Fracture-Dislocation of Fifth Metacarpal

Prereduction X-Ray

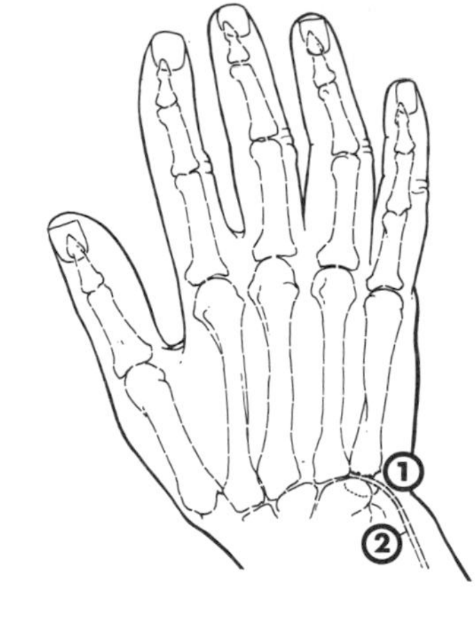

1. Fracture-dislocation of the base of the fifth metacarpal with volar displacement.
2. Motor branch of the ulnar nerve is involved by the injury.

Note: Always test for ulnar nerve function with this type of injury. Surgical decompression of the nerve is necessary to stabilize the fracture and prevent permanent intrinsic paralysis.

Operative Decompression of the Ulnar Nerve

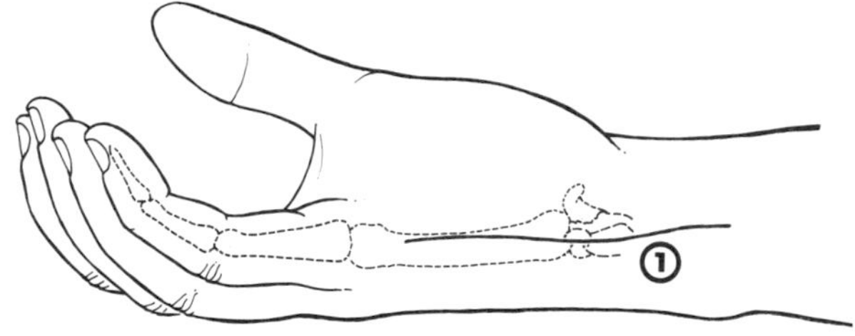

1. Medial approach is used along the distal ulna and carpus.

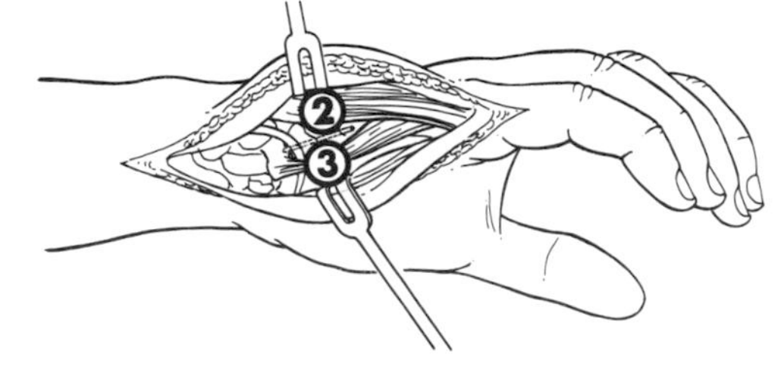

2. Motor branch of the ulnar nerve is identified, which is trapped in the fracture site.
3. After the nerve is released from the fracture site, the fracture-dislocation of the metacarpal is reduced and fixed with a threaded Kirschner wire.

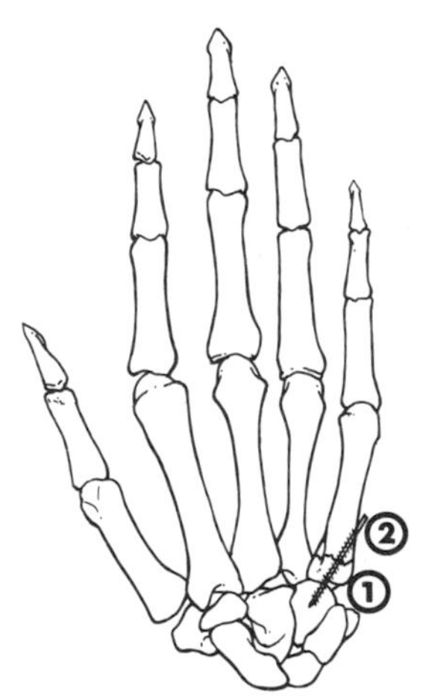

Postreduction X-Ray

1. Volar displacement of the fifth metacarpal is corrected.
2. Fragments are stabilized by a smooth Kirschner wire.

Subsequent Management

The hand is supported in a compression hand dressing or boxing glove dressing until the swelling subsides. Subsequently, a short-arm cast is applied for 3 weeks. The pin is then removed, and the patient is allowed actively to regain function and grip strength in the injured hand.

Fractures of the Metacarpals

REMARKS

Of all hand fractures, metacarpal fractures are second in frequency only to phalangeal fractures. They result commonly from direct blows, as when a clenched fist hits a firm object and the fifth metacarpal head fractures. A crushing injury to the dorsum of the hand frequently causes multiple metacarpal fractures.

In a hand with severe swelling after fracture, a compression hand dressing and continuous elevation for 2–3 days are necessary to eliminate edema.

Most metacarpal fractures are stable because of the support from surrounding intraosseous muscles. These fractures can be readily treated with closed reduction and plaster cast-splint support.

The aim of treatment is to provide sufficient stability by either external or internal fixation to allow early movement. There should be little justification for immobilizing these fractures longer than 3 weeks. Significant loss of hand function, even with relatively minor fractures, is likely to follow longer immobilization.

Rotational realignment is critical and should be ensured during the early phase of treatment by careful observation and by splinting the injured finger to the adjacent uninjured one.

Only rarely are metacarpal fractures sufficiently unstable to warrant internal fixation. The types that are likely to be unstable result from direct crushing injury that fractures more than one metacarpal and causes comminution or bone loss.

The most common fracture involves the head and neck of the fifth metacarpal. Dorsal angulation of this bone may usually be accepted. Vigorous operative or nonoperative treatment of this common injury frequently produces greater disability than does the fracture itself.

Dorsal angulation of the stable second and third metacarpals is less readily acceptable because these bones provide power grip, which can be impaired by displacement of the metacarpal heads into the palm.

Mechanism of Fracture

1. "Boxer's fracture" is usually produced by a violent self-inflicted blow when the fist is struck against a wall, with the fifth metacarpal head absorbing most of the force.
2. True boxers use the second and third metacarpals, which are the stable metacarpals of the fist, and are less likely to be broken than the more mobile fourth and fifth metacarpals.

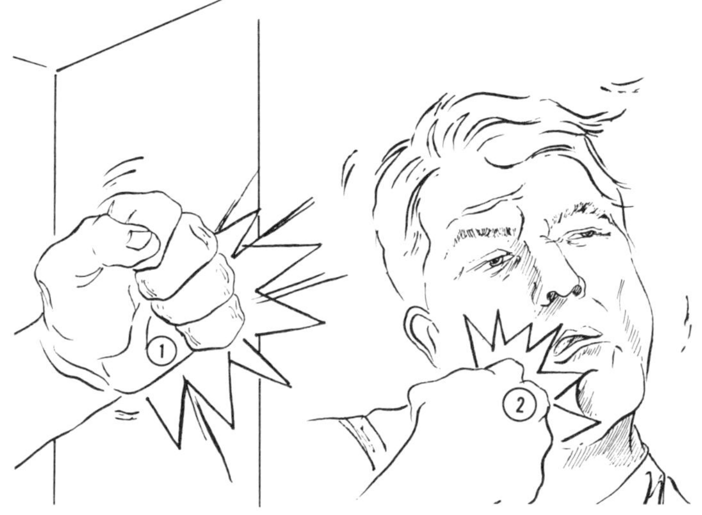

1. *Caution*: Beware of a fracture of the metacarpal or any fracture of the hand sustained by a human bite. These are extremely contaminated wounds and are almost universally infected. They require complete cleansing, debridement, and antibiotic treatment to avoid serious infection.

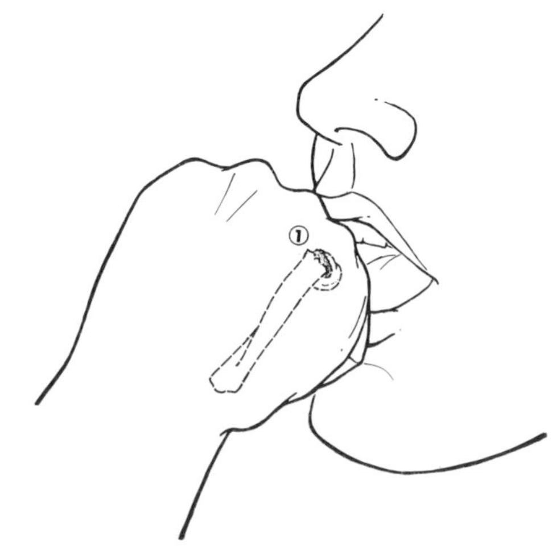

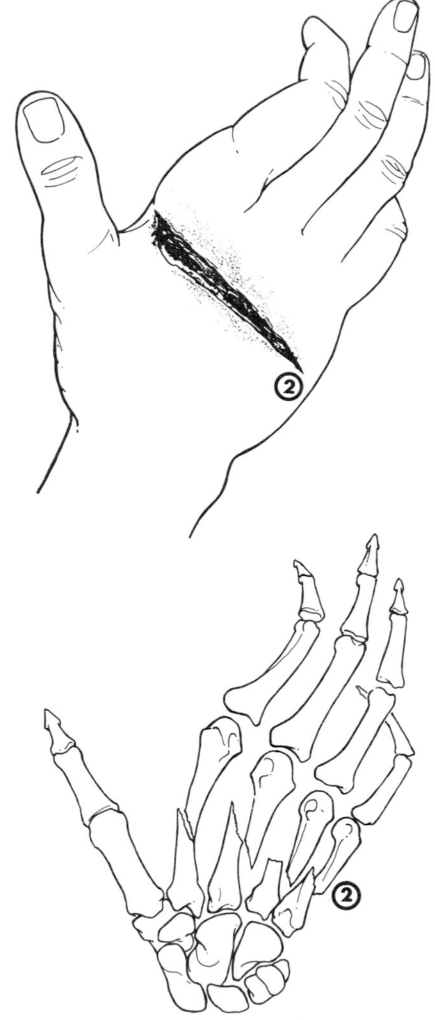

2. Crushing injury produces soft tissue damage and multiple metacarpal fractures with or without comminution.

Mechanism of Deformity

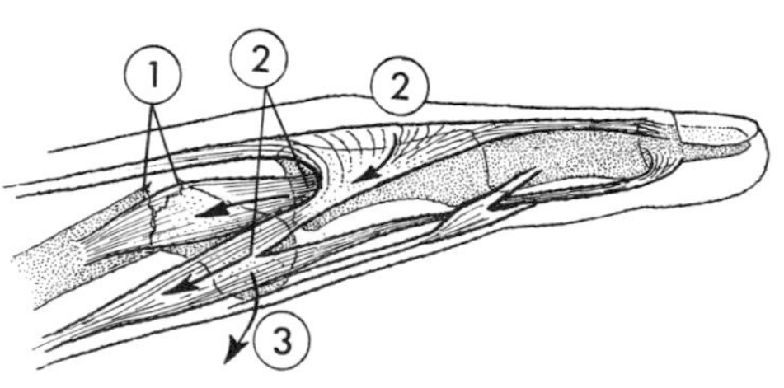

1. Fracture of the metacarpal neck or shaft produces a
2. Tightening of the extensor communis tendon, causing hyperextension of the MP joint.
3. Pull of the lumbricals accentuates the volar displacement of the distal fragment.

Reduction

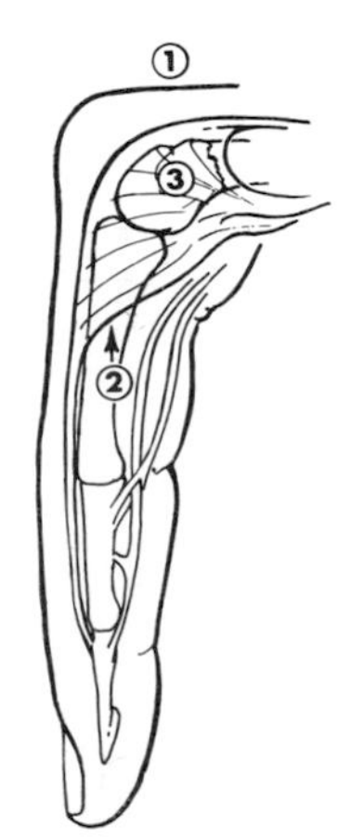

1. Flexion of the MP joint relaxes the lumbrical and permits
2. Correction of the deformity by upward redirection of the metacarpal head.
3. Flexion of the MP joint and correction of the deformity permits the extensor to stabilize the fracture.

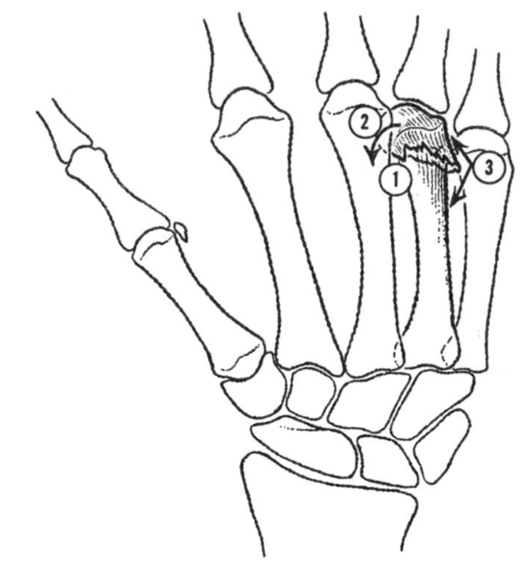

Stable Fracture of the Neck of the Metacarpal of the Finger

Prereduction X-Ray

1. Fracture of the fourth metacarpal.
2. Head of the metacarpal is tilted volarly into the palm.
3. Fracture is angulated dorsally.

Reduction

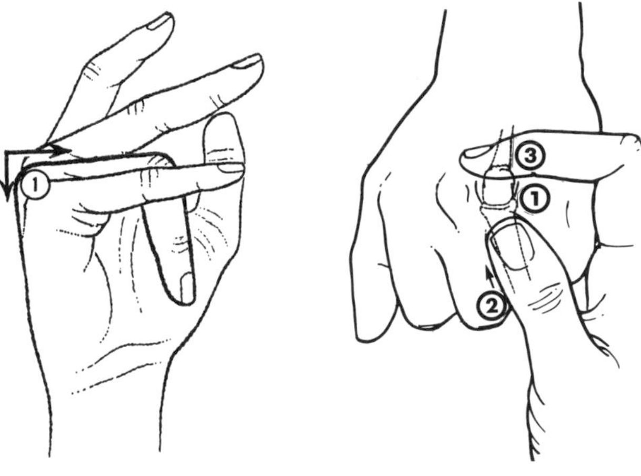

This procedure is performed with the patient under local anesthesia.

1. Flex the MP joint to a right angle.
2. With the MP joint flexed, push the proximal phalanx upward so as to redirect the distal metacarpal head.
3. Push the proximal fragment down by direct pressure.

Note: Although the fracture may be reduced by this maneuver, it tends to be unstable, and the angulation is likely to recur. This does not cause anything more than a small prominence over the metacarpal head. Therefore, with the exception of multiple fractures, repeated attempts at anatomic reduction should be avoided.

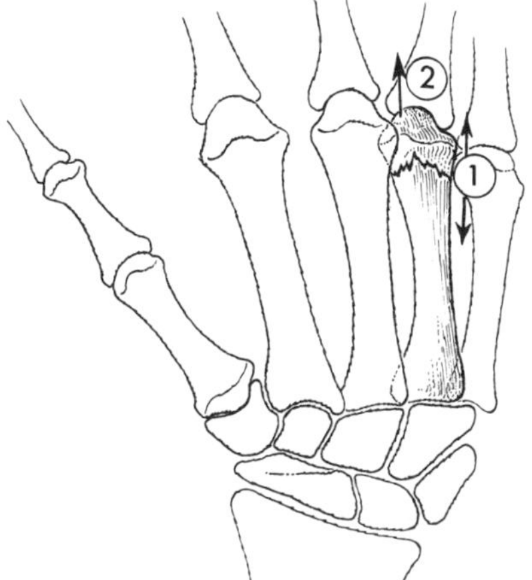

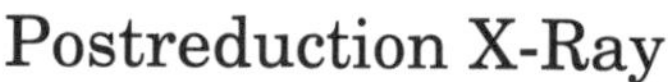

Postreduction X-Ray

1. Dorsal angulation is corrected.
2. Head of the metacarpal is directed along the long axis of the finger.

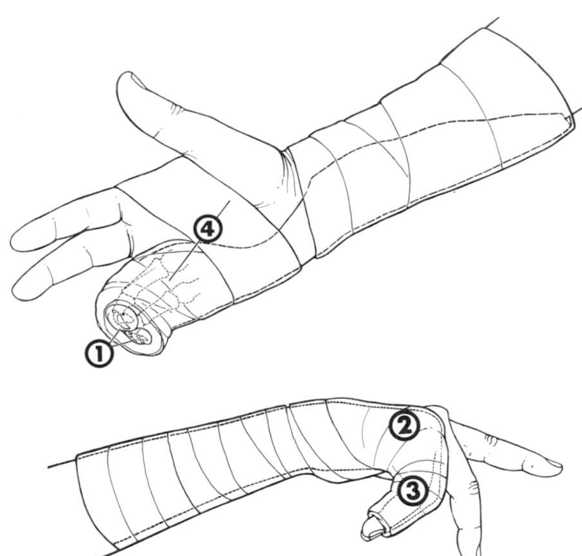

Immobilization

Apply a plaster cast-splint.

1. Incorporate the fracture and the adjacent, unfractured metacarpal.
2. MP joint is flexed 70°.
3. IP joints are in slight flexion.
4. Tips of the fingers are aligned to point toward the scaphoid tuberosity for correct rotational alignment.

Note: The key to holding reduction is to maintain maximal flexion of the MP joints to tighten the extensor hood around the fracture.

Postreduction Management

Encourage the patient to exercise the nonimmobilized fingers actively.

Remove the splint at 10 days, and have the patient begin active exercises in warm water three times a day.

Reapply the splint if the fracture is still tender and the patient is likely to injure the hand.

Some redisplacement, up to 40°, may be accepted without remanipulation.

Discard the splint no later than 3 weeks. Immobilization longer than 3 weeks is likely to cause prolonged stiffness.

Angulation of these fractures causes little clinical deformity and does not interfere with normal use of the hand.

Rotational malalignment, however, should not be accepted because it produces overlapping fingers in flexion.

Unstable Fractures of the Neck of the Metacarpal of the Finger

REMARKS

Rarely, dorsal angulation of the metacarpals cannot be satisfactorily corrected by closed means. This is particularly true with multiple fractures.

Persistent displacement of middle metacarpal heads into the palm may impair grip. Internal fixation may be necessary to reduce and hold the fracture.

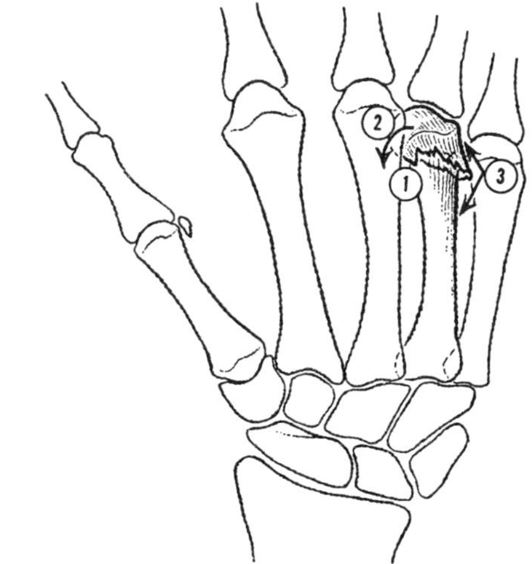

X-Ray After Unsuccessful Closed Reduction

1. Fracture of the neck of the fourth metacarpal.
2. Head of the metacarpal remains tilted into the palm.
3. Fracture is angulated dorsally.

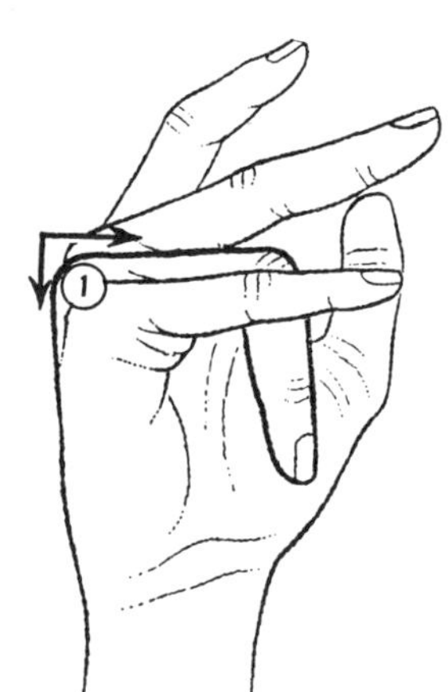

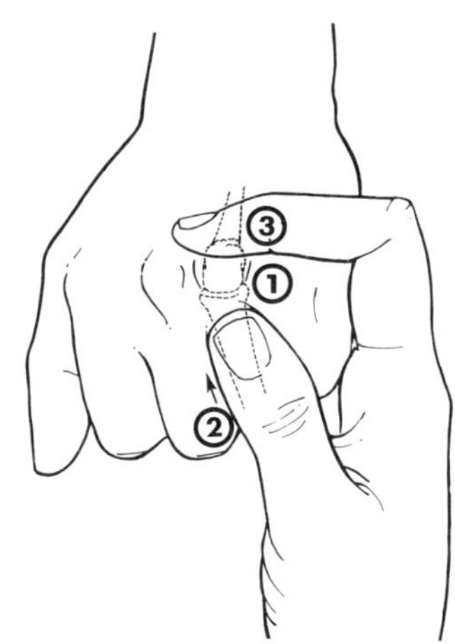

Reduction and Fixation

1. Flex the MP joint maximally.
2. Reduce the fracture by direct upward pressure on the distal fragment and
3. Downward pressure on the proximal phalanx.

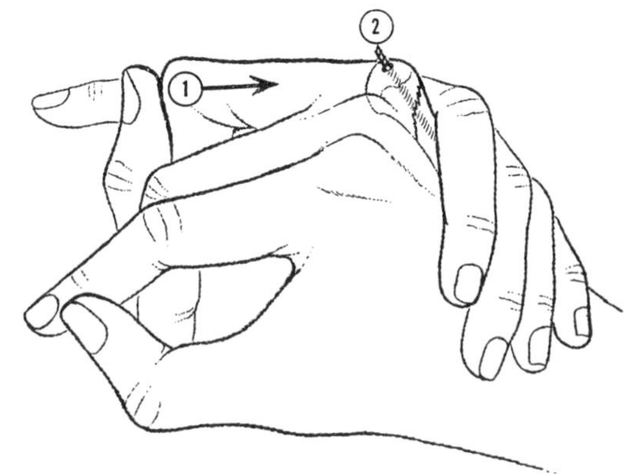

1. While an assistant maintains flexion of the MP joint and reduction of the fracture,
2. Pass a fine threaded pin through the lateral condyle of the metacarpal head and across the fracture.

Cut the wire 1 cm from the skin.

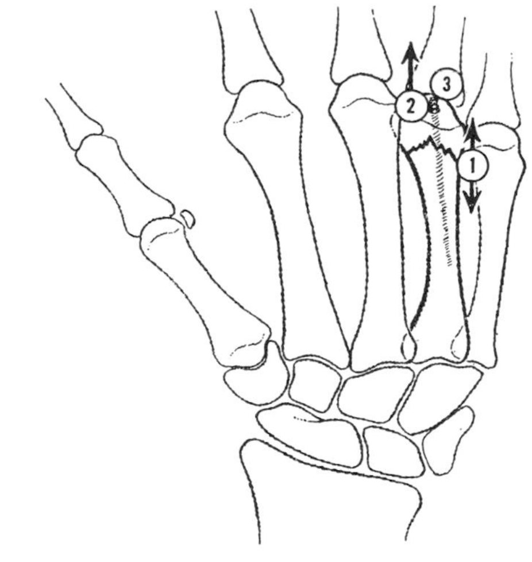

Postreduction X-Ray

1. Dorsal angulation is corrected.
2. Head of the metacarpal is redirected along the long axis of the finger.
3. Wire passes lateral to the MP joint.

Caution: One of the most common sources of delayed union and nonunion of fractures of the fingers or metacarpals is Kirschner wire fixation, which distracts the fracture. If there is evidence that the pin is maintaining a fracture gap, it should be removed, and alternative means of fixation should be used.

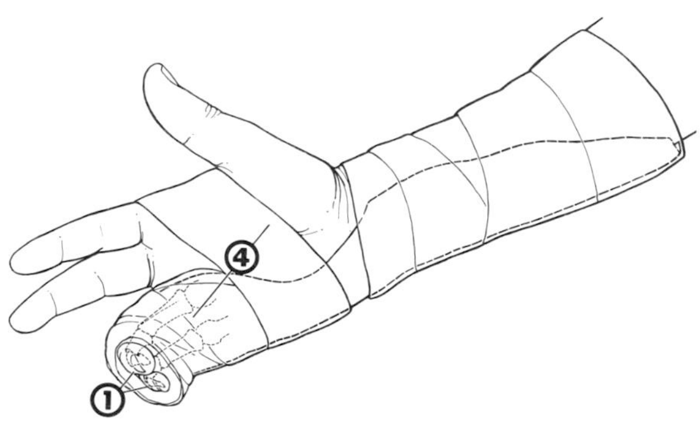

Immobilization

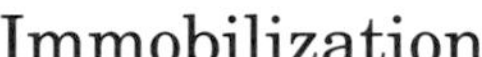

Apply a plaster cast-splint.

1. Incorporate the fractured metacarpal and the adjacent, uninjured metacarpal.
2. MP joint is flexed 70°.
3. PIP joints are in slight flexion.
4. Tips of the fingers are aligned to point toward the scaphoid tuberosity for correct rotational alignment.

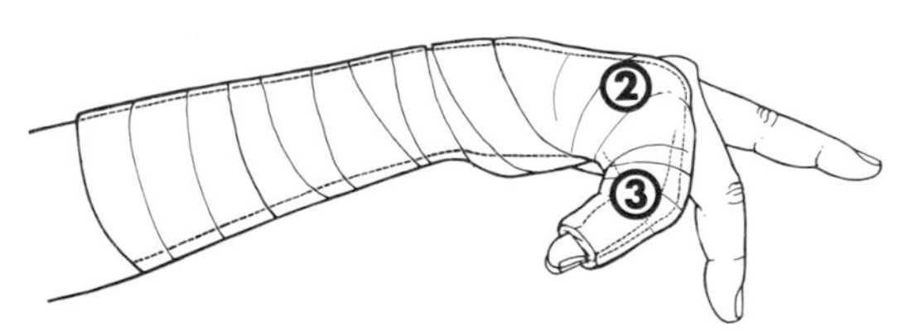

Postreduction Management

Remove the wire by 10 days to 2 weeks. The patient may then begin active range of motion two to three times a day in warm water.

When the patient is not exercising, the gutter splint should be worn. Discard the splint completely by the end of 3 weeks because immobilization for longer than this time is likely to cause permanent stiffness.

Fracture of the Shaft of the Metacarpal of the Finger

REMARKS

Most shaft fractures are injuries of one metacarpal. Splinting by the surrounding interosseous muscles and adjacent metacarpals prevents significant displacement, except for malrotation.

Single metacarpal fractures can be reduced and held in a functional position, and a guarded exercise program can be begun at 10–14 days.

Multiple metacarpal shaft fractures are usually produced by direct crushing trauma to the dorsum of the hand. These tend to be unstable.

With multiple metacarpal fractures, the first priority is to eliminate edema by a hand compression dressing and elevation.

Internal fixation can later be used to provide stability and permit early functional exercise.

Stable Fracture of the Shaft of the Metacarpal

Appearance on X-Ray

NO DISPLACEMENT

1. Spiral fracture of the second metacarpal with no displacement.

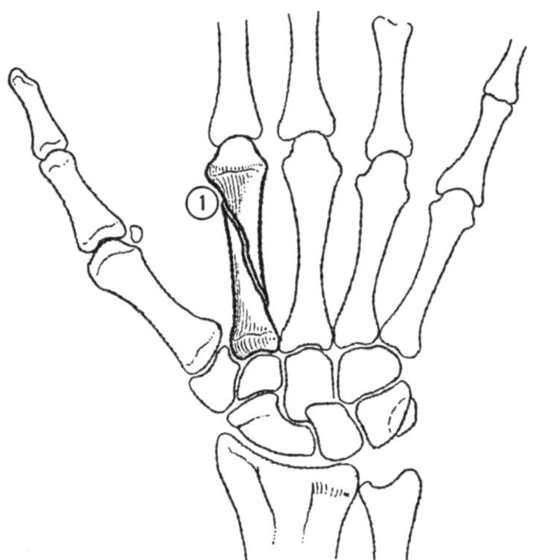

MINIMAL DISPLACEMENT

1. Spiral fracture of the third and fourth metacarpal with minimal displacement and shortening.

Note: This amount of shortening is acceptable.

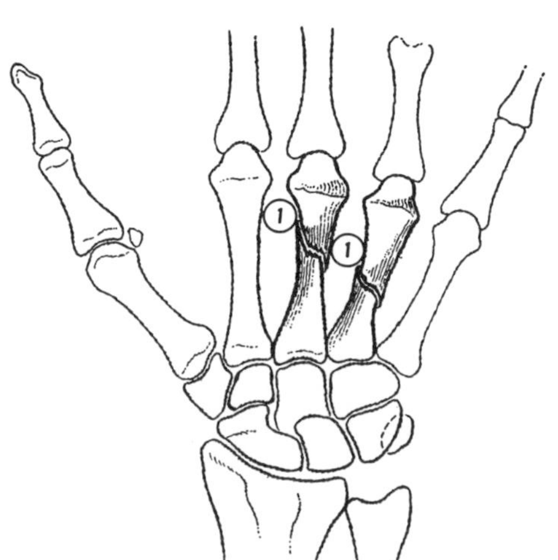

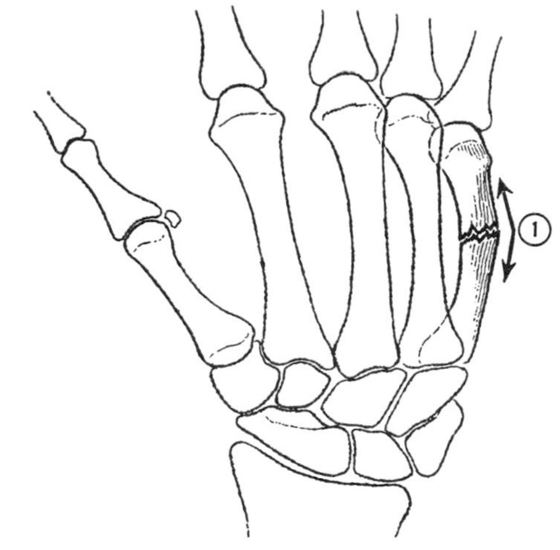

MINIMAL DISPLACEMENT

1. Fracture of the fifth metacarpal with slight posterior angulation.

Note: This degree of angulation is usually acceptable. It causes only mild clinical deformity that does not interfere with the use of the hand or cause patient dissatisfaction.

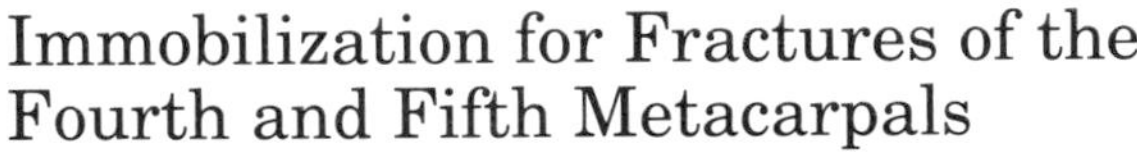

Immobilization for Fractures of the Fourth and Fifth Metacarpals

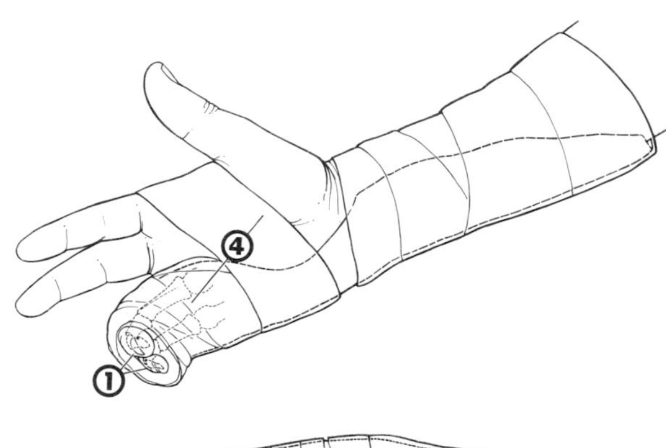

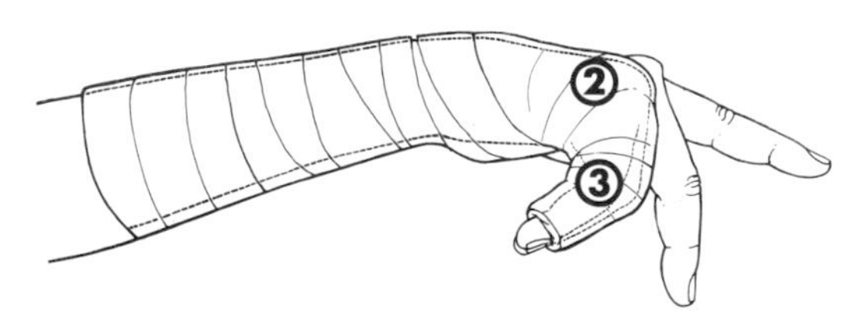

Note: For extensive swelling, apply a compression hand dressing for 2–3 days, and elevate the limb. When swelling subsides, apply a plaster cast-splint.

1. Incorporate the fractured finger and the adjacent, uninjured finger.
2. MP joint is flexed 70°.
3. IP joint is in slight flexion.
4. Finger tips are directed toward the scaphoid tuberosity to ensure rotational realignment.

Note: The key to achieving and maintaining reduction is to hold the MP joint in maximal flexion to tighten the extensor apparatus.

Alternative Method—Management of Metacarpal Fractures With the Clam Shell Plaster Method

The clam shell plaster method is designed to maintain maximal flexion of the MP joint while allowing motion of the MP and IP joints.

The wrist should be extended, and the patient should be encouraged to excercise the fingers actively to maintain mobility and diminish swelling.

1. Well-padded 3-in (7.5-cm) plaster splint is applied to the dorsal surface of the forearm and wrist with the
2. Wrist extended.
3. Plaster is molded to maintain the MP joints in maximal flexion. To achieve this, the palm should not be heavily padded.
4. IP joints are allowed to flex slightly and are held in the position of function.

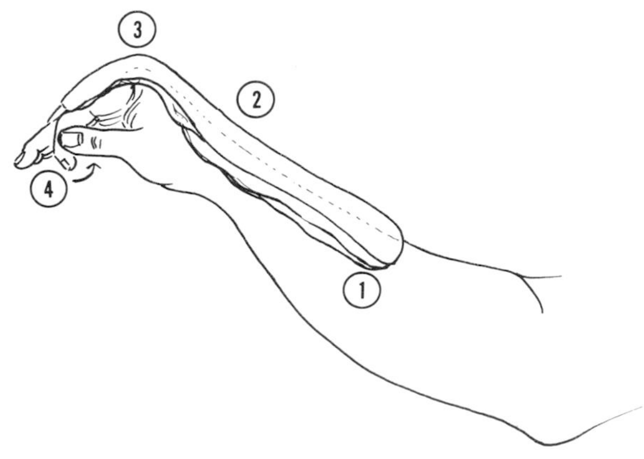

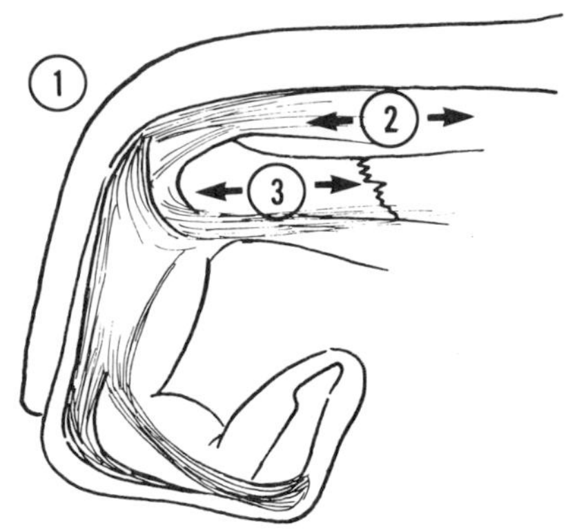

Mechanism of Stabilization With Clam Shell Plaster

1. Dorsal clam shell splint maintains the MP joint in maximal flexion.
2. Intact dorsal mechanism serves as a tension band.
3. This promotes compression of the palmar corticals at the surface of the fracture during active flexion of the finger.

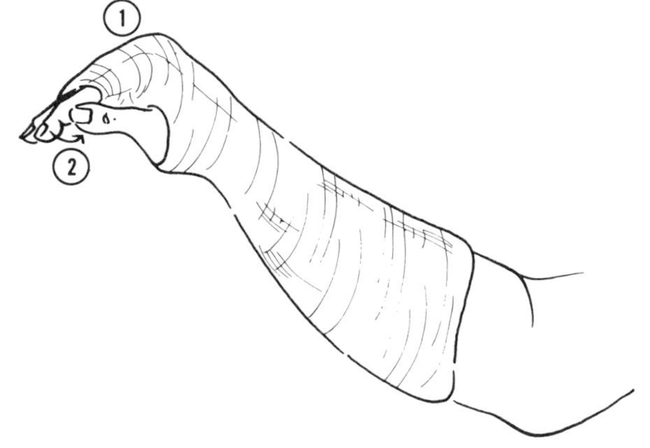

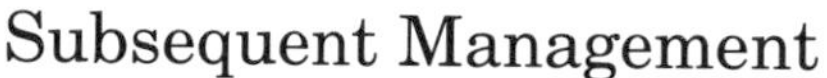

Subsequent Management

1. Clam shell plaster splint is incorporated in a short-arm cast.
2. As the acute swelling subsides, the patient begins active flexion of the fingers. Extension should be avoided until the fracture heals by 3 weeks when the cast is removed.

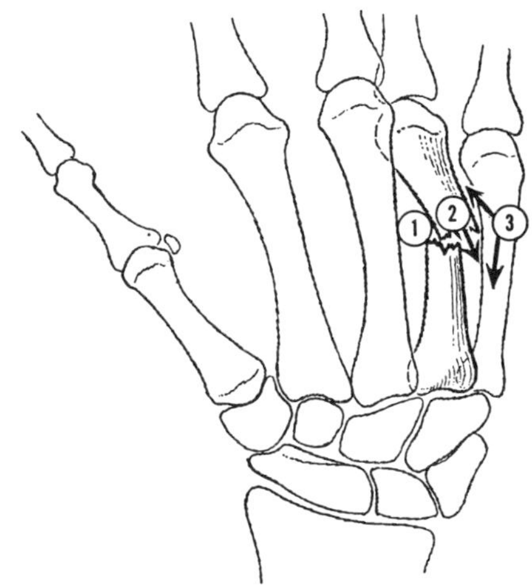

Unstable Fractures of Metacarpals

Prereduction X-Ray: Unacceptable Displacement

1. Transverse fracture of the fourth metacarpal.
2. Head of the metacarpal is displaced volarly.
3. Posterior angular deformity is marked.

Note: This much shortening and angulation is liable to impair intrinsic hand function or cause rotational malalignment.

Reduction

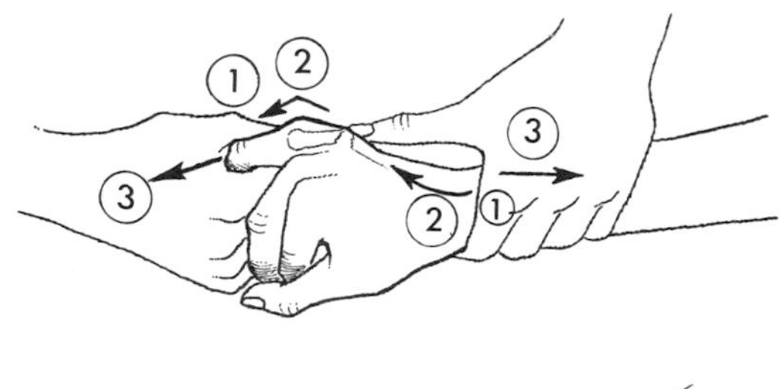

1. One hand of the operator encircles the patient's wrist while the other hand grasps the finger of the fractured metacarpal.
2. Wrist is dorsiflexed, and the MP joint is flexed 70°.
3. Apply traction to the injured finger to restore the metacarpal length.

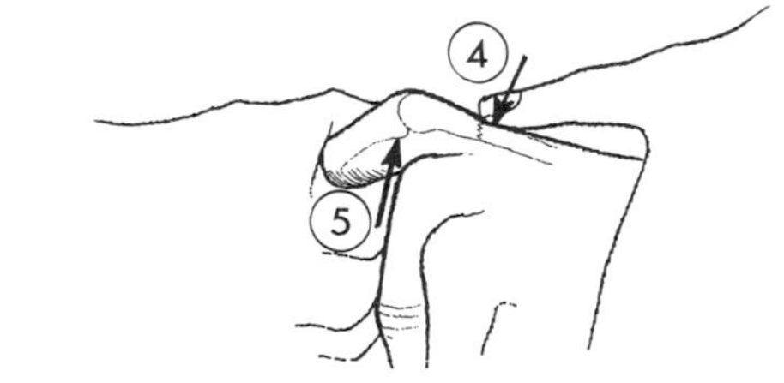

4. Apply direct pressure to the apex of the deformity.
5. With the MP joint flexed, push the distal fragment dorsally.

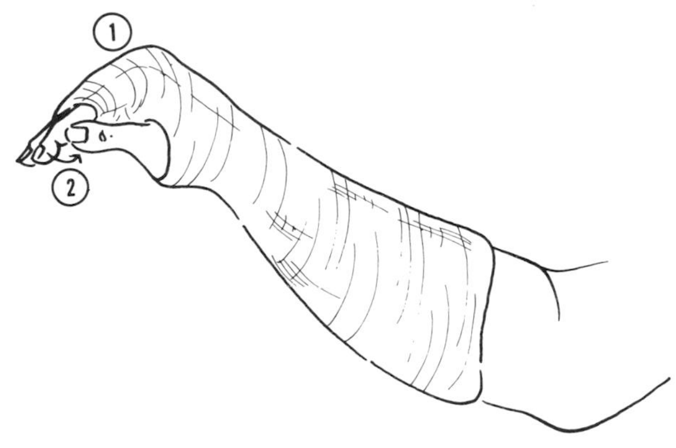

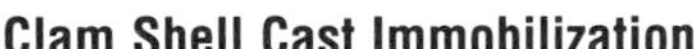

Clam Shell Cast Immobilization

1. The clam shell plaster cast immobilizes the fracture as previously described, with the MP joints maximally flexed. This maintains reduction by means of the dorsal mechanism, which serves as a tension band.
2. The patient is allowed to flex the fingers actively as soon as the acute pain subsides.

The cast is removed at 3–4 weeks. After this time, active extension exercises are carried out.

Internal Fixation of Unstable Fractures of the Metacarpals

REMARKS

Internal fixation need rarely be necessary for fractures of the hand unless the fracture cannot be reduced by closed methods, as previously described, or there are multiple fractures that make closed reduction less effective.

It is estimated that only 5–10 per cent of fractures of the hand should be considered candidates for operative treatment because, by far, most of them do well with closed methods. Kirschner wire fixation is sometimes associated with persistent fracture gap and a high incidence of delayed union and non-union.

If the injured hand is extremely swollen, elevate the limb for 2–3 days in a hand compression dressing before attempting internal fixation.

The objective of any internal fixation technique is to allow early resumption of functional exercises to restore normal gliding between the tendons and joint structures of the hand.

Indications for Internal Fixation

THIRD METACARPAL FRACTURE

1. Oblique fracture of the third metacarpal with posterior bowing.
2. Shaft of the metacarpal is shortened.

Note: Shortening or angulation of the second or third metacarpals is a problem because these are the stabilizing metacarpals of the arches of the hand and, therefore, are best reduced as anatomically as possible.

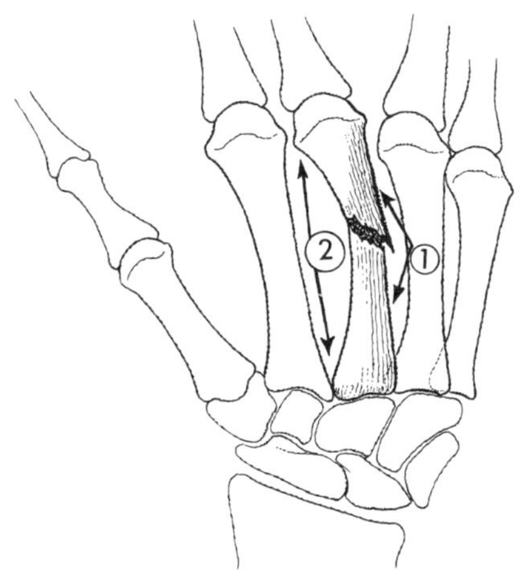

Prereduction X-Rays

FOURTH METACARPAL FRACTURE

1. Transverse fracture of the fourth metacarpal.
2. Distal fragment is displaced volarly and proximally, forming a
3. Posterior angular deformity.

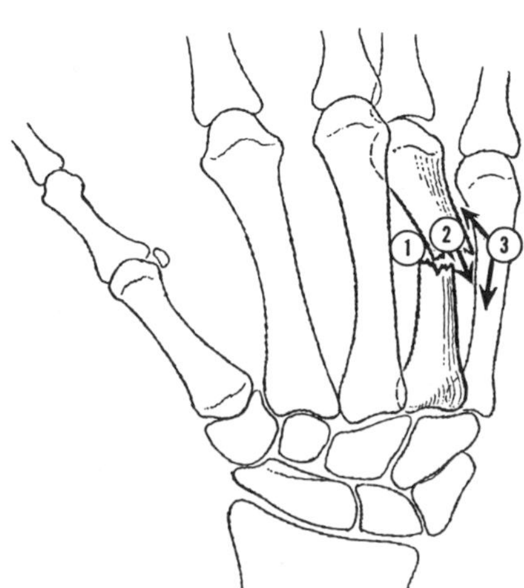

Preferred Method of Fixation for Unstable Metacarpal Fractures

1. Oblique fracture of the metacarpal may be fixed by open reduction, with small fragment screws applied perpendicular to the fracture site.
2. Transverse fracture is best fixed by a small fragment plate fixation technique. (Alternatively, an intramedullary pin could be used.)

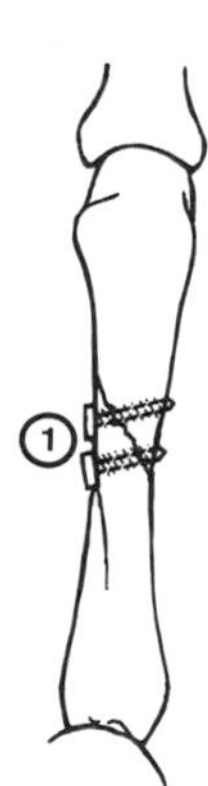

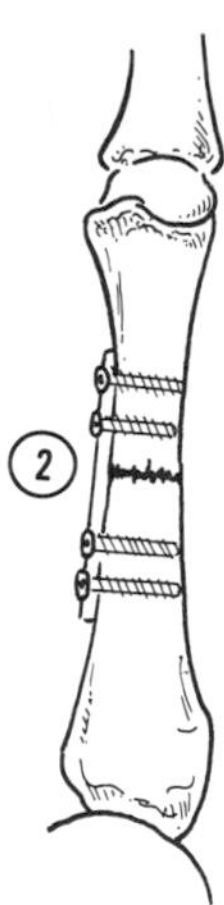

Alternative Method for Displaced Fractures of the Metacarpals: Intramedullary Fixation

REMARKS

Fractures of the metacarpal may also be reduced closed and fixed with intramedullary pins.

Care should be taken that these pins do not distract the fracture site but allow adequate stabilization.

Prereduction X-Ray

DISPLACED FRACTURE

1. Oblique fracture of the fifth metacarpal.
2. Volar displacement of the head.
3. Posterior angulation of the fragments.

Reduction and Transfixion

1. Assistant flexes the MP joint to a right angle and,
2. With the patient's finger flexed, applies direct pressure upward on the metacarpal head in the long axis of the proximal phalanx.
3. At the same time, strong downward pressure is applied over the apex of the deformity.

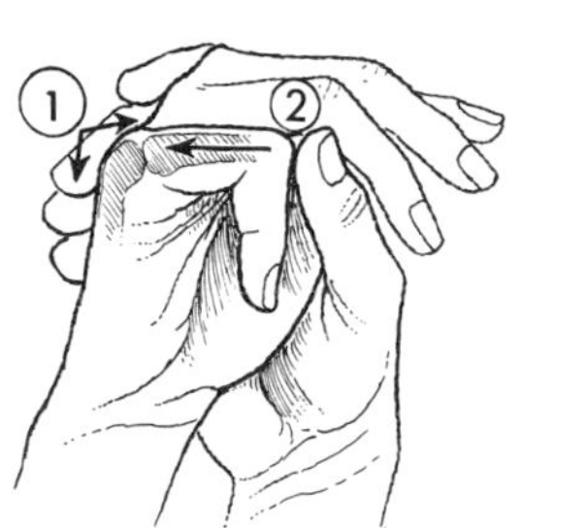

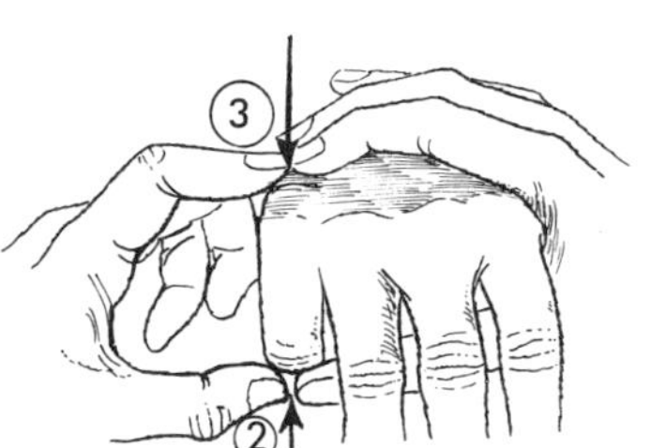

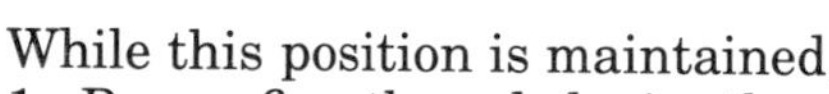

While this position is maintained,

1. Pass a fine threaded wire through the metacarpal head and into the distal fragment. Cut the wire 0.5 cm from the skin.

Note: With multiple unstable fractures, two intramedullary pins may be necessary.

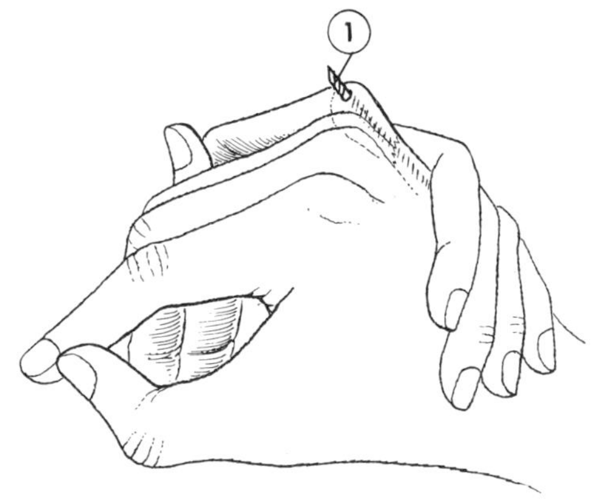

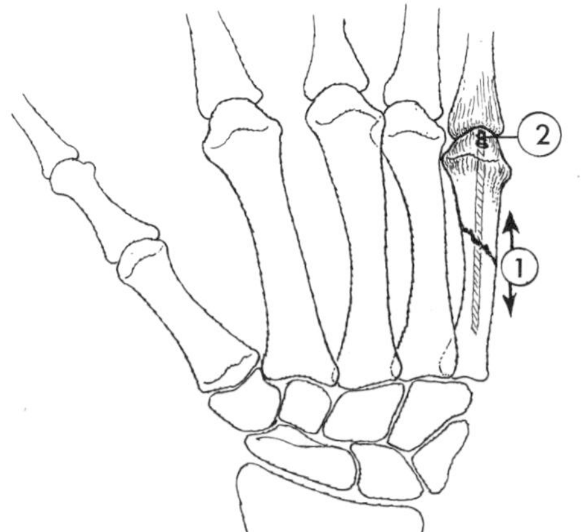

Postreduction X-Rays

DISPLACED FRACTURE

1. Dorsal angulation of the fracture is corrected.
2. Intramedullary wire has restored length to the metacarpal.

Immobilization

After intramedullary fixation, apply the clam shell plaster cast.

This allows the fingers to be exercised actively as soon as the acute swelling subsides and assists in stabilizing the fracture until healing occurs at 2–3 weeks.

After 2–3 weeks, remove the clam shell plaster and pin and allow continued active exercise.

Multiple Metacarpal Fractures With Open Wounds

1. This is usually the result of a crush injury to the dorsum of the hand, producing an open wound with involvement of tendons and bone.
2. Multiple metacarpal fractures produce an extremely unstable injury. This is best stabilized with either small fragment plates or intramedullary Kirschner wires to allow tendon repair and resumption of active function.

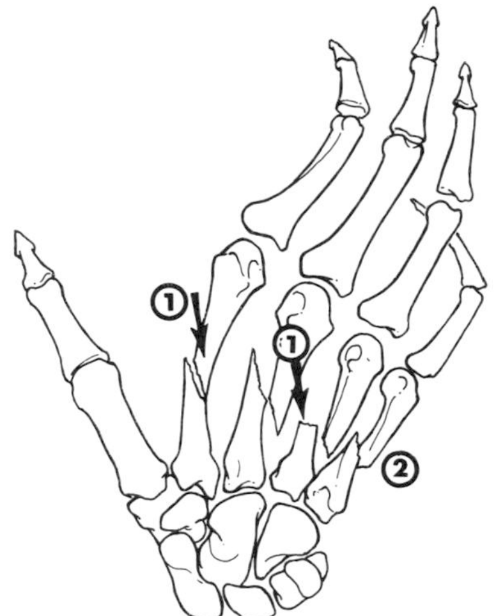

Multiple Fractures With Open Wounds

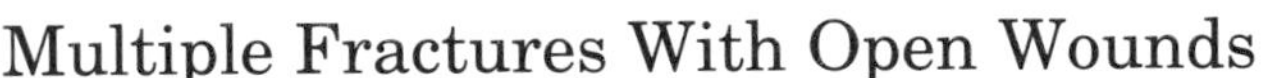

1. Two Kirschner wires in each metacarpal may be necessary to stabilize the fracture.
2. Stabilization of the skeletal injury aids significantly in the management of the soft tissue wound.

Note: Fasciotomy may be necessary to relieve any swelling of the dorsal compartments associated with these multiple fractures. See also discussion of open wrist injuries in Chapter 16.

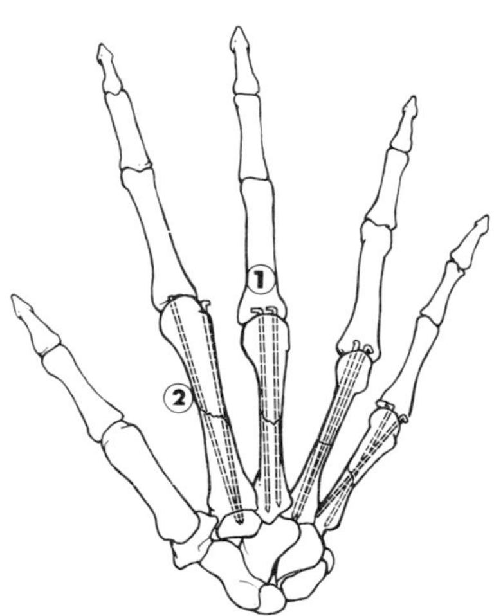

Fractures of the Bases of the Metacarpals

REMARKS

The bases of the metacarpals are firmly bound together by palmar and dorsal ligaments. Consequently, displacement of any fracture fragments rarely occurs except when there is a carpal-metacarpal dislocation.

Many of these fractures are impacted, and visualization with standard x-ray can be difficult. Consequently, routine x-ray of the hand often does not demonstrate the fracture despite swelling and pain in the region.

Under these circumstances, where the injury at the base of the metacarpal is suspected, a CT evaluation is usually justified to determine whether the metacarpal is dislocated (see page 1517).

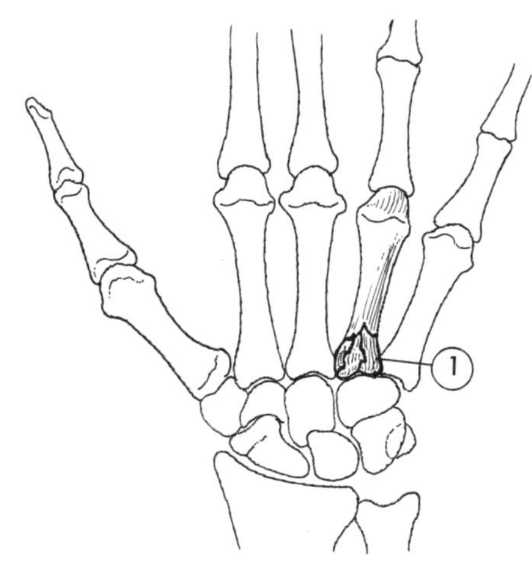

Appearance on X-Ray

1. Comminuted fracture of the fourth metacarpal.

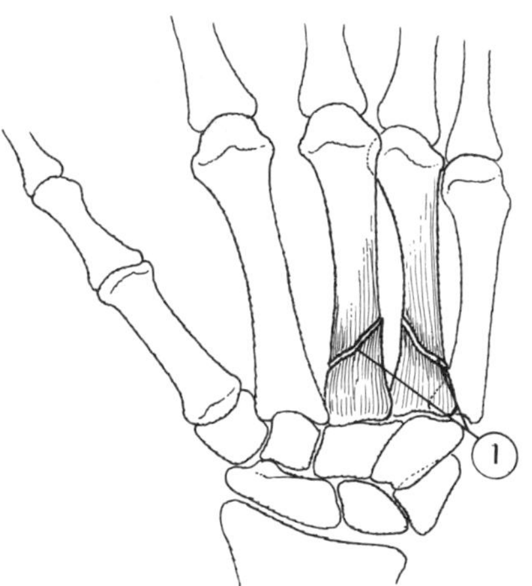

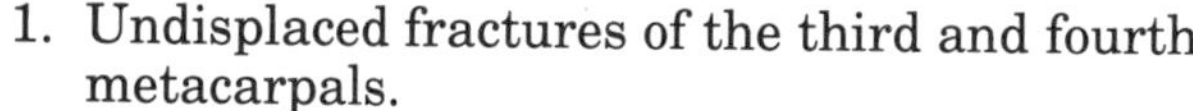

1. Undisplaced fractures of the third and fourth metacarpals.

Note: Evaluate these fractures carefully on x-ray or CT scan for any dissociation of the CM joint. Volar displacement of the fracture may involve the motor branch of the ulnar nerve and may require open reduction with internal fixation.

Management

After careful evaluation (including CT scan, if necessary), if the fracture at the base of the metacarpal is not associated with dislocation, closed treatment with splint immobilization is indicated.

If there is evidence of subluxation or dislocation, the injury is reduced by manipulation and can usually be stabilized by percutaneous fixation.

For the injury that is not recognized initially or for the injury that may involve the motor branch of the ulnar nerve, open reduction with internal stabilization is indicated.

Immobilization

If the hand is swollen, apply a compressive hand dressing for several days.

Most of these undisplaced fractures can be treated by immobilization in a short arm cast for 2–3 weeks.

1. Fingers are free.
2. Patient is able to exercise the MP joints actively.
3. Wrist is slightly dorsiflexed.

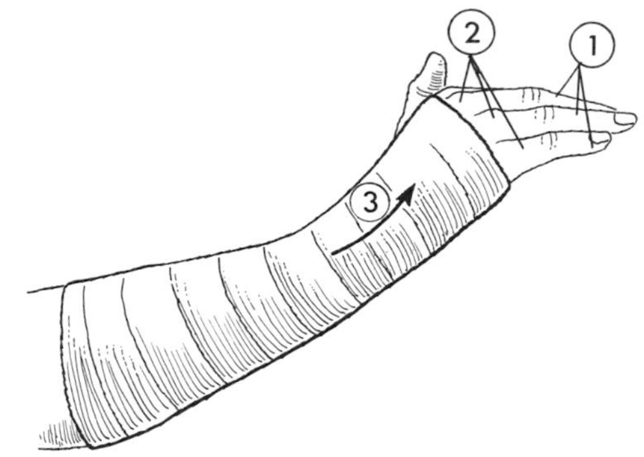

Injuries of the Metacarpophalangeal Joints of the Fingers

REMARKS

Dislocations of the MP joints may be surprisingly difficult to recognize unless adequate true lateral x-ray views are obtained.

The injury usually occurs in either the index or the small finger. Visual examination of the finger can be deceiving in that it merely appears short and deviated slightly to the ulnar side.

A lateral x-ray will show the hyperextended position of the simple dislocation, but a complex dislocation may not be so apparent.

Like dislocations of the MP joint of the thumb, these injuries may be either simple or complex, depending on whether or not the volar plate has become trapped in the joint.

Reduction is possible by closed methods when the dislocation is simple, but open reduction is always necessary for complex dislocation.

Repeated attempts at reduction inflict further damage to joint structures. Avoid more than two attempts at closed reduction.

Surgical exposure is best done by a volar approach. The key to reduction is to release the transverse metacarpal ligament attachment to the volar plate to allow it to be removed from the joint.

Occasionally, with a chronic dislocation, a dorsal extension of the incision is also necessary to free the lateral capsular structures.

Simple Dislocation

Prereduction X-Ray

1. Base of the phalanx sits on the dorsum of the head of the metacarpal at a right angle.

Note: When the phalanx is in this position, it can be assumed that the anterior capsule is not interposed between the bones. This is far less common than a complex dislocation with capsular interposition.

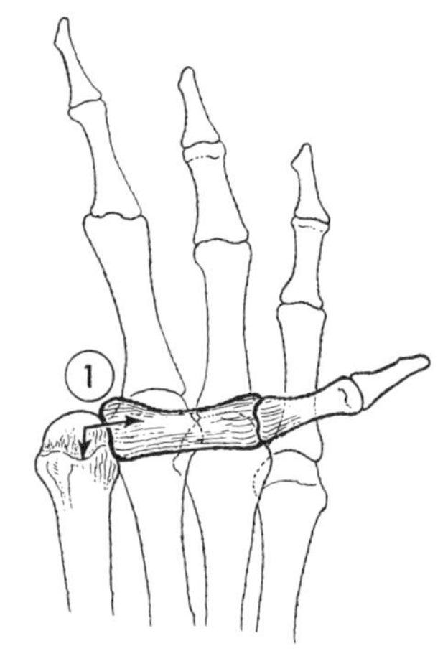

Manipulative Reduction

1. Bandage is first looped around the patient's finger and then around the operator's hand.
2. Grasp the finger with your thumb and index finger, and apply traction along the axis of the hyperextended phalanx (not along the axis of the metacarpal).
3. While traction is maintained, push the base of the dislocated phalanx distalward to a position opposite the head of the metacarpal.
4. Flex the MP joints.

Note: The key to reduction is to *push* the hyperextended dislocated phalanx volarly over the metacarpal head. Trying to reduce the dislocation by pulling the finger will trap the volar plate in the joint and produce a complex dislocation.

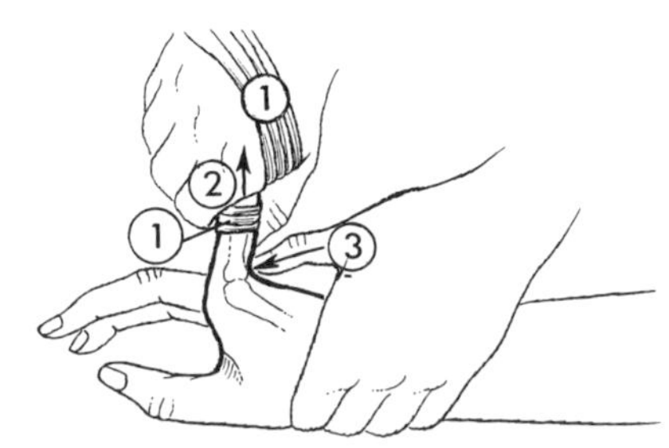

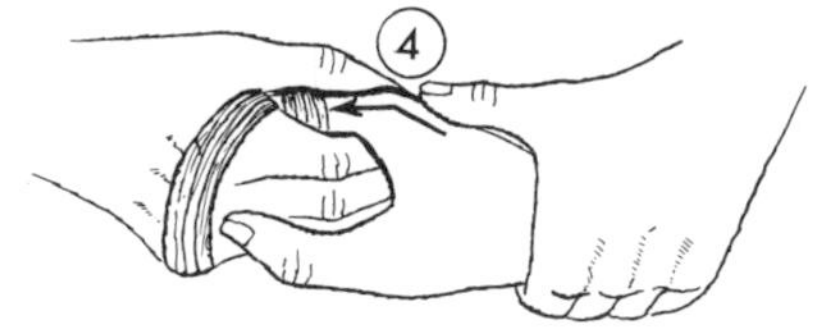

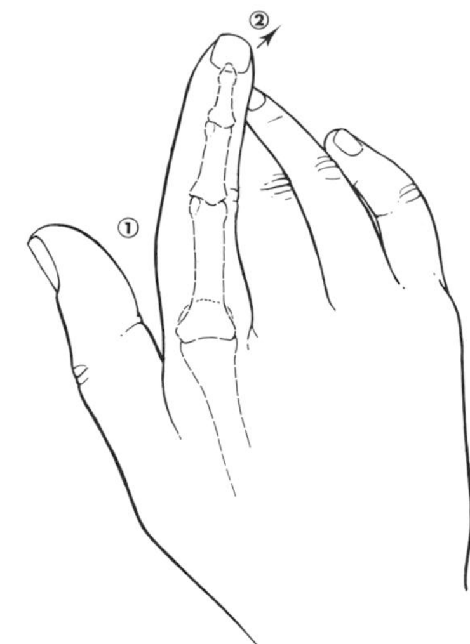

Complex Dislocation

Clinical Appearance

Clinical appearance can be deceiving about the extent of injury.
1. Finger looks a little short.
2. There is slight ulnar deviation.

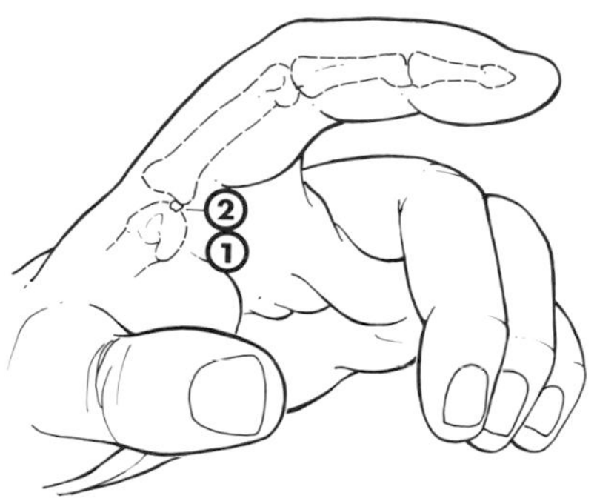

Clues to a complex dislocation.
1. Dimpling in the palm.
2. Inclusion of a sesamoid bone in the joint on x-ray.

Avoid mistaking this for a chip fracture.

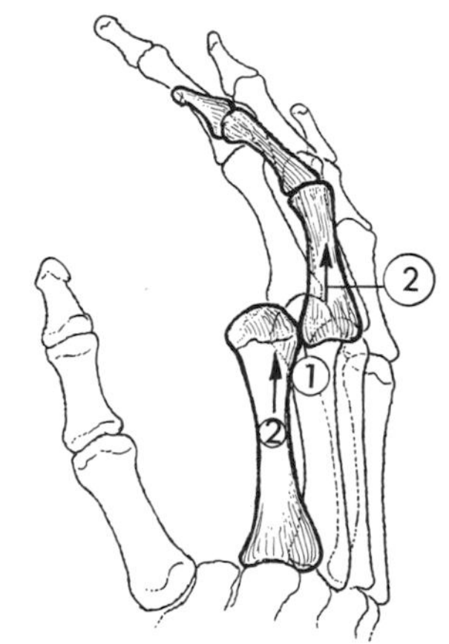

Prereduction X-Ray

1. Base of the phalanx lies on the dorsal surface of the head of the metacarpal.
2. Axis of the phalanx is almost parallel to that of the metacarpal.

Note: When the phalanx lies in this position, it can be assumed that the anterior palmar ligament is interposed between the bones.

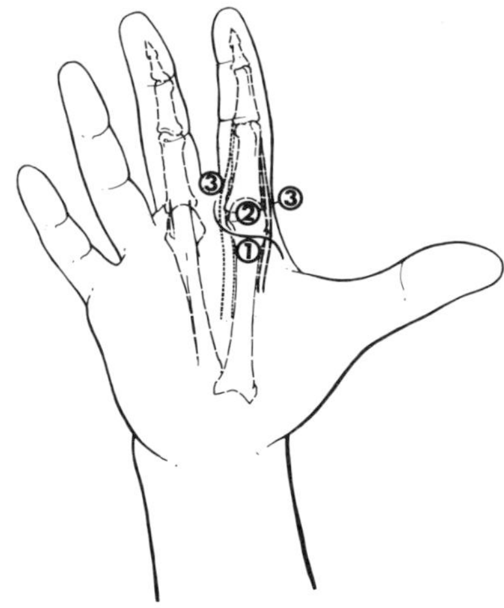

Surgical Reduction of a Complex MP Dislocation of the Index or Small Finger

1. Dislocation is exposed through a curved palmar skin incision.
2. Metacarpal head is directly beneath the skin.
3. Flexor tendon and neurovascular structures are displaced as a result of the metacarpal head dislocation and must be carefully protected.

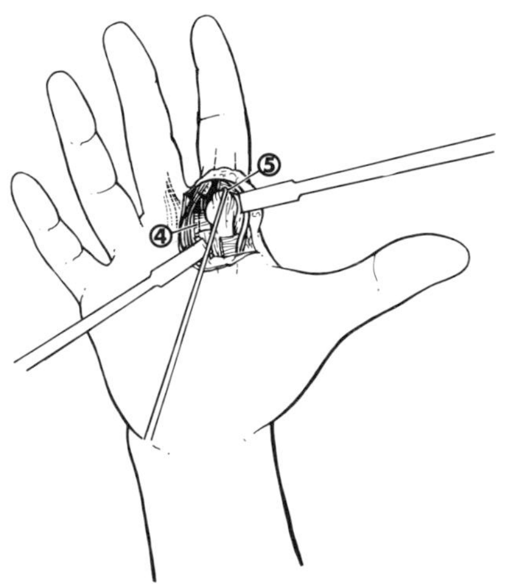

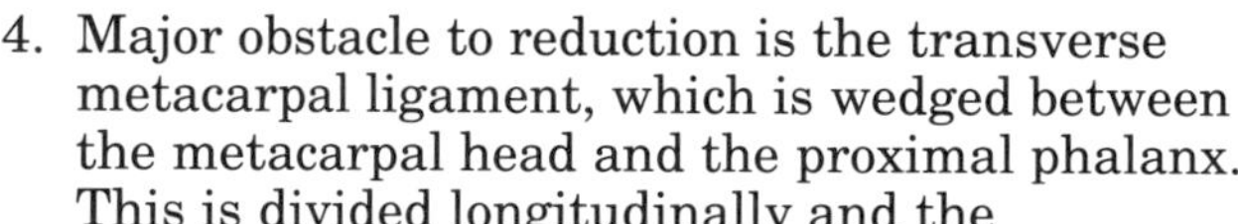

4. Major obstacle to reduction is the transverse metacarpal ligament, which is wedged between the metacarpal head and the proximal phalanx. This is divided longitudinally and the
5. Volar capsule is then removed from the joint with a small hook.

Immobilization

A simple MP dislocation treated by closed reduction can be splinted with buddy-taping of the finger to the adjacent, uninjured finger. The patient is allowed to begin active exercises, and the tape is removed after 3–5 days.

If open reduction of a complex dislocation has been carried out, the joint is usually stable.

Stability of the joint should be confirmed at the time of surgery by passively moving the finger through a full range of motion.

After open reduction of the MP dislocation, the hand is immobilized and elevated for 3 days to diminish edema. Active exercise is permitted when the edema has subsided, usually by 3–5 days.

Immobilization of the hand after these injuries for longer than 10 days contributes nothing except further stiffening of the joint.

Fracture-Dislocations of the Metacarpophalangeal Joint

Appearance on X-Ray

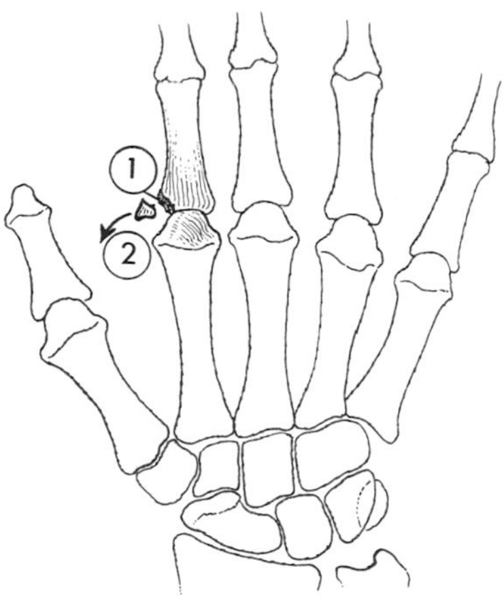

SMALL DISPLACED FRAGMENT

1. Small avulsed fragment from the base of the phalanx.
2. Fragment is displaced.

Note: This fragment may be removed at the time of open reduction and the torn ligament repaired.

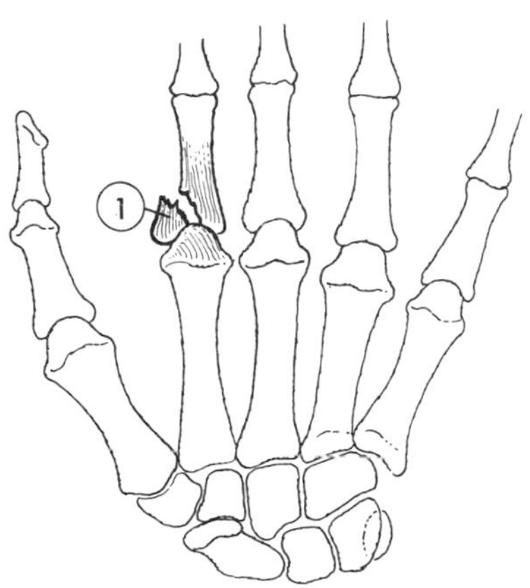

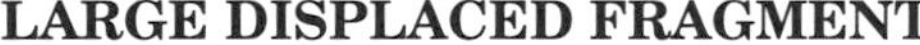

LARGE DISPLACED FRAGMENT

1. Large triangular fragment from volar aspect of the base of the phalanx.

Note: Reduce the dislocation and this fragment, which involves more than one third of the articular surface, and fix it with a small fragment screw.

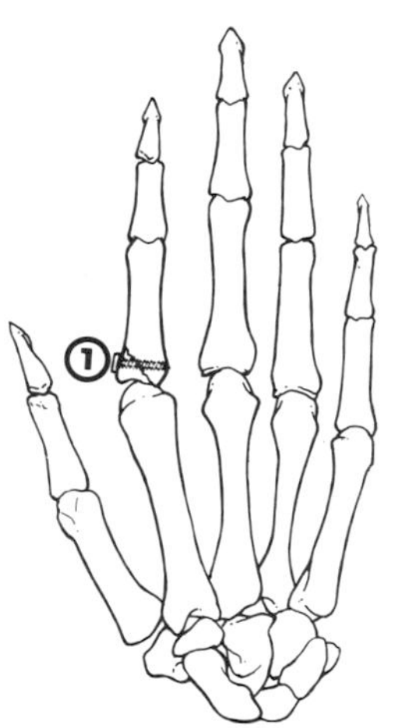

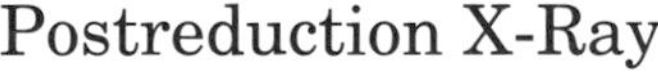

Postreduction X-Ray

1. Fragment is fixed in its normal position with a small fragment screw.

Fractures of the Phalanges

REMARKS

Phalangeal fractures, which can range from minor to severe, are the most common of all hand fractures.

The disability they cause depends on the degree of initial injury and the treatment.

Direct injury to the finger frequently produces open comminuted fractures. All open fractures must be thoroughly cleansed, and the fracture must be immobilized by either internal or external means.

The objective of fracture treatment should be to provide sufficient stability by either external or internal fixation to permit early movement of the finger's joints and muscles.

Fracture reduction should be as close to anatomic as possible, with particular attention given to rotational realignment.

Most phalangeal shaft fractures are stable injuries that can be effectively managed by buddy-taping to the adjacent finger. This stabilizes the fracture and ensures correct rotational alignment while permitting joint and tendon motion.

Splinting the fractured finger alone is likely to accentuate rotational malalignment. Displaced, unstable phalangeal fractures can frequently be successfully treated by closed reduction and cast-splint immobilization with the finger in the intrinsic-plus position.

Although most phalangeal fractures can be effectively treated by closed means, knowledge of the deformities common with these injuries is important to select the most appropriate means of treatment.

Anatomic Causes of Fracture Deformities

Fractures of the shaft of the proximal phalanx are characterized by volar angulation of the fragments. Such angulation is due to the action of the extrinsic and intrinsic muscles, which buckles the fragments.

1. Fracture of the middle of the shaft of the proximal phalanx.
2. Pull of the intrinsic muscles flexes the proximal fragment while the central slip attachment to the PIP joint hyperextends the distal fragment.

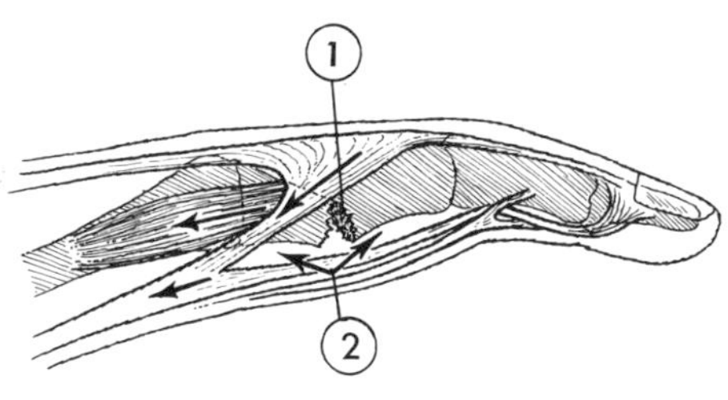

1. Fracture of the middle phalanx.
2. Central slip of the extensor tendon extends the proximal fragment.
3. Flexor digitorum sublimis flexes the distal fragment, producing
4. Dorsal angulation of the fragments.

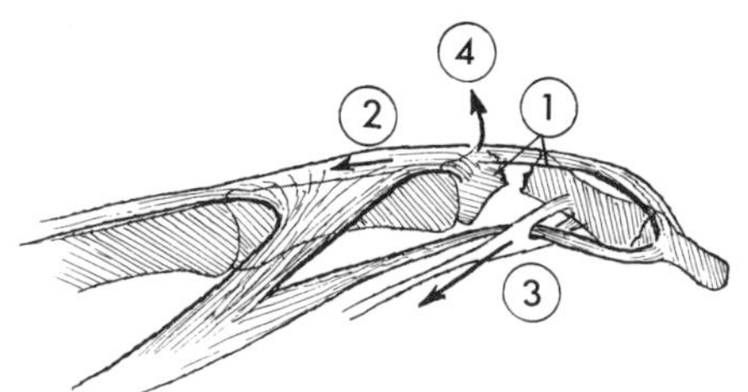

1. Fracture of the middle phalanx distal to the insertion of the flexor digitorum sublimis tendon.
2. Proximal fragment is flexed.
3. Distal fragment is extended, producing
4. Volar angulation of the fragments.

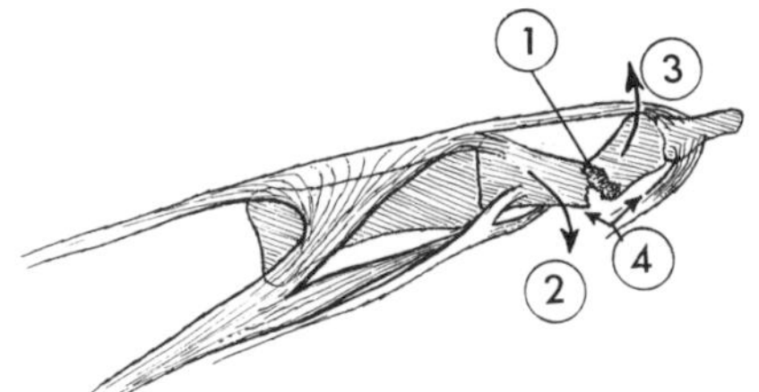

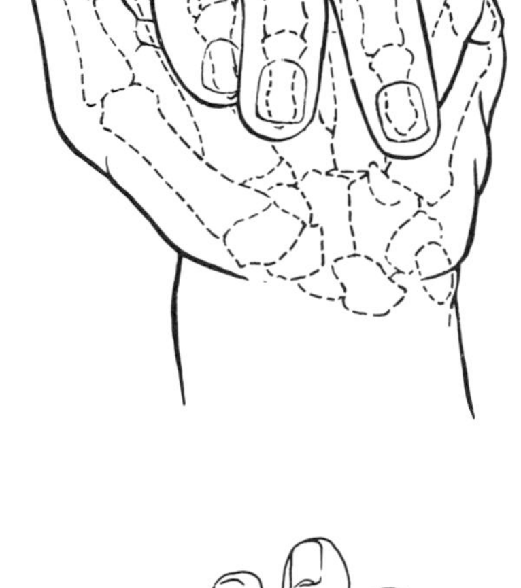

Malrotation of the finger is particularly likely if the fracture is produced by rotation.

1. Persistent malrotation of the phalangeal fracture can impair function because of overlapping of the fingers during grasp.

1. Avoid immobilizing a phalangeal fracture in single isolated splintage. This makes it difficult to assess rotational malalignment.

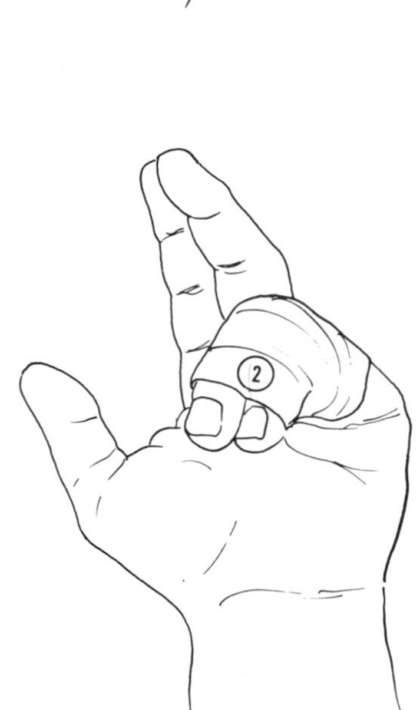

2. Preferred method of immobilizing isolated phalangeal fractures is with buddy-splinting, which allows the adjacent finger to support the fractured finger and aids in proper rotational alignment of the injured finger.

Undisplaced Fractures of the Proximal Phalanx

REMARKS

Undisplaced fractures of the proximal phalanx need only immobilization by buddy-taping to the adjacent, uninjured finger.

This method permits correct rotational alignment while allowing the patient to exercise the joints and tendons of the injured finger actively.

If the finger is initially too swollen to apply buddy-taping, use the clam shell plaster method previously described for metacarpal fractures. Subsequently, as the swelling subsides by 5–7 days, buddy-taping may be used.

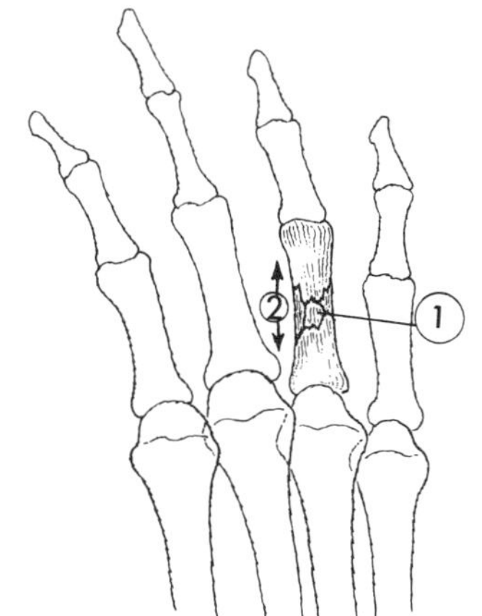

Appearance on X-Ray

1. Comminuted fracture of the proximal phalanx.
2. There is no diplacement of the fragments.

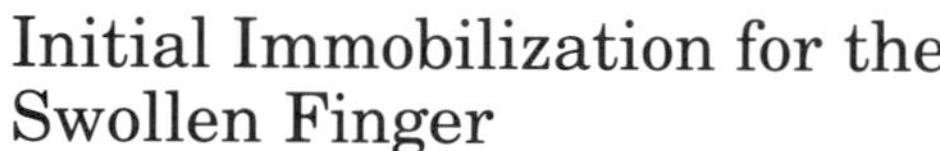

Initial Immobilization for the Swollen Finger

1. Apply a clam shell plaster with the MP joints of the fingers in maximal flexion (see page 1529).
2. Elevate the hand for several days, and encourage active range of motion during this time. Subsequently, as the swelling subsides by 7–10 days, the clam shell plaster may be removed, and buddy-taping may be applied.

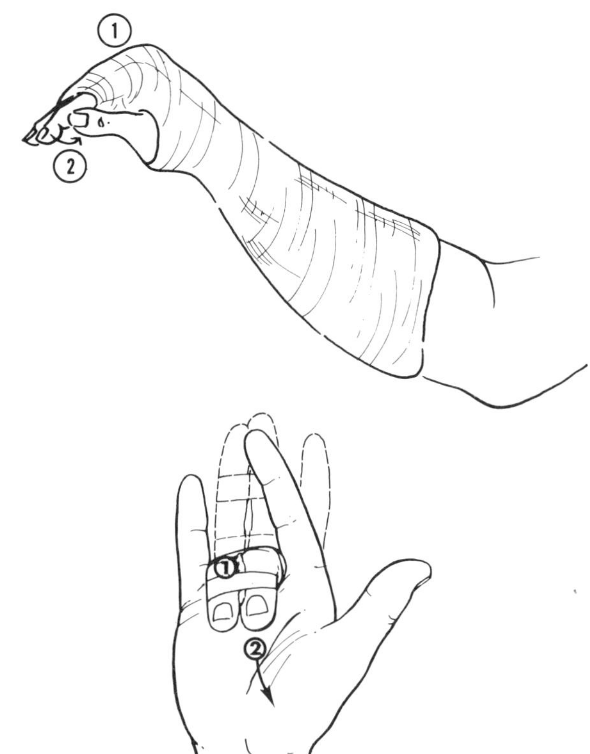

Buddy-Taping Immobilization

1. Tape the injured finger to the adjacent, uninjured one with a small amount of cast padding applied between the fingers.
2. Ensure correct rotational alignment by directing the finger tips toward the scaphoid tuberosity.

Subsequent Management

Allow the patient to exercise the taped fingers actively.

The taping may be removed by 10–14 days, and active exercises should be continued.

Avoid prolonging immobilization beyond 3 weeks because this adds significantly to the likelihood of impaired finger function.

Displaced Fractures of the Proximal Phalanx

REMARKS

Displaced fractures of the proximal phalanx are among the most deceptive and difficult to treat phalangeal fractures.

They are deceptive because the usual anteroposterior and oblique x-rays in this area are obscured by the overlap of the adjacent fingers. Consequently, the fracture may appear undisplaced on superficial review of the x-ray, but on the true lateral x-ray, the typical volar angulation may be evident.

Fractures of the proximal phalanx should be carefully evaluated by x-ray, including a lateral view focused on the finger itself and not on all the fingers.

Closed manipulation is possible, and the fracture may be stable if the MP joint is held in maximal flexion.

The unstable fracture of this area occasionally requires stabilization either with intramedullary Kirschner wire or small fragment screws. Internal fixation can be difficult and is best reserved for fixation of unstable fractures or fractures in multiple fingers. It is best carried out by individuals skilled in the technique.

For the most part, the safest method of handling these fractures is by closed technique with early finger mobilization and functional casting.

Prereduction X-Rays

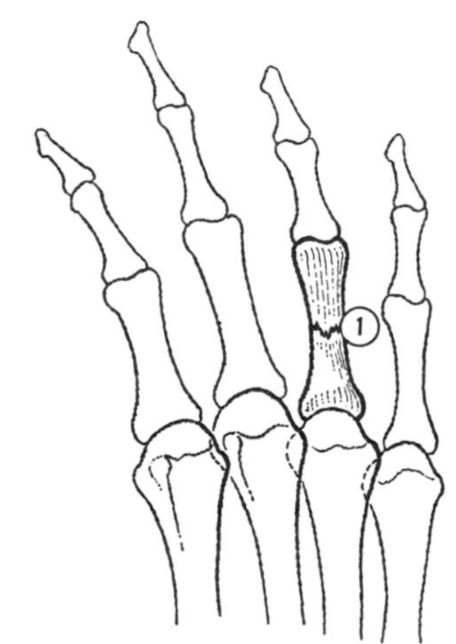

1. Initial x-ray taken in the anteroposterior view appears to show an undisplaced fracture of the proximal phalanx.

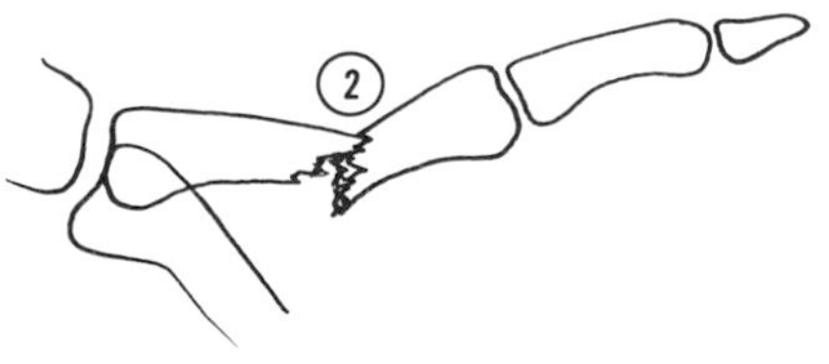

2. True lateral view is essential to demonstrate the extent of volar angulation, which should be corrected.

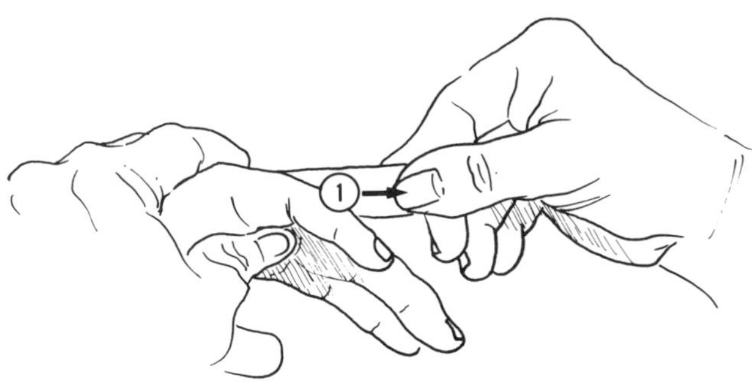

Manipulative Reduction

1. Under adequate local or intravenous anesthesia, the angulated proximal phalanx is reduced by longitudinal traction.

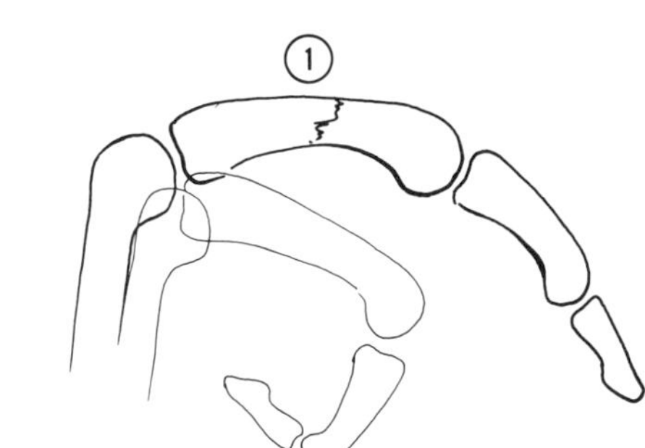

2. Alignment is achieved by maintaining traction with the metacarpal joint in maximal flexion.

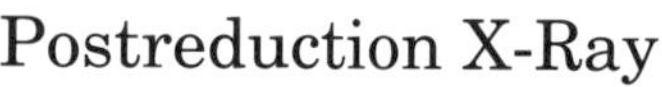

Postreduction X-Ray

1. True lateral x-ray should be obtained. The lateral x-ray can be difficult to visualize unless the adjacent fingers are held away from the injured finger. Slight bayonet apposition can be accepted provided early flexion of the IP joint is allowed to achieve satisfactory motion of the adjacent joints and tendons.

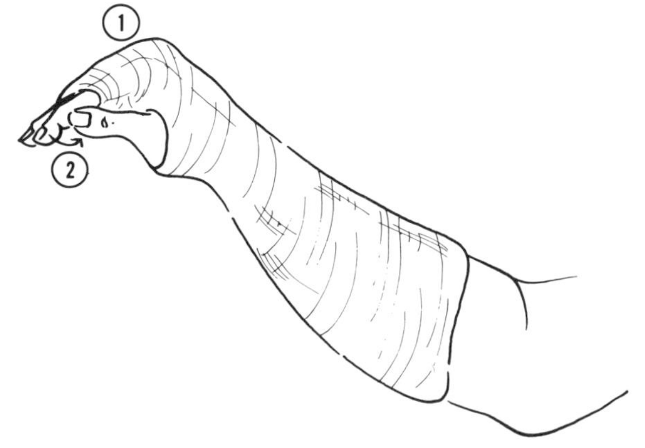

Subsequent Immobilization

1. Clam shell plaster cast is applied, which maintains the desired position of maximal MP flexion (see page 1529).
2. This also allows active interphalangeal joint flexion, which produces a compression effect on the fracture of the proximal phalanx.

Subsequent Management

The clam shell plaster cast is continued for 3 weeks.

During this time, x-rays are repeated on the fifth and tenth day to ensure that alignment has been maintained.

Active exercise is strongly encouraged to use flexion of the IP joints to maintain tendon motion and aid in aligning the fractured phalanx.

Alternative Method of Fixation for Unstable Phalangeal Fractures: Intramedullary Kirschner Wire Fixation

If the phalangeal fracture remains unstable or displaces after initial reduction, stabilization can be accomplished by several methods.

Technique of Manipulation and Kirschner Wire Fixation

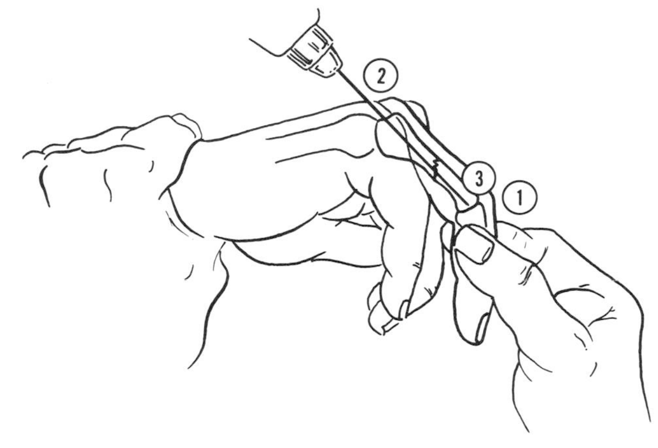

1. Fracture is reduced under adequate anesthesia by longitudinal traction with the MP joint flexed.
2. Reduction is assessed under x-ray fluoroscopic control and stabilized with a Kirschner wire.
3. This is introduced into the proximal phalanx at the MP joint under fluoroscopic control and is driven down to the subchondral bone in the neck.

Alternative Method: Stabilization With Percutaneous Kirschner Wires

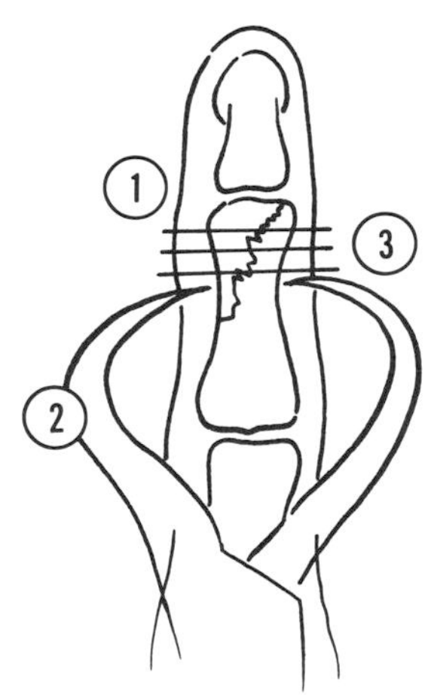

1. Fracture is reduced under fluoroscopic control using longitudinal traction with the MP joint flexed.
2. Reduction is held with clamps or reduction forceps.
3. Fixation is then achieved with Kirschner wires passed percutaneously across the fracture site. These are cut outside the skin, and the fractured hand is then immobilized in the previously described clam shell plaster cast.

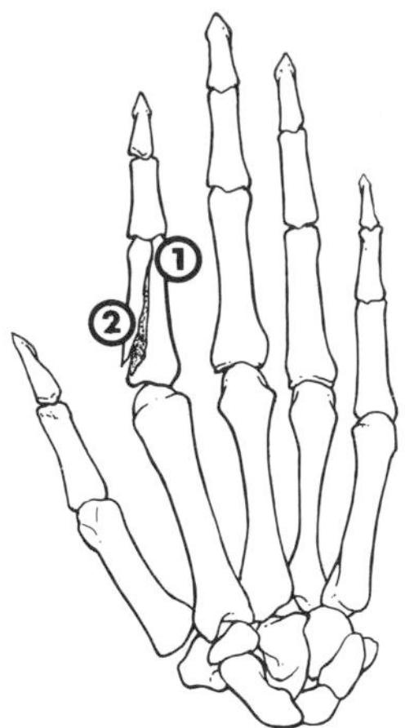

Alternative Method for Oblique Fractures of the Proximal Phalanx

1. Fracture may extend to involve most of the length of the proximal phalanx.
2. Oblique fracture tends to shorten and displace, thereby impeding tendon motion and gliding. This may occasionally require stabilization.

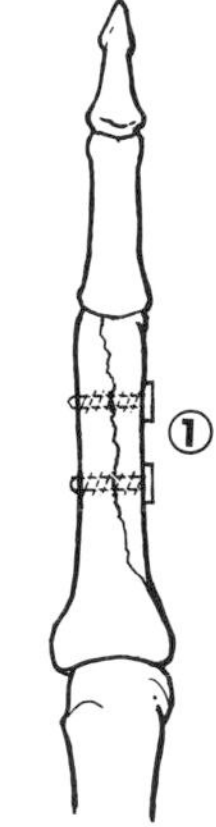

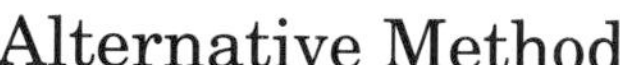

Alternative Method

1. Spiral oblique fracture may also be stabilized with small fragment screws. These may be preferable, particularly for the open fracture, and should be inserted to encourage early range-of-motion exercises.

Postoperative Management

The hand is elevated until the swelling subsides, and by 2–3 days, active exercise is encouraged.

A clam shell plaster cast is continued for support for 2–3 weeks.

The Kirschner wires are generally removed as an office procedure by 3 weeks to encourage range-of-motion exercises further.

Condylar Fractures of the Distal End of the Proximal Phalanx

REMARKS

Condylar fractures of the distal end of the proximal phalanx are fairly common problems that present and can cause significant difficulty and stiffening of the PIP joint.

The condylar fragments are best reduced anatomically and fixed percutaneously if at all possible.

An alternative method would be open reduction and screw fixation if the fracture cannot be reduced by closed manipulation.

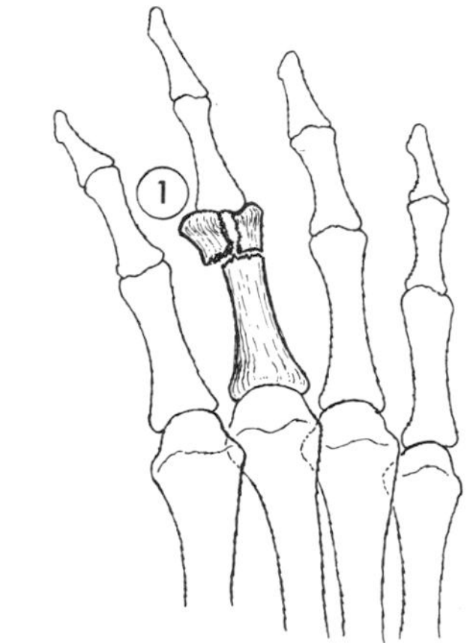

Prereduction X-Ray

1. T-shaped fracture of the end of the proximal phalanx of the third finger.

Technique of Manipulation and Percutaneous Screw Fixation

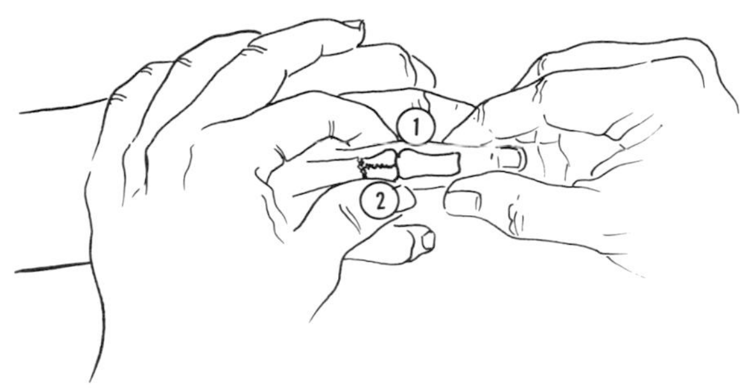

1. Under adequate anesthesia, the fracture can be reduced by longitudinal traction with the finger in extension.
2. Displaced condyle is palpated and molded back to articulate with the remaining portion of the phalanx.

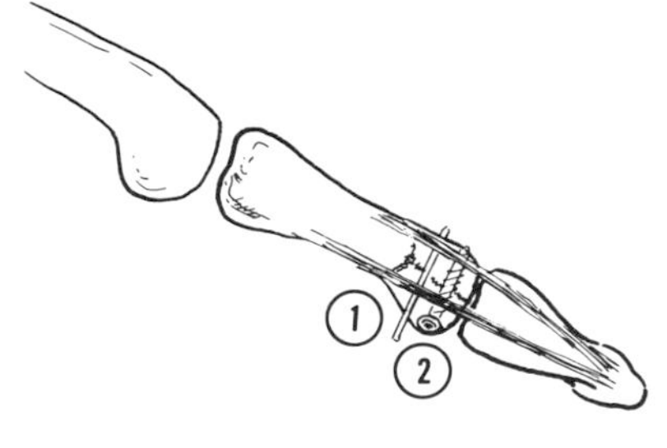

1. When adequate reduction is achieved, percutaneous fixation is carried out using a Kirschner wire.
2. A second Kirschner wire or percutaneous screw is inserted to aid in further alignment of the fracture.

Note: This technique may also be used for T-shaped condylar fractures, although occasionally, small fragment plates are needed.

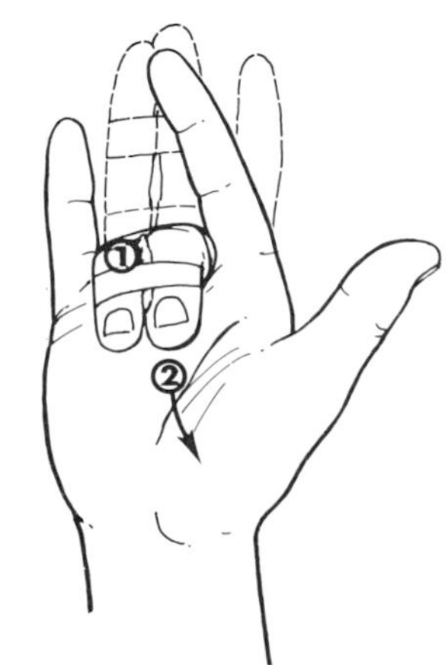

Immobilization

After swelling has subsided, use external support by means of buddy-taping or a plaster cast-splint.

1. Injured finger is taped to the adjacent, uninjured finger, and cast padding is applied between the fingers.
2. Finger tips are aligned to point toward the scaphoid tuberosity.

Impacted Fractures of the Proximal Phalanx in Children and Adults

REMARKS

Fractures of the base of the phalanx occur most often in children and are epiphyseal injuries that should be reduced.

A similar fracture can occur at the base of the phalanx in adults and can cause significant volar angulation. This volar angulation may be difficult to estimate unless a true lateral x-ray is obtained.

Reduction of these injuries can usually be accomplished by closed manipulation and stabilized by clam shell plaster cast immobilization.

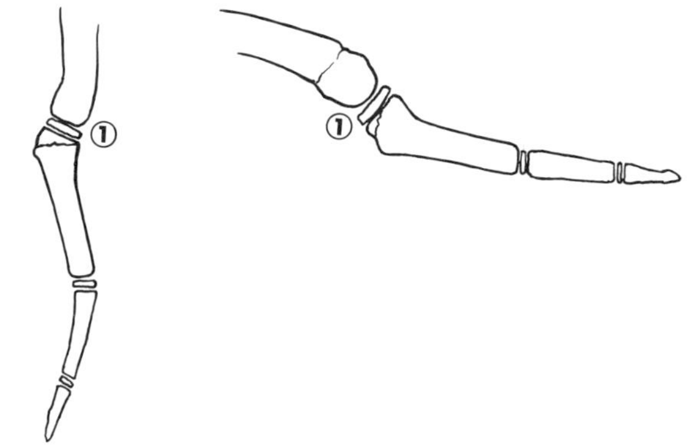

1. Impacted proximal epiphyseal fracture causes rotational malalignment of the finger.

Proximal Phalangeal Fracture

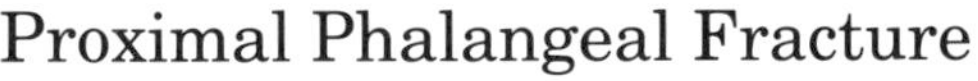

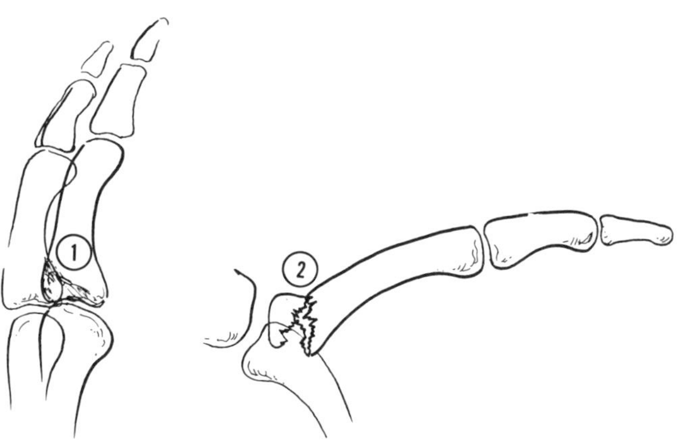

1. Proximal phalangeal fracture in the adult may look undisplaced in the routine anterior posterior oblique view of the finger.
2. Careful assessment is necessary with a true lateral view to determine that there is usually significant volar angulation that requires reduction.

Technique of Reduction

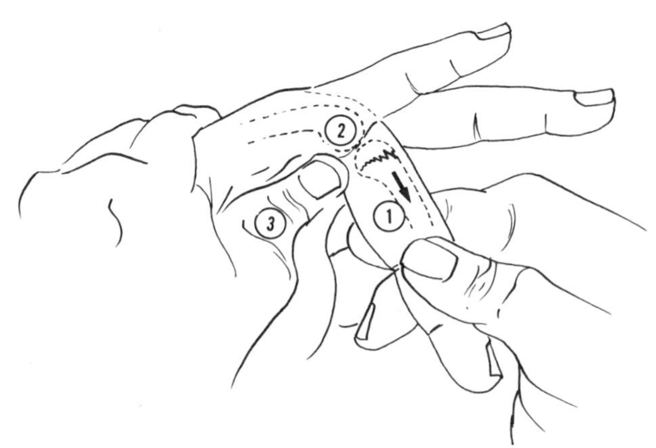

1. Reduction is achieved by applying longitudinal traction.
2. MP joint is maintained in flexion while traction is applied.
3. Pressure is applied to the volar angulation to correct the alignment.

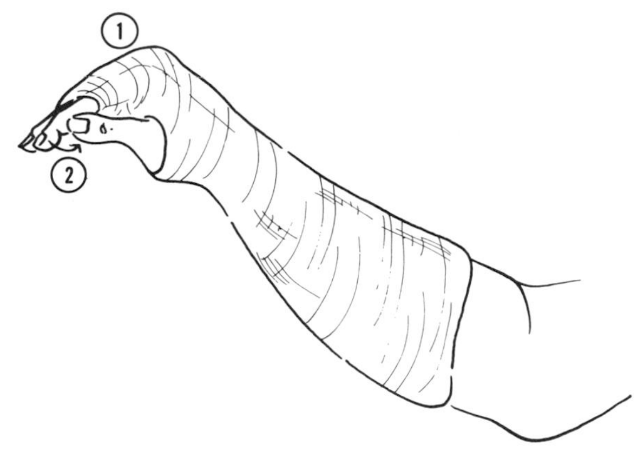

Immobilization

1. Immobilization is carried out with the clam shell plaster cast or gutter splint technique, as previously described (see page 1529).
2. Active flexion of the fingers encourages a tension band effect, maintaining the reduction of the proximal phalangeal fracture.

Subsequent Management

The patient is encouraged to exercise the fingers actively in the clam shell plaster cast as the swelling subsides.

The splint immobilization can be discarded by 2–3 weeks because these fractures are usually stable.

When the clam shell cast is removed, active extension of the MP joint is usually regained within a few weeks.

Fractures of the Shaft of the Middle Phalanx

REMARKS

Transverse fractures of the middle phalanx are displaced in the direction of the pull of the flexor digitorum sublimis.

Angulation of the fracture may be in either a volar or a dorsal direction, depending on whether the fracture is proximal or distal to the insertion of this muscle.

In either instance, the fracture can be reduced by flexing the MP joint of the finger to a maximal degree, thereby relaxing the pull of the flexor digitorum sublimis and tightening the extensor hood.

Oblique, longitudinal fractures of the middle phalanx may cause difficulty by shortening and impinging on tendinous structures. These fractures are frequently best stabilized with percutaneous Kirschner wires.

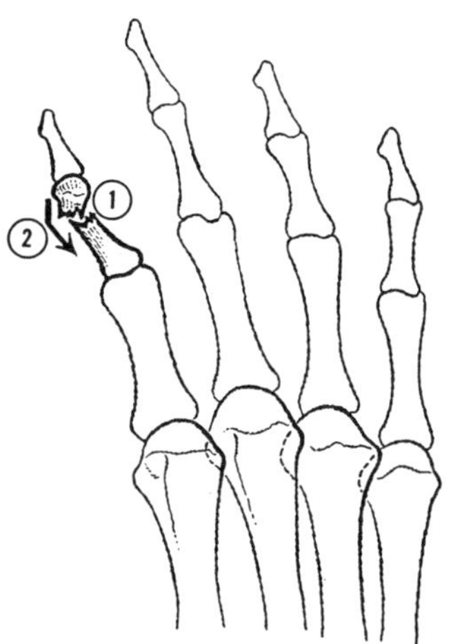

Prereduction X-Ray

VOLAR ANGULATION

1. Fracture of the middle phalanx distal to the insertion of the flexor digitorum sublimis.
2. Volar angulation results from pull of this muscle on the proximal fragment.

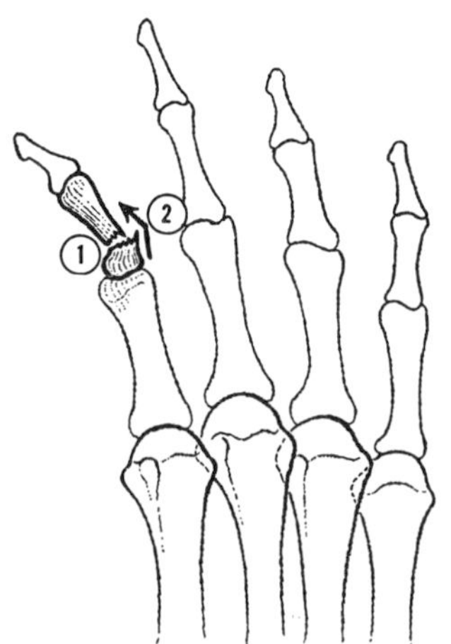

DORSAL ANGULATION

1. Fracture of the middle phalanx proximal to the flexor digitorum sublimis insertion.
2. Dorsal angulation results from pull of this muscle on the distal fragment.

Reduction and Immobilization

1. Both of these fractures may be reduced by immobilizing the fingers in the intrinsic-plus position with the clam shell plaster cast technique.
2. Patient is encouraged to flex the fingers actively in the clam shell cast after the swelling subsides. This encourages impaction of the fracture and also normal gliding of the tendon and joint structures.

Postreduction X-Ray

1. Fracture distal to the flexor digitorum sublimis insertion has been reduced by relaxing the tendon pull on the proximal fragment.

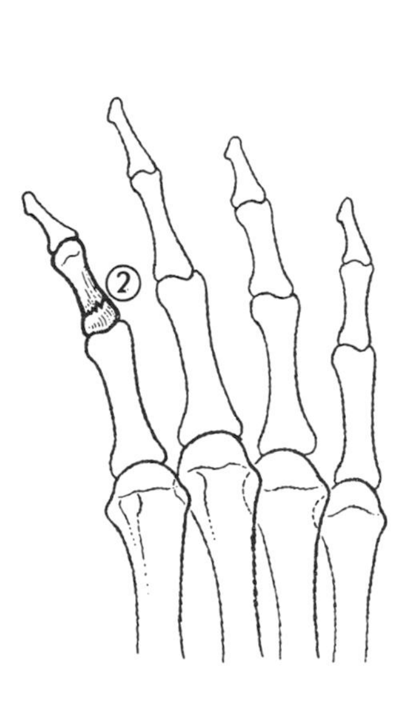

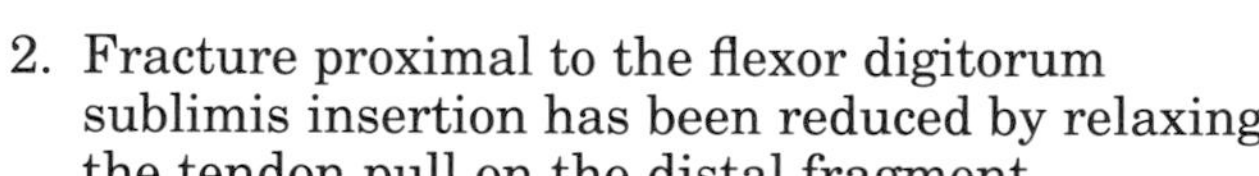

2. Fracture proximal to the flexor digitorum sublimis insertion has been reduced by relaxing the tendon pull on the distal fragment.

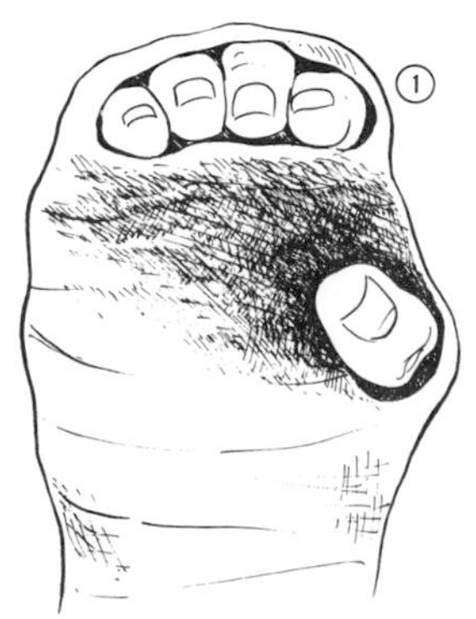

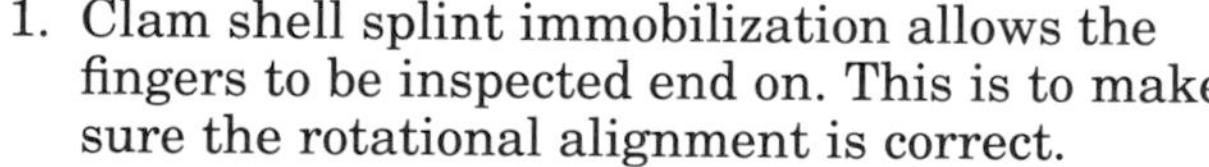

1. Clam shell splint immobilization allows the fingers to be inspected end on. This is to make sure the rotational alignment is correct.

Note: Clam shell splint immobilization for the unstable fracture is usually only necessary for 2–3 weeks. After this time, the splint may be removed, and active exercise is encouraged.

Oblique Fractures of the Middle Phalanx

REMARKS

Oblique fractures of the middle phalanx may sometimes be best reduced and held with percutaneous Kirschner wire fixation to allow early restoration of function.

This is particularly true if the fracture is displaced and shortened and likely to cause impingement on the intrinsic or extrinsic tendons.

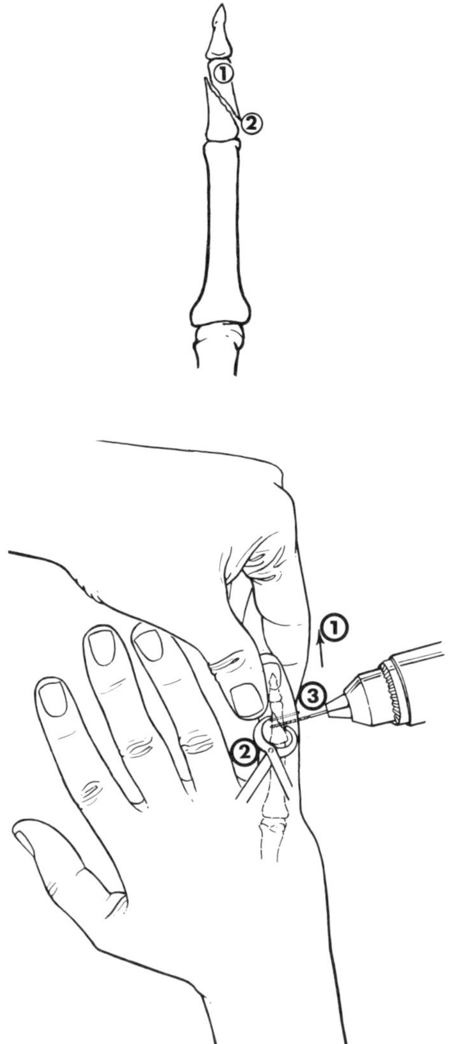

Appearance on X-Ray

1. Oblique fracture of the middle phalanx has shortened and angulated.
2. Unreduced fracture prominence will impale intrinsic and extrinsic tendons.

Technique of Closed Reduction and Percutaneous Kirschner Wire Fixation (Under Local Anesthesia)

1. Traction is maintained by an assistant to keep the fracture reduced.
2. Padded clamp is used to compress the spiral fracture fragments together.
3. Two fine Kirschner wires are drilled percutaneously through the fracture fragments and are bent outside of the skin.

Note: Subsequent management is the same as that described for fractures of the proximal phalanx with clam shell plaster or other splints.

Postreduction Management

The fractured finger or fingers are further stabilized with clam shell plaster splinting for 2–3 weeks.

The Kirschner wires are removed by 3 weeks, and the patient is encouraged to work vigorously at restoring full flexion and extension.

Fracture of the Distal Phalanx

REMARKS

Comminution of the distal phalanx occurs frequently if the finger tip is crushed or caught in a door. Usually, there is minimal or no displacement of the fragments.

In children and adolescents, the distal phalangeal epiphysis becomes separated and requires reduction.

The nail over the injury should be left in place if at all possible because it serves as an effective splint for the displaced epiphysis.

Occasionally, fractures of the distal phalanx will be so displaced that internal fixation with a Kirschner wire or Riordan pin may be necessary.

Frequently, the tip of the finger is amputated, and the fractured bone is exposed. The most effective method of management for most of these tip amputations is simple continuous cast protection. Local skin grafting or flaps are usually not necessary, particularly in children.

Appearance on X-Ray

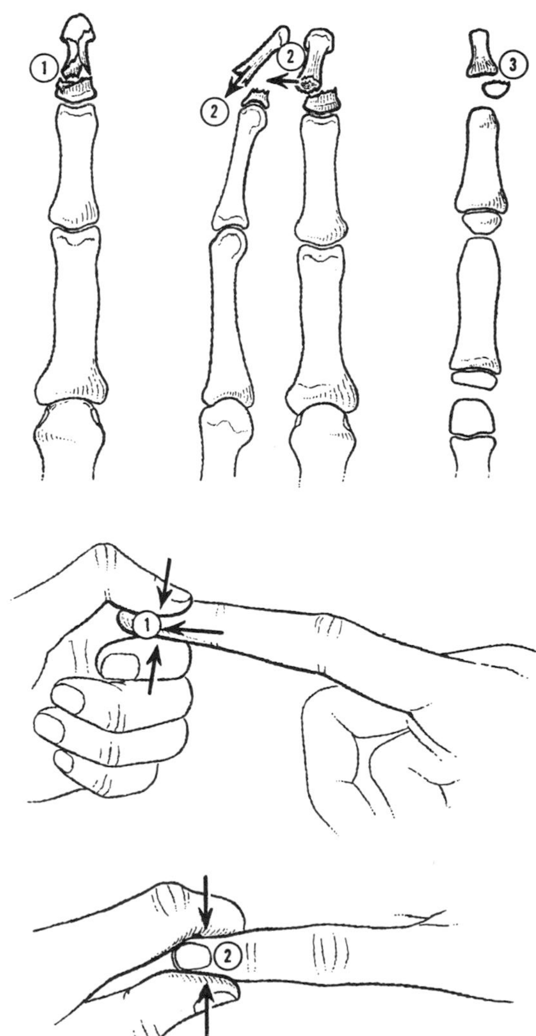

1. Severe comminution of the distal phalanx with minimal displacement of fragments.

Note: This fracture requires no reduction.

2. Fracture of the terminal phalanx with upward, backward, and lateral displacement of the distal fragment.

Note: This fracture should be reduced.

3. Epiphyseal separation of the terminal phalanx of the index finger.

Note: This epiphyseal fracture should be reduced. The nail bed serves as an effective splint after the fracture is reduced.

Manipulative Reduction

1. Apply traction, and mold the fragments by squeezing the end of the finger between your thumb and index finger.

2. Correct the lateral displacement by compressing the lateral borders of the terminal phalanx between your index finger and thumb.

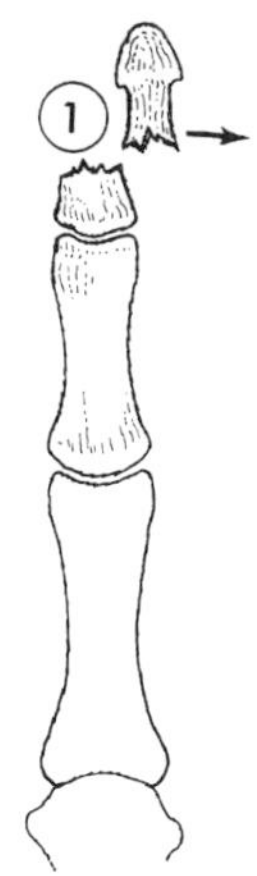

Prereduction X-Rays

1. Fracture of the shaft with lateral displacement of the distal fragment.

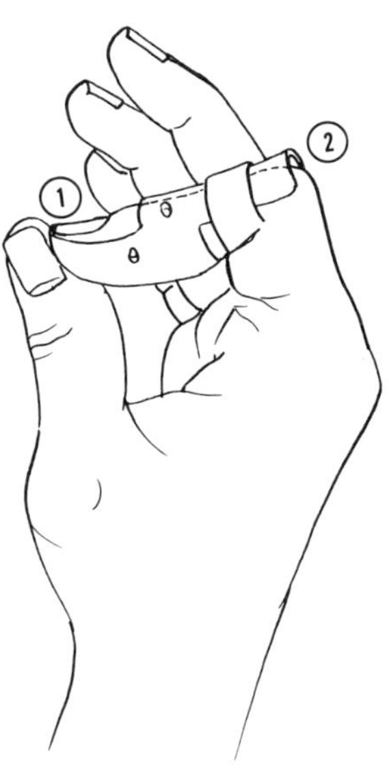

Immobilization

Apply a protective finger splint to support the soft tissue and skeletal injury.

1. MP joint should be free.
2. PIP joint should also be free for most stable fractures of the distal phalanx.

Note: A Stax splint (Richards Co., Memphis, TN) or other similar type of commercially available splint serves the purpose of immobilizing the phalangeal fractures effectively.

Subsequent Management

The splint is usually continued for 2–3 weeks until the symptoms of pain and swelling subside.

If the patient wishes to engage in heavy mechanical work, it is best to protect the finger for an additional 2–3 weeks and treat the problem symptomatically thereafter.

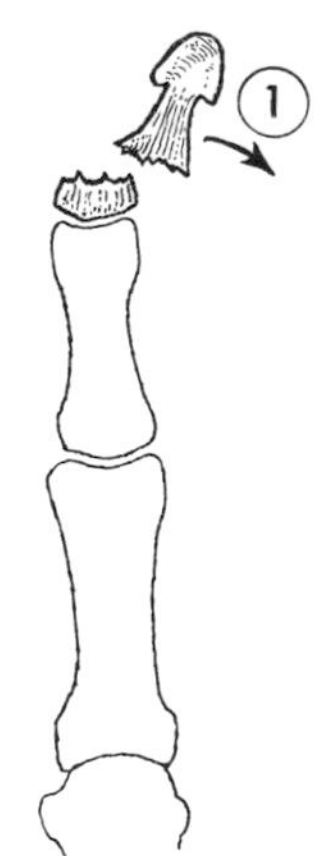

Unstable Fracture of the Shaft of the Distal Phalanx With Lateral Displacement of the Fragment

Prereduction X-Ray

1. Fracture through the base of the phalanx with lateral deviation of the distal fragment.

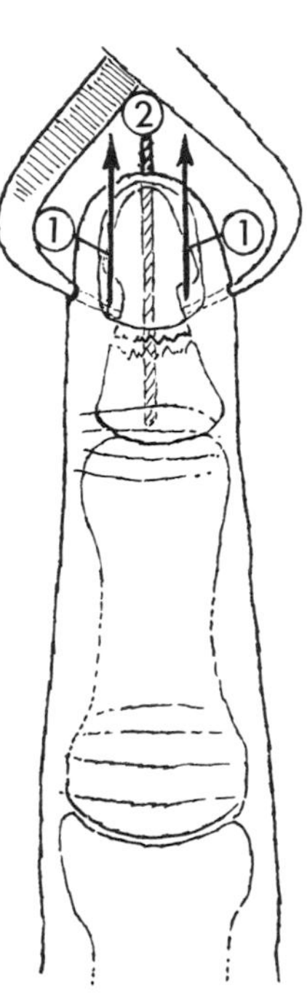

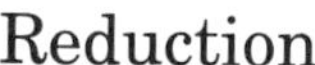

Reduction

1. Grasp the distal fragment with a towel clip, and apply straight traction. This realigns the fragments.
2. Pass a threaded wire through the distal end of the finger into the proximal fragment.

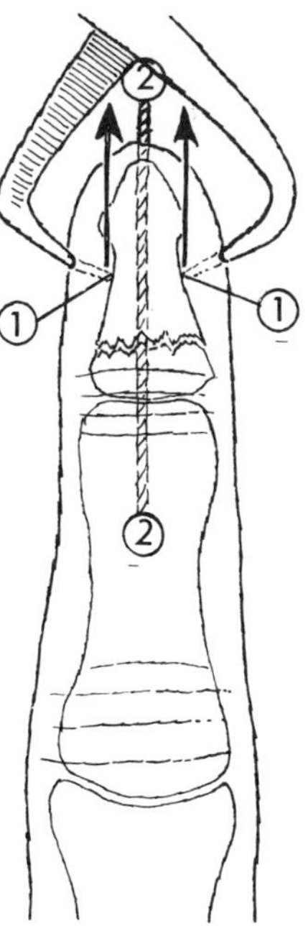

Alternative Method for Fractures Near the Joint

REDUCTION

1. Grasp the distal fragment with a towel clip and make straight traction.
2. Pass a threaded wire through both fragments, across the distal joint, and into the middle phalanx.

Subsequent Management

The pin is continued for 4–6 weeks, depending on the amount of instability.

Frequently, these fractures are associated with avulsion of the tendons and, therefore, should be treated as described for mallet finger deformity, which requires immobilization for at least 6 weeks.

If the tendon is intact, the fracture usually heals by 3 weeks, and the Kirschner wire and immobilization may be discontinued.

OPEN HAND FRACTURES AND DISLOCATIONS

REMARKS

The most common open hand fracture is an amputation of the finger tip through the distal phalanx. These most often are produced by crushing injuries when the finger tip is caught in a closing car door. The typical patient is a young child.

The most treacherous open hand injury is a human bite sustained in a brawl during which the knuckle, usually the MP joint, strikes the opponent's tooth. This wound is always severely contaminated, despite its frequently benign appearance. Severe infections, resulting in digit or even hand amputations, have been reported from this type of open hand fracture-dislocation.

Open fractures and dislocations may also result from crushing injuries or high-velocity gunshot wounds to the hand. These require carefully planned management to provide the best chance for maximal restoration and function.

Finger Tip Amputation

REMARKS

Finger tip amputation is seen commonly in the emergency room, particularly in young children; however, adults may also sustain these open fractures as a result of crushing injury to the finger tip.

Treatment should consist of thorough cleansing and debridement of the wound, including any protruding bone fragments.

In general, grafts or local flaps are not indicated, particularly in children. Such attempts at acute closure of the wound can produce a poor eschar and sometimes a painful finger tip.

The most effective method for most of these finger tip amputations, particularly in young individuals, is simple cast immobilization for 3 weeks.

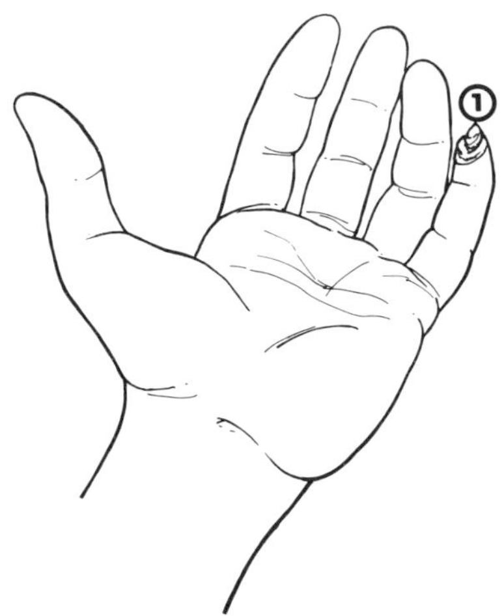

1. Typical amputation of the finger tip with exposed, fractured bone in a young patient.

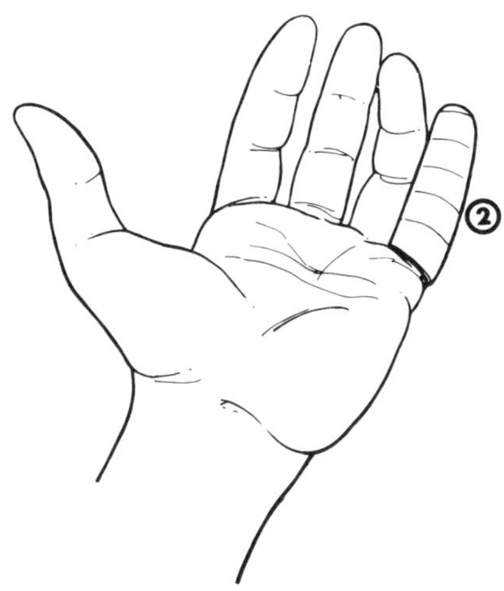

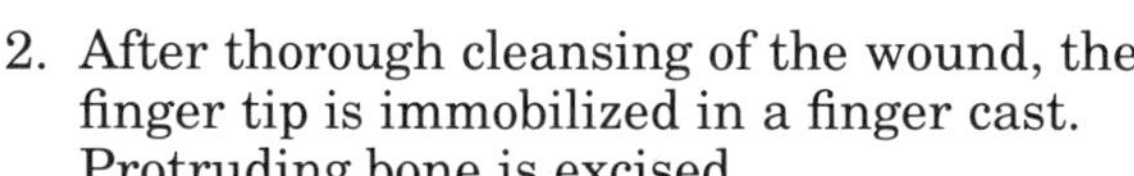

2. After thorough cleansing of the wound, the finger tip is immobilized in a finger cast. Protruding bone is excised.

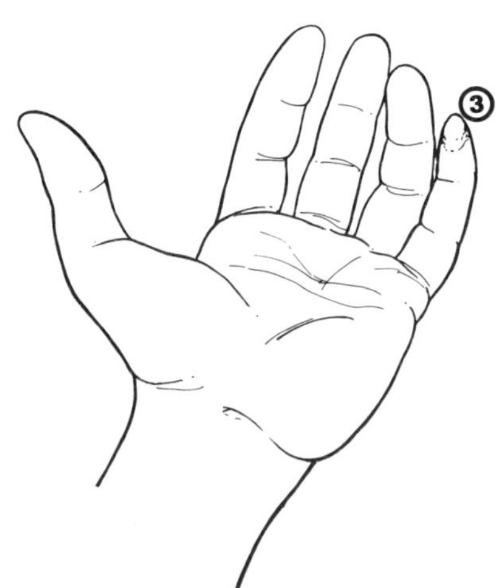

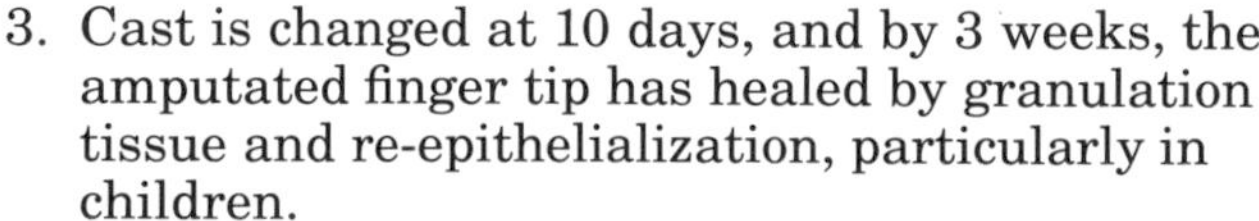

3. Cast is changed at 10 days, and by 3 weeks, the amputated finger tip has healed by granulation tissue and re-epithelialization, particularly in children.

Note: This continuous cast immobilization provides an occlusive dressing that allows natural wound intussusception to shrink the scar down to minimal size. Skin grafting may be necessary in adults if the wound has not healed at 10 days.

Open Injuries From Human Bites to the Hand

REMARKS

The typical presentation for human bites to the hand is a transverse laceration over the dorsal surface of the MP joint. The typical mechanism is impaction of the knuckle against an opponent's tooth.

The patient initially may not remember how the injury was sustained or deny it was the result of a fight. However, any laceration of this type over the knuckles should be suspected of human bite origin and is a potential source of infection.

The penetration of the tooth into the joint can introduce a wide variety of bacterial pathogens in this area.

Frequently, the patient ignores the injury initially and may not present to the physician for several days when infection is obvious.

An alternative problem is that the patient denies the origin of the injury and the superficial laceration may be sutured closed in the emergency room or physician's office with subsequent infection from anaerobic organisms.

The diagnosis is suspected with any laceration or avulsion injury of the finger in the individual after a fight.

X-rays are usually not helpful, although occasionally, a chip fracture or broken tooth fragment may be evident in the soft tissues about the joint.

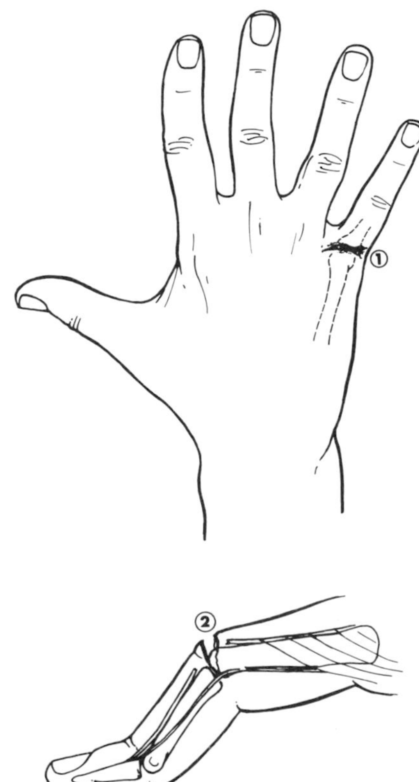

1. Open wound over the MP of the knuckle is frequently caused by a human bite. This may appear relatively benign but is usually extremely contaminated and will become infected if closed primarily.

2. Occasionally, the laceration involves the PIP joint or is an avulsion-type injury as a result of somebody purposely biting the finger in a fight.

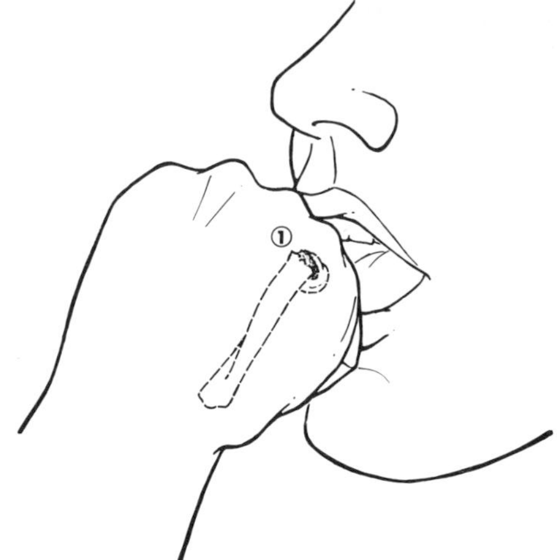

1. Suspect that any laceration over the knuckle may be the result of a human bite, even if this is initially denied by the patient. These can cause severe infections and even amputations of the digit or hand if the infection spreads throughout the compartments of the hand.

Management

The laceration from a human bite demands wound debridement and opening rather than closure.

Avoid suturing any wound that is suspected of having a human bite origin. Rather, perform a thorough irrigation and debridement down into the depths of the laceration to be sure that all bacterial contamination has been removed as far as possible.

In addition, a culture should be taken from the depths of the wound, and appropriate antibiotics should be started and adjusted according to the type of bacteria growing in the wound.

The patient should be cautioned that this is an extremely contaminated wound and that high-dose antibiotics are generally needed if there is any evidence of infection.

Aggressive early debridement and antibiotic treatment of these injuries can prevent serious complications as a result of this notorious type of injury to the hand.

Open Contaminated Wounds of the Hand

Open contaminated wounds of the hand can result from high-velocity gunshot wounds such as those sustained in Vietnam or in civilian combat casualties or they can be produced by crushing injury sustained at work when the hand is caught in machinery.

These generally cause severe compromise of soft tissue and bony structures and require carefully planned and staged treatment.

The method worked out by Burkhalter and coworkers from their experience in Vietnam is still helpful in managing these problems by a staged approach.

Management by Delayed Primary Closure (After Burkhalter and Coworkers)

REMARKS

Open hand wounds are usually contaminated from several sources, either at the time of gunshot injury or when sustained at work.

A high-velocity missile causes considerable debris to be sucked into the depths of the wound.

The injury at work is usually sustained in a greasy, dirty environment, and frequently, oil, grease, or other substances are driven into the wound.

Severe injuries such as these should be treated as initially infected when first seen in the emergency room. A compression dressing should be applied, and the wound should not be explored until the patient is in the operating room.

X-rays are obtained while the patient is awaiting surgery and the hand is elevated.

Intravenous fluid, containing high-dose penicillin or other appropriate antibiotics, are given, and tetanus toxoid is also administered.

Surgical debridement is then carried out after careful skin preparation. All foreign bodies and necrotic tissue should be removed.

In addition to initial debridement, Burkhalter and coworkers emphasize removal of necrotic tissue and foreign bodies. Additional procedures are then carried out at 5–7 days to achieve delayed primary closure if the wound permits.

1. Typical injury is a high-velocity missile wound to the hand that is sustained in war or, frequently, in "civilian combat."

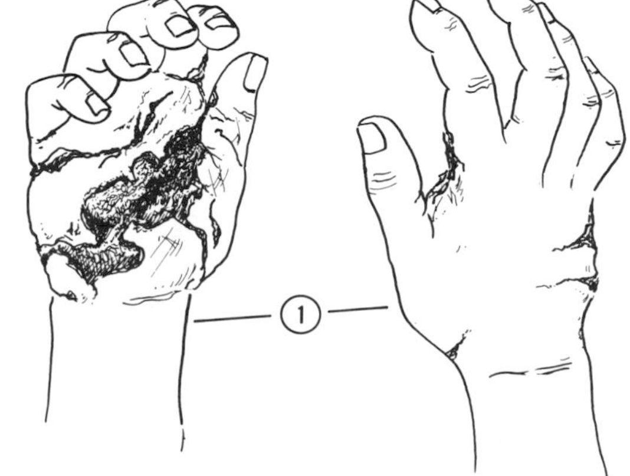

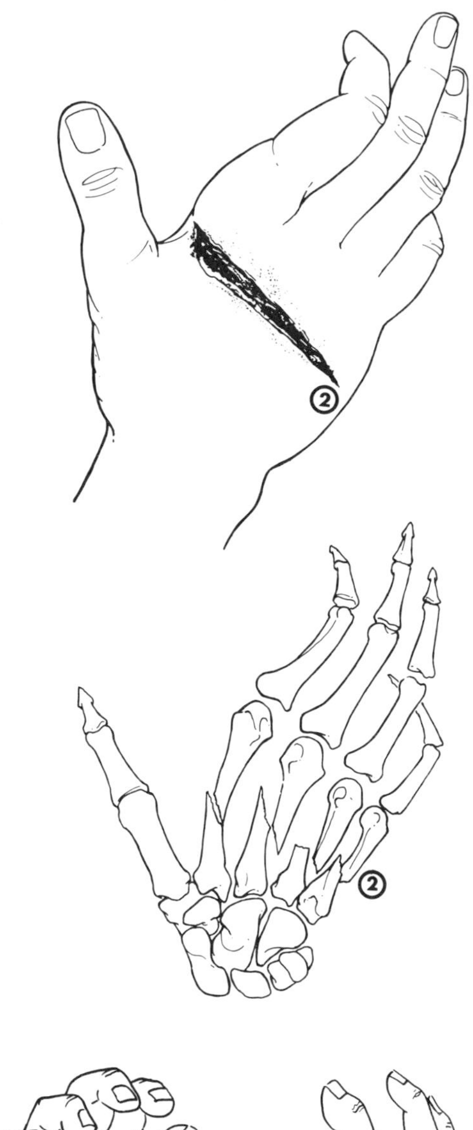

2. Crush injury to the hand can produce soft tissue damage on the dorsal surface. This usually results in multiple metacarpal fractures or phalangeal fractures and injuries to the tendons and soft tissue structures.

Initial Debridement

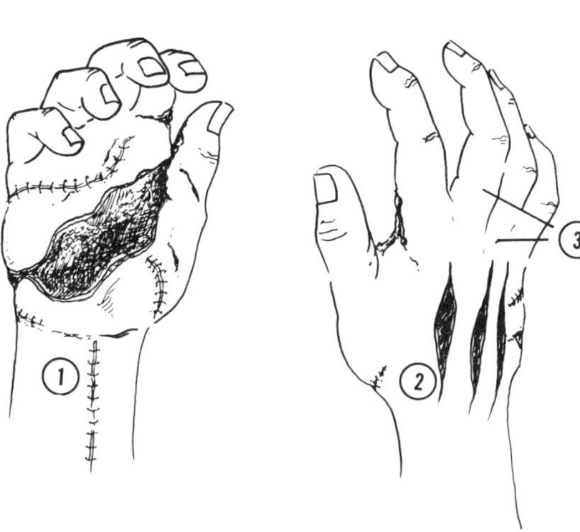

1. When the injury is severe and associated with carpal fractures, the volar carpal ligament is opened to decompress the median nerve. The wounds are debrided but not closed primarily.
2. For massive swelling, a fasciotomy of the intermetacarpal compartments is performed. These are best carried out through dorsal incisions longitudinally.
3. All structures such as tendons and nerves that are thought in the preoperative examination to be nonfunctional are examined, and their injuries are noted in the operative record for secondary repair.

Postdebridement Management

After debridement, the tourniquet is released, and any bleeding vessels are ligated.

A bulky hand dressing (boxing glove type) is applied with the hand in the position of function. The splinted hand is elevated for several days to diminish swelling.

Antibiotics are continued and modified, depending on the cultures obtained during debridement.

Immobilization of the Swollen Hand by Compressive Dressing

It is important to eliminate swelling and edema from the injured hand as quickly as possible before and after treatment.

This can be best accomplished by using a compressive dressing and elevating the hand.

1. Wrist is slightly extended, and the MP and IP joints are immobilized in the intrinsic-plus position.
2. Thumb is in apposition with the fingers.
3. Soft tissue fluffs are applied liberally in the palm between the fingers.
4. Rolled gauze is wrapped around the soft tissue from the elbow to the finger tips.
5. Light plaster is applied with the rolled gauze.

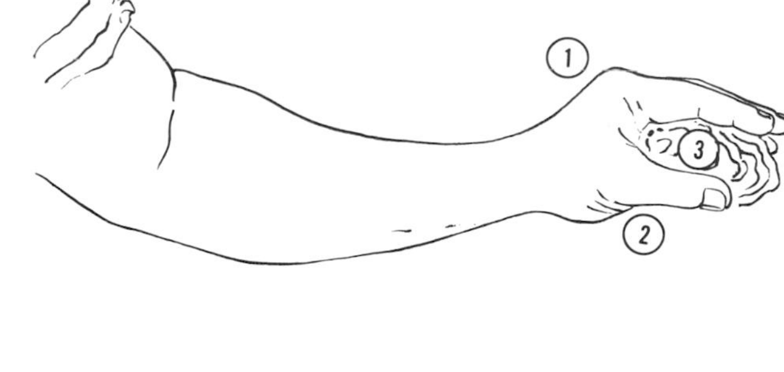

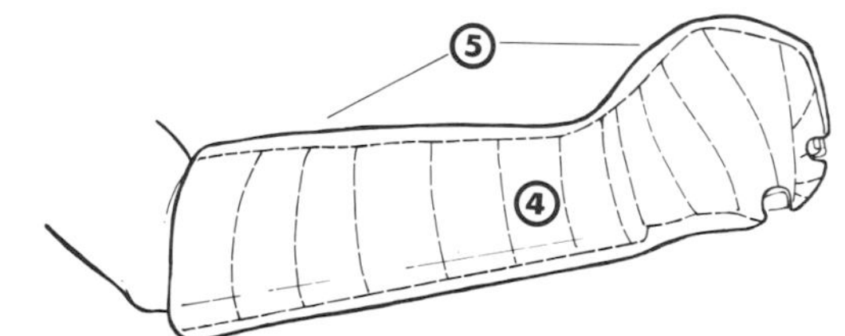

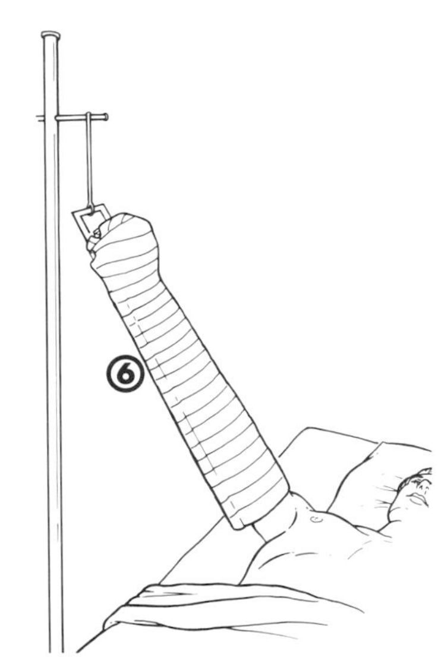

6. Limb is elevated above the level of the heart on an armrest.

Subsequent Management

When the swelling subsides, the second stage of the operative treatment is carried out, usually by 5–7 days.

Secondary debridement of the original marginal tissue is done as necessary to remove all devitalized tissue.

Secondary closure of the wound or skin grafting can then usually be performed on a good granulation bed over the injured hand.

A split-thickness skin graft is usually adequate to cover most of these injuries.

Fractures and dislocations can be stabilized at the same time with Kirschner wire techniques.

Closure should be avoided, however, if the wound is frankly infected.

This method of staged wound management has been used in numerous severe hand injuries by Burkhalter and by ourselves. It has been effective in providing a hand that is ready for rehabilitation and any definitive reconstruction procedures within 2 weeks after the wound has been incurred.

INJURIES OF INTERPHALANGEAL JOINTS OF THE FINGERS

"Jammed Fingers" From Sprains, Fractures, Dislocations, or Tendon Avulsions

REMARKS

Dislocations and fracture-dislocations of the IP joints are common injuries that are usually produced by lateral or hyperextension overload of the joint structures.

An injury to the proximal IP joint is particularly treacherous and is often considered a jammed finger; however, such injuries need to be carefully evaluated to avoid permanent and significant limitation of function.

Only careful assessment will detect injuries likely to cause significant impairment of finger function.

Evaluation of the jammed finger should include careful direct palpation for areas of tenderness, adequate x-rays to show small fractures or signs of instability, and active and passive stress testing of joint stability.

Common Mechanisms of Injury

Mechanisms

1. Jammed finger commonly occurs from athletic injuries in which a tip of the finger is struck by a ball or other object.
2. Injury can produce an avulsion fracture of the attachment of the extensor tendon.
3. The result is a chronic mallet finger deformity.

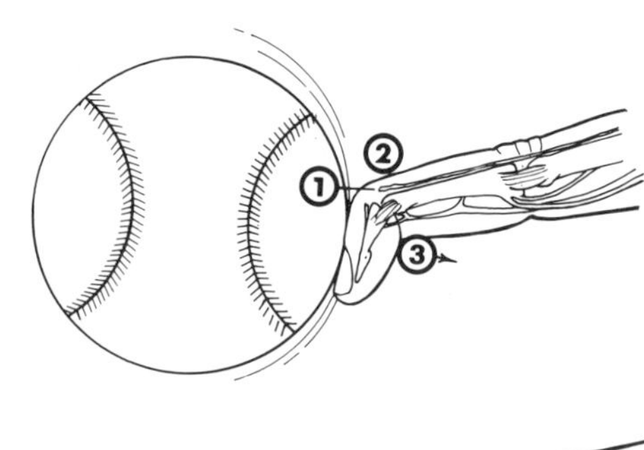

Other Mechanisms Include Avulsion of the Flexor Digitorum Profundus

1. Forceful hyperextension of the ring or long finger occurs while grasping a lunging individual.
2. Resultant loss of active DIP flexion from disruption of the flexor digitorum profundus may not be initially detected.

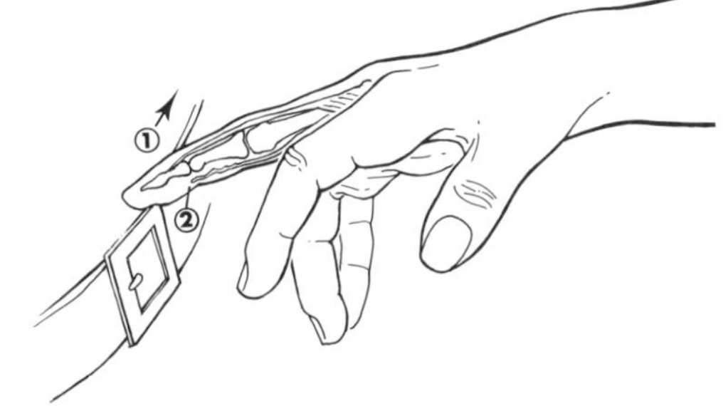

Normal Finger

1. Common extensor tendons form the central slip, which inserts at the base of the middle phalanx and extends the PIP joint.
2. Intrinsic tendons pass beneath the axis of the MP joint as flexors.
3. Lateral bands pass slightly dorsal to the PIP joint to insert on the base of the distal phalanx. They supplement the central slip for extension of the PIP joint and also extend the DIP joint.

Mallet Finger Deformity

1. Rupture of the extensor tendon inserting into the distal phalanx, causing flexion deformity of the DIP joint.
2. Contracture of lateral bands, producing hyperextension of the PIP joint.

Boutonnière Deformity

1. Central slip rupture causes loss of extension of the PIP joint.
2. Gradual displacement of the lateral bands volar to the axis of the PIP joint may occur after several weeks. The result is flexion deformity of the PIP joint and
3. Hyperextension of the DIP joint.

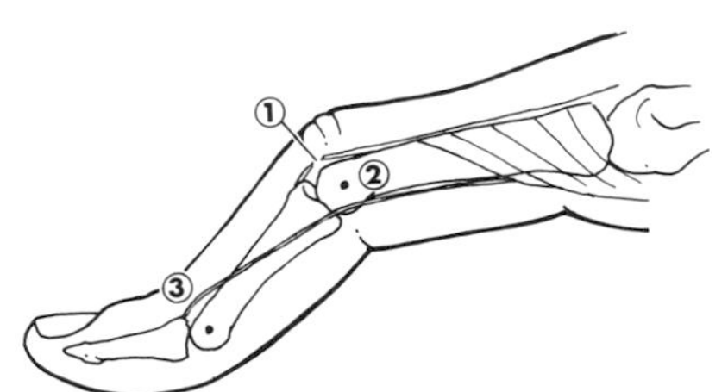

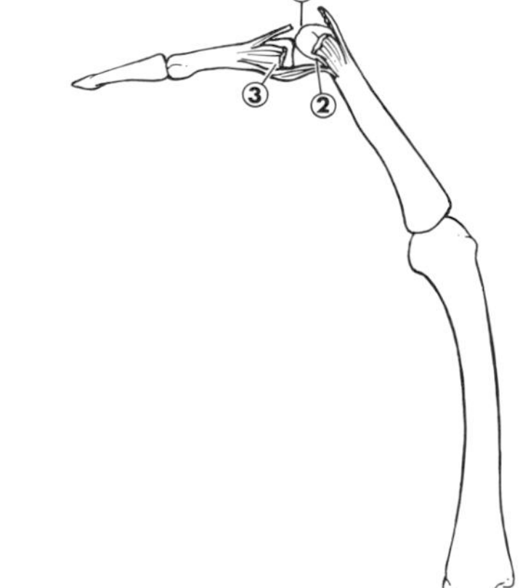

Boutonnière Deformity From Anterior Dislocation of the PIP Joint

1. Anterior displacement of the PIP joint ruptures the central slip and
2. Tears the volar plate.
3. Usually, the collateral ligament is also torn.

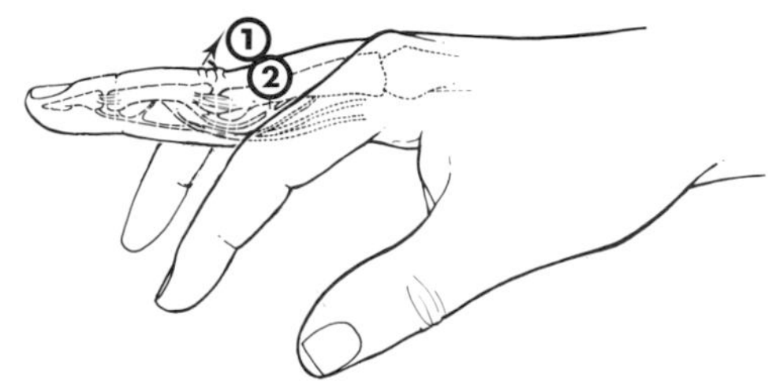

Pseudoboutonnière Deformity

1. Hyperextension injury to the PIP joint disrupts the
2. Proximal attachment of the volar capsule and volar plate to proximal phalanx.

This results gradually in

1. Bone spur formation at the capsular attachment and
2. Fixed flexion contracture of the PIP joint from scarring in the capsule and at least one lateral band.
3. Slight hyperextension of the DIP joint is not as marked or as fixed as a true boutonnière deformity because only one lateral band is usually contracted.

Note: This most often occurs in athletic injuries, particularly football injuries to the little finger.

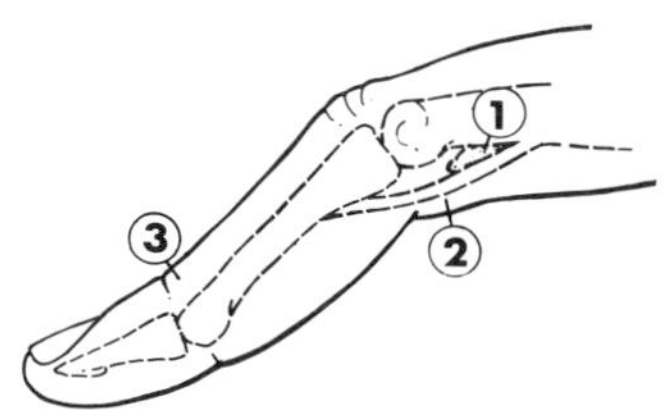

Reverse Boutonnière or Swan-Neck Deformity: Volar Plate Injury With Hyperextension Deformity

Hyperextension of the PIP joint results from

1. Disruption of the volar plate attachment to the middle phalanx or fracture of the middle phalanx.
2. Relaxation of the extensor mechanism permits the unapposed flexor digitorum profundus pull to draw the distal phalanx into slight flexion.

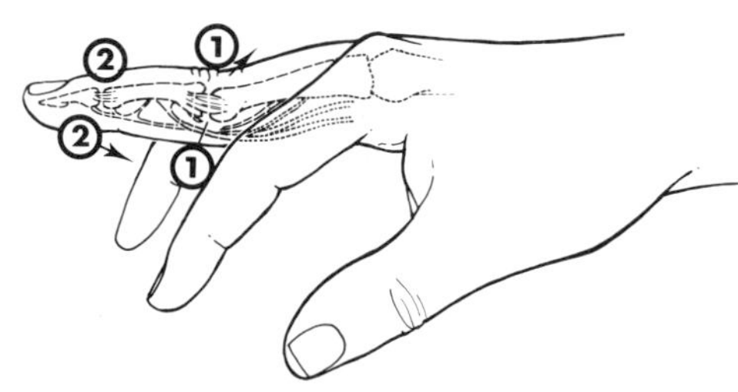

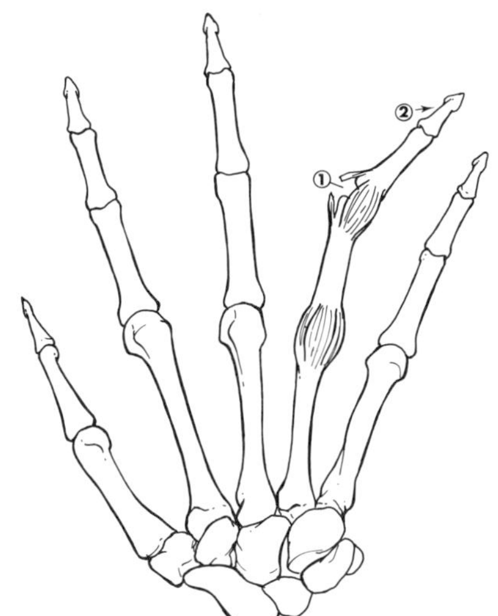

Lateral Instability of the PIP Joint

Most often, this results from acute or chronic disruption of the radial collateral ligament after a lateral dislocation. Always check for collateral instability after reduction of an IP joint dislocation, particularly one that does not reduce with a definite "click."

1. Disruption of the radial collateral ligament from dislocation produces
2. Gross clinical and radiographic instability.

Assessment of the "Jammed Finger"

Evaluate the patient's ability to move the finger actively through a full range. If necessary, use local digital anesthetic to relieve pain.

Should a joint deformity recur with active motions, there is significant instability that requires adequate splinting. If the joint is functionally stable and the patient is able to flex fully and extend without redisplacement, splinting may be minimized.

If redisplacement of the joint occurs in an anterior (palmar) direction, the disrupted dorsal capsule and central slip require splinting in extension to prevent boutonnière deformity. If anterior displacement is associated with a dorsal chip fracture from the midphalanx, operative repair is usually indicated primarily.

If the joint is unstable and displaces dorsally, treatment with an extension block splint is generally indicated. If a fracture involving more than 40 per cent of the joint's surface is causing the dorsal instability, operative stabilization is necessary.

Chronic disruption of the volar capsule from the middle phalanx will produce a swan-neck deformity, which requires treatment by surgical advancement of the volar capsule.

Chronic disruption of the volar capsule from its attachment on the proximal phalanx leads to scarring and a pseudoboutonnière deformity.

The injured or swollen joint should also be stressed in a lateral direction to determine if disruption of the collateral ligament has occurred. Lateral instability of the IP joint can generally be treated by closed splinting methods, provided that the instability is recognized soon after injury.

Early recognition of dorsal, volar, or lateral instability offers enormous advantage because it generally permits closed treatment and satisfactory functional healing. Delay in recognition for longer than 3 weeks usually necessitates open treatment with variable prognosis for functional return.

Be suspicious of any jammed finger. Evaluate it thoroughly by palpation, by active and passive stress testing, and by adequate anteroposterior and lateral x-rays centered on the finger, not the hand.

Physical Examination

Palpation

Palpate the entire swollen finger for the precise areas of tenderness to identify common injuries, such as

1. Collateral ligament injury.
2. Volar plate disruption.
3. Injury to the central slip.
4. Avulsion of extensor tendon insertion on distal phalanx.
5. Avulsion of flexor digitorum profundus tendon. This is tender at the point to which the tendon has retracted, either in the sheath or up in the palm.
6. Fracture or fracture-dislocation of the MP joint.

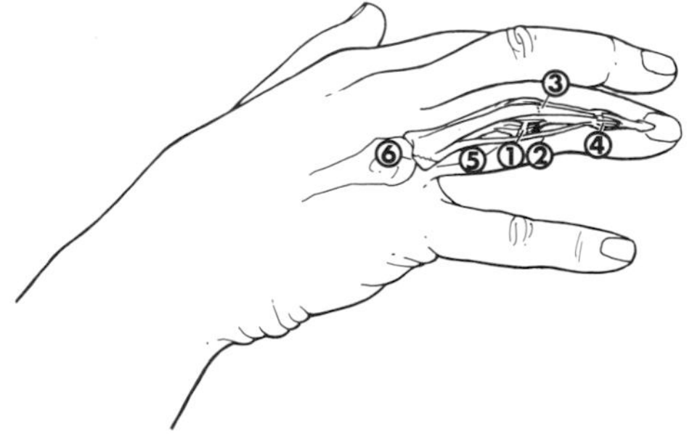

Active Testing of Functional Stability (Under Local Anesthesia)

PROXIMAL INTERPHALANGEAL JOINT

Have the patient move the injured point actively through a full range to evaluate stability. This may require digital nerve block to determine if the PIP joint is unstable.

1. Dorsally from volar plate injury or

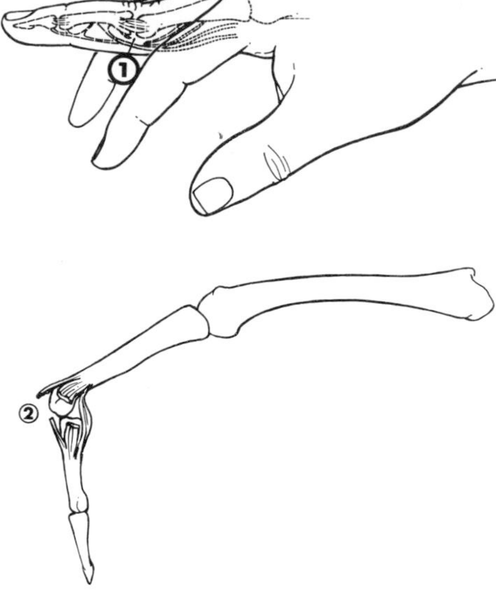

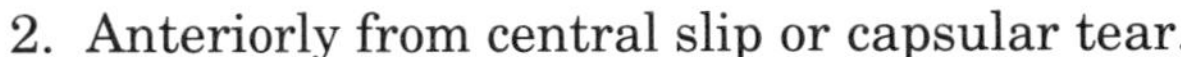

2. Anteriorly from central slip or capsular tear.

DISTAL INTERPHALANGEAL JOINT

Evaluate motion of the DIP joint for

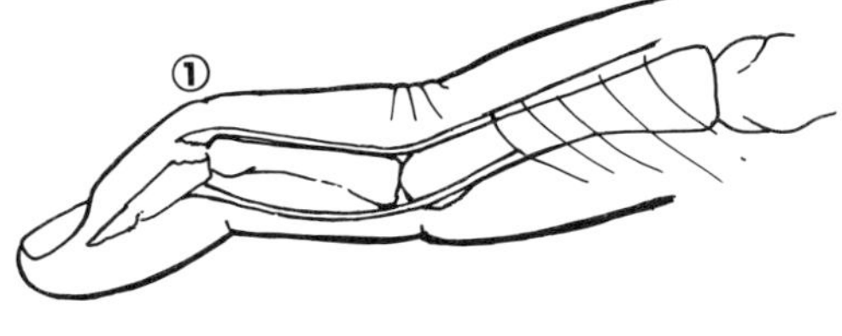

1. Loss of full extension caused by mallet finger.

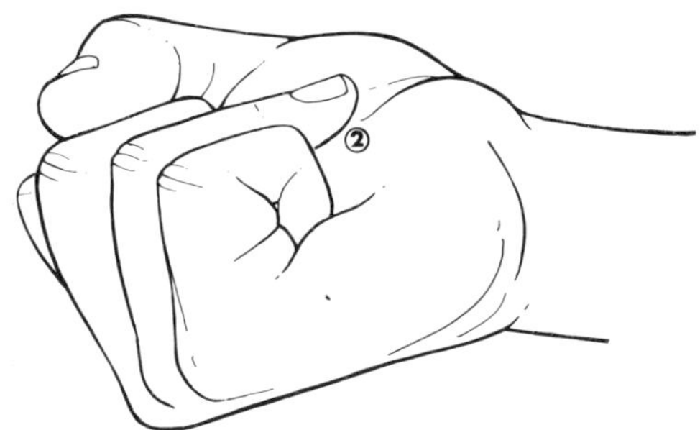

2. Loss of flexion as a result of avulsion of the flexor digitorum profundus.

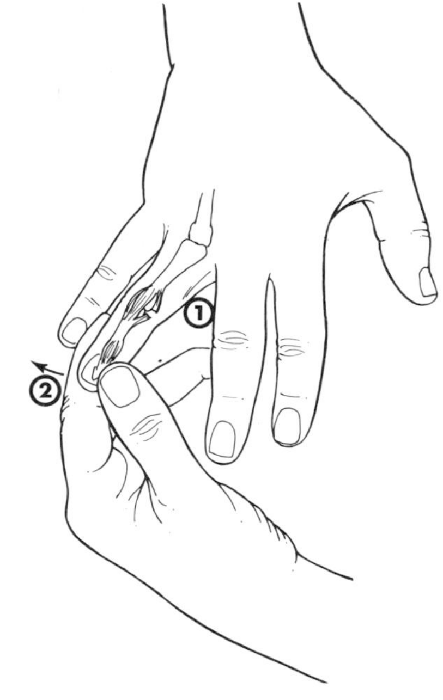

Passive Stress Testing

After the patient has carried out active functional testing, evaluate the joints for collateral stability by passive stress testing.

1. Finger is extended.
2. Lateral instability may be evident with gentle stressing.

Radiographic Evaluation

The x-ray view should be centered on the finger and not the hand to detect subtle changes, such as the following.

1. Small fractures associated with PIP dislocation.

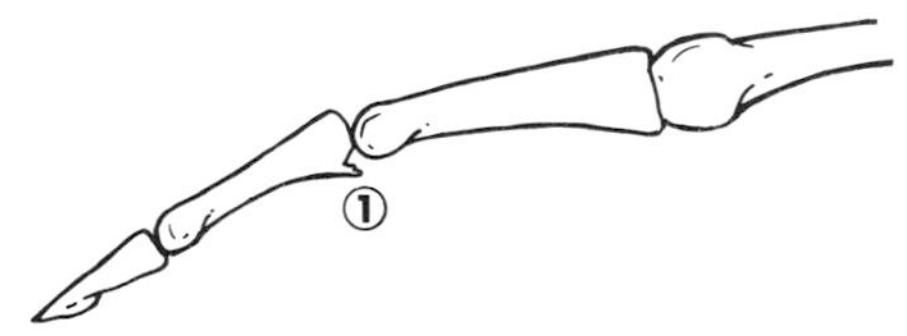

2. Avulsed bone fragments from hyperextension injury.

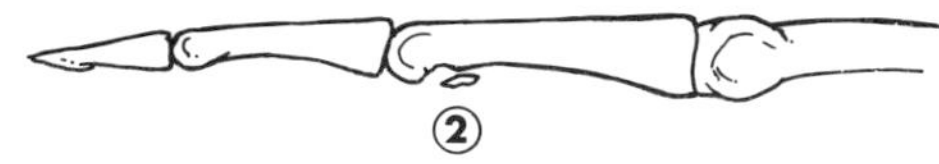

3. Avulsed bone fragments from mallet finger.

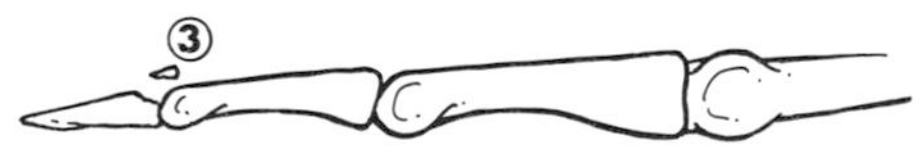

4. Avulsion of flexor digitorum profundus tendon.

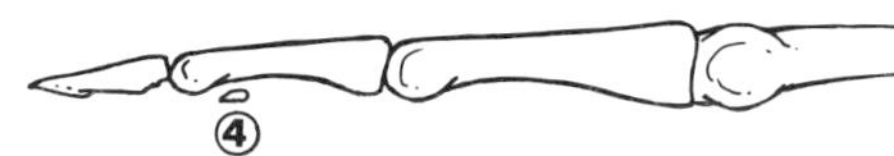

Management of Lateral Dislocations of the Interphalangeal Joints

REMARKS

In lateral dislocation of the IP joint, the collateral ligament is generally ruptured on the side to which the force was applied.

Dislocation usually is reduced by the patient or a bystander soon after injury.

Be wary of a joint that is unusually swollen or tender. This frequently indicates extensive damage to the collateral ligament and requires immobilization until the pain and swelling subside.

Evaluate the injury carefully by physical examination and x-ray to determine precisely the extent of the damage.

Prereduction X-Ray

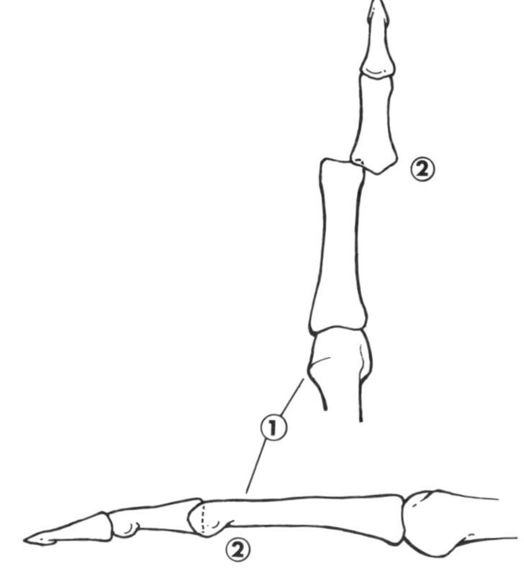

1. X-ray views should include true anteroposterior and lateral views of the finger and not just the hand to rule out small fractures.
2. Lateral dislocation of the PIP joint has occurred without anterior or posterior displacement.

Note: For the acute dislocation, it is preferable to reduce the painful injury first before the x-rays are obtained because the diagnosis is usually obvious and the x-ray is not essential. If there is a question about a fracture associated with dislocation, x-ray is indicated.

Manipulative Reduction

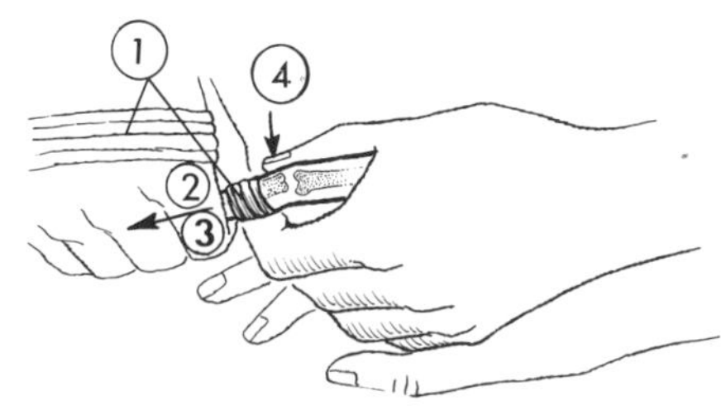

1. Loop a gauze bandage around the end of the injured finger and around the operator's hand.
2. Grasp the end of the finger with your thumb and index finger.
3. Apply steady traction along the axis of the finger.
4. While traction is being maintained, bring the distal phalanx in line with the proximal phalanx.

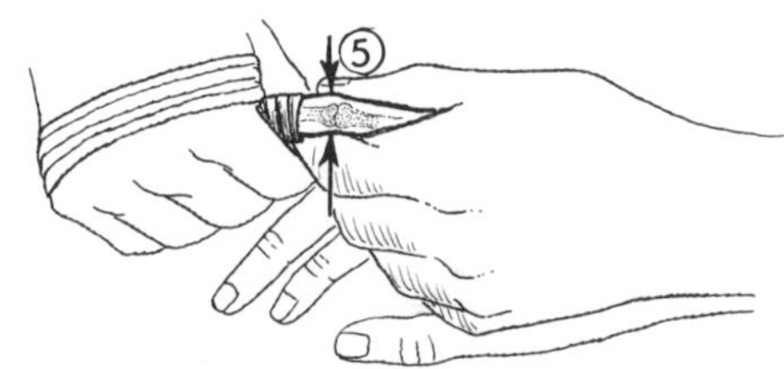

5. Squeeze the sides of the joint to correct any residual lateral displacement.

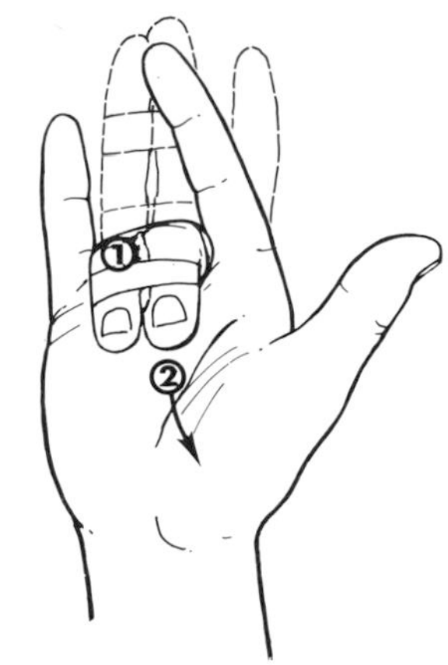

Postreduction Management for Usual Injury

In most instances, the dislocated joint requires only brief support by buddy-taping to the adjacent finger.

1. Apply tape to the fingers with the interdigital area padded.
2. Allow active flexion and extension.

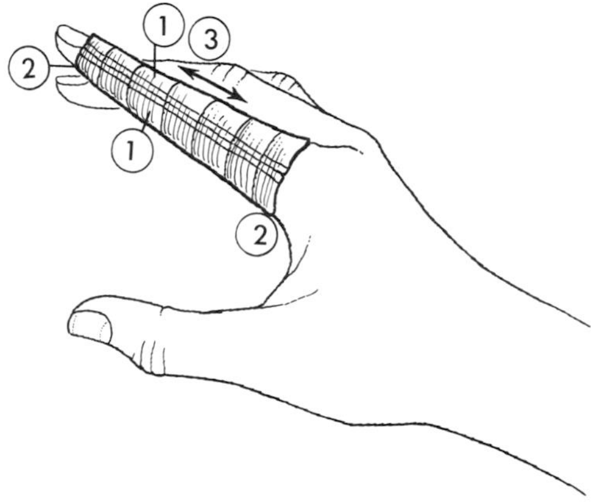

Postreduction Management for Unstable Injury

Evaluate functional stability and stress stability as described previously.

If the joint is swollen, tender, or unstable, the finger should be immobilized in a finger cast-splint.

1. Apply anterior and posterior splints designed to accommodate for swelling.
2. Plaster extends from the MP joint to the base of the nail.
3. IP joints are in almost full extension to keep the ligaments stretched to length.

Hyperextension Dislocation of the Proximal Interphalangeal Joints

REMARKS

Hyperextension dislocation is a common injury of the PIP joint and can cause disability far out of proportion to the apparent magnitude of the initial injury.

The usual presentation is a jammed finger from football or other sports.

These jammed fingers can include significant injury to the central slip dorsally, which allows anterior displacement of the middle phalanx.

Avulsion injury of the volar capsule from the middle phalanx can lead to dislocation and a chronic swan-neck or hyperextension deformity.

Volar plate avulsion from the proximal phalanx can cause a flexion contracture of the joint and a pseudoboutonnière deformity.

Prereduction X-Ray

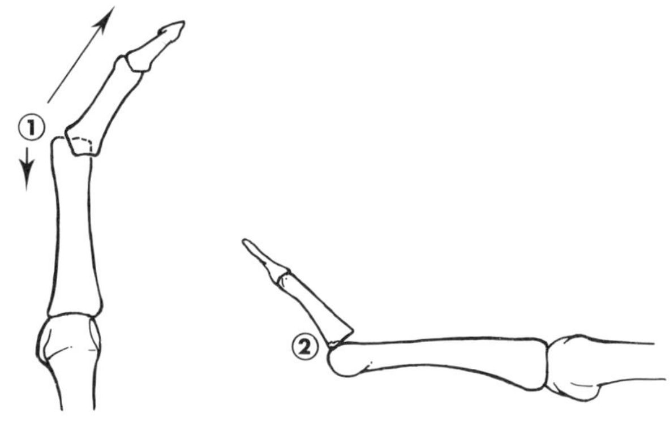

1. X-ray view should be centered on the injured finger, not the hand.
2. Lateral view shows PIP joint has dislocated dorsally. A small avulsion fracture is evidence for damage to the volar plate attachment.

Manipulative Reduction

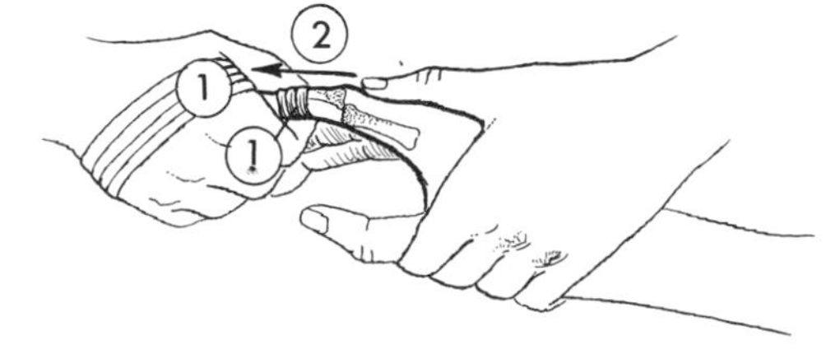

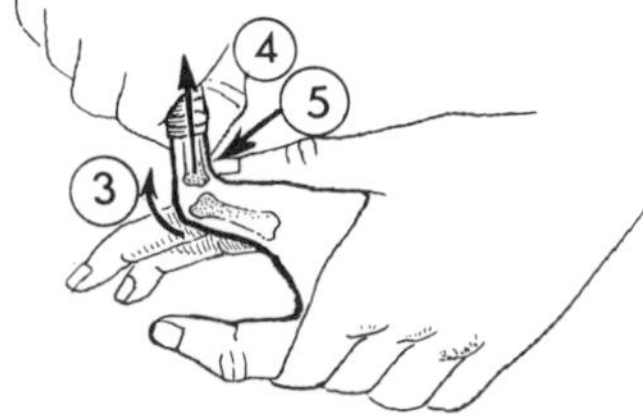

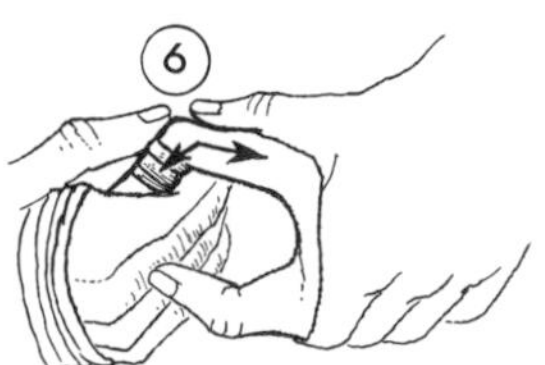

This is performed after injection of local anesthetic.

1. Bandage is first looped around the end of the injured finger and then around the operator's hand.
2. Grasp the dislocated finger with your thumb and index finger and apply gentle traction along the axis of the dislocated phalanx; at the same time,
3. Bring the phalanx into the hyperextended position.
4. While traction is being maintained,
5. Slide the base of the phalanx distalward to a position opposite the head of the proximal phalanx; then,
6. Flex the IP joint.

Postreduction X-Ray

After reduction by the patient or the physician, evaluate carefully for functional stability. Look particularly for

1. Dorsal instability caused by avulsion of the volar plate from the middle phalanx.

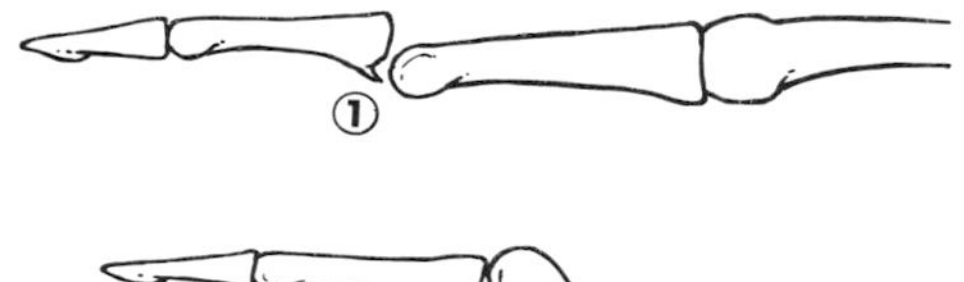

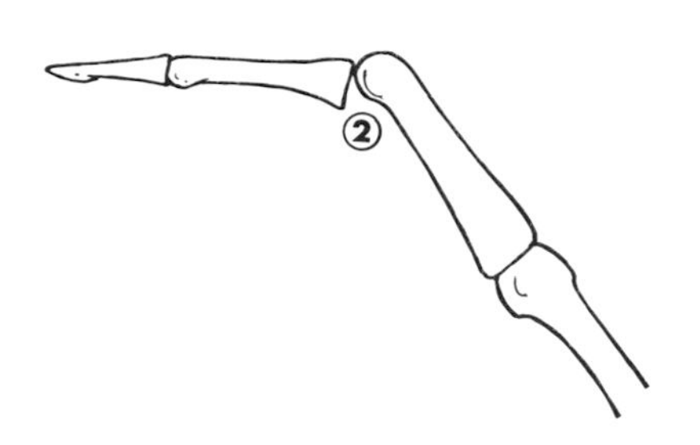

2. Anterior instability as a result of central slip and capsular damage.

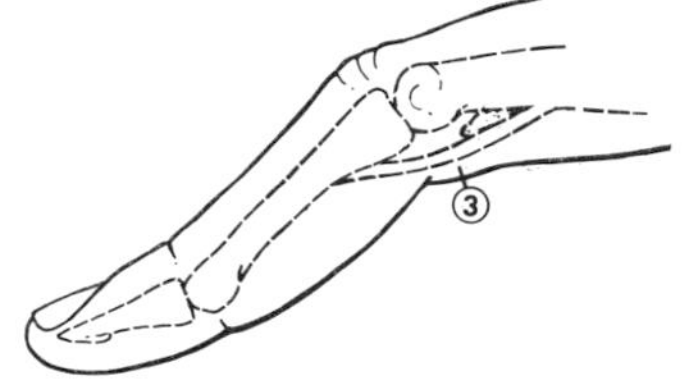

3. Avulsion of the volar capsule from the proximal phalanx causing pseudoboutonnière deformity.

Fracture-Dislocation of the Proximal Interphalangeal Joint

REMARKS

The usual force applied to the PIP joint disrupts the palmar base of the middle phalanx, by either fracturing the phalanx or tearing the capsule. The consequence is that the PIP joint dislocates dorsally into extension.

An alternative mechanism of injury may be a direct blow to the dorsal surface, which disrupts the dorsal capsule and central slip and allows dislocation to occur volarly. This is less frequent than a dorsal dislocation, however.

If the injury fractures more than 30 per cent of the support of the middle phalanx, a stable reduction is difficult to maintain.

The dilemma in the treatment of the unstable dislocation or fracture-dislocation of the PIP joint is to stabilize the joint while minimizing its tendency to become stiff.

A variety of methods have been devised to stabilize the unstable PIP joint. These include percutaneous pinning and extension block splintage. The simplest method is percutaneous dorsal pinning for no more than 3 weeks.

If this is not possible to achieve stability, extension block splinting should be considered.

For larger fractures that produce instability of the joint, open reduction and small fragment screw fixation may rarely be the treatment of choice.

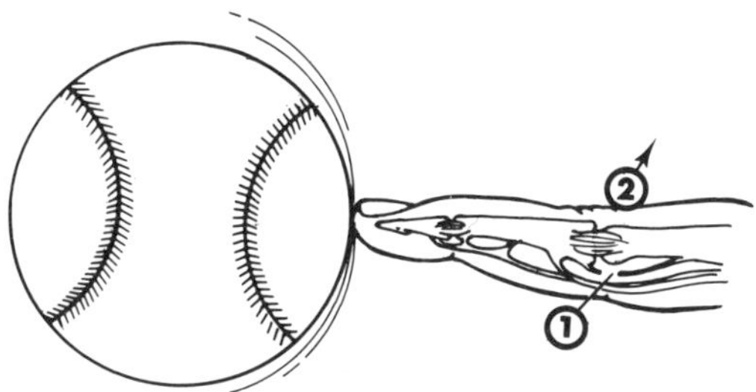

1. Rupture of the volar plate from the middle phalanx produces
2. Hyperextension deformity of the PIP joint.

Appearance on X-Ray

UNDISPLACED FRACTURE

1. Small undisplaced fracture of the palmar aspect of the base of the middle phalanx.

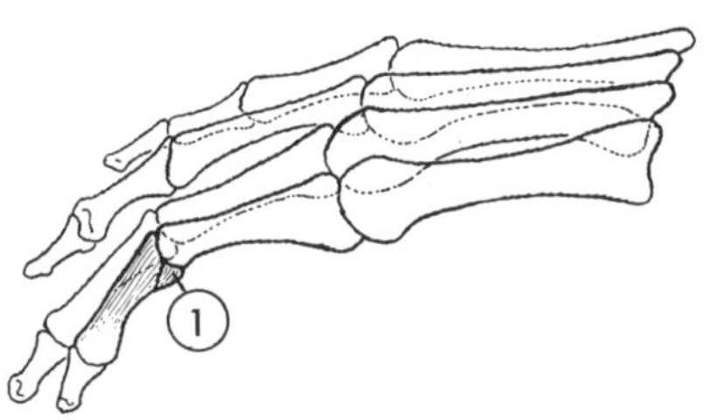

Note: Evaluate stability carefully by palpation, x-ray, functional testing, and stress testing. If there is any evidence of dorsal instability, treat with an extension block splint. Usually, they can be managed by buddy-taping. However, percutaneous pinning may be necessary if the joint is unstable.

Percutaneous Pinning for Fracture-Subluxation of the Proximal Interphalangeal Joint

Barton described a percutaneous Kirschner wire fixation technique for fracture-subluxations of the PIP joint.

The technique is basically the same as that used for a Bennett fracture-dislocation of the thumb metacarpal.

Small Displaced Fracture With Subluxation

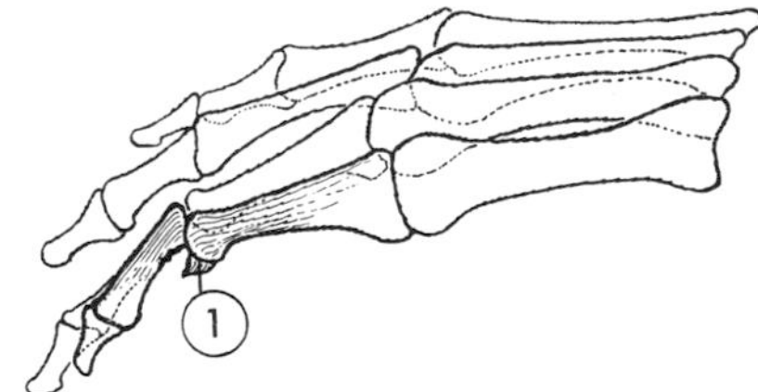

1. Small marginal fracture of the ulnar aspect of the base of the middle phalanx.

Technique of Percutaneous Pinning

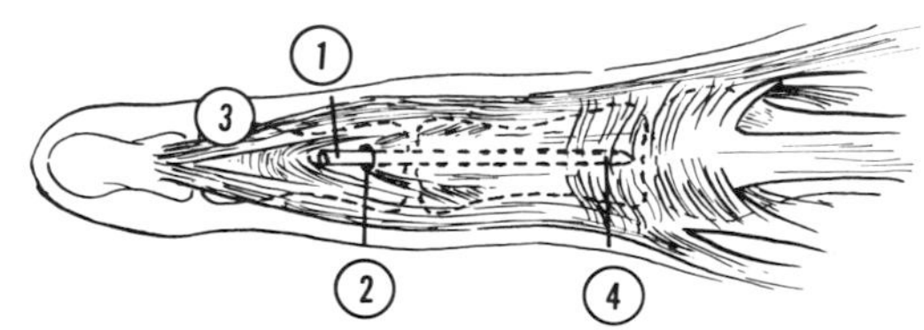

1. Kirschner wire is inserted through the dorsal aspect of the base of the middle phalanx
2. Distal to the insertion of the central slip but
3. Proximal to the joining of the lateral slips.
4. Joint is reduced and stabilized by passing the pin into the head of the proximal phalanx.

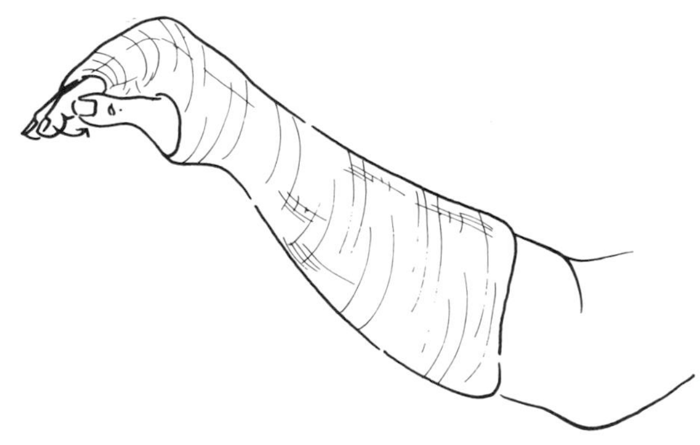

Subsequent Management

The finger is supported and protected in an extension block splint or clam shell plaster device.

The wire is removed at 2–3 weeks, and active motion is allowed. If the wire is inserted without impinging on the central slip or lateral bands, motion can be regained fairly rapidly.

Alternative Method of Managing Fracture-Dislocations of the Proximal Phalanx: Extension Block Splinting

REMARKS

Extension block splinting may be used for the fracture-dislocation that cannot be reduced by percutaneous pinning of the joint in flexion.

If more than 40 per cent of the joint surface has been fractured, open reduction and internal fixation should be considered.

The concept of the extension block splint is to allow the joint to heal in a flexed position to prevent dorsal redislocation and slowly to bring the joint up into extension as the volar capsule and fracture fragments heal. This method can be used for the unstable fracture but requires careful monitoring on a weekly basis to determine the alignment of the fracture-dislocation.

1. Apply a plaster gauntlet cast with a dorsal splint.
2. Maintain the MP joint in the position of full flexion.
3. Splint blocks extension of the PIP joint 10°–15° short of the point where subluxation occurs.
4. Proximal phalanx is taped to the splint.
5. Full flexion of the PIP joint is allowed from the beginning.

Note: If more than 40 per cent of the proximal phalangeal articular surface is fractured, open reduction and internal fixation may be necessary. This procedure may be followed by postoperative use of the dorsal extension block splint.

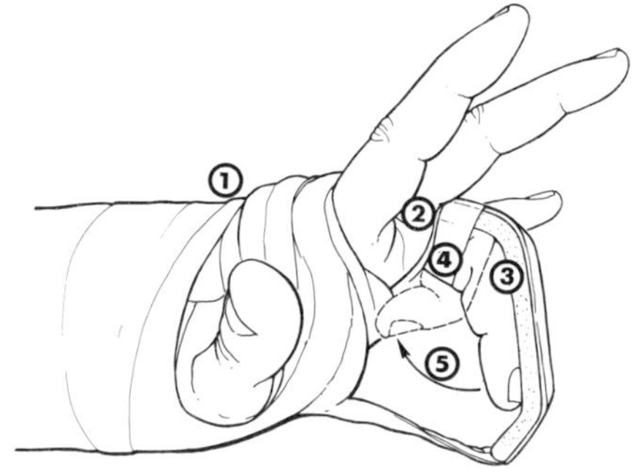

Subsequent Management

Decrease the angle of the extension block 25 per cent each week.

The patient should be able to flex the joint 70°–90° by the third week.

Continue to block full extension for 6–12 weeks, depending on the degree of initial instability.

Alternative Method of Management: Open Reduction and Internal Fixation

If the fracture fragment is sufficiently large or cannot be reduced and stabilized by the closed technique, open reduction may be necessary.

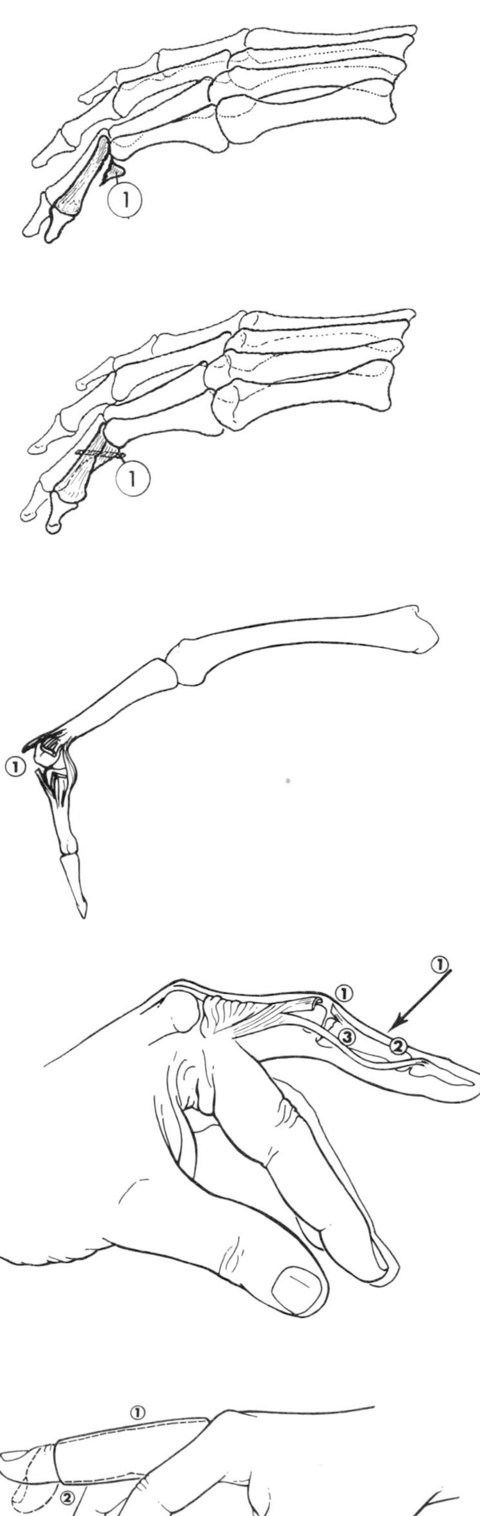

Prereduction X-Ray

1. Large triangular fragment from the palmar aspect of the middle phalanx caused the IP joint to remain unstable despite attempted closed reduction.

Postoperative X-Ray

1. Fragment is reduced and fixed with a Kirschner wire or with a small fragment screw.

Note: Stabilizing this articular fracture is necessary to permit treatment with active joint motion using a dorsal extension block splint.

Management of Acute Anterior Instability or Dislocation

1. Anterior dislocation of the PIP joint is unusual and indicates significant disruption of the central slip attachment. Capsular and collateral ligament structures are also frequently damaged.

1. The consequence of chronic anterior instability is a boutonnière disruption with chronic subluxation of the PIP joint.
2. Disruption of the central slip contracts the DIP joint and limits flexion of the DIP joint in a true boutonnière deformity.
3. In a pseudoboutonnière caused by injury to the volar capsule of the PIP joint, a fixed flexion deformity develops at the PIP joint, but the DIP joint remains mobile.

The complication of boutonnière deformity after this injury should be anticipated and prevented.

1. PIP joint is immobilized in a finger cast or splint.
2. DIP joint flexes actively.

Subsequent Management

Six weeks of continuous immobilization in extension are usually sufficient.

If the patient desires to return to sports or vigorous activities, protect the PIP joint with a dorsal splint for 4–6 weeks longer.

Note: For acute injuries with extreme instability, large fracture fragments, or open injuries, early operative repair is indicated.

Pseudoboutonnière Deformity

REMARKS

A pseudoboutonnière deformity develops as a chronic residual problem after acute disruption of the volar capsular attachment to the proximal phalanx. This can be prevented by anticipation of the complication and treatment with adequate immobilization.

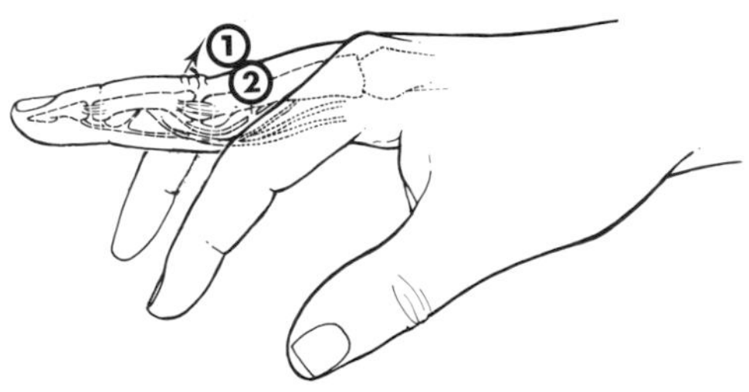

1. Hyperextension injury to the PIP joint may occasionally
2. Disrupt the capsular attachment from the proximal phalanx, eventually producing flexion contracture of the joint.

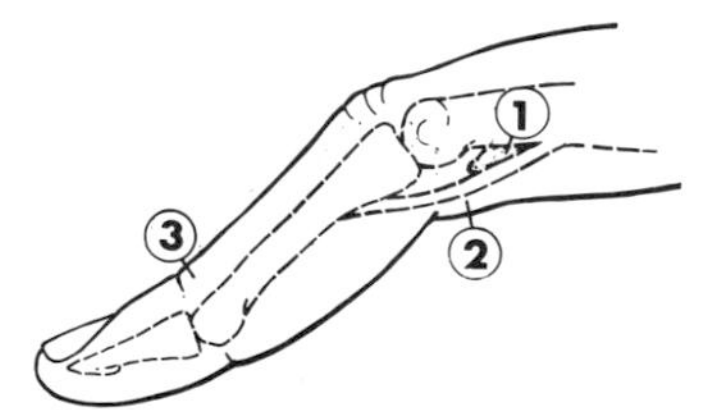

1. A small avulsed fragment of bone from the proximal phalanx may be a clue to the site of injury.
2. Chronic flexion contracture of the capsule produces pseudoboutonnière deformity.
3. DIP joint is usually not fixed in extension because both lateral bands are usually not involved. This is in contrast to a true boutonnière deformity.

If you suspect, on the basis of tenderness or of an avulsion fracture from the proximal phalanx, that the hyperextension injury is likely to progress to a pseudoboutonnière deformity, immobilize the finger as in a true boutonnière deformity.

1. PIP joint is immobilized in a finger cast or splint in extension.
2. DIP joint is allowed to flex actively.

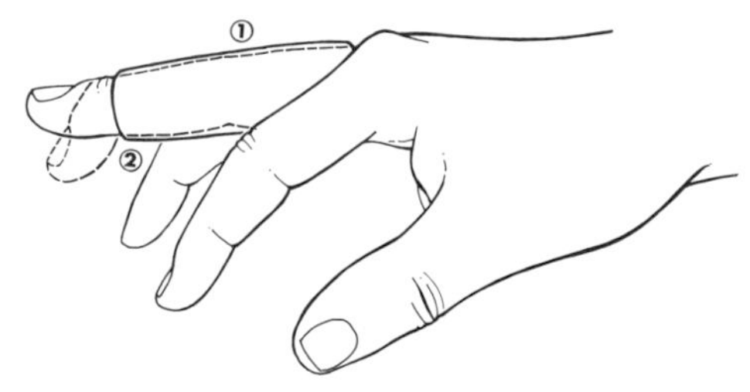

Note: Cast immobilization for the boutonnière deformity is usually necessary for 6 weeks. After cast removal, the patient should be advised to observe the finger for any recurrence of the deformity, which would require repeat cast immobilization.

■ The "Jammed Finger"—Tendon Avulsions With or Without Fractures

Mallet Finger Deformity: Subluxation of the Distal Interphalangeal Joint

REMARKS

A mallet finger is among the most common injuries to the tendon and joint structures of the digit.

The mechanism is the result of a blow to the end of the finger, causing hyperflexion of the DIP joint and avulsion of the extensor tendon with or without fracture.

Secondarily, the PIP joint becomes hyperextended as the extensor mechanism retracts dorsally and proximally.

Closed treatment using a dorsal splint for 5–6 weeks is usually most effective for these injuries with or without fracture. Closed treatment can be attempted for most mallet fingers even when they are seen 6 weeks or more after injury.

Mallet fingers with fracture-dislocations in which the joint cannot be reduced generally require open reduction and internal fixation. However, if the subluxation can be reduced in the splint, closed treatment is preferable.

Mechanism

1. Blow to the tip of the finger causes hyperflexion and avulsion of the extensor tendon.
2. Swelling and pain over the extensor insertion.
3. Deformity of the DIP joint varies, but the patient cannot actively extend the distal phalanx.

Note: In all injuries of this type to the distal phalanx, tendon avulsion should be suspected and treated.

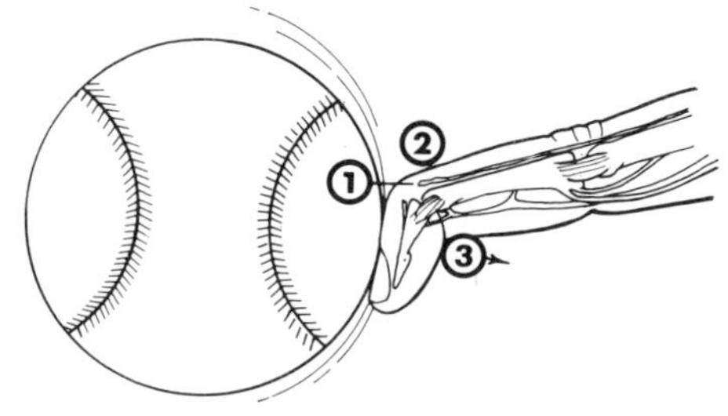

Prereduction X-Ray

1. Avulsion fracture is evident, producing the mallet finger deformity.
2. DIP joint has subluxated volarly.

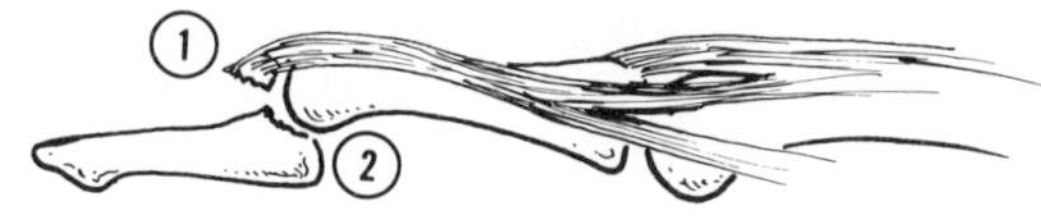

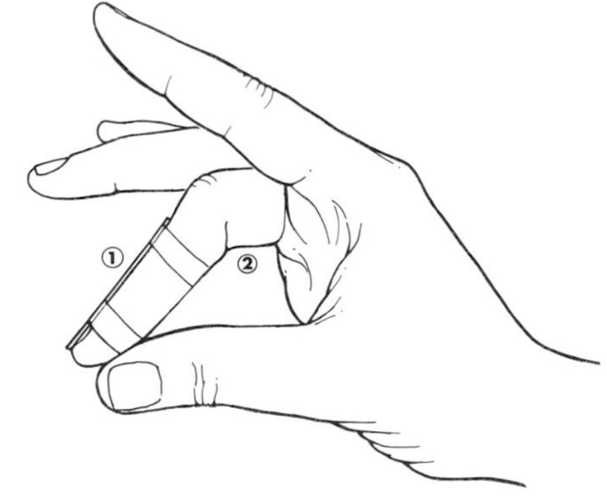

Management of a Mallet Finger

1. Apply dorsal splint with the DIP joint extended but not hyperextended.
2. Leave the PIP joint free and encourage active motion.

Postreduction

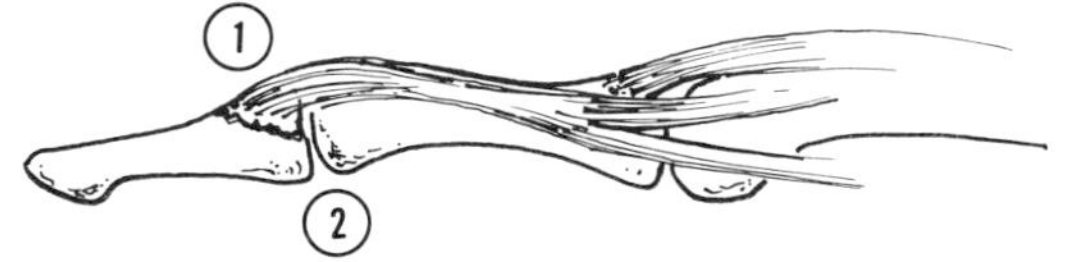

1. Avulsion fracture has been replaced at the base of the proximal phalanx, but this need not be anatomically reduced.
2. It is important that the subluxation of the DIP joint is reduced to allow restoration of function. If the subluxation cannot be reduced, operative treatment and internal stabilization is necessary.

Subsequent Management

Continue splint immobilization for 4–5 weeks.

The splint tape may be changed carefully during this time to prevent skin maceration, but the patient must maintain extension of the joint.

After 4–5 weeks, the patient may remove one strip of tape to allow active, gentle flexion of the joint. The tape is reapplied when the patient is not exercising.

When active joint motion reaches 40° of flexion and full extension, the splint may be discarded.

Management of a Mallet Finger Deformity With an Avulsion Fracture and Persistent Subluxation of the Distal Interphalangeal Joint

Prereduction X-Ray

1. Large avulsion fragment is evident at the base of the distal phalanx.
2. DIP joint remains subluxated despite attempted reduction with a dorsal splint. Persistent dislocation of the DIP joint is generally an indication for open reduction and stabilization.

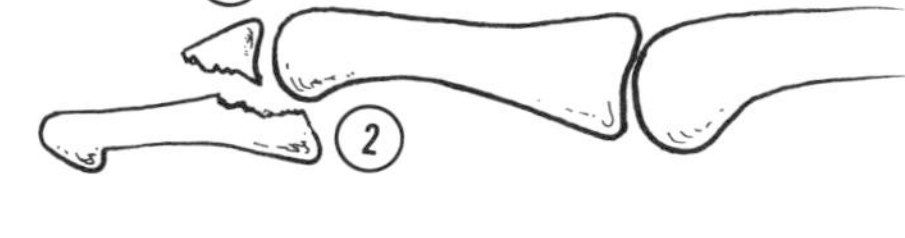

Riordan Pin* Fixation for Open Reduction of Mallet Finger Deformity

A useful way to manage the occasional mallet finger that is unstable or associated with a dorsal wound is by transarticular pin fixation.

External splint support is still needed to prevent breakage or pin migration.

1. Dorsal laceration involves the extensor tendon and DIP joint.

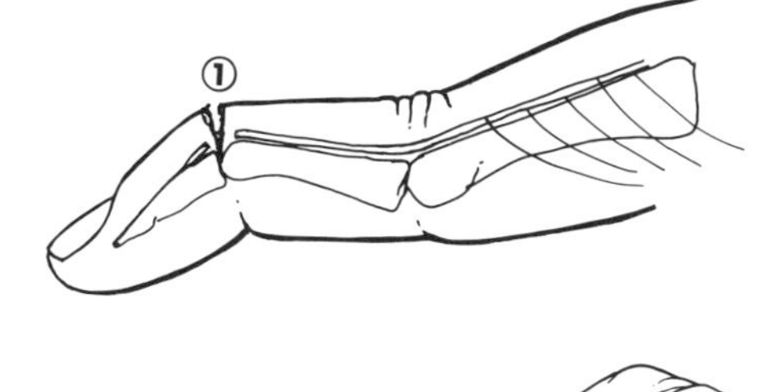

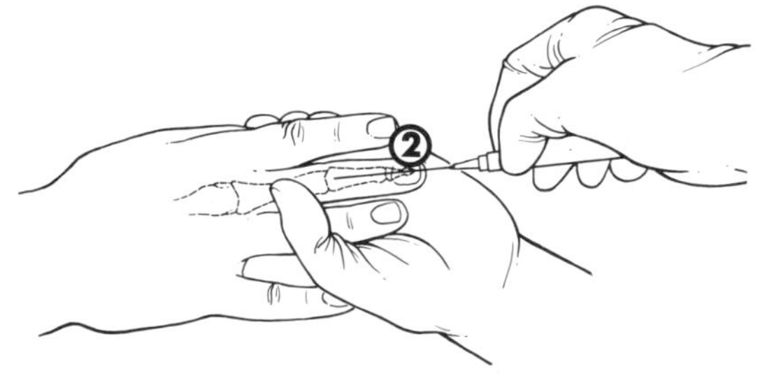

2. After thorough wound cleansing, a Riordan pin is inserted transarticularly to support the tendon reattachment.

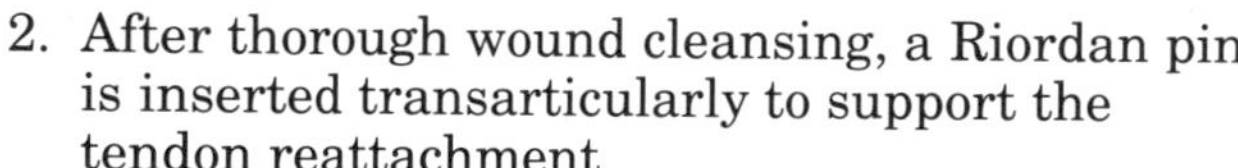

3. Tendon is reattached, and the skin laceration is closed by a figure-of-eight suture through both skin and tendon.

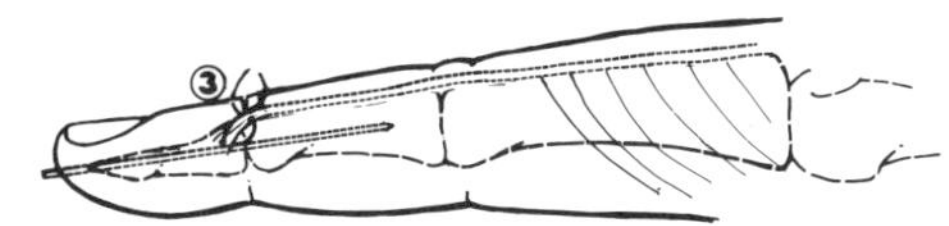

Subsequent Management

Additional external support with a dorsal splint is necessary during the healing phase.

Remove the pin at 5–6 weeks.

Continue external splinting, but allow the patient to begin active exercises of the DIP joint.

When active flexion has reached 40° and the patient has maintained active extension, the splint may be discarded.

---

*Available from Zimmer-U.S.A. (Warsaw, IN).

Avulsion of Flexor Digitorum Profundus Insertion With or Without Fracture

REMARKS

Another frequently unrecognized injury that presents as a swollen, jammed finger is avulsion of the flexor digitorum profundus tendon insertion. This commonly results from the act of grasping the shirt of an individual, such as a football player, as the person lunges forward. The injury may also occur in older individuals who avulse the tendon while lifting heavy objects.

The resultant complete disruption of the flexor insertion, which is most commonly from the ring finger or small finger, is frequently treated as a jammed finger.

If the injury is unrecognized, the tendon will retract proximally in its sheath or completely up into the palm.

Be alert to this commonly missed but significant problem in any individual who sustains a grasping injury.

The diagnosis can be made easily by the loss of active flexion of the DIP joint. Always check DIP and PIP joint motion.

Occasionally, the position of the tendon will be indicated on the x-ray by a small fragment of bone avulsed with it.

Consistently, the point of tenderness is at the end of the retracted tendon, usually over the PIP joint but, occasionally, in the palm.

Repair of this injury should be performed only by a surgeon experienced in flexor tendon surgery, including tendon grafting.

Unsuccessful surgery will impair the function of the uninjured flexor digitorum sublimis tendon.

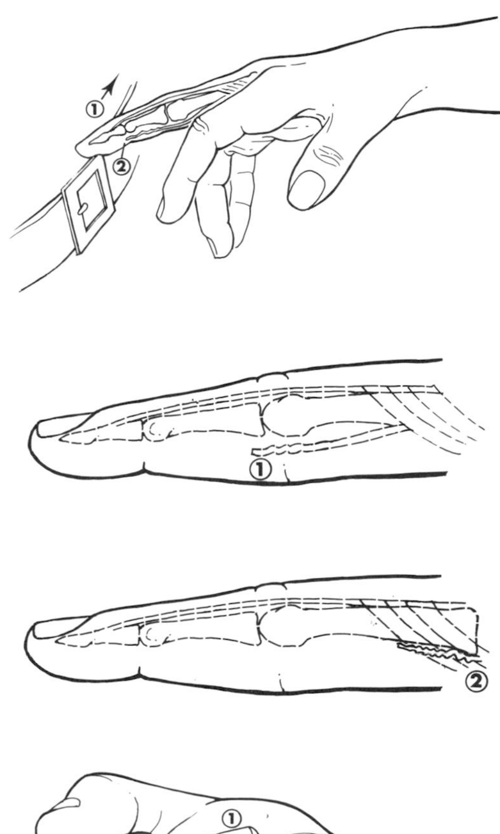

1. Avulsion of the flexor digitorum profundus is most commonly produced by forceful grasping.
2. Occasionally, a small fragment of bone is seen on x-ray to be displaced within the tendon.

The area of tenderness is localized directly to the tendon either
1. Adjacent to the PIP joint or
2. In the palm.

The diagnosis can be readily made on the basis of
1. Loss of active flexion of the DIP joint.

Note: If the diagnosis of flexor digitorum profundus avulsion is made immediately after injury, immobilize the finger to prevent further tendon retraction. Prompt repair should be carried out by an individual skilled in tendon surgery.

Boutonnière Deformity

REMARKS

Commonly, a direct laceration over the PIP joint produces a rupture of the central slip attachment to the middle phalanx. Another common cause of this injury is a closed crushing injury that forces the joint into passive flexion while it is being actively extended.

Frequently, the significance of injury to the extensor mechanism goes unrecognized or is treated with brief immobilization of the joint in flexion until the soft tissue wound heals.

The flexion immobilization permits the apex of the joint to prolapse through the "buttonhole" defect created by the disrupted central slip.

The disruption between the central slip and the lateral bands permits the lateral tendons to fall gradually beneath the axis of PIP motion. The result is that the intrinsics become flexors of the joint rather than extensors.

The typical boutonnière deformity may develop gradually several weeks or months after the initial injury.

To avoid the difficulties of treatment of a chronic PIP deformity, all lacerations and direct injuries to the PIP knuckle must be carefully evaluated. A laceration through the tendon can usually be repaired by a simple figure-of-eight removable stitch of stainless steel wire that closes both the tendon and the skin.

The joint should be immobilized in the extended position for 4–6 weeks to ensure adequate healing of the tendon. This also prevents flexion displacement of the lateral bands.

Even if seen 6–12 weeks after initial injury, closed treatment can be used.

The major indications for operative repair of a boutonnière deformity are avulsion fractures of the middle phalanx, long-standing deformities in young persons, or anterior dislocation with gross instability of the joint.

1. Laceration through the middle slip of the long extensor.
2. Apex of the joint buttonholes through the defect created by the laceration.
3. Longitudinal tearing allows the lateral bands to become flexors of the PIP joint and hyperextensors of DIP joint.

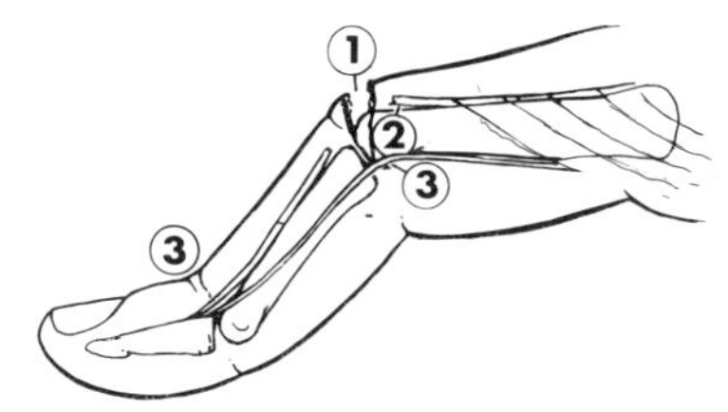

Treatment

1. Both the tendon and the
2. Skin laceration may be repaired by a simple figure-of-eight wire.

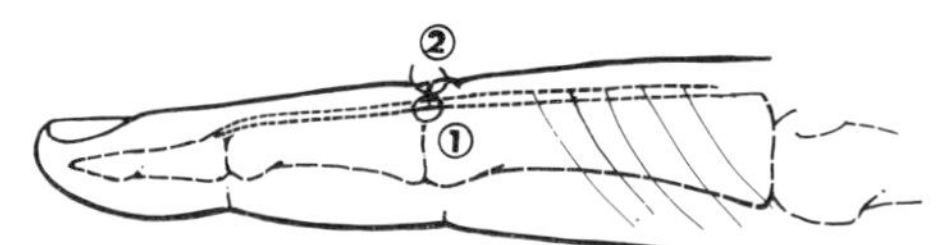

Immobilization in Extension

1. Finger cast is applied from the MP joint while keeping the PIP joint in extension.
2. DIP joint is allowed free motion.

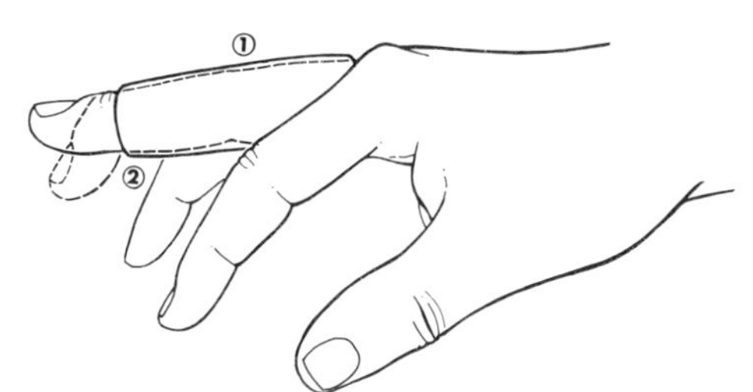

Subsequent Management

The cast is maintained for 6 weeks and then is removed.

A protective dorsal splint should be used if the patient is going to use the finger vigorously.

Apply another extension cast for 3 more weeks if the flexion deformity of the PIP joint recurs.

Occasionally, with chronic boutonnière deformities, a preliminary period of dynamic extension splinting is necessary to correct flexion contractures and permit closed treatment.

Management of Chronic Dorsal Instability of the Proximal Interphalangeal Joint (Swan-Neck Deformity)

REMARKS

A chronic dorsal subluxation of the PIP joint may develop after a "sprain" treated by taping the finger to a tongue depressor.

If the torn volar capsule is allowed to heal in a lengthened position, it will permit dorsal displacement of the middle phalanx.

Treatment of the chronic condition requires excision of the volar plate and reconstruction by means of a strip from the collateral ligament (Kleinert procedure).

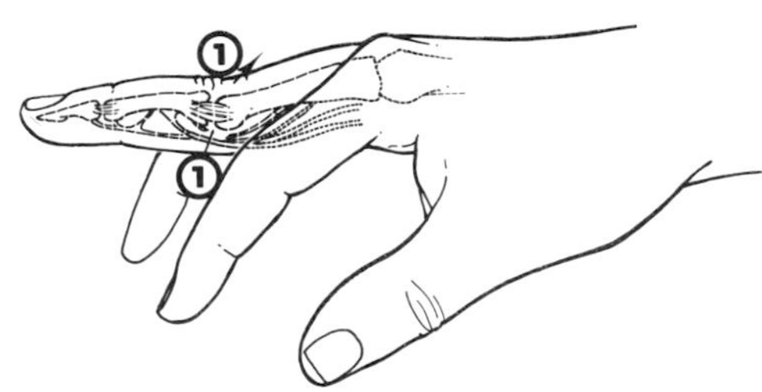

1. Chronic dorsal instability impairs function of the entire finger. It should be corrected by surgical reconstruction done by a skilled hand surgeon.

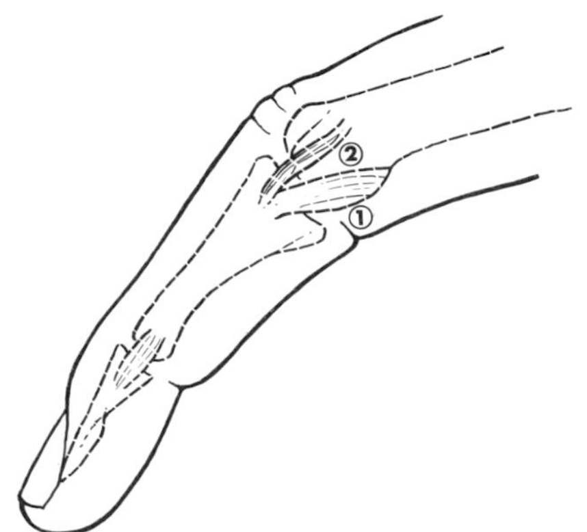

Kleinert Procedure for Chronic Dorsal Subluxation

1. Scarred and lengthened volar capsule is excised.
2. Proximal and volar portion of the collateral ligament is shifted volarly to stabilize the joint.

BIBLIOGRAPHY

Agee JM: Unstable fracture-dislocations of the proximal interphalangeal joint of the fingers. Clin Orthop 214:101, 1987.

Barton NJ: Fractures of the hand. J Bone Joint Surg Br 66:159, 1984.

Belsole R: Physiologic fixation of displaced and unstable fractures of the hand. Orthop Clin North Am 11:393, 1980.

Burkhalter WE, Butler B, Metz W, et al: Experience with delayed primary closure of war wounds of the hand in Viet Nam. J Bone and Joint Surg Am 50:945, 1968.

Burkhalter W, Reyes P: Closed treatment of fractures in the hand. Bull Hosp Joint Dis Orthop Inst 44:145, 1984.

Burton RI, Eaton RG: Common hand injuries in the athlete. Orthop Clin North Am 4:809, 1973.

Cannon S, Dowd G, Gore DR: Carpometacarpal dislocation producing compression of the deep branch of the ulnar nerve. J Bone Joint Surg Am 53:1387, 1971.

Cannon S, Dowd G, Williams D, et al: A long-term study following Bennett's fracture. J Hand Surg Br 11:426, 1986.

Carroll RE, Match RM: Avulsion of the flexor profundus tendon insertion. J Trauma 10:1109, 1970.

Charnley J: The Closed Treatment of Common Fractures, pp 143–150. Edinburgh: Churchill Livingstone, 1981.

Coonrad RW, Pohlman MH: Impacted fractures in the proximal portion of the proximal phalanx of the finger. J Bone Joint Surg Am 51:1291, 1969.

Dobyns J, Lunscheid R, Cooney W: Fractures and dislocations of the wrist and hand, then and now. J Hand Surg Am 8:687, 1983.

Fox J, Golden G, Rodeheaver G, et al: Nonoperative management of fingertip pulp amputation by occlusive dressings. Am J Surg 133:255, 1977.

Gore DR: Carpometacarpal dislocation producing compression of the deep branch of the ulnar nerve. J Bone Joint Surg Am 53:1387, 1971.

Green DP, Anderson JR: Closed reduction and percutaneous pin fixation of fractured phalanges. J Bone Joint Surg Am 55:1651, 1973.

Green DP, Terry GC: Complex dislocation of the metacarpophalangeal joint. J Bone Joint Surg Am 55:1480, 1973.

Gunter GS: Traumatic avulsion of the insertion of the flexor digitorum profundus insertion in athletes. J Hand Surg Am 4:461, 1979.

Hastings H II: Unstable metacarpal and phalangeal fracture treatment with screws and plates. Clin Orthop 214:37, 1987.

Hazlett JW: Carpometacarpal dislocations other than the thumb: A report of 11 cases. Can J Surg 11:315, 1968.

Holm A, Zachariae L: Fingertip lesions. An evaluation of conservative treatment versus free skin grafting. Acta Orthop Scand 45:382, 1974.

Hunter JM, Cowen NJ: Fifth metacarpal fracture in a compensation clinic population. J Bone Joint Surg Am 52:1159, 1970.

James JIP: Fractures of the proximal and middle phalanges of the fingers. Acta Orthop Scand 32:401, 1962.

James JIP: The assessment and management of the injured hand. Hand 2:97, 1970.

Jones WW: Biomechanics of small bone fixation. Clin Orthop 214:11, 1987.

Jupiter JB, Koniuch M, Smith RJ: The management of delayed unions and nonunions of the tubular bones of the hand. J Hand Surg Am 4:457, 1985.

Kaplan EB: Dorsal dislocation of the metacarpophalangeal joint of the index finger. J Bone Joint Surg Am 39:1081, 1957.

Kleinert HE, Kasdan ML: Reconstruction of chronically subluxated proximal interphalangeal finger joint. J Bone Joint Surg Am 47:958, 1965.

Kleinman WB, Grantham SA: Multiple volar carpometacarpal joint dislocation. J Hand Surg Am 3:377, 1978.

Lawlis JF, Gunther SF: Carpometacarpal dislocations. J Bone Joint Surg Am 73:56, 1991.

Malerich MM, Eaton RG: Complete dislocation of a little finger metacarpophalangeal joint treated by closed technique. J Trauma 20:424, 1980.

McCue F, Honner R, Marriott C, et al: Athletic injuries of the proximal interphalangeal joint requiring surgical treatment. J Bone Joint Surg Am 52:937, 1970.

McElfresh EL, Dobyns JH, O'Brien ET: Management of fracture-dislocation of the proximal interphalangeal joint by extension-block splinting. J Bone Joint Surg Am 54:1705, 1972.

McElfresh EC, Dobyns JH: Intra-articular metacarpal head fractures. J Hand Surg Am 8:383, 1983.

McLaughlin HL: Complex "locked" dislocation of the metacarpophalangeal joints. J Trauma 5:683, 1965.

Peterson P, Sack S: Fracture-dislocation of the base of the fifth metacarpal associated with injury to the deep motor branch of the ulnar nerve: A case report. J Hand Surg Am 11:525, 1986.

Pollen A: The conservative treatment of Bennett's fracture-subluxation of the thumb metacarpal. J Bone Joint Surg Br 50:91, 1968.

Reyes F, Latta L: Conservative management of difficult phalangeal fractures. Clin Orthop 214:23, 1987.

Shah J, Patel M: Dislocation of the carpometacarpal joint of the thumb. A report of four cases. Clin Orthop 175:166, 1983.

Stener B: Displacement of the ruptured ulnar collateral ligament of the metacarpophalangeal joint of the thumb. J Bone Joint Surg Br 44:869, 1962.

Strickland JW, Steichen JB, Showalter JF: Phalangeal fractures in a hand surgery practice: A statistical review and in-depth study of the management of proximal phalangeal shaft fractures. J Hand Surg Am 4:285, 1979.

Wright TA: Early mobilization in fractures of the metacarpals and phalanges. Can J Surg 11:491, 1968.

Index

Note: Page numbers in *italics* refer to illustrations.

ISBN 0-7216-6619-1